CONTRIBUTORS

Anne W. Alexandrov, PhD, RN, CCRN, FAAN
Professor
School of Nursing
University of Alabama
Tuscaloosa, Alabama
Program Director
NET SMART
Health Outcomes Institute
Fountain Hills, Arizona
*Chapter 23: Integrative Review of Outcomes and Performance
    Improvement Research on Advanced Practice Nursing*

Rhonda L. Babine, MS, ACNS-BC
Clinical Nurse Specialist, Geriatrics
Maine Medical Center
Portland, Maine
Chapter 8: Guidance and Coaching

Sally D. Bennett, MSN, RN, FNP-BC
Camden Healthcare Associates, Inc.
Kingsland, Georgia
Chapter 19: Business Planning and Reimbursement Mechanisms

Karen A. Brykczynski, DNSc, RN, FNP-BC, FAANP, FAAN
Professor
School of Nursing
University of Texas Medical Branch
Galveston, Texas
Chapter 4: Role Development of the Advanced Practice Nurse

Margaret Faut Callahan, PhD, CRNA, FNAP, FAAN
Dean and Professor
College of Nursing
Marquette University
Milwaukee, Wisconsin
Chapter 18: The Certified Registered Nurse Anesthetist

Michael Carter, DNSc, DNP, FNP/GNP-BC, FAAN
University Distinguished Professor
College of Nursing
University of Tennessee Health Science Center
Memphis, Tennessee
Chapter 12: Collaboration

Cathy C. Cartwright, MSN, RN, PCNS
Pediatric Clinical Nurse Specialist
Neurosurgery
Children's Mercy Hospital
Kansas City, Missouri
Chapter 14: The Clinical Nurse Specialist

Garrett K. Chan, PhD, APRN, FAEN, FPCN, FAAN
Lead Advanced Practice Professional
Emergency Department
Stanford Hospital
Stanford, California
Associate Adjunct Professor
Department of Physiological Nursing
University of California
San Francisco, California
Chapter 14: The Clinical Nurse Specialist

Anne Z. Cockerham, PhD, CNM, WHNP-BC
Clinical Coordinator
Frontier Nursing University
Chantilly, Virginia
*Chapter 1: A Brief History of Advanced Practice Nursing
    in the United States*

Sarah A. Delgado, MSN, RN, ACNP
Chronic Care Nurse Practitioner
Bright Health Physicians/Presbyterian Intercommunity Hospital
Whittier, California
Chapter 13: Ethical Decision Making

Michelle Rene Frazelle, MS, RN, CCRN
Assistant Director, Nursing
CJW Medical Center
HCA Virginia Health System
Richmond, Virginia
*Chapter 5: Evolving and Innovative Opportunities for Advanced
    Practice Nursing*

**Mikel Gray, PhD, FNP-BC, PNP-BC, CUNP, CCCN,
    FAANP, FAAN**
Clinical Professor
Department of Urology
University of Virginia
Charlottesville, Virginia
Chapter 10: Evidence-Based Practice

Jane Guttendorf, MSN, CRNP, APRN,BC, CCRN
Acute Care Nurse Practitioner
Department of Critical Care Medicine, CTICU
University of Pittsburgh Medical Center Presbyterian
Pittsburgh, Pennsylvania
Chapter 16: The Acute Care Nurse Practitioner

Ann B. Hamric, PhD, RN, FAAN
Associate Dean for Academic Programs
Professor
School of Nursing
Virginia Commonwealth University
Richmond, Virginia
Chapter 3: A Definition of Advanced Practice Nursing
Chapter 13: Ethical Decision Making

Charlene Hanson, EdD, FNP-BC, FAAN
Professor Emerita
School of Nursing
Georgia Southern University
Statesboro, Georgia
Chapter 11: Leadership
Chapter 12: Collaboration
Chapter 19: Business Planning and Reimbursement Mechanisms
Chapter 20: Marketing and Negotiation
Chapter 21: Understanding Regulatory, Legal, and Credentialing
    Requirements

Marilyn Hravnak, PhD, ACNP-BC, FCCM, FAAN
Associate Professor
School of Nursing
University of Pittsburgh
Pittsburgh, Pennsylvania
Chapter 16: The Acute Care Nurse Practitioner

Jean E. Johnson, PhD, RN, FAAN
Dean
School of Nursing
The George Washington University
Washington, DC
Chapter 22: Health Policy Issues in Changing Environments

Tsui-Sui Annie Kao, PhD, FNP-BC
Assistant Professor
School of Nursing
University of Michigan
Ann Arbor, Michigan
Chapter 15: The Primary Care Nurse Practitioner

Arlene W. Keeling, PhD, RN, FAAN
School of Nursing
University of Virginia
Charlottesville, Virginia
Chapter 1: A Brief History of Advanced Practice Nursing
    in the United States

Maureen A. Kelley, PhD, RN, CNM
Independence Chair
Clinical Associate Professor
Nell Hodgson Woodruff School of Nursing
Emory University
Atlanta, Georgia
Chapter 17: The Certified Nurse-Midwife

Ruth M. Kleinpell, PhD, APRN, BC, FAAN, CCRN
Professor
Adult Health Nursing
College of Nursing
Rush University
Chicago, Illinois
Chapter 16: The Acute Care Nurse Practitioner
Chapter 23: Integrative Review of Outcomes and Performance
    Improvement Research on Advanced Practice Nursing

Michael J. Kremer, PhD, CRNA, FAAN
Professor
Adult Health and Gerontological Nursing
Director
Nurse Anesthesia Program
Co-Director
Rush University Simulation Lab
Rush University College of Nursing
Chicago, Illinois
Chapter 18: The Certified Registered Nurse Anesthetist

Kathy S. Magdic, MSN, APRN,BC
Coordinator
Acute Care Nurse Practitioner Program
University of Pittsburgh
Pittsburgh, Pennsylvania
Chapter 16: The Acute Care Nurse Practitioner

Vicky A. Mahn-DiNicola, RN, MS, CPHQ
Vice President
Clinical Analytics and Regulatory Reporting
ACS Healthcare Provider Services
Midas+ Solutions
Tucson, Arizona
Chapter 24: Using Health Care Information Technology to
    Evaluate and Improve Performance and Patient Outcomes

Jane E. Mashburn, CNM, MN, FACNM
Director
Clinical Associate Professor
Nurse Midwifery Program
Nell Hodgson Woodruff School of Nursing
Emory University
Atlanta, Georgia
Chapter 17: The Certified Nurse-Midwife

Allison Barker Morse, ScM, ANP-BC, WHNP, AOCNP
Nurse Practitioner
Steward Division of Gynecologic Oncology
Steward Health Care System
Boston, Massachusetts
Lecturer
School of Nursing and Health Studies
Simmons College
Boston, Massachusetts
Chapter 9: Consultation

Eileen T. O'Grady, PhD, RN, ANP
Visiting Professor
Leinhard School of Nursing
Pace University
New York, New York
Policy Editor
AJNP and *NP World News*
Monroe Township, New Jersey
Certified Nurse Practitioner and Wellness Coach
Private Practice
McLean, Virginia
Chapter 22: Health Policy Issues in Changing Environments

Barbara C. Phillips, MN, GNP-BC, FNP-BC
Beachwater Health Associates
Olympia, Washington
Chapter 20: Marketing and Negotiation

Joanne M. Pohl, PhD, ANP-BC, FAAN, FAANP
Professor Emerita
PI, Institute for Nursing Centers
The University of Michigan School of Nursing
Ann Arbor, Michigan
Chapter 15: The Primary Care Nurse Practitioner

Joyce A. Pulcini, PhD, PNP-BC, FAAN, FAANP
Professor
School of Nursing
George Washington University
Washington, DC
*Chapter 6: International Development of Advanced
    Practice Nursing*

Jeanne Salyer, PhD, RN
Associate Professor
Adult Heath Nursing
Virginia Commonwealth University
Richmond, Virginia
*Chapter 5: Evolving and Innovative Opportunities for Advanced
    Practice Nursing*

Judith A. Spross, PhD, RN, FAAN
Professor
College of Science, Technology and Health
University of Southern Maine
Portland, Maine
Chapter 2: Conceptualizations of Advanced Practice Nursing
Chapter 8: Guidance and Coaching

Julie Vosit-Steller, DNP, FNP-BC, AOCN
Associate Professor of Practice
School of Nursing and Health Sciences
Simmons College
Boston, Massachusetts
Consultant
Steward Division of Gynecologic Oncology
Boston, Massachusetts
Palliative Care Consultant
Home and Hospice Care of Rhode Island
Providence, Rhode Island
Chapter 9: Consultation

Mary Fran Tracy, PhD, RN, CCNS, FAAN
Critical Care Clinical Nurse Specialist
University of Minnesota Medical Center
Minneapolis, Minnesota
Chapter 7: Direct Clinical Practice
Chapter 11: Leadership

Contributors to Teaching/ Learning Resources

Karen Brykczynski, DNSc, RN, FNP-BC, FAANP, FAAN
Professor
School of Nursing
University of Texas Medical Branch
Galveston, Texas

Margaret Faut Callahan, PhD, CRNA, FNAP, FAAN
Dean and Professor
College of Nursing
Marquette University
Milwaukee, Wisconsin

Susan K. Rice, PhD, RN, CPNP, CNS
Professor
College of Nursing
University of Toledo-HSC
Toledo, Ohio

Joanne M. Pohl, PhD, ANP-BC, FAAN, FAANP
Professor Emerita
PI, Institute for Nursing Centers
The University of Michigan School of Nursing
Ann Arbor, Michigan

Jeanne Salyer, PhD, RN
Associate Professor
Adult Heath Nursing
Virginia Commonwealth University
Richmond, Virginia

Julie Vosit-Steller, DNP, FNP-BC, AOCN
Associate Professor of Practice
School of Nursing and Health Sciences
Simmons College
Boston, Massachusetts
Consultant
Steward Division of Gynecologic Oncology
Boston, Massachusetts
Palliative Care Consultant
Home and Hospice Care of Rhode Island
Providence, Rhode Island

Mary Fran Tracy, PhD, RN, CCNS, FAAN
Critical Care Clinical Nurse Specialist
University of Minnesota Medical Center
Minneapolis, Minnesota

REVIEWERS

Nancy F. Altice, DNP, RN, CCNS, ACNS-BC
Cardiology Clinical Nurse Specialist
Carilion Clinic
Roanoke, Virginia

Karen Cummins, PhD, MSN, FNP-BC, CNE
Director
FNP Program
CRNP—Infectious Disease Services
Carlow University
VA Pittsburgh Healthcare System
Pittsburgh, Pennsylvania

Robin Donohoe Dennison, DNP, APRN, CCNS, CEN, CNE
Associate Professor
Georgetown University
Washington, DC

Joanne T. Ehrmin, PhD, CNS, RN
Professor
College of Nursing
University of Toledo
Toledo, Ohio

William Mark Enlow, DNP, ACNP, CRNA
Assistant Director
Assistant Professor
School of Nursing
Columbia University
New York, New York

Kathleen Farrell, DNSc, ACNP-BC, CCNS
Associate Professor Nursing
Murray State University
Murray, Kentucky

Lynne A. Frost, APRN, DNP, CPNP
Pediatric Nurse Practitioner
Clinical Preceptor for DNP students
University of Portland
Portland, Oregon

Jessica Lynn Haddy, RN, CNM, MSW
Clinical Instructor
University of Colorado at Denver
Aurora, Colorado

Leslie Corrine Trischank Hussey, PhD, RN
Contributing Faculty
Walden University
School of Nursing
Minneapolis, Minnesota

Rita Marie John, EdD, DNP, CPNP, PMHS
Associate Professor of Clinical Nursing
School of Nursing
Columbia University
New York, New York

Jill Johnson, DNP, APRN, FNP-BC, CCRN, CEN, CFRN
Market Manager
Clinic Operation
Take Care Health Systems
Alton, Illinois
Graduate Nursing Faculty
Chamberlain College of Nursing
Downers Grove, Illinois
Family Nurse Practitioner
Team Health Emergency Services
Lexington, Kentucky

Evelyn J. Norton, RN, DNP, CNL, NEA-BC, PMHNP-BC
Assistant Professor of Nursing
Saint Xavier University
Chicago, Illinois

Camille Payne, PhD, RN
Professor
WellStar School of Nursing
Kennesaw State University
Kennesaw, Georgia

Chad Rittle, DNP, MPH, RN
Assistant Professor
Nursing and Pathways coordinator
Chatham University
Pittsburgh, Pennsylvania

Margaret (Peggy) Slota, DNP, RN, FAAN
Director
Associate Professor
DNP and Graduate Nursing Leadership Programs
Carlow University
Pittsburgh, Pennsylvania

Joanne Spetz, PhD
Professor
University of California
San Francisco, California

Sheila Cox Sullivan, PhD, RN, VHA-CM
Associate Nurse Executive
Central Arkansas Veterans Healthcare System
Little Rock, Arkansas
Adjunct Associate Professor
University of Arkansas for Medical Sciences
Little Rock, Arkansas

Michele J. Upvall, PhD, RN, CRNP
Professor of Nursing
Carlow University
Pittsburgh, Pennsylvania

M. Terese Verklan, PhD, CCNS, RNC, FAAN
Professor
Neonatal clinical nurse specialist
University of Texas Medical Branch
Galveston, Texas

Since the first edition of *Advanced Practice Nursing: An Integrative Approach* was published in 1996, advanced practice nursing has continued its rapid evolution. Although there continue to be divergent perspectives, a unified and integrative understanding of advanced practice nursing and its core competencies is emerging both within and outside of the profession. Advanced practice nursing has continued to flourish as evidence mounts that this critically important level of nursing practice is good for patients/consumers. Indeed, the number of advanced practice nurses (APNs) in the United States increased 55% between 1996 and 2008 (the most recent report available), with sustained growth in all APN groups except clinical nurse specialists (CNSs). The APN role that has grown the most dramatically is the nurse practitioner (NP) role, which has experienced a 225% growth during that period (HHS, 2010).

These increases have occurred against a backdrop of dynamic national changes that represent significant opportunities for APNs. Notable recent developments that are incorporated in this edition of *Advanced Practice Nursing* include the Consensus Model for Advanced Practice Registered Nurse (APRN) Regulation (NCSBN, 2008), now fully implemented in 7 U.S. states, with additional states in various stages of adoption as of this writing; the passage of the Patient Protection and Affordable Care Act (PPACA) (HHS, 2011); and the Institute of Medicine (IOM) Report on *The Future of Nursing* (2011). The last two initiatives in particular have caused a re-examination of physician-dominated primary care, and primary and specialty care provided by APNs have achieved significant gains in the health care marketplace. The Doctor of Nursing Practice (DNP) degree spearheaded by the American Association of Colleges of Nursing (AACN, 2006) is now being offered in more than 200 U.S. Schools of Nursing, with more than 100 programs for this new degree in the planning stages (AACN, 2013). All of these developments have created uncertainties and chaos even as they have opened significant opportunities for the future of advanced practice nursing. These initiatives provided the impetus for this latest edition of *Advanced Practice Nursing*.

Purpose

Since its inception, this book has issued a clarion call for nursing leaders, educators, and practicing clinicians to reach greater consensus regarding an integrated understanding of and preparation for advanced practice nursing and the roles that APNs assume. This understanding asserts that advanced practice nursing is not medical substitution, but a value-added complement to patient care distinct from traditional medical practice. Clarity regarding advanced practice nursing is a professional imperative, as we must speak with increasing authority and consistency to policymakers, to those in other disciplines, and to one another. While the Editors are encouraged by the progress being made and the use of our work in this progress, the profession has not yet achieved clarity at all levels. Hence, our goal remains to describe an integrated understanding of advanced practice nursing that provides clarity and structure for students, faculty, practicing APNs, and the profession at large.

We believe this fifth edition defines and strengthens our understanding of advanced practice nursing—the competencies, roles, environmental complexity, and issues facing APNs—with clarity and authority that have strengthened with each revision. As with the previous edition, we have woven DNP competencies and expectations throughout the book *as they apply to and support this core understanding of advanced practice nursing*. However, the book remains equally useful for both master's- and DNP-level APN educational programs. An additional purpose with this edition is to describe and include international developments in advanced practice nursing. Some of the most exciting and active literature on APN roles is coming from countries outside of the United States, and is reflected in multiple chapters throughout the book.

Underlying Premises

We have deliberately elected to continue using the term "advanced practice nurse" or APN when discussing professional issues, even though the regulatory term "advanced practice registered nurse" or APRN is increasingly being adopted by states to conform to the Consensus Model for Regulation (NCSBN, 2008) and is seen frequently in the literature. The term *APRN* is an appropriate regulatory title, which we use when discussing legal and regulatory issues. However, regulation by the states does not constitute the full understanding of the advanced practice of nursing. We believe that advanced practice nursing is much broader than the "three Ps" (physical assessment, pathophysiology, and pharmacology; see

Chapter 3) and mastering expanded direct practice, as important as these elements are. Indeed, as discussed in Chapter 3, advanced practice nursing is a larger concept; regulation usually centers on the primary criteria for advanced practice nursing (graduate education, APN specialty certification, and a patient/family-focused practice) and thus does not incorporate the full professional understanding of this level of practice. The primary criteria, core APN competencies, and environmental elements affecting advanced practice embody this more complete understanding of advanced practice nursing and remain the focus of this text.

Several premises underlie our conviction that APN in this larger definitional sense holds great promise for improving patient care and the systems within which that care occurs:

- Improving the U.S. health care system requires simultaneous pursuit of the Institute of Healthcare Innovation's Triple Aim: improving the experience of health care, improving the health of populations, and reducing per capita costs of health care (IHI, 2013). APNs are unequivocally qualified to achieve these aims.

- For certain patient populations, APNs are the best providers for delivering quality care at a reasonable cost. As the PPACA unfolds, with added patients and increasing morbidities, the skill set of APNs, especially those practicing within community settings, will be essential. The recommendations of the IOM Report for nursing need to become a national priority in order to be realized. Other provider groups, particularly physicians, need to come to consensus around these key recommendations to achieve the synergy necessary to support health care reform; such consensus remains elusive at the time of this writing (Donelan, DesRoches, Dittue & Buerhaus, 2013; Iglehart, 2013).

- A uniform definition of advanced practice nursing and standards for educating and credentialing that are consistent across APN groups is a baseline requirement for advanced practice nursing to be fully implemented. Defining advanced practice for regulation has been the major contribution of the Consensus Model, but this understanding has not yet been enacted in all states. In the absence of a consistent definition and education for practice, the instability of the health care system and increased competition among providers pose a threat to the legitimacy of all APNs as providers. Such threats may lead to the loss of hard-won legal and regulatory battles. Similarly, the need for a consistent definition is clearly seen when looking at the international evolution of advanced practice nursing (see Chapter 6).

- A consistent definition of core competencies for APNs is essential in order to standardize APN education and to evaluate the outcomes of APN care across roles. It is also imperative that APNs practice these competencies in order to demonstrate the value-added component that they bring to care delivery and to ensure that advanced practice nursing is not confused with physician substitution.

- A uniform definition is essential for interprofessional teamwork. Administrators, physicians, and other providers must be able to rely on a core set of role expectations to design and implement cost-effective health care delivery systems that fully utilize all APN roles.

- Advanced practice nursing is good for patients; APNs represent important alternative providers in the health care system of the future. This conviction is strengthened by the PPACA mandates around nurse-managed clinics, accountable care organizations, APNs leading Medical Homes, and APNs serving as primary care providers of record.

Organization

As were previous editions, this fifth edition of *Advanced Practice Nursing: An Integrative Approach* has been extensively updated and revised to reflect current literature and trends. Particular attention has been paid to updating regulatory, credentialing, and emerging professional issues facing all APN roles. We have significantly increased the number of exemplars throughout the text to better demonstrate advanced practice nursing in action. In addition, the fifth edition contains the following major revisions:

In Part I, "Historical and Developmental Aspects of Advanced Practice Nursing," Chapter 1 has been revised to focus on each established APN role. Newly added historical photographs provide the context in which specialty nurse pioneers practiced. We have moved the chapter on "Evolving and Innovative Opportunities for Advanced Practice Nursing" into this section to reflect APN opportunities in new specialties, and have added a new Chapter 6 on advanced practice nursing's dramatic international evolution. In Part II, "Competencies of Advanced Practice Nursing," the seven core competencies are examined. The stability of the seven core APN competencies throughout the five editions of this text is noteworthy, even though elements of various competencies continue to be refined. One major change we have made in this edition is to modify the "Research" competency to clarify its focus on "Evidence-Based Practice" (see Chapter 3). This change reflects the central emphasis of this competency; APNs are sophisticated users of research evidence in making and sustaining practice change. Chapter 10 has been extensively rewritten to explore the continuum of evidence-based practice and practical strategies used by APNs in enacting this competency. Chapter 11 strengthens the Leadership competency to meet the needs of DNP graduate students. Chapter 12 has an in-depth focus on interprofessional collaboration to meet the challenges of the PPACA and the IOM Report.

The chapters in Part III, "Advanced Practice Roles: The Operational Definitions of Advanced Practice Nursing," continue to explicitly incorporate the core competencies and demonstrate how these competencies are played out in current APN practices. Features unique to each APN role, as well as the latest professional and policy changes relevant to the specific role, are described. The CNS chapter (Chapter 14) has been significantly updated to discuss the opportunities and challenges experienced by nurses in this role, along with strategies for strengthening the role going forward. The primary care NP chapter (Chapter 15) has been revised to explore the opportunities presented by the PPACA for new and innovative primary care practices. All of the changes in the APN roles chapters reflect the movement toward DNP education for APNs. Part IV, "Critical Elements in Managing Advanced Nursing Practice Environments," continues to explore key environmental factors affecting APN practice. Each chapter incorporates the social, political, and organizational contexts that APNs must manage for success. Chapter 22 on health policy incorporates an expanded discussion of political issues, a review of how the PPACA will likely impact APN practice, and the numerous opportunities and challenges health care reform poses for APNs. The final two chapters focus on outcomes and the critical contributions of APNs to improved patient and system outcomes. Chapter 23 presents an integrative review of the past 10 years of APN outcomes research. This chapter provides a wealth of evidence and APN-sensitive measures useful to both APN students and practitioners. Chapter 24 is essentially a new chapter for this edition, given the dramatic changes in health information technology and its use in clinical practice. The chapter author gives APNs the tools needed to use data and information technology to improve practice so that they are prepared to meet agency expectations for achieving clinical and institutional outcomes. In addition, the chapter describes strategies for strengthening APN performance evaluation through foci of quality improvement and outcomes evaluation.

Audience

This book is intended for graduate nursing students, practicing APNs in all roles, and educators, administrators, and leaders in the nursing profession. For students in any APN graduate program, whether master's or doctoral, this text provides a comprehensive resource that will be useful throughout their program of study. Initial clarity about the definition and competencies of advanced practice nursing can guide students as they enter their clinical coursework. We strongly recommend the book's use early in the program of study—in theory, research, policy, and APN role courses. This text is a valuable tool for use throughout clinical courses as students see the various APN roles and related competencies in action and as they begin practicing their chosen APN role. The critical focus on information technology and outcomes attributable to APN practices can help students in clinical courses begin to identify outcomes they will use to measure their success. Students who are nearing graduation, in role transition or capstone courses, will appreciate the role development chapter, the in-depth information on evidence-based practice, and the content in Part IV that explores business practices and environmental issues that they must be prepared to manage in the workplace.

For practicing APNs, the book updates both theoretical and practical content to guide role implementation. Individuals interested in strengthening or changing their roles will find many strategies for accomplishing these changes. The exploration of current issues in the health care environment makes the book particularly useful to practicing clinicians who face challenges within a marketplace that changes daily. The interprofessional, collaborative focus in many chapters may be useful to clinicians and educators in other fields. For example, interprofessional teams could benefit from discussions of the chapters that address guidance and coaching, collaboration, ethical decision-making skills, and health care policy. Administrators will appreciate the descriptions of various APN roles and the strategies for justifying and supporting APN positions.

For educators, the book will serve as a comprehensive curricular resource in preparing APNs for practice. It also serves as a guide to designing relevant courses on all the facets of advanced practice nursing. An exciting feature for faculty is the Instructor Resources on Evolve, which accompany the text. The Instructor Resources include more than 900 PowerPoint slides that are organized by chapter and include concepts and illustrations from the book. Also included are an electronic Image Collection containing all images from the book and an Instructor's Manual that provides strategies for effectively teaching the content of each chapter along with discussion questions that can be used for both classroom and online discussion. It is available on the Evolve website at http://evolve. elsevier.com/Hamric/).

Approach

We continue to describe advanced practice nursing at its best—as it is being enacted by APNs throughout the United States and around the world. There is still much work to be done: not all APN students are educated to practice with the competencies described here; too many nurses are in APN roles without the necessary credentials or core competencies, and thus true advanced practice nursing is not demonstrated; and there is still too much "alphabet soup" in role titles (for example, CNSs are variously called clinical coordinators, outcomes managers, educators, or consultants).

Roles continue to evolve as nursing matures in its enactment of advanced practice. In order to continue flourishing, however, advanced practice nursing must be distinct, recognizable, and describable. It will be clear to the reader that although the diverse roles described in Part III share the core criteria and competencies of advanced practice nursing, they are different and distinct from one another in their role enactment. This should be a cause for celebration as nursing recognizes its strength and range in meeting patient/client needs.

Creating this new edition has once again been a challenging undertaking. We are grateful for the hard work of our contributors, who substantially revised their chapters to portray a cutting-edge understanding of advanced practice nursing. We are privileged to participate with them in shaping this ever-changing area of nursing practice. Advanced practice nursing is a relatively young idea in the profession's evolution. We continue to be impressed by the complex process of integrating and incorporating the perspectives of all APN specialties. Not all groups have addressed the core concepts of advanced practice nursing or the competencies of APNs in a complete or consistent manner. The literature from the various advanced practice specialty groups remains unfortunately separated, and clinicians and educators tend to read and cite only their own group's literature. One of the major contributions of this book is an effort to solidify this integrative conceptualization of advanced practice nursing and to struggle with the complexities of all APN roles. Adopting this integrative approach, as challenging as it continues to be, has enriched this work immeasurably.

As a growing and critical component of present and future health care delivery systems, APNs are, and must continue to be, active participants in solving various pressing problems in health care delivery. We remain convinced that advanced practice nursing is essential to improving the health and well-being of individuals and populations across the globe. Increasing numbers of competent, well-prepared APNs will be invaluable as this century unfolds.

Transitions

The Editors wish to extend our thanks to Judy Spross, who retired from the Editor team after the publication of the 4th Edition. Although she did not participate as an Editor for the 5th Edition, she asked to share her reflections with our readers. Judy writes:

> I was a CNS graduate student when I met Ann Hamric in 1976—I was transformed by her teaching. A few years later, she, I, and, later Charlene "Chuckie" Hanson, would write together, leading and shaping contemporary advanced practice nursing. As editors, we were committed to a text that was reality-based—grounded in the day-to-day experiences of APNs. Writing from this perspective meant synthesizing empirical evidence and codifying our personal, experiential knowing related to the subject. Readers needed to recognize or imagine themselves in the text. In this vein, there are two things of which I am particularly proud. First, my Model of APN Guidance and Coaching reflects this synthesis and codification—starting with my experience with Ann as a teacher (before the term coaching was used), application of early empirical literature on APNs' teaching/coaching, my own work with patients and students, and then tacking back and forth between the literature and experience for every revision. Second, when Chuckie and I worked on the collaboration chapter in the first edition, I complained that dictionary definitions were inadequate and did not do justice to the great clinical and professional experiences we had had. Together we came up with a definition that is, I believe, more robust, aspirational, and timely as we move toward full realization of interprofessional practice. Perhaps someday it will make it into a dictionary! I am grateful for having been part of this endeavor and for colleagues and students who wrote for, edited, reviewed, or otherwise inspired and nurtured each edition."

As part of continued succession planning, Dr. Eileen O'Grady and Dr. Mary Fran Tracy have joined the Editor team for the 5th Edition. We welcome them and look forward to their contributions to future editions.

Ann B. Hamric
Charlene M. Hanson
Mary Fran Tracy
Eileen O'Grady

References

American Association of Colleges of Nursing (AACN). (2006). *The essentials of doctoral education for advanced nursing practice*. Washington, DC: Author.

AACN. (2013). DNP Fact Sheet. (http://www.aacn.nche.edu/media-relations/fact-sheets/dnp).

Institute of Healthcare Innovation (IHI). (2013). IHI triple aim initiative. (http://www.ihi.org/offerings/Initiatives/TripleAim/Pages/default.aspx).

Donelan, K., DesRoches, C. M., Dittus, R. S., & Buerhaus, P. (2013). Perspectives of physicians and nurse practitioners on primary care practice. *New England Journal of Medicine, 368*, 1898–1906.

Iglehart, J. K. (2013). Expanding the role of advanced nurse practitioners—risks and rewards. *New England Journal of Medicine, 368*, 1935–1941.

Institute of Medicine (IOM). (2011). *The future of nursing: Leading change, advancing health*. Washington, DC: National Academies Press.

NCSBN (National Council of State Boards of Nursing). (2008). Consensus model for APRN regulation: Licensure, accreditation, certification & education (APRN Consensus Work Group and NCSBN APRN Advisory Committee). Available from https:www.ncsbn.org/july_2008_consensus_model_for_aprn_regulation.pdf.

U.S. Department of Health and Human Services (HHS), Division of Nursing. (2010). *The registered nurse population, March 2008. Findings from the national sample survey of registered nurses*. Washington, DC: Author.

U.S. Department of Health and Human Services (HHS). (2011). Patient Protection and Affordable Care Act (PPACA). (http://www.healthcare.gov/law/full/index.html).

CONTENTS

CHAPTER

1

A Brief History of Advanced Practice Nursing in the United States

Anne Z. Cockerham • Arlene W. Keeling

CHAPTER CONTENTS

To understand the challenges facing advanced practice nursing today and determine a path for the future, it is essential to look to the past (see Box 1-1). This chapter presents some highlights of the history of advanced practice nursing in the United States, from the late nineteenth century to the present. It examines four established advanced practice roles—certified registered nurse anesthetists (CRNAs), certified nurse-midwives (CNMs), clinical nurse specialists (CNSs), and nurse practitioners (NPs)—in the context of the social, political, and economic environment of the time and within the context of the history of medicine, technology, and science. Legal issues and issues related to gender and health care manpower are considered. Although sociopolitical and economic context is critical to understanding nursing history, only historical events specifically relevant to the history of advanced practice nursing are included. The reader is encouraged to consult the references of this chapter for further information.

A brief comment on terminology:

The use of the term *specialist* in nursing can be traced to the turn of the twentieth century, when it was used to designate a nurse who had completed a postgraduate course in a clinical specialty area or who had extensive experience and expertise in a particular clinical practice area. With the introduction of the NP role during the 1960s and 1970s, the terms *expanded role* and *extended role* were used, implying a horizontal movement to encompass expertise from medicine and other disciplines. The more contemporary term, *advanced practice,* which began to be used in the 1980s, reflects a more vertical or hierarchical movement encompassing graduate education within nursing, rather than a simple expansion of expertise by the development of knowledge and skills used by other disciplines. Since the 1980s, the term *advanced practice nurse* (APN) has increasingly been used to delineate CRNAs, CNMs, CNSs, and NPs. In the last decade, state nursing practice acts have increasingly adopted the term *advanced practice registered nurse* (APRN). These professional and regulatory influences served to unite the advanced practice specialty roles conceptually and legislatively, thereby promoting collaboration and cohesion among APNs.

BOX 1-1   Timeline

1751   Pennsylvania Hospital opens in Philadelphia
1820   Florence Nightingale born
1860   *Notes on Nursing* published in the United States
1861   Dorothea Dix appointed Superintendent of Female Nurses of the Union Army
1861   Catholic Sisters deliver chloroform anesthesia during American Civil War
1873   Bellevue Hospital Training School and Connecticut Training School founded
1879   Mary Eliza Mahoney, first black graduate nurse, completes training program
1880-1900 Rapid proliferation of hospital nursing schools, from 15 schools to more than 400
1881   Clara Barton and others establish American Red Cross
1893   Nightingale pledge first recited in Detroit
1893   American Society of Superintendents of Training Schools for Nurses (precursor to National League for Nursing [NLN]) founded at Chicago World's Fair
1900   *American Journal of Nursing* first published
1901   Nurse Corps becomes permanent (became Army Nurse Corps in 1908)
1903   North Carolina passes first nurse registration law in United States
1908   National Association of Colored Graduate Nurses established
1910   Florence Nightingale dies
1910   Flexner Report criticizes quality of medical education
1912   National Organization of Public Health Nursing founded
1915   Lakeside Hospital School of Anesthesia opens in Cleveland, Ohio
1917   Frank v. South (Kentucky) upholds nursing anesthesia
1918-1919 Influenza epidemic and World War I
1922   Sigma Theta Tau formalized
1923   Goldmark Report criticizes quality of nursing education

1923   Yale School of Nursing becomes first autonomous school of nursing in the United States
1925   Kentucky Committee for Mothers and Babies, precursor to Frontier Nursing Service, founded
1931   American Association of Nurse Anesthetists (AANA) founded
1938   Chalmers Frances v. Nelson; practice of nurse anesthesia made legal
1943-1948 U.S. Cadet Nurse Corps supports nursing education to prepare nurses for military
1945   AANA develops and implements Certified Registered Nurse Anesthetists (CRNA) certification examination
1946   Hill Burton Act enacted, providing funds to construct hospitals
1947   Army-Navy Nurse Act secures commission status for military nurses
1950   NLN assumes responsibility for administering first national state board examination
1955   American College of Nurse-Midwives incorporated
1964   Nurse Training Act passed
1965   Medicare legislation enacted
1965   Pediatric Nurse Practitioner (PNP) certification program opens in Colorado
1975   American Nurses Association (ANA) holds ceremony to honor first certified nurses
1979   Nursing Doctorate (ND), first clinical doctorate program, established at Case Western Reserve University
1984   All states recognize nurse-midwifery
1985   American Academy of Nurse Practitioners (AANP) founded
1995   National Association of Clinical Nurse Specialists formed
2004   American Association of Colleges of Nursing recommends that all advanced practice nurses earn Doctorate in Nursing Practice (DNP)

Nurse Anesthetists

The roots of nurse anesthesia in the United States can be traced to the late nineteenth century. During the 1860s, two key events converged—the widespread use of the newly discovered chloroform anesthesia and the demand for such treatment for wounded soldiers during the American Civil War (1861 to 1865). In 1861, except for Catholic sisters and Lutheran deaconesses, there were few professional nurses in the United States. There were only a handful of nurse training schools[1] in the country and, for the most part, laywomen cared for families and friends when they were ill. When the first shots were fired on Fort Sumter and Civil War broke out, thousands of laywomen from the North and South volunteered to nurse. Because of social restrictions, these women actually did little hands-on nursing. Instead, they helped by reading to patients, serving them broths and stimulants such as tea,

---

[1]The word *training* was commonly used to describe nursing education in this era.

coffee, and alcohol, and assisting with the preparation of food in diet kitchens. Catholic sisters who nursed were given more freedom to provide direct care; their work included assisting in surgery, particularly with the administration of chloroform. Because the administration of chloroform was a relatively simple procedure in which the anesthetizer poured the drug over a cloth held over the patient's nose and mouth, the nuns quickly mastered this technique, providing the surgeons with invaluable assistance during the war (Jolly, 1927; Wall, 2005).

In the decade following the Civil War, hospitals throughout the United States opened nurse training schools modeled according to Florence Nightingale's school at St. Thomas Hospital in London. By the late nineteenth century, most U. S. hospitals used student nurses for staffing, rather than employing graduate nurses. One exception to this trend was the increasing use of graduate nurses as nurse anesthetists. Surgeons readily accepted them, valuing the fact that unlike the medical students who usually assisted them in giving anesthesia and spent much of the time observing the surgery itself rather than the patient's response to anesthesia, nurse anesthetists concentrated on administering the chloroform and observing the patient.

Anesthesia at Mayo Clinic

At St. Mary's Hospital in Rochester, Minnesota, Dr. William Worrall Mayo was among the first physicians in the country to recognize and train nurse anesthetists formally. In 1889, Dr. W.W. Mayo hired Edith Granham to be his anesthetist and office nurse. Subsequently, he hired Alice Magaw (later referred to as the "mother of anesthesia"; Keeling, 2007). Magaw kept excellent records of her results and, in 1900, published them in the *St. Paul's Medical Journal*. Reporting her "Observations on 1,092 Cases of Anesthesia from January 1, 1899 to January 1, 1900," she wrote:

> In that time, we administered an anesthetic 1,092 times; ether alone 674 times; chloroform 245 times; ether and chloroform combined, 173 times. I can report that out of this number, 1,092 cases, we have not had an accident; we have not had occasion to use artificial respiration once; nor one case of ether pneumonia; neither have we had any serious renal results. Tongue forceps were used but once, the operation was on the jaw and it was quite necessary (p. 306).

Between 1899 and 1901, the Doctors Mayo added several other nurse anesthetists to their surgical teams. Soon, Mayo Clinic would become world renowned for its nurse anesthesia training program.

During the 1910s, nurse anesthetists faced obstacles and new opportunities. Early in the decade, as the specialty of anesthesia was on the rise, the medical profession began to question a nurse's right to administer anesthesia, claiming that these nurses were practicing medicine without a license. In 1911, the New York State Medical Society argued (unsuccessfully) that the administration of an anesthetic by a nurse violated state law (Thatcher, 1953). A year later, the Ohio State Medical Board passed a resolution specifying that only physicians could administer anesthesia. Despite this resolution, nurse anesthetist Agatha Hodgins established the Lakeside Hospital School of Anesthesia in Cleveland, Ohio, in 1915. The challenge culminated in a lawsuit brought against the Lakeside Hospital program by the state medical society. This lawsuit was unsuccessful and resulted in an amendment to the Ohio Medical Practice Act protecting the practice of nurse anesthesia. However, medical opposition to the practice of nurse anesthesia continued in Kentucky and another lawsuit (Frank v. South) against nurse anesthetists was filed in 1917. In that case, the Kentucky appellate court ruled that anesthesia provided by nurse anesthetist Margaret Hatfield did not constitute the practice of medicine if it was given under the orders and supervision of a licensed physician (in this case, Dr. Louis Frank). The significance of this decision was that the courts declared nurse anesthesia legal but "subordinate" to the medical profession. It was a landmark decision, one that would have lasting implications for nurse anesthetists' practice. Later in the century it would also affect all advanced practice nurses (Keeling, 2007).

Wartime Opportunities

Opportunities for nurse anesthetists increased when the United States entered World War I in 1917. That year, more than 1000 nurses were deployed to Britain and France, including nurse anesthetists, some of whom had trained at Mayo and Cleveland Clinics. The realities of the front were gruesome; shrapnel created devastating wounds and mustard gas destroyed lungs and caused profound burns (Beeber, 1990). The resulting need for pain relief and anesthesia care for the wounded soldiers created an immediate demand for nurse anesthetists' knowledge and skills (Keeling, 2007).

It also created opportunities for research and physicians and nurses began investigating new methods of administering anesthesia. At the well-established Lakeside Hospital anesthesia program, Dr. George Crile and nurse anesthetist Agatha Hodgins experimented with combined nitrous oxide–oxygen administration. They also investigated the use of morphine and scopolamine as adjuncts to anesthesia. Also, as anesthesia practice became more complicated and scientific, physicians became interested in naming it as a medical specialty. As they did, some medical anesthesia groups again claimed that nurse anesthetists were practicing medicine without a license and once again initiated legal battles. Interprofessional conflict over disciplinary boundaries seemed inescapable.

After the war, opportunities for the employment of nurse anesthetists were mixed. For example, in 1922, Samuel Harvey, a Yale professor of surgery, hired Alice M. Hunt as an instructor of anesthesia with university rank at the Yale Medical School, a significant and prestigious appointment for a nurse (Thatcher, 1953). In contrast to Hunt's experience, however, many other nurse anesthetists struggled to find practice opportunities. Medicine was becoming increasingly complex, scientific, and controlled by organized medical specialties. See Box 1-2 for information on the Goldmark report.

It was soon clear that nurse anesthetists needed to organize and, in 1931, at Lakeside Hospital, Hodgins established the American Association of Nurse Anesthetists (AANA) and served as the organization's first president. At the first meeting of the association, the group voted to affiliate with the American Nurses Association (ANA). However, the ANA denied the request, probably because the ANA was afraid to assume legal responsibility for a group that could be charged with practicing medicine without a license (Thatcher, 1953).

The ANA's fears were not unfounded. During the 1930s, the devastation of the national economy made jobs scarce and the tension between nurse anesthetists and their physician counterparts continued, with more legal challenges to the practice of nurse anesthesia. In California, the Los Angeles County Medical Association sued nurse anesthetist Dagmar Nelson in 1934 for practicing medicine without a license; Nelson won. According to the judge, "The administration of general anesthetics by the defendant Dagmar A. Nelson, pursuant to the directions and supervision of duly licensed physicians and surgeons, as shown by the evidence in this case, does not constitute the practice of medicine or surgery...." (McGarrel, 1934).

In response, Dr. William Chalmers-Frances filed another suit against Nelson in 1936, which again resulted in a judgment for Nelson (Chalmers-Frances v. Nelson, 1936). In 1938, the physician appealed the case to the California Supreme Court, which again ruled in favor of Nelson. The case became famous. The courts established legal precedent—the practice of nurse anesthesia was legal and within the scope of nursing practice, as long as it was done under the guidance of a supervising physician.

While World War II provided opportunities for young nurses in Europe to learn the skills necessary to administer anesthesia, it also was the period in which anesthesia grew into a medical specialty (Waisel, 2001). In 1939, just

---

BOX 1-2   Goldmark Report

As nursing and nurses' training developed in the late nineteenth and early twentieth centuries, many accused the widely used apprentice system of lacking academic rigor. With mounting pressure to examine the state of nursing education, the Rockefeller Foundation supported the formation of the Committee for the Study of Nursing Education. Yale University public health professor Charles-Edward Amory Winslow chaired the committee on which six nurses served, including Adelaide Nutting, Annie Goodrich, and Lillian Wald. The committee's secretary and survey research leader was social worker and author Josephine Goldmark.

The survey included a sample of 23 schools and was intended to be representative of the more than 1800 nurse training schools then in existence. In 1923, the committee released their findings, known as the Goldmark Report. The major recommendations included increasing educational standards in nursing schools, focusing student time on education rather than on providing labor for hospital wards, moving educational programs to universities, and requiring that nurse educators have advanced education (Goldmark, 1923).

Although some changes in nursing education became apparent after publication of the Goldmark Report, notably the establishment of Yale University's autonomous nursing school, the hoped for widespread elevation of nursing education did not occur. Hospital administrators strenuously resisted elimination of the free labor that nursing students provided to hospitals. Physicians argued that nurses were overtrained to provide the services that nurses needed to give. Fueled by disagreements among nurses themselves, state laws setting out requirements for nursing education varied drastically. The continued variability in nursing education stood in contrast to the medical profession's response to the Flexner Report, issued in 1910, which resulted in standardization of medical education at the postgraduate level.

---

before the United States entered the war, the first written examination for board certification in medical anesthesiology was given, but the specialty still sought legitimacy. Meanwhile, demands for anesthetists, advances in the types of anesthesia available, and continuing education in the field increasingly stimulated physicians' interest in the specialty. The medical journal *Anesthesiology,* established in 1940, further strengthened medicine's claim to anesthesia practice. In particular, the use of the new drug sodium pentothal required specialized knowledge of physiology and pharmacology, underscoring the emerging view that only physicians could provide anesthesia. In fact, the administration of anesthesia was becoming more complex, and anesthesiologists demonstrated their expertise not only in administering sodium pentothal but also in performing endotracheal intubation and regional blocks (Waisel, 2001). Clearly, medicine was strengthening its hold on the specialty.

At the same time, World War II increased the demand for anesthetists on the battlefield. Despite profound shortages of anesthetists early in the war, the U.S. military would not grant nurse anesthetists a specific designation within the military, and experienced nurse anesthetists were required to accept general nurse status. Later, when shortages became even more severe, staff nurses were trained to administer anesthesia.

◎ EXEMPLAR 1-1   **Nurse Anesthetists in the 8th Evacuation Hospital, Italy, 1942-1945**

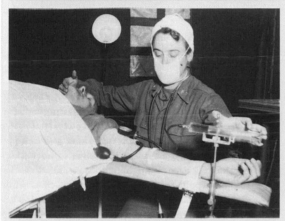

(Courtesy University of Virginia, Center for Nursing Historical Inquiry.)

During World War II, the University of Virginia sponsored the 8th Evacuation Hospital, a 750-bed mobile hospital a few miles from the front lines in North Africa and Italy. Conditions were demanding and the work overwhelming; surgical teams sometimes operated round the clock despite air raids, heavy rains, and blackouts. There, Dorothy Sandridge Gloor, a young surgical nurse, was trained on the job to give anesthesia. The unit had only one trained anesthesiologist and two nurse anesthetists on staff, and it soon became apparent that more help was needed if the team was to keep up with the "endless stream of battle casualties requiring surgery" (Kinser, 2011, p. 11). Gloor and other nurse anesthetists worked side by side with the surgeons for 16-hour shifts, collaborating with their colleagues to save the injured soldiers. She learned new skills and the specialty knowledge necessary to deliver anesthesia, noting how she learned to start IVs and make critical observations of the patient on which to base the administration of anesthesia (Kinser, 2011). Working with patients to calm their fears prior to surgery, and explaining what would happen in the operating suite, Gloor and her colleagues demonstrated expertise in coaching the critically injured men; see Box 1-3.

After the war, the specialty of nurse anesthesia continued to take steps to increase its legitimacy. The AANA instituted mandatory certification for CRNAs in 1945. This formal credentialing of CRNAs specified the requirements that a nurse had to meet to practice as a nurse anesthetist, preceded credentialing of nurses in the other specialties, and marked a significant milestone. Meanwhile, during the 1950s, increasing numbers of physicians were choosing anesthesia as a specialty. However, nurse anesthetists were not to be deterred. In 1952, the AANA established an accreditation program to monitor the quality of nurse anesthetist education. Soon, the United States was once again at war, this time with Korea and, once again, war provided a setting in which opportunities abounded for nurse anesthetists, particularly for those who were male. By the end of the decade, the army had established nurse anesthesia education programs, including one at Walter Reed General Hospital, which graduated its first class in 1961—but this class consisted only of men. Later, the Letterman General Hospital School of Anesthesia in San Francisco also graduated an all-male class. This significant movement of men into a nursing specialty was unprecedented and would continue in the next decade when the United States entered the war in Vietnam.

As was the case in wars of other eras, the war in Vietnam (1955-1975) provided nurses with opportunities to stretch the boundaries of the discipline as they treated thousands of casualties in evacuation hospitals and aboard hospital ships. Not surprisingly, nurse anesthetists played an active role at the front, providing vital services in the prompt surgical treatment of the wounded. According to one account (Jenicek, 1967):

The nurse anesthetist suddenly became a part of a new concept in the treatment of the severely wounded. The Dust-Off helicopter brings medical aid to severely wounded casualties who formerly would have died before or perhaps during evacuation. ... Very often it is a nurse anesthetist who first is available to intubate a casualty, and by so doing may avoid the need for tracheostomy (p. 348).

EXEMPLAR 1-1　　**Nurse Anesthetists in the 8th Evacuation Hospital, Italy, 1942-1945—*cont'd***

Opportunity was not without cost. Of the 10 nurses killed in Vietnam, two were nurse anesthetists (Bankert, 1989).

At home in the United States, the 1970s proved to be a difficult decade for nurse anesthetists. In 1972, years after the inception of nurse anesthesia as a specialty role, only four state practice acts specifically mentioned them. Nevertheless, some progress was made in interprofessional relations that year. The AANA and the American Society of Anesthesiologists (ASA) issued a "Joint Statement on Anesthesia Practice," promoting the concept of the anesthesia team. However, a few years later, in 1976, the ASA Board of Directors voted to withdraw support from the 1972 statement, endorsing one that explicitly supported physician control over CRNA practice (Bankert, 1989).

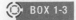 BOX 1-3　**Growth of Hospitals, Scientific Nursing, and the GI Bill**

In the period after World War II, optimism about the possibilities of research and scientific knowledge permeated the United States. Without a doubt, specialization and a scientific approach to medical care had captured the interest of Americans. These two factors would set the stage for dramatic changes in health care. Another important factor was economic as federally funded hospital construction reshaped the setting in which physicians and nurses practiced. In 1946, Congress passed the Hill-Burton Act, which provided large-scale funding to modernize aging hospitals and build new ones. The new hospital spaces changed how care was given because the sickest patients were grouped together in the ICU (Fairman & Lynaugh, 1998). This trend contributed to an increase in specialization in nursing while simultaneously accelerating nursing's invisibility when the costs of nursing care were included with the room rate.

In addition to funding new hospitals, the federal government provided funds for nurse education in the postwar years. Nurses returning from World War II were eligible to pursue advanced education under the GI Bill and many took advantage of the opportunity to return to school. Prompted by the Brown Report of 1948, the National League of Nursing Education (NLNE) established a committee that catalogued all nursing programs, including those leading to a master's degree, in a 1949 issue of AJN (Donahue, 1996).

graduate degree did, in fact, promote nurse anesthesia eduction. In 1973, the University of Hawaii opened the first master's degree program for nurse anesthesia, moving the role forward in the evolving criteria of advanced practice nursing.

Reimbursement for CRNA practice was not as clearcut. In fact, third-party payment had its own set of issues. Beginning in 1977, the AANA led a long and complex effort to secure third-party reimbursement under Medicare so that CRNAs could bill for their services. The organization would finally succeed in 1989. Meanwhile, the financial threat posed by CRNAs to physicians was the source of continued interprofessional conflicts with medicine. During the second half of the twentieth century, tensions escalated, particularly in relation to malpractice policies, antitrust, and restraint of trade issues. In 1986, Oltz v. St. Peter's Community Hospital established the right of CRNAs to sue for anticompetitive damages when anesthesiologists conspired to restrict practice privileges. A second case, Bhan v. NME Hospitals, Inc. (1985), established the right of CRNAs to be awarded damages when exclusive contracts were made between hospitals and physician anesthesiologists. Undeniably, CRNAs were winning the legal battles and overcoming practice barriers erected by hospital administrators and physicians.

The 1990s saw a significant growth in CRNA education programs, although many of the programs were very small. As the decade opened, there were 17 master's programs in nurse anesthesia; by 1999, there were 82 (Bigbee & Amidi-Nouri, 2000). As of 1998, all accredited programs in nurse anesthesia were required to be at the master's level; however, they were not uniformly located in schools of nursing. Instead, they were housed in a variety of disciplines, including schools of nursing, medicine, allied health, and basic science, a fact that is still true today. Today, with the American Association of Colleges of Nursing (AACN) pushing for the Doctor of Nursing Practice (DNP), these programs face a new challenge—redesigning their curricula to meet the requirements for CRNAs set by AANA while simultaneously meeting those

Education and Reimbursement

Later in the decade, with the new requirement that CRNAs have a master's degree, the number of nurse anesthesia education programs declined significantly, largely because of the closure of many small certification programs. However, the new requirement that programs offer a for DNP (AACN, 2006). Nonetheless, in 2007, the AANA affirmed its support that the Doctor of Nurse Anesthesia Practice (DNAP) be the entry for nurse anesthesia practice by 2025 (AANA, 2007).

Nurse-Midwives

Like nurse anesthesia, the origins of nurse-midwifery in America can be traced to the preprofessional work of women. Throughout the eighteenth and nineteenth centuries, lay midwives, rather than professional nurses or physicians, assisted women in childbirth. Midwives who were brought to the United States with the slave trade in 1619, and others who arrived later with waves of European immigration, were respected community members. In the late nineteenth and early twentieth centuries however, these untrained midwives would lose respect as scientific, hospital-based deliveries became the norm. Meanwhile, women in isolated communities throughout the country, particularly in rural settings, continued to employ lay midwives for deliveries well into the twentieth century.

In the early twentieth century, national concern about high maternal-infant mortality rates led to heated debates surrounding issues of midwife licensing and control; lay midwives would soon be blamed for the high maternal and infant mortality rates that plagued the United States. In 1914, Dr. Frederick Taussig, speaking at the annual meeting of the National Organization of Public Health Nursing (NOPHN) in St. Louis, proposed that the creation of "nurse-midwives" might solve the "midwife question" and suggested that nurse-midwifery schools be established to train graduate nurses (Taussig, 1914). Later in the decade, the Children's Bureau called for efforts to instruct pregnant women in nutrition and recommended that public health nurses teach principles of hygiene and prenatal care to so-called granny midwives (Rooks, 1997). In 1918, responding to a study conducted by the New York City Health Commissioner that indicated the need for comprehensive prenatal care, the Maternity Center Association (MCA) was established. It soon served as the central organization for a network of community-based maternity centers throughout the city.

The midwife problem was not easily solved, however. The use of midwives varied along ethnic, geographic, race, and class lines. With the rise in scientific medicine, many upper and middle class urban white women began to use obstetricians to deliver their babies in hospital delivery rooms (Rinker, 2000). However, nationality and other issues continued to influence women's choices. For example, many urban European immigrants continued to employ midwives to deliver their babies at home. Geographic location and access to physicians' services also played a part. For example, in rural southern states such as Mississippi, in which 50% of the population was black, most women (80% of African American and 8% of white women) relied on African American granny midwives to deliver their babies (Smith, 1994). Soon, a pattern could be identified: physicians delivered women of higher socioeconomic status in hospitals. Midwives attended the poor in the women's homes.

Nurse-Midwifery Education and Organization

Aside from two tiny, short-lived, nurse-midwifery schools, about which little is documented (Manhattan Midwifery School in New York City and Preston Retreat Hospital in Philadelphia), the earliest school to educate nurse-midwives was the School of the Association for the Promotion and Standardization of Midwifery (APSM) in New York City (Burst & Thompson, 2003). Affiliated with the Maternity Center Association (MCA), the APSM opened in 1932. More commonly known as the Lobenstine Midwifery School, in honor of Ralph Waldo Lobenstine, chairman of the MCA's medical board, the APSM graduated its first class in 1933. In 1939, the entry of Britain into World War II proved to be the catalyst for the establishment of the second major school for nurse-midwifery in the United States, the Frontier Graduate School of Midwifery (FGSM). That year, the Kentucky FNS lost many of its British nurse-midwives when they returned to England to work; in response, FNS leader Mary Breckinridge established the FGSM (Buck, 1940; Cockerham & Keeling, 2012).[2]

While the United States was at war, nurse-midwives continued their work on the home front. Key to their development in the 1940s was the establishment of a formal organization of practicing nurse-midwives, the American Association of Nurse-Midwives (AANM), which incorporated in 1941 under the leadership of Mary Breckinridge. By July 1942, the AANM had a "membership of 71 graduate nurses" who had specialty training in midwifery (News Here and There, 1942, p. 832). Three years later, in 1944, the National Organization of Public Health Nurses established a section for nurse-midwives[3] within their organization.

This group prepared a roster of all midwives in the country and defined their practice, making it clear that

---

[2]This program was for nurses who already had a degree in nursing (i.e., registered nurses), but was not a graduate program in the modern sense of the term.

[3]Expanded preparation for nurse-midwives also influenced the practice of lay midwives. As the CNMs gained knowledge, they began to share it with the lay midwives. During this decade, minority nurses were also encouraged to become CNMs, albeit in segregated institutions. On March 13, 1942, "the first class of three Negro nurse midwives graduated from the midwifery school operated at the Tuskegee Institute under the auspices of the Macon County Health Department" (Negro Nurse-Midwives, 1942, p. 705).

EXEMPLAR 1-2   The Frontier Nursing Service: A New Model for Nurse-Midwifery

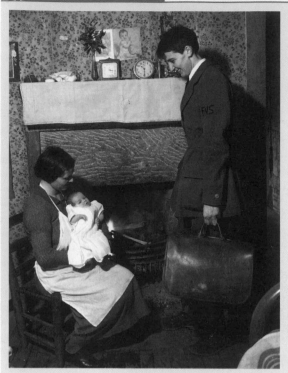

(Courtesy Frontier Nursing Service.)

In 1925, nurse-midwife Mary Breckinridge founded the Frontier Nursing Service (FNS) in an economically depressed, rural mountainous area of southeastern Kentucky. British nurse-midwives and American public health nurses provided midwifery and nursing care through a decentralized network of nurse-run clinics (Breckinridge, 1981; Rooks, 1997). Because there were few roads in the mountainous region, the nurses traveled by horseback to attend births, carrying their supplies in saddlebags. One FNS nurse described the bags and their

standing orders, or Medical Routines, whereby a physician committee supervised their practice:

> The whole of the district work of the FNS in the Kentucky mountains is done with the aid of two pairs of saddlebags ... In these bags we have everything needed for a home delivery .... In one of the pockets we carry our *Medical Routines* which tells us what we may—and may not—do. A very treasured possession! (pp. 1183-1184).

From the outset, FNS nurses carefully maintained records of their work and their outcomes were stellar. Reflecting on her work in later years, Breckinridge (1981) noted that "trained statisticians were to come later, through a grant from the Carnegie Corporation, but from the start we had records and report sheets and kept them carefully" (p. 166). When the Metropolitan Life Insurance Company analyzed the findings in 1951, they found that FNS staff members had attended 8596 births, with 6533 of those occurring in patients' homes, since 1925. More importantly, the FNS maternal mortality rate of 1.2/1000 was significantly lower than the national average of 3.4/1000 during the same period (Varney, 2004). Throughout the service's existence, the FNS nurses' documentation of the outcomes of their care would serve to advance their cause.

Despite exemplary clinical outcomes of the FNS, by midcentury, nurse-midwives were experiencing some of the same tensions with physicians that nurse anesthetists had faced. Changes in leadership on the advisory board, an increase in medical knowledge, the rapid development of new drugs, and a changing economic climate all played a part in accounting for these stricter controls over FNS nursing practice. The FNS medical advisory board reinforced traditional disciplinary boundaries on nursing's scope of practice (Keeling, 2007).

nurse-midwives would continue to practice under physician authority.

Move Toward Natural Childbirth

The renewed public interest in natural childbirth that stemmed from the women's movement was particularly beneficial to the practice of nurse-midwifery in the 1970s; the demand for nurse-midwifery services increased dramatically during that decade. In addition, sociopolitical developments, including the increased employment of CNMs in federally funded health care projects and the

increased birth rate resulting from baby boomers reaching adulthood, converged with inadequate numbers of obstetricians to foster the rapid growth of CNM practice (Varney, 2004). In 1971, only 37% of CNMs who responded to an American College of Nurse-Midwives (ACNM) survey were employed in clinical midwifery practice. By 1977, this number increased to 51%. Not surprisingly, the earlier pattern continued; most CNMs practiced in the rural underserved areas of the Southwest and southeastern United States, including Appalachia.

At the national level, physician support for CNM practice became official. In 1971, the ACNM, the American

EXEMPLAR 1-3   Jean Fee: Public Health Nurse, Nurse-Midwife, and Nurse Practitioner

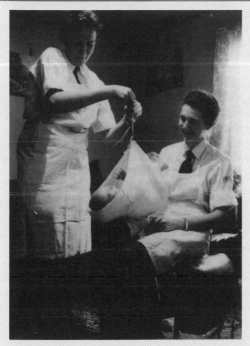

(From Frontier Nursing University)

Jean Fee, born in rural Alberta, Canada, arrived in Hyden, Kentucky, in 1958 eager to become a district nurse and pursue her passion to do public health work. Dismayed to find that only those with nurse-midwifery training were permitted to work on [sic] the districts, Fee enrolled in the Frontier Graduate School of Midwifery. She soon discovered the excitement and fulfillment of combining public health nursing and nurse-midwifery. Fee recalled, "I absolutely detested obstetrics in [nursing] training. I did the midwifery course [at Frontier] in self-defense so that I could work on the district, and in the meantime I learned that midwifery was a whole different ball game, much more up my alley" (Cockerham, 2012). After graduation from the midwifery training program in 1959, Fee remained in Kentucky, serving as district nurse-midwife for several different districts for 18 months. During that time, Fee demonstrated her expertise in clinical practice as she traveled around the districts on her horse, attending births and caring for the health needs of entire families. Several decades after leaving the FNS, and having worked in a variety of capacities in different areas, Fee wanted to apply for a family nurse practitioner position but needed official recognition of her preparation in primary care of families during her time at Frontier. According to Fee (Cockerham, 2012):

I had found ways to challenge the exam for nurse practitioner ... My English midwifery instructor, Molly Lee, still at FNS ... she got up into the attic and found the curriculum for the year that we were there. At FNS we did full care; we didn't just do midwifery and we were primary care nurse practitioners from 1925 on. The title hadn't been thought up at the time, but the job description was there and we had it! I won the right to sit that exam. In 1980, I was able to certify as a Family Nurse Practitioner.

College of Obstetricians and Gynecologists, and the Nurses' Association of the American College of Obstetricians and Gynecologists issued a joint statement supporting the development and employment of nurse-midwives in obstetric teams directed by a physician. The joint statement, which was critical to the practice of nurse-midwifery, reflected some resolution of the interprofessional tension that had existed through much of the twentieth century. However, it did not provide for autonomy for CNMs. Later in the decade, the ACNM revised its definitions of CNM practice and its philosophy, emphasizing the distinct midwifery and nursing origins of the role (ACNM, 1978a, b). This conceptualization of nurse-midwifery as the combination of two disciplines, nursing and midwifery, was unique among the advanced practice nursing specialties. It served to align nurse-midwives with non–nurse midwives, thereby broadening their organizational and political base. Philosophically controversial, even within nurse-midwifery, the conceptualization created some distance from other APN specialties that saw advanced practice roles as based solely in the discipline of nursing. This distinction would continue to isolate CNMs from some APNs for the next several decades.

By the 1980s, the public's acceptance of nurse-midwives had grown, and demand for their services had increased among all socioeconomic groups. By the middle of 1982, there were almost 2600 CNMs, most located on the East Coast. "Nurse-midwifery had become not only acceptable but also desirable and demanded. Now the problem was that, after years during which nurse-midwives struggled for existence, there was nowhere near the supply to meet the demand" (Varney, 1987, p. 31).

Meanwhile, conflict with the medical profession increased as obstetricians perceived a growing threat to their practices. The denial of hospital privileges, attempts to deny third-party reimbursement, and state legislative battles over statutory recognition of CNMs ensued. In particular, problems concerning restraint of trade emerged. In 1980, Congress and the Federal Trade Commission (FTC) conducted a hearing to determine the extent of the restraint of trade issues experienced by CNMs. In two cases, one in Tennessee and one in Georgia, the FTC obtained restraint orders against hospitals and insurance companies attempting to limit the practice of CNMs (Diers, 1991), in essence ensuring that CNMs they could practice. Third-party reimbursement for CNMs was a second issue. In 1980, CNMs, working under the Civilian Health and Medical Program of the Uniformed Services (CHAMPUS; now Tricare) for military dependents, were the first to receive approval for reimbursement. Third-party payment for CNMs was also included under Medicaid. Statutory recognition by state legislatures was a third problem that would be addressed in the 1980s. By 1984, all 50 states had recognized nurse-midwifery in their state laws or regulations (Varney, 1987).

During the 1990s, increasing demand for CNM services resulted in the gradual expansion in the scope of nurse-midwifery practice. CNMs began to provide care to women with relatively high-risk pregnancies in collaboration with obstetricians in some of the nations' academic tertiary care centers (Rooks, 1997). During this decade, two practice models emerged, the CNM service model, in which CNMs were responsible for the care of a caseload of women determined to be eligible for midwifery care, and the CNM-MD team model. Nurse-midwives continued making progress in establishing laws and regulations needed to support their practice. However, the struggle for prescriptive authority continued until 2007, when Pennsylvania's nurse-midwives, the last in the country, finally received the right to prescribe (ACNM, 2007).

Clinical Nurse Specialists

The roots of the clinical nurse specialist role lie in the area of psychiatric nursing, which had its origins in the Quaker reform movement initiated earlier in mid–nineteenth century England. In the United States, these Quaker reformers challenged the brutal treatment of the insane and advocated "moral treatment," emphasizing gentler methods of social control in a domestic setting (D'Antonio, 1991, p. 411).

The first American training program for psychiatric nurses was founded in 1880 at McLean Hospital in Massachusetts (Critchley, 1985). According to Linda Richards, a 1873 graduate of the New England Hospital School of Nursing, the McLean Hospital maintained high standards and demonstrated "the value of trained nursing for the many persons afflicted with mental disease" (Richards, 1911, p. 109). Richards served as superintendent of nurses

at the Taunton Insane Hospital for 4 years, beginning in 1899. She subsequently organized a nursing school for the preparation of psychiatric nurses at the Worcester Hospital for the Insane and finally went to the Michigan Insane Hospital in Kalamazoo, where she remained until 1909 (Richards, 1911). Because of this work, Richards is credited with founding the specialty of psychiatric nursing.

The first decades of the twentieth century witnessed growth in all specialties, including the area of psychiatry. During this period, Harry Stack Sullivan's classic writings and the work of Sigmund Freud changed psychiatric nursing dramatically. The emphasis on interpersonal interaction with patients and milieu treatment supported the movement of nurses into a more direct role in the psychiatric care of hospitalized patients.

Because of an increased public awareness of psychiatric problems in returning soldiers, (Critchley, 1985), World War II influenced the specialty of psychiatric nursing. During the 1940s, new treatments were introduced for the care of the mentally ill, including the widespread use of electroshock therapy. The new treatments would require the assistance of nurses who had specialized knowledge and training in the area. According to a 1942 *American Journal of Nursing* (AJN) article, "Only the nurse skilled in her profession and with additional psychiatric background has a place in mental hospitals today" (Schindler, 1942, p. 861). By 1943, three postgraduate programs in psychiatric nursing had been established. As nurse educator Frances Reiter later reflected on her career, she recalled having first used the term *nurse clinician* in a speech in 1943 to describe a nurse with advanced "curative" knowledge and clinical competence committed to providing the highest quality of direct patient care (Reiter, 1966). In 1946, after Congress passed the National Mental Health Act designating psychiatric nursing as a core discipline in mental health, federal funding for graduate and undergraduate educational programs and research became available, and programs in psychiatric and mental health were included in schools of nursing throughout the United States. Psychiatric nursing knowledge was now widely accepted as essential content in the nursing curriculum. Psychiatric nursing was also becoming established as a graduate level specialty, one that would lead the way for clinical nurse specialization in the next decade.

Psychiatric nursing blossomed as a specialty in the 1950s. In 1954, Hildegarde E. Peplau, Professor of Psychiatric Nursing, established a master's program in psychiatric nursing in the United States at Rutgers University in New Jersey. Considered the first CNS education program, this program, and the growth of specialty knowledge in psychiatric nursing that ensued, provided support for psychiatric nurses to begin exploring new leadership roles in the care of patients with mental illness in inpatient and outpatient settings. Scholarship in psychiatric nursing also flourished, including Peplau's conceptual framework for psychiatric nursing. Her book, *Interpersonal Relations in Nursing: A Conceptual Frame of Reference for Psychodynamic Nursing* (1952), provided theory-based practice for the specialty. Clearly, the link between academia and specialization was becoming stronger and the psychiatric specialty was leading the way.

The 1960s are most often noted as the decade in which clinical nurse specialization took its modern form. Peplau (1965) contended that the development of areas of specialization is preceded by three social forces: (1) an increase in specialty-related information; (2) new technologic advances; and (3) a response to public need and interest. In addition to shaping most nursing specialties, these forces had a particularly strong effect on the development of the psychiatric CNS role in the 1960s. The Community Mental Health Centers Act of 1963, as well as the growing interest in child and adolescent mental health care, directly enhanced the expansion of that role in outpatient mental health care.

Psychiatric nursing was not the only nursing specialty developing after mid–twentieth century. After the enactment of the 1964 Nurse Training Act, numerous CNS master's programs were created. These new, clinically focused graduate programs were instrumental in developing and defining the CNS role.

Coronary Care Unit: A New Era of Specialization

With the establishment of the Bethany Hospital Coronary Care Unit (CCU) in Kansas City, Kansas, in 1962 and a second unit at the Presbyterian Hospital in Philadelphia, coronary care nursing emerged as a new clinical specialty. As CCUs proliferated across the country with the support of federally funded regional medical programs, nurses and physicians acquired specialized clinical knowledge in the area of cardiology. Together, these nurses and physicians discussed clinical questions and negotiated responsibilities (Lynaugh & Fairman, 1992). In so doing, CCU nurses also expanded their scope of practice. Identifying cardiac arrhythmias, administering IV medications, and defibrillating patients who had lethal ventricular fibrillation, CCU nurses blurred the invisible boundary separating the disciplines of nursing and medicine. These nurses were diagnosing and treating patients in dramatic life-saving situations, thereby challenging the very definition of nursing that had been published by the ANA only a few years earlier (Keeling, 2004, 2007; Box 1-4). However, they did not differentiate specialization from advanced practice nursing. That would come later, as nursing faculty developed master's programs to prepare cardiovascular CNSs and, after that, nurse practitioners.

 BOX 1-4   **American Nurses Association Defines Nursing Practice (c. 1950s)**

The seminal work of nurse scholar Virginia Henderson on scientifically based, patient-centered care laid the foundation for changes in nursing that would occur in the second half of the twentieth century. Influenced by Henderson and Peplau, innovative nurses such as Frances Reiter at New York Medical College initiated a clinical nurse graduate curriculum designed to provide nurses with an intellectual clinical component based on a liberal arts education, in effect, supporting a broader role for nurses (Fairman, 2001). However, although academic nursing was making strides toward establishing specialty education and expanding the nurse specialist's scope of practice, the ANA developed a model definition of nursing that would unduly restrict nursing practice for the next several decades. The definition, prepared in 1955 and adopted by many states, read as follows (ANA, 1955):

> The practice of professional nursing means the performance for compensation of any act in the observation, care and counsel of the ill … or in the maintenance of health or prevention of illness … or the administration of medications and treatments as prescribed by a licensed physician. … The foregoing shall not be deemed to include acts of diagnosis or prescription of therapeutic or corrective measures.

Although the ANA may simply have been seeking clarity in defining the discipline's boundaries, its exclusion of the acts of diagnosis and prescription stifled the development of advanced practice nursing. Discussing the impact of the ANA's restrictions on diagnosis and prescription, law professor Barbara Safriet (1992) argued: "Even at the time the ANA's model definition was issued … it was unduly restrictive when measured by then current nursing practice." Nurses had been assessing patients for more than 50 years. According to historian Bonnie Bullough (1984), "The fascinating thing about the disclaimer [regarding diagnosis and prescription] is that it was made *not* by the American Medical Association, but the American Nurses Association. … In effect, organized nursing surrendered without any battle over boundaries." The ANA's 1955 definition of nursing would restrict the expansion of nurses' scope of practice for the rest of the twentieth century as the profession struggled with the dichotomy of care versus cure and of medical versus nursing diagnoses. In essence, the definition reversed years of hard-won gains in expanding the scope of nursing practice.

EXEMPLAR 1-4   **Expanding Role of the Nurse in the 1960s**

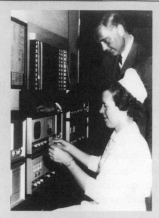

(Courtesy University of Virginia, Center for Nursing Historical Inquiry.)

In 1962, Dr. Lawrence Meltzer, of the Presbyterian Hospital in Philadelphia, proposed that the role of the nurse would be central to the new system of coronary care. The nurse would be present in the CCU 24 hours a day. When the research project began on January 15, 1963, about 8 months after the Hartford CCU opened in Kansas City, Meltzer immediately faced the challenge of staffing it. Rose Pinneo, RN, MSN, a graduate of both Johns Hopkins School of Nursing and the University of Pennsylvania, agreed to be the nursing director. In July 1963, 6 months after agreeing to accept the job, Pinneo, a small-framed, unassuming professional, took on the nursing leadership role in the new unit, implementing the new role for nurses (Pinneo, 1967).

In the coronary care units in the 1960s, clinical expertise on the part of the nurse would be invaluable. As she described it, "The nurses' role is more complex than that of the usual hospital nurse" and went on to explain it further (Pinneo, 1972):

Utilizing the unique combination of clinical assessment and cardiac monitoring, the nurse makes independent decisions. She determines those situations requiring her immediate intervention to save life prior to the physicians' arrival or those situations that warrant calling the physicians and waiting for his evaluation. It is in these precious moments that the patient's life may literally be in the hands of the nurse (p. 4).

Collaboration with physicians at the grassroots level would be key to the CCU nurses' success. Pinneo and other nurses who worked in the first CCUs worked closely with cardiologists (Keeling, 2004) interprofessional on the job training was the norm. These changes in setting, technology, and expectations of the nurse exemplify stage 1 in the transition of specialties into advanced practice nursing (see Chapter 5).

The creation of the CCU initiated a new era for nurses. The changes that occurred in the clinical setting of the CCU helped establish collegial relationships between nurses and physicians that would be important for APNs in the decades to follow. In intensive care units (ICUs) and CCUs, collaborative practice was essential. "Most importantly, nurses and physicians learned to trust each other … ." (Lynaugh & Fairman, 1992, p. 24).

Defining the Clinical Nurse Specialist's Role

The rapid proliferation of CNS programs and jobs, as well as the emerging role ambiguity and confusion that accompanied them, defined the 1970s for CNSs. During this decade, psychiatric CNSs continued to provide leadership in the educational and clinical arenas while federal funding from the Professional Nurse Traineeship Program provided fiscal support to new programs. The specialties of critical care and oncology nursing also grew during the 1970s. The American Association of Critical Care Nurses (AACCN), established by a small group of concerned nurses at the end of the previous decade, organized further to meet the continuing educational needs of new specialists in the areas of coronary care and intensive care nursing. Only f4 years later, after the ANA and American Cancer Society (ACS) sponsored the first National Cancer Nursing Research Conference, a group of oncology nurses

met to discuss the need for a national organization to support their specialty. Officially incorporated in 1975, the Oncology Nursing Society (ONS) provided a forum for issues related to cancer nursing and supported the growth of advanced practice nursing in this specialty (ONS, 2011).

By the middle of the 1970s, the ANA officially recognized the CNS role, defining the CNS as an expert practitioner and change agent. Of particular significance, the ANA's definition specified a master's degree as a requirement for the CNS (ANA Congress of Nursing Practice, 1974). As with the other advanced nursing specialties, the development of the CNS role included early evaluation research that served to validate and promote the innovation. Georgopoulos and colleagues (Georgopoulos & Christman, 1970; Georgopoulos & Jackson, 1970; Georgopoulos & Sana, 1971) conducted studies evaluating

◆ BOX 1-5 **Building Credibility and Defining Practice (1970s)**

The 1970s ushered in a period of rapid growth and development for nursing. It was a decade in which selected roles would become firmly established. According to historians Lynaugh and Brush (1996), "What was historically unique ... was the emerging [public] consensus that nursing, the largest single health care group, should expand its scope of practice to provide direct services to patients, including services previously considered solely in the physician's domain." Recognizing the need for leadership in the area, the ANA Congress of Nursing Practice (1974) published educational standards, described the NP and CNS roles, and attempted to define the expanding scope of nursing practice.

the effect of CNS practice on nursing process and outcomes in inpatient adult health care settings. These and other evaluative studies (Ayers, 1971; Girouard, 1978; Little & Carnevali, 1967) demonstrated the positive effect of the CNS on improving nursing care and patient outcomes. Moreover, with the increasing demand from society to cure illness using the latest scientific and technologic advances, hospital administrators willingly supported specialization in nursing and hired CNSs, particularly in the revenue-producing ICUs. Box 1-5 presents more information on the growth and development of nursing in the 1970s.

The CNS role continued to be the dominant APN role in the 1980s, with CNSs representing 42% of all APNs (U.S. Department of Health and Human Services, 1996). The ANA's Social Policy Statement (1980), clearly delineating the criteria required to assume the title of CNS, was of particular significance to the maturation of the CNS role during this decade. According to that statement,

> The specialist in nursing practice is a nurse who, through study and supervised clinical practice at the graduate level (masters or doctorate), has become expert in a defined area of knowledge and practice in a selected clinical area of nursing. ... Upon completion of a graduate program degree in a university graduate program with an emphasis on clinical specialization, the specialist in nursing practice should meet the criteria for specialty certification through nursing's professional society (p. 23).

Nurse executives were eager to hire CNSs, and the demand for programs increased. In February 1983, the executive committee of the ANA's Council of Clinical Nurse Specialists met and provided a forum for CNSs

and a general repository for documents and information about the role. By 1984, the NLN had accredited 129 programs for the preparation of CNSs (NLN, 1984). However, at about that time, the increasing concerns over health care cost containment raised concerns about the future of the CNS role (Hamric, 1989). Concurrently, some nurse researchers once again studied the outcomes related to CNS practice. In 1987, for example, McBride and colleagues demonstrated that nursing practice, particularly in relation to documentation, improved as a result of the introduction of a CNS in an inpatient psychiatric setting.

By the late 1980s, many CNSs shifted the focus of their practice away from the clinical area and instead focused on the educational and organizational aspects of the CNS role. This shift was supported by the view that CNSs were too valuable to spend their time on direct patient care (Wolff, 1984). Meanwhile, others who asserted that the essence of the CNS role was clinical expertise were publishing articles and books on the topic (Hamric & Spross, 1983, 1989; Sparacino, 1990). In addition, articles describing CNS practice and consensus reports on this APN role began to appear in critical care, oncology, and other nursing specialty journals. These publications helped lay the groundwork for curriculum development in APN specialties.

Also during the 1980s, the ANA Council of Clinical Nurse Specialists (CCNS) and Council of Primary Health Care Nurse Practitioners (CPHCNP) began to explore the commonalities of the two roles. In 1988, the councils conducted a survey of all NP and CNS graduate programs and identified considerable overlap in curricula. Subsequently, between 1988 and 1990, the two councils discussed a proposal to merge and, in 1991, the Council of Nurses in Advanced Practice was formed. Unfortunately, the merger was short-lived because of the restructuring of the ANA during the early 1990s. Nevertheless, it was an important step in the organizational coalescence of advanced practice nursing (ANA, 1991).

The 1990s began with cutbacks in employment opportunities for CNSs because of the financial problems in hospitals and closed with the federal government's recognition of Medicare reimbursement for CNS services. Nationwide, in the opening years of the decade, CNS programs were the most numerous of all master's nursing programs, serving more than 11,000 students (NLN, 1994). The largest area of specialization was adult health–medical-surgical nursing; Box 1-6 presents more information on specialization in nursing. With the increasing emphasis on primary care in the mid 1990s, the rapid growth of NP programs, financial challenges faced by hospital administrators, and introduction of the ACNP role in tertiary care centers, the number of CNS positions in

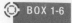

Defining the Concept of Advanced Practice Nursing

BOX 1-6

Defining specialization and later coming to grips with a definition of advanced practice nursing would more or less demand the profession's attention at various times over the course of the twentieth century. The use of the term *specialist* in nursing can be traced to the turn of the twentieth century, when hospitals offered postgraduate courses in various specialty areas, including anesthesia, tuberculosis, operating room, laboratory, and dietetics. In the first issue of the AJN, in an article entitled "Specialties in Nursing," Katherine Dewitt (1900) described specialty practice and the specialist's need for continuing education:

Those who devote themselves to one branch of nursing often do so because of the keen interest they feel in it. The specialist can and should reach greater perfection in her sphere when she gives her entire time to it. Her studies should be continued in that direction, she should try constantly to keep up with the rapid advances in medical science ... The nurse who is a specialist can often supplement the doctor's work to a great extent. ...

Specialists in nursing were important to patients and physicians. The educational requirements for specialization, the nature of specialty practice, and the definition of a nurse specialist were all issues that the profession would later have to address.

hospitals declined sharply. Consequently, there was also a decrease in the number of nurses interested in pursuing a master's degree for the CNS role.

The 1996 Sample Survey of Registered Nurses revealed that a significant number (7802) of CNSs were also prepared as NPs. According to that report, these dual-role–prepared APNs were more likely to be employed as NPs rather than as CNSs. By that time, of the 61,601 CNSs in the United States, only 23% were practicing in CNS-specific positions (U.S. Department of Health and Human Services, 1996). This low percentage may have reflected the fact that CNSs accepted different positions—for example, as administrators or staff educators. It may also have reflected the decline in the number of CNS positions available because of budget cutbacks.

Clinical Nurse Specialist Certification, Organization, and Prescriptive Authority

Certification for CNS practice was particularly complicated. In many specialties, existing certification examinations were targeted to nurses who were experts by experience, not graduates of master's programs that specifically trained them for specialty practice. Advanced-level certification for the CNS was slow to emerge. For example, it was not until 1995 that the ONS administered the first certification examination for advanced practice in oncology nursing. A further complication was that not all states recognized these examinations for APN regulatory purposes.

The creation of the National Association of Clinical Nurse Specialists (NACNS), followed by third-party reimbursement for their services, represented two major steps for the CNS. NACNS was formed In 1995, promoting organization of the role at the national level. Soon thereafter, in 1997, the Balanced Budget Act (Public Law 105-33) specifically identified the CNS as eligible for Medicare reimbursement (Safriet, 1998). The law, providing Medicare Part B direct payment to NPs and CNSs, regardless of their geographic area of practice, allowed both types of APNs to be paid 85% of the fee paid to physicians for the same services. Moreover, the law's inclusion and definition of CNSs corrected the previous omission of this group for reimbursement (Safriet, 1998). The possibility of reimbursement for services was an important step in the continuing development of the CNS role because hospital administrators would continue to focus on the cost of having APNs provide patient care.

Some CNS roles require prescription of medications and the ability of a CNS to prescribe depends on state regulations. As of January 2012, CNSs have independent prescriptive authority in 11 states and in Washington, DC, no prescribing authority in 15 states, and noninde-pendent prescriptive authority in the remaining 24 states (National Council of State Boards of Nursing, 2012).

Nurse Practitioners

Early Public Health Nurses' Role in Direct Care

The idea of using nurses to provide what we now refer to as primary care services dates to the late nineteenth century. During this period of rapid industrialization and social reform, public health nurses played a major role in providing care for poverty-stricken immigrants in cities throughout the country. In 1893, Lillian Wald, a young graduate nurse from the New York Training School for Nurses, established the Henry Street Settlement (HSS) House on the Lower East Side of Manhattan. Its purpose was to address the needs of the poor, many of whom lived in overcrowded, rat-infested tenements. For several decades, the HSS visiting nurses, like other district nurses, visited thousands of patients with little interference in their work (Wald, 1922). The needs of this disadvantaged community were limitless. According to one account (Duffus, 1938):

> There were nursing infants, many of them with the summer bowel complaint that sent infant mortality soaring during the hot months; there were children with measles, not quarantined; there were children with ophthalmia, a contagious eye disease; there were children scarred with vermin bites; there were adults with typhoid; there was a case of puerperal septicemia, lying on a vermin-infested bed without sheets or pillow cases; a family consisting of a pregnant mother, a crippled child and two others living on dry bread … a young girl dying of tuberculosis amid the very conditions that had produced the disease … (p. 43).

In addition to making home visits, the HSS nurses saw patients in the nurses' dispensary in the settlement house. There they treated "simple complaints and emergencies not requiring referral elsewhere" (Buhler-Wilkerson, 2001). For a time, their work usually went unnoticed, but interprofessional conflict was inevitable. According to nurse historian Karen Buhler-Wilkerson (2001):

> As the number of ambulatory visits grew, the settlement risked attracting the unwelcome attention of the increasingly disagreeable "uptown docs." The New York Medical Society's recent success in attaching a clause to the Nursing Registration Bill prohibiting nurses from practicing medicine gave the society a new opportunity to disrupt the settlement's neighborly activities … By 1904 … Lavinia Dock [a colleague of Lillian Wald] wrote to Wald about doctors' concerns that nurses were "carrying ointments and even giving pills" outside the strict control of physicians (p. 110).

To resolve this problem, the HSS nurses obtained standing orders for emergency medications and treatments from a group of Lower East Side physicians (Buhler-Wilkerson, 2001; Keeling, 2007). Nonetheless, conflicts with medicine surfaced again when the HHS nurses expanded their visits to areas of the city outside the Lower East Side. The situation came to a head with the collapse of the stock market in 1929, when uptown physicians apparently saw the nurses as an economic threat. That year, the Westchester Village Medical Group accused the nurses of practicing medicine. Angered by the accusation, Elizabeth Mackenzie, Associate Director of Nurses at Henry Street Settlement, defended the HSS nurses in her reply (MacKenzie, 1929):

> My dear Dr. Black:
> Your letter … addressed to Miss Elizabeth Neary, Supervisor of our Westchester Office, has been referred to me for reply. May I call the attention of your group to the fact that in administering the work in that office, Miss Neary does so as a representative of the HSS Visiting Nurse Service and in accord with definite policies in effect throughout the entire city-wide service. It has been the unvarying policy of the organization over the 35 years of its service to work in close cooperation with the medical profession doing nursing and preventive health work entirely and avoiding any semblance of the "practice of medicine" in competition with the doctors. … We will call a meeting … to which the members of your group will be invited for a frank discussion of our common problems.

Although the records about this meeting are no longer available, one can assume that the meeting happened and the nurses continued to practice, because HSS remained active until the 1950s. Nonetheless, as apparent in these two scenarios, from early in the twentieth century there was evidence of interprofessional conflicts with medicine as nurses began to expand their scope of practice. There is also evidence of emerging collaboration between the professions as physicians and nurses negotiated solutions to the boundary problems. What is clear, even in those early years, is that nurses were considered "good enough" to care for the poor, whereas physicians would care for those who could pay.

Primary Care in Appalachia—the Frontier Nursing Service

In addition to providing midwifery services, FNS nurses in Leslie County, Kentucky, informally modeled what would later become the primary care NP role. During the 1930s, the FNS continued the work that Breckinridge had started in 1925, providing most of the primary health care needed by people living in rural Appalachia. Working out of eight centers that covered 78 square miles in remote mountainous regions, the FNS nurses had considerable autonomy. They made diagnoses and treated patients, dispensing herbs and medicines (including morphine) with the permission of their medical advisory committee. Working from standing orders written by that committee, the nurses also dispensed medicines such as aspirin, ipecac, cascara, and castor oil at their own discretion (FNS, 1948). That unprecedented autonomy in practice was not always recognized, however, even by the FNS nurses themselves. During an interview in 1978, FNS nurse Betty Lester reflected on her work as assistant field supervisor in Leslie county in the 1930s (Keeling, 2007):

> See, we nurses don't prescribe and we don't diagnose. We can make a tentative diagnosis and we can give that to the doctor, and if there's anything wrong then he'll tell us how to treat it. So they [the doctors] gave us this routine of things that we could use and the things we could do—and the things we couldn't do (p. 49).

Lester denied the extent of the practice autonomy she had had. Like other registered nurses of the era, she had been socialized to defer to physicians' judgment and orders. So, recalling her practice later in her life, Lester acknowledged only that she and her colleagues had made "tentative" diagnoses. In reality, she had practiced on her own because there were few telephones in the isolated community and even fewer physicians available for personal consultation. For all practical purposes, the diagnoses she had made were the only diagnoses, and the treatment she had given was the only treatment (Keeling, 2007).

During the 1930s, in addition to the FNS nurses, other nurses working among the poor in rural areas also practiced with exceptional autonomy. In particular, the Farm Security Administration (FSA) nurses "were given unusual latitude in their clinical roles" (Grey, 1999, p. 94) in migrant health clinics across the United States. According to historian Michael Grey (1999), who chronicled the history of rural health programs established by President Franklin D. Roosevelt during the Great Depression, an event that began in 1929 and lasted through approximately 1940:

With the verbal approval of the camp doctor, they [FSA nurses] could write prescriptions and dispense drugs from the clinic formulary. … They staffed well baby clinics, coordinated immunization programs … decided whether a sick migrant required referral to a physician … and provided emergency care (p. 94).

Like the FNS nurses, FSA nurses practiced according to standing orders issued by the FSA medical offices and approved by local physicians. As Dr. H. Daniels recalled in a 1984 interview, "Nurses functioned pretty autonomously. They were able to do a lot of what NPs do after a lot of training, but these nurses did it through experience" (Grey, 1999, p. 96). Essential to this practice autonomy for the FNS and FSA nurses was the tacit requirement that the patients be poor, marginalized, and have little access to physician-provided medical care.

The same requirements held true for the field nurses working with the Bureau of Indian Affairs (BIA) in the first half of the twentieth century, who often found themselves traveling the reservations alone, making diagnoses and treating patients. In addition to making home visits, BIA nurses conducted well-baby "nursing conferences," the initial intent of which was health education and disease prevention, not treatment. In actuality, these conferences became what we refer to today as nurse-run clinics; Navajo mothers would bring in sick infants and children to be seen by the nurse (Keeling, 2007). Reporting on her work at Teec Nos Pas in the Northern Navajo region in May 1931, nurse Dorothy Williams described the reality of providing much-needed care of ear infections, sore throats, skin infections, and other

---

⊙ EXEMPLAR 1-5   Migrant Camp Nursing (circa 1930s)

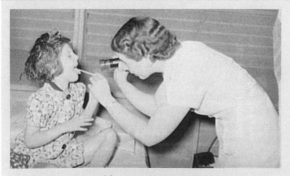

(Courtesy Library of Congress 8b24752r; FSA photographs.)

As thousands of people from the Dust Bowl states lost their farms to foreclosure or lost their jobs to the new farm machines, they followed crops in search of work. Some went west to the coastal states of California, Oregon, and Washington. Others headed east, beginning in Florida and following crops up the East Coast as seasonal harvests demanded. In 1938, the FSA established its first camps, known as farm workers communities, in Californian counties in which the migrants concentrated.

Among these was the Brawley migratory camp, the camp to which public health nurse Mary Sears was first assigned. There she worked with unprecedented autonomy, using her clinical expertise to assess patients' conditions and collaborate with local physicians, social workers, and nutritionists to provide care (Keeling, 2011).

commonly occurring problems. Williams referred to the conferences as "clinics":

> Five clinics held this week, three general and two baby clinics. Mothers bathed their babies and were given material to cut out and make gowns for baby. Preschool children were weighed, inspected and mothers advised about diets for underweights [sic] … Fifty treatments given. … (Williams, 2007).

Although the NP role had been modeled informally in the FNS in the 1930s, it was during the 1960s that the role was first described formally and implemented in outpatient pediatric clinics, originating in part as a response to a shortage of primary care physicians. As the trend toward medical specialization drew increasing numbers of physicians away from primary care, many areas of the country were designated underserved with respect to the numbers of primary care physicians. "Report after report issued by the AMA [American Medical Association] and the Association of American Medical Colleges decried the shortage of physicians in poor rural and urban areas" (Fairman, 2002, p. 163). At the same time, consumers across the nation were demanding accessible, affordable, and sensitive health care while health care delivery costs were increasing at an annual rate of 10% to 14% (Jonas, 1981).

Pediatric Nurse Practitioners Pave the Way

The event marking the inception of the modern NP role was the establishment of the first pediatric NP (PNP) program by Loretta Ford, RN, and Henry Silver, MD, at the University of Colorado in 1965. This demonstration project, funded by the Commonwealth Foundation, was designed to prepare professional nurses to provide comprehensive well-child care and manage common childhood health problems. The 4-month program, which certified registered nurses (RNs) as PNPs without requiring master's preparation, emphasized health promotion and the inclusion of the family. A study evaluating the project demonstrated that PNPs were highly competent in assessing and managing 75% of well and ill children in community health settings. In addition, PNPs increased the number of patients served in private pediatric practice by 33% (Ford & Silver, 1967). Like early nurse-midwife and nurse anesthetist studies, these positive findings demonstrated support for this new nursing role.

The PNP role was not without significant intraprofessional controversy, particularly with regard to educational preparation. Early on, certificate programs based on the Colorado project rapidly sprang into existence. According to Ford (1991), some of these programs shifted

the emphasis of PNP preparation from a nursing to a medical model. As a result, one of the major areas of controversy in academia was over the fact that NPs made medical diagnoses and wrote prescriptions for medications, essentially stepping over the invisible medical boundary into the realm of curing. Because of this, some nurse educators and other nurse leaders questioned whether the NP role could be conceptualized as being within the discipline of nursing, a profession that had historically been ordered to care (Rogers, 1972; Reverby, 1987).

While nursing professors debated the educational preparation of NPs (Rogers, 1972; Keeling, 2007), the NP role attracted considerable attention from professional groups and policymakers. Health policy groups such as the National Advisory Commission on Health Manpower issued statements in support of the NP concept (Moxley, 1968). At the grassroots level, physicians accepted the new role and hired nurse practitioners. The NP role had already appeared in the practice setting.

In the 1970s, nurse practitioners continued to enhance their visibility in the health care system, negotiating with physicians to expand their scope of practice, and demonstrating their cost-effectiveness in providing quality care. Nevertheless, it was also a period characterized by intraprofessional conflict because some leaders in the nursing community continued to reject the role. In contrast, state legislatures increasingly recognized these expanded roles of RNs and a group of pro-NP nursing faculty, already teaching in NP programs, held their first national meeting in Chapel Hill, North Carolina, in 1974. This meeting would lay the foundation for the formation of the National Organization of Nurse Practitioner Faculties (NONPF).

National Reports and Federal Funding

In the early 1970s, U.S. Department of Health, Education, and Welfare (HEW) Secretary Elliott Richardson established the Committee to Study Extended Roles for Nurses. This group of health care leaders was charged with evaluating the feasibility of expanding nursing practice (Kalisch & Kalisch, 1986). They concluded that extending the scope of the nurse's role was essential to providing equal access to health care for all Americans. According to an editorial in the AJN, "The kind of health care Lillian Wald began preaching and practicing in 1893 is the kind the people of this country are still crying for" (Schutt, 1971, p. 53). The committee urged the establishment of innovative curricular designs in health science centers and increased financial support for nursing education. It also advocated standardizing nursing licensure and national certification and developed a model nurse practice law suitable for national application. In addition, the committee called for further research related to cost-benefit analyses and attitudinal surveys to assess the impact of the NP role (HEW, 1972). This report resulted in increased federal support for training programs for the preparation of several types of NPs, including family NPs, adult NPs, and emergency department NPs.

Controversy and Support for the Nurse Practitioner's Role

Conflict and discord about the NP role continued to characterize relationships between NPs and other nurses. Some members of academia who believed that NPs were not practicing nursing continued to pose resistance to the role (Ford, 1982). Nurse theorist Martha Rogers, one of the most outspoken opponents of the NP concept, argued that the development of the NP role was a ploy to lure nurses away from nursing to medicine, thereby undermine nursing's unique role in health care (Rogers, 1972). Subsequently, nurse leaders and educators took sides for and against the establishment of educational programs for NPs in mainstream master's programs. Over time, the standardization of NP educational programs at the master's level, initiated by the group of faculty who formed NONPF, would serve to reduce intraprofessional tension.

Despite the resistance to NPs in nursing, physicians increasingly accepted NPs in individual health care practices. Working together in local practices, NPs and MDs established collegial relationships, negotiating with each other to construct work boundaries and reach agreement about their collaborative practice. "In the NP-MD dyad, negotiations centered on the NP's right to practice an essential part of traditional medicine: the process or skill set of clinical thinking ... to perform a physical examination, elicit patient symptoms, ... create a diagnosis, formulate treatment options, prescribe treatment and make decisions about prognosis" (Fairman, 2002, pp. 163–164). The proximity of a supervising physician was thought to be key to effective practice, and on-site supervision was the norm. Grassroots acceptance of the role was dependent on tight physician supervision and control of the protocols under which NPs practiced. That supervision was not without benefit to the newly certified, inexperienced NPs. According to Corene Johnson, "Initially, we had to always have a physician on site. ... I didn't resent that. Actually, I needed the backup" (Fairman, 2002, p. 164).

During the 1980s, the concept of advanced nursing practice began to be defined and used in the literature. In 1983, Harriet Kitzman, an associate professor at the University of Rochester, explored the interrelationships between CNSs and NPs (Kitzman, 1983). She used the term *advanced practice* throughout her discussion, applying the term not only to advanced education, but also to CNS and NP practice. She noted, "Recognition for advanced practice competence is already established for both NPs and CNSs through the profession's certification programs .... advanced nursing practice cannot be setting-bound, because nursing needs are not exclusively setting-restricted" (Kitzman, 1983, pp. 284, 288). In 1984, an associate professor at the University of Wisconsin–Madison, Joy Calkin, proposed a model for advanced nursing practice, specifically identifying CNSs and NPs with master's degrees as APNs (Calkin, 1984). By the end of the decade, the nursing literature was increasingly using the term. Published in 1996, the first edition of this text included CRNA and CNM roles as advanced practice nursing, reflecting an integrative vision of advanced practice that was increasingly being seen in the literature.

Although physicians and NPs collaborated at the local level, organized medicine began to increase its resistance to the NP role. One of the most contentious areas of interprofessional conflict involved prescriptive authority for nursing. As one author so aptly noted, "Nursing's efforts to obtain the legal authority to prescribe may be seen as the second chapter in the struggle over the use of the word 'diagnosing' in Nurse Practice Acts" (Hadley, 1989, p. 291). Basically, prescriptive authority, regarded as a delegated medical act, was dependent on NPs' legal right to provide treatment. In 1971, Idaho became the first state to recognize diagnosis and treatment as part of the scope of practice of specialty nurses (Idaho Code 54-1413, 1971). However, "As path-breaking as the statute was, it was still rather restrictive in that any acts of diagnosis and treatment had to be authorized by rules and regulations promulgated by the Idaho State Boards of Medicine and Nursing" (Safriet, 1992, p. 445). Moreover, the Drug Enforcement Act required that practitioners wishing to prescribe controlled substances obtain U.S. Drug Enforcement Agency (DEA) registration numbers, and only those practitioners with broad prescriptive authority (e.g., physicians and dentists) could obtain these numbers. In spite of these barriers, by the end of the 1970s, PNPs obtained legal authority to prescribe drugs for infants and children using standing protocols developed by physicians[4] (Ford, 1982).

The increasing emphasis on cost containment in the 1980s produced legislative and economic changes that affected advanced practice nursing and the health care delivery system as a whole (Box 1-7). In particular, the establishment of a prospective payment system in 1983 was a landmark event.. This payment system, which used

---

[4]Alaska and North Carolina authorized PNPs to write prescriptions in 1975.

BOX 1-7 **Access to Cost-Effective, Quality Health Care For All Americans**

The need to provide cost-effective, quality health care to U.S. citizens prompted the Senate Committee on Appropriations to request a report on the contributions of NPs, CNMs, and physician assistants (PAs) in meeting the nation's health care needs. The report, released in 1986, entitled "Nurse Practitioners, Physician Assistants, and Certified Nurse-Midwives," was based on an analysis of numerous studies that assessed quality of care, patient satisfaction, and physician acceptance. It concluded that "within their areas of competence NPs ... and CNMs provide care whose quality is equivalent to that of care provided by physicians" (Office of Technology Assessment, 1986). However, while the Office of Technology Assessment was conducting this study, the AMA House of Delegates, threatened by the possibility of competition from APNs, passed a resolution to "oppose any attempt at empowering non-physicians to become unsupervised primary care providers and be directly reimbursed" (Safriet, 1992).

 BOX 1-8 **The Fight for APRN Prescriptive Privileges**

The fight for prescriptive authority for NPs spanned the latter decades of the twentieth century. By 1983, only Oregon and Washington granted NPs statutory, independent prescriptive authority. Other states granting prescriptive authority to NPs did so with the provision that the NP be directly supervised by a licensed physician. How prescriptions were handled depended on the availability of the physician, negotiated boundaries of the individual physician-NP team, and state in which practice occurred. In some cases, that meant that physicians presigned a pad of prescriptions for the NP to use at her or his discretion; in remote area clinics, such as those in the Frontier Nursing Service, a physician would countersign NP prescriptions once a week and, in other cases, the physician would write and sign a prescription at the request of the NP. With the exception of the latter, these practices were of questionable legality (Keeling, 2007).

diagnosis-related groups (DRGs) to classify billing for hospitalized Medicare recipients, represented an effort to control rising costs and reimbursement to hospitals by shifting reimbursement from payment for services provided to payment by case (capitation). As a result, hospital administrators put increasing pressure on nurses and physicians to save money by decreasing how long patients remained in the hospital. The emphasis on cost containment also heralded budget cuts for hospitals, which forced nursing administrators to evaluate the cost-effectiveness of CNSs carefully, then the most commonly employed APNs. The result was the elimination of some CNS positions by the end of the decade.

The cost of health care was a constant concern and, by 1992, when Bill Clinton was elected President of the United States, the country was in serious need of health care reform. Determined to take a proactive stance in the movement, the ANA wrote its Agenda for Health Care Reform (1992). The plan focused on restructuring the U.S. health care system to reduce costs and improve access to care. Although the Clinton administration's efforts for health care reform failed, radical changes were made by the private sector in which the once-dominant fee for service insurance plans were overtaken by managed care organizations (Safriet, 1998). The changing marketplace created new challenges for APNs as they struggled not only with restrictive outdated state laws on prescriptive authority, but also with "non-governmental, market-based

impediments" to their practices (Safriet, 1998, p. 25). In this environment, APNs continued to expand their roles, educational programs, and practice settings (Box 1-8).

Growth in Nurse Practitioner Numbers and Expanded Scope of Practice

Significant growth in the numbers of NPs in practice and the fight for prescriptive authority for NPs characterized the 1980s. NP practice increased immeasurably during the 1980s as new types of NPs developed, the most significant of which were the emergency NP, neonatal NP, and family NP. By 1984, approximately 20,000 graduates of NP programs were employed, for the most part, in settings "that the founders envisioned" (Kalisch & Kalisch, 1986, p. 715): outpatient clinics, health maintenance organizations, health departments, community health centers, rural clinics, schools, occupational health clinics, and private offices. By the late 1980s, however, based on their success in neonatal intensive care units, NPs with specialty preparation were increasingly being used in tertiary care centers (Silver and McAtee, 1988).

During this period, the multiple roles for NPs created competing interests that would affect their ability to speak with one voice on legislative issues. In an attempt to rectify this situation, the ANA established the Primary Health Care Nurse Practitioner Council. At about the same time, the Alliance of Nurse Practitioners was established as an umbrella organization for all the various NP associations.

Throughout the 1980s, NPs worked tirelessly to convince state legislatures to pass laws and establish reimbursement policies that would support their practice. Interprofessional conflicts with organized medicine, and to a lesser extent with pharmacists, centered on control issues and the degree of independence the NP was allowed. These conflicts intensified as NPs moved beyond the physician extender model to a more autonomous one. In a 1980 seminal case, Sermchief v. Gonzales (1983), the Missouri medical board charged two women's health care NPs with practicing medicine without a license (Doyle & Meurer, 1983). The initial ruling was against the NPs but, on appeal, the Missouri Supreme Court overturned the decision, concluding that the scope of practice of APNs could evolve without statutory constraints (Wolff, 1984). In essence, this case provided a model for new state nurse practice acts to address issues related to APN practice with very generalized wording, a change that allowed for expansion in the roles and functions of APNs.

In the early 1990s, federal legislation regulating narcotics in the Controlled Substances Act (1991 and 1992) would be of major significance to NP progress in implementing prescriptive authority. As NPs began to gain prescriptive authority for controlled substances in different states, they required a parallel authority granted by the DEA. In 1991, the DEA first responded to this situation by proposing registration for "affiliated practitioners" (56FR 4181). This proposal called for those NPs who had prescriptive authority pursuant to a practice protocol or collaborative practice agreement to be assigned a registration number for controlled substances tied to the number of the physician with whom they worked. This proposal received much criticism specifically related to the restriction of access to health care and the legal liability of the prescribers, and the proposal was revoked in 1992. Later that year, the DEA amended its regulations by adding a category of "mid-level providers" (MLPs) who would be issued individual provider DEA numbers as long as they were granted prescriptive authority by the state in which they practiced. The MLP's number would begin with an M for mid-level provider, rather than an A or B. The MLP provision took effect in 1993, significantly expanding NPs' ability to prescribe.

During the 1990s, the number of NPs increased dramatically in response to increasing demand, the national emphasis on primary care, and the concomitant decrease in the number of medical residencies in the subspecialties. In 1990, there were 135 master's degree and 40 certificate NP programs. Between 1992 and 1994, the number of institutions offering NP education more than doubled, from 78 to 158. In 1994, most

institutions offered several tracks, which led to a total of 384 NP tracks in master's programs throughout the United States. By 1998, the number of institutions offering NP education again doubled, representing a total of 769 distinct NP specialty tracks (NONPF, 1997; AACN, 1999). Most of these programs were at the master's or post–master's level. By 1998, only 12 post–basic RN certificate programs remained in existence. This rapid expansion created concern about the need for so many programs and the quality of the programs. In the end, most nurse educators supported the master's degree as the educational requirement for NP practice, and most used the NONPF guidelines in determining their curricula (NONPF, 1997).

Neonatal and Acute Care Nurse Practitioners

One of the newer types of NPs to emerge was the neonatal NP. Originating in the late 1970s in response to a shortage of neonatologists coinciding with restrictions in the total time pediatric residents could devote to neonatal intensive care, the neonatal NP was the forerunner of the acute care NP of the 1990s. These highly skilled, experienced neonatal nurses assumed a wide range of new responsibilities formerly undertaken by pediatric residents, including interhospital transport of critically ill infants and newborn resuscitation (Clancy & Maguire, 1995).

Like the earlier neonatal NP role, the adult acute care NP (ACNP) role grew in response to residency shortages in ICUs, although this time the shortage was because of decreases in the number of residents available to work in the medical subspecialties. In addition, increasingly complicated tertiary care systems lacked coordination of care. Advanced practice nursing responded quickly to this need, building on the earlier work of Silver and McAtee (1988) to create a role that promoted quality patient care and nursing's leadership in health care delivery (Daly, 1997). University of Pennsylvania professors Anne Keane and Theresa Richmond (1993) were among those who documented the emergence of the tertiary NP (TNP):

> The TNP is an advanced practice nurse educated at the master's level with both a theoretical and experiential focus on complex patients with specialized health needs … There is precedent for the NP in tertiary care. For example, neonatal nurse practitioners are central to the provision of care in many intensive care nurseries … It is our belief that the TNP can provide clinically expert specialized care in a holistic manner in a system that is often typified by fragmentation, lack of communication among medical specialists, and a loss of recognition of the patient and patient's needs as central to the care delivered (p. 282).

From 1992 to 1995, ACNP tracks in master's programs proliferated across the country.[5] Soon, questions abounded concerning the content of the curriculum. To resolve these, educators met annually at ACNP consensus conferences, beginning in 1993. ANCC administered the first ACNP certification examination in December 1995. By 1997, there were 43 programs nationwide that prepared ACNPs at the master's or post–master's level (Kleinpell, 1997). In 2002, ACNP formally merged with the American Academy of Nurse Practitioners (AANP), with the goal of uniting primary care and acute care NPs under an umbrella organization. By this time, ACNPs were employed in multiple specialties, including cardiology, cardiovascular surgery, neurosurgery, emergency and trauma, internal medicine, and radiology services (Daly, 2002).

During this decade, the growth in the number of NP programs, increase in prescriptive authority for NPs, and autonomy that NPs found in their practice settings, converged to make the NP role enticing and increasing numbers of nurses who wanted to be APNs chose the NP role. The problem was that there were a number of organizations speaking for the various types of NPs. In the mid-1990s, NPs attempted to unify their organizational voice by establishing the AANP. Membership in this organization included national organizational affiliates, state NP organizations, and individuals. Supposedly, the focus of the organization was to address public policy issues that affected all NPs. However, NPs never unified. Throughout this period, many were angry about the establishment of the AANP. The Alliance of Nurse Practitioners continued to be active and the American College of Nurse Practitioners was founded. In addition, PNPs formed the National Association of Pediatric Nurse Associates and Practitioners (NAPNAP; nurses interested in women's' health issues formed the Association of Women's Health, Obstetric, and Neonatal Nurses (AWHONN). These groups soon offered their own certification examinations in competition with those offered by the ANA's Credentialing Center (ANCC). Overall, dissention about which group should speak for NPs would continue well into the twenty-first century. One thing they did agree on, however, was education for practice. In August 1993, representatives of 63 of 66 tricouncil organizations attending a national nursing summit agreed to require master's education for the NP role (Cronenwett, 1995).

American Association of Colleges of Nursing and Doctor of Nursing Practice

A primary example of an attempt to address current issues in the profession and in the United States is the DNP developed by the AACN in 2001. Initially, this initiative was aimed at ensuring adequate educational preparation for APNs and was developed in response to the reality of ever-increasing curricular requirements in master's programs throughout the country (Keeling, Kirschgessner & Brodie, 2010). As originally proposed by the AACN, the DNP would standardize practice entry requirements for all APNs by the year 2015, assuring the public that each APN would have had 1000 supervised clinical hours prior to entering the practice setting. (The DNP has also broadened to include nurses with specialties such as informatics, administration, and public health. See Chapter 3 for further discussion of DNP education for non-APNs.) Moreover, the proposed curriculum for DNPs would include competencies deemed essential for nursing practice in the twenty-first century, including the following: (1) scientific underpinnings for practice; (2) organizational and systems leadership; (3) clinical scholarship and analysis for evidence-based practice; (4) information systems technology; (5) health care policy; (6) interprofessional collaboration; and (7) clinical prevention and population health (AACN, 2006). Although it is too early to evaluate this initiative from a historical perspective, the national dialogue to move APN education to a practice doctorate offers significant opportunity for the profession to connect scientific evidence and practice (Magyary, Whitney, & Brown, 2006). Expanded educational preparation could position APNs to be vital players in the translation of research evidence at the point of care, help nursing education achieve parity with physician education, and potentially decrease interprofessional tensions.

Conclusion

This review of the history of advance practice nursing in the twentieth century encompasses several themes:

1. Throughout the century, APNs have been permitted by organized medicine and state legislative bodies to provide care to the underserved poor, particularly in rural areas of the nation. However, when that care competes with physicians' reimbursement for their services, there has been significant resistance from organized medicine, which resulted in interprofessional conflict.

2. Documentation of the outcomes of practice helped establish the earliest nursing specialties and continues to be of critical importance to the survival of APN practice.

---

[5]The University of Pittsburgh, Case Western Reserve University, University of Connecticut, University of Rochester, Rush Presbyterian University, and University of Pennsylvania were among the first university schools of nursing to embrace the idea and implement programs, most of which were originally at the post–master's level (Daly, 2002).

3. The efforts of national professional organizations, national certification, and the move toward graduate education as a requirement for advanced practice have been critical to enhancing the credibility of advanced practice nursing.
4. Intraprofessional and interprofessional resistance to expanding the boundaries of the nursing discipline continue to recur.
5. Societal forces, including wars, the economic climate, and health care policy, have influenced APN history.

Providing care to people in underserved areas has, by default, been assigned to nursing throughout the twentieth and early twenty-first centuries. Moreover, history is clear that the concept of expanding the scope of practice for nurses was inextricably entwined with that assignment. HSS visiting nurses cared for poor immigrants of the Lower East Side unopposed by physicians until MDs perceived them as a threat. FNS nurses made diagnoses and treated patients in remote areas of Appalachia with the blessings of the physician committee who supervised them and BIA nurses cured, as best they could, native American Indians in their communities. In other cases, if one considers time as place, so-called after midnight nurses expanded their scope of practice by defibrillating patients in CCUs across the nation, and army nurses did whatever needed to be done on the battlefield (Keeling, 2004). Only when APNs threatened physicians' practice and income did organized medicine accuse them of practicing medicine without a license. Moreover, organized nursing itself was responsible for resisting the expansion of the scope of practice of nursing. However, it is also clear that when nurses and physicians focused on providing quality care for their patients, they were capable of working collaboratively and interdependently throughout the twentieth century.

Further analysis of the history of advanced practice nursing demonstrates the importance of evaluative research in documenting the contributions of APNs to the health care system and patients' well-being. As evidenced by nurse anesthetist Alice Magaw's 1900 publication on outcomes, the early "APNs" were particularly visionary in their use of data to document their effectiveness. Throughout the century, evaluative research based on measurable outcomes served as a tool for the profession to argue its position to health care policymakers and the medical profession (Brooten, Kumar, Brown, et al., 1986; Hamric, Lindbak, Jaubert, & Worley, 1998; Mitchell-DiCenso, Guyatt, Marrin, et al., 1996; Shah, Brutlomesso, Sullivan, & Lattanzio, 1997). As Beck (1995) stated, "It is inconsistent for a state medical association to maintain a position that quality health care is their objective … [while] … disregarding data demonstrating the positive impact of APNs on health care" (p. 15).

The powerful influence of organizational efforts also emerges as a theme. National organization has been key to progress for advanced practice nursing. Within the development of each of the advanced practice specialties, several common features have emerged. Strong national organizational leadership has been clearly demonstrated to be of critical importance in enhancing the growth and protection of the specialty. On the basis of the experience of the two oldest specialties, nurse anesthesia and nurse-midwifery, the process of establishing an effective national organization has taken a minimum of 3 decades. The history of these specialties reveals that specialty organizations have also played a critical role in the credentialing process for individuals in the specialty. The strength, unity, and depth of the organizational development of the two oldest advanced nursing specialties continue to serve as models for the younger developing specialties.

An additional theme to emerge is the importance of professional unity regarding the requisite education of APNs. Early in the twentieth century, specialty education was considered to be postgraduate with a heavy component of on the job training; however, that education was commonly postdiploma, not postbaccalaureate, and did not result in a master's degree. These early programs were of variable length and quality. The establishment of credible and stable educational programs has been a crucial step in the evolution of advanced practice nursing. As educational programs moved from informal, institutionally based models with a strong apprenticeship approach to more formalized graduate education programs, the credibility of APN roles has increased. State regulations also influenced the evolution of advanced practice as an increasing number of states mandated a master's degree as a prerequisite for APN licensure.

The influence of interprofessional struggles is apparent in all the advanced specialties, with the possible exception of the CNS. The legal battles between nursing and organized medicine are long-standing, particularly in relation to nurse anesthesia and nurse-midwifery. Most of these tensions have revolved around issues of control, autonomy, and economic competition. However, the issues are complex, with isolated examples of physician support of expanding nursing practice, such as physicians' support of early nurse anesthesia practice and Melzer's collaboration with Pineo in expanding CCU nurse practice. In all, outcomes of the legal battles have mostly proven to be positive for nursing and have helped legitimize APN roles.

Nurse anesthetists, nurse-midwives, and NPs have specifically challenged the boundaries between nursing and medical practice. When they did, organized medicine responded and, today, these predictable responses should not be unexpected or underestimated. According to Inglis and Kjervik (1993), "It should be noted that organized medicine, largely through lobbying, has played a central role in creating and perpetuating the states' contradictory and constraining provisions of APN practice" (p. 196).

Controversy within the nursing community was also a strong theme as the specialties developed. CRNAs, and to some extent NPs, developed outside of mainstream nursing whereas, from the start, CNSs developed within the mainstream. Nevertheless, each specialty has had to deal with resistance from other nurses. These intraprofessional struggles can be understood within the context of change—each of the APN specialties represented innovations that challenged the status quo of the nursing establishment and the health care system.

Throughout the twentieth and twenty-first centuries, prescriptive authority for advanced practice nursing, inextricably linked to economic and boundary issues between medicine and nursing, has been a particularly volatile legislative issue. Today, in most states, NPs, CNMs, and CRNAs can prescribe drugs with varying degrees of physician involvement and supervision. Although CNSs can prescribe in many states, they have not received the full recognition that has been granted to the other APN groups. Thus, despite a great deal of progress in the roles of APNs over the last century and gradual changes in state legislation and third-party reimbursement, APNs have not reached their full potential to fulfill U.S. health care needs. Barriers to enhancement of prescriptive authority for APNs include the following: (1) exclusive reimbursement patterns; (2) anticompetitive practices and resistance of organized medicine; (3) variable state regulation and practice acts; and (4) restrictive DEA registration laws (Beck, 1995; Keeling 2007). Hopefully, the recent APRN regulatory model (Stanley, 2009) will have a positive effect on these issues.

Societal forces have clearly influenced the development of advanced practice nursing. Gender issues have affected all the specialties to some degree because of the unique position of nursing as a female-dominated profession. The specialties of nurse anesthesia and nurse practitioner have been the exceptions, with more men entering these fields. Within nurse-midwifery, the status of women and women's health were powerful forces in the establishment and development of the specialty. Overall, war has served as a catalyst to the development of advanced practice nursing, education, and professional organizations. Finally, economic changes, particularly in relation to health care financing, have had a powerful effect on the development of advanced practice nursing. The dramatic growth of managed care systems in the 1990s, in particular, has presented new challenges and opportunities for APNs related to reimbursement, scope of practice, and autonomy (Safriet, 1998). Current efforts at health care reform mandated in the Patient Protection and Affordable Care Act (2010) may lead to more fundamental changes in health care financing and delivery.

With unremitting changes in nursing and health care, it is apparent that APN specialties will continue to evolve and diversify. As new roles emerge, the history of advanced practice nursing continues to be written. Today, particularly in light of the DNP initiative, the profession is at a critical juncture in which it must decide whether it will mandate doctoral level preparation for all APN roles. Agreement on master's preparation for all APNs is relatively new and disagreements about the requirement of the doctorate (Cronenwett, Dracup, Grey, et al., 2011) may continue to impede progress on the adoption of standardized educational criteria in the future. Undoubtedly, as law professor Safriet (1998) has argued, consistency in the definition of advanced practice nursing and in the criteria for licensure as an APRN is critical to autonomy in practice.

Thus, what remains to be seen is whether the profession can unite on issues related to the definition of advanced practice nursing and standardized criteria for educational preparation to ensure that APNs are permitted to practice with the autonomy experienced by other professionals. If that can be done, as the recent Institute of Medicine *Future of Nursing* report (2010) suggested, APNs could make a significant contribution to the transformation of health care in the twenty-first century.

References

American Association of Colleges of Nursing. (1999). *Enrollment and graduations in baccalaureate and graduate programs in nursing.* Washington, DC: Author.

American Association of Colleges of Nursing. (2006). *Essentials of doctoral education for advanced practice nursing.* Washington, DC: Author.

American Association of Nurse Anesthetists. (2007). *AANA announces support of doctorate for entry into nurse anesthesia practice by 2025.* Park Ridge, IL: Author.

American College of Nurse-Midwives. (1978a). *Definition of a certified nurse-midwife.* Washington, DC: Author.

American College of Nurse-Midwives. (1978b). *Philosophy.* Washington, DC: Author.

American College of Nurse-Midwives. (2007). *News release: Pennsylvania midwives are granted prescriptive authority.* Washington, DC: Author.

American Nurses Association. (1955). ANA board approves a definition of nursing practice. *American Journal of Nursing, 5,* 1474.

American Nurses Association. (1980). *Nursing: A social policy statement.* Kansas City, MO: Author.

American Nurses Association. (1991). *Report of the Congress on Nursing Practice to ANA Board of Directors on the merger of the*

Council of Clinical Nurse Specialists and the Council of Primary Health Care Nurse Practitioners into the Council of Nurses. Washington, DC: Author.

American Nurses Association. (1992). *Agenda for health care reform.* Washington, DC: Author.

American Nurses Association Congress for Nursing Practice. (1974). *Definition: Nurse practitioner, nurse clinician and clinical nurse specialist.* Kansas City, MO: American Nurses Association.

Ayers, R. (1971). Effects and development of the role of the clinical nurse specialist. In R. Ayers (Ed.), *The clinical nurse specialist: An experiment in role effectiveness and role development* (pp. 32–49). Duarte, CA: City of Hope National Medical Center.

Bankert, M. (1989). *Watchful care: A history of America's nurse anesthetists.* New York: Continuum.

Beck, M. (1995). Improving America's health care: Authorizing independent prescriptive privileges for advanced practice nurses. *University of San Francisco's Law Review, 29,* 951.

Beeber, L. S. (1990). To be one of the boys: Aftershocks of the WWI nursing experience. *Advances in Nursing Science, 12,* 32–43.

Bhan v. NME Hospitals, Inc., et al., 772 F.2d 1467 (9th Cir. 1985).

Bigbee, J., & Amidi-Nouri, A. (2000). History and evolution of advanced nursing practice. In A. B. Hamric, J. A. Spross, & C. M. Hanson (Eds.), *Advanced nursing practice: An integrative approach* (pp. 3–32, 2nd ed.). Philadelphia: W. B. Saunders.

Breckinridge, M. (1981). *Wide neighborhoods: A story of the Frontier Nursing Service.* Lexington, KY: University Press of Kentucky.

Brooten, D., Kumar, S., Brown, L. P., Butts, P., Finkler, S. A., Bakewell-Sachs, S., et al. (1986). A randomized clinical trial of early hospital discharge and home follow-up of very-low-birth-weight infants. *New England Journal of Medicine, 315,* 934–939.

Buck, D. F. (1940). The nurses on horseback ride on. *American Journal of Nursing, 40,* 993–995.

Buhler-Wilkerson, K. (2001). *No place like home: A history of nursing and home care in the United States.* Baltimore: Johns Hopkins University Press.

Bullough, B. (1984). The current phase of the development of nurse practice acts. *St. Louis Law Journal, 28,* 365–395.

Burst, H. V., & Thompson, J. E. (2003). Geneologic origins of nurse-midwifery education programs in the United States. *Journal of Midwifery and Women's Health, 48,* 464–472.

Calkin, J. D. (1984). A model for advanced nursing practice. *Journal of Nursing Administration, 14,* 24–30.

Chalmers-Frances v. Nelson, 6 Cal.2d 402 (1936).

Clancy, G. T., & Maguire, D. (1995). Advanced practice nursing in the neonatal intensive care unit. *Critical Care Nursing Clinics of North America, 7,* 71–76.

Cockerham, A. Z. (2012). Personal communication.

Cockerham, A. Z., & Keeling, A. W. (2012). *Rooted in the mountains, reaching to the world: Stories of nursing and midwifery at Kentucky's Frontier School.* Louisville, KY: Butler Books.

Critchley, D. L. (1985). Evolution of the role. In D. L. Critchley & J. T. Maurin (Eds.), *The clinical specialist in psychiatric mental health nursing* (pp. 5–22). New York: John Wiley.

Cronenwett, L. R. (1995). Modeling the future of advanced practice nursing. *Nursing Outlook, 43,* 112–118.

Cronenwett, L., Dracup, K., Grey, M., McCauley, L., Meleis, A., & Salmon, M. (2011). The doctor of nursing practice: A national workforce perspective. *Nursing Outlook, 59,* 9–17.

Daly, B. (1997). *The acute care nurse practitioner.* New York: Springer.

Daly, B. (2002). ACNP 2002: "Where we've been and where we're going." Original manuscript, keynote address, presented at the April 2002 ACNP Consensus Conference, Charlottesville, VA; the Keeling Collection, Center for Nursing Historical Inquiry, UVA.

D'Antonio, P. (1991). Staff needs and patient care: Seclusion and restraint in a nineteenth-century insane asylum. *Transactions and Studies of the College of Physicians of Philadelphia, 13*(4), 411–423.

Dewitt, K. (1900). Specialties in nursing. *American Journal of Nursing, 1,* 14–17.

Diers, D. (1991). Nurse-midwives and nurse anesthetists: The cutting edge in specialist practice. In L. H. Aiken & C. M. Fagin (Eds.), *Charting nursing's future: Agenda for the 1990s* (pp. 159–180). New York: J. B. Lippincott.

Donahue, P. M. (1996). *Nursing, the finest art: An illustrated history.* 2nd ed. St. Louis, MO: Mosby.

Doyle, E., & Meurer, J. (1983). Missouri legislation and litigation: Practicing medicine without a license. *Nurse Practitioner, 8,* 41–44.

Drug Enforcement Agency. (1991). Definition and exemption of affiliated practitioners, 56 Fed. Reg. 4181.

Duffus, R. L. (1938). *Lillian Wald: Neighbor and crusader.* New York: Macmillan.

Fairman, J. (2001). Delegated by default or negotiated by need? Physicians, nurse practitioners, and the process of clinical thinking. In E. Baer, P. D Antonio, S. Rinker, & J. Lynaugh (Eds.), *Enduring issues in American nursing* (pp. 309–333). New York: Springer.

Fairman, J. (2002). The roots of collaborative practice: Nurse practitioner pioneers' stories. *Nursing History Review, 10,* 159–174.

Fairman, J., & Lynaugh, J. (1998). *Critical care nursing: A history.* Philadelphia: University of Pennsylvania.

Ford, L. C. (1982). Nurse practitioners: History of a new idea and predictions for the future. In L. H. Aiken (Ed.), *Nursing in the 80s* (pp. 231–248). Philadelphia: J. B. Lippincott.

Ford, L. C. (1991). Advanced nursing practice: Future of the nurse practitioner. In L. H. Aiken & C. M. Fagin (Eds.), *Charting nursing's future: Agenda for the 1990s* (pp. 287–299). New York: J. B. Lippincott.

Ford, L. C., & Silver, H. K. (1967). The expanded role of the nurse in child care. *Nursing Outlook, 15,* 43–45.

Frank et al. v. South et al., 175 KY. 416-428 (1917).

Frontier Nursing Service. (1948). *Medical routines.* Lexington, KY: University of Kentucky, Frontier Nursing Service Collection.

Georgopoulos, B. S., & Christman, L. (1970). The clinical nurse specialist: A role model. *American Journal of Nursing, 70,* 1030–1039.

Georgopoulos, B. S., & Jackson, M. M. (1970). Nursing Kardex behavior in an experimental study of patient units with and without clinical specialists. *Nursing Research, 19,* 196–218.

Georgopoulos, B. S., & Sana, M. (1971). Clinical nursing specialization and intershift report behavior. *American Journal of Nursing, 71,* 538–545.

Girouard, S. (1978). The role of the clinical nurse specialist as change agent. An experiment in preoperative teaching. *International Journal of Nursing Studies, 15,* 57–65.

Goldmark, J. (1923). *Nursing and nursing education in the United States.* New York: Macmillan.

Grey, M. (1999). *New Deal medicine: The rural health programs of the Farm Security Administration.* Baltimore: Johns Hopkins University.

Hadley, E. (1989). Nurses and prescriptive authority: A legal and economic analysis. *American Journal of Law and Medicine, 15*(213), 245–299.

Hamric, A., Lindbak, S., Jaubert, S., & Worley, D. (1998). Outcomes associated with advanced nursing practice prescriptive authority. *Journal of the American Academy of Nurse Practitioners, 10,* 113–118.

Hamric, A. B. (1989). History and overview of the CNS role. In A. B. Hamric & J. A. Spross (Eds.), *The clinical nurse specialist in theory and practice* (pp. 3–18, 2nd ed.). Philadelphia: W. B. Saunders.

Hamric, A. B., & Spross, J. (Eds.), (1983). *The clinical nurse specialist in theory and practice.* New York: Grune & Stratton.

Hamric, A. B., & Spross, J. A. (Eds.), (1989). *The clinical nurse specialist in theory and practice* (2nd ed.). Philadelphia: W. B. Saunders.

Idaho Code 54-1413 (1971).

Inglis, A. D., & Kjervik, D. K. (1993). Empowerment of advanced practice nurses: Regulation reform needed to increase access to care. *Journal of Law, Medicine and Ethics, 21* (2), 193–205.

Institute of Medicine. (2010). *The future of nursing: leading change, advancing health.* Washington, DC: National Academy of Science Press.

Jenicek, J. (1967). Vietnam—new challenges for the army nurse anesthetist. *Journal of the American Association of Nurse Anesthetists, 67,* 347–352.

Jolly, E. (1927). *Nuns of the battlefield.* Providence, RI: Providence Visitor Press.

Jonas, S. (1981). *Health care delivery in the United States.* New York: Springer.

Kalisch, P. A., & Kalisch, B. J. (1986). *The advance of American nursing* (2nd ed.). Boston: Little, Brown and Company.

Keane, A. & Richmond, T. (1993). Tertiary nurse practitioners. *Image: Journal of Nursing Scholarship, 25,* 281–284.

Keeling, A. (2004). Blurring the boundaries between medicine and nursing: Coronary care nursing, circa the 1960s. *Nursing History Review, 12,* 139–164.

Keeling, A. (2007). *Nursing and the Privilege of Prescription.* Columbus: Ohio State University Press.

Keeling, A., Kirschgessner, J., & Brodie, B. (2010). *The voice of professional nursing education: A 40-year history of the AACN.* Washington, DC: Author.

Keeling, A. (2011). Clinics in the "suitcase camps": Nursing the migrants during the Great Depression, 1938–1941. *Windows in Time, Newsletter of University of Virginia School of Nursing Center for Historical Inquiry,* 8–11.

Kinser, P. (2011). "We were all in it together": Medicine and nursing in the 8th Evacuation Hospital, 1942–1945. *Windows in Time, Newsletter of University of Virginia School of Nursing Center for Historical Inquiry,* 7–13.

Kitzman, H. J. (1983). The CNS and the nurse practitioner. In A. B. Hamric & J. A. Spross (Eds.), *The clinical nurse specialist in theory and practice* (pp. 275–290). New York: Grune & Stratton.

Kleinpell, R. M. (1997). Acute care nurse practitioners: Roles and practice profiles. *AACN Clinical Issues, 8,* 156–162.

Little, D. E., & Carnevali, D. (1967). Nurse specialist effect on tuberculosis. *Nursing Research, 16,* 321–326.

Lynaugh, J. E., & Brush, B. L. (1996). *American nursing: From hospitals to health systems.* Hoboken, NJ: Wiley-Blackwell.

Lynaugh, J. E., & Fairman, J. (1992). New nurses, new spaces: A preview of the AACN history study. *American Journal of Critical Nursing, 1*(1), 19–24

Magaw, A. (1900). Observations on 1092 cases of anesthesia from January 1, 1899 to January 1, 1900. *St. Paul's Medical Journal,* 306–311.

MacKenzie, E. (1929). *"Report of the Associate Director, Henry Street Visiting Nurses Service," December 15, 1928-January 15, 1929. Lillian Wald Collection,* New York: Columbia University.

Magyary, D., Whitney, J., & Brown, M. (2006). Advancing practice inquiry: Research foundations of the practice doctorate in nursing. *Nursing Outlook, 543,* 139–151.

McBride, A. B., Austin, J. K., Chestnut, E. E., Main, C. S., Richards, B. S., & Roy, B. A. (1987). Evaluation of the impact of the clinical nurse specialist in a state psychiatric hospital. *Archives of Psychiatric Nursing, 1,* 55–61.

McGarrel, A. (1934). *Transcript on appeal, volume 1. William Chalmers-Francis and the Anesthesia Section of the LA County Medical Association v. Dagmar A. Nelson and St. Vincent's Hospital.* Chicago: AANA Executive Office, Historical Files.

Mitchell-DiCenso, A., Guyatt, G., Marrin, M., Goeree, R., Willan, A., Southwell, D., et al. (1996). A controlled trial of nurse practitioners in neonatal intensive care. *Pediatrics, 98,* 1143–1148.

Moxley, J. (1968). The predicament in health manpower. *American Journal of Nursing, 68,* 1489–1492.

National Council of State Boards of Nursing. (2012). CNS prescriptive authority by state. (http://www.nacns.org/docs/RxAuthorityTable.pdf).

National League for Nursing. (1984). *Master's education in nursing: Route to opportunities in contemporary nursing, 1984–1985.* New York: Author.

National League for Nursing. (1994). *Graduate education in nursing, advanced practice nursing.* New York: Author.

National Organization of Nurse Practitioner Faculties. (1997). *Criteria for evaluation of nurse practitioner programs.* Washington, DC: National Task Force on Quality Nurse Practitioner Education.

Negro nurse-midwives. (1942). *American Journal of Nursing, 42,* 705.

News here and there: American Association of Nurse-Midwives. (1942). *American Journal of Nursing, 42,* 832.

Office of Technology Assessment. (1986). *Nurse practitioners, physicians assistants and certified nurse-midwives: A policy analysis*. Washington, DC: Author.

Oltz v. St. Peter's Community Hospital, CV 81-271-H-Res (D. Mont. 1986).

Oncology Nursing Society. (2011). About ONS (http://www.ons.org/about).

Patient Protection and Affordable Care Act (PPACA) (2010). Pub. L. No. 111-148, 124 Stat. 119.

Peplau, H. E. (1952). *Interpersonal relations in nursing: A conceptual frame of reference for psychodynamic nursing*. New York: Putnam.

Peplau, H. E. (1965). Specialization in professional nursing. *Nursing Science, 3*, 268–287.

Pinneo, R. (1967). A new dimension in nursing: Intensive coronary care. *American Association of Industrial Nurses Journal, 15*, 7–10.

Pinneo, R. (1972). Mastering monitoring. *Nursing, 72, 2*, 22–25.

Reiter, F. (1966). The nurse-clinician. *American Journal of Nursing, 66*, 274–280.

Reverby, S. M. (1987). *Ordered to care: The dilemma of American nursing, 1850-1945*. New York: Cambridge University Press.

Richards, L. (1911). *Reminiscences of America's first trained nurse*. Boston: Whitcomb and Barrows.

Rinker, S. (2000). To cultivate a feeling of confidence: The nursing of obstetric patients, 1890-1940. *Nursing History Review, 8*, 117–142.

Rogers, M. E. (1972). Nursing: To be or not to be. *Nursing Outlook, 20*, 42–46.

Rooks, J. (1997). *Midwifery and childbirth in America*. Philadelphia: Temple University Press.

Safriet, B. J. (1992). Health care dollars and regulatory sense: The role of advance practice nursing. *Yale Journal on Regulation, 9*, 417–488.

Safriet, B. J. (1998). Still spending dollars, still searching for sense: Advanced practice nursing in an era of regulatory and economic turmoil. *Advanced Practice Nursing Quarterly, 4*, 24–33.

Schindler, F. (1942). Nursing in electro-shock therapy. *American Journal of Nursing, 42*, 858–861.

Schutt, B. (1971). A prophet honored. Lillian D. Wald. *American Journal of Nursing, 71*, 53.

Sermchief v. Gonzales, 660 S.W.2d 683 (1983).

Shah, H., Brutlomesso, K., Sullivan, D., & Lattanzio, J. (1997). An evaluation of the role and practices of the acute care nurse practitioner. *AACN Clinical Issues, 8*, 147–155.

Silver, H. K., & McAtee, P. (1988). Speaking out: Should nurses substitute for house staff? *American Journal of Nursing, 88*, 1671–1673.

Smith, S. (1994). White nurses, black midwives, and public health in Mississippi, 1920-1950. *Nursing History Review, 2*, 29–49.

Sparacino, P. (1990). A historical perspective on the development of the CNS role. In P. Sparacino, D. M. Cooper, & P. A. Minarik (Eds.), *The CNS: Implementation and impact* (Chapter 1, pp. 3–10), Norwalk, CT: Appleton and Lange.

Spross, J., & Hamric, A. B. (1983). A model for future clinical specialist practice. In A. B. Hamric & J. Spross (Eds.), *The clinical nurse specialist in theory and practice* (pp. 291–306). New York: Grune & Stratton.

Stanley, J. M. (2009). Reaching consensus on a regulatory model: What does this mean for APRNs? *Journal for Nurse Practitioners, 5*, 99–104.

Taussig, F. J. (1914) The nurse-midwife. *Public Health Quarterly*, 33–39.

Thatcher, V. S. (1953). *A history of anesthesia: With emphasis on the nurse specialist*. Philadelphia: J. B. Lippincott.

U.S. Department of Health, Education, & Welfare Secretary's Committee to Study Extended Roles for Nurses. (1972). *Extending the scope of nursing practice: A report of the Secretary's Committee* (pp. 3–6). Washington, DC: U.S. Government Printing Office.

U.S. Department of Health and Human Services. (1996). *The registered nurse population March 1996: Findings from the National Sample Survey of Registered Nurses*. Washington, DC: Author.

Varney, H. (1987). *Nurse-midwifery* (2nd ed.). Boston: Blackwell Scientific.

Varney, H., Kriebs, J. M., & Gegor, C. L. (2004). *Nurse-midwifery* (4th ed.). Boston: Blackwell Scientific.

Waisel, D. (2001). The role of World War II and the European theater of operations in the development of anesthesiology as a physician specialty in the USA. *Anesthesiology, 94*, 907–912.

Wald, L. (1922). *The origin and development of Henry Street Settlement*. New York: Lillian Wald Papers, New York Public Library.

Wall, B. (2005). *Unlikely entrepreneurs: Catholic Sister and the hospital marketplace, 1863-1925*. Columbus: The Ohio State University Press.

Williams, D. (2007). Field nurses' narrative report, May 1931. In A. Keeling (Ed.), *Nursing and the privilege of prescription, 1893-2000*. Columbus: Ohio State University Press.

Wolff, M. A. (1984). Court upholds expanded practice roles for nurses. *Journal of Law, Medicine and Ethics, 12*, 26–29.

Conceptualizations of Advanced Practice Nursing

Judith A. Spross

CHAPTER CONTENTS

Why are conceptualizations of advanced practice nursing important for students and practicing advanced practice nurses (APNs) to understand? The content may seem dry to students, who are otherwise excited about learning new ways of caring for individuals, through their APN education. Concepts, models, and theories seem remote from the real work of eliciting histories, performing physicals, planning treatment, evaluating outcomes, and otherwise helping patients and families improve their health, cope with illnesses, and die with dignity. Whether one does so consciously, all these advanced practice activities are guided by some model or framework. Novices may rely more frequently on rules and guidelines to accomplish their work. Expert APNs may not consult rules and guidelines for common problems, but can improvise new ways of thinking (models)

when faced with novel situations. Regardless of years of experience, APNs rely on common processes and language in their communications with colleagues about patient care and recognize when they must explain a clinical situation to someone unfamiliar with the patient. Similarly, it is important for the nursing profession and for individual APNs to understand the language of advanced practice nursing to communicate with each other, clients, and stakeholders. Currently, converging forces in the United States are moving rapidly, requiring the profession to advance a common understanding of advanced practice nursing, which is likely to inform future conceptualizations of advanced practice nursing.

The development of a common language and conceptual framework for communication and for guiding and evaluating practice, education, policy, research, and theory is fundamental to sound progress in any practice discipline. Given the evolving changes in the U.S. health care system, such a foundation is particularly crucial at this stage in the development of advanced practice nursing. Since the last edition, a professional consensus on advanced practice nursing regulation has been reached in the United States—the Consensus Model for APRN Regulation (2008) and is being implemented. In addition, the Institute of Medicine [IOM] (2011) has called for integrating advanced practice nursing more completely into the U.S. health care delivery system. Other forces driving a common understanding of advanced practice nursing are the expansion of programs offering the Doctorate of Nursing Practice (DNP), the Patient Protection and Affordable Care Act (PPACA, 2010), accountable care organizations, and the promulgation of interprofessional competencies (Canadian Interprofessional Health Collaborative [CIHC], 2010; Health Professions Networks, Nursing and Midwifery, & Human Resources for Health, 2010; Interprofessional Education Collaborative [IPEC] Expert Panel, 2011) and education (see Chapters 12 and 22). Understanding what advanced practice nursing is, what APNs do, similarities and differences among APNs, and how APNs contribute to affordable, accessible, and effective care is central to the redesign of U.S. health care. It is important for readers to understand that because of the dynamic and evolving nature of health care reform and nursing organizations' activities in this arena, nationally and globally, the content in this chapter is changing quickly. Readers are encouraged to consult the websites cited in this chapter for up to date information.

Internationally, there have been efforts to clarify, establish, and/or regulate advanced practice roles within the nursing profession in other countries (e.g., Canadian Nurses Association [CNA] 2007, 2008, 2009a, b; International Council of Nurses [ICN] (2009). In countries in which APN roles exist, in addition to studies of the distinctions among roles (Gardner, Chang, & Duffield, 2007; Gardner, Gardner, Middleton, et al., 2010), efforts are underway to establish educational programs (Wong, Peng, Kan, et al., 2009) or develop frameworks that clarify education, scope of practice, registration and licensing, and/or credentialing that are country-specific (e.g., Fagerström, 2009). Statements by national organizations such as the CNA and ICN and articles on conceptualizations of advanced practice nursing proposed by authors from other countries (e.g., Ball & Cox, 2004; CNA, 2007, 2008, 2009a, b; DiCenso, Martin-Misener, Bryant-Lukosius, et al., 2010; Gardner, Chang, & Duffield, 2007; Gardner et al., 2010; Mantzoukas & Watkinson, 2007; McMurray, 2011; Pringle, 2010) have been reviewed. Although contextual factors may differ from those in the United States, there are global opportunities for clarifying and advancing advanced practice nursing and these

should be specific to a country's culture, health system, professional standards, and regulatory requirements. Content from articles about advanced practice in other countries is used to present models or illuminate certain conceptual issues; they also inform the discussion of recommendations and future directions. For a more complete discussion of global perspectives on advanced practice nursing, see Chapter 6.

In reviewing the literature for this edition, searches were conducted using the terms *advanced practice nursing, model,* or *theory,* and the four APN roles. In addition, a search was done of the authors of models cited in the prior edition. Few new curricular models were identified (Fagerström, 2009; Perraud, Delaney, Carlson-Sabelli, et al., 2006; Wong et al., 2009), but several types of articles related to model development, model testing, and models used in advanced practice nursing were identified. These models may be characterized as follows:

- Curriculum models (e.g., Fagerström, 2009; Perraud et al., 2006; Wong et al., 2009)
- Administrative or organizational models (e.g., Ackerman, Mick, & Witzel, 2010; Scarpa & Connelly, 2011; Skalla & Caron, 2008)
- Models that differentiate among advanced practice roles (e.g., Gardner, Chang, & Duffield, 2007)
- Models of the nature of advanced practice nursing (e.g., Ball & Cox, 2003; Brown, 1998; Hamric, 1996, 2009, and see Chapter 3; Mantzoukas & Watkinson, 2007; Styles & Lewis, 2000)
- Models that differentiate between basic and advanced practice nursing (e.g., Calkin, 1984; Oberle & Allen, 2001)
- Models of role development of APNs (see Chapter 4)
- Models of APN regulation and credentialing (e.g., the APRN [Advanced Practice Registered Nurse] Consensus Model, 2008; CNA, 2007, 2008, 2009a, b; Stanley, Werner, & Apple, 2009; Styles, 1998);
- Models of interdisciplinary practice (Dunphy & Winland-Brown, 1998; Dunphy, Winland-Brown, Porter, Thomas, & Gallagher, 2011);
- Models that APNs would find useful include the following:
  ○ Application or testing of grand and middle-range theories to APN practice (e.g., Musker, 2011; Newcomb, 2010);
  ○ Models of role implementation (Ball & Cox, 2004; Bryant-Lukosius, DiCenso, Browne, & Pinelli, 2004) and APN care delivery (Mahler, 2010; McAiney, Haughton, Jennings, et al., 2008; Dunphy & Winland-Brown, 1998; Dunphy, Winland-Brown, Porter, Thomas, & Gallagher, 2011; Curley, 1998; American Association of Critical Care Nurses, 2012)

- Models to evaluate outcomes of advanced nursing practice (see Chapters 23 and 24).

In addition, professional organizations with interests in licensing, accreditation, certification, and educational (LACE) issues regarding APNs can be viewed as operating from some conceptualization of advanced practice nursing, whether implicit or explicit. In this chapter, the following types of models will be discussed: those promulgated by APN stakeholder organizations, models that describe the nature of advanced practice and/or differentiate between advanced and basic practice, and selected models that APNs may find useful in practice.

In previous editions, problems associated with lack of a unified definition of advanced practice and imperatives for undertaking this important work were identified. When practicable, consensus on advanced practice nursing models should be beneficial for patients, society, and the profession. Although the APRN Consensus Model (2008) has brought needed conceptual clarity to regulation of advanced practice nursing in the United States, there is still work to be done with regard to other aspects of conceptualizing advanced practice nursing, such as APN competencies, differentiating basic and advanced nursing practice, and differentiating the advanced practice of nursing from the practices of other disciplines. This work has become more urgent given the impacts of other U.S. initiatives that are unfolding. I have reviewed published documents from national professional organizations and the literature and focused selectively on models of APN practice. This review is not exhaustive. For example, in limiting the scope of this chapter, statements on advanced practice nursing by specialty organizations have not been examined. Thus, the purposes of this chapter are as follows:

1. Lay the foundation for thinking about the concepts underlying advanced practice nursing by describing the nature, purposes, and components of conceptual models.
2. Identify conceptual challenges in defining and operationalizing advanced practice nursing.
3. Describe selected conceptualizations of advanced practice nursing.
4. Make recommendations for assessing existing models and developing, implementing, and evaluating conceptual frameworks for advanced practice.
5. Outline future directions for conceptual work on advanced practice nursing.

Readers are invited to debate and enlarge on the models, issues, and thinking put forward in this chapter.

Nature, Purposes, and Components of Conceptual Models

A conceptual model is one part of the structure, or holarchy, of nursing knowledge. This structure consists of metaparadigms (most abstract), philosophies, conceptual models, theories, and empirical indicators (most concrete; Fawcett, 2005). Traditionally, key concepts in the metaparadigm of nursing, which nursing theories are expected to address in their conceptual underpinnings, are humans, the environment, health, and nursing (Fawcett, 2005). Although some theorists have proposed additional or expanded concepts, Fawcett's ideas inform this discussion. At this stage of the evolution, conceptual models of advanced practice nursing remain an appropriate focus.

- What is a conceptual model?
- What purposes does it serve?
- What are its components?

A number of answers to these questions are in the nursing literature. Fawcett (2005) has identified a conceptual model as "a set of relatively abstract and general concepts that address the phenomena of central interest to a discipline, the propositions that broadly describe these concepts, and the propositions that state relatively abstract and general relations between two or more of the concepts" (p. 16).

Fawcett (2005) also noted that a conceptual model is "a distinctive frame of reference…that tells [adherents] how to observe and interpret the phenomenon of interest to the discipline" and "provide alternative ways to view the subject matter of the discipline; there is no 'best' way." Although there is no best way to view a phenomenon, evolving a more uniform and explicit conceptual model of advanced practice nursing is likely to benefit patients, nurses, and other stakeholders (IOM, 2011) and have practical benefits. It can facilitate communication, reduce conflict, ensure consistency of advanced practice nursing, when relevant and appropriate, across APN roles, and offer a "systematic approach to nursing research, education, administration, and practice" (Fawcett, 2005). Thus, conceptual models serve many purposes.

Models may help APNs articulate professional role identity and function, serving as a framework for organizing beliefs and knowledge about their professional roles and competencies, providing a basis for further development of knowledge. In clinical practice, APNs use conceptual models in the delivery of their holistic, comprehensive, and collaborative care (e.g., Carron & Cumbie, 2011; Dunphy & Winland-Brown, 1998; Dunphy et al., 2011; Musker, 2011). Models may also be used to differentiate among levels of nursing practice—for example, between staff nursing and advanced practice nursing (Calkin, 1984; ANA, 2010b). In research and other scholarly activities, investigators use conceptual models to guide research and theory development. An investigator could decide to focus on the study of one concept or examine relationships among select concepts to elucidate testable theories. For example, research by Fenton (1985) and Brykczynski (1989) has elucidated new domains of practice for clinical nurse specialists (CNSs) and nurse practitioners (NPs), respectively. In education, faculty use conceptual models to plan curricula, identify important concepts and the relationships among them, and make choices about course content and clinical experiences for preparing APNs (Perraud et al. 2006; Wong et al., 2009).

Fawcett and colleagues (Fawcett, Newman, & McAllister, 2004; Fawcett & Graham, 2005) have raised additional conceptual questions about advanced practice:

- What do APNs do that makes their practice "advanced?"
- To what extent does incorporating activities traditionally done by physicians qualify nursing practice as "advanced?"
- Are there nursing activities that are also advanced?

Because direct clinical practice is viewed as the central APN competency, one could also ask: "What does the term *clinical* mean? Does it refer only to hospitals or clinics?" These questions are becoming more important given the APRN Consensus Model and given the role that APNs are expected to play across the continua of health care as a result of the PPACA and its reforms. From a regulatory standpoint, the emphasis on a specific population as a focus of practice will lead, when appropriate, to reconceptualizing curricula to ensure that graduates are prepared to succeed in new or revised certification examinations. Hamric (see Chapter 3) has noted that some APN competencies are likely to be performed by nurses in other roles but suggests that the expression of these competencies by APNs is different. For example, all nurses collaborate but a unique aspect of APN practice is that APNs are authorized to initiate referrals and prescribe treatments that are implemented by others (e.g., physical therapy). Innovations and reforms arising from the PPACA will ensure that APNs are explicitly engaged in the delivery of care across care settings, including in nursing clinics and palliative care settings, and as full participants in interprofessional teams. Changes in regulations and in the delivery of health care must and should lead to new or revised conceptualizations of advanced practice nursing, such as defining theoretical and evidence-based differences between APN care and the care offered by other providers and clinical staff, the role of APNs in interprofessional teams, and specialization and subspecialization in advanced practice nursing. This work will enable nursing leaders and health policy makers to design a health care system that delivers high-quality care at reasonable cost based on disciplinary and interdisciplinary competencies, outcomes, effectiveness, efficacy, and costs. Indeed, this textbook reflects a consistent effort to evaluate and revise the authors' conceptualizations of advanced practice

nursing based on current contextual factors. The conceptualization advanced in this text has been remarkably stable since it was first proposed in 1996 and has required modest modifications as APN roles and health care have evolved.

In addition to a pragmatic reevaluation of advanced practice nursing concepts based on the evolution of APN regulation and health care reform, writers in the United States and abroad are raising important theoretical questions about conceptualizations of advanced practice, including the following: the epistemologic, philosophical, and ontologic underpinnings of advanced practice (Arslanian-Engoren, Hicks, Whall, & Algase, 2005); the nature of advanced practice knowledge, discerning the differences between and among the notions of specialty, advanced practice, and advancing practice (Allan, 2011; Christensen, 2009, 2011; Macdonald, Herbert, & Thibeault, 2006; Thoun, 2011); and the extent to which APNs are prepared to study and apply nursing theories in their practices (Algase, 2010; Arslanian-Engoren, Hicks et al., 2005; Karnick, 2011).

In summary, questions arising from a changing health policy landscape and from theorizing about advanced practice nursing point to the need for well thought-out, robust conceptual models to help individuals answer important questions about the phenomenon—in this case, advanced practice nursing. The need for clarity about advanced practice nursing, what it is and is not, is becoming more important, not only for patients and those in the nursing profession but for evolving initiatives such as interprofessional education (CIHC, 2010; Health Professions Networks, 2010; IPEC Expert Panel, 2011), practice (American Association of Nurse Anesthetists, 2012), and creation of accountable care organizations, efforts to build teams and systems in which effective communication, collaboration, and coordination lead to quality care and improved patient, institutional, and fiscal outcomes.

Conceptualizations of Advanced Practice Nursing: Problems and Imperatives

Despite the usefulness and benefits of conceptual models, some difficulties are apparent in the literature when the clinical and professional issues inherent to advanced practice nursing are examined. Although there is increasing conceptual clarity about advanced practice nursing, five issues of conceptual confusion or uncertainty in the evolution of advanced practice nursing can still be identified.

Despite improvements in the area of regulation, the first issue remains the absence of well-defined and consistently applied terms of reference. A core stable vocabulary, a lingua franca, is needed for definition and model building. The lack of a consistent stable vocabulary can be seen in the literature. Shuler and Davis (1993a) have stated that "One of the greatest barriers to using nursing models in [nurse practitioner] practice relates to vocabulary and communication...." Despite progress, this challenge remains. For example, in the United States, *advanced practice nursing* is the term that is used but the ICN and CNA use the term *advanced nursing practice*. Furthermore, the role and functions of APNs could be better conceptualized. Although the use of competency is becoming more common, concepts about APN work are variously termed *roles, hallmarks, competencies, functions, activities, skills,* and *abilities*. Few models of APN practice address nursing's metaparadigm (person, health, environment, nursing) comprehensively. The problem in comparing, refining, or developing models is that terms are used with no universal meaning or frame of reference; occasionally, no definition is offered at all, or terms are used inconsistently. This instability and inconsistency are evident in many models cited in this chapter. It is rightly anticipated that conceptual models of the field and its practice change over time. However, the evolution of advanced practice nursing and its comprehension by nurses, policymakers, and others will be enhanced if scholars and practitioners in the field agree on the use and definition of fundamental terms of reference.

The second issue is that many attempts to articulate models of advanced practice nursing fail to consider extant literature that is directly relevant to such conceptualizing activities. In part, this may be a result of the lag between the conceptualizing effort and its ultimate publication, the knowledge explosion, and the role of the Internet and social media in the generation and dissemination of knowledge. For example, some recently published articles reviewed for this chapter cited work from the 1980s and 1990s; revised publications of these earlier cited works, although apparently available, were not cited. This caution should be considered when proposing, evaluating, or refining advanced practice nursing models.

The third issue is a lack of clarity regarding conceptualizations that differentiate between and among levels of clinical practice:

- Does the practice of APNs differ from the practice of registered nurses (RNs) who are experts by experience (i.e., no graduate degree in advanced practice)?
- How does the practice of an APN certified in a subspecialty such as oncology differ from the practice of a non–master's prepared clinician who is certified at the basic level in the oncology subspecialty?
- With the definition of population foci and subspecialty advanced in The APRN Consensus Model, how does certification in one or more subspecialties influence the quality and outcomes of care?

- How does the care provided by an adult health NP with a subspecialty APN certification in oncology or critical care differ from one who is certified in adult health only?

Although many authors who write about advanced practice nursing cite Benner's model of expert practice (1984), they rarely indicate that the model was derived from the study of nurses who were primarily experts by experience, not APNs. Certainly, Benner's model is relevant to efforts to conceptualize advanced practice nursing, as demonstrated by Fenton's (1985) and Brykczynski's (1989) work. Given that clinical practice is why the profession of nursing exists and is central to advanced practice nursing, models that help the profession differentiate levels of practice are needed.

The fourth issue is the need to clarify the differences between advanced practice nursing and medicine (see Chapter 3). Graduate APN students struggle with this issue as part of role development (see Chapter 4). This lack of conceptual clarity is apparent in advertisements that invite NPs or physician assistants to apply for the same job. As noted in Chapters 21 and 22, organized medicine expends resources in trying to limit or discredit advanced practice nursing, even as some physician leaders work on behalf of advocating for APNs. Hamric, in Chapter 3, asserts that advanced practice nursing is not the junior practice of medicine, an assertion supported by the seven competencies of advanced practice nursing (Chapters 7 through 13). Fawcett, a well-respected nursing leader, has asked, "What does it mean to blend nursing and medicine?" (Fawcett et al., 2004; Fawcett & Graham, 2005). Finally, little is understood about the impact of APN-physician collaboration on practice or about strategies for matching the level of knowledge and skill to the needs of patient populations (Brooten & Youngblut, 2006; Calkin, 1984).

The fifth issue is interprofessional education and practice, a concept that is central to accountable, collaborative, coordinated, and high-quality care. The development of interprofessional competencies for health professionals (CIHC, 2010; Health Professions Networks, 2010; IPEC Expert Panel, 2011) suggests that the more important questions now are *not* about "blending" APN and physician practice, but questions such as "How do we ensure that despite differing disciplinary backgrounds, patients, colleagues, and other observers recognize the behavioral expressions of interprofessional competencies?" Also, how do we undertake the conceptual, curricular, credentialing, and other work that will be needed to make interprofessional practice and effective teamwork the gold standard of quality care? The existence of interprofessional competencies and emergence of promising conceptualizations of interprofessional work. (e.g., Barr, Freeth, Hammick, et al., 2005; Reeves, Goldman, Gilbert, et al., 2011) are critical contextual factors for elucidating and advancing conceptualizations of advanced practice nursing. See Chapter 12.

Among many imperatives for reaching a conceptual consensus on advanced practice nursing, most important are the interrelated areas of policymaking, licensing and credentialing, and practice, including competencies. In the policymaking arena, for example, not all APNs are eligible to be reimbursed by insurers, and even those activities that are reimbursable are often billed incident to a physician's care, rendering the work of APNs invisible. The APRN Consensus Model (2008), the PPACA, and the IOM's call for changes to enable APNs to work within their full scope of practice (IOM, 2011). will make it easier for U.S. policymakers to recommend and adopt changes to policies and regulations that now constrain APN practice, eventually making the contributions of APNs to quality care visible and reimbursable. Agreement on vocabulary and concepts such as competencies that are common to all APN roles will maximize the ability of APNs to work within their full scope of practice.

Although some progress has been made, there are compelling reasons for continuing dialogue and activity aimed at clarifying advanced practice nursing and the concepts and models that help stakeholders understand the nature of APN work and their contributions. Reaching consensus on concepts and vocabulary will serve theoretical, practical, and policymaking purposes. As the work of health care reform and implementing interprofessional competencies, education, and practice moves forward, there will be opportunities for the profession to conceptualize advanced practice nursing more clearly. Clarification and consensus on conceptualization of the nature of advanced practice nursing will lead to the following outcomes:

1. Clear differentiation of advanced practice nursing from other levels of clinical nursing practice.
2. Clear differentiation between advanced practice nursing and the clinical practice of physicians and other non-nurse providers within a specialty.
3. Clear understanding of the roles and contributions of APNs on interprofessional teams, enabling employers to create teams and accountable care organizations that can meet institutions' clinical and fiduciary outcomes.
4. Clear delineation of the similarities and differences among APN roles and the ability to match APN skills and knowledge to the needs of patients.
5. Regulation and credentialing of APNs that protects the public and ensures equitable treatment of all APNs.
6. Clear articulation of international, national, state, and local health policies that do the following:

   a. Recognize and make visible the substantive contributions of APNs to quality, cost-effective health care, and patient outcomes.
   b. Ensure the public's access to APN care.
   c. Ensure explicit and appropriate mechanisms to bill and pay for APN care.
7. A maximum social contribution by APNs in health care, including improvement in health outcomes and health-related quality of life for the people to whom they provide care.
8. The actualization of practitioners of advanced practice nursing, enabling APNs to reach their full potential, personally and professionally.

Conceptualizations of Advanced Practice Nursing Roles: Organizational Perspectives

Practice with individual clients or patients is the central work of the field; it is the reason for which nursing was created. The following questions are the kinds of questions a conceptual model of advanced practice nursing should answer:

- What is the scope and purpose of advanced practice nursing?
- What are the characteristics of advanced practice nursing?
- Within what settings does this practice occur?
- How do APNs' scopes of practice differ from those of other providers offering similar or related services?
- What knowledge and skills are required?
- How are these different from other providers?
- What patient and institutional outcomes are realized when APNs deliver care? how are these outcomes different from other providers?
- When should health care systems employ APNs and what types of patients particularly benefit from APN care?
- For what types of pressing health care problems are APNs a solution in terms of improving outcomes, quality of care, and cost-effectiveness?

Some conceptual models reviewed in this chapter are more narrowly focused than others. Some advanced practice models are more homogeneous and some are mixed with respect to the phenomenon studied. Some could be seen as micromodels in terms of the unit of analysis and others could be seen as metamodels, incorporating a number of conceptual frameworks. Some models explain systems; others explain relationships between and among systems. All these foci are important, depending on the purposes to be served. However, in the development of conceptual models, the phenomenon to be modeled must be carefully defined. For example, is the model intended to encompass the entire field of advanced practice nursing, or is it confined to distinctive concepts such as collaborative practice between physicians and APNs? Is advanced nursing practice different from advanced practice nursing? If a phenomenon and its related concepts are not clearly defined, the model could be so inconsistent as to be confusing or so comprehensive that its impact will be diluted.

In addition to describing concepts and how they are related, assumptions about the philosophy, values, and practices of the profession should be reflected in conceptual models. The present discussion of conceptualizations of advanced practice nursing is guided by three assumptions:

1. Each model, at least implicitly, addresses the four elements of nursing's metaparadigm—persons, health and illness, nursing, and the environment.
2. The development and strengthening of the field of advanced practice nursing depends on professional agreement regarding the nature of advanced practice nursing (a conceptual model) that can inform APN program accreditation, credentialing, and practice.
3. That APNs meet the needs of society for advanced nursing care.
4. Advanced practice nursing will reach its full potential to the extent that foundational conceptual components of any model of advanced practice nursing framework are delineated and agreed on.

In the next section, the implicit and explicit conceptualizations of advanced practice nursing promulgated by professional organizations concerned with defining APN practice and with clarifying particular APN roles are discussed. Organizations such as the Oncology Nursing Society and the American Association of Critical-Care Nurses [AACN]) have addressed advanced practice nursing in their specialties. Although specialty models and standards are important to students and APNs, they are not addressed in this chapter. As students and readers consider their own APN practices, they may want to review the history of advanced practice nursing (see Chapter 1) and evolving advanced practice nursing roles (see Chapter 5) to inform their efforts to conceptualize their own practices.

Although not all the documents described in this section are conceptual models, many imply, describe, or reference a conceptual framework. The APRN Consensus Model (2008) represents a major step forward in promulgating a uniform definition of advanced practice nursing, for the purposes of regulation, in the United States. This accomplishment is informing efforts by other organizations; even so, some problems with the absence of a core vocabulary noted earlier are apparent as one reads the different approaches taken by other professional organizations; therefore, comparisons are difficult to make because terms of reference and their meanings vary. To help the

---

BOX 2-1   Definition of Terms

Competent Having requisite or adequate ability or qualities; legally qualified or adequate; having the capacity to function or develop in a particular way (sufficient)

Competence, competency The quality or state of being competent; the knowledge that enables a person to speak and understand a language

Component A constituent part; ingredient

Domain A sphere of knowledge, influence, or activity

Role A socially expected behavior pattern usually determined by an individual's status in a particular society

Hallmark Distinguishing characteristic, trait, or feature

Sphere An area or range over or within which someone or something acts, exists, or has influence or significance

Scope Space or opportunity for unhampered motion, activity, or thought; extent of treatment, activity, or influence

Standard Something established by authority, custom, or general consent as a model or example; something set up and established by an authority as a rule for the measure of quantity, weight, extent, value, or quality

Adapted from Mish, F.C. (Ed.). (2001). *Merriam-Webster's collegiate dictionary*. (10th ed.). Springfield, MA: Merriam-Webster International; and American Association of Colleges of Nursing (AACN). (2006). The essentials of doctoral education for advanced nursing practice (http://www.aacn.nche.edu/publications/position/DNPEssentials.pdf).

---

reader appreciate the challenge of developing a common language to characterize advanced practice nursing, dictionary definitions of terms used in conceptualizations of advanced practice nursing are found in Box 2-1. In spite of differences in terminology, the efforts of the profession to deal with a definition of advanced practice nursing are evident in the documents reviewed here. Reflection on and discussion of the various terms used, and debate about interpreting terms such as *roles, domains,* and *competencies,* may contribute to the clarification of conceptual models and the emergence of a common language. The descriptions of each model in the following sections are necessarily limited. The reader is encouraged to refer to the original documents and organizations' websites to understand advanced practice nursing as described by organizations and individual authors more fully. Website addresses for national APN organizations are found in Chapter 21. The APRN Consensus Model, the result of collaboration of many organizations, is described first, because it will continue to guide and influence conceptualizations of advanced practice, at least with regard to regulation and credentialing, for the near future.

Consensus Model for Advanced Practice Registered Nurse Regulation

In 2004, an APN Consensus Conference was convened, based on a request from the American Association of Colleges of Nursing (AACN) and the National Organization of Nurse Practitioner Faculties (NONPF) to the Alliance for APRN Credentialing. The purpose was to develop a process for achieving consensus regarding the credentialing of APNs (APRN Consensus Model, 2008; Stanley, Werner, & Apple 2009) and the development of a regulatory model for advanced practice nursing. Independently, the APRN Advisory Committee for the National Council of State Boards of Nursing (NCSBN) was charged by the NCSBN board of directors with a similar task of creating a future model for APRN regulation and, in 2006,

disseminated a draft of the APRN Vision Paper (NCSBN, 2006), a document that generated debate and controversy. Within a year, these groups came together to form the APRN Joint Dialogue Group, with representation from numerous stakeholder groups, including AACN, NCSBN, and organizations representing APNs. The outcome was the APRN Consensus Model (2008).

The APRN Regulatory Model includes important definitions, the roles and titles to be used, and population foci. Furthermore, it defines specialties and describes how to make room for the emergence of new APRN roles and population foci within the regulatory framework. In addition, a timeline for adoption and strategies for implementation were proposed, and progress has been made in these areas (see Chapter 21 for further information; only the model is discussed here). Figure 2-1 depicts

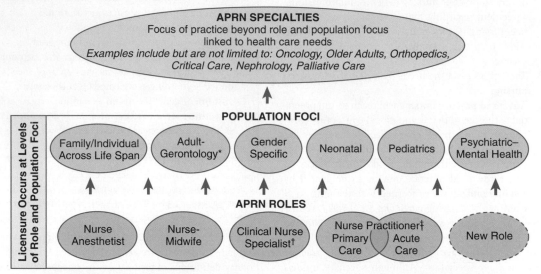

FIG 2-1 Consensus model for APRN regulation. This model was based on the work of the APRN Consensus Work Group and the NCSBN APRN Advisory Committee. *(From APRN Joint Dialogue Group. [2008]. Consensus Model for APRN Regulation. [http://www.aacn.nche.edu/education-resources/APRNReport.pdf]).*

*The population focus *Adult-Gerontology* encompasses the young adult to the older adult, including the frail elderly. APRNs educated and certified in the Adult-Gerontology population are educated and certified across both areas of practice and will be titled Adult-Gerontology CNP or CNS. In addition, all APRNs in any of the four roles providing care to the adult population (e.g. Family or Gender Specific) must be prepared to meet the growing needs of the older adult population. Therefore the education program should include didactic and clinical education experiences necessary to prepare APRNs with these enhanced skills and knowledge.

†The clinical nurse specialist (CNS) is educated and assessed through national certification processes across the continuum from wellness through acute care.

‡The certified nurse practitioner (CNP) is prepared with the acute care CNP competencies and/or the primary care CNP competencies. At this point in time the acute care and primary care CNP delineation applies only to the Pediatrics and Adult-Gerontology CNP population foci. Scope of practice of the primary care or acute care CNP **is not setting-specific** but is based on patient care needs. Programs may prepare individuals across both the primary care and acute care CNP roles. If programs prepare graduates across both roles, the graduate must be prepared with the consensus-based competencies for both roles and must successfully obtain certification in both the acute and the primary care CNP roles.

the components of the APRN Consensus Model, the four recognized APN roles and six population foci. The term *advanced practice registered nurse* (APRN) refers to all four APN roles. An APRN is defined as a nurse who meets the following criteria (APRN Consensus Model, 2008):

- Completes an accredited graduate-level education program preparing him or her for one of the four recognized APRN roles and a population focus (see discussion in Chapter 3)
- Passes a national certification examination that measures APRN role and population-focused competencies and maintains continued competence by national recertification in the role and population focus
- Possesses advanced clinical knowledge and skills preparing him or her to provide direct care to patients; the defining factor for *all* APRNs is that a significant component of the education and practice focuses on direct care of individuals
- Builds on the competencies of RNs by demonstrating greater depth and breadth of knowledge and greater synthesis of data by performing more complex skills and interventions and by possessing greater role autonomy
- Is educationally prepared to assume responsibility and accountability for health promotion and/or maintenance, as well as the assessment, diagnosis, and management of patient problems, including the use and prescription of pharmacologic and nonpharmacologic interventions
- Has sufficient depth and breadth of clinical experience to reflect the intended license
- Obtains a license to practice as an APRN in one of the four APRN roles

The definition of the components of the APRN Consensus Model begins to address some of the questions about advanced practice posed earlier in this chapter. An important agreement was that providing direct care to individuals is a defining characteristic of all APRN roles. This agreement affirms a position long held by editors of this text—that when there is no direct practice component, one is not practicing as an APN. It also has important implications for LACE and for career development of APNs.

Graduate education for the four APRN roles was described in the consensus document. It must include completion of at least three separate, comprehensive graduate courses in advanced physiology and pathophysiology, health assessment, and advanced pharmacology, consistent with requirements for the accreditation of APN education programs. In addition, curricula must address three other areas—the principles of decision making for the particular APN role, preparation in the core competencies

identified for the role, and role preparation in one of the six population foci.

The Consensus Model asserts that licensure must be based on educational preparation for one of the four existing APN roles and a population focus; certification must be within the same area of study; and that the four separate processes of LACE are necessary for the adequate regulation of APRNs (APRN Consensus Model, 2008; see Chapter 21). The six population foci displayed in Figure 2-1 include the individual and family across the life span, including adult, gerontologic, neonatal, pediatric, women's health/gender-specific, and psychiatric and mental health populations. Preparation in a specialty, such as oncology or critical care, cannot be the basis for licensure. Specialization "indicates that an APRN has additional knowledge and expertise in a more discrete area of specialty practice. Competency in the specialty area could be acquired either by educational preparation or experience and assessed in a variety of ways through professional credentialing mechanisms (e.g., portfolios, examinations)" (APRN Consensus Model, 2008, p. 12). This was a critical decision for the group to reach, given the numbers of specialties and APN specialty examinations in place when the document was prepared.

With this brief overview of the APRN Consensus Model, one can ask how this model has advanced the conceptualization of advanced practice nursing. It is helpful for many reasons. First, for the United States, it affirms that there are four APN roles. Second, it is advancing a uniform approach to LACE and advanced practice nursing that will have many practical and policymaking effects, including better alignment between and among APN curricula and certification examinations. Although not comprehensively described, it begins to address the issue of differentiating between RNs and APNs and will be foundational to future efforts to differentiate among nursing roles. By addressing the issue of specialization, the model offers a reasoned approach for the following: (1) avoiding confusion that would arise from a proliferation of specialty certification examinations; (2) ensuring that because of a limited and parsimonious focus (four roles and six populations), there will be sufficient numbers of APNs for the relevant examinations to ensure psychometrically valid data on test results; and (3) allowing for the development of new APN roles or foci to meet society's needs.

What are the limits of this conceptualization of advanced practice nursing? First, competencies that are common across APN roles are not addressed beyond defining an APRN and indicating that students must be prepared "with the core competencies for one of the four APRN roles across at least one of the six population foci" (APRN Consensus Model, 2008). However, as the Hamric Model suggests (see Chapter 3), there are core competencies that all APNs should possess. In addressing specialization, the model also leaves open the issue of the importance of educational preparation, in addition to experience, for advanced practice in a specialty. Experience in an area is certainly a factor that leads to the emergence of new specialties, but will experience alone be sufficient for the APN who specializes in oncology or critical care (or another specialty) to achieve desired outcomes in timely and cost-effective ways? These are specialties in which the population's needs are many and complex and the scope of research knowledge is similarly broad and deep. These are important conceptualization questions that are probably best addressed by the ANA and specialty professional nursing organizations, rather than by a group with a regulatory focus.

Numerous efforts are underway to implement this model in the United States; NCSBN has an extensive toolkit to help educators, APNs, consumers, and policymakers implement the new APRN regulatory model (NCSBN, 2012; https://www.ncsbn.org/2276.htm). The work undertaken to produce the APRN Consensus Model (2008) illustrates the power of interorganizational collaboration and is a promising example of how a model can, as Fawcett (2005) has suggested, reduce conflicts and facilitate communication within the profession, across professions, and with the public.

American Nurses Association

As the "only full-service professional organization representing the interests of the nation's 3.1 million registered nurses through its constituent and state nurses associations and its organizational affiliates," the American Nurses Association (ANA) and its constituent organizations have also been active in developing and promulgating documents that address advanced practice nursing. Two of these are particularly important as we consider contemporary conceptualizations of advanced practice nursing. Since 1980, ANA has periodically updated its Social Policy Statement (ANA, 2010a). Specialization, expansion, and advancement have consistently been identified as concepts that can differentiate advanced practice nursing from basic nursing practice. The most recent edition notes that specialization ("focusing on a part of the whole field of professional nursing") can occur at basic or advanced levels and that APNs use expanded and specialized knowledge and skills in their practices. According to the 2010 statement, expansion, specialization, and advanced practice were defined as follows (ANA, 2010a):

> *Expansion* refers to the acquisition of new practice knowledge and skills, including the knowledge and skills that

authorize role autonomy within areas of practice that may overlap traditional boundaries of medical practice.

> *Specialization* is concentrating or delimiting one's focus to part of the whole field of nursing such as ambulatory care, pediatric, maternal-child, psychiatric, palliative care, or oncology nursing.

> *Advanced practice* is characterized by the integration of a broad range of theoretical, research-based, and practical knowledge that occurs as part of graduate education. Advanced practice registered nurses hold master's or doctoral degrees and are licensed, certified, and/or approved to practice in their expanded roles (p. 9).

ANA's definitions of specialization and advanced practice are consistent with the APRN Consensus Model.

ANA also establishes and promulgates standards of practice and competencies for RNs and APNs. In the second edition of their text, *Nursing: Scope and Standards of Practice* (ANA, 2010b), six standards of practice and 16 standards of professional performance are described. Of the 22 standards, one standard outlines additional expectations for APNs compared with RNs; Standard 5, "Implementation," addresses the consultation and prescribing responsibilities of APRNs. Each standard is associated with competencies. It is in the description of the competencies that RN practice is differentiated from APNs and nurses prepared in a specialty at the graduate level. This document is must reading for APN students, practitioners, and others wishing to understand how basic, advanced, and specialized practice differ.

In addition to these documents, ANA, together with the American Board of Nursing Specialties (ABNS), convened a task force on CNS competencies. For many reasons, including the recognition that developing psychometrically sound certifications for numerous specialties, especially for clinical nurse specialists (CNSs), would be difficult as the profession moved toward implementing the APRN Consensus Model, the ANA and ABNS convened a group of stakeholders in 2006 to develop and validate a set of core competencies that would be expected of CNSs entering practice (National Association of Clinical Nurse Specialists [NACNS]/National CNS Core Competency Task Force, 2010). This group was charged with identifying core, entry-level competencies that are common in CNS practice, regardless of specialty. This work is discussed later in this chapter in the section on NACNS.

ANA continues to make numerous contributions to promoting clarity about all nursing roles, including advanced practice nursing. Its definitions of expansion, specialization, and advanced practice have remained consistent over time. ANA's *Nursing: Scope and Standards of*

BOX 2-2   **Essentials of Doctoral Education for Advanced Nursing Practice**

I.   Scientific underpinnings for practice
II.   Organizational and systems leadership for quality improvement and systems thinking
III. Clinical scholarship and analytical methods for evidence-based practice
IV.   Information systems and technology and patient care technology for the improvement and transformation of health care
V.   Health care policy for advocacy in health care
VI.   Interprofessional collaboration for improving patient and population health outcomes
VII. Clinical prevention and population health for improving the nation's health
VIII. Advanced nursing practice

From American Association of Colleges of Nursing (AACN) (2006). The essentials of doctoral education for advanced nursing practice (http://www.aacn.nche.edu/publications/position/DNPEssentials.pdf).

Practice (2010), should inform theoretical and empirical work that aims to differentiate nursing roles.

American Association of Colleges of Nursing

Over the last decade, the AACN has undertaken two nursing education initiatives aimed at transforming nursing education. In 2006, AACN called for all APN preparation to take place at the doctoral level in practice-based programs (DNP), with master's level education being refocused on generalist preparation for roles such as clinical nurse leaders (CNLs) and staff and clinical educators. CNLs are not APNs (AACN, 2005, 2012a; Spross, Hamric, Hall, et al., 2004) and, therefore, are not included in this discussion of conceptualizations. Through these initiatives, and to the extent that the AACN and Commission on Collegiate Nursing Education (CCNE) influence accreditation, the DNP may become the preferred degree for most APNs, although this goal is controversial. Since the last edition, despite lingering disagreements, DNP education has advanced considerably. In 2006, there were 20 DNP programs; in 2011, there were 182. Similarly, enrollments in and graduation from DNP programs have also risen substantially (AACN, 2012).

The *DNP Essentials* (AACN, 2006) are comprised of eight competencies for DNP graduates (Box 2-2). Graduates are expected to demonstrate the eight essentials on graduation. For APNs, "Essential VIII specifies the foundational practice competencies that cut across specialties and are seen as requisite for DNP practice" (AACN, 2006, p. 16; Box 2-3). Recognizing that DNP programs will prepare nurses for roles other than APN roles, the AACN

BOX 2-3   **Essential VIII: Advanced Nursing Practice Competencies**

I.   Conduct a comprehensive and systematic assessment of health and illness parameters in complex situations, incorporating diverse and culturally sensitive approaches.
II.   Design, implement, and evaluate therapeutic interventions based on nursing science and other sciences.
III. Develop and sustain therapeutic relationships and partnerships with patients (individual, family, or group) and other professionals to facilitate optimal care and patient outcomes.
IV.   Demonstrate advanced levels of clinical judgment, systems thinking, and accountability in designing, delivering, and evaluating evidence-based care to improve patient outcomes.
V.   Guide, mentor, and support other nurses to achieve excellence in nursing practice.
VI.   Educate and guide individuals and groups through complex health and situational transitions.
VII. Use conceptual and analytical skills in evaluating the links among practice, organizational, population, fiscal, and policy issues.

From American Association of Colleges of Nursing (AACN). (2006). The essentials of doctoral education for advanced nursing practice (http://www.aacn.nche.edu/publications/position/DNPEssentials.pdf).

---

acknowledged that organizations representing APNs are expected to develop Essential VIII as it relates to specific advanced practice roles and "to develop competency expectations that build upon and complement DNP Essentials 1 through 8" (AACN, 2006, p. 17). These Essentials affirmed that the advanced practice nursing core includes the three Ps (three separate courses)—advanced health and physical assessment, advanced physiology and pathophysiology, and advanced pharmacology—and is specific to APNs. The specialty core must include content and clinical practice experiences that help students acquire the knowledge and skills essential to a specific advanced practice role. These requirements were reconfirmed in the Consensus Model (2008).

The DNP has been described as a "disruptive innovation" (Hathaway, Jacob, Stegbauer, et al., 2006) and a natural evolution for NP practice. Although the DNP remains controversial (Avery & Howe, 2007; American College of Nurse-Midwives [ACNM], 2012b; Dreher & Smith Glasgow, 2011; Irvin-Lazorko, 2011; NACNS, 2009a), the proposal to make the DNP required for entry into advanced practice nursing is one of several national initiatives that have contributed to a broader discussion and may lead the profession to a clearer definition of advanced practice nursing. One outcome of the national DNP discussion is that APN organizations have promulgated practice competencies for doctorally prepared APNs (e.g., ACNM, 2011c; NACNS, 2009b) or have proposed a practice doctorate, even though it may not be the DNP (AANA, 2007). The National Organization of Nurse Practitioner Faculties (2012) now has one set of core competencies for NPs. Organizational positions on doctoral education are briefly explored in the discussion of APN organizations (see later). Readers can consult Chapters 14 through 18 and are urged to visit stakeholder organizations' websites for the history and up to date information on organizational responses to AACN's DNP position paper (AACN, 2004) and the *DNP Essentials* (AACN, 2006).

Although not a conceptual model per se, the AACN's publication, *DNP Essentials* (2006) addresses concepts and content that are now evident in many other documents that address standards of APN practice and education. The fact that Essential VIII affirms a set of common competencies across APN roles is an important contribution to conceptual clarity about advanced practice in the United States. Because these Essentials, with the exception of Essential VIII, are intended to address DNP preparation for any nursing role, its contribution to conceptual clarity regarding advanced practice nursing specifically is limited. Eventually, the evolution of the DNP may lead to more conceptual clarity about advanced practice nursing and the role of APNs. However, it is possible that the rapid expansion of this degree may contribute to less clarity in the short term about the nature of advanced nursing practice and the centrality of direct care of patients to APN work, particularly because the DNP will prepare people for other, nonclinical nursing roles. In the next section, in addition to discussing the organizations' conceptualizations of APN practice, the extent to which their responses to the DNP proposal might influence conceptual clarity on advanced nursing practice is addressed.

National Organization of Nurse Practitioner Faculties

The mission of the NONPF is to provide leadership in promoting quality NP education. Since 1990, NONPF has fulfilled this mission in many ways, including the development, validation, and promulgation of NP competencies. As of 2012, there is only one set of NP core competencies in use (NONPF, 2012); the 2002 and 2006 competencies are available on the website but are no longer active. A brief history of the development of competencies for NPs

is presented, in part because their development has influenced other APN models.

In 1990, NONPF published a set of domains and core competencies for primary care NPs based on Benner's (1984) domains of expert nursing practice and the results of Brykczynski's (1989) study of the use of these domains by primary care NPs (Price et al., 1992; Zimmer et al., 1990). Within each domain were a number of specific competencies. Until the 2011 competencies were published, these validated domains and core competencies served as a framework for primary care NP education and practice.

After endorsing the DNP as entry level preparation for the NP role, and consistent with the recommendations in the APRN Consensus Model (2008), new NP core competencies were developed in 2011 and amended in 2012 (http://www.nonpf.com/displaycommon.cfm?an=1& subarticlenbr=14). Each of the nine core competencies is accompanied by specific behaviors that all graduates of NP programs, whether master's or DNP-prepared, are expected to demonstrate. The document includes a glossary of key terms. Population-specific competencies for specific NP roles, together with the nine core competencies, are intended to inform curricula and ensure that graduates will meet certification and regulatory requirements.

From a conceptual perspective, these NP core and population-specific competency documents are notable for several reasons: (1) the competencies for NPs were developed collaboratively by stakeholder organizations; (2) empirical validation is used to affirm the competencies; (3) overall, the competencies are conceptually consistent with statements in the APRN Consensus Model, the *DNP Essentials* (2006), and ANA's *Nursing: Scope and Standards* (2010); and (4) the revised competencies are responsive to society's needs for advanced nursing care and the contextual factors that will shape NP practice for at least the next decade. In the amended 2011 NONPF competencies (2011, 2012), one also sees an appropriate emphasis on practice that is not in the APRN Consensus Model (2008)—patient-centered care, interprofessional care, and independent or autonomous NP practice, clearly responsive to health care reform initiatives, are addressed.

National Association of Clinical Nurse Specialists

The NACNS published the *Statement on Clinical Nurse Specialist Practice and Education* in 1998 and revised it in 2004. Although acknowledging the early conceptualization of CNS practice as subroles proposed by Hamric and Spross (1983, 1989), the authors of the NACNS statement believed that this conceptualization, although delineating competencies, failed to differentiate CNS practice from

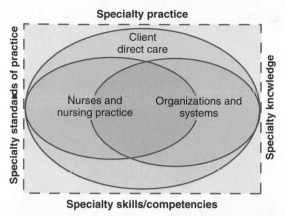

FIG 2-2 National Association of Clinical Nurse Specialists model. CNS practice conceptualized as core competencies in three interacting spheres is shown, as actualized in specialty practice and guided by specialty knowledge and standards. *(From National Association of Clinical Nurse Specialists. [2004]. Statement on clinical nurse specialist practice and education. Harrisburg, PA: Author.) N.B. This model predates the Consensus Model of APRN Regulation and the definitions of specialization and population foci in the Consensus Model.*

that of other APNs and proposed their statement to resolve the ambiguity about this particular APN role. Three spheres of influence are posited: patient, nurses and nursing practice, and organization or system, each of which requires a unique set of competencies (NACNS, 2004; Fig. 2-2). In addition, the statement outlined expected outcomes of CNS practice for each sphere and competencies that parallel those of the nursing process. Thus, CNSs have sphere-specific competencies of assessment, diagnosis, intervention, and evaluation.

As work on the APRN Consensus Model neared completion, NACNS and the APRN Consensus Work Group asked the ANA and the ABNS to "convene and facilitate the work of a National CNS Competency Task Force..." using a standard process to develop nationally recognized education standards and competencies (NACNS/National Core Competency Task Force, 2010). The process of developing and validating the competencies is described in the document. Figure 2-3 illustrates the model of CNS competencies that emerged from this work, a synthesis of NACNS' spheres of influence, Hamric's seven APN competencies, and the Synergy Model. Subsequently, new criteria for evaluating CNS education programs were developed, based on the competencies (Validation Panel of the NACNS, 2011). It is important to note that the APRN Consensus Model, as discussed in Chapter 3, has had more impact on certification for CNS roles than for other APN roles.

The 2004 statement and the new CNS competencies are not entirely parallel. Some aspects of the 2004 statement were more comprehensive with regard to theoretical elements, such as the inclusion of assumptions and theoretical roots in nursing. The 2010 document has an appendix that includes definitions of key concepts such as nurses and nursing practice, spheres of influence, and competencies. An underlying assumption of the 2008 competencies, which has empirical validation (e.g., Lewandowski & Adamle, 2009; see Chapter 23), is that CNSs have an impact on patients, nursing practice, and institutional outcomes. From a conceptual standpoint, the CNS competencies document brought needed clarity on several fronts: (1) ensuring that all CNSs would be eligible for credentialing under the APRN Consensus Model so that CNSs could take a psychometrically valid examination on their core competencies, because these examinations could not be developed for every existing area of specialization; (2) advanced the work of NACNS in ensuring consistency among programs preparing CNSs; and (3) because CNSs' work often looks very different from that of other APNs (e.g., fewer responsibilities for prescribing but more responsibilities for clinical and systems leadership) facilitated the profession's ability to speak about what is common across APN roles. At least two areas will need further clarification. One is the relationship between the 2004 statement and the 2010 competencies, because both documents are available and CNS authors still refer to the 2004 statement. Both are being used, which is understandable; there is content in the statement that is not in the new competencies document, including, in addition to the 2004 competencies, relevant history, a description of CNS practice, and recommendations for graduate programs. The second area will be the ongoing need for clarity regarding specialty as defined in the Consensus Model (the population focus, not specialization, is the basis for regulation). From a regulatory standpoint, it would seem that a CNS's specialty is his or her population focus as defined in the Consensus Model.

In 2005, NACNS published a white paper on the DNP in which a number of concerns were raised and the leaders called for extensive dialogue with stakeholders. NACNS reaffirmed the position taken in 2005, which is "a position of neutrality [in which] the board neither endorses oropposes the DNP degree as an option for [CNS] education" (NACNS, 2009a). Recognizing that some CNSs would pursue advanced clinical doctorates, core competencies for doctoral level practice were published by NACNS; these are to be used in conjunction with the 2010 CNS competency document and the *DNP essentials* "to inform education programs and employer expectations" (NACNS' CNS Practice Doctorate Competencies Taskforce, 2009b).

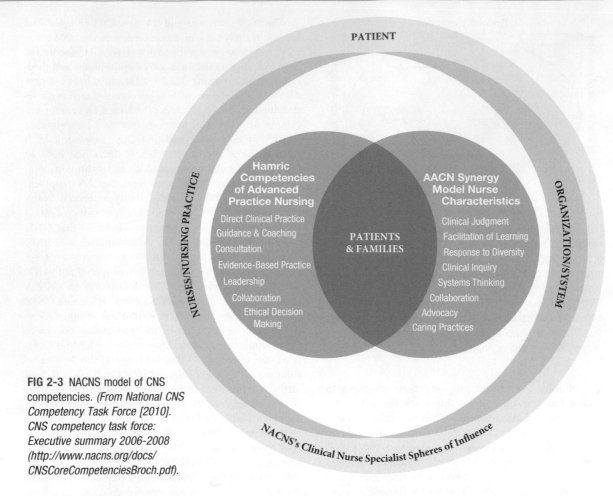

PATIENT

NURSES/NURSING PRACTICE

ORGANIZATION/SYSTEM

Hamric Competencies of Advanced Practice Nursing

Direct Clinical Practice

Guidance & Coaching

Consultation

Evidence-Based Practice

Leadership

Collaboration

Ethical Decision Making

PATIENTS & FAMILIES

AACN Synergy Model Nurse Characteristics

Clinical Judgment

Facilitation of Learning

Response to Diversity

Clinical Inquiry

Systems Thinking

Collaboration

Advocacy

Caring Practices

NACNS's Clinical Nurse Specialist Spheres of Influence

FIG 2-3 NACNS model of CNS competencies. *(From National CNS Competency Task Force [2010]. CNS competency task force: Executive summary 2006-2008 (http://www.nacns.org/docs/ CNSCoreCompetenciesBroch.pdf).*

In 2012, NACNS published a *Statement on the APRN Consensus Model Implementation*, outlining a number of concerns and recommendations, in particular the importance of grandfathering currently practicing CNSs and monitoring implementation of the Consensus Model to ensure that adoption of the model does not negatively affect the ability of CNSs to practice. Although the details of the statement are beyond the scope of this chapter, the fact that there are concerns may have implications for a professional consensus on conceptualization of advanced practice nursing. For further information, see the NACNS website and Chapters 14 and 21.

American Association of Nurse Anesthetists and American College of Nurse-Midwives

Certified registered nurse anesthetists (CRNAs) and certified nurse-midwives (CNMs) have been recognized as APNs and are recognized as such in the APRN Consensus Model. Advanced practice competencies, as described in the *DNP Essentials*, ANA Scope and Standards, and APN

competencies identified in this text, are evident in the official statements of the AANA (2010a, b) and the ACNM (2008, 2011a, b). These statements include scopes of practice, standards for practice, and ethics. See Chapters 17 and 18 for a thorough discussion of CNM and CRNA practice, respectively.

American Association of Nurse Anesthetists

The CRNA's scope of practice was defined in the most recent revision of the AANA's *Scope and Standards for Nurse Anesthesia Practice* (2010a). The scope is followed by 10 items that can be characterized as clinical competencies or responsibilities (e.g., managing a patient's airway)—the direct clinical practice of CRNAs. CRNAs have seven additional responsibilities that are within the CRNA's scope of practice that can be characterized as leadership behaviors, including participation in research. Eleven standards and an interpretation for each are also listed. The purposes of the standards are as follows: (1) assist the profession in evaluating CRNA care; (2) provide a common foundation on which CRNAs can develop a quality practice; (3) help the public understand what they can expect from CRNAs; and (4) support and preserve the basic rights of patients.

Initially, the AANA did not support the DNP for entry into CRNA practice and established a task force to evaluate doctoral preparation further. Subsequently, AANA issued a position statement (2007) requiring doctoral preparation for nurse anesthesia practice by the year 2025. The position statement did not specify the type of doctoral degree. This likely reflects the diversity of existing practice doctorates for nurse anesthesia practice in addition to the DNP, such as Doctor of Nurse Anesthesia Practice (DNAP) and Doctor of Management of Practice in Nurse Anesthesia (DMPNA) (Dreher & Smith Glasgow, 2011; Hawkins & Nezat, 2009). The Council of Accreditation (COA) of Nurse Anesthesia Educational Programs revised their 2004 accreditation standards for nurse anesthesia education (2012a). Notably, the standards include a requirement for the "three P" courses, consistent with requirements specified in the APRN Consensus document. The standards also distinguish between competencies expected for graduates of practice doctorate (referencing both DNP and DNAP as examples) and research-oriented doctorate programs. In addition, the first draft of accreditation standards have been developed for the practice doctorate in nurse anesthesia (COA, 2012b), which are expected to be effective in 2015 (personal communication, Barbara Farkas, MAdEd, COA, July 5, 2012). Both the revised 2012 standards and the draft practice doctorate standards have competencies that align with those in the DNP Essentials. Although these are not cited in either document, throughout there is consistent reference to "commonly accepted national standards," a phrase defined in the glossary.

American College of Nurse-Midwives

The scope of practice for CNMs (and certified midwives [CMs] who are not nurses) has been defined in four ACNM documents: "Definition of midwifery and scope of practice of CNMs and CMs" (ACNM, 2011a), the "Core competencies for basic midwifery practice" (ACNM, 2012a), "Standards for the practice of midwifery" (ACNM, 2011), and a "Code of ethics" (ACNM, 2008). The core competencies are organized into sixteen hallmarks that describe the art and science of midwifery and the components of midwifery care. The components of midwifery care include professional responsibilities, midwifery management processes, fundamentals, primary health care of women, and the childbearing family, within which are prescribed competencies. According to the definition, "CNMs are educated in two disciplines: nursing and midwifery" (ACNM, 2011a). Competencies "describe the fundamental knowledge, skills and behaviors of a new practitioner" (ACNM, 2012a). The hallmarks, components, and associated core competencies are the foundation on which midwifery curricula and practice guidelines are based.

In addition to the competencies, there are eight ACNM standards that midwives are expected to meet (ACNM, 2011b) and a code of ethics (ACNM, 2008). The standards address issues such as qualifications, safety, patient rights, assessment, documentation, and expansion of midwifery practice. Three ethical mandates related to its mission to promote the health and well-being of women and newborns in their families and communities are identified in the ethics code.

As of 2010, CNMs entering practice must earn a graduate degree, complete an accredited midwifery program, and pass a national certification examination (see Chapter 17 for detailed requirements; ACNM, 2011a), the type of graduate degree is not specified. ACNM does recognize the value of doctoral education as a valid and valuable path for CNMs, evidenced by a statement on a practice doctorate in midwifery, including competencies (2011c). Although not cited, these competencies are in alignment with those in the DNP Essentials; ACNM recognizes that there are other paths for a practice doctorate in midwifery. ACNM does not support the DNP as a requirement for entry into nurse-midwifery practice because of the following: (1) midwifery practice is safe, based on the rigor of their curriculum standards and outcome data; (2) evidence is insufficient to justify the DNP as a mandatory requirement for CNM; and (3) the costs of attaining such a degree could limit the applicant pool and access to midwifery care (ACNM, 2012b, 2012c). Midwifery organizations have recently addressed the aspects of the 2008 Consensus Model that they support and identified those that are of concern (ACNM et al., 2011d).

International Organizations and Conceptualizations of Advanced Practice Nursing

International perspectives on advanced practice nursing are covered in Chapter 6. In this section, I highlight issues with regard to a common language and conceptual frameworks for advanced practice nursing.

In 2009, the ICN defined the NP-APN "as a registered nurse who has acquired the expert knowledge base, complex decision-making skills and clinical competencies for expanded practice, the characteristics of which are shaped by the context and/or country in which s/he is credentialed to practice." A master's degree is recommended for entry level (ICN, 2009). Based on the definition, key concepts include educational preparation, the nature of practice, and regulatory mechanisms. The statement is necessarily broad, given the variations in health systems, regulatory mechanisms, and nursing education programs in individual countries.

In 2008, the CNA published *Advanced Nursing Practice: A National Framework,* which defined advanced nursing practice, described educational preparation and regulation, identified the two APN roles (NP and CNS), and specified competencies in clinical practice, research, and leadership. In addition, they have issued position statements on advanced nursing practice (CNA, 2007), which affirm the key points in the national framework document and defined and described the roles and contributions to health care of nurse practitioners (2009a) and clinical nurse specialists (2009b). Furthermore, leaders have undertaken an evidence-based, patient-centered, coordinated effort (called a decision support synthesis) to develop, implement, and evaluate the APN roles of the CNS and NP in Canada (DiCenso, Martin-Meisener, Bryant-Lukosius, et al., 2010), a process different from the one used to advance APN roles in the United States. This process included a review of 468 published and unpublished articles and interviews conducted with 62 key informants and four focus groups that included a variety of stakeholders. The purpose of this work was to "describe the distinguishing characteristics of CNSs and NPs relevant to Canadian contexts," identify barriers and facilitators to effective development and use of APN roles, and inform the development of evidence-based recommendations that individuals, organizations, and systems can use to improve the integration of APNs into Canadian health care.

Section Summary: Implications for Advanced Practice Nursing Conceptualizations

From this overview of organizational statements that clarify and advance APN practice, it is clear that nationally and internationally, stakeholders are engaged in a more active dialogue about advanced practice nursing and progress has been made in this area since the last edition. Progress includes global agreement that there is a type of clinical nursing practice that is advanced and builds on basic nursing education, requiring additional education and characterized by additional competencies and responsibilities. In the United States, the consensus on an approach to APRN regulation was critical for the following reasons: (1) clarifying what is an APN and the role of graduate education and certification in licensing APRNs; (2) ensuring that APNs are fully recognized and integrated in the delivery of health care; (3) reducing barriers to mobility of APNs across state lines; (4) fostering and facilitating ongoing dialogue among APN stakeholders; and (5) offering common language regarding regulation.

Although there may not be agreement on the DNP as the requirement for entry into advanced practice nursing,

the promulgation of the document fostered dialogue nationally and within APN organizations on the clinical doctorate (whether or not it is the DNP) as a valid and likely path for APNs to pursue. As a result, each APN organization has taken a stand on the role of the clinical doctorate for those in the role and has developed or is developing doctoral level clinical competencies. In doing so, it appears that the needs of their patients, members, other constituencies, and contexts have been considered. Until the time when a clinical doctorate becomes a requirement for entry into practice for all APN roles, the development of doctoral level competencies for APN roles will help stakeholders distinguish between master's- and doctorate-prepared APNs with regard to competencies.

MacDonald, Herbert, & Thibeault (2006) have suggested that a common identity for advanced practice nurses is worth pursuing. It will most likely be through regulatory mechanisms that a consistent definition of advanced practice nursing and authority to practice, in particular APN roles, will be established in the United States. However, it will be important to heed the caution of NACNS to ensure that the APRN Consensus Model is not implemented selectively (NACNS, 2012). Although important differences exist between roles and across countries, a common identity for APNs will most likely result from policy and regulatory initiatives and should facilitate communication within and outside the profession, consistent with assertions by Styles (1998) and Fawcett (2005) on the purposes of models. There are important differences among APN organizations regarding such issues as doctoral preparation, which is also consistent with Fawcett's assertion that there is not one best model.

The level of consensus regarding regulation in the United States reflects considerable and laudable progress, paving the way for policies and health care system transformations that will enable APNs to be used fully to ensure access to health care and improve its quality. The processes that have led to this juncture in the United States have required openness, civility, a willingness to disagree, and wisdom. Finally, there are at least two different approaches (collaborative policymaking in the United States and an evidence-based approach in Canada) to determine how best to assess contributions of APNs and develop ways to integrate them into health care infrastructures and to maximize benefits to patients and populations. The global APN community can examine these processes for insights on how to adapt them to suit their particular context.

In conclusion, the organizational models described enable the reader to understand who engages in advanced practice nursing and the nature of the respective APN practices. These models primarily address professional roles, licensing, accreditation, certification, education,

TABLE 2-1 Comparison of AANA, ACNM, NACNS, and NONPF Statements on Primary Criteria and APN Competencies*

	PRIMARY CRITERIA			COMPETENCIES						
Organization	Graduate Education	Certification (if available)	Practice Focused on Patient and Family	Direct Care	Guidance and Coaching	Collaboration	Consultation	Evidence-based Practice	Leadership	Ethical Decision Making
AANA	Y	Y	Y	Y	Y	Y	Y	Y	Y	Y
ACNM	Y	Y	Y	Y	Y	Y	Y	Y	Y	Y
NACNS	Y	Qualified yes[†]	Y	Y	Y	Y	Y	Y	Y	Y
NONPF	Y	Y	Y	Y	Y	Y	Y	Y	Y	Y

*Each organization's current primary statements on advanced practice competencies were used to complete the grid as follows: AANA (2010a); ACNM (2008); NACNS (2004, 2010); NONPF (2011, 2012).

[†]Several CNS examinations, including the ANCC examination for CNS core competencies have been retired. NACNS (NACNS.org, accessed 10/30/12) notes under current initiatives that they are working with ANCC on CNS certification examinations. Readers are encouraged to visit the ANCC website for the latest information on available CNS certifications (e.g., adult, gerontology) http://www.nursecredentialing.org/certification.aspx#specialty. See also discussion in Chapter 3.

competencies, and clinical practice, some of the purposes of models identified earlier. The descriptive statements about APN roles and competencies demonstrate that common elements exist across all APN roles. These include a central focus on and accountability for patient care, knowledge and skills specific to each APN role, and a concern for patient rights. Using Hamric's Model of primary criteria and the seven competencies, Table 2-1 was constructed based on the content of official statements of the AANA, ACNM, NACNS, and NONPF to illustrate commonalities across the four roles. The published definitions, standards, and competencies offer models against which differences among APN roles and practices can be distinguished, educational programs can be developed and evaluated, knowledge and behaviors can be measured for certification purposes, practitioners can understand, examine, and improve their own practice, and job descriptions can be developed. As advanced practice nursing moves forward in the United States and globally, the profession will continue to have opportunities to define those situations in which a conceptual consensus will serve the public and the profession and those situations in which alternative conceptualizations are needed for the same reasons—serving the public and our profession.

Conceptualizations of the Nature of Advanced Practice Nursing

The APN role-specific models promulgated by professional organizations naturally lead to the following questions:

- What is common across APN roles?
- Can an overarching conceptualization of advanced practice nursing be articulated?
- How can one distinguish among basic, expert, and advanced levels of nursing practice?

Some authors have attempted to discern the nature of advanced practice nursing and address these questions. The extent to which they considered all existing APN roles is not always clear; some authors have considered only the CNS and NP roles.

In this section, the focus is on those frameworks that address the nature of advanced practice nursing. The term *role* is used loosely and variably, sometimes seeming to describe functions (e.g., management, teaching, research, consultation) and sometimes taking a psychological or sociologic perspective on developing social roles in relation to environment. Dictionary definitions add to the confusion by using the terms *role, function, occupation,* and *duties* to define one another. For example, *role* is generally used to refer to titles appearing in legal documents, certification programs, or job descriptions. From this perspective, the CNS, NP, CNM, and CRNA designations represent advanced practice roles. From the present review of a number of frameworks, domain and competency may be the most commonly used concepts in explaining nursing practice and advanced practice nursing. However, meanings are not consistent. Hamric's Model, which uses the terms roles and competencies, is the only one that is integrative—that is, it explicitly considers all four APN roles. Because it is integrative, has remained relatively stable since 1996, has informed the development of the *DNP Essentials* and CNS competencies, and is widely cited, it will be discussed first, enabling the reader to consider the extent to which important concepts are addressed by other models. Otherwise, the models are discussed in chronologic order. In most cases, new literature on the models discussed here were not found in literature searches in the *Cumulative Index to Nursing and Allied Health Literature* (CINAHL), which included using the "cited references" function.

Hamric's Integrative Model of Advanced Practice Nursing

One of the earliest efforts to synthesize a model of advanced practice that would apply to all APN roles was developed by Hamric (1996). Hamric, whose early conceptual work was done on the CNS role (Hamric & Spross, 1983, 1989), proposed an integrative understanding of the core of advanced practice nursing, based on literature from all APN specialties (Hamric, 1996, 2000, 2005, 2009; see Chapter 3). Hamric proposed a conceptual definition of advanced practice nursing and defining characteristics that included primary criteria (graduate education, certification in the specialty, and a focus on clinical practice with patients) and a set of core competencies (direct clinical practice, collaboration, guidance and coaching, evidence-based practice, ethical decision making, consultation, and leadership). This early model was further refined, together with Hanson and Spross in 2000 and 2005, based on dialogue among the editors. Key components of the model (Fig. 2-4) include the primary criteria for advanced nursing practice, seven advanced practice competencies with direct care as the core competency on which the other competencies depend, and environmental and contextual factors that must be managed for advanced practice nursing to flourish.

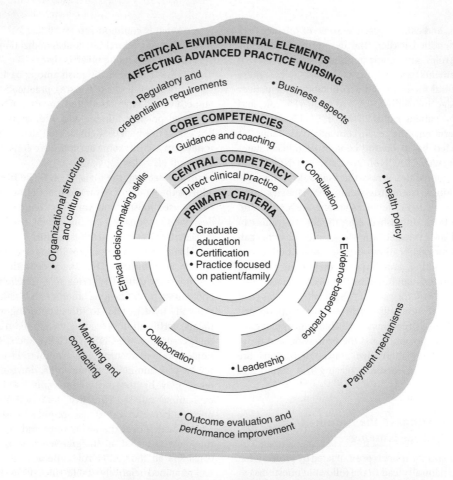

FIG 2-4 Hamric's model of advanced practice nursing.

The revisions to the Hamric Model since 1996 highlight the dynamic nature of a conceptual model; at the same time, the fact that essential features remain the same demonstrates the inherent stability and robustness of Hamric's Model, particularly when many potentially transformative advanced practice nursing initiatives are being developed. Models are refined over time according to changes in practice, research, and theoretical understanding. This model forms the understanding of advanced practice nursing used throughout this text and has provided the structure for each edition of the book. Using Hamric's Model, some contributors to this text have further elaborated on the specific competencies proposed (see Chapter 3) by describing and graphically depicting concepts relevant to the specific competency. These include guidance and coaching (Spross, 2009; see Chapter 8), consultation (see Chapter 9), and ethical decision making (see Chapter 13). In addition, as noted, it has informed the development of the *DNP Essentials* and the revised CNS competencies and is widely cited in the advanced practice literature, evidence of its contribution to conceptualizing advanced practice nursing.

Integrative reviews of the literature provide further support for Hamric's integrative conceptualization of advanced practice nursing. The purpose of the review by Mantzoukas and Watkinson (2007) was to identify "generic features" of advanced nursing practice. They identified seven generic features: (1) use of knowledge in practice; (2) critical thinking and analytic skills; (3) clinical judgment and decision making; (4) professional leadership and clinical inquiry; (5) coaching and mentoring; (6) research skills; and (7) changing practice. The first three generic features are consistent with the direct care competency in Hamric's Model; three of the seven characteristics seem directly related to clinical practice, which supports the notion that direct care is a central competency. The remaining four features are consistent with the three competencies of leadership, guidance and coaching, and evidence-based practice competency in Hamric's Model.

An integrative review of the literature on CNS practice (Lewandowski & Adamle, 2009) similarly affirmed direct care, collaboration, consultation, systems leadership, and coaching (patient and staff education) competencies in the Hamric Model. Ten countries were represented in their review, which included 753 anecdotal articles, 277 research articles, and 62 dissertations or theses. Their findings were organized using NACNS's three spheres of influence. Within the first sphere, management of complex or vulnerable populations, they found three essential characteristics—expert direct care, coordination of care, and collaboration. In the sphere of educating and supporting interdisciplinary staff, substantive areas of CNS practice were education, consultation, and collaboration. Within the system sphere of influence, CNSs facilitate

innovation and change. These findings lend support for the integration of the Hamric Model with the NACNS model in the CNS core competencies (2008).

Fenton's and Brykczynski's Expert Practice Domains of the Clinical Nurse Specialist and Nurse Practitioner

Fenton's and Brykczynski's studies of APNs were based on Benner's model of expert nursing practice (1984). To appreciate the contributions of Fenton (1985) and Brykczynski (1989) to the understanding of advanced practice, it is important to highlight some of Benner's key findings about nurses who are experts by experience. Although many have used Benner's seminal work (1984), *From Novice to Expert,* in their conceptualizations of advanced practice nursing, it is important to note that Benner has not studied advanced practice nurses. Fenton's and Brykczynski's studies represent an appropriate extension of Benner's findings and theories to advanced practice nursing. Benner and colleagues continue to study how nurses (not APNs) acquire clinical expertise; these findings are interesting and APNs are likely to find them useful. However, because APNs were not subjects, the later findings are not presented here (Benner, Tanner, & Chesla, 2009).

The early work of Benner and associates informed the development of the first NONPF competencies, graduate curricula in schools of nursing, models of practice (e.g., the Synergy Model, discussed later) and the standards for clinical promotion (APNs may be identified at senior levels in these schema by employers). Most importantly, as the authors noted, this early work "put into words what they had always known about their clinical nursing expertise but had difficulty articulating" (Benner, et al., 2009). It is perhaps this impact that has led to the sustained integration of Benner's studies of experts by experience into the APN literature, including descriptions and development of competencies.

Through the analysis of clinical exemplars discussed in interviews, Benner derived a range of competencies that resulted in the identification of seven domains of expert nursing practice. Within this lexicon, these domains are a combination of roles, functions, and competencies, although the three were not precisely differentiated. The seven domains are as follows (Benner, 1984): the helping role, administering and monitoring therapeutic interventions and regimens, effective management of rapidly changing situations, diagnostic and monitoring function, teaching and coaching function, monitoring and ensuring the quality of health care practices, and organizational and work role competencies.

Fenton (1985) and Brykczynski (1989) each independently applied Benner's Model of expert practice to APNs, examining the practice of CNSs and NPs, respectively. In a later publication, Fenton and Brykczynski (1993) compared their earlier research findings to identify similarities and differences between CNSs and NPs. Fenton and Brykczynski verified that nurses in advanced practice were indeed experts, as defined by Benner, but that they demonstrated that APNs possess something more than being experts by experience. They identified additional domains and competencies (Fig. 2-5). Across the top of this figure are the seven domains identified by Benner and the additional domain found in CNS practice (Fenton, 1985), that of consultation provided by CNSs to other nurses (*rectangular dotted box, top right*). Under this box, there are two new CNS competencies (*hexagonal boxes*). The third (rounded) box is a new NP competency identified by Brykczynski in 1989. In this study of NPs, Brykczynski also identified an eighth domain, the management of health and illness in ambulatory care settings. It would seem that rather than identify it as a ninth domain, Brykczynski recognized this as a qualitatively different expression of the first two domains identified by Benner; for NPs, the new competencies identified are a result of the integration of the diagnostic-monitoring and administering-monitoring domains. A close examination of Figure 2-5 also reveals the new competencies identified by Fenton and Brykczynski's work. In the hexagonal boxes, new CNS competencies are identified under the organization and work role domain (e.g., providing support for nursing staff) and the helping role, in addition to the consulting domain and competencies. Similarly, in the rectangles with rounded edges, one sees additional NP competencies under seven of the eight domains (e.g., detecting acute or chronic disease while attending to illness under the diagnostic-administering domains). Their findings further illuminate why Benner's work has influenced descriptions of advanced practice. By examining the extent to which APNs demonstrate the seven domains found in experts by experience and uncovering differences, the findings offer a possible explanation of the differences between expert and advanced practice. In addition, they also describe ways in which two advanced practice nursing roles, CNSs and NPs, may be different with regard to practice domains and competencies.

Even though these studies are older, the findings suggest that a deeper understanding of advanced practice could be beneficial to understanding ("giving words to") and conceptualizing. advanced nursing practice. Benner's methods could be applied to studies of advanced practice nursing, with the following aims: (1) to confirm Fenton and Brykczynski's findings in CNS and NP roles and identify new domains and competencies across all four APN roles; (2) to understand how APN competencies develop in direct entry graduate and RN graduate students; and (3) to

compare the non–master's-prepared clinician's competencies with the APN's competencies to distinguish components of expert versus advanced practice nursing further. Also, studies focused on how APNs acquire expertise in APN and interprofessional competencies could inform future conceptualizations of advanced practice nursing.

Calkin's Model of Advanced Nursing Practice

Calkin's model (1984) was the first to distinguish explicitly the practice of experts by experience from advanced practice nursing as practiced by CNSs and NPs. Calkin developed the model to help nurse administrators differentiate advanced practice nursing from other levels of clinical practice in personnel policies, and proposed that this could be accomplished by matching patient responses to health problems with the skill and knowledge levels of nursing personnel. In Calkin's model, three curves were overlaid on a normal distribution chart. Calkin depicted the skills and knowledge of novices, experts by experience, and APNs in relation to knowledge required to care for patients whose responses to health care problems (i.e., health care needs) ranged from simple and common to complex and complicated (Fig 2-6). A closer look at Figure 2-6, *A,* shows, as one would expect, that there are many more human responses (the highest and widest curve) than a beginning nurse would have the knowledge and skill to manage. The impact of experience is illustrated in Figure 2-6, *B.* The highest and widest curve is effectively the same, but because of experience, expert nurses have more knowledge and skill; the curves are higher and somewhat wider, but their additional skill and knowledge do not yet match the range of responses that they may encounter in the patients for whom they care. In Figure 2-6, *C,* APNs, by virtue of education and experience, have knowledge and skills that enable them to respond to a wider range of human problems. The three curves in Figure 2-6, *C,* parallel each other; this suggests that even as less common human responses arise in clinical practice, APNs have the knowledge and skill to respond creatively and effectively to these unusual problems.

Calkin used the framework to explain how APNs perform under different sets of circumstances—when there is a high degree of unpredictability, new conditions, new patient population, or new sets of problems, and a wide variety of health problems requiring the services of "specialist generalists." What APNs do in terms of functions were also defined. For example, when patients' health problems elicit a wide range of human responses with continuing and substantial unpredictable elements, the APN should do the following (Calkin, 1984):

- Identify and develop interventions for the unusual by providing direct care.

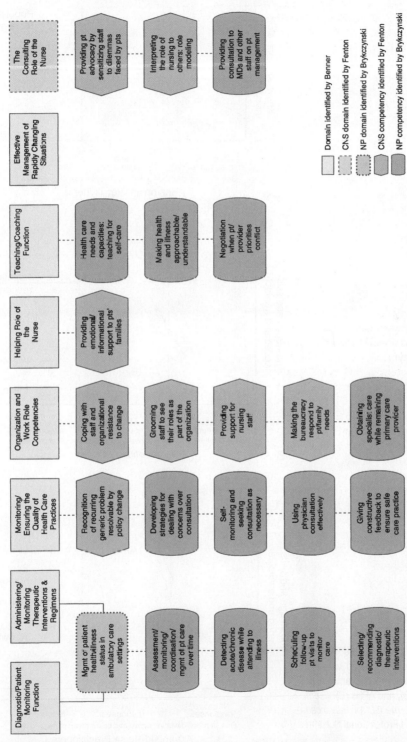

FIG 2-5 Fenton's and Brykczynski's expert practice domains of the CNS and NP. *(From Fenton, M.V., & Brykczynski, K.A. [1993]. Qualitative distinctions and similarities in the practice of clinical nurse specialists and nurse practitioners. Journal of Professional Nursing, 9, 313–326.)*

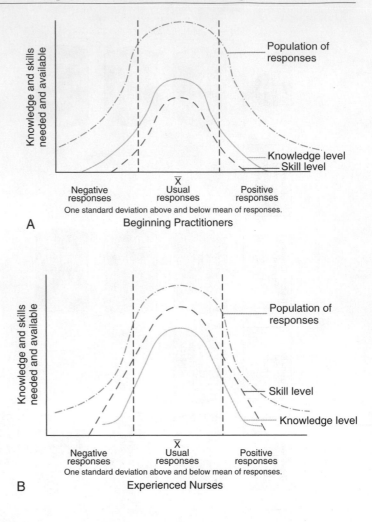

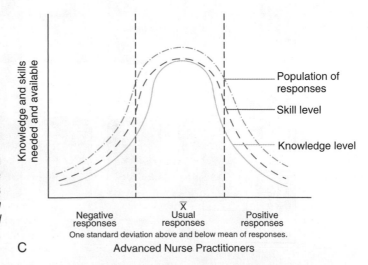

FIG 2-6 Calkin's model of advanced nursing practice. Patient responses correlated with the knowledge and skill of beginning practitioners **(A)**, experienced nurses **(B)**, and APNs **(C)**. *(From Calkin, J. D. [1984]. A model for advanced nursing practice.* Journal of Professional Nursing, *14, 24–30.)*

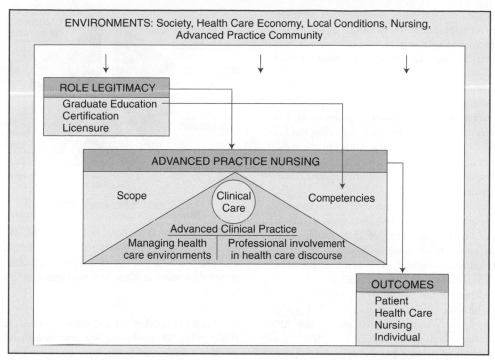

FIG 2-7 Brown's framework for advanced practice nursing. *(From Brown, S. J. [1998]. A framework for advanced practice nursing.* Journal of Professional Nursing, 14, *157–164.)*

- Transmit this knowledge to nurses and, in some settings, to students.
- Identify and communicate the need for research or carry out research related to human responses to these health problems.
- Anticipate factors that may lead to unfamiliar human responses.
- Provide anticipatory guidance to nurse administrators when the changes in the diagnosis and treatment of these responses may require altered levels or types of resources.

A principal advantage to Calkin's model is that the skills, education, and knowledge of the nurses needed are considered based on patient needs. It provides a framework for scholars to use in studying the function of APNs in a variety of work situations and should be a useful conceptualization for administrators who must maximize a multilevel interprofessional workforce and need to justify the use of APNs. In today's practice environments, this conceptualization could be modified and applied in other settings:

- Which situations require APNs or RNs?
- Which mix of professional staff and support staff is needed when settings have a high degree of predictability versus those routinely characterized by clinical uncertainty?

The model has been left for others to test; although Calkin's thinking remains relevant, no new applications of the work were found. However, Brooten's and Youngblut's work (2006) on the concept of nurse dose, based on years of empirical research, offers a similar understanding of the differences among beginners, experts by experience, and APNs. They proposed, as did Calkin, that one needs to understand patients' needs and responses and the expertise, experience, and education of nurses to match nursing care to the needs of patients, but they did not cite Calkin's work. Similarly, the Synergy Model in critical care is based, in part, on an understanding of patient and nurse characteristics consistent with Calkin's ideas.

Brown's Framework for Advanced Practice Nursing

Brown (1998) developed a conceptual framework for the entire field of advanced practice nursing, including the environments that surround and impact upon practice (Fig. 2-7). Studies were synthesized to propose a conceptual framework that included 4 main and 17 specific concepts (specific concepts are in parentheses): environments (society, health care economy, local conditions, nursing, advanced practice community); role legitimacy (graduate education, certification, licensure); advanced practice nursing (scope, clinical care, competencies, managing health care environments, professional involvement in health care discourse); and outcomes (patient, health care system, the nursing profession, individual APN outcomes).

The central concept, conceptually and visually, is advanced practice nursing. Brown (1998) proposed a definition of advanced practice nursing: "professional health care activities that (1) focus on clinical services rendered at the nurse-client interface, (2) use a nursing orientation, (3) have a defined but dynamic and evolving scope, and (4) are based on competencies that are acquired through graduate nursing education."

This comprehensive model is one of the few that explicates the relevant components of a conceptual framework, as described in the beginning of this chapter. Brown defined the concepts or building blocks of the model, articulated assumptions, and proposed linkages among concepts that could be tested. The model is comprehensive in that it addressed the nature of the practice and the context in which the practice occurs. The importance of a nursing orientation was noted, particularly when APNs perform activities traditionally done by physicians. Brown noted that scope is "defined but dynamic and evolving," an observation that reflects the rapidity with which knowledge accrues and practice changes. The model is sufficiently explicated that it could be used for all the purposes that conceptual models can serve—differentiating practice, designing curricula, and evaluating advanced practice. Like the early NONPF competencies, Brown used domains and competencies to describe the work of APNs. Brown's model has been cited in later theoretical and research investigations on advanced practice (e.g., Gardner et al., 2007).

Strong Memorial Hospital's Model of Advanced Practice Nursing

APNs at Strong Memorial Hospital developed a model of advanced practice nursing (Ackerman, Clark, Reed, et al., 2000; Ackerman, Norsen, Martin, et al., 1996; Mick & Ackerman, 2000). The model evolved from the delineation of the domains and competencies of the acute care NP (ACNP) role, conceptualized as a role that "combines the clinical skills of the NP with the systems acumen, educational commitment, and leadership ability of the CNS" (Ackerman et al., 1996, p. 69). The five domains are direct comprehensive patient care, support of systems, education, research, and publication and professional leadership. All domains have direct and indirect activities associated with them. In addition, necessary unifying threads influence each domain, which are illustrated as circular and continuous threads in Figure 2-8:

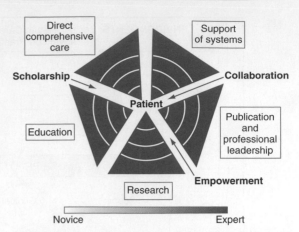

FIG 2-8 The Strong Memorial Hospital's model of advanced practice nursing. *(From Ackerman, M. H., Norsen, L., Martin, B., Wiedrich, J., & Kitzman H. J. [1996]. Development of a model of advanced practice.* American Journal of Critical Care, *5, 68–73.)*

collaboration, scholarship, and empowerment (Ackerman et al., 1996). These threads are operationalized in each practice domain. Ackerman and colleagues (2000) noted that the model is based on an understanding of the role development of APNs; the concept of novice (APN) to expert (APN) is foundational to the Strong Model (see later).

Direct comprehensive care includes a range of assessments and interventions performed by APNs, including history taking, physical assessment, requesting and/or performing diagnostic studies, performing invasive procedures, interpreting clinical and laboratory data, prescribing medications and other therapies, and case management of complex, critically ill patients. The support of systems domain includes indirect patient care activities that support the clinical enterprise and serve to improve the quality of care. These activities include consultation, participating or leading strategic planning, quality improvement initiatives, establishing and evaluating standards of practice, precepting students, and promoting APN practice. The education domain includes a variety of activities, such as evaluating educational programs, providing formal and informal education to staff, educating patients and families, and identifying and disseminating educational resources. The research domain addresses the use and conduct of research. The publication and professional leadership domain includes those APN functions involved with disseminating knowledge about the ACNP role, participating in professional organizations as a member or leader, influencing health and public policy, and publishing. APNs are expected to exert influence within and outside their institution.

The unifying threads of collaboration, scholarship, and empowerment are attributes of advanced practice that exert influence across all five domains and characterize the professional model of nursing practice. Collaboration ensures that the contributions of all caregivers are valued. APNs are expected to create and sustain a culture that supports scholarly inquiry, whether it is questioning a common nursing practice or developing and disseminating an innovation. APNs support the empowerment of staff, ensuring that nurses have authority over nursing practice and opportunities to improve practice.

The Strong Model is a parsimonious model that has many similarities with other advanced practice conceptualizations. For example, its domains are consistent with the competencies delineated in the Hamric Model. Unlike the Hamric Model, which posits direct care as the central competency that informs all other advanced nursing practice competencies, all domains of practice in the Strong Model, including direct care, are considered "mutually exclusive of each other and exhaustive of practice behaviors" (Ackerman et al., 1996). Like the Synergy Model, discussed later, role development is incorporated within the model (novice to expert). As described in the original article, the Strong Model emerged from consideration of the ACNP as a combined CNS-NP role. It is notable that this model was the result of a collaborative effort between practicing APNs and APN faculty members. One could infer that such a model would be useful for guiding clinical practice and planning curricula, two of the purposes of conceptual models outlined earlier in this chapter. The Strong Model has informed studies of advanced practice nursing in critical care since its publication (e.g., Mick & Ackerman, 2000; Becker, Kaplow, Muenzen, & Hartigan, 2006; Chang, Gardner, Duffield, & Ramis, 2010). More recently, Ackerman and coworkers (2010) have proposed an administrative model for managing APNs.

Oberle and Allen: The Nature of Advanced Practice Nursing

At the time that they wrote, Oberle and Allen (2001) asserted that conceptualizations of advanced practice nursing were limited; particular gaps were the lack of clear distinctions between the expert practice of experienced nurses and of APNs, as well as the lack of nursing theories to address such levels of practice. The authors noted that, although the literature on expert nursing is mostly focused on expertise as it unfolds in the context of relationships, the literature on advanced practice nursing seems to focus more on expertise as "skills acquisition and critical thinking abilities."

According to Oberle and Allen (2001), any conceptualization of advanced practice nursing should be embedded in a conceptual understanding of nursing, so the authors first proposed a conceptualization of nursing practice. They refer to practice by the term *praxis,* which captures the values-oriented, reflective, and creative nature of the work of nurses. They conceive of nursing as a dialectic (back and forth) process between the nurse's knowledge and his or her experiences and relationships with patients. In this process, the nurse considers general and particular knowledge, synthesizes this knowledge, and generates options for care that can be offered to the patient. By this, they mean that experiences with patients (and, presumably, reflection on these experiences) extend nurses' knowledge, this new knowledge informs their practice with subsequent patients, and experiences with applying the new knowledge gained from experience and reflection again inform and extend their thinking, a dialectic process that occurs repeatedly. As nurses accumulate experience, this dialectic process that occurs in relationships with patients contributes to developing expertise.

The conceptualization of advanced practice nursing proposed by Oberle and Allen (2001) is illustrated in Figure 2-9. Each of the elements in the model is described in Box 2-4. Oberle and Allen (2001) differentiated between experts by experience and APNs as follows: "The inherent difference between expert and advanced practice is that the expert nurse's knowledge base is largely experientially acquired, whereas the APN has a greater store of theoretical knowledge acquired through graduate study" (p. 151).

Although Figure 2-9 is meant to illustrate advanced practice nursing, the elements in the model are the same as those used for the authors' textual description of experts by experience; there are no separate illustrations of the two levels of practice. Differences between experts by experience and APNs are described in the text. Oberle and Allen (2001) proposed that graduate education is a process in which students (presumably experts by experience) have experiences that lead to transformations in self and in practice, a dialectic process that results in "transformative practice." Although the notion of transformative practice is provocative and likely to resonate with students and faculty, neither the model nor the text helps the reader understand the nature of this transformative practice and how it differs from the practice of experts by experience.

Oberle and Allen (2001) acknowledged that they did not consider the specifics of advanced practice and did not address environment or contexts of practice, which is a limitation of their model. Environment is a significant theoretical concept for nursing in general and for advanced practice nursing in particular, a concept that is addressed, for example, in Brown's and Hamric's models. Another limitation of Oberle and Allen's model is the assumption of significant practical experience in nursing prior to graduate school. With more and more career changers

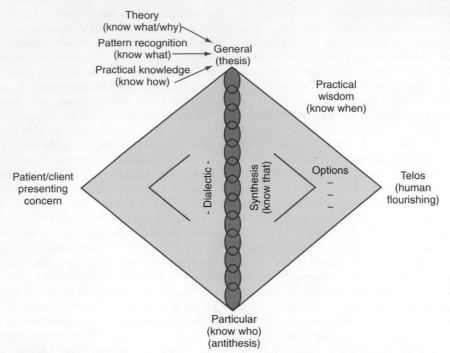

FIG 2-9 Oberle and Allen's conceptualization of advanced practice. *(From Oberle, K., & Allen, M. [2001]. The nature of advanced practice nursing. Nursing Outlook, 49, 148–153.)*

entering nursing through direct-entry programs that prepare APNs, future conceptualizations of advanced practice nursing will need to take into account how non-nursing experience helps graduate nursing students experience the dialectic process that is at the heart of praxis and helps them develop the practical wisdom essential to effective nursing practice. Graduate APN students who do not have nursing experience prior to graduate school are encouraged to reflect and expand on this model, considering how their life and professional experiences account for their experience of transformation and their mastery of advanced practice nursing.

Shuler's Model of Nurse Practitioner Practice

This model is complex and the review for this edition found no additional reports using this model. Because of its historical importance as an early NP model, the Shuler model (Shuler & Davis, 1993a) is briefly discussed. Readers should refer to the original article to see the full model.

Shuler's experience integrating nursing and medical knowledge skills into the NP role led to the development of a conceptual model that would make apparent the unique contributions of NPs, purposefully addressing the

need for a model that reflects the acquisition of expertise by the NP in two health care disciplines, nursing and medicine. Shuler's Nurse Practitioner Practice Model is a complex systems model that is holistic and wellness-oriented. It is definitive and detailed in terms of how the NP-patient interaction, patient assessment, intervention, and evaluation should occur (Shuler & Davis, 1993a). It is complex and its value for understanding NP practice may not become clear until one is in practice. Table 2-2 outlines key model constructs and related theories, many of which should be familiar to students. Knowing that these familiar concepts are embedded in this comprehensive model may help readers appreciate its potential usefulness.

Shuler's model is intended "to impact the NP domain at four levels: theoretical, clinical, educational, and research" (Shuler & Davis, 1993a). A close review of the model indicates that it addresses important components of a model of advanced practice nursing, such as the following: (1) nursing's metaparadigm (person, health, nursing, and environment); (2) the nursing process; (3) assumptions about patients and nurse practitioners; and (4) theoretical concepts relevant to practice. The model could be characterized as a network or system of frameworks.

BOX 2-4 **Elements of Oberle and Allen's Conceptualization of Advanced Practice Nursing**

Patient-client presenting concern—problem or potential problem for which an individual needs nursing care

General and particular knowledge—nurses move back and forth between global knowledge (e.g., the features of an illness or the nursing care that usually works for a particular problem) and specific knowledge (specifics about the individual patient or situation).

General Knowledge

- Theory—know what and know why.
- Pattern recognition—know what.
- Practical knowledge—know how.

Particular Knowledge

- Client's meanings, desired outcomes, and acceptable actions—know who.
- *Dialectic*—the process whereby nurses consider general and particular knowledge and synthesize this information to generate options and propose actions to the patient to move the patient toward his or her goals.
- *Synthesis*—know that (a particular action is called for in a specific situation).
- *Practical wisdom*—know when (a particular action ought to be taken). The dialectic process and experience with synthesis, informed by praxis, lead to the development of practical wisdom.
- *Telos*—human flourishing (the object of nursing care, of which health is a part—health is a resource for human flourishing.
- *Options*—possibilities for actions identified by nurse.

From Oberle, K., & Allen, M. (2001). The nature of advanced practice nursing. *Nursing Outlook*, 49, 148–153.

Clinical application of the Shuler Model is intended to describe the NP's combined functions (i.e., nursing and medicine), benefits for practitioner and patient, and a framework whereby NP services can be evaluated (Shuler & Davis, 1993b). Shuler and Davis (1993b) published a lengthy template for conducting a visit. Although it is difficult to imagine ready implementation into today's busy NP practices, Shuler and colleagues published clinical applications of the model (Shuler & Davis, 1993b; Shuler, 2000; Shuler, Huebscher, & Hallock, 2001). In the current health care environment, the Circle of Caring Model (Dunphy, Winland-Brown, Porter, et al., 2011) may be more useful for addressing some of the issues that led Shuler to create the model—integrating nursing and medical skills while learning the NP role and retaining her or his nursing focus while providing complex diagnostic and therapeutic interventions.

Ball and Cox: Restoring Patients to Health— A Theory of Legitimate Influence

One of the few empirical international studies of advanced practice nursing was a grounded theory study of NPs, CNSs, and *clinical nurse consultants*—a term used in Australia for those in CNS-like positions (Ball & Cox, 2003, 2004). Subjects (*N* = 36) from the United States, Canada, United Kingdom, and Australia participated; they were required to be master's-prepared or graduate students preparing for an advanced practice role. The investigators conducted interviews and made observations of the participants over a 3-year period. The theory of legitimate influence emerged from this study (Fig. 2-10). The figure illustrates the range of activities in which APNs engage to "enhance patient stay" and "improve patient outcomes." This study provided empirical support for many of the competencies described in the models reviewed in this chapter. For example, findings from their work are consistent with the competencies in Hamric's model (Table 2-3). Ball and Cox's work suggests that the activities of APNs, in this case NPs and CNSs, are strategic and focused and that some activities involve direct service to patients, whereas others are aimed at communication and system issues.

Section Summary: Implications for Advanced Practice Nursing Conceptualizations

When one considers conceptualizations of advanced practice nursing described by professional organizations and individual authors, similarities and differences emerge. Many conceptual models address competencies that APNs must possess. All are in agreement that the direct care of patients is central to APN practice. Most models affirm two or more competencies identified by Hamric and some models emphasize some competencies more than others. Some models (e.g., the Calkin and Strong models) address the issue of skill mix as it relates to APNs, an issue of concern to administrators who hire APNs. A notable difference across models is the extent to which the concept of environment as it relates to APN practice is addressed. In the next section, selected models, which APNs may find useful as they develop and evaluate their own practices, are described. Models of APN role development are explored in Chapter 4.

TABLE 2-2 Model Constructs and Underlying Theoretical Concepts Included in Shuler's Model of Nurse Practitioner Practice

Model Constructs	Holistic Patient Needs	Nurse Practitioner– Patient Interaction	Self-Care	Health Prevention	Health Promotion	Wellness
Underlying theoretical concepts	Basic needs Wellness activities Health and illness Psychological health Family Culture Social support Environmental health Spirituality	Contracting Role modeling Self-care activities Teaching/ learning Contracting Culture Family Social support Environmental health	Wellness activities Preventive health activities Health promotion activities Compliance Problem solving Teaching/ learning Contracting Culture Family Social support Environmental health	Primary prevention Secondary prevention Tertiary prevention Preventive health behavior Family Culture Environmental health	Health promotion behavior Wellness Family Culture Environmental health Social support	Self-care activities Wellness activities Disease prevention activities Health promotion activities Family Culture Social support Environmental health Spirituality Contracting Teaching/ learning

From Shuler, P. A., & Davis, J. E. (1993a). The Shuler nurse practitioner practice model: A theoretical framework for nurse practitioner clinicians, educators, and researchers, Part 1. *Journal of the American Academy of Nurse Practitioners, 5*, 11–18.

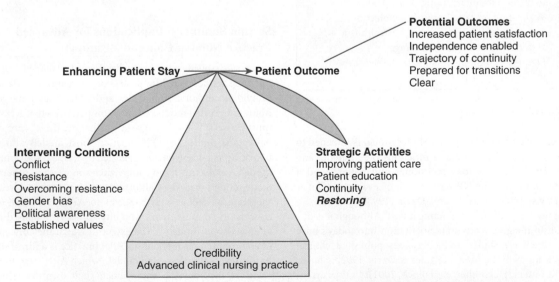

FIG 2-10 Ball and Cox's theory of legitimate influence. *(From Ball, C., & Cox, C. L. [2003]. Restoring patients to health: Outcomes and indicators of advanced nursing practice in adult critical care, Part 1.* International Journal of Nursing Practice, 9, *356–367.)*

TABLE 2-3	Comparison of Concepts in Ball and Cox's Theory* and Hamric's Competencies†
Hamric Competency	**Ball and Cox Concept**
Direct care	Credibility; advanced clinical practice; restoring "to health outcomes"
Guidance and coaching	Patient education; continuity
Consultation	Legitimate influence; credibility
Evidence-based practice	Improving patient care
Collaboration	Conflict
Leadership	Improving patient care; addressing or overcoming resistance; recognizing and/or addressing gender bias; political awareness; legitimate influence
Ethical decision making	Established values

*Ball and Cox's Theory of Legitimate Influence.
†Hamric's Seven Advanced Practice Nurse Competencies.

Models Useful for Advanced Practice Nurses in Their Practice

American Association of Critical-Care Nurses' Synergy Model

The American Association of Critical-Care Nurses created the Synergy Model (2003; Fig. 2-11) to link nursing practice with patient outcomes (Curley, 1998). Components of the model are patient's characteristics, nurse's competencies, and patient, nurse, and system level outcomes. Patients' capacity for health and their vulnerability to illness are influenced by biologic, genetic, psychological, and socioecologic determinants. The Synergy Model posits a unique cluster of personal characteristics that arise from these determinants and exist along a continuum that parallels health and illness states—stability, complexity, predictability, resiliency, vulnerability, participation in decision making and care, and resource availability (Table 2-4). An important function of the nurse is to ensure the patient's safe passage through the health care system.

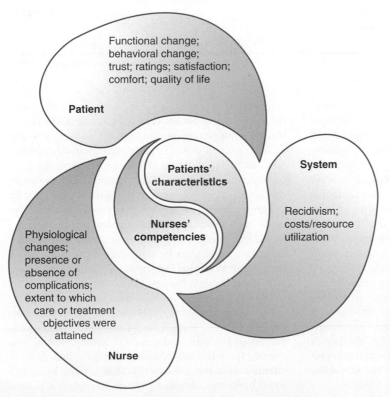

FIG 2-11 American Association of Critical-Care Nurses Synergy Model. The Synergy Model delineates three levels of outcomes—those derived from the patient, those derived from the nurse, and those derived from the health care system. *(From Curley, M. A. Q. [1998]. Patient-nurse synergy: Optimizing patient's outcomes.* American Journal of Critical Care, 7, *64–72.)*

TABLE 2-4	The Synergy Model: The Seven Continua of Patient Characteristics				
	1	**2**	**3**	**4**	**5**
Minimally resilient					Highly resilient
Highly vulnerable					Minimally vulnerable
Minimally stable					Highly stable
Minimally complex					Highly complex
Not predictable					Highly predictable
Few resources available					Many resources available
No participation in decision making and care					Full participation in decision making and care

Adapted from American Association of Critical-Care Nurses. (2003). The AACN Synergy Model for patient care (http://www.aacn.org/WD/Certifications/Docs/SynergyModelforPatientCare.pdf).

TABLE 2-5	The Synergy Model: The Eight Continua of Nurse Characteristics and Nursing Competencies				
	1	**2**	**3**	**4**	**5**
Clinical judgment	Competent				Expert
Advocacy, moral agency	Competent				Expert
Caring practices	Competent				Expert
Collaboration	Competent				Expert
Systems thinking	Competent				Expert
Response to diversity	Competent				Expert
Clinical inquiry or innovator, evaluator	Competent				Expert
Facilitator of patient and family learning	Competent				Expert

Adapted from American Association of Critical-Care Nurses. (2003). The AACN Synergy Model for patient care (http://www.aacn.org/WD/Certifications/Docs/SynergyModelforPatientCare.pdf).

Nursing competencies are derived from the needs of patients and also exist along a continuum. The eight nursing competencies are clinical judgment, advocacy and moral agency, caring practices, facilitation of learning, collaboration, systems thinking, diversity of responsiveness, and clinical inquiry (Table 2-5). These range from competent (level 1) to expert (level 5). However, a discussion of the interpretation of these levels is beyond the scope of this chapter. The reader is referred to the American Association of Critical-Care Nurses website (http://www.aacn.org) and other publications (American Association of Critical-Care Nurses, 2012; Curley, 1998).

Outcomes are conceptualized as being derived from the patient, nurse, and/or system. For example, trust of the caregiver and patient satisfaction are patient outcomes that arise or are derived from the patient. Physiologic outcomes are derived from the nurse (i.e., the nurse's interventions). Systems level outcomes are derived from the hospital or insurer (e.g., readmission to the hospital for a preventable complication).

The model is interesting for several reasons. From the perspective of patient-centered care, the model recognizes the importance of nurse-patient relationships and patients' trust in their caregivers. Certification examinations, including those for APNs, are based on the conceptualization of levels of competency and represent conceptual coherence between the nature of the practice and how a person's knowledge of the practice is tested. The model has shown considerable stability, informing practice (a regular column in their publications) and changes in certification. As can be seen, there is overlap between the Synergy Model and Hamric Model, both of which have been integrated into the new CNS competencies.

Finally, the model has been used to document differences among critical care APN roles (Becker et al., 2006). Like the NACNS, Hamric, and DNP conceptualizations, the Synergy Model addresses the patient, nurse, and system. Since the last edition, there have been several publications using the Synergy Model, often by APNs, about basic and advanced practice to explain a patient phenomenon or guide clinical care (e.g., Smith, 2006). Other evaluations of the Synergy Model may lead to identifying differences between expert and advanced practice nurses in critical care (e.g., Brewer, Wojner-Alexandrov, Triola, et al., 2007; Scarpa & Connelly, 2011).

Advanced Practice Nursing Transitional Care Models

There are several models of transitional care in which care is provided by APNs; some of these are discussed in Chapter 8. Early work by Brooten and colleagues (1988) continues to inform these models of APN care (e.g., Partiprajak, Hanucharurnkul, Piaseu, et al., 2011). Brooten's model is important because it illustrates how a theory of clinical care can be studied to obtain a better understanding of the work of APNs; it is a model that has evolved but has resulted in steady contributions to understanding and improving APN practice. This theoretical and empirical steadfastness has had a significant influence on the new policies evolving as the United States undergoes health care reform.

Brooten and colleagues (1988) used a conceptual framework proposed by Doessel and Marshall (1985). They integrated this framework into their evaluation of outcomes of APN transitional care with different clinical populations. APN transitional care was defined as "comprehensive discharge planning designed for each patient group plus APN home follow-up through a period of normally expected recovery or stabilization" (Brooten et al., 2002). Brooten's model was intended to address outlier patient populations (e.g., those whose care, for clinical reasons, was likely to cost more). Across all studies, care was provided by NPs and/or CNSs whose clinical expertise was matched to the needs of the patient population. In these studies, APN care was associated with improved patient outcomes and reduced costs (see Chapters 8 and 23).

Research by Brooten, Naylor (e.g., Bradway, Trotta, Bixby, et al., 2012), and others who have studied transitional care by APNs has provided empirical support for several elements important to a conceptualization of advanced practice nursing. In a summary of the studies conducted, the investigators identified several factors that contribute to the effectiveness of APNs: content expertise, interpersonal skills, knowledge of systems, ability to implement change, and ability to access resources (Brooten, Youngblut, Deatrick, et al., 2003). This finding provides empirical support for the importance of the APN competencies of direct care, collaboration, coaching, and systems leadership.

Two other important findings were the existence of patterns of morbidity within patient populations and an apparent dose effect (i.e., outcomes seemed to be related to how much time was spent with patients, how many interactions APNs had with patients, and numbers and types of APN interventions; Brooten et al., 2003). Subsequently, based on this finding of a dose effect, Brooten and Youngblut (2006) proposed a conceptual explanation of nurse dose. Their explanation suggests that nurse dose depends on patient and nurse characteristics. For the nurse, differences in education and experience can influence the dose of nursing needed.

The concept of nurse dose, which has empirical support, may enable the profession to differentiate more clearly among novice, expert, and advanced levels of nursing practice. Taken together, findings from this program of research suggest that characteristics of patients and characteristics and dose of APN interventions are likely to be important to any conceptualization of advanced practice nursing, an idea consistent with the relationships posited in the Synergy Model. Finally, the fact that this program of research has used NPs and CNSs to intervene with patients provides support for a broad conceptual model of APN practice that encompasses APN characteristics, competencies, patient factors, environment, and other concepts that can inform role-specific models.

Although there have been other studies of APNs providing transitional care (see Chapter 8), Brooten's work is highlighted because of the additional analyses that were done and the ultimate influence on health policy of this program of research (e.g., Naylor, Aiken, Kurtzman, et al., 2011). The findings help us understand the APN characteristics and interventions that have contributed to the success of the interventions and a model of care that evolved from the skilled care provided by APNs.

Dunphy and Winland-Brown's Circle of Caring: A Transformative, Collaborative Model

A central premise of Dunphy and Winland-Brown's model (1998) is that the health care needs of individuals, families, and communities are not being met in a health care system that is dominated by medicine and one in which medical language (i.e., the International Classification of Disease Codes [ICD-10-CM]) is the basis for reimbursement. They proposed the "Circle of Caring: A Transformative Model" to foster a more active and visible nursing presence in the health care system and to explain and promote medical-nursing collaboration. Dunphy and Winland-Brown's transformative model, which has been slightly revised since its original publication (Dunphy, Winland-Brown, Porter, et al., 2011; Fig. 2-12) is a synthesized problem-solving approach to advanced practice nursing that builds on nursing and medical models (Dunphy & Winland-Brown, 1998).

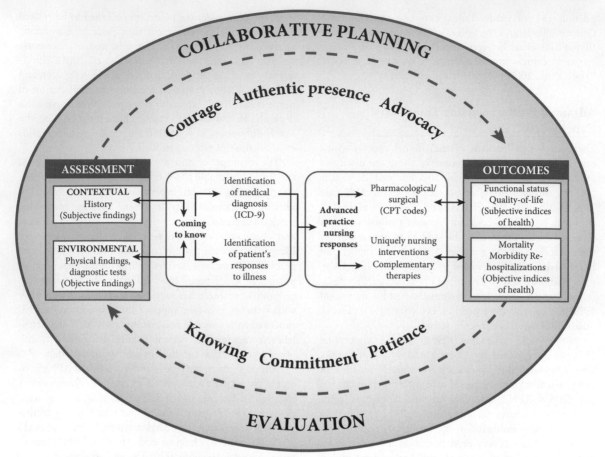

FIG 2-12 Dunphy and Winland-Brown's Circle of Caring model. *(From Dunphy, L. M., Winland-Brown, J. E., Porter, B. O., et al. [2011]. Primary care in the twenty-first century: A Circle of Caring. In L. M. Dunphy, J. E. Winland-Brown, B. O. Porter, & D. J. Thomas [Eds.]. Primary care: The art and science of advanced practice nursing [3rd ed., pp. 3–18]. Philadelphia: F. A. Davis.)*

When first proposed, the authors argued that a model such as theirs was needed because nursing and medicine have two different traditions, with the medical model being viewed as primarily reductionistic and nursing being regarded as primarily humanistic. Neither model, by itself, provided a structure that allowed APNs to be recognized for their daily practice and the positive patient health outcomes that can be attributed to APN care. The model's authors viewed the development of nursing diagnoses as an attempt to differentiate nursing care from medical care, but because few nursing diagnoses are recognized by current reimbursement systems, the nursing in APN care was rendered invisible.

The Circle of Caring Model was proposed to incorporate the strengths of medicine and nursing in a transforming way. The conceptual elements are the processes of assessment, planning, intervention, and evaluation, with a feedback loop. Integrating a nursing model with a traditional medical model permits the following to occur:

- The assessment and evaluation are contextualized, incorporating subjective and environmental elements into traditional history taking and physical examination.
- The approach to therapeutics is broadened to include holistic approaches to healing and makes nursing care more visible.
- Measured outcomes include patients' perceptions of health and care, not just physiologic outcomes and resource use.

The assessment-planning-intervention-evaluation processes in linear configuration are encircled by caring. Caring is actualized through interpersonal interactions with patients and caregivers to which NPs bring patience, courage, advocacy, authentic presence, commitment, and knowing (Dunphy & Winland-Brown, 1998; Dunphy, et al., 2011). Conceptual definitions of these terms would add to the understanding of how these processes interact with and affect the caregiving of APNs. The authors suggested that the model promotes the incorporation of the lived experience of the patient into the provider-patient interaction, and that the process of caring is a prerequisite to APNs providing effective and meaningful care to patients.

The Circle of Caring is an integrated model of caregiving that incorporates the discrete strengths of nursing and medicine. This is an important concern for many graduate students. They struggle with integrating their nursing expertise and philosophy with new knowledge and skills that were traditionally viewed as medicine. Although the authors regard the concept of caring as a way to bridge the gap between advanced practice nursing and medicine and raise awareness, the model provides no clear guidance on how faculty can help students or how students themselves can use the model to bridge the gap.

Several issues remain to be considered. For example, if one goal of proposing the model is to resolve differences about the diagnostic language used by medicine and nursing to obtain reimbursement, no specific mechanism is offered for APNs to resolve this issue using the model. The model does not seem to be described in enough detail to guide policymaking. The conceptual significance of encircling the four practice processes with the six caring processes is unclear, although their recent work devotes a chapter to caring in the nurse practitioner role (Boykin & Schoenhofer, 2011). Given today's health policy context, the value of this model, with its emphasis on the APN-patient relationship and caring processes, could inform practice evaluation and research on APN practices. Since it was first proposed, it is only recently that publications informed by this model have appeared. For example, the Circle of Caring Model has been used for the development of an online risk assessment of mental health (McKnight, 2011), evaluation of medication adherence (Palardy & March, 2011), and neonatal transport (Thomas, 2011). In addition, their primary care textbook (Dunphy, Winland-Brown, Porter, & Thomas, 2011) is informed by their Circle of Caring Model.

Given the emphasis on interprofessional education and efforts to distinguish advanced practice from medical practice, empirical testing of this model is warranted. This testing would help determine whether the model has the following features: (1) applicability to all advanced practice nursing roles; (2) potential to be used to distinguish expert by experience practice from advanced practice; (3) viewed by other disciplines as having an interdisciplinary focus that would promote collaboration; and (4) result in more visibility for NPs and other APNs in the health care system.

Recommendations and Future Directions

It is understandable that students may feel confused by the variety of conceptualizations and inconsistency in terminology. The challenge for students and practicing APNs is to find a model that works for them, that enables them to understand and evaluate their practices and attend to the profession's efforts to create a coherent, stable, and robust conceptualization of advanced practice nursing.

Conceptualizations of Advanced Practice Nursing

This review of extant models of advanced practice nursing is necessarily cursory, primarily focused on U.S. literature, and may be incomplete. It is more a survey or overview than a review of the literature. Although there is some agreement on selected elements of advanced practice, there has generally been no comprehensive synthesis of existing work and limited evidence that new conceptualizations have built on earlier work. To promote a unified conceptualization of advanced practice nursing, I suggest that the following be undertaken:

1. A rigorous content analysis of the statements published by national and international professional organizations that describe the advanced practice nursing of recognized APNs (CNMs, CNSs, CRNAs, CNPs). This would be a natural evolution of the work done by the APRN Consensus Work Group, NCSBN APRN Advisory Committee, and CNA, among others, to inform future work. As part of this analysis, an assessment of the extent to which nursing's metaparadigmatic concepts are integrated into the statements about advanced practice that organizations make about the nature of advanced practice nursing should be undertaken.

2. A similar content analysis of statements that address advanced practice nursing promulgated by specialty organizations.

3. A review of recent role delineation studies of the four APN roles.

4. A comprehensive integrative review of the advanced practice literature (building on the work of Mantzoukas and Watkinson [2007] and Lewandowski and Adamle [2009]). This could be modeled on the work of Reeves, Goldman, Gilbert, et al. (2011) and their work on the conceptualization of interprofessional education, identifying

concepts and relationships that need further development.

5. Based on recommendations 1 through 4, a synthesis of results should be generated that could be used to propose a definition of the phenomenon—advanced practice nursing.

6. Informed by these analyses, a common structure for organizational statements about APNs could be developed that ensures common nursing concepts are included, such as the following:
   - Definition of nursing and advanced practice nursing
   - Specification of assumptions
   - Incorporating the metaparadigmatic elements of persons, health and illness, nursing, and the environment, into scopes and introductions to key documents
   - Referencing documents such as ANA's social policy statement and ICN's statements on nursing

7. Evolving a similar structure for developing statements that define advanced practice nursing would make clear the foundational and philosophical underpinnings of each organization's approach to defining advanced practice nursing.

8. Using the results of 1 through 5 to inform revisions of the DNP *Essentials,* standards, and other documents that address APN LACE issues for existing and new APN roles. Future revision of documents regarding APNs should be informed by a clear conceptualization of advanced practice nursing and empirical evidence.

9. Because the terms *advanced practice nursing* and *advanced nursing practice* are being used to refer to APN work, revisit the work on definitions of these terms done by Styles (Styles & Lewis, 2000; Styles, 1998) and clarify these definitions as they relate to APNs.

Consensus Building Around Advanced Practice Nursing

A collaboratively developed conceptualization of advanced practice nursing and what is common across APN roles is a prerequisite for building consensus among APNs, stakeholder organizations, and policymakers; this is a priority for the profession. This work is critical to ensuring that patients will continue to benefit from advanced practice nursing. The APRN Consensus Model represents substantial progress in the area with regard to regulation. Studies are underway worldwide (see Chapter 6) that could inform efforts to refine conceptualizations of advanced nursing practice. Ongoing development of consensus on advanced practice nursing should involve the following:

- Now that there is a common language regarding the regulation of U.S. advanced practice nursing, periodic updates on the progress of nationwide implementation of the regulatory model—successes and challenges—will be important (note that NCSBN periodically updates state by state maps on its website).

- Because U.S. nurse anesthetists and nurse-midwives operate under different accrediting and certification bodies and mechanisms than CNSs and NPs, their experience may be helpful in countries in which nurses and midwives are regulated separately, or where nurse anesthesia is not a practice role.

- Define common terms used in documents describing APN practice. It is evident from this review that there is still a need for common language to describe advanced practice nursing. There is no clear articulation of the differences among terms such as *essentials, competencies, hallmarks,* and *standard of care* as they are used by various organizations. Such clarity would be helpful to those in the profession and other stakeholders.

The responses of NACNS, NONPF, ACNM, and AANA to the DNP initiative and concerns about selective implementation of the APRN Consensus Model are likely to influence the evolution of advanced practice nursing in the next decade. The extent to which we reach agreement within the profession will affect policy related to advanced practice and whether the public recognizes and requests the services of APNs. Disagreement on the nature and credentialing of advanced practice nursing should be resolved by continued efforts to foster true consensus by the following:

- Addressing the legitimate concerns of these organizations (e.g., impact on access to care, concerns about certification or grandfathering existing APNs)

- Establishing priorities for negotiation and resolution by stakeholder groups and initiating a process to find common ground and address disagreements.

- In the face of disagreements, working toward agreement on a common identity to facilitate public understanding of APN roles.

These consensus-building efforts are needed if our profession is to remain attractive to new nurses and new APNs and make room for evolving APN roles.

Consensus on Key Elements of Practice Doctorate Curricula

With the promulgation of AACN's DNP essentials and the increasing numbers of practice doctorate programs in nursing, there may be less disagreement on the need for APNs prepared at the doctoral level, but disagreements about elements of the curricula are emerging. Several authors have expressed concern that the DNP may not be demanding enough with regard to theory and research methods, which may be just as important for evaluating practice and testing practice models as they are in nursing PhD programs. Although NACNS and ACNM do not support the practice doctorate for entry into practice and AANA has delayed doctoral preparation for entry into practice until 2025, APN organizations have prepared doctoral level competencies that are consistent with those proposed in the DNP. One question that will need to be addressed is whether regulations will specify which type of nursing practice doctorate will be needed when, and if, a doctorate becomes the entry level credential for APNs because, as Dreher and Smith Glasgow (2011) have noted, there are other practice doctorates in nursing.

Research on Advanced Practice Nurses and Their Contributions to Patient, Team, and Systems Outcomes

Theory-based research on APNs' contributions to improved patient outcomes and cost-effectiveness is needed to inform and validate the conceptualizations of advanced practice nursing. Increased knowledge about advanced practice nursing is critical (see Chapter 24). The worth of any service depends on the extent to which practice meets the needs and priorities of health care systems, the public policy arena, and society in general. In addition to research that links advanced practice nursing with outcomes, I recommend the following:

1. Promising conceptual models of advanced practice nursing should be refined based on research that validates key concepts and tests theoretical propositions associated with these models.
2. Research on APNs should examine the interpersonal processes used in the course of coaching patients and collaborating with colleagues within and across disciplines; across many of the models reviewed in this chapter, the APN's skill in communication and collaboration is considered important. I hypothesize that advanced communication skills contribute to APNs' effectiveness (Spross, 2009; see Chapter 8). APNs can contribute descriptive data on the interpersonal strategies that they use in practice through case studies and other practice analyses to enable researchers to examine links between these less tangible aspects of APN care and patient outcomes.
3. Studies should be undertaken to examine advanced practice nursing across APN roles and between physician and APN practices with regard to processes and outcomes. The studies conducted across APN roles can determine whether the assumption

that a core set of competencies is used by all APNs is valid, and the activities that differentiate one APN role from another. The studies of APNs and physicians can identify the factors that distinguish APNs from physicians as a basis for understanding differences in outcomes and developing proposals about how best to use these providers to achieve high quality, cost-effective care.
4. As conceptualizations of interprofessional teams evolve, the roles and contributions of APNs and their interdisciplinary colleagues to outcomes should be studied.

When there is a better empirical understanding of the similarities and differences across APN roles and between physicians and APNs, this knowledge must be packaged and presented to colleagues in other disciplines, policymakers, and the public. This information is important to educating physicians, consumers, and policymakers about the meaning and relevance of advanced practice nursing to the health of our society.

For a further discussion of research directions relevant to advanced practice nursing, see Chapter 23.

Conclusion

Conceptual models serve many purposes for the fields that they seek to describe. If the nursing profession can achieve consensus on a conceptual model of advanced practice nursing, considerable progress will have been made. The future of advanced practice nursing depends on the extent to which practice meets the needs and priorities of society, health care systems, and the public policy arena. A stable robust model of advanced practice nursing will serve to guide the development of advanced practice nursing and ensure that patients will have access to APN care.

I have identified problems and imperatives related to conceptualizing advanced practice nursing, reviewed a number of models, and made some recommendations for future work on conceptualizing advanced practice nursing that address problems and imperatives. The nursing profession, nationally and internationally, remains at a critical juncture with regard to advanced practice nursing. In each country in which APNs practice, the need to move forward with one voice on this issue is urgent if APNs and the nursing profession as a whole are to fulfill their social contract with the individuals, institutions, and communities we serve. A unified conceptualization of advanced practice nursing focuses the efforts of the profession on preparing APNs, promulgating policies, and fostering research to enable the realization of the outcomes stated at the beginning of this chapter, including maximizing the social contribution of APNs to the health needs of society and promoting the actualization of APNs.

References

Ackerman, M., Clark J., Reed, T., Van Horn, L., & Francati, M. (2000). A nurse practitioner–managed cardiovascular intensive care unit. In J. Hickey, R. Ouimette, & S. Venegoni (Eds.), *Advanced practice nursing: Changing roles and clinical applications* (pp. 470–480). Philadelphia: Lippincott.

Ackerman, M. H., Mick, D., & Witzel, P. (2010). Creating an organizational model to support advanced practice. *Journal of Nursing Administration, 40,* 63–68. doi: 10.1097/NNA.0b013e3181cb9f71

Ackerman, M. H., Norsen, L., Martin, B., Wiedrich, J., & Kitzman, H. J. (1996). Development of a model of advanced practice. *American Journal of Critical Care, 5,* 68–73.

Algase, D. L. (2010). Essentials of scholarship for the DNP: Are we clear yet? *Research & Theory for Nursing Practice, 24,* 91–93. doi: 10.1891/1541-6577.24.2.91

Allan, H. (2011). A commentary on Christensen M (2011). Advancing nursing practice: Redefining the theoretical and practical integration of knowledge. *Journal of Clinical Nursing, 20,* 873–881. doi: 10.1111/j.1365-2702.2011.03837.x

American Association of Colleges of Nursing (AACN). (2004). AACN position statement on the practice doctorate in nursing. (http://www.aacn.nche.edu/publications/position/DNPpositionstatement.pdf).

American Association of Colleges of Nursing (AACN). (2005). Fact sheet: The clinical nurse leader. (http://www.aacn.nche.edu/cnl/CNLFactSheet.pdf).

American Association of Colleges of Nursing (AACN). (2006). Essentials of doctorate education for advanced nursing practice. (http://www.aacn.nche.edu/DNP/pdf/Essentials.pdf).

American Association of Colleges of Nursing (AACN). (2012a). Clinical nurse leader (CNL): Frequently asked questions. (http://www.aacn.nche.edu/cnl/CNLFAQ.pdf).

American Association of Colleges of Nursing (AACN). (2012b). Growth in doctoral programs 2006-2011. (http://www.aacn.nche.edu/membership/members-only/presentations/2012/12doctoral/Potempa-Doc-Programs.pdf).

American Association of Critical-Care Nurses. (2012). The AACN Synergy Model for patient care. (http://www.aacn.org/WD/Certifications/Docs/SynergyModelforPatientCare.pdf).

American Association of Nurse Anesthetists. (2007). AANA position on doctoral preparation for nurse anesthetists. (http://www.aana.com/ceandeducation/educationalresources/Documents/AANA_Position_DTF_June_2007.pdf).

American Association of Nurse Anesthetists (AANA). (2010a). Scope and standards for nurse anesthesia practice. (http://www.aana.com/resources2/professionalpractice/Documents/PPM%20Scope%20and%20Standards.pdf).

American Association of Nurse Anesthetists. (2010b). Nurse anesthesia education. (http://www.aana.com/aboutus/Documents/naeducation.pdf).

American Association of Nurse Anesthetists. (2012). Position statement number 1.12 Patient-centered care: CRNAs and the interprofessional team. (http://www.aana.com/Search/Pages/DefaultResults.aspx?k=Position%20Statement%201.12).

American College of Nurse Midwives. (2008). ACNM Code of Ethics. (http://www.midwife.org/siteFiles/descriptive/code_of_ethics_2008.pdf).

American College of Nurse Midwives. (2011a). Definition of midwifery and scope of practice of certified nurse-midwives and certified midwives. (http://www.midwife.org/ACNM/files/ACNMLibraryData/UPLOADFILENAME/000000000266/Definition%20of%20Midwifery%20and%20Scope%20of%20Practice%20of%20CNMs%20and%20CMs%20Feb%202012.pdf).

American College of Nurse Midwives. (2011b). Standards for the practice of midwifery. (http://www.midwife.org/ACNM/files/ACNMLibraryData/UPLOADFILENAME/000000000051/Standards_for_Practice_of_Midwifery_Sept_2011.pdf).

American College of Nurse Midwives. (2011c). The practice doctorate in midwifery. (http://www.midwife.org/ACNM/files/ACNMLibraryData/UPLOADFILENAME/000000000260/Practice%20Doctorate%20in%20Midwifery%20Sept%202011.pdf).

American College of Nurse Midwives, Accreditation Commission for Midwifery Education, & American Midwifery Certification Board. (2011d). Midwifery in the United States and the Consensus Model for APRN regulation. (http://www.midwife.org/ACNM/files/ccLibraryFiles/Filename/000000001458/LACE_White_Paper_2011.pdf).

American College of Nurse Midwives. (2012a). Core competencies for basic midwifery practice. (http://www.midwife.org/ACNM/files/ACNMLibraryData/UPLOADFILENAME/000000000050/Core%20Competencies%20June%202012.pdf).

American College of Nurse Midwives. (2012b) Position statement: Midwifery education and the Doctor of Nursing Practice (DNP). (http://www.midwife.org/ACNM/files/ACNMLibraryData/UPLOADFILENAME/000000000079/Midwifery%20Ed%20and%20DNP%20Position%20Statement%20June%202012).

American College of Nurse Midwives. (2012c). Position statement: Mandatory degree requirements for entry into midwifery practice. (http://www.midwife.org/ACNM/files/ACNMLibraryData/UPLOADFILENAME/000000000076/Mandatory%20Degree%20Requirements%20Position%20Statement%20June%202012.pdf).

American Nurses Association (ANA). (2010a). *Nursing's social policy statement* (3rd ed.). Silver Spring, MD: Author.

American Nurses Association (ANA). (2010b). *Nursing: Scope and standards of practice* (2nd ed.). Silver Spring, MD: Author.

APRN Joint Dialogue Group Report. (2008). Consensus Model for APRN regulation: Licensure, accreditation, certification & education. (http://www.aacn.nche.edu/education-resources/APRNReport.pdf).

Arslanian-Engoren, C., Hicks, F. D., Whall, A. L., & Algase, D. L. (2005). An ontological view of advanced practice nursing. *Research & Theory for Nursing Practice, 19,* 315–322

Avery, M., & Howe, C. (2007). The DNP and entry into midwifery practice: An analysis. *Journal of Midwifery and Women's Health, 52,* 14–22.

Ball, C., & Cox, C. (2003). Restoring patients to health—outcomes and indicators of advanced nursing practice in adult critical care, Part 1. *International Journal of Nursing Practice, 9,* 356–367.

Ball, C., & Cox, C. (2004). The core components of legitimate influence and the conditions that constrain or facilitate advanced nursing practice in adult critical care, Part 2. *International Journal of Nursing Practice, 10,* 10–20.

Barr, H., Freeth, D., Hammick, M., Koppel, I., & Reeves, S. (2005). The evidence base and recommendations for interprofessional education in health and social care. In H. Barr, I. Koppell, S. Reeves, M. in Barr, I. Koppell, S. Reeves, M. Hammick, et al (Eds.), *Effective interprofessional education: Argument, assumption and evidence* (pp. 2–4). Oxford: Blackwell.

Becker, D., Kaplow, R., Muenzen, P., & Hartigan, C. (2006). Activities performed by acute and critical care advanced practice nurses: American Association of Critical Care Nurses study of practice. *American Journal of Critical Care, 2,* 130–148.

Benner, P. (1984). *From novice to expert.* Menlo Park, CA: Addison-Wesley.

Benner, P., Tanner, C., & Tesla, C. (2009). *Expertise in nursing practice: Caring, clinical judgment and ethics.* New York: Springer Publishing Company.

Boykin, A., & Schoenhofer, S. O. (2011). Caring and the advanced practice nurse. In L. M. Dunphy, J. E. Winland-Brown, B. O. Porter, & D. J. Thomas (Eds.), *Primary care: The art and science of advanced practice nursing* (3rd ed., pp. 19–23). Philadelphia: F. A. Davis.

Bradway, C., Trotta, R., Bixby, M., McPartland, E., Wollman, M., Kapustka, H., et al. (2012). A qualitative analysis of an advanced practice nurse-directed transitional care model intervention. *Gerontologist, 52,* 394–407.

Brewer, B. B., Wojner-Alexandrov, A. W., Triola, N., Pacini, C., Cline, M., Rust, J. E., et al. (2007). AACN Synergy Model's characteristics of patients: psychometric analyses in a tertiary care health system. *American Journal of Critical Care, 16,* 158–167.

Brooten, D., Brown, L., Munro, B., York, R., Cohen, S., Roncoli, M., et al. (1988). Early discharge and specialist transitional care. *Image: Journal of Nursing Scholarship, 20,* 64–68.

Brooten, D., Naylor, M., York, R., Brown, L., Munro, B., Hollingsworth, A., et al. (2002). Lessons learned from testing the quality cost model of advanced practice nursing (APN) transitional care. *Journal of Nursing Scholarship, 34,* 359–375.

Brooten, D., & Youngblut, J. (2006). Nurse dose as a concept. *Journal of Nursing Scholarship, 38,* 94–99.

Brooten, D., Youngblut, J., Deatrick, J., Naylor, M., & York, R. (2003). Patient problems, advanced practice nurse (APN) interventions, time and contacts among five patient groups. *Journal of Nursing Scholarship, 35,* 73–79.

Brown, S. J. (1998). A framework for advanced practice nursing. *Journal of Professional Nursing, 14,* 157–164.

Bryant-Lukosius, D., DiCenso, A., Browne, G., & Pinelli, J. (2004). Advanced practice nursing roles: Development, implementation and evaluation. *Journal of Advanced Nursing, 48,* 519–529.

Brykczynski, K. A. (1989). An interpretive study describing the clinical judgment of nurse practitioners. *Scholarly Inquiry for Nursing Practice, 3,* 75–104.

Calkin, J. D. (1984). A model for advanced nursing practice. *Journal of Nursing Administration, 14,* 24–30.

Canadian Interprofessional Health Collaborative (CIHC). (2010). A national interprofessional competency framework. (http://www.cihc.ca/files/CIHC_IPCompetencies_Feb1210.pdf).

Canadian Nurses Association. (2007). Position statement: Advanced nursing practice. (http://www2.cna-aiic.ca/CNA/documents/pdf/publications/PS60_Advanced_Nursing_Practice_2007_e.pdf).

Canadian Nurses Association. (2008). Advanced nursing practice: A national framework. (http://www2.cna-aiic.ca/CNA/documents/pdf/publications/ANP_National_Framework_e.pdf).

Canadian Nurses Association. (2009). Position statement: The nurse practitioner. (http://www2.cna-aiic.ca/CNA/documents/pdf/publications/PS_Nurse_Practitioner_e.pdf)

Canadian Nurses Association. (2009). CNA position on clinical nurse specialist. (http://www2.cna-aiic.ca/CNA/documents/pdf/publications/PS104_Clinical_Nurse_Specialist_e.pdf).

Carron, R., & Cumbie, S. A. (2011). Development of a conceptual nursing model for the implementation of spiritual care in adult primary healthcare settings by nurse practitioners. *Journal of the American Academy of Nurse Practitioners, 23,* 552–560. doi: 10.1111/j.1745-7599.2011.00633.x

Chang, A. M., Gardner, G. E., Duffield, C., & Ramis, M. (2010). A Delphi study to validate an Advanced Practice Nursing tool. *Journal of Advanced Nursing, 66,* 2320–2330. doi: 10.1111/j.1365-2648.2010.05367.x

Christensen, M. (2009). Advancing practice in critical care: A model of knowledge integration. *Nursing in Critical Care, 14,* 86–94. doi: 10.1111/j.1478-5153.2008.00318.x

Christensen, M. (2011). Advancing nursing practice: Redefining the theoretical and practical integration of knowledge. *Journal of Clinical Nursing, 20,* 873–881. doi: 10.1111/j.1365-2702.2010.03392.x

Council on Accreditation of Nurse Anesthesia Educational Programs. (2012a). *Standards for accreditation of nurse anesthesia educational programs.* Park Ridge, IL: Author. http://home.coa.us.com/accreditation/Documents/Standards%20for%20Accreditation%20of%20Nurse%20Anesthesia%20Education%20Programs.pdf Accessed November 3, 2012.

Council on Accreditation Standards Revision Task Force. (2012b). *Standards for accreditation of nurse anesthesia education programs: Practice Doctorate (Draft 1, February 2012).* Park Ridge, IL: Council on Accreditation of Nurse Anesthesia Educcational Programs.

Curley, M. A. Q. (1998). Patient-nurse synergy: Optimizing patients' outcomes. *American Journal of Critical Care, 7,* 64–72.

DiCenso, R., Martin Misener, D., Bryant Lukosius, I., Bourgeault, K., Kilpatrick, F., Donald, S., et al. (2010). Advanced practice nursing in Canada: Overview of a decision support synthesis. *Nursing Leadership, 23*(special Issue), 15–34.

Doessel, D., & Marshall, J. (1985). A rehabilitation of health outcomes in quality assessment. *Social Science and Medicine, 21,* 1319–1328.

Dreher, H. M., & Smith Glasgow, M. E. (2011). Global perspectives on the professional doctorate. *International*

Journal of Nursing Studies, 48, 403–408. doi: 10.1016/j.ijnurstu.2010.09.003

Dunphy, L. M., & Winland-Brown, J. E. (1998). The circle of caring: A transformative model of advanced practice nursing. *Clinical Excellence for Nurse Practitioners, 2,* 241–247.

Dunphy, L. M., Winland-Brown, J. E., Porter, B. O., Thomas, D. J., & Gallagher. L. M. (2011). Primary care in the twenty-first century: A Circle of Caring. In L. M. Dunphy, J. E. Winland-Brown, B. O. Porter, & D. J. Thomas (Eds.), *Primary care: The art and science of advanced practice nursing* (3rd ed., pp. 3–18). Philadelphia: F. A. Davis.

Dunphy, L. M., Winland-Brown, J. E., Porter, B. O., & Thomas, D. J. (Eds.). (2011). *Primary care: The art and science of advanced practice nursing* (3rd ed.). Philadelphia: F. A. Davis.

Fagerström, L. (2009). Developing the scope of practice and education for advanced practice nurses in Finland. *International Nursing Review, 56,* 269–272. doi: 10.1111/j.1466-7657.2008.00673.x

Fawcett, J. (2005). *Contemporary nursing knowledge: Analysis and evaluation of nursing models and theories* (2nd ed.). Philadelphia: F. A. Davis.

Fawcett, J., & Graham, I. (2005). Advanced practice nursing: Continuation of the dialogue. *Nursing Science Quarterly, 18,* 37–41.

Fawcett, J., Newman, D., & McAllister, M. (2004). Advanced practice nursing and conceptual models of nursing. *Nursing Science Quarterly, 17,* 135–138.

Fenton, M. V. (1985). Identifying competencies of clinical nurse specialists. *Journal of Nursing Administration, 15,* 31–37.

Fenton, M. V., & Brykczynski, K. A. (1993). Qualitative distinctions and similarities in the practice of clinical nurse specialists and nurse practitioners. *Journal of Professional Nursing, 9,* 313–326.

Gardner, G., Chang, A., & Duffield, C. (2007). Making nursing work: Breaking through the role confusion of advanced practice nursing. *Journal of Advanced Nursing, 57,* 382–391. doi: 10.1111/j.1365-2648.2007.04114.x

Gardner, G., Gardner, A., Middleton, S., Della, P., Kain, V., & Doubrovsky, A. (2010). The work of nurse practitioners. *Journal of Advanced Nursing, 66,* 2160–2169. doi: 10.1111/j.1365-2648.2010.05379.x

Hamric, A. B. (1996). A definition of advanced practice nursing. In A. B. Hamric, J. A. Spross, & C. M. Hanson (Eds.), *Advanced nursing practice: An integrative approach* (pp. 25–41). Philadelphia: WB Saunders.

Hamric, A. B. (2009). A definition of advanced practice nursing. In A. B. Hamric, J. A. Spross, & C. M. Hanson (Eds.), *Advanced nursing practice: An integrative approach* (4th ed., pp.75–94). St. Louis: Saunders Elsevier.

Hamric, A. B., & Spross, J. A. (1983). A model for future clinical specialist practice. In A. B. Hamric & J. A. Spross (Eds.), *The clinical nurse specialist in theory and practice* (pp. 291–306). New York: Grune & Stratton.

Hamric, A. B., & Spross, J. A. (1989). *The clinical nurse specialist in theory and practice* (2nd ed.). Philadelphia: WB Saunders.

Hathaway, D., Jacob, S., Stegbauer, C., Thompson, C., & Graff, C. (2006). The practice doctorate: Perspectives of early adopters. *Journal of Nursing Education, 45,* 487–496.

Hawkins, R., & Nezat, G. (2009). Doctoral education: Which degree to pursue? *AANA Journal, 77,* 92–96.

Health Professions Networks, Nursing and Midwifery, & Human Resources for Health. (2010). Framework for action on interprofessional education and collaborative practice. (http://whqlibdoc.who.int/hq/2010/WHO_HRH_HPN_10.3_eng.pdf).

Institute of Medicine. (2011). *The future of nursing: Leading change, advancing health.* Washington, DC: National Academies Press.

Interprofessional Education Collaborative Expert Panel. (2011). *Core competencies for interprofessional collaborative practice: Report of an expert panel.* Washington, DC: Interprofessional Education Collaborative.

International Council of Nurses. (2009). Fact sheet: Nurse practitioner/advanced practice nurse: Definition and characteristics (http://www.icn.ch/images/stories/documents/publications/fact_sheets/1b_FS-NP_APN.pdf).

Irvin-Lazorko, P. A. (2011). I am the doctor: Conflicts and tensions of a professional doctorate as a labour market qualification. (http://wblearning-ejournal.com/currentIssue/E3007%20rtb.pdf).

Karnick, P. M. (2011). Theory and advanced practice nursing. *Nursing Science Quarterly, 24,* 118–119. doi: 10.1177/0894318411399470

Lewandowski, W., & Adamle, K. (2009). Substantive areas of clinical nurse specialist practice: A comprehensive review of the literature. *Clinical Nurse Specialist: The Journal for Advanced Nursing Practice, 23,* 73–92. doi: 10.1097/NUR.0b013e31819971d0

MacDonald, J., Herbert, R., & Thibeault, C. (2006). Advanced practice nursing: Unification through a common identity. *Journal of Professional Nursing, 3,* 172–179.

Mahler, A. (2010). The clinical nurse spcialist role in developing a geropalliative model of care. *CNS: The Journal for Advanced Nursing Practice, 24,* 18–23.

Mantzoukas, S., & Watkinson, S. (2007). Review of advanced nursing practice: The international literature and developing the generic features. *Journal of Clinical Nursing, 16,* 28–37.

McAiney, C. A., Haughton, D., Jennings, J., Farr, D., Hillier, L., & Morden, P. (2008). A unique practice model for Nurse Practitioners in long-term care homes. *Journal of Advanced Nursing, 62,* 562–571. doi: 10.1111/j.1365-2648.2008.04628.x

McKnight, S. (2011). Risk assessment in the electronic age: Application of the Circle of Caring Model (ojni.org/issues/?p=911).

McMurray, R. (2011). The struggle to professionalize: An ethnographic account of the occupational position of Advanced Nurse Practitioners. *Human Relations, 64,* 801–822. doi: 10.1177/0018726710387949

Mick, D., & Ackerman, M. (2000). Advanced practice nursing role delineation in acute and critical care: Application of the Strong Model of advanced practice. *Heart & Lung, 29,* 210–221.

Musker, K. P. (2011). Nursing theory-based independent nursing practice: A personal experience of closing the theory-practice gap. *Advances in Nursing Science January March, 34,* 67–77.

National Association of Clinical Nurse Specialists (NACNS). (2004). *Statement on clinical nurse specialist practice and education* (2nd ed.). Harrisburg, PA: Author.

National Association of Clinical Nurse Specialists. (2009a). Position statement on the nursing practice doctorate. (http://www.nacns.org/docs/PositionOnNursingPracticeDoctorate.pdf).

National Association of Clinical Nurse Specialists' Doctoral Competency Task Force. (2009b). Core practice doctorate clinical nurse specialist (CNS) competencies. (http://www.nacns.org/docs/CorePracticeDoctorate.pdf).

National Association of Clinical Nurse Specialists/National CNS Competency Task Force. (2010). Clinical nurse specialist core competencies: Executive summary 2006-2008. (http://www.nacns.org/docs/CNSCoreCompetenciesBroch.pdf).

National Association of Clinical Nurse Specialists. (2012). National Association of Clinical Nurse Specialists' Statement on the APRN Consensus Model Implementation. (http://www.nacns.org/docs/NACNSConsensusModel.pdf).

National Council of State Boards of Nursing (NCSBN). (2006). The future regulation of advanced practice nurses. (http://www.ncsbn.org/Draft_APRN_Vision_Paper.pdf).

National Council of State Boards of Nursing (NCSBN). (2012). APRN Consensus Model toolkit. (https://www.ncsbn.org/2276.htm).

National Organization of Nurse Practitioner Faculties. (2011). Nurse practitioner entry level competencies. (http://www.nonpf.com/associations/10789/files/IntegratedNPCoreCompsFINALApril2011.pdf).

National Organization of Nurse Practitioner Faculties. (2012). Nurse practitioner entry level competencies. (http://www.nonpf.com/associations/10789/files/NPCoreCompetenciesFinal2012.pdf).

Naylor, M. D., Aiken, L. H., Kurtzman, E. T., Olds, D. M., & Hirschman, K. B. (2011). The importance of transitional care in achieving health reform. *Health Affairs*, *30*, 746–754. doi:10.1377/hlthaff.2011.0041

Newcomb, P. (2010). Using symptom management theory to explain how nurse practitioners care for children with asthma. *Journal of Theory Construction & Testing*, *14*, 40–44.

Oberle, K., & Allen, M. (2001). The nature of advanced practice nursing. *Nursing Outlook*, *49*, 148–153.

Palardy, L. G., & March, A. L. (2011). The Circle of Caring Model: Medication adherence in cardiac transplant patients. *Nursing Science Quarterly*, *24*, 120–125. doi: 10.1177/0894318411399463

Partiprajak, S., Hanucharurnkul, S., Piaseu, N., Brooten, D., & Nityasuddhi, D. (2011). Outcomes of an advanced practice nurse-led type 2 diabetes support group. *Pacific Rim International Journal of Nursing Research*, *15*(4), 288–304.

Patient Protection and Affordable Care Act (PPACA) (2010). Pub. L. No. 111-148. 124 Stat. 119.

Perraud, S., Delaney, K. R., Carlson, S. L., Johnson, M. E., Shephard, R., & Paun, O. (2006). Advanced practice psychiatric mental health nursing, finding our core: the therapeutic relationship in the 21st century. *Perspectives in Psychiatric Care*, *42*, 215–226.

Price, M. J., Martin, A. C., Newberry, Y. G., Zimmer, P. A., Brykczynski, K. A., & Warren, B. (1992). Developing national guidelines for nurse practitioner education: An overview of the product and the process. *Journal of Nursing Education*, *31*, 10–15.

Pringle, D. (Ed.). (2010). Special issue on advanced practice nursing in Canada. *Canadian Journal of Nursing Leadership*, *23*, 1–259.

Reeves, S., Goldman, J., Gilbert, J., Tepper, J., Silver, I., Suter, E., et al. (2011). A scoping review to improve conceptual clarity of interprofessional interventions. *Journal of Interprofessional Care*, *25*, 167–174. doi: 10.3109/13561820.2010.529960

Scarpa, R., & Connelly, P. E. (2011). Innovations in performance assessment: A criterion-based performance assessment for advanced practice nurses using a synergistic theoretical nursing framework. *Nursing Administration Quarterly 35*, 164–173. doi: 10.1097/NAQ.0b013e31820fface

Shuler, P. A. (2000). Evaluating student services provided by school-based health centers: Applying the Shuler Nurse Practitioner practice model. *Journal of School Health*, *70*, 348–352.

Shuler, P. A., & Davis, J. E. (1993a). The Shuler nurse practitioner practice model: A theoretical framework for nurse practitioner clinicians, educators, and researchers, Part 1. *Journal of the American Academy of Nurse Practitioners*, *5*, 11–18.

Shuler, P. A., & Davis, J. E. (1993b). The Shuler nurse practitioner practice model: Clinical application, Part 2. *Journal of the American Academy of Nurse Practitioners*, *5*, 73–88.

Shuler, P. A., Huebscher, R., & Hallock, J. (2001). Providing wholistic health care for the elderly: Utilization of the Shuler nurse practitioner practice model. *Journal of the American Academy of Nurse Practitioners*, *13*, 297–303.

Skalla, K. A., & Caron, P. A. (2008). Leadership & professional development. Building a collaborative hematology/oncology advanced nursing practice: part I. *Oncology Nursing Forum*, *35*, 29–32. doi: 10.1188/08.onf.29-32

Smith, A. R. (2006). Using the Synergy Model to provide spiritual nursing care in critical care settings. *Critical Care Nurse*, *26*(4), 41–47.

Spross, J. A. (2009). Expert coaching and guidance. In A. B. Hamric, J. A. Spross, & C. M. Hanson (Eds.), *Advanced nursing practice: An integrative approach* (4th ed., pp. 159–190). St. Louis: Saunders Elsevier.

Spross, J. A., Hamric, A. B., Hall, G., Minarik, P., Sparacino, P. S. A., & Stanley, J. M. (2004). *Working statement comparing the clinical nurse leader and clinical nurse specialist roles: Similarities, differences, and complementarities*. Washington, DC: American Association of Colleges of Nursing.

Stanley, J. M., Werner, K. E., & Apple, K. (2009). Positioning advanced practice registered nurses for health care reform: Consensus on APRN regulation. *Journal of Professional Nursing*, *25*, 340–348. doi: 10.1016/j.profnurs.2009.10.001

Styles, M. (1998). An international perspective: APN credentialing. *Advanced Practice Nursing Quarterly*, *4*(3), 1–5.

Styles, M. M., & Lewis, C. (2000). Conceptualizations of advanced nursing practice. In A. B. Hamric, J. A. Spross, & C. M. Hanson (Eds.), *Advanced nursing practice: An integrative approach* (2nd ed., pp. 25–41). Philadelphia: WB Saunders.

Thomas, J. (2011). The Circle of Caring Model for neonatal transport. *Neonatal Network*, *30*(1), 14–20.

Thoun, D. S. (2011). Specialty and advanced practice nursing: Discerning the differences. *Nursing Science Quarterly*, *24*, 216–222. doi: 10.1177/0894318411409436

Validation Panel of the National Association of Clinical Nurse Specialists. (2011). Criteria for the evaluation of clinical nurse specialist, master's, practice doctorate, and post-graduate certificate educational programs. (http://www.nacns.org/docs/CNSEducationCriteria.pdf).

Wong, F. K. Y., Peng, G., Kan, E. C., Li, Y., Lau, A., Zhang, L., et al. (2009). Description and evaluation of an initiative to develop advanced practice nurses in mainland China. *Nurse Education Today*, 30, 344–349. doi: 10.1016/j.nedt.2009.09.004

Zimmer, P., Brykczynski, K., Martin, A., Newberry, Y., Price, M., & Warren, B. (1990). *National guidelines for nurse practitioner education*. Seattle: National Organization of Nurse Practitioner Faculties.

A Definition of Advanced Practice Nursing

Ann B. Hamric

CONTENTS

This chapter considers two central questions that provide the foundation for this text:

- Why is it important to define carefully and clearly what is meant by the term *advanced practice nursing?*
- What distinguishes the practices of advanced practice nurses (APNs) from those of other nurses and other health care providers?

Advanced practice nursing is considered here as a concept, not a role, a set of skills, or a substitution for physicians. Rather, it is a powerful idea, the origins of which date back more than a century. Such a conceptual definition provides a stable core understanding for all APN roles (see Chapter 2), it promotes consistency in practice that can aid others in understanding what this level of nursing entails, and it promotes the achievement of value-added patient outcomes and improvement in health care delivery processes. Advanced practice nursing is a relatively new concept in nursing's evolution (see Chapter 1). Although debates and dissention are necessary and even healthy in forging consensus, ultimately the profession must agree on the key issues of definition, education, credentialing, and practice. This agreement is critically important to the survival, much less the growth, of advanced practice nursing. In this chapter, advanced practice nursing is defined and the scope of practice of APNs is discussed. Various APN roles are

differentiated and key factors influencing advanced practice in health care environments are identified. The importance of a common and unified understanding of the distinguishing characteristics of advanced practice nursing is emphasized.

The advanced practice of nursing builds on the foundation and core values of the nursing discipline. APN roles do not stand apart from nursing; they do not represent a separate profession, although references to "the nurse practitioner (NP) profession," for example, are seen in the literature. It is the nursing core that contributes to the distinctiveness seen in APN practices. According to the American Nurses Association (ANA, 2010), contemporary nursing practice has seven essential features:

… provision of a caring relationship that facilitates health and healing; attention to the range of human experiences and responses to health and illness within the physical and social environments; integration of assessment data with knowledge gained from an appreciation of the patient or the group; application of scientific knowledge to the processes of diagnosis and treatment through the use of judgment and critical thinking; advancement of professional nursing knowledge through scholarly inquiry; influence on social and public policy to promote social justice; and, assurance of safe, quality, and evidence-based practice (p. 9).

These characteristics are equally essential for advanced practice nursing. Core values that guide nurses in practice include advocating for patients, respecting patient and family values and informed choices, viewing individuals holistically within their environments, communities, and cultural traditions, and maintaining a focus on disease prevention, health restoration, and health promotion (ANA, 2001; Creasia & Friberg, 2011; Hood, 2010). These core professional values also inform the central perspective of advanced practice nursing.

Efforts to standardize the definition of advanced practice nursing have been ongoing since the 1990s (American Association of Colleges of Nursing [AACN], 1995, 2006; ANA, 1995, 2003, 2010; Hamric, 1996, 2000, 2005, 2009; National Council of State Boards of Nursing [NCSBN], 1993, 2002, 2008). However, full clarity regarding advanced practice nursing has not yet been achieved, even as this level of nursing practice spreads around the globe. The growing international use of APNs with differing understandings in various countries has only complicated the picture (see Chapter 6). Different interpretations of advanced practice (AACN, 2006; ANA, 2005), debates about who is and is not an APN, and discrepancies in educational preparation for APNs remain issues for the international community, even as they are being standardized within countries.

In spite of this lack of clarity (Ruel and Motyka, 2009; Pearson, 2011), emerging consensus on key features of the concept is increasingly evident. The definition that I have developed has been relatively stable throughout the five editions of this book. The primary criteria used in this definition are now standard elements used in the United States and, increasingly, elsewhere to regulate APNs. Similarly, consensus is growing in understanding advanced practice nursing in terms of core competencies. Even authors who deny a clear understanding of the concept propose competencies—variously called attributes, components, or domains—that are generally consistent with, although not always as complete as, the competencies proposed here.

It is important to distinguish the conceptual definition of advanced practice nursing from regulatory requirements for any APN role (in the regulatory arena, the alternative term *advanced practice registered nurse* [APRN] is most commonly used; NCSBN, 2008). Of necessity, regulatory understandings focus on the more basic and measurable primary criteria of graduate educational preparation, advanced certification in a particular population focus, and practice in one of the four common APN roles: nurse practitioner (NP), clinical nurse specialist (CNS), certified registered nurse anesthetist (CRNA), and certified nurse-midwife (CNM). This approach is clearly seen in the APRN definition outlined in the Consensus Model

(NCSBN, 2008) and has been very helpful and influential in standardizing state requirements for APRN licensure across the United States. Although necessary for regulation, however, this approach does not constitute an adequate understanding of advanced practice nursing. Limiting the profession's understanding of advanced practice nursing to regulatory definitions can lead to a reductionist approach that results in a focus on a set of concrete skills and activities, such as diagnostic acumen or prescriptive authority. Understanding the advanced practice of the nursing discipline requires a definition that encompasses broad areas of skilled performance (the competency approach). As Chapter 2 notes, conceptual models and definitions are also useful for providing a robust framework for graduate APN curricula and for building an APN professional role identity.

Distinguishing Between Specialization and Advanced Practice Nursing

Before the definition of advanced practice nursing can be explored, it is important to distinguish between specialization in nursing and advanced practice nursing. Specialization involves the development of expanded knowledge and skills in a selected area within the discipline of nursing. All nurses with extensive experience in a particular area of practice (e.g., pediatric nursing, trauma nursing) are specialized in this sense. As the profession has advanced and responded to changes in health care, specialization and the need for specialty knowledge have increased. Thus, few nurses are generalists in the true sense of the word (Kitzman, 1989). Although family NPs traditionally represented themselves as generalists, they are specialists in the sense discussed here because they have specialized in one of the many facets of health care—namely, primary care. As Cockerham and Keeling note in Chapter 1, early specialization involved primarily on-the-job training or hospital-based training courses, and many nurses continue to develop specialty skills through practice experience and continuing education. Examples of currently evolving specialties include genetics nursing, forensic nursing, and clinical research nurse coordination. As specialties mature, they may develop graduate-level clinical preparation and incorporate the competencies of advanced practice nursing for their most advanced practitioners (Hanson & Hamric, 2003; also see Chapter 5); examples include critical care, oncology nursing, and palliative care nursing.

The nursing profession has responded in various ways to the increasing need for specialization in nursing practice. The creation of specialty organizations, such as the American Association of Critical-Care Nurses and the Oncology Nursing Society, has been one response.

The creation of APN roles—the CRNA and CNM roles early in nursing's evolution and the CNS and NP roles more recently—has been another response. A third response has been the development of specialized faculty, nursing researchers, and nursing administrators. Nurses in all these roles can be considered specialists in an area of nursing (e.g., education, research, administration); some of these roles may involve advanced education in a clinical specialty as well. However, they are not necessarily advanced practice nursing roles.

Advanced practice nursing includes specialization but also involves expansion and educational advancement (ANA, 1995, 2003; Cronenwett, 1995). As compared with basic nursing practice, APN practice is further characterized by the following: (1) acquisition of new practice knowledge and skills, particularly theoretical and evidence-based knowledge, some of which overlap the traditional boundaries of medicine; (2) significant role autonomy; (3) responsibility for health promotion in addition to the diagnosis and management of patient problems, including prescribing pharmacologic and non-pharmacologic interventions; (4) the greater complexity of clinical decision making and leadership in organizations and environments; and (5) specialization at the level of a particular APN role and population focus (ANA, 1996; 2003; NCSBN, 2008).

It is necessary to distinguish between specialization as understood in this chapter and the term *population focus*. The framers of the Consensus Model for APRN regulation were interested in licensing and regulating advanced practice nursing in two broad categories. The first was regulation at the level of role—CNS, NP, CRNA, or CNM. The second category was termed *population focus* and, although not explicitly defined, six population foci were identified: family and individual across the life span, adult-gerontology, pediatrics, neonatal, women's health and gender-related, and psychological and mental health. These foci are at different levels of specialization; for example, family and individual across the life span is broad, while neonatal is a subspecialty designation under the specialty of pediatrics. Therefore, this term is not synonymous with specialization and should not be understood in the same light. As the Consensus Model states (NCSBN, 2008):

> Education, certification, and licensure of an individual must be congruent in terms of role and population foci. APRNs may specialize but they cannot be licensed solely within a specialty area. In addition, specialties can provide depth in one's practice within the established population foci. Education and assessment strategies for specialty areas will be developed by the nursing profession, i.e., nursing organizations and special interest groups.

Education for a specialty can occur concurrently with APRN education required for licensure or through postgraduate education. Competence at the specialty level will not be assessed or regulated by boards of nursing but rather by the professional organizations.

Distinguishing Between Advanced Nursing Practice and Advanced Practice Nursing

The terms *advanced practice nursing* and *advanced nursing practice* have distinct definitions and cannot be seen as interchangeable. In particular, recent definitions of advanced nursing practice do not clarify the clinically focused nature of advanced practice nursing. For example, ANA's 2010 edition of *Nursing's Social Policy Statement* defines the term *advanced nursing practice* as "characterized by the integration and application of a broad range of theoretical and evidence-based knowledge that occurs as part of graduate nursing education." This broad definition has evolved from the American Association of Colleges of Nursing's "Position Statement on the Practice Doctorate in Nursing" (AACN, 2004), which recommended doctoral-level educational preparation for individuals at the most advanced level of nursing practice. The Doctor of Nursing Practice (DNP) position statement (AACN, 2004) advanced a broad definition of advanced nursing practice as the following:

> … any form of nursing intervention that influences health care outcomes for individuals or populations, including the direct care of individual patients, management of care for individuals and populations, administration of nursing and health care organizations, and the development and implementation of health policy.

A definition this broad goes beyond advanced practice nursing to include other advanced specialties not involved in providing direct clinical care to patients, such as administration, policy, informatics, and public health. One reason for such a broad definition was the desire to have the DNP degree be available to nurses practicing at the highest level in many varied specialties, not only those in APN roles. A decision was reached by the original Task Force (AACN, 2004) that the DNP degree was not to be a clinical doctorate, as was advocated in early discussions (Mundinger, Cook, Lenz, et al., 2000) but, rather, a practice doctorate in an expansive understanding of the term *practice*. The AACN's *The Essentials of Doctoral Education for Advanced Nursing Practice* (2006) distinguishes between roles with an aggregate, systems, and organizational focus (advanced specialties) and roles with a direct clinical practice focus (APN roles of CNS, NP, CRNA, and CNM), while recognizing that these two groups share some essential competencies. It is important to understand that the DNP is a *degree,* much as is the Master's of Science in Nursing (MSN), and not a *role;* DNP graduates can assume varied roles, depending on the specialty focus of their program. Some of these roles are not APN roles as advanced practice nursing is defined here.

The end result of this work requires a distinction to be made between the terms *advanced nursing practice* and *advanced practice nursing.* Advanced practice nursing is a concept that applies to nurses who provide direct patient care to individual patients and families. As a consequence, APN roles involve expanded clinical skills and abilities and require a different level of regulation than non-APN roles. This text focuses on advanced practice nursing and the varied roles of APNs. Graduate programs that prepare students for APN roles will have different curricula from those preparing students for administration, informatics, or other specialties that do not have a direct practice component (AACN, 2006).

Defining Advanced Practice Nursing

As noted, the concept of advanced practice nursing continues to be defined in various ways in the nursing literature. The *Cumulative Index to Nursing and Allied Health Literature* defines advanced practice broadly as anything beyond the staff nurse role: "The performance of additional acts by registered nurses who have gained added knowledge and skills through post-basic education and clinical experience..." (Advanced Nursing Practice, 2012). As noted with the DNP definition, a definition this broad incorporates many specialized nursing roles, not all of which should be considered as advanced practice nursing.

Advanced practice nursing is often defined as a constellation of four roles: the NP, CNS, CNM, and CRNA (NCSBN, 2002, 2008; Stanley, 2011). For example, the ANA's *Scope and Standards of Practice,* Third Edition (2010) does not provide a definition of advanced practice nursing but uses a regulatory definition of APRNs:

> A nurse who has completed an accredited graduate-level education program preparing her or him for the role of certified nurse practitioner, certified registered nurse anesthetist, certified nurse-midwife, or clinical nurse specialist; has passed a national certification examination that measures the APRN role and population-focused competencies; maintains continued competence as evidenced by recertification; and is licensed to practice as an APRN.

In the past, some authors discussed advanced practice nursing only in terms of selected roles such as NP and CNS (Lindeke, Canedy, & Kay, 1997; Rasch & Frauman,

1996) or the NP role exclusively (Hickey, Ouimette, & Venegoni, 2000; Mundinger, 1994). Defining advanced practice nursing in terms of particular roles limits the concept and denies the reality that some nurses in these four APN roles are not using the core competencies of advanced practice nursing in their practice. These definitions are also limiting because they do not incorporate evolving APN roles. Thus, although such role-based definitions are useful for regulatory purposes, it is preferable to define and clarify advanced practice nursing as a concept without reference to particular roles.

Core Definition of Advanced Practice Nursing

The definition proposed in this chapter builds on and extends the understanding of advanced practice nursing proposed in the first four editions of this text. Important assertions of this discussion are as follows:

- Advanced practice nursing is a function of educational and practice preparation and a constellation of primary criteria and core competencies.
- Direct clinical practice is the central competency of any APN role and informs all the other competencies.
- All APNs share the same core criteria and competencies, although the actual clinical skill set varies, depending on the needs of the APN's specialty patient population.

A definition should also clarify the critical point that advanced practice nursing involves advanced nursing knowledge and skills; it is not a medical practice, although APNs perform expanded medical therapeutics in many roles. Throughout nursing's history, nurses have assumed medical roles. For example, common nursing tasks such as blood pressure measurement and administration of chemotherapeutic agents were once performed exclusively by physicians. When APNs begin to transfer new skills or interventions into their repertoire, they become nursing skills, informed by the clinical practice values of the profession.

Actual practices differ significantly based on the particular role adopted, specialty practiced, and organizational framework within which the role is performed. In spite of the need to keep job descriptions and job titles distinct in practice settings, it is critical that the public's acceptance of advanced practice nursing be enhanced and confusion decreased. As Safriet (1993, 1998) noted, nursing's future depends on reaching consensus on titles and consistent preparation for title holders. The nursing profession must be clear, concrete, and consistent about APN titles and their functions in discussions with nursing's larger constituencies: consumers, other health care professionals, health care administrators, and health care policymakers.

Conceptual Definition

> Advanced practice nursing is the patient-focused application of an expanded range of competencies to improve health outcomes for patients and populations in a specialized clinical area of the larger discipline of nursing.[1]

The term *competencies* refers to a broad area of skillful performance; seven core competencies combine to distinguish nursing practice at this level. Competencies include activities undertaken as part of delivering advanced nursing care directly to patients. Some competencies are processes that APNs use in all dimensions of their practice, such as collaboration and leadership. At this stage of the development of the nursing discipline, competencies may be based in theory, practice, or research. Although the discipline is expanding its research-based evidence to guide practice, an expanded ability to use theory also is a key distinguishing feature of advanced practice nursing. In addition, a strong experiential component is necessary to develop the competencies and clinical practice expertise that characterize APN practice. Graduate education and in-depth clinical practice experience work together to develop the APN. The definition also emphasizes the patient-focused and specialized nature of advanced practice nursing. APNs expand their capability to provide and direct care, with the ultimate goal of improving patient and specialty population outcomes; this focus on outcome attainment is a central feature of advanced practice nursing and the main justification for differentiating this level of practice. Finally, the critical importance of ensuring that any type of advanced practice is grounded within the larger discipline of nursing is made explicit.

Certain activities of APN practice overlap with those performed by physicians and other health care professionals. However, the experiential, theoretical, and philosophical perspectives of nursing make these activities advanced nursing practice when they are carried out by an APN. Advanced practice nursing further involves highly developed nursing skill in areas such as guidance and coaching, as well as the performance of select medical therapies. Particularly with regard to physician practice, the nursing profession needs to be clear that advanced practice nursing is embedded in the nursing discipline—

the advanced practice of nursing is not the junior practice of medicine.

Advanced practice nursing is further defined by a conceptual model integrating three primary criteria and seven core competencies, one of them central to the others. This discussion and the chapters in Part II isolate each of these core competencies to clarify them. The reader should recognize that this is only a heuristic device for clarifying the conceptualization of advanced practice nursing used in this text. In reality, these elements are integrated into an APN's practice; they are not separate and distinct features. The concentric circles in Figures 3-1 through 3-3 represent the seamless nature of this interweaving of elements. In addition, an APN's skills function synergistically to produce a whole that is greater than the sum of its parts. The essence of advanced practice nursing is found not only in the primary criteria and competencies demonstrated, but also in the synthesis of these elements into a unified composite practice that conforms to the conceptual definition just presented.

Primary Criteria

Certain criteria (or qualifications) must be met before a nurse can be considered an APN. Although these baseline criteria are not sufficient in and of themselves, they are necessary core elements of advanced practice nursing. The three primary criteria for advanced practice nursing are shown in Figure 3-1 and include an earned graduate degree with a concentration in an advanced practice nursing role and population focus, national certification at an advanced level, and a practice focused on patients and their families. As noted, these criteria are most often the ones used by states to regulate APN practice because they are objective and easily measured (see Chapter 21).

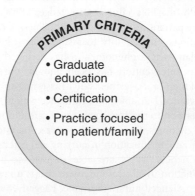

FIG 3-1 Primary criteria of advanced practice nursing.

---

[1]The term *patient* is intended to be used interchangeably with *individual* and *client*.

Graduate Education

First, the APN must possess an *earned graduate degree with a concentration in an APN role.* This graduate degree may be a master's or a DNP. Advanced practice students acquire specialized knowledge and skills through study and supervised practice at the graduate level. Curricular content includes theories and research findings relevant to the core of a particular advanced nursing role, population focus, and relevant specialty. For example, a CNS interested in palliative care will need coursework in CNS role competencies, the adult population focus, and the palliative care specialty. Because APNs assess, manage, and evaluate patients at the most independent level of clinical nursing practice, all APN curricula contain specific courses in advanced health and physical assessment, advanced pathophysiology, and advanced pharmacology (the so-called three Ps; AACN, 1995, 2006, 2011). Expansion of practice skills is acquired through faculty-supervised clinical experience, with master's programs requiring a minimum of 500 clinical hours and DNP programs requiring 1000 hours. As noted earlier in the ANA definition, there is consensus that a master's education in nursing is a baseline requirement for advanced practice nursing (nurse-midwifery was the latest APN specialty to agree to this requirement; see ACNM, 2009).

Why is graduate educational preparation necessary for advanced practice nursing? Graduate education is a more efficient and standardized way to inculcate the complex competencies of APN-level practice than nursing's traditional on the job or apprentice training programs (see Chapter 5). As the knowledge base within specialties has grown, so too has the need for formal education at the graduate level. In particular, the skills necessary for evidence-based practice (EBP) and the theory base required for advanced practice nursing mandate education at the graduate level.

Some of the differences between basic and advanced practice in nursing are apparent in the following: the range and depth of APNs' clinical knowledge; APNs' ability to anticipate patient responses to health, illness, and nursing interventions; their ability to analyze clinical situations and explain why a phenomenon has occurred or why a particular intervention has been chosen; the reflective nature of their practice; their skill in assessing and addressing nonclinical variables that influence patient care; and their attention to the consequences of care and improving patient outcomes. Because of the interaction and integration of graduate education in nursing and extensive clinical experience, APNs are able to exercise a level of discrimination in clinical judgment that is unavailable to other experienced nurses (Spross & Baggerly, 1989).

Professionally, requiring at least master's-level preparation is important to create parity among APN roles so that all can move forward together in addressing policy-making and regulatory issues. This parity advances the profession's standards and ensures more uniform credentialing mechanisms. Moving toward a doctoral-level educational expectation may also enhance nursing's image and credibility with other disciplines. Decisions by other health care providers, such as pharmacists, physical therapists, and occupational therapists, to require doctoral preparation for entry into their professions have provided compelling support for nursing to establish the practice doctorate for APNs to achieve parity with these disciplines (AACN, 2006). Nursing has a particular need to achieve greater credibility with medicine. Organized medicine has historically been eager to point to nursing's internal differences in APN education as evidence that APNs are inferior providers.

The new clinical nurse leader (CNL) role represents a new and different understanding of the master's credential. Historically, master's education in nursing was, by definition, specialized education (see Chapter 1). However, the master's-prepared CNL is described as a generalist, a staff nurse with expanded leadership skills at the point of care (AACN, 2003). AACN's recent revision of *The Essentials of Master's Education in Nursing* (2011) was developed for this generalist practice, whereas the DNP *Essentials* (2008) are aligned more with the understanding of advanced practice nursing described here. Even though CNLs have expanded leadership skills and graduate-level education, they are clearly not APNs. APN graduate education is highly specialized and involves preparation for an expanded scope of practice, neither of which characterizes CNL education. The existence of generalist and APN specialty master's programs has the potential to confuse consumers, institutions, and nurses alike; it is incumbent on educational programs to differentiate clearly the curricula for generalist CNL versus specialist APN roles to avoid role confusion for these graduates.

AACN's proposed 2015 deadline for APNs to be prepared at the DNP level continues to be debated (Cronenwett, Dracup, Grey, et al., 2011) and undoubtedly will not be realized, even though DNP programs are increasing dramatically in number (from 20 programs in 2006 to 182 by 2011 [http://www.aacn.nche.edu/membership/members-only/presentations/2012/12doctoral/Potempa-Doc-Programs.pdf]. As a result, master's-level programs that prepare APNs are continuing.

Certification

The second primary criterion is professional certification for practice at an advanced level within a clinical population focus. The continuing growth of specialization has dramatically increased the amount of knowledge and experience required to practice safely in modern health care settings. National certification examinations have been developed by specialty organizations at two levels. The first level that was developed tested the specialty knowledge of experienced nurses and not knowledge at the advanced level of practice. More recently, organizations have developed APN-specific certification examinations in a specialty. CNM and CRNA organizations were farsighted in developing certifying examinations for these roles early in their history (see Chapter 1). As regulatory groups, particularly state boards of nursing, increasingly use the certification credential as a component of APRN licensure, the certification landscape continues to change. As noted, the Consensus Model has mandated regulation of APRNs at a role and population focus level (NCSBN, 2008), accelerating the development of more broad based APN certification examinations.

National certification at an advanced practice level is an important primary criterion for advanced practice nursing. Continuing variability in graduate curricula make sole reliance on the criterion of graduate education insufficient to protect the public. Although standardization in educational requirements for each APN role has improved over the last decade, it is difficult to argue that graduate education alone can provide sufficient evidence of competence for regulatory purposes. National certification examinations provide a consistent standard that must be met by each APN to demonstrate beginning competency for an advanced level of practice in his or her role. Finally, certification enhances title recognition in the regulatory arena, which promotes the visibility of advanced practice nursing and enhances the public's access to APN services.

Table 3-1 lists the numbers of APNs and numbers certified in the United States from 2000 through 2008. Certification percentages have increased for all APN groups except CNSs, with CRNAs and CNMs having the consistently highest percentage of certified practitioners.

It is critically important that certifying organizations work to clarify the certification credential as appropriate only for currently practicing APNs. Given the centrality of the direct clinical practice component to the definition of advanced practice nursing, certification examinations must establish a significant number of hours of clinical practice as a requirement for maintaining APN certification. Some faculty and nursing leaders who do not maintain a direct clinical practice component in their positions have been allowed to sit for certification examinations and represent themselves as APNs. Statements such as "Once a CNS, always a CNS," which are heard with NPs and CNMs as well, perpetuate the mistaken notion that an APN title is a professional attribute rather than a practice role. Such a misunderstanding is confusing inside and outside of nursing; by definition, these individuals are no longer APNs.

As noted, the Consensus Model focuses regulatory efforts on these broad role and population foci rather than on particular specialties, although some specialties are represented (e.g., neonatal NPs). This decision not to recognize established APN certification examinations in specialties such as oncology or critical care for state licensure purposes has challenged the CNS role more than other APN specialties. The American Nurses' Credentialing Center (ANCC) has become the dominant certifying organization for State Board of Nursing–supported CNS examinations; the number of examination options for CNSs is decreasing as the Consensus Model is being implemented (see the ANCC website for a listing of currently available CNS examinations—www. nursecredentialing.org). Even though APRN regulation is becoming more standardized, a need exists for the continued development of specialty examinations at the advanced practice nursing level, particularly for CNS specialties; as it stands now, many CNSs have to take the broad-based certification examination recognized by their state in addition to an APN-level specialty certification examination necessary for their practice. Another unintended consequence of the limitations set by recognizing only six population foci is that educational programs have closed CNS concentrations given the lack of a sanctioned certification examination in the specialty. Although other factors also influenced these decisions, not recognizing specialty examinations for regulatory purposes is a key factor in these closures.

The limited population foci sanctioned at present can be seen as a first step in standardizing regulation; the Consensus Model report notes the expectation that additional population foci will evolve. Even with these transitional issues, the Consensus Model represents an important standardization of APRN regulation and has helped cement the primary criterion of certification as a core regulatory requirement for APRN licensure.

Practice Focused on Patient and Family

The third primary criterion is a practice focused on patients and their families. As noted in describing DNP graduates, the AACN DNP Essentials Task Force differentiated APNs from other roles using this primary criterion. They noted two general role categories (AACN, 2006): "roles which specialize as an advanced practice nurse (APN) with a focus on care of individuals; and roles that specialize in practice at an aggregate, systems, or organizational level. This distinction is important as APNs face different licensure, regulatory, credentialing, liability, and reimbursement issues than those who practice at an aggregate, systems, or organizational level." This criterion does not imply that direct practice is the only activity that APNs undertake, however. APNs also educate others,

TABLE 3-1   Number of Advanced Practice Nurses in the United States

APN Category	2000*			2004†			2008‡		
	Total No.	Currently in Nursing (%)	Nationally Certified (%)	Total No.	Currently in Nursing (%)	Nationally Certified (%)	Total No.	Currently in Nursing (%)	Nationally Certified (%)
CRNA	29,844	85.7	84.4	32,523	89.6	95.3	34,821	91.5	90.9
CNM	9,232	85.7	88.4	13,684	89.3	93.7	15,328	84.3	89.7
CNS	54,374	87	36.5	57,832	85.1	44.7	42,400	84	39.7
NP	88,186	89	74	126,520	87.7	77.6	141,978	89.2	83.8
Blended CNS-NP preparation (not included in CNS or NP numbers)	14,654	95.7	73.4	14,689	93.4	Not reported	16,370	88.1	Not reported

*From U.S. Department of Health and Human Services (HHS), Division of Nursing. (2002). *The registered nurse population March 2000: Findings from the national sample survey of registered nurses.* Washington, DC: Author.
†From HHS, Division of Nursing. (2006). *The registered nurse population March 2004: Findings from the seventh national sample survey of registered nurses.* Washington, DC: Author.
‡From HHS, Division of Nursing. (2010). *The registered nurse population: Findings from the March 2008 national sample survey of registered nurses.* Washington, DC: Author.

participate in leadership activities, and serve as consultants (Brown, 1998); they understand and are involved in practice contexts to identify and effect needed system changes; and, they work to improve the health of their specialty populations (AACN, 2006). But to be considered an APN role, the patient/family direct practice focus must be primary.

Historically, APN roles have been associated with direct clinical care. Recent work is solidifying this understanding. The Consensus Model (NCSBN, 2008) has made clear that the provision of direct care to individuals as a significant component of their practice is *the* defining factor for all APRNs. The centrality of direct clinical practice is further reflected in the core competencies presented in the next section.

This requirement for a patient-focused practice puts some community health nurses in a gray area between advanced practice nursing and specialized practices of program development or consultation. Some APNs in community-based practices take a community view of their practice and consider the community to be their patient or client. Certainly, the broad perspective of the APN encompasses the community and society in which care is provided (AACN, 2006; Davies & Hughes, 1995); effecting positive outcomes for populations of patients is an important expectation for APNs in general. The National Organization of Nurse Practitioner Faculties (NONPF) has integrated community health concepts into NP education and considers them to be a core competency of NP practice (NONPF, 2000).

However, advanced practice nursing is focused on and realized at the level of clinical practice with patients and families. As long as APNs in community health practices maintain a direct clinical practice focused on patients and their families, in addition to program or consulting responsibilities, they are APNs by this definition. Community and public health specialists who do not have a patient-focused practice but focus on community assessment, monitoring community health status, and developing policies and program plans are more appropriately considered advanced specialty nurses rather than APNs (AACN, 2006; Hanson & Hamric, 2003). Community and public health nursing leaders have differentiated their specialty from this understanding of advanced practice nursing in two reports (ANA, 2005; Association of Community Health Nursing Educators Task Force on Community and Public Health Master's Level Preparation, 2000). The competencies listed for the community and public health specialty differ from the core APN competencies outlined here, particularly with regard to direct clinical practice. This specialty's movement away from the direct clinical practice requirement of advanced practice nursing is similarly reflected in the ANCC's change of the certification credential from community health CNS to advanced public health nurse (http://www.nursecredentialing.org/Certification/Nurse Specialties/AdvPublicHealth.html).

Why limit the definition of advanced practice nursing to roles that focus on clinical practice to patients and families? There are many reasons. Nursing is a practice profession. The nurse-patient interface is at the core of nursing practice; in the final analysis, the reason that the profession exists is to render nursing services to individuals in need of them. Clinical practice expertise in a given specialty develops from these nurse-patient encounters and lies at the heart of advanced practice nursing. In addition, ongoing direct clinical practice is necessary to maintain and develop an APN's expertise. Without regular immersion in practice, the cutting edge clinical acumen and expertise found in APN practices cannot be sustained. In addition, the knowledge base needed for APN roles differs from that for non-APN roles.

If every specialized role in nursing were considered advanced practice nursing, the term would become so broad as to lack meaning and explanatory value. Distinguishing between APN roles and other specialized roles in nursing can help clarify the concept of advanced practice nursing to consumers, other health care providers, and even other nurses. In addition, the monitoring and regulation of advanced practice nursing are increasingly important issues as APNs work toward more authority for their practices (see Chapter 21). If the definition of advanced practice nursing included nonclinical roles, development of sound regulatory mechanisms would be impossible.

It is critical to understand that this definition of advanced practice nursing is not a value statement but, rather, a differentiation of one group of nurses from other groups for the sake of clarity within and outside the profession. Some nurses with specialized skills in administration, research, and community health have viewed the direct practice requirement as a devaluing of their contributions. Some faculty who teach clinical nursing but do not themselves maintain an advanced clinical practice have also thought themselves to be disenfranchised because they are not considered APNs by virtue of this primary criterion. Perhaps this problem has been exacerbated with use of the term *advanced,* because this term can inadvertently imply that nurses who do not fit into the APN definition are not advanced (i.e., are not as well prepared or highly skilled as APNs).

The contention advanced in this text is that no value difference exists between nurses in non-APN specialties and APNs; both groups are equally important to the overall growth and strengthening of the profession. The profession must be able to differentiate its various roles without such differentiation being viewed as a disparagement of any one group. Thus, it is critical to understand that this definition of advanced practice nursing is not a value statement but a differentiation of one group of nurses from other groups for the sake of clarity within and outside the profession. We must be able to say what advanced practice nursing is not, as well as what it is, if we are to clarify the concept. As the ANA (1995) has noted, all nurses—whether their focus is clinical practice, educating students, conducting research, planning community programs, or leading nursing service organizations—are valuable and necessary to the integrity and growth of the larger profession. However, all nurses, particularly those with advanced degrees, are not the same, nor are they necessarily APNs. Historically, the profession has had difficulty differentiating itself and has struggled with the prevailing lay notion that "a nurse is a nurse is a nurse." This antiquated view does not match the reality of the health care arena, nor does it celebrate the diverse contributions of all the various nursing roles and specialties.

Seven Core Competencies of Advanced Practice Nursing

Direct Clinical Practice: The Central Competency

As noted earlier, the primary criteria are necessary but insufficient elements of the definition of advanced practice nursing. Advanced practice nursing is further defined by a set of seven core competencies that are enacted in each APN role. The first core competency of direct clinical practice is central to and informs all of the others (Fig. 3-2). In one sense, it is "first among equals" of the seven core competencies that define advanced practice

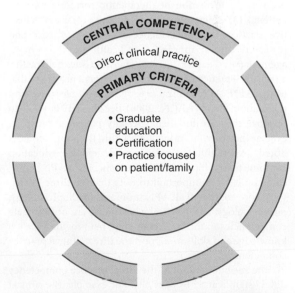

FIG 3-2 Central competency of advanced practice nursing.

nursing. Although APNs do many things, excellence in direct clinical practice provides the foundation necessary for APNs to execute the other competencies, such as consultation, guidance and coaching, and leadership within organizations.

However, clinical expertise alone should not be equated with advanced practice nursing. The work of Patricia Benner and colleagues (Benner, 1984; Benner, Hooper-Kyriakidis, & Stannard, 1999; Benner, Tanner, & Chesla, 1996) is a major contribution to an understanding of clinically expert nursing practice. These researchers extensively studied expert nurses in acute care clinical settings and described the engaged clinical reasoning and domains of practice seen in clinically expert nurses. Although some of the participants in this research were APNs (in the most recent report [Benner et al., 1999], 16% of the nurse participants were APNs), most were nurses with extensive clinical experience who did not have APN preparation. Calkin (1984) has characterized these latter nurses as "experts by experience." (See Chapter 2 for a discussion of Calkin's conceptual differentiation between levels of nursing practice.) Benner and colleagues did not discuss differences in the practices of APNs as compared with other nurses that they have studied. They stated that "'Expert' is not used to refer to a specific role such as an advanced practice nurse. Expertise is found in the practice of experienced clinicians and advanced practice nurses" (Benner et al., 1999).

Although clinical expertise is a central ingredient of an APN's practice, the direct care practice of APNs is distinguished by six characteristics: (1) use of a holistic perspective; (2) formation of therapeutic partnerships with patients; (3) expert clinical performance; (4) use of reflective practice; (5) use of evidence as a guide to practice; and (6) use of diverse approaches to health and illness management (see Chapter 7). These characteristics help distinguish the practice of the expert by experience from that of the APN. APN clinical practice is also informed by a population focus (AACN, 2006) because APNs work to improve the care for their specialty patient population, even as they care for individuals within the population. As noted, experiential knowledge and graduate education combine to develop these characteristics in an APN's clinical practice. It is important to note that the three Ps that form core courses in all APN programs (pathophysiology, pharmacology, and physical assessment) are not separate competencies in this understanding, but provide baseline knowledge and skills to support the direct clinical practice competency.

The specific content of the direct practice competency differs significantly by specialty. For example, the clinical practice of a CNS dealing with critically ill children differs from the expertise of an NP managing the health maintenance needs of older adults or a CRNA administering anesthesia in an outpatient surgical clinic. In addition, the amount of time spent in direct practice differs by APN specialty. CNSs in particular may spend most of their time in activities other than direct clinical practice (see Chapter 14). Thus, it is important to understand this competency as a central defining characteristic of advanced practice nursing rather than as a particular skill set or expectation that APNs only engage in direct clinical practice.

Additional Advanced Practice Nurse Core Competencies

In addition to the central competency of direct clinical practice, six additional competencies further define advanced practice nursing regardless of role function or setting. As shown in Figure 3-3, these additional core competencies are as follows:

- Guidance and coaching
- Consultation
- Evidence-based practice
- Leadership
- Collaboration
- Ethical decision making

These competencies have repeatedly been identified as essential features of advanced practice nursing. In addition, each role is differentiated by some unique competencies (see the specific role chapters in Part III). The nature of the patient population receiving APN care, organizational expectations, emphasis given to specific competencies, and practice characteristics unique to each role distinguish the practice of one APN group from others. Each APN role organization publishes role-specific competencies on their websites (CNS—www.nacns.org; NP—www.nonpf.com; CNM—www.acnm.org; CRNA—www.aana.com). There is a dynamic interplay between the core APN competencies and each role; role-specific expectations grow out of the core competencies and similarly serve to inform them as APNs practice in a changing health care system. In addition, competencies promoted by other professional groups become important to the understanding of advanced practice nursing; for example, the Interprofessional Education Collaborative (IPEC) competencies on interprofessional practice are helping shape the understanding of collaboration (IPEC Expert Panel, 2011; see Chapter 12).

It is also important to understand that each of the competencies described in Part II of this text have specific definitions in the context of advanced practice nursing. For example, leadership has clinical, professional, and systems expectations for the APN that differ from those for a nurse executive or staff nurse. These unique definitions of each competency help distinguish practice at the

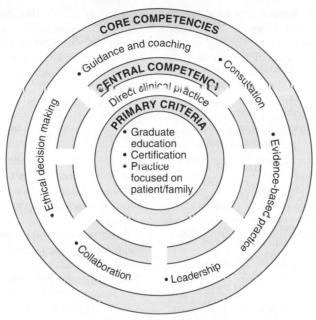

FIG 3-3 Core competencies of advanced practice nursing.

advanced level. Similarly, certain competencies are important components of other specialized nursing roles. For example, collaboration and consultation are important competencies for nursing administrators. The uniqueness of advanced practice nursing is seen in the synergistic interaction between direct clinical practice and this constellation of competencies. In Figure 3-3, the openings between the central practice competency and these additional competencies represent the fact that the APN's direct practice skill interacts with and informs all the other competencies. For example, APNs consult with other providers who seek their practice expertise to plan care for specialty patients. They are able to provide expert guidance and coaching for patients going through health and illness transitions because of their direct practice experience and insight.

The core competencies are not unique to APN practices. Physicians and other health care providers may have developed some of them. Experienced staff nurses may master several of these competencies with years of practice experience. These nurses are seen as exemplary performers and are often encouraged to enter graduate school to become APNs. What distinguishes APN practice is the *expectation* that every APN's practice encompasses all these competencies and seamlessly blends them into daily practice encounters. This expectation makes APN practice unique among that of other providers.

These complex competencies develop over time. No APN emerges from a graduate program fully prepared to enact all of them. However, it is critical that graduate programs provide exposure to each competency in the form of didactic content and practical experience so that new graduates can be tested for initial credentialing and be given a base on which to build their practices. These key competencies are described in detail in subsequent chapters and are not further elaborated here.

Scope of Practice

The term *scope of practice* refers to the legal authority granted to a professional to provide and be reimbursed for health care services. The ANA (2010) defined the scope of nursing practice as "The description of the *who, what, where, when, why,* and *how* of nursing practice." This authority for practice emanates from many sources, such as state and federal laws and regulations, the profession's code of ethics, and professional practice standards. For all health care professionals, scope of practice is most closely tied to state statutes; for nursing in the United States, these statutes are the nurse practice acts of the various states. As previously discussed, APN scope of practice is characterized by specialization, expansion of services provided, including diagnosing and prescribing, and autonomy to practice (NCSBN, 2008). The scopes of practice also differ among the various APN roles; various APN organizations have provided detailed and specific descriptions for their particular role. Carving out an adequate scope of APN practice authority has been an historic struggle for most of the advanced practice groups (see Chapter 1) and this continues to be a hotly debated issue among and within the health professions. Significant variability in state practice acts continues, such that APNs can perform certain activities in some states, notably prescribing certain medications and practicing without physician supervision, but may be constrained from performing these same activities in another state (Lugo, O'Grady, Hodnicki, & Hanson, 2007). The Consensus Model's proposed regulatory language can be used by states to achieve consistent scope of practice language and standardized APRN regulation (NCSBN, 2008).

The Pew Commission's Taskforce on Health Care Workforce Regulation (Finocchio, Dower, Blick, et al., 1998) noted that the tension and turf battles between professions and the increased legislative activities in this area "clog legislative agendas across the country." These battles are costly and time-consuming and lawmakers' decisions related to scope of practice are frequently distorted by campaign contributions, lobbying efforts, and political power struggles rather than being based on empirical evidence. More recently, the Institute of Medicine report, *The Future of Nursing* (2011), made a number of recommendations to expand the scope of APN practice in the primary care arena, including one entire recommendation devoted to supporting the Consensus Model and efforts to remove scope of practice barriers across the various states (see Chapter 21 for further discussion). Encouraging progress is being made on these issues, particularly in regard to interdisciplinary scopes of practice (NCSBN, Association of Social Work Boards, Federation of State Boards of Physical Therapy, Federation of State Medical Boards, National Association of Boards of Pharmacy, & National Board for Certification in Occupational Therapy, 2006), although much remains to be done.

Differentiating Advanced Practice Roles: Operational Definitions of Advanced Practice Nursing

As noted earlier, it is critical to the public's understanding of advanced practice nursing that APN roles and resulting job titles reflect actual practices. Because actual practices differ, job titles should differ. The following corollary is also true—if the actual practices do not differ, the job titles should not differ. For example, some institutions have retitled their CNSs as *clinical coordinators* or *clinical educators*, even though these APNs are practicing consistent

with that of a CNS. This change in job title renders the CNS practice less clearly visible in the clinical setting and thereby obscures CNS role clarity. As noted, differences among roles must be clarified in ways that promote understanding of advanced practice nursing, and the Consensus Model (NCSBN, 2008) clarifies appropriate titling for APNs.

Workforce Data

Table 3-1 provides U.S. sample survey data on RNs prepared to practice as APNs from 2000 to 2008. As of 2008, an estimated 250,527 RNs, or 8.2% of the RN population, were prepared in at least one APN role (U.S. Department of Health & Human Services [HHS], 2010). Almost 17% of these individuals were from racial or ethnic minority backgrounds, a percentage comparable to that of the overall RN population (16.8%). This represents a substantial increase compared with 2004, when only 8% of APNs were from minority backgrounds. However, the diversity of the RN population remains lower than the U.S. population, of whom 34.4% are from racial or ethnic minority backgrounds. The overall number of RNs prepared as APNs represents a 4.2% increase as compared with 2004 data. When changes in APN group numbers are compared over time, different patterns are evident. CRNA numbers show a 7% increase from 2004 to 2008. CNMs experienced 12% growth, although this is based on a small sample, and only 55.5% of CNMs reported graduate preparation. CNSs were the only APN role to experience a decrease, declining 18.3% between 2004 and 2008. However, there was an increase of 11.4% in the number of RNs prepared as both NPs and CNSs. Even so, this represents a net 7% decrease in the total number of RNs educated as CNSs.

The APN role that continues to show the most significant growth is the NP. Although the rate of growth slowed between 2004 and 2008, the number of RNs educated as NPs increased by 12.3% (excluding dual-prepared CNS and NP) and more than doubled from 1996 to 2008. The number of RNs with dual preparation as a CNS and NP showed an 11.4% increase, as noted earlier; most of these nurses reported working as NPs. The 2008 National Sample Survey noted that there are APNs with additional role preparation, notably combining NP and CNM credentials; these APNs represent 17% of nurse-midwives. The breakdown of various APN roles is shown in Figure 3-4.

Four Established Advanced Practice Nurse Roles

Advanced practice nursing is applied in the four established roles and in emerging roles. These APN roles can

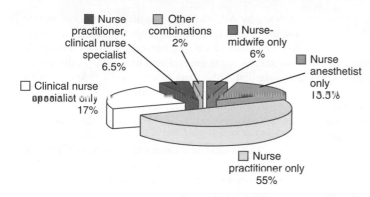

FIG 0 4 Registered nurses prepared for advanced practice, March 2008. *(From U.S. Department of Health and Human Services [HHS], Division of Nursing. [2010].* The registered nurse population March 2008: Findings from the national sample survey of registered nurses. *Washington, DC: Author.)*

be considered to be the operational definitions of the concept of advanced practice nursing. Although each APN role has the common definition, primary criteria, and competencies of advanced practice nursing at its center, it has its own distinct form. Some of these distinctive features of the various roles are listed here. Differences and similarities among roles are further explored in Part III.

The National Association of Clinical Nurse Specialists (NACNS, 2004) has distinguished CNS practice by characterizing "spheres of influence" in which the CNS operates. These include the patient-client sphere, the nursing personnel sphere, and the organization-network sphere (see Chapter 14). A CNS is first and foremost a clinical expert who provides direct care to patients with complex health problems and not only learns consultation processes, as do other APNs, but also functions as a formal consultant to nursing staff and other care providers within his or her organization. Developing, supporting, and educating nursing staff and other interprofessional staff to improve the quality of patient care is a core part of the nursing personnel sphere. Managing system change in complex organizations to build teams and improve nursing practices, and effecting system change to enable better advocacy for patients, are additional role expectations of the CNS. Expectations regarding sophisticated evidence-based practice activities have been central to this role since its inception.

NPs, whether in primary care or acute care, possess advanced health assessment, diagnostic, and clinical management skills that include pharmacology management (see Chapters 15 and 16). Their focus is expert direct care, managing the health needs of individuals and their families. Incumbents in the classic NP role provide primary health care focused on wellness and prevention; NP practice also includes caring for patients with minor, common acute conditions and stable chronic conditions. The acute care NP (ACNP) brings practitioner skills to a specialized patient population within the acute care

setting. The ACNP's focus is the diagnosis and clinical management of acutely or critically ill patient populations in a particular specialized setting. Acquisition of additional medical diagnostic and management skills, such as interpreting computed tomography (CT) and magnetic resonance imaging (MRI) scans, inserting chest tubes, and performing lumbar punctures, also characterize this role.

The CNM (see Chapter 17) has advanced health assessment and intervention skills focused on women's health and childbearing. CNM practice involves independent management of women's health care. CNMs focus particularly on pregnancy, childbirth, the postpartum period, and neonatal care, but their practices also include family planning, gynecologic care, primary health care for women through menopause, and treatment of male partners for sexually transmitted infections (ACNM, 2012). The CNM's focus is on providing direct care to a select patient population.

CRNA practice (see Chapter 18) is distinguished by advanced procedural and pharmacologic management of patients undergoing anesthesia. CRNAs practice independently, in collaboration with physicians, or as employees of a health care institution. Like CNMs, their primary focus is providing direct care to a select patient population. Both CNM and CRNA practices are also distinguished by well-established national standards and certification examinations in their specialties.

These differing roles and their similarities and distinctions are explored in detail in subsequent chapters. It is expected that other roles may emerge as health care continues to change and new opportunities become apparent. This brief discussion underscores the rich and varied nature of advanced practice nursing and the necessity for retaining and supporting different APN roles and titles in the health care marketplace. At the same time, the consistent definition of advanced practice nursing described here undergirds each of these roles, as will be seen in Part III of this text.

Critical Elements in Managing Advanced Practice Nursing Environments

The health care arena is increasingly fluid and changeable; some would even say it is chaotic. Advanced practice nursing does not exist in a vacuum or a singular environment. Rather, this level of practice occurs in an increasing variety of health care delivery environments. These diverse environments are complex admixtures of interdependent elements. The term *environment* refers to any milieu in which an APN practices, ranging from a community-based rural health care practice for a primary care NP to a complex tertiary health care organization for an ACNP. Certain core features of these environments dramatically shape advanced practice and must be

managed by APNs in order for their practices to survive and thrive (Fig. 3-5). Although not technically part of the core definition of advanced practice nursing, these environmental features are included here to frame the understanding that APNs must be aware of these key elements in any practice setting. Furthermore, APNs must be prepared to contend with and shape these aspects of their practice environment to be able to enact advanced practice nursing fully.

The environmental elements that affect APN practice include the following:

- Managing payment mechanisms and business aspects of the practice
- Dealing with marketing and contracting considerations

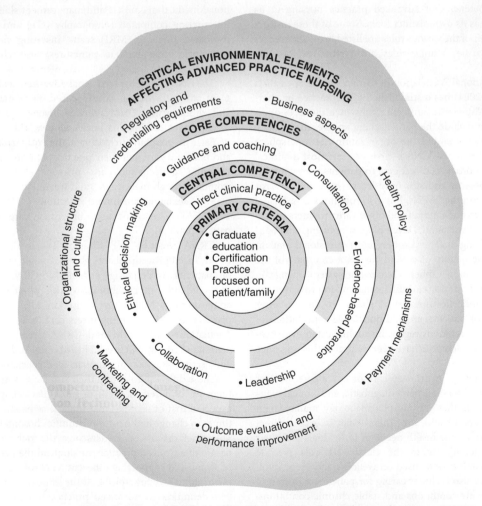

FIG 3-5 Critical elements in advanced nursing practice environments.

- Understanding legal, regulatory, and credentialing requirements
- Understanding and shaping health policy considerations
- Strengthening organizational structures and cultures to support advanced practice nursing
- Enabling outcome evaluation and performance improvement

With the exception of organizational structures and cultures, Part IV of this text explores these elements in depth. Discussion of organizational considerations are presented in Chapter 4 and woven throughout the chapters in Part III.

Common to all these environmental elements is the increasing use of technology and the need for APNs to master various new technologies to improve patient care and health care systems. The ability to use information systems and technology and patient care technology is an essential element of master's and DNP curricula (AACN, 2006, 2011). Electronic technology is changing health care practice in documentation formats, coding schemas, communications, Internet use, and provision of care across state lines through telehealth practices. These changes, in turn, are reshaping all seven APN core competencies. Proficiency in the use of new technologies is increasingly necessary to support clinical practice, implement quality improvement initiatives, and provide leadership to evaluate outcomes of care and care systems (see Chapter 24).

Managing the business and legal aspects of practice is increasingly critical to APN survival in the competitive health care marketplace. All APNs must understand current reimbursement issues, even as changes related to the Patient Protection and Affordable Care Act (2010) are being instituted. Payment mechanisms and legal constraints must be managed, regardless of setting. Given the increasing competition among physicians, APNs, and nonphysician providers, APNs must be prepared to market their services assertively and knowledgeably. Marketing oneself as a new NP in a small community may look different from marketing oneself as a CNS in a large health system, but the principles are the same. Marketing considerations often include the need to advocate for and actively create positions that do not currently exist. Contract considerations are much more complex at the APN level and all APNs, whether newly graduated or experienced, must be prepared to enter into contract negotiations.

Health policy at the state and federal levels is an increasingly potent force shaping advanced practice nursing; regulations and policies that flow from legislative actions can enable or constrain APN practices. Variations in the strength and number of APNs in various states attest to the power of this environmental factor. Organizational structures and cultures, whether those of a community-based practice or a hospital unit, are also important facilitators of or barriers to advanced practice nursing; APN students must learn to assess and intervene to build organizations and cultures that strengthen APN practice. Finally, APNs are accountable for the use of evidence-based practice to ensure positive patient and system outcomes. Measuring the favorable impact of advanced practice nursing on these outcomes and effecting performance improvements are essential activities that all APNs must be prepared to undertake, because continuing to demonstrate the value of APN practice is a necessity in chaotic practice environments.

Special mention must be made of health care quality. As quality concerns have escalated, more attention is being paid to quality metrics for all settings (see Chapter 24). APNs are an important part of the solution to ensuring quality outcomes for their specialty populations. Quality is not itself a competency or an environmental element, but is an important feature that should be evident in the processes that APNs use and the outcomes that they achieve. For example, coaching for wellness should demonstrate the quality processes of a therapeutic nurse-patient relationship and the patient being a partner with the APN in achieving wellness outcomes. The importance of APN involvement in quality initiatives can be seen in the work of the Nursing Alliance for Quality Care, a national partnership of organizations, consumers, and other stakeholders in the safety and quality arena (http://www.gwumc.edu/healthsci/departments/nursing/naqc/).

Implications of the Definition of Advanced Practice Nursing

A number of implications for education, regulation and credentialing, practice, and research flow from this understanding of advanced practice nursing. The Consensus Model (NCSBN, 2008) makes the important point that effective communication between legal and regulatory groups, accreditors, certifying organizations, and educators (LACE) is necessary to advance the goals of advanced practice nursing. Decisions made by each of these groups affect and are affected by all the others. Historically, advanced practice nursing has been hampered by the lack of consensus in APN definition, terminology, educational and certification requirements, and regulatory approaches. The Consensus Model process, by combining stakeholders from each of the LACE areas, has taken a giant step forward toward the profession's achieving needed consensus on APN practice, education, certification, and regulation.

Implications for Advanced Practice Nursing Education

Graduate programs should provide anticipatory socialization experiences to prepare students for their chosen APN role. Graduate experiences should include practice in all the competencies of advanced practice nursing, not just direct clinical practice. For example, students who have no theoretical base or guided practice experiences in consultative skills or clinical, professional, and systems leadership will be ill-equipped to demonstrate these competencies on assuming a new APN role. In addition, APN students need to understand the critical elements in health care environments, such as the business aspects of practice and health care policy that must be managed if their practices are to survive and grow.

All APN roles require at least a specialty master's education; master's programs are continuing even as the DNP degree is being developed in many institutions. The profession has embraced a wide variety of graduate educational models for preparing APNs, including direct-entry programs for non-nurse college graduates and RN to MSN programs. It is highly unlikely that doctoral preparation for advanced practice nursing will supplant these various master's programs by 2015, as originally proposed by the AACN. Debate on the issue of the DNP continues (Marion et al., 2003; Dracup, Cronenwett, Meleis, & Benner, 2005; Fulton & Lyon, 2005; Cronenwett, Dracup, Grey, et al., 2011; see also Part III for views of leaders in each APN role). Ensuring quality and standardization of APN education in the various specialties is imperative if the profession is to guarantee a highly skilled, uniformly educated APN to the public. The definition of advanced practice nursing used here can serve as a guide for developing quality courses and clinical practice experiences that prepare APN students to practice at an advanced level.

Implications for Regulation and Credentialing

Clarifying the definition of advanced practice nursing helps explain the concept to nursing's external stakeholders, such as legislators, insurers, and those in other disciplines. Significant progress has been made toward an integrative view of APRN regulation over the past decade, culminating in the LACE regulatory framework detailed in the Consensus Model. In particular, the primary criteria of graduate education, advanced certification, and focus on direct clinical practice for all APN roles proposed in this definition have been affirmed as the key elements in regulating and credentialing APRNs (NCSBN, 2008). Such internal cohesion can go a long way toward removing barriers to the public's access to APN care.

The Consensus Model has been an important unifying force within the APN community. The regulatory clarity in this document has increasingly been seen in other national statements and the work was highlighted in the IOM Report on the Future of Nursing (IOM, 2011). The NCSBN has embarked on the "Campaign for APRN Consensus" (https://www.ncsbn.org/aprn.htm), a nationwide effort to have this model enacted in all the states.

In addition, the IOM Report has given rise to action coalitions, funded by the Robert Wood Johnson Foundation, in numerous states (http://www.thefutureofnursing.org). The Campaign for Action has a dual focus, implementing solutions to the challenges facing the nursing profession and strengthening nurse-based approaches to transform how Americans receive quality health care. Although the Campaign for Action is broader in scope than just advanced practice nursing, many of the solutions for transforming health care involve APNs being able to practice to the full extent of their education. It is critically important for all APNs to be aware of and involved in these efforts.

One implication for credentialing flows from the diverse specialty and role base of advanced practice nursing. Just as no APN can be characterized as a generalist, no one APN program can prepare students for the full depth and breadth of advanced practice nursing. As a consequence, APNs must practice and be certified in the specific population focus and role for which they have been educated. APNs who wish to change their specialty, population focus, or APN role need to return to school for education targeted to that area. The days are past when a primary care NP could take a job in a specialized acute care practice without further education to prepare for that specialty. This issue of aligning APN job expectations with education and certification is not always well understood by practice environments, educators, or even APNs themselves. However, the need to ensure congruence among particular APN specialties and roles and education, certification, and subsequent practice has been identified by regulators, and more stringent regulations regarding this issue are being promulgated (NCSBN, 2008).

Implications for Research

As noted in Chapter 10, one of the core competencies of advanced practice nursing is the use of evidence-based practice in an APN's practice and in changing the practice environment to incorporate the use of evidence. The practice doctorate initiative identified the increased need for leadership in evidence-based practice and application of knowledge to solve practice problems and improve health outcomes as reasons for moving to the DNP degree for APN practice (AACN, 2006). If research is to be relevant to health care delivery and to nursing practice at all levels, APNs must be involved. APNs need to recognize the importance of advancing the profession's and health care system's knowledge about effective patient care practices and to realize that they are a vital link in building and translating this knowledge in clinical practice.

Related to this research involvement is the necessity for more research differentiating basic and advanced practice nursing and identifying the patient populations that benefit most from APN intervention. For example, there is compelling empirical evidence that APNs can effectively manage chronic disease—preventing or mitigating complications, reducing rehospitalizations, and increasing patients' quality of life. This evidence is presented in the chapters in Part III and in Chapter 23. Linking advanced practice nursing to specific patient outcomes remains a major research imperative for this century. It is interesting to note the increasing research being conducted in international settings as more countries implement advanced practice nursing and study the effectiveness of these new practitioners; discussions of this research are woven throughout the chapters of this book.

Similarly, research is needed on the outcomes of the different APN educational pathways in terms of APN graduate experiences and patient outcomes. Such data would be invaluable in continuing to refine advanced practice education. Outcomes achieved by graduates from DNP programs need similar study in comparison to master's-level APN graduates; in critiquing the need for the DNP degree, Fulton and Lyon (2005) noted the absence of research data on whether there are weaknesses in current master's-level graduates.

Implications for Practice Environments

Because of the centrality of direct clinical practice, APNs must hold onto and make explicit their direct patient care activities. They must also articulate the importance of this level of care for patients. In addition, it is important to identify those patients who most need APN services and ensure that they receive this care.

APN roles require considerable autonomy and authority to be fully enacted. Practice settings have not always structured APN roles to allow sufficient autonomy or accountability for achievement of the patient and system outcomes that are expected of advanced practitioners. It is equally important to emphasize that APNs have expanded responsibilities—expanded authority for practice requires expanded responsibility for practice. APNs must demonstrate a higher level of responsibility and accountability if they are to be seen as legitimate providers of care and full partners on provider teams responsible for patient populations. This willingness to be accountable for practice will

also promote consumers' and policymakers' perceptions of APNs as credible providers in line with physicians.

The APN leadership competency mandates that APNs serve as visible role models and mentors for other nurses (see Chapter 11). Leadership is not optional in APN practice; it is a requirement. APNs must be a visible part of the solution to the health care system's problems. For this goal to be realized, each APN must practice leadership in his or her daily activities. In practice environments, APNs need structured time and opportunities for this leadership, including mentoring activities with new nurses.

New APNs require a considerable period of role development before they can master all the components and competencies of their chosen role, which has important implications for employers of new APNs. Employers should provide experienced preceptors, some structure for the new APN, and ongoing support for role development (see Chapter 4 for further recommendations).

Finally, APN roles must be structured in practice environments to allow APNs to enact advanced nursing skills rather than simply substitute for physicians. It is certainly necessary for APNs to gain additional skills in medical diagnosis and therapeutic interventions, including the knowledge needed for prescriptive authority. However, *advanced practice nursing is a value-added complement to medical practice, not a substitute for it.* This is particularly an imperative in the primary care arena; it may well be that substituting APNs for physicians in classic, medically driven primary care configurations is not the best use of APN skills. Because APN competencies include those of partnering with patients, use of evidence, and coaching skills, APNs may be more effectively used in wellness programs, working with chronically ill patients to strengthen their self-management and adherence and designing and implementing educational programs for patients with complex management needs. New models are needed that are more collaborative and configure teams in innovative ways to minimize fragmentation of care and make the best use of the APN as a value-added complement to the traditional medical team.

As physician shortages increase, particularly the number of physicians prepared in family practice and the new hospitalist practices, this distinction between advanced practice nursing and medical practice must be clear in the minds of employers, insurers, and APNs themselves. As advanced practice nursing evolves, it is becoming clear that APNs represent a choice and an alternative for patients seeking care. Consequently, understanding what APNs bring to health care must be articulated to multiple stakeholders to enable informed patient choice. A competency-based definition of advanced practice nursing aids in this articulation, so that APNs are not just seen as physician substitutes.

Conclusion

Since the first edition of this text in 1996, substantial progress has been made toward clarifying the definition of advanced practice nursing. This progress is enabling APNs, educators, administrators, and other nursing leaders to be clear and consistent about the definition of advanced practice nursing so that the profession speaks with one voice.

This is a critical juncture in the evolution of advanced practice nursing as national attention on nursing and recommendations for nursing's central role in redesigning the health care system are increasing. APNs must continue to clarify that the advanced practice of nursing is not the junior practice of medicine but represents an important alternative practice that complements rather than competes with medical practice. In some cases, patients need advanced nursing and not medicine; identifying these situations and matching APN resources to patients' needs are important priorities for transforming the current health care system. APNs must be able to articulate their defining characteristics clearly and forcefully so that their practices will survive and thrive amidst continued cost cutting in the health care sector.

For a profession to succeed, it must have internal cohesion and external legitimacy, and have them at the same time (Safriet, 1993). Clarity about the core definition of advanced practice nursing and recognition of the primary criteria and competencies necessary for all APNs enhance nursing's internal cohesion. At the same time, clarifying the differences among APNs and showcasing their important roles in the health care system enhance nursing's external legitimacy.

References

Advanced Nursing Practice. (2012). *Cumulative index to nursing and allied health literature.* Retrieved from the index on October 26, 2012.

American Association of Colleges of Nursing (AACN). (1995). *The essentials of master's education for advanced practice nursing.* Washington, DC: Author.

American Association of Colleges of Nursing (AACN). (2003). *White paper on the role of the clinical nurse leader.* Washington, DC: Author.

American Association of Colleges of Nursing (AACN). (2004). *Position statement on the practice doctorate in nursing.* Washington, DC: Author.

American Association of Colleges of Nursing (AACN). (2006). *The essentials of doctoral education for advanced nursing practice.* Washington, DC: Author.

American Association of Colleges of Nursing (AACN). (2011). *The essentials of master's education in nursing.* Washington, DC: Author.

American College of Nurse-Midwives (ACNM). (2009). *Position statement: Mandatory degree requirements for entry into midwifery practice.* Washington, DC: Author.

American College of Nurse-Midwives (ACNM). (2012). Core competencies for basic midwifery practice (http://www.midwife.org/ACNM/files/ACNMLibraryData/UPLOADFILENAME/000000000050/Core Competencies Dec 2012.pdf).

American Nurses Association (ANA). (1995). *Nursing's social policy statement.* Washington, DC: Author.

American Nurses Association (ANA). (1996). *Scope and standards of advanced practice registered nursing.* Washington, DC: Author.

American Nurses Association (ANA). (2001). *Code of ethics for nurses with interpretive statements.* Washington, DC: Author.

American Nurses Association (ANA). (2003). *Nursing's social policy statement* (2nd ed.). Washington, DC: Author.

American Nurses Association (ANA). (2005). *Public health nursing: Scope and standards of practice.* Washington, DC: Author.

American Nurses Association (ANA). (2010). *Nursing's social policy statement* (3rd ed.). Washington, DC: Author.

Association of Community Health Nursing Educators Task Force on Community and Public Health Master's Level Preparation. (2000). *Graduate education for advanced community and public health nursing practice.* Louisville, KY: Author.

Benner, P. (1984). *From novice to expert.* Menlo Park, CA: Addison-Wesley.

Benner, P., Hooper-Kyriakidis, P., & Stannard, D. (1999). *Clinical wisdom and interventions in critical care.* Philadelphia: Saunders.

Benner, P., Tanner, C. A., & Chesla, C. A. (1996). *Expertise in nursing practice: Caring, clinical judgment, and ethics.* New York: Springer.

Brown, S. J. (1998). A framework for advanced practice nursing. *Journal of Professional Nursing, 14,* 157–164.

Calkin, J. D. (1984). A model for advanced nursing practice. *Journal of Nursing Administration, 14,* 24–30.

Creasia, J. L. & Friberg, E. E. (Eds.) (2011). Conceptual foundations: The bridge to professional nursing practice (5th ed.). St. Louis: Mosby.

Cronenwett, L. R. (1995). Molding the future of advanced practice nursing. *Nursing Outlook, 43,* 112–118.

Cronenwett, L., Dracup, K., Grey, M., McCauley, L., Meleis, A., & Salmon, M. (2011). The Doctor of Nursing Practice: A national workforce perspective. *Nursing Outlook, 59,* 9–17. doi:10.1016/j.outlook.2010.11.003.

Davies, B., & Hughes, A. M. (1995). Clarification of advanced nursing practice: Characteristics and competencies. *Clinical Nurse Specialist, 9,* 156–160.

Dracup, K., Cronenwett, L., Meleis, A. I., & Benner, P. E. (2005). Reflections on the doctorate of nursing practice. *Nursing Outlook, 53,* 177–182.

Finocchio, L. J., Dower, C. M., Blick, N. T., Gragnola, C. M., & the Taskforce on Health Care Workforce Regulation. (1998). *Strengthening consumer protection: Priorities for health care workforce regulation.* San Francisco: Pew Health Professions Commission.

Fulton, J. S., & Lyon, B. L. (2005). The need for some sense making: Doctor of nursing practice. *Online Journal of Issues in Nursing, 10*, 4.

Hamric, A. B. (1996). A definition of advanced nursing practice. In A. B. Hamric, J. A. Spross, & C. M. Hanson (Eds.), *Advanced nursing practice: An integrative approach* (pp. 42–56). Philadelphia: WB Saunders.

Hamric, A. B. (2000). A definition of advanced nursing practice. In A. B. Hamric, J. A. Spross, & C. M. Hanson (Eds.), *Advanced nursing practice: An integrative approach* (pp. 53–73; 2nd ed.). Philadelphia: Saunders.

Hamric, A. B. (2005). A definition of advanced practice nursing. In A. B. Hamric, J. A. Spross, & C. M. Hanson (Eds.), *Advanced practice nursing: An integrative approach* (pp. 85–108; 3rd ed.). Philadelphia: Saunders.

Hamric, A. B. (2009). A definition of advanced practice nursing. In A. B. Hamric, J. A. Spross, & C. M. Hanson (Eds.), *Advanced nursing practice: An integrative approach* (pp. 75–94; 4th ed.). Philadelphia: Saunders.

Hanson, C. M., & Hamric, A. B. (2003). Reflections on the continuing evolution of advanced practice nursing. *Nursing Outlook, 51*, 203–211.

Hickey, J. V., Ouimette, R. V., & Venegoni, S. L. (2000). *Advanced practice nursing: Changing roles and clinical applications* (2nd ed.). Philadelphia: Lippincott.

Hood, L. J. (2010). *Leddy and Pepper's conceptual bases of professional nursing* (7th ed.). Philadelphia: Lippincott Williams & Wilkins.

Institute of Medicine. (2011). *The Future of Nursing: Leading Change, Advancing Health*. Washington, DC: The National Academies Press.

Interprofessional Education Collaborative Expert Panel. (2011). *Core competencies for interprofessional collaborative practice: Report of an expert panel*. Washington DC: Interprofessional Education Collaborative.

Kitzman, H. (1989). The CNS and the nurse practitioner. In A. B. Hamric & J. A. Spross (Eds.), *The clinical nurse specialist in theory and practice* (pp. 379–394; 2nd ed.). Philadelphia: WB Saunders.

Lindeke, L. L., Canedy, B. H., & Kay, M. M. (1997). A comparison of practice domains of clinical nurse specialists and nurse practitioners. *Journal of Professional Nursing, 13*, 281–287.

Lugo, N. R., O'Grady, E. T., Hodnicki, D. R., & Hanson, C. M. (2007). Ranking state nurse practitioner regulation: Practice environment and consumer health care choice. *American Journal of Nurse Practitioners, 11*, 8–24.

Marion, L., Viens, D., O'Sullivan, A., Crabtree, K., Fontana, S., & Price, M. (2003). The practice doctorate in nursing: Future or fringe? (http://www.doctorsofnursingpractice.org/cmsAdmin/uploads/Marion_Viens2003.pdf).

Mundinger, M. O. (1994). Advanced practice nursing: Good medicine for physicians? *New England Journal of Medicine, 330*, 211–214.

Mundinger, M., Cook, S., Lenz, E., Piacentini, K., Auerhahn, C., & Smith J. (2000). Assuring quality and access in advanced practice nursing: A challenge to nurse educators. *Journal of Professional Nursing, 16*, 322–329.

National Association of Clinical Nurse Specialists (NACNS). (2004). *Statement on clinical nurse specialist practice and education* (2nd ed.). Glenview, IL: Author.

National Council of State Boards of Nursing (NCSBN). (1993). *Position paper on the regulation of advanced nursing practice.* Chicago: Author.

National Council of State Boards of Nursing (NCSBN). (2002). *Position paper on the regulation of advanced practice nursing.* Chicago: Author.

NCSBN (National Council of State Boards of Nursing). (2008). *Consensus model for APRN regulation: Licensure, accreditation, certification & education* (APRN Consensus Work Group and NCSBN APRN Advisory Committee). Available from https://www.ncsbn.org/july_2008_consensus_model_for_aprn_regulation.pdf

National Council of State Boards of Nursing (NCSBN), Association of Social Work Boards, Federation of State Boards of Physical Therapy, Federation of State Medical Boards, National Association of Boards of Pharmacy, & National Board for Certification in Occupational Therapy. (2006). *Changes in healthcare professions' scope of practice: Legislative considerations.* (Brochure). Chicago: Authors.

National Organization of Nurse Practitioner Faculties (NONPF). (2000). *Challenges and opportunities for integrating community health in nurse practitioner programs.* Washington DC: Author.

Patient Protection and Affordable Care Act (PPACA). (2010). Pub. L. No. 111-148, 124 Stat. 119.

Pearson, H. (2011). Concepts of advanced practice: what does it mean? *British Journal of Nursing, 20*, 184–185.

Rasch, R. F. R., & Frauman, A. C. (1996). Advanced practice in nursing: Conceptual issues. *Journal of Professional Nursing, 12*, 141–146.

Ruel, J., & Motyka, C. (2009). Advanced practice nursing: a principle-based concept analysis. *Journal of the American Academy of Nurse Practitioners, 21*, 384–392.

Safriet, B. J. (1993). *Keynote address: One strong voice.* Presented at the National Nurse Practitioner Leadership Summit, Washington DC, February 1993.

Safriet, B. J. (1998). Still spending dollars, still searching for sense: Advanced practice nursing in an era of regulatory and economic turmoil. *Advanced Practice Nursing Quarterly, 4*, 24–33.

Spross, J. A., & Baggerly, J. (1989). Models of advanced practice. In A. B. Hamric & J. A. Spross (Eds.), *The clinical nurse specialist in theory and practice* (pp. 19–40; 2nd ed.). Philadelphia: Saunders.

Stanley, J. M. (Ed.), (2011). *Advanced practice nursing: Emphasizing common roles* (3rd ed.). Philadelphia: F. A. Davis.

U.S. Department of Health and Human Services (HHS), Division of Nursing. (2010). *The registered nurse population March 2008. Findings from the national sample survey of registered nurses.* Washington, DC: Author.

Role Development of the Advanced Practice Nurse

Karen A. Brykczynski

CHAPTER CONTENTS

What is it like to become an advanced practice nurse (APN)? Role development in advanced practice nursing is described here as a process that evolves over time. The process is more than socializing and taking on a new role. It involves transforming one's professional identity and the progressive development of the seven core advanced practice competencies (see Chapter 3). The scope of nursing practice has expanded and contracted in response to societal needs, political forces, and economic realities (Levy, 1968; Safriet, 1992; see Chapter 1). Historical evidence suggests that the expanded role of the 1970s was common nursing practice during the early 1900s (DeMaio, 1979). However, the core of nursing is not defined by the tasks nurses perform. This task-oriented perspective is inadequate and disregards the complex nature of nursing.

In the current cost-constrained environment, the pressure to be cost-effective and to make an impact on outcomes is greater than ever, but studies have shown that the initial year of practice is one of transition (Brown & Olshansky, 1998; Brykczynski, 2009; Kelly & Mathews, 2001) and an APN's maximum potential may not be realized until after approximately 5 or more years in practice (Cooper & Sparacino, 1990). This chapter explores the complex processes of APN role development, with the objectives of providing the following: (1) an understanding of related concepts and research; (2) anticipatory guidance for APN students; (3) role facilitation strategies for new APNs, APN preceptors, faculty, administrators, and

interested colleagues; and (4) guidelines for continued role evolution. This chapter consolidates literature from all the APN specialties—including clinical nurse specialists (CNSs), nurse practitioners (NPs), certified nurse-midwives (CNMs), and certified registered nurse anesthetists (CRNAs)—to present a generic process relevant to all APN roles. Some of this literature is foundational to understanding issues of role development for all APN roles and, although dated, remains relevant. This chapter has been expanded to include international APN role development experiences.

The discussion is separated into (1) the educational component of APN role acquisition and (2) the occupational or work component of role implementation. This division in the process of role development is intended to clarify and distinguish the changes occurring during role transitions experienced during the educational period (role acquisition) and the changes occurring during the actual performance of the role after program completion (role implementation). Strategies for enhancing APN role development are described. The chapter concludes with summary comments and suggestions to facilitate future APN role development and evolution.

Perspectives on Advanced Practice Nurse Role Development

Professional role development is a dynamic ongoing process that, once begun, spans a lifetime. The concept of graduation as commencement, whereby one's career begins on completion of a degree, is central to understanding the evolving nature of professional roles in response to personal, professional, and societal demands (Gunn, 1998). Professional role development literature in nursing is abundant and complex, involving multiple component processes, including the following: (1) aspects of adult development; (2) development of clinical expertise; (3) modification of self-identity through initial socialization in school; (4) embodiment of ethical comportment (Benner, Sutphen, Leonard, & Day, 2010); (5) development and integration of professional role components; and (6) subsequent resocialization in the work setting. Similar to socialization for other professional roles, such as those of attorney, physician, teacher, and social worker, the process of becoming an APN involves aspects of adult development and professional socialization. The professional socialization process in advanced practice nursing involves identification with and acquisition of the behaviors and attitudes of the advanced practice group to which one aspires (Waugaman & Lu, 1999, p. 239). This includes learning the specialized language, skills, and knowledge of the particular APN group, internalizing its values and norms, and incorporating these into one's professional nursing identity and other life roles (Cohen, 1981).

Novice to Expert Skill Acquisition Model

Acquisition of knowledge and skill occurs in a progressive movement through the stages of performance from novice to expert, as described by Dreyfus and Dreyfus (1986, 2009), who studied diverse groups, including pilots, chess players, and adult learners of second languages. The skill acquisition model has broad applicability and can be used to understand many different skills better, ranging from playing a musical instrument to writing a research grant. The most widely known application of this model is Benner's (1984) observational and interview study of clinical nursing practice situations from the perspective of new nurses and their preceptors in hospital nursing services. Although this study included several APNs, it did not specify a particular education level as a criterion for expertise. As noted in Chapter 3, there has been some confusion about this criterion. The skill acquisition model is a situation-based model, not a trait model. Therefore, the level of expertise is not an individual characteristic of a particular nurse but is a function of the nurse's familiarity with a particular situation in combination with his or her educational background. This model could be used to study the level of expertise required for other aspects of advanced practice, including guidance and coaching, consultation, collaboration, evidence-based practice ethical

decision making, and leadership (see Brykczynski [2009] for a detailed discussion of the Dreyfus model).

Figure 4-1 shows a typical APN role development pattern in terms of this skill acquisition model. A major implication of the novice to expert model for advanced practice nursing is the claim that even experts can be expected to perform at lower skill levels when they enter new situations or positions. Hamric and Taylor's report (1989) that an experienced CNS starting a new position experiences the same role development phases as a new graduate, only over a shorter period, supports this claim.

The overall trajectory expected during APN role development is shown in Figure 4-1; however, each APN experiences a unique pattern of role transitions and life transitions concurrently. For example, a professional nurse who functions as a mentor for new graduates may decide to pursue an advanced degree as an APN. As an APN graduate student, she or he will experience the challenges of acquiring a new role, the anxiety associated with learning new skills and practices, and the dependency of being a novice. At the same time, if this nurse continues to work as a registered nurse, his or her functioning in this work role will be at the competent, proficient, or expert level, depending on experience and the situation. On graduation, the new APN may experience a limbo period, during which the nurse is no longer a student and not yet an APN, while searching for a position and meeting certification requirements (see later). Once in a new APN position, this nurse may experience a return to the advanced beginner stage as he or she proceeds through the phases of role implementation. Even after making the transition to an APN role, progression in role implementation is not a linear process. As Figure 4-1 indicates, there are discontinuities, with movement back and forth as the trajectory begins again. Years later, the APN may decide to pursue yet another APN role. The processes of role acquisition, role implementation, and novice to expert skill development will again be experienced—although altered and informed by previous experiences—as the postgraduate student acquires additional skills and knowledge. Role development involves multiple, dynamic, and situational processes, with each new undertaking being characterized by passage through earlier transitional phases and with some movement back and forth, horizontally or vertically, as different career options are pursued.

Direct-entry students who are non-nurse college graduates (NNCGs) and APN students with little or no experience as nurses before entry into an APN graduate program would be expected to begin their APN role development at the novice level (see Fig. 4-1). Some evidence indicates that although these inexperienced nurse students may lack the intuitive sense that comes with clinical experience,

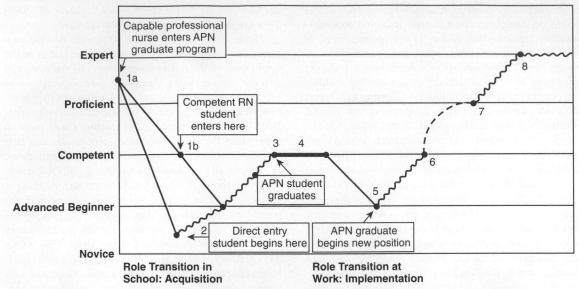

FIG 4-1 Typical APN role development pattern. *1a,* APN students may begin graduate school as proficient or expert nurses. *1b,* Some enter as competent RNs, with limited practice experience. Depending on previous background, the new APN student will revert to novice level or advanced beginner level on assuming the student role. *2,* A direct-entry APN student or NNCG student with no experience would begin the role transition process at the novice level. *3,* The graduate from an APN program is competent as an APN student but has no experience as a practicing APN. *4,* A limbo period is experienced while the APN graduate searches for a position and becomes certified. *5,* The newly employed APN reverts to the advanced beginner level in the new APN position as the role trajectory begins again. The imposter phenomenon may be experienced here (Arena & Page, 1992; Brown & Olshansky, 1998). *6,* Some individuals remain at the competent level. There is a discontinuous leap from the competent to the proficient level. *7,* Proficiency develops only if there is sufficient commitment and involvement in practice along with embodiment of skills and knowledge. *8,* Expertise is intuitive and situation-specific, meaning that not all situations will be managed expertly. See text for details.

Noᴛᴇ: Refer to the Dreyfus skill acquisition model for further details (Benner, 1984; Benner, Tanner, & Chesla, 2009; Dreyfus & Dreyfus, 1986; 2009). For the purpose of illustration, this figure is more linear than the individualized role development trajectories that actually occur.

they avoid the role confusion associated with letting go of the traditional RN role commonly reported with experienced nurse students (Heitz, Steiner, & Burman, 2004). This finding has implications for APN education as the profession moves toward the Doctor of Nursing Practice (DNP) as the preferred educational pathway for APN preparation (American Association of Colleges of Nursing [AACN], 2006).

Another significant implication of the Dreyfus model (Dreyfus & Dreyfus, 1986, 2009) for APNs is the observation that the quality of performance may deteriorate when performers are subjected to intense scrutiny, whether their own or that of someone else (Roberts, Tabloski, & Bova, 1997). The increased anxiety experienced by APN students during faculty on-site clinical evaluation visits or during videotaped testing of clinical performance in

simulated situations is an example of responding to such intense scrutiny. A third implication of this skill acquisition model for APNs is the need to accrue experience in actual situations over time, so that practical and theoretical knowledge are refined, clarified, personalized, and embodied, forming an individualized repertoire of experience that guides advanced practice performance. As the profession encourages new nurses to move more rapidly into APN education, students, faculty, and educational programs must search for creative ways to incorporate the practical and theoretical knowledge necessary for advanced practice nursing. Discussing unfolding cases is a useful approach for teaching the clinical reasoning in transition so essential for clinical practice (Benner, Sutphen, Leonard, & Day, 2010; Day, Cooper, & Scott, 2012).

TABLE 4-1 Selected Role Concepts

Concept	Definition	Examples
Role stress	A situation of increased role performance demand	Returning to school while maintaining work and family responsibilities
Role strain	Subjective feeling of frustration, tension, or anxiety in response to role stress	Feeling of decreased self-esteem when performance is below expectations of self or significant others
Role stressors	Factors that produce role stress	Financial, personal, or academic demands and role expectations that are ambiguous, conflicting, excessive, or unpredictable
Role ambiguity	Unclear expectations, diffuse responsibilities, uncertainty about subroles	Some degree of ambiguity in all professional positions because of the evolving nature of roles and expansion of skills and knowledge
Role incongruity	A role with incompatibility between skills and abilities and role obligations or between personal values, self-concept, and role obligations	An adult NP in a role requiring pediatric skills and knowledge
Role conflict	Occurs when role expectations are perceived to be mutually exclusive or contradictory	Role conflict between APNs and other nurses and between APNs and physicians
Role transition	A dynamic process of change over time as new roles are acquired	Changing from a staff nurse role to an APN role
Role insufficiency	Feeling inadequate to meet role demands	New APN graduate experiencing the imposter phenomenon (Arena & Page, 1992; Brown & Olshansky, 1998)
Role supplementation	Anticipatory socialization	Role-specific educational components in a graduate program

Adapted from Hardy, M.E., & Hardy, W.L. (1988). Role stress and role strain. In M.E. Hardy & M.E. Conway (Eds.), *Role theory: Perspectives for health professionals* (pp. 159–239, 2nd ed.). Norwalk, CT: Appleton & Lange; and Schumacher, K.L., & Meleis, A.I. (1994). Transitions: A central concept in nursing. *Image: The Journal of Nursing Scholarship, 26,* 119–127.

Role Concepts and Role Development Issues

This discussion of professional role issues incorporates role concepts described by Hardy and Hardy (1988) along with the concept that different APN roles represent different subcultural groups within the broader nursing culture (Leininger, 1994). Building on Johnson's (1993) conclusion that NPs have three voices, Brykczynski (1999a) described APNs as tricultural and trilingual. They share background knowledge, practices, and skills of three cultures—biomedicine, mainstream nursing, and everyday life. They are fluent in the languages of biomedical science, nursing knowledge and skill, and everyday parlance. Some APNs (e.g., CNMs) are socialized into a fourth culture as well, that of midwifery. Others are also fluent in more than one everyday language.

The concepts of role stress and strain discussed by Hardy and Hardy (1988) are useful for understanding the dynamics of role transitions (Table 4-1). Hardy and Hardy described *role stress* as a social structural condition in which role obligations are ambiguous, conflicting, incongruous, excessive, or unpredictable. *Role strain* is defined as the subjective feeling of frustration, tension, or anxiety experienced in response to role stress. The highly stressful nature of the nursing profession needs to be recognized as the background within which individuals seek advanced education to become APNs (Aiken, Clarke, Sloan, et al., 2002; Dionne-Proulz & Pepin, 1993). Role strain can be minimized by the identification of potential role stressors, development of coping strategies, and rehearsal of situations designed for application of those strategies. However, the difficulties experienced by neophytes in new positions cannot be eliminated. As noted, expertise is holistic, involving embodied perceptual skills (e.g., detecting qualitative distinctions in pulses or types of anxiety), shared background knowledge, and cognitive ability. A school-work, theory- practice, ideal-real gap will remain because of the nature of human skill acquisition.

Bandura's (1977) social cognitive theory of self-efficacy may be of interest to APNs in terms of understanding what motivates individuals to acquire skills and what builds confidence as skills are developed. Self-efficacy theory, a person's belief in their ability to succeed, has been used widely to further understanding of skill acquisition with patients (Burglehaus, 1997; Clark & Dodge, 1999; Dalton & Blau, 1996). Self-efficacy theory has also been applied to mentoring APN students (Hayes, 2001) and training health care professionals in skill acquisition (Parle, Maguire, & Heaven, 1997).

Role Ambiguity

Role ambiguity (see Table 4-1) develops when there is a lack of clarity about expectations, a blurring of responsibilities, uncertainty regarding role implementation, and the inherent uncertainty of existent knowledge. According to Hardy and Hardy (1988), role ambiguity characterizes all professional positions. They have noted that role ambiguity might be positive in that it offers opportunities for creative possibilities. It can be expected to be more prominent in professions undergoing change, such as those in the health care field. Role ambiguity has been widely discussed in relation to the CNS role (Bryant-Lukosius, Carter, Kilpatrick, et al, 2010; Hamric, 2003; see also Chapter 14), but is also a relevant issue for other APN roles (Kelly & Mathews, 2001), particularly as APN roles evolve (Stahl & Myers, 2002).

Role Incongruity

Role incongruity is intrarole conflict, which Hardy and Hardy (1988) described as developing from two sources. Incompatibility between skills and abilities and role obligations is one source of role incongruity. An example of this is an adult APN hired to work in an emergency department with a large percentage of pediatric patients. Such an APN will find it necessary to enroll in a family NP or pediatric NP program to gain the knowledge necessary to eliminate this role incongruity. This is a growing issue as NP roles become more specialized. Another source of role incongruity is incompatibility among personal values, self-concept, and expected role behaviors. An APN interested primarily in clinical practice may experience this incongruity if the position that she or he obtains requires performing administrative functions. An example comes from Banda's (1985) study of psychiatric liaison CNSs in acute care hospitals and community health agencies. She reported that they viewed consultation and teaching as their major functions, whereas research and administrative activities produced role incongruity.

Role Conflict

Role conflict develops when role expectations are perceived to be contradictory or mutually exclusive. APNs may experience conflict with varying demands of their role, as well as intraprofessional and interprofessional role conflict.

Intraprofessional Role Conflict

APNs experience intraprofessional role conflict for a variety of reasons. The historical development of APN roles has been fraught with conflict and controversy in nursing education and nursing organizations, particularly for CNMs (Varney, 1987), NPs (Ford, 1982), and CRNAs (Gunn, 1991; see also Chapter 1). Relationships among these APN groups and nursing as a discipline have improved markedly in recent years, but difficulties remain (Fawcett, Newman, & McAllister, 2004). The degree to which APN roles demonstrate a holistic nursing orientation as opposed to a more disease-specific medical orientation remains problematic (see value-added discussion under collaboration, later).

Communication difficulties that underlie intraprofessional role conflict occur in four major areas: (1) at an organizational level; (2) in educational programs; (3) in the literature; and (4) in direct clinical practice. Kimbro (1978) initially described these communication difficulties in reference to CNMs, but they are relevant for all APN roles. The fact that CNSs, NPs, CNMs, and CRNAs each have specific organizations with different certification requirements, competencies, and curricula creates boundaries and sets up the need for formal lines of communication. Communication gaps occur in education when courses and textbooks are not shared among APN programs, even when more than one specialty is offered in the same school. Specialty-specific journals are another formal communication barrier because APNs may read primarily within their own specialty and not keep abreast of larger APN issues. In clinical settings, some APNs may be more concerned with providing direct clinical care to individual patients, whereas staff nurses and other APNs may be more concerned with 24-hour coverage and smooth functioning of the unit or institution. These differences may set the stage for intraprofessional role conflict.

During the 1980s and 1990s, when there was more confusion about the delineation of roles and responsibilities between RNs and NPs, RNs would sometimes demonstrate resistance to NPs by refusing to take vital signs, obtain blood samples, or perform other support functions for patients of NPs (Brykczynski, 1985; Hupcey, 1993; Lurie, 1981), and they were not admonished by their supervisors for these negative behaviors. These behaviors are suggestive of horizontal violence (a form of hostility), which may be more common during nursing shortages (Thomas, 2003). Roberts (1983) first described horizontal violence among nurses as oppressed group behavior wherein nurses who were doubly oppressed as women and as nurses demonstrated hostility toward their own less powerful group, instead of toward the more powerful oppressors. Recognizing that intraprofessional conflict among nurses is similar to oppressed group behavior can be useful in the development of strategies to overcome these difficulties (Bartholomew, 2006; Brykczynski, 1997; Farrell, 2001, Freshwater, 2000, Roberts, 1996, Rounds, 1997; see Chapter 11). According to Rounds (1997), horizontal violence is less common among NPs as a group than among RNs generally. Over the years, as the NP role has become more accepted by nurses, there appear to be fewer cases of these hostile passive-aggressive behaviors, often currently referred to as bullying, toward NPs. However, they are still reported in APN transition literature (Heitz et al., 2004; Kelly & Mathews, 2001).

One way to address these issues would be to include APN position descriptions in staff nurse orientation programs. Curry's claim (1994) that thorough orientation of staff nurses to the APN role, including clear guidelines and policies regarding responsibility issues, is an important component of successful integration of NP practice in an emergency department setting is also applicable to other roles and settings. Another significant strategy for minimizing intraprofessional role conflict is for the new APN, and APN students, to spend time getting to know the nursing staff to establish rapport and learn as much as possible about the new setting from those who really know what is going on—the nurses. This action affirms the value and significance of nurses and nursing and sets up a positive atmosphere for collegiality and intraprofessional role cooperation and collaboration. In Kelly and Mathews' study (2001) of new NP graduates, such a strategy was exactly what new NPs regretted not having incorporated into their first positions.

Interprofessional Role Conflict

Conflicts between physicians and APNs constitute the most common situations of interprofessional conflict. Major sources of conflict for physicians and APNs are the perceived economic threat of competition, limited resources in clinical training sites, lack of experience working together, and the historical hierarchy. The relationship between anesthesiologists and CRNAs is an ongoing exemplar for examination of the issues of interprofessional role conflict between physicians and APNs.

One way to promote positive interprofessional relationships is to provide education and practice experiences that include APN students, medical students, and both physician and APN faculty to enhance mutual understanding of both professional roles (Kelly & Mathews, 2001). Developing such interprofessional education (IPE) experiences is difficult because of different academic calendars and clinical schedules. However, these obstacles can be overcome if these interdisciplinary activities are considered essential for improved health care delivery and

---

 EXEMPLAR 4-1   **Interprofessional Role Conflict: The Case of Certified Registered Nurse Anesthetists and Anesthesiologists**

For many years, nurse anesthetists have provided high-quality anesthesia care in a variety of settings. They are the primary anesthesia providers in rural U.S. hospitals (www.aana.com). According to the American Association of Nurse Anesthetists (AANA, 2012), more than 42,000 certified registered nurse anesthetists provide quality anesthesia care to more than 65% of all patients undergoing surgical or other medical interventions that necessitate the services of an anesthetist (see Chapter 18). The fact that nurse anesthetists predated the first physician anesthesiologists by many years (see Chapter 1) may partly explain why the relationship between anesthesiologists and CRNAs has historically been interpreted by anesthesiologists as one of direct competition, thus creating an adversarial stance. Over the years, this relationship might be characterized as a cold war with overt offensives mounted periodically by anesthesiologists.

In 1970, CRNAs outnumbered anesthesiologists by a ratio of 1.5:1. By 2000, anesthesiologists outnumbered CRNAs (Blumenreich, 2000). This is one of the factors underlying conflicts over CRNA autonomy (see the AANA website, www.aana.com, for updates on this issue). Another factor is the decision made by the Centers for Medicare and Medicaid Services, after study of the available evidence in 1997, to reimburse nurse anesthetists directly under Medicare (Kleinpell, 2001). In response, anesthesiologists and the American Medical Association (AMA) launched a major campaign against CRNA autonomy in the operating room, claiming that supervision of CRNAs by physicians is essential for public safety (Federwisch, 1999; Kleinpell, 2001; Stein, 2000; see also Chapter 18). This struggle with physicians over limiting the scope of practice of CRNAs is ongoing and reflects the experiences of other advanced practice nurse (APN) groups as well. An example of this continuing struggle is the Scope of Practice Partnership (SOPP), a coalition recently formed by the AMA with other physician organizations, to mount initiatives to limit the scope of practice of nonphysician clinicians (Waters, 2007).

if they have sufficient administrative support. Some programs attempt to overcome these scheduling issues by mandating IPE for APNs while it remains an elective experience for medical students, thereby reinforcing an optional and not important perspective among medical students.

The issues of professional territoriality and physician concern about being replaced by APNs were reported by Lindblad and colleagues (2010) from an ethnographic study of the first four APNs to graduate in 2005 from the first CNS program in Sweden. The APNs and general practitioners (GPs) agreed that the usefulness of the APNs would have been greater if the APNs had been able to prescribe medications and order treatments. After working with the APNs, the GPs saw them more as an additional resource and complement rather than a threat. By 2009, there were 16 APNs working in the new role in primary health care. Further clarification and definition of APN role responsibilities and collaboration will be forthcoming from Sweden.

The complementary nature of advanced practice nursing to medical care is a foreign concept for some physicians, who view all health care as an extension of medical care and see APNs simply as physician extenders. This misunderstanding of advanced practice nursing underlies physicians' opposition to independent roles for nurses because they believe that APNs want to practice medicine without a license (see Chapters 1 and 3). In fact, numerous earlier studies of APN practice have demonstrated that advanced practice roles incorporate a holistic approach that blends elements of nursing and medicine (Brown, 1992; Brykczynski, 1999a, b; Fiandt, 2002; Grando, 1998; Johnson, 1993). However, when APNs are viewed by physicians as direct competitors, it is understandable that some physicians would be reluctant to be involved in assisting with APN education (National Commission on Nurse Anesthesia Education, 1990). In addition, some nurse educators have believed that physicians should not be involved in teaching or acting as preceptors for APNs. Improved relationships between APNs and physicians will require redefinition of the situation by both groups. The Interprofessional Education Collaborative's (IPEC, 2011) advocacy for an interprofessional vision for all health professionals and the Institute of Medicine's (IOM, 2003) recommendation that the health professional workforce be prepared to work in interdisciplinary teams underscore the imperative of interprofessional collaboration (see Chapter 12). Competency in interprofessional collaboration is critical for APNs because it is central to APN practice. This content is incorporated into the leadership and interprofessional partnership components of *The Essentials of*

Doctoral Education for Advanced Nursing Practice (AACN, 2006).

Some interesting research has recently emerged on this issue in Canada and Europe. A participatory action research study conducted in British Columbia, Canada (Burgess & Purkis, 2010) indicated that NPs viewed collaboration as both a philosophy and a practice. "They cultivated collaborative relations with clients, colleagues, and health care leaders to address concerns of role autonomy and role clarity, extend holistic client-centered care and team capacity, and create strategic alliances to promote innovation and system change" (p. 300). Of particular importance is the fact that the NP participants described themselves as being nurses first and practitioners second. This is significant because when role emphasis is on physician replacement and support rather than on the patient-centered, health-focused, holistic nursing orientation to practice, the nursing components of the role become less valued and invisible (Bryant-Lukosius, DiCenso, Browne, & Pinelli, 2004). Medically driven and illness-oriented health systems tend to devalue these value-added components of APN roles and reimbursement mechanisms for including these aspects of care are lacking. Fleming and Carberry (2011) reported on a grounded theory study of expert critical care nurses transitioning to the role of APN in an intensive care unit (ICU) setting in Scotland. Initial perceptions were that the APN role was closely aligned with medical practice, but later perceptions supported earlier studies that the APN role was characterized by an integrated, holistic, patient-centered approach to care, which was close to the medical model, but different because it was carried out within an expert nursing knowledge base. They identified that further research is needed to explore the outcomes of this integrated practice. This is the research imperative for APNs—to demonstrate the impact of the holistic nursing approach to care on patient outcomes.

Nurse-midwives have been in the forefront of developing collaborative relationships with physicians for many years. All APN groups would benefit from attention to the progress that CNMs have made in collaboration with physicians. The joint practice statement of the American College of Nurse Midwives (ACNM) and the American College of Obstetricians and Gynecologists (ACOG) can be used as a model for other APN groups (ACOG/ACNM, 2011). It highlights key principles for improving communication, working relationships, and seamlessness in the provision of women's health services (see also the ACNM's website, www.acnm.org). Problems with previous joint practice statements were that they included varying interpretations of physician supervision. According to the most recent statement, "OB-GYNs and CNMs/

CMs are experts in their respective fields of practice and are educated, trained, and licensed, independent providers who may collaborate with each other based on the needs of their patients. Quality of care is enhanced by collegial relationships characterized by mutual respect and trust, as well as professional responsibility and accountability" (ACOG/ACNM, 2011).

Role Transitions

Role transitions are defined here as dynamic processes of change that occur over time as new roles are acquired (see Table 4-1). Five essential factors influence role transitions (Schumacher & Meleis, 1994): (1) personal meaning of the transition, which relates to the degree of identity crisis experienced; (2) degree of planning, which involves the time and energy devoted to anticipating the change; (3) environmental barriers and supports, which refer to family, peer, school, and other components; (4) level of knowledge and skill, which relates to prior experience and school experiences; and (5) expectations, which are related to such factors as role models, literature, and media. The role strain experienced by individuals in response to role insufficiency (see Table 4-1 for definitions) that accompanies the transition to APN roles can be minimized, although certainly not completely prevented, by individualized assessment of these five essential factors, development of strategies to cope with them, and rehearsal of situations designed for application of these strategies. Entering graduate school may be associated with a ripple effect of concurrent role transitions in family, work, and other social arenas (Klaich, 1990).

Advanced Practice Nurse Role Acquisition in Graduate School

The personal meaning of role transitions was a major focus of literature in nursing role development in the United States from the 1970s through 2005. This topic is currently more prevalent in the international APN literature as APN roles are being established in different countries. In a review of APN role development literature from certificate and graduate NP programs, alterations in self-identity and self-concept emerged as a consistent theme, with role acquisition experiences commonly described as identity crises (see Brykczynski [1996] for a detailed discussion of this earlier work).

In their study of NP students, Roberts and colleagues (1997) reported findings similar to those observed decades earlier by Anderson, Leonard, and Yates (1974). Anderson and colleagues described the process of role development observed in three NP programs (a graduate program, post-baccalaureate certificate program, and continuing education program), whereas Roberts and associates described a current graduate NP program. Anderson and colleagues' (1974) description of NP students' progression from dependence to interdependence being accompanied by regression, anxiety, and conflict was found to be similar to observations made by Roberts and coworkers (1997) in graduate NP students over a period of 6 years (Table 4-2). For many years, my NP faculty colleagues and I have observed similar role transition processes in teaching role and clinical courses for graduate NP students. In a discussion of role transition experiences for neonatal NPs, Cusson and Viggiano (2002) made the important point that even positive transitions are stressful.

Roberts and colleagues (1997) observed 100 NP graduate students and reviewed their student clinical journals. They identified three major areas of transition as students progressed from dependence to interdependence: (1) development of professional competence; (2) change in role identity; and (3) evolving relationships with preceptors and faculty. The lowest level of competence coincided with the highest level of role confusion. This occurred at the end of the first semester and the beginning of the second semester in the three-semester program examined (Roberts et al., 1997). The most intense transition period seemed to come at the end of the students' first clinical immersion experience.

Roberts and colleagues (1997) described the first transition as involving an initial feeling of loss of confidence and competence accompanied by anxiety (see Table 4-2, stage I). Initial clinical experiences were associated with the desire to observe, rather than provide care, the inability to recall simple facts, the omission of essential data from history taking, feelings of awkwardness with patients, and difficulty prioritizing data. The students' focus at this time was almost exclusively on acquiring and refining assessment skills and continued development of physical examination techniques. By the end of the first semester, students reported returning feelings of confidence and the regaining of their former competence in interpersonal skills. Although they were still tentative about diagnostic and treatment decisions, students reported feeling more comfortable with patients as some of their basic nursing abilities began to return (see Table 4-2, stage II).

Transitions in nursing role identity occurring during the first two stages were associated with feelings of role confusion. Students were dismayed at how slowly and inefficiently they were performing in clinical situations and reported feelings of self-doubt and lack of confidence in their abilities to function in the real world of health care. They sought shortcuts in attempts to increase their efficiency. They reported profound feelings of

⚙ **TABLE 4-2**   Role Acquisition Process in School

Stage	Definition	Descriptive Features
I	Complete dependence	Immersion in learning medical components of care; role transition associated with role confusion and anxiety; decreased appreciation for psychosocial components of health and illness concerns; loss of confidence in clinical skills; feelings of incompetence
II	Developing competence	Ongoing clinical preceptorship experiences; didactic classes that incorporate medical diagnostic and nursing and medical therapeutic components, along with personal experience of illness components; renewed sense of appreciation for the value of nursing knowledge and skills; more realistic self-expectations of clinical performance, although still uncomfortable about accountability; increased confidence in ability to succeed in learning and making a valid contribution to care; initial formation of own philosophy and standards of practice
III	Independence	Comfortable with ability to conduct holistic assessments (physical and psychosocial); concentration on intervention and management options; conflicts with preceptors as student and preceptor challenge one another; conflicts with faculty relate to management options, clinical evaluations, examination questions, concern over not being taught all there is to know
IV	Interdependence	Renewed appreciation for interdependence of nursing and medicine; development of individualized version of advanced practice role

Adapted from Anderson, E.M., Leonard, B.J., & Yates, J.A. (1974). Epigenesis of the nurse practitioner role. *American Journal of Nursing,* 10, 12–16; and Roberts, S.J., Tabloski, P., & Bova, C. (1997). Epigenesis of the nurse practitioner role revisited. *Journal of Nursing Education,* 36, 67–73.

responsibility regarding diagnostic and treatment decisions and, at the same time, increasingly realized the limitations of clinical practice when they were confronted with the real-life situations of their patients. They recalled finding it easy to second-guess physicians' decisions in their previous nursing roles, but now they found those decisions more problematic when they were responsible for making them. They joked about feeling like adolescents. This is the point that Cusson and Viggiano (2002) were making when they commented, in reference to neonatal NPs, that the infant really does look different when viewed from the head of the bed rather than the side of the bed. They explained that "rather than taking orders, as they did as staff nurses, neonatal NPs must synthesize incredibly complex information and decide on a plan of action. Experienced neonatal nurses often guide house staff regarding care decisions and writing orders to match the care that is being given. However, the shift in responsibility to actually writing the orders can be very intimidating" (p. 24).

Roberts and colleagues (1997) observed that a blending of the APN student and the former nurse developed during stage II as students renewed their appreciation for their previous interpersonal skills as teachers, supporters, and collaborators and again perceived their patients as unique individuals in the context of their life situations. Students developed increased awareness of the uncertainty involved in the process of making definitive diagnostic and treatment decisions. In spite of current attempts to reduce diagnostic and treatment uncertainty through evidence-based practice, a basic degree of uncertainty is still inherent in clinical practice. Although these insights served to demystify the clinical diagnostic process, the students' anxiety about providing care increased. Learning about strategies to cope with clinical decision making in situations of uncertainty, such as ruling out the worst case scenario, seeking consultation, and monitoring patients closely with phone calls and follow-up visits, can decrease anxiety and promote increased confidence (Brykczynski, 1991).

The transition in the relationships between students and preceptors and students and faculty in the study by Roberts and colleagues (1997) involved students feeling anxious that they were not learning enough and would never know enough to practice competently. Students felt frustrated and perceived that faculty and preceptors were not providing them with all the information they needed. During the third stage (see Table 4-2), as they felt more confident and competent, students began to question the clinical judgments of their preceptors and faculty. This process is thought to help students advance from independence to interdependence—the last stage of the transition process. Much of the conflict at this juncture appeared to derive from students' feelings of "ambivalence about giving up dependence on external authorities" (Roberts et al., 1997, p. 71) such as preceptors and faculty and assuming responsibility for making independent judgments based on their own assessments from their clinical and educational experiences and the literature. The relevance of these role acquisition processes for other APN roles has not been reported. This is another area in which research would be helpful.

Until recently, the literature on APN role acquisition in school has focused exclusively on individuals who were already nurses. A commonly held assumption among nurses is "the more clinical experience, the better" for acquiring the necessary knowledge and skill to take on complex APN roles. At least 1 year of nursing practice is typically preferred for admission to APN programs. The process of role acquisition for students in direct-entry APN master's programs that admit NNCGs may differ because these individuals were not functioning as nurses before they entered the program. For additional information regarding this topic, see the qualitative study reported by Rich and Rodriguez (2002). In their qualitative study of family nurse practitioner (FNP) role transition, Heitz and colleagues (2004) found differences in role acquisition experiences between FNP students who were inexperienced nurses and FNP students who were experienced nurses. Feelings of insecurity, inadequacy, vulnerability, and being overwhelmed were typical, but role confusion was reported primarily by the more experienced RN students as they went through the letting go process of the RN role and taking on the FNP role. It will be interesting to observe whether this finding holds true for BSN to DNP students.

Strategies to Facilitate Role Acquisition

The anticipatory socialization to APN roles that occurs in graduate education is analogous to a process that Kramer (1974) described for undergraduate RNs called "immunization." The overall objective is to expose role incumbents to as many real-life experiences as possible during the educational program to minimize reality shock and role insufficiency on graduation and initial role implementation. Role content can be incorporated into APN curricula in a variety of ways, including the following: (1) in the overall framework for designing an APN curriculum; (2) in a specific role course; (3) as part of specific assignments; and (4) in role seminars that span an entire curriculum. Hamric and Hanson (2003) asserted that it is an ethical mandate for all APN educators, regardless of specialty, to provide graduates with up to date knowledge of professional role and regulatory issues in addition to concentration on clinical competence. The importance of explicit role preparation for the complex and challenging roles of graduates of DNP programs is recognized in the curriculum proposed by the American Association of Colleges of Nursing (AACN, 2006). If there is not a separate role course, careful attention must be paid to this curriculum component so that it does not become integrated out of existence.

Specific strategies for facilitating role acquisition can be categorized according to three major purposes: (1) role rehearsal; (2) development of clinical knowledge and skills, including strategies for dealing with uncertainty; and (3) creation of a supportive network. For adequate role rehearsal, APN students should experience all aspects of the core competencies (see Chapter 3) directly while faculty and fellow students are available to help them process or debrief these experiences. Faculty can help students by identifying role acquisition periods of high stress in their particular program so that support can be built in during those periods. APN students should be cautioned that other nurses, physicians, other providers, and administrators in the work setting may value only clinical expertise and not the other core competencies. Strategies for enhancing understanding of how the core competencies are embedded in each APN role include preparation of short-term and long-term goals to use as guides in the development of professional portfolios, analysis of existing position descriptions, and development of the ideal position description. These are also helpful for guiding students in their search for an initial APN position.

The development of clinical knowledge and skills for APN role acquisition can be promoted by planning for realistic clinical experiences with the support of faculty and preceptors nearby. Emphasis on realism and a holistic situational perspective are important in clinical experiences for helping students understand that the complex clinical judgments involved in APN assessment and management of patient situations over time are not simply technical medical knowledge, but a hybrid of nursing and medical knowledge and experience. Teaching and learning experiences for all the APN role components should integrate elements of research and theory and be incorporated into specialty APN courses to build on the knowledge gained in the traditional graduate core and clinical support courses in the curriculum. New APN graduates can benefit from familiarity with role transition processes by not expecting to be able to demonstrate all APN role components fully and expertly immediately on graduation.

Clinical mentoring by preceptors is an important component of ensuring realistic clinical learning experiences (Hayes, 2001; Heitz, et al., 2004; Kelly & Mathews, 2001; Kleinpell-Nowell, 2001). A survey of 258 graduating NP students at 10 institutions indicated that students who selected their own preceptor scored higher on mentoring and self-efficacy than those whose preceptors were assigned by faculty (Hayes, 1998). In addition, students with non-nurse preceptors scored lower than those with nurse preceptors. These findings need to be considered in planning preceptor arrangements. A mix of APN and non-nurse preceptors during the program can be valuable. Hayes (2001) observed that requiring students to locate their own preceptors can be problematic for some students who may not have the necessary professional connections to identify a qualified preceptor.

Anticipatory planning for the first APN position after program completion is important. Reports of the transition experiences of new NP graduates during their first year after graduation suggested that the first position can be critical in terms of solidifying the NP's career (Brown & Olshansky, 1997; Heitz et al., 2004; Kelly & Mathews, 2001). Preparation of students for assuming APN roles on graduation should be a collaborative effort of students, faculty, and preceptors. The need for position descriptions that clearly outline roles and responsibilities has been emphasized as essential for smooth role transition (Cooper & Sparacino, 1990; Hamric & Taylor, 1989; McMyler & Miller, 1997). The transition to the first position is a process, not an event, that may take 6 months to 2 years (Steiner et. al., 2004). It needs to be a focus of role content in APN programs (Hamric & Hanson, 2003; Hunter, Bormann, & Lops, 1996). Some APN faculty share the belief that frequent position changes or staying in the same registered nurse job after graduation from an APN program reflects role disillusionment. Substantive role courses are critical to smooth the path to full APN role implementation (Hamric & Hanson, 2003; Hunter et al., 1996).

Finally, and perhaps most importantly, an overall strategy for enhancing APN clinical knowledge and skill is for faculty to maintain competency in clinical practice. Clinical competency enhances the faculty's ability to evaluate students clinically, discuss clinically relevant examples in classes, serve as preceptors for students, and evaluate the care provided in clinical preceptorship sites. The clinical competence of faculty is important to prevent a wide gap between education and practice, enhance faculty credibility, and foster realistic expectations for new APN graduates.

Establishing a peer support system, planning social functions with faculty and preceptors, and creating a virtual community can facilitate the development of a support network. Computer literacy is critical for networking and access to the high-quality materials available on websites (Table 4-3), in literature searches, and on smartphones. The importance of forming a support network was emphasized by study findings (Kelly & Mathews, 2001; Kleinpell-Nowell, 2001). The establishment of a system for self-directed learning activities during the first few years after program completion forms the basis for maintaining competence throughout one's career (Gunn, 1998). The establishment of a process for lifelong learning should be initiated during the APN

TABLE 4-3   Useful Internet Sites for Creating a Support Network

Website	Organization	Highlights
www.aahcdc.org	Association of Academic Health Centers	Interdisciplinary education and practice in prevention; resources for building a practice
www.nonpf.com	National Organization of Nurse Practitioner Faculties	NP competencies, publications, resource centers
www.aanp.org	American Association of Nurse Practitioners*	Certification, legislative news, research, continuing education
www.nacns.org	National Association of Clinical Nurse Specialists	Position statement on CNS practice and education
www.nursingworld.org	American Nurses Association	Credentialing center; patient safety, advocacy
www.napnap.org	National Association of Pediatric Nurse Practitioners	Scope of practice for PNPs, healthy eating initiative, immunization education
www.aana.com	American Association of Nurse Anesthetists	Click on "Resources" for professional practice documents
www.acnm.org	American College of Nurse-Midwives	Click on "About Midwives" for Scope of practice
www.ncsbn.org	National Council of State Boards of Nursing	Click on "Nursing Policy" for APRN consensus model

*The American Academy of Nurse Practitioners and the American College of Nurse Practitioners merged to form the American Association or Nurse Practitioners in 2013.

educational program as students create a computer-based, self-monitoring system that includes clinical and role transition experiences over time to serve as a reality check or timetable. On graduation, continuing education program attendance could be incorporated into this monitoring system to facilitate compilation of necessary documentation for certification, along with ongoing self-evaluation and role development.

Advanced Practice Nursing Role Implementation at Work

After successfully emerging from the APN educational process, new APN graduates face yet another transition, from the student role to the professional APN role (see Fig. 4-1). APN graduates can be expected to experience attitudinal, behavioral, and value conflicts as they move from the academic world, in which holistic care is highly valued, to the work world, in which organizational efficiency is paramount. Anticipatory guidance is needed for role transition yet again. The process of APN role implementation is an example of a situational transition (Schumacher & Meleis, 1994), which has been described as a progressive movement through phases. There is general agreement that significant overlap and fluidity exist among the phases. However, for purposes of discussion, the phases will be considered sequentially.

Hamric and Taylor's (1989) study of CNS role development and Brown and Olshansky's (1997) study of NP role transition are two major U.S. investigations of APN role implementation processes. Additional U.S. studies that have contributed to an understanding of the transitional processes as APNs implement their roles include the following: the longitudinal survey of acute care NP practice (Kleinpell-Nowell, 1999, 2001; Kleinpell, 2005), in which the first six cohorts to take the adult acute care national certification examination were followed annually for 5 years; Kelly and Mathews' (2001) qualitative focus group study of 21 recent NP graduates; Heitz and colleagues' (2004) qualitative study of nine FNPs' role transition experiences; and Steiner and colleagues' (2008) follow-up of the study by Heitz and associates. Reports of role implementation studies from other countries will also be integrated into the discussion.

Hamric and Taylor (1989) described seven phases of CNS role development, along with associated characteristics and developmental tasks derived from the analysis of questionnaires returned by 100 CNSs (Table 4-4). Of 42 CNSs in their first positions for 3 years or less, 40 experienced progression through the first three phases (identical to those phases identified by Baker [1979]). Most of the CNS respondents went through these three phases within 2 years. Phase 1, the orientation phase, is characterized by enthusiasm, optimism, and attention to mastery of clinical skills. The second phase, the frustration phase, is associated with feelings of conflict, inadequacy, frustration, and anxiety. Arena and Page (1992) identified the imposter phenomenon as a feature of CNS practice that could interfere with effective role implementation. In retrospect,

it appears that the imposter phenomenon is one of the distressing features of the frustration phase. The next phase, the implementation phase, is described as one of role modification in response to interactions with others. This phase is associated with a renewed or returning perspective.

CNSs with more than 3 years of experience described their role development experiences in terms very different from Baker's (1979) phases. Content analysis of these data led to a description of four additional phases (see Table 4-4). Experienced CNSs identified the integration phase, which was characterized by "self-confidence and assurance in the role, high job satisfaction, an advanced level of practice, and signs of recognition and respect for expertise within and outside the work setting" (Hamric & Taylor, 1989, p. 56). Only 10% of the CNSs with less than 5 years of experience in the role met the criteria for this phase, whereas 50% of those with more than 6 years of experience could be categorized as being in this phase. The integration phase was typically reached after 3 to 5 years in the CNS role. This fourth phase, of integration—thought to be reached only after successful transition through the earlier phases—is characterized by refinement of clinical expertise and integration of role components appropriate for the particular situation.

Llahana and Hamric (2011) reported on a nationwide study of the role development experiences of diabetes specialist nurses (DSNs) conducted in 2001 in the United Kingdom, which was based on Hamric and Taylor's (1989) work. Although the 334 DSNs were not all master's prepared, most held postgraduate qualification in diabetes care. The findings indicated that role development phases were similar to those in the earlier study, with the addition of a transition phase associated with the orientation phase when a competent DSN moved to a different practice site. The anxiety experienced during the transition phase was related to orienting to a new work setting rather than to knowledge or competence in the role.

Hamric and Taylor (1989) also described three negative phases not evident in previous literature. The frozen phase is described as being associated with frustration, anger, and lack of career satisfaction. Restructuring of role responsibilities and changing organizational expectations characterize the reorganization phase. The complacent phase is characterized by comfort, stability, and maintenance of the status quo. Unlike the integration phase, these additional phases share a negative nonproductive character. It is of interest that there was a higher proportion of nurses in negative phases (58%) in the UK study (Llahana & Hamric, 2011) than reported in the original Hamric and Taylor study (1989) (27%). One might speculate that APNs experiencing these negative phases would

TABLE 4-4   Phases of Advanced Practice Nurse Role Development

Phase	Features	Developmental Tasks	Facilitation Strategies
Orientation	Enthusiasm, optimism, eager to prove self to setting; anxious about ability to meet self- and institutional expectations; expects to make change	Learn formal and informal organizations. Learn key players; begin establishing relationship and power base. Explore expectations to see whether compatible with own. Identify and clarify role to self and others.	Structure an orientation plan. Establish mutually agreed on role expectations. Circulate literature on APN role. Meet with key individuals. Network with peers. Identify with a role model or mentor. Set reasonable 3- to 6-mo goals. Concentrate on clinical mastery. Postpone recommendations for major changes. Join key committees.
Frustration*	Discouragement and questioning as a result of unrealistic expectations (either self or employer); difficult and slow-paced change; resistance encountered; feelings of inadequacy in response to the overwhelming problems encountered, pressure to prove worth	Develop more realistic expectations. Work on time management and setting priorities. Develop short-term goals or projects to obtain tangible results and feedback. Develop support system within and/or outside of work setting.	Schedule debriefing sessions. Practice time management. Review initial logs. Update professional portfolio. Continue seeking peer and mentor support. Maintain communication with administrators. Consult with experts. Organize resources for easy accessibility.
Implementation	Returning optimism and enthusiasm as positive feedback received and expectations realigned; organization and reorganization of role tasks, modified in response to feedback; implementing and balancing new subroles; regaining sense of perspective; may focus on specific project(s)	Enhance visibility and power base within informal and formal organizations; build coalitions and networks. Identify tangible accomplishments. Complete transition to advanced practice level, if necessary. Continue to reassess and refocus direction.	Reassess demands, priorities, and goals. Plan for performance and outcome evaluation. Sustain communication with peers, administrators, and others.
Integration	Self-confident and assured in role; rates self at advanced level of practice; activities reflect wide recognition, influence in area of specialty; continuously feels challenged, takes on new projects; expands practice; moderately or very satisfied with present position; congruence between personal and organizational goals and expectations	Continue role evolution and skill development to strengthen all role components and competencies. Share expertise and experience with others through publications, research, and professional activities. Maintain flexible approach. Be alert for signs of complacency or boredom.	Continue debriefing sessions. Plan for role expansion and refinement. Schedule performance and outcome evaluations. Develop broader professional interests. Formulate short- and long-term goals for further development.

TABLE 4-4 Phases of Advanced Practice Nurse Role Development—*cont'd*

Phase	Features	Developmental Tasks	Facilitation Strategies
Frozen	Self-confident, assured in role; rates self at intermediate or advanced practice level; experiences anger, frustration reflecting experience; conflict between self-goals and those of organization or supervisor; reports sense of being unable to move forward because of forces outside of self	Obtain feedback from supervisor and peers. Reevaluate self-goals in relation to CNS role and organization. Objective assessment of organization—is there potential for compatibility? Attempt to redesign or renegotiate the role. Consider career move or change. If unsuccessful, consider change in position or career direction.	Self-assessment and early recognition of problems. Conflict resolution and role clarification discussions. Appraisal of APN goals in relation to organizational goals. Renegotiate role expectations.
Reorganization	Reports earlier experiences that represent integration; organization experiencing major changes; pressure to change role in ways that are incongruent with own concept of CNS role and/or personal goals	Have open discussion with change agents. Attempt compromise to preserve integrity of role and still meet needs of organization. If unsuccessful, change position or title, or negotiate job change.	
Complacent	Experiences self in role as settled and comfortable; variable job satisfaction; questionable impact on organization	Need to reenergize; reconfigure role to allow growth by identifying changing needs of patient population or institution.	

*The imposter phenomenon (Arena & Page, 1992) may be experienced during the frustration phase. Adapted by Brykczynski, K.A. from Hamric, A.B., & Taylor, J.W. (1989). Role development of the CNS. In A.B. Hamric & J.A. Spross (Eds.), *The clinical nurse specialist in theory and practice* (p. 48, 2nd ed.). Philadelphia: WB Saunders.

be more vulnerable to position changes in today's cost-constrained health care system.

The complexity of APN role development processes is further demonstrated by findings from Brown and Olshansky's (1997) longitudinal grounded theory study of the role transition experiences of 35 novice NPs conducted at 1, 6, and 12 months for two different cohorts of graduates during their first year of practice. They described a four-stage process of moving from "limbo to legitimacy" during the first year of practice, outlined in Table 4-5. Related developmental tasks and strategies included in this table were specifically developed for this chapter. The first stage, laying the foundation, was not described in previous literature. During this stage, new graduates take certification examinations, obtain necessary recognition or licensure from state boards of nursing, and look for positions. This stage has been shortened because of the availability of certification examinations by computer.

The second stage, the launching stage, was defined as beginning with the first NP position and lasting at least 3 months. During this stage, the new graduate NP experiences the anxiety associated with the crisis of confidence and competence that accompanies taking on a new position and the return to the advanced beginner skill level (Benner et al., 2009; Dreyfus & Dreyfus, 1986, 2009). As the advanced beginner becomes increasingly aware of the number of elements relevant to actual performance in the role, he or she may become overwhelmed with the complexity of the skills required for the role and exhausted by the effort required for mastery. New NPs in Kelly and Mathews' (2001) study described similar experiences of exhaustion and frustration with lack of control over time. This is the at-work version of the crisis of confidence and competence experienced during stage I of the in-school role acquisition process (see Table 4-2).

The feeling of being "an imposter" or "a fake," described by Brown and Olshansky (1997), Arena and Page (1992), and Huffstutler and Varnell (2006), was first reported in the psychological literature in reference to high-achieving women (Clance & Imes, 1978). Clinical symptoms associated with this phenomenon—generalized anxiety, lack of self confidence, depression, frustration—are commonly reported by APNs experiencing the frustration or launching phase. It is related to feeling unable to meet one's own expectations and those of others (Clance & Imes, 1978)

TABLE 4-5   Transition Stages in First Year of Primary Care Practice

Stage	Features	Developmental Tasks	Facilitation Strategies
Laying the foundation	Period of role identity confusion immediately after graduation; not yet an NP, but no longer a student; feelings of worry, confusion, and insecurity about ability to practice successfully as an NP	Recuperate from school. Initiate a job search and secure a position. Obtain certification.	Take time out to recuperate from the pressures of school. Plan rewards for self. Maintain peer support network. Refine professional portfolio and use it to analyze available positions in terms of future goals.
Launching	Discomfort of advanced beginner level of knowledge and skills; feelings of unreality, insecurity—the imposter phenomenon; pervasive performance anxiety; daily stress; time pressure	Develop realistic expectations. Incorporate feeling of legitimacy into NP role identity. Cope with anxiety. Mobilize problem-solving skills. Work on time management and setting priorities. Develop support system.	Plan for longer appointments initially. Anticipate need for time to feel comfortable in new role. Realize that the transition process is time-limited. Schedule debriefing sessions with experienced MD or APN. Seek peer and mentor support regularly. Learn time-saving tips. Clarify appropriate patient problems to work with initially. Monitor internal self-talk; be positive.
Meeting the challenge	Decreased anxiety; increased feeling of legitimacy; increased confidence develops, along with increased competence; increased acceptance and comfort with the uncertainty inherent in primary care	Expand recognition of practice concerns to include the work environment. Gain situational knowledge and skill in managing clinical problems. Identify tangible accomplishments. Develop individualized style of approaching patients and organizing care.	Schedule a 6-mo evaluation. Maintain communication with peers, administrators, and others. Modify expectations to be more realistic. Learn from repetitive practice. Structure work situation so that resources are readily available. Practice strategies to manage uncertainty. Gain ability to handle uncertainty.
Broadening the perspective	Feeling of enhanced self-esteem; solid feeling of legitimacy and competence; realistic and positive feelings about future practice	Acknowledge strengths and identify ways to incorporate additional challenges. Identify larger system problems and seek solutions.*	Schedule a 12-mo evaluation to reflect on progress and accomplishments. Continue to seek verification and feedback from colleagues. Make changes in work situation to increase support and effectiveness. Inform staff and colleagues about NP role. Affirm self-worth.[†]

*All the developmental tasks from the integration phase in Table 4-4 would be appropriate here also.
[†]Facilitation strategies from the Integration phase of Table 4-4 would be useful here also)
Data from Brown, M.A., & Olshansky, E. (1997). From limbo to legitimacy: A theoretical model of the transition to the primary care nurse practitioner role. *Nursing Research*, 46, 46–51; and Brown, M.A., & Olshansky, E. (1998). Becoming a primary nurse practitioner: Challenges of the initial year of practice. *Nurse Practitioner, 23*, 46, 52–56. Adapted from Hamric, A.B., & Taylor, J.W. (1989). Role development of the CNS. In A.B. Hamric & J.A. Spross (Eds.), *The clinical nurse specialist in theory and practice* (2nd ed., p. 48). Philadelphia: WB Saunders.

and feelings of inadequacy and constantly being tested (Arena & Page, 1992). This phenomenon is typically a temporary experience associated with taking on a new role or beginning a new job. Heitz and colleagues' (2004) study related similar role transition experiences of self-doubt, disillusionment, and turbulence and also reported that engaging in positive self-talk was helpful. They suggested that issues of gender and age may underlie differing perceptions of personal commitments and sacrifices as obstacles to surmount in role transition.

Although Brown and Olshansky (1997, 1998) did not relate their findings about NP role transition to Hamric and Taylor's (1989) findings about CNS role development, there appear to be many similarities in the results of the two studies. The characteristics of the launching stage are similar to those described by Hamric and Taylor (1989) for the frustration phase. Brown and Olshansky's (1997, 1998) third stage, meeting the challenge, is associated with feelings of regaining confidence and increasing competence. This stage has much in common with Hamric and Taylor's (1989) implementation phase, which is noted for returning optimism and enthusiasm as expectations are realigned. The last stage, broadening the perspective, is characterized by feelings of legitimacy and competency as NPs. This last stage is similar to Hamric and Taylor's (1989) fourth stage of integration, during which the role is expanded and refined.

Fleming and Carberry (2011) studied expert critical care nurses transitioning to APN roles in an ICU setting in Scotland. The core category of steering the course to advanced practice and the phases of finding a niche, coping with the pressures, feeling competent to do, and internalizing the role share many similarities with the findings from the studies of Hamric and Taylor (1989) and Brown and Olshansky's (1997). Fleming and Carberry observed that the extreme anxiety provoked by moving from expert to novice and back to expert again was similar to findings reported in previous studies of this process in critical care settings (Ball & Cox, 2004; Cussons & Strange, 2008).

Rich (2005) investigated the relationship between duration of experience as an RN and NP clinical skills in practice among NPs who graduated within 4 years from three universities in the Northeast. These graduates, 150 NPs, completed the self-report instrument assessments of their clinical skills (a response rate of 21%), and 60% of the collaborating physicians completed assessments of their NP clinical skills. Findings from the NP self-report data indicated that duration of practice experience as an RN was not correlated with level of competency in NP practice skills. "An unexpected finding was that there was a significant negative correlation between years of experience as an RN and NP clinical practice skills as assessed by the collaborating physicians" (Rich, 2005, p. 55). Data describing which role development phase the NP participants were experiencing would have been helpful for enhancing understanding of the findings. The finding that collaborating physicians rated the NPs as more clinically competent than the NPs rated themselves (Rich, 2005) would be expected for NPs in the frustration or launching phase (see Tables 4-4 and 4-5). Inclusion of assessments of role development and clinical competency in APN

follow-up studies would be helpful for building on the existing knowledge base.

Strategies to Facilitate Role Implementation

The seven major developmental phases identified by Hamric and Taylor (1989) to describe CNS role development are combined with strategies for facilitating APN role implementation (see Table 4-4). Table 4-5 lists the four stages of NP role implementation and their characteristics, as identified by Brown and Olshansky (1997), and includes developmental tasks and strategies for facilitating NP role development in an attempt to link this study with those findings from the Hamric and Taylor (1989) study. The reader is encouraged to compare and contrast Tables 4-4 and 4-5 to glean relevant content for their particular APN role.

The phases described by Hamric and Taylor (1989) are used here to structure discussion of strategies to facilitate role implementation. The importance of being patient and recognizing that it takes time to develop fully in a new APN role was stressed by NPs in Kleinpell-Nowell's surveys (1999, 2001). A strategy to facilitate role implementation for all APNs during the orientation phase is development of a structured orientation plan. Brown and Olshansky (1997, 1998) noted the importance of clarification of values, needs, and expectations and of recognition that transitional experiences are time-limited. They also noted the importance of anticipatory guidance and realizing that these transition experiences follow a common pattern in new graduates. An APN in a new position, whether experienced in the role or not, needs to be aware of the importance of being informed about the organizational structure, philosophy, goals, policies, and procedures of the agency.

Networking was emphasized by NPs in Kleinpell-Nowell's surveys (1999, 2001). Peer support within and outside of the work setting is important, as noted by Hamric and Taylor (1989). New NPs stressed the importance of getting to know other nurses in the work setting, gaining their respect, and forming key alliances with them to enhance optimal functioning in their new position (Kelly & Mathews, 2001). Designating a more experienced APN in the work setting as a mentor would be helpful and would provide support for all APNs new to a position. APNs who serve as preceptors for students might be particularly effective mentors for new graduates (Hayes, 2005). The importance of careful selection of a mentor was reported by NPs in the study by Kelly and Mathews (2001). Additional strategies suggested for networking within the system include developing peer support groups, being accessible to colleagues by phone or email, and getting involved in interdisciplinary committees (Page & Arena, 1991). APNs should be encouraged to join local APN groups for peer support, legislative and political updates, and networking opportunities. Numerous Internet sites are also available for networking, as noted earlier.

Page and Arena (1991) recommended that CNSs schedule and devote the major portion of their time during the orientation phase to direct patient care to substantiate the clinical expert role. They also suggested making appointments with nursing leaders, physicians, and other health care professionals during this phase to garner administrative support. They recommended distributing business cards and making the job description available for discussion. They also counseled new CNSs to withhold suggestions for change until they have had the opportunity to assess the system more fully. When a new APN joins the staff of an organization, the administrator should send a letter describing the APN's background experiences and new position to key people in the organization.

Hamric and Taylor (1989) observed that the frustration phase might come and go and may overlap other phases. They noted that painful affective responses are typical of this difficult phase. They suggested that monthly sessions for sharing concerns with a group of peers and an administrator might facilitate movement through this phase. Strategies identified as helpful for energizing movement from the frustration phase to the implementation phase include the following: obtaining assistance with time management (Allen, 2001); participating in support groups to ameliorate feelings of inadequacy; engaging in discussions for conflict resolution and role clarification; reassessing priorities and setting realistic expectations; and focusing on short-term, visible goals.

Page and Arena (1991) suggested keeping a work portfolio to document activities so that APN progress is more readily visible and accessible. This can be an expansion of the portfolio and self-monitoring system initiated during the APN program. Brown and Olshansky (1997) noted that organized sources of support such as phone calls, seminars, planned meetings with mentors, and scheduled time for consultation can significantly decrease feelings of anxiety. They noted that recognition of the discomfort arising from moving from expert back to novice and the realization that previous expertise can be valuable in the new role may help reduce feelings of inadequacy. They suggested that new APNs request reasonable time frames for initial patient visits because novices take longer than experienced practitioners, and this may be key to successful adjustment to a new position.

During the implementation phase, it is important for the APN to reassess demands to prevent feeling overwhelmed. Priorities may need to be readjusted and short-term goals may need to be reformulated. Brown and Olshansky (1997, 1998) observed that competence and confidence are fostered through repetition. They also recommend scheduling a formal evaluation after approximately 6 months in which feedback about areas of strength and those needing improvement can be ascertained. Strategies mentioned as important during this time include seeking administrative support through involvement in meetings, maintaining visibility in clinical areas, and developing in-service programs with input from staff (Page & Arena, 1991). After some time in the implementation phase, APNs may plan and execute small-scale projects to demonstrate their effectiveness in their new role.

Hamric and Taylor's (1989) survey data indicated that CNSs maximize their role potential during the integration phase. Satisfactory completion of the earlier phases appears to be essential for passage into this phase. One strategy for enhancing and maintaining optimal role implementation during this phase is having a trusted colleague who can act as a safe sounding board for "feedback, constructive criticism, and advice" (Hamric & Taylor, 1989, p. 79). During this phase, it is important to have a plan to guide continued role expansion and refinement, such as the portfolio mentioned earlier. Seeking appointment to key committees is important to increase recognition of APNs in the organization. Administrative support and constructive feedback from a trusted mentor continue to be important. Development of a promotional system that offers professional advancement in the APN practice role remains a challenge for practitioners and administrators. Page and Arena (1991) observed that less time is required for establishing relationships and assessing the system during this phase; therefore, more time can be devoted to areas of scholarly interest. Brown and Olshansky (1997, 1998) noted the importance of formulating short-term goals to further development.

Whether the frozen, reorganization, and complacent phases are distinct developmental phases or variations of the implementation and integration phases, they are clearly negative resolutions for APNs and their organizations. Table 4-4 includes strategies described by Hamric and Taylor (1989) for enhancing role development in these phases (see the earlier editions of this text for further discussion of these phases). APNs should engage in periodic self-assessment so that they recognize beginning signs associated with these phases, such as feelings of anger or dissatisfaction, conflict between self-goals and those of the organization or supervisor, feeling pressure to change one's APN role in ways that are incongruent with one's concept of the role, and feelings of complacency. Early recognition of problems and taking proactive steps to deal with organizational changes can help prevent or ameliorate the negative feelings associated with these phases.

Further analysis of the relationships between the stages described by Brown and Olshansky (1997, 1998) for NPs and the phases described by Hamric and Taylor (1989) for CNSs is needed. The relevance of these frameworks for transition processes experienced by other APNs also needs study. Further refinement of these findings could promote their incorporation into APN teaching, research, and practice. The following are questions of interest:

1. Is the laying the foundation stage common to other APN groups?
2. Do the negative phases—frozen, reorganization, and complacent—appear after 3 years of practice in APN groups other than CNSs?
3. How do role acquisition and role implementation experiences of APN graduates of DNP programs compare with those reported here for master's-prepared APNs?

International Experiences with Advanced Practice Nurse Role Development and Implementation: Lessons Learned and A Proposed Model for Success

Over the last decade, as APN roles have been introduced in other countries, there has been increasing interest in APN role development and implementation internationally. The most recent research on APN roles has been conducted in countries outside the United States. The Canadian experience provides significant lessons learned and suggestions for successful APN role implementation worldwide. CNS and NP roles have existed in Canada for 40 years, but their implementation has been sporadic because of numerous system-level factors (DiCenso, Martin-Misnener, Bryant-Lukosius, et al., 2010; Sangster-Gormley, Martin-Misener, Downe-Wamboldt, & DiCenso, 2011). A decreased demand for APN roles in Canada resulted from many factors, including lack of legislative and regulatory authority of APN roles, multiple titles and conflicting definitions, absence of reimbursement mechanisms, opposition from the medical profession, and inconsistent curriculum requirements, which subsequently led to the gradual closure of most NP and CNS programs by the late 1980s (Sangster-Gormley, et al, 2011). Recently, there has been renewed interest in APN roles as a way to promote changes in the Canadian health care system (DiCenso et al., 2010.)

Although external factors such as supports and barriers were addressed, the major focus of APN role development and implementation research has been on the micro level, with a focus on personal experiences of the individual clinician taking on a new role. A new framework for role implementation developed in Canada is noteworthy in that it takes a macro perspective and involves stakeholders (e.g., administrators, patients, advocacy groups, support staff, professional organizations) in the APN role implementation process. It specifically addresses barriers to role implementation at the system, organizational, and practice setting levels (Bryant-Lukosius & DiCenso, 2004). The participatory, evidence-based, patient-focused process for advanced practice nursing role development, implementation and evaluation (PEPPA) framework (Bryant-Lukosius & DiCenso, 2004) recognizes the complexity of the system factors involved in implementing a new role into an existing system. The PEPPA framework (Fig. 4-2) incorporates the principles of participatory action research (PAR) "to promote more equitable distribution of power and enhance the contributions of nurses, patients, and other stakeholders in APN role development" (Bryant-Lukosius & DiCenso, 2004, p. 531). It was developed to guide APN role implementation and has been used effectively in a variety of practice settings in Canada (McNamara 2009; McAiney, 2008; & Martin-Misener, 2010).

Facilitators and Barriers in the Work Setting

Aspects of the work setting exert a major influence on APN role definitions and expectations, thereby affecting role ambiguity, role incongruity, and role conflict. Findings from a survey by McFadden and Miller (1994) of CNSs identify access to support services, such as computers, statistical consultation, and secretarial and library services, as facilitators of role development. Factors found to promote NP role development include the following: being recognized as a primary care provider; having one's own examination room; and being supported by coworkers, administrators, and patients (Andrews, Hanson, Maule, & Snelling, 1999; Hupcey, 1993; Kelly & Mathews, 2001). This need for ongoing peer and administrative support is a theme throughout the literature on role development, beginning with the student experience and extending into practice.

Practical strategies identified by Bonnel and associates (2000) for initiating NP practice in nursing facilities included proactive communication, developing a consistent system for visits, setting up the physical environment, and building a team approach to care. Factors found to impede NP role development include pressure to manage care for large numbers of patients, resistance from staff nurses, and lack of understanding of the NP role (Andrews et al., 1999; Hupcey, 1993; Kelly & Mathews, 2001). More recent constraints operating in today's health care settings that affect not only APNs but also other providers and office staff include new billing and coding guidelines,

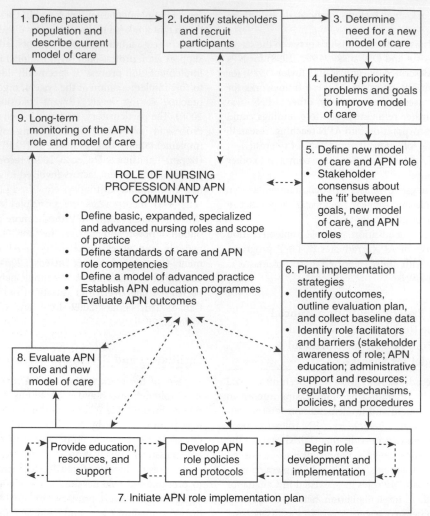

FIG 4-2 PEPPA framework. *(From Bryant-Lukosius, D., & DiCenso, A. (2004). A framework for the introduction and evaluation of advanced practice nursing roles. Journal of Advanced Nursing, 48, 532.)*

Health Insurance Portability and Accountability Act (HIPAA) regulations, monitoring for fraud and abuse, sexual harassment, and demands to integrate technology into practice.

Keating, Thompson, and Lee (2010) reported on a study of perceived barriers to progression and sustainability of NP roles in emergency departments 10 years after they were introduced in Victoria, Australia. The main barriers identified were lack of organizational support, legislative constraints, and lack of ongoing funding for APN education. They noted that some organizations successfully increased their numbers of NPs by using measures such as reallocation of resources and creating a common nursing and medical budget. They encouraged

continued exploration of role implementation issues and development of methods to address them to realize the potential benefits of NP practice to the health care delivery system.

The ability to incorporate teaching and counseling into the patient encounter may be a function of skill development gained with experience in the APN role. This observation may be used as a rationale for structuring more time for visits and fewer total patients for new APNs, with gradual increases in caseloads as experience is accrued. Older research has indicated that NPs incorporate counseling and teaching into the flow of patient visits—capturing the teachable moment (Brykczynski, 1985; Johnson, 1993; Lurie, 1981). Future plans to redesign primary care payment systems to blend monthly patient panel fees with fee for service charges and include incentives for patient-centered care performance are promising for APNs because these payment systems highlight and support the additional dimensions of care that APNs can provide (Davis, Schoenbaum, & Audet, 2005).

Administrative factors that should be considered include whether APNs are placed in line or staff positions, whether they are unit-based, population-based, or in some other arrangement, who evaluates them, and whether they report to administrative or clinical supervisors. Baird and Prouty (1989) maintained that the organizational design should have enough flexibility to change as the situation changes. The placements of various APN positions may differ, even within one setting, depending on size, complexity, and distribution of the patient population (Andrews et al., 1999; Baird & Prouty, 1989; Nevidjon & Simonson, 2009). Issues of professional versus administrative authority underlie the importance of the structural placement of the APN within the organization. Effectiveness of the APN role is enhanced when there is a mutual fit between the goals and expectations of the individual and the organization (Nevidjon & Simonson, 2009). Clarification of goals and expectations before employment and periodic reassessments can minimize conflict and enhance role development and effectiveness.

Continued Advanced Practice Nurse Role Evolution

CNMs, CRNAs, NPs, and CNSs have attained positive recognition and support in clinical positions in many settings in the United States. However, in spite of the increasing familiarity and popularity of these APN roles, some health care settings have used few, if any, APNs and some staff members have had minimal experience working with APNs. In some areas of the United States, physicians or physician assistants are preferred over APNs. Even experienced APNs can expect to encounter resistance to full implementation of their roles if they seek positions in institutions with no history of employing APNs. Andrews and colleagues (1999) described their experiences introducing the NP role into a large academic teaching hospital. They delineated helpful strategies for marketing a new NP role to staff, patients, and the surrounding community, as well as ways to set up the necessary infrastructure to support the new role in the institution. They referred to this process as evolutionary.

The meaning of the evolution of established APN roles varies according to the type of APN role. For example, for CNMs, role evolution refers to broadening the scope of practice to include primary health care (Kinsley, 2005). For over a decade, midwifery has encompassed primary care management of women in their core competencies for basic midwifery practice (ACNM, 2012; see also the ACNM's website, www.acnm.org). The emphasis on cost containment in the health care delivery system has led to the trend of having acute care NPs staff intensive care units to compensate for the shortage of house staff physicians (Rosenfeld, 2001; Sechrist & Berlin, 1998; see also Chapter 16). Evolution of APN roles is also reflected in the expansion of practice to multiple areas or sites. Although responsibility for multiple areas in the same facility has been typical of many CNS roles for years, it is an evolutionary process for most other APN roles. Multi-site roles might signify practice responsibilities at different sites or multiple areas of responsibility in the same site, and they may combine inpatient and outpatient responsibilities (Stahl & Myers, 2002). Stahl and Myers' clinical practices (see Exemplar 4-2) are models for APN practice evolving to multiple sites, which constitute a strategy for

---

◉ EXEMPLAR 4-2   Evolving APN Roles in Multisite Practices

Stahl is a CNS whose practice has evolved from the full range of CNS practice for four medical cardiac units at a tertiary care center to also include support primarily in education, consultation, and program development at two additional hospitals. Myers is an adult NP who directs a hepatitis C program for a specialty physician group with 11 physicians at nine practice locations, and she also provides direct care for patients at four of the sites.

The complexity of multisite roles can be overwhelming if the APN does not develop a certain degree of comfort with ambiguity. Stahl and Myers relied on Quinn's (1996) wisdom for developing the leader within by expecting to "build the bridge as you walk on it" (p. 83) and learning "how to get lost with confidence" (p. 86). Their commitment to being continuous learners is a useful model for APNs to follow as they experience the situational transitions that are inevitable as clinical practices evolve. Stahl and Myers used the National Association of Clinical Nurse Specialists' (NACNS, 1998) position statement (an updated version is now available on the NACNS website; see Table 4-3) describing three spheres of CNS influence to stimulate creativity and guide their APN practices as they evolve into new and multiple practice settings.

extending APN resources and trying to use them more efficiently.

As individual APNs mature into their respective roles and become comfortable and confident in all role components, greater concentration on the unique nature of APN practice can be expected. In their study of CNSs, Hamric and Taylor (1989) found that freedom to develop their unique APN role, availability of feedback from a mentor, support to broaden their influence and take on new projects, and recognition of their contributions enabled experienced CNSs to stay energized in their clinical practice roles. As Peplau (1997) advocated, nurse leaders must emphasize what nurses do for patients. The claim that APN practice incorporates patient education, family assessment, involvement, and support, and community awareness and connections (Neale, 1999) needs to be documented. For example, Kelly and Mathews (2001) found that graduates with 1 to 7 years of experience as NPs found it difficult to adhere to ideals of holistic care and health promotion, given the pressures of the clinical situation. Continued research that demonstrates positive outcomes of APN care is essential for APN practice to make an impact on health care policy (Brooten et al., 2002; Murphy-Ende, 2002; Russell, VorderBruegge, & Burns, 2002; Ryden et al., 2000; see also Chapter 23). Rashotte (2005) advocated for dialogical forms of research to evoke the more holistic and humanistic aspects of what it means to be an APN to complement the predominant instrumental and economic perspectives underlying most APN research. Brykczynski's (2012) interpretive phenomenologic study of how NP faculty incorporate holistic aspects of care into teaching NP students is an example of such dialogical research. More research activity and increasing involvement in the larger arena of health policy may also represent continuing role evolution for APNs.

Evaluation of Role Development

Evaluation is fundamental to enhancing role implementation (see Chapter 24). Development of a professional portfolio to document APN accomplishments can be useful for performance and impact (process and outcome) evaluation. Performance evaluation for APNs should include self-evaluation, peer review, and administrative evaluation (Cooper & Sparacino, 1990; Hamric & Taylor, 1989). Use of a competency profile can be helpful for organizing evaluation in a dynamic way that allows for changes in role implementation over time as expertise, situations, and priorities change (Callahan & Bruton-Maree, 1994). The competency profile can be used to assess performance in each of the core APN competencies. APN programs need to include content and skill development regarding self-evaluation and peer evaluation of role implementation so that individuals can learn to monitor their practice and identify difficulties early to avoid moving into negative developmental phases (Hamric & Hanson, 2003).

Outcome evaluation is important to demonstrate the effectiveness of each APN role. Ongoing development of appropriate outcome evaluation measures, particularly for patient outcomes, is important (Ingersoll, McIntosh, & Williams, 2000; see Chapter 23). The existence of a reward system to provide for career advancement through a clinical ladder program and accrual of additional benefits is particularly important for retaining APNs in clinical roles. In less structured situations, APNs can negotiate for periodic reassessments and salary increases through options such as profit sharing.

The evaluation process broadens to incorporate interdisciplinary review when APN practice includes hospital privileges, prescriptive privileges, and third-party reimbursement. This expansion of the evaluation process has positive and negative aspects. Advantages to the review process associated with securing and maintaining hospital privileges include the many factors considered in the evaluation, variety of perspectives, and visibility afforded APNs. APNs should seek key positions on hospital review committees to promote APN roles within the organization. A major difficulty in implementing interdisciplinary peer review is lack of interaction between and among the incumbents of the various health professional groups during their formative educational programs. The resurgence of interest in developing and implementing IPE experiences between nursing students and medical students is encouraging (AACN, 2006; Hamric & Hanson, 2003; Institute of Medicine [IOM], 2003; Interprofessional Education Collaborative Expert Panel [IPEC], 2011; also see websites listed in Table 4-3).

Conclusion

Role development experiences for APNs are described as a two-phase process that consists of role acquisition in school and role implementation after graduation. The limits of the educational process in preparing graduates for the realities of the work world are acknowledged. Students, faculty, preceptors, and administrators need to be informed about the human skill acquisition process and its stages, processes of adult and professional socialization, identity transformation, role acquisition, role implementation, and overall career development. Knowing (theoretical knowledge) and actually experiencing (practical knowledge) are different phenomena, but at least students and new graduates can be forewarned about the transition experiences in school and the turbulence that can be expected during the first year of practice. Anticipatory guidance can be provided through role rehearsal experiences, such as clinical preceptorships and role seminars. Students need to be encouraged to begin networking with practicing APNs through local, state, and national APN groups. This networking is especially important for APNs who will not be practicing in proximity to other APNs. Experienced APNs and new APN graduates can form mutually beneficial relationships.

Although anticipatory socialization experiences in school can facilitate role acquisition, they cannot prevent the transition that occurs with movement into a new position and actual role implementation. APN programs should have a firm foundation in the real world. However, a certain degree of incongruence or conflict between academic ideals and work world reality will continue to exist (Ormond & Kish, 2001). APNs must take a leadership role in guiding and directing planned change and guard against the mere maintenance of the status quo.

Establishing mentor programs for new APNs in the work setting is one way to develop and maintain support for the positive developmental phases of role implementation described in this chapter.

APN role development has been described as dynamic, complex, and situational. It is influenced by many factors, such as experience, level of expertise, personal and professional values, setting, specialty, relationships with coworkers, aspects of role transition, life transitions, and organizational, system, and political realities. Frameworks for understanding APN role development processes have been discussed, along with strategies for facilitating role acquisition and role implementation. Ongoing evolution of APN roles in response to organizational and health care system changes and demands will continue. Future research studies to assess the applicability of this information to all APN specialty groups and for APN graduates of DNP programs are needed to further the understanding of APN role development and the impact of APN practice on health care outcomes.

References

Aiken, L. H., Clarke, S. P., Sloan, D. M., Sochalski, J., & Silber, J. H. (2002). Hospital nurse staffing and patient mortality, nurse burnout, and job dissatisfaction. *JAMA: The Journal of the American Medical Association, 288*, 1987–1995.

Allen, D. (2001). *Getting things done: The art of stress-free productivity.* New York: Penguin Books.

American Association of Colleges of Nursing (AACN). (2006). *The essentials of doctoral education for advanced nursing practice.* (http://www.aacn.nche.edu/DNP/pdf/Essentials.pdf).

American Association of Nurse Anesthetists (AANA). (2012). Qualifications and capabilities of the certified registered nurse anesthetist. (http://www.aana.com/ceandeducation/becomeacrna/ Pages/Qualifications-and-Capabilities-of-the-Certified-Registered-Nurse-Anesthetist-.aspx).

American College of Obstetricians and Gynecologists (ACOG/ American College of Nurse Midwives (ACNM). (2011). Joint statement of practice relations between obstetrician-gynecologists and certified nurse-midwives/certified midwives. (http://www.acog.org/~/media/News%20Releases/nr2011-03-31.pdf).

American College of Nurse-Midwives (ACNM). (2012). Core competencies for basic midwifery practice. (www.midwife.org/ ACNM/files/ACNMLibrary).

Anderson, E. M., Leonard, B. J., & Yates, J. A. (1974). Epigenesis of the nurse practitioner role. *American Journal of Nursing, 74,* 1812–1816.

Andrews, J., Hanson, C., Maule, S., & Snelling, M. (1999). Attaining role confirmation in nurse practitioner practice. *Clinical Excellence for Nurse Practitioners, 3,* 302–310.

Arena, D. M., & Page, N. E. (1992). The imposter phenomenon in the clinical nurse specialist role. *Image: The Journal of Nursing Scholarship, 24,* 121–125.

Baird, S. B., & Prouty, M. P. (1989). Administratively enhancing CNS contributions. In A. B. Hamric & J. A. Spross (Eds.), *The clinical nurse specialist in theory and practice* (pp. 261–283; 2nd ed.). Philadelphia: WB Saunders.

Baker, V. (1979). Retrospective explorations in role development. In G. V. Padilla (Ed.), *The clinical nurse specialist and improvement of nursing practice* (pp. 56–63). Wakefield, MA: Nursing Resources.

Ball, C., & Cox, C. L. (2004). Part two: The core components of legitimate influence and the conditions that constrain or facilitate advanced nursing practice in adult critical care. *International Journal of Nursing Practice, 10,* 10–20.

Banda, E. E. (1985). *Role problems, role strain: Perception and experience of clinical nurse specialist.* Boston: Unpublished master's thesis, Boston University School of Nursing.

Bandura, A. (1977). Self-efficacy: Toward a unifying theory of behavioral change. *Psychological Review, 84,* 191–215.

Bartholomew, K. (2006). *Ending nurse to nurse hostility: Why nurses eat their young and each other.* Mission, KS: Opus Communications.

Benner, P. (1984). *From novice to expert: Excellence and power in clinical nursing practice.* Menlo Park, CA: Addison-Wesley.

Benner, P., Sutphen, M., Leonard, V., & Day, L. (2010). *Educating nurses. A call for radical transformation.* Stanford, CA: Carnegie Foundation for the Advancement of Teaching.

Benner, P., Tanner, C. A., & Chesla, C. A. (2009). *Expertise in nursing practice: Caring, clinical judgment and ethics* (2nd ed.). New York: Springer.

Blumenreich, G. A. (2000). Legal briefs: Supervision. *AANA Journal, 68,* 404–409.

Bonnel, W., Belt, J., Hill, D., Wiggins, S., & Ohm, R. (2000). Challenges and strategies for initiating a nursing facility practice.

Journal of American Academy of Nurse Practitioners, 12, 353–359.

Brooten, D., Naylor, M. D., York, R., Brown, L. P., Munro, B. H., Hollingsworth, A. O., et al. (2002). Lessons learned from testing the quality cost model of advanced practice nursing (APN) transitional care. *Journal of Nursing Scholarship, 34,* 369–375.

Brown, M. A., & Olshansky, E. F. (1997). From limbo to legitimacy: A theoretical model of the transition to the primary care nurse practitioner role. *Nursing Research, 46,* 46–51.

Brown, M. A., & Olshansky, E. F. (1998). Becoming a primary care nurse practitioner: Challenges of the initial year of practice. *The Nurse Practitioner, 23*(46), 52–66.

Brown, S. J. (1992). Tailoring nursing care to the individual client: Empirical challenge of a theoretical concept. *Research in Nursing and Health, 15,* 39–46.

Bryant-Lukosius, D., Carter, N., Kilpatrick, K., Martin-Misener, R., Donald, F., Kaasalaninen, S., et al. (2010). The clinical nurse specialist role in Canada. *Nursing Leadership, 23,* 140–166.

Bryant-Lukosius, D., & DiCenso, A. (2004). A framework for the introduction and evaluation of advanced practice nursing roles. *Journal of Advanced Nursing, 48,* 530–540.

Bryant-Lukosius, D., DiCenso, A., Browne, G., & Pinelli, J. (2004). Advanced practice nursing roles: Development, implementation and evaluation. *Journal of Advanced Nursing, 48,* 519–529.

Brykczynski, K. A. (1985). Exploring the clinical practice of nurse practitioners. *Scholarly Inquiry for Nursing Practice: An International Journal, 3,* 75–104.

Brykczynski, K. A. (1991). Judgment strategies for coping with ambiguous clinical situations encountered in family primary care. *Journal of the Academy of Nurse Practitioners, 3,* 79–84.

Brykczynski, K. A. (1996). Role development of the advanced practice nurse. In A. B. Hamric, J. A. Spross, & C. M. Hanson (Eds.), *Advanced practice nursing: An integrative approach,* (pp. 89–95). Philadelphia: Saunders.

Brykczynski, K. A. (1997). Holism: A foundation for healing wounds of divisiveness among nurses. In P. B. Kritek (Ed.), *Reflections on healing. A central nursing construct* (pp. 234–241). New York: National League for Nursing.

Brykczynksi, K. A. (1999a). Reflections on clinical judgment of nurse practitioners. *Scholarly Inquiry for Nursing Practice: An International Journal, 13,* 175–184.

Brykczynski, K. A. (1999b). An interpretive study describing the clinical judgment of nurse practitioners. *Scholarly Inquiry for Nursing Practice: An International Journal, 13,* 141–166.

Brykczynski, K. A. (2009). Role development of the advanced practice nurse. In A. B. Hamric, J. A. Spross, & C. M. Hanson (Eds.), *Advanced practice nursing: An integrative approach* (pp. 95–120, 4th ed.). Philadelphia: Saunders.

Brykczynski, K. A. (2012). Clarifying, affirming, and preserving the nurse in NP education and practice. *Journal of the Academy of Nurse Practitioners, 24,* 554–564. doi: 10.1111/j.1745-7599.2012.00738.x.

Burgess, J., & Purkis, M. E. (2010). The power and politics of collaboration in nurse practitioner role development. *Nursing Inquiry, 17,* 297–308.

Burglehaus, M. (1997). Physicians and breastfeeding: Beliefs, knowledge, self-efficacy and counseling practices. *Canadian Journal of Public Health, 88,* 383–387.

Callahan, L., & Bruton-Maree, N. (1994). Establishing measures of competence. In S. D. Foster & L. M. Jordan (Eds.), *Professional aspects of nurse anesthesia practice* (pp. 275–290). Philadelphia: FA Davis.

Clance, P., & Imes, S. (1978). The imposter phenomenon in high achieving women: Dynamics and therapeutic intervention. *Psychotherapy: Theory, Research and Practice, 15,* 241–247.

Clark, N., & Dodge, J. (1999). Exploring self-efficacy as a predictor of disease management. *Health Education & Behavior, 26,* 72–89.

Cohen, H. A. (1981). *The nurse's quest for a professional identity.* Menlo Park, CA: Addison-Wesley.

Cooper, D. M., & Sparacino, P. S. A. (1990). Acquiring, implementing, and evaluating the clinical nurse specialist role. In P. S. A. Sparacino, D. M. Cooper, & P. A. Minarik (Eds.), *The clinical nurse specialist: Implementation and impact* (pp. 41–75). Norwalk, CT: Appleton & Lange.

Curry, J. L. (1994). Nurse practitioners in the emergency department: Current issues. *Journal of Emergency Nursing, 20,* 207–215.

Cusson, R. M., & Viggiano, N. M. (2002). Transition to the neonatal nurse practitioner role: Making the change from the side to the head of the bed. *Neonatal Network: NN, 21,* 21–28.

Cusson, R., & Strange, S. (2008). Neonatal nurse practitioner role transition: The process of reattaining expert status. *Journal of Perinatal and Neonatal Nursing, 22,* 329–337.

Dalton, J., & Blau, W. (1996). Changing the practice of pain management: An examination of the theoretical basis of change. *Pain Forum, 5,* 266–272.

Davis, K., Schoenbaum, S. C., & Audet, A. (2005). A 20-20 vision of patient-centered primary care. *Journal of General Internal Medicine, 20,* 953–957.

Day, L., Cooper, P. L., & Scott, W. M. (2012). Using unfolding cases in primary care coursework for nurse practitioner students: Prepared to certify or prepared to practice? Presentation abstract, National Organization of Nurse Practitioner Faculties (NONPF) 38th Annual Meeting, Charleston, SC.

DeMaio, D. (1979). The born-again nurse. *Nursing Outlook, 27,* 272–273.

DiCenso, A., Martin-Misener, R., Bryant-Lukosius, D., Bourgeault, I., Kilpatrick, K., Donald, F., et al. (2010). Advanced practice nursing in Canada: Overview of a decision support synthesis. *Canadian Journal of Nursing Leadership, 23,* 15–34.

Dionne-Proulx, J., & Pepin, R. (1993). Stress management in the nursing profession. *Journal of Nursing Management, 1,* 75–81.

Dreyfus, H. L., & Dreyfus, S. E. (1986). *Mind over machine: The power of human intuition and expertise in the era of the computer.* New York: Free Press.

Dreyfus, H. L., & Dreyfus, S. E. (2009). The relationship of theory and practice in the acquisition of skill. In P. Benner, C. A. Tanner, & C. A. Chesla, *Expertise in nursing practice: Caring, clinical judgment and ethics* (pp. 1–23, 2nd ed.). New York: Springer.

Farrell, G. A. (2001). From tall poppies to squashed weeds: Why don't nurses pull together more? *Journal of Advanced Nursing, 35*, 26–33.

Fawcett, J., Newman, D. M. L., & McAllister, M. (2004). Advanced practice nursing and conceptual models of nursing. *Nursing Science Quarterly, 17*, 135–138.

Federwisch, A. (1999). CRNA autonomy: Nurse anesthetists fight latest skirmish (http://www.nurseweek.com/features/99-1/crna.html).

Fiandt, K. (2002). Finding the nurse in nurse practitioner practice: A pilot study of rural family nurse practitioner practice. *Clinical Excellence for Nurse Practitioners, 5*, 13–21.

Fleming, E., & Carberry, M. (2011). Steering a course towards advanced nurse practitioner: A critical care perspective. *Nursing in Critical Care, 16*, 67–76.

Ford, L. C. (1982). Nurse practitioners: History of a new idea and predictions for the future. In L. H. Aiken (Ed.), *Nursing in the 1980s: Crises, opportunities, challenges* (pp. 231–247). Philadelphia: JB Lippincott.

Freshwater, D. (2000). Crosscurrents: Against cultural narration in nursing. *Journal of Advanced Nursing, 32*, 481–484.

Grando, V. T. (1998). Articulating nursing for advanced practice nursing. In T. J. Sullivan (Ed.). *Collaboration: A health care imperative* (pp. 499–514). New York: McGraw-Hill.

Gunn, I. P. (1991). The history of nurse anesthesia education: Highlights and influences. Report of the National Commission on Nurse Anesthesia Education. *Journal of the American Association of Nurse Anesthetists, 59*, 53–61.

Gunn, I. P. (1998). Setting the record straight on nurse anesthesia and medical anesthesiology education. *CRNA: The Clinical Forum for Nurse Anesthetists, 9*, 163–171.

Hamric, A. B. (2003). Defining our practice: A personal perspective [letter to the editor]. *Clinical Nurse Specialist, 17*, 75–76.

Hamric, A. B., & Hanson, C. M. (2003). Educating advanced practice nurses for practice reality. *Journal of Professional Nursing, 19*, 262–268.

Hamric, A. B., & Taylor, J. W. (1989). Role development of the CNS. In A. B. Hamric & J. Spross (Eds.), *The clinical nurse specialist in theory and practice* (pp. 41–82, 2nd ed.). Philadelphia: WB Saunders.

Hardy, M. E., & Hardy, W. L. (1988). Role stress and role strain. In M. E. Hardy & M. E. Conway (Eds.), *Role theory: Perspectives for health professionals* (pp. 159–239, 2nd ed,). Norwalk, CT: Appleton & Lange.

Hayes, E. (1998). Mentoring and nurse practitioner student self-efficacy. *Western Journal of Nursing Research, 20*, 521–525.

Hayes, E. (2005). Mentoring research in the NP preceptor/student relationship. In L. Rauckhorst (Ed.), *Mentoring: Ensuring the future of NP practice and education*. Washington, DC: National Organization of Nurse Practitioner Faculties.

Hayes, E. F. (2001). Factors that facilitate or hinder mentoring in the nurse practitioner preceptor/student relationship. *Clinical Excellence for Nurse Practitioners, 5*, 111–118.

Heitz, L. J., Steiner, S. H., & Burman, M. E. (2004). RN to FNP: A qualitative study of role transition. *Journal of Nursing Education, 43*, 416–420.

Huffstutler, S. Y., & Varnell, G. (2006). The imposter phenomenon in new nurse practitioner graduates. (http://www.medscape.com/viewarticle/533648).

Hunter, L. P., Bormann, J. E., & Lops, V. R. (1996). Student to nurse-midwife role transition process: Smoothing the way. *Journal of Nurse-Midwifery, 41*, 328–333,

Hupcey, J. E. (1993). Factors and work settings that may influence nurse practitioner practice. *Nursing Outlook, 41*, 181–185.

Ingersoll, G. L., McIntosh, E., & Williams, M. (2000). Nurse-sensitive outcomes of advanced practice. *Journal of Advanced Practice, 32*, 1272–1281.

Institute of Medicine (IOM). (2003). *Health professions education: A bridge to quality*. Washington, DC: National Academies Press.

Interprofessional Education Collaborative Expert Panel (IPEC). (2011). *Core competencies for interprofessional collaborative practice: Report of an expert panel*. Washington, DC: Interprofessional Eduction Collaborative.

Johnson, R. (1993). Nurse practitioner-patient discourse: Uncovering the voice of nursing in primary care practice. *Scholarly Inquiry for Nursing Practice: An International Journal, 7*, 143–157.

Keating, S. F. J., Thompson, J. P., & Lee, G. A. (2010). Perceived barriers to the sustainability and progression of nurse practitioners. *International Emergency Nursing, 18*, 147–153.

Kelly, N. R., & Mathews, M. (2001). The transition to first position as nurse practitioner. *Journal of Nursing Education, 40*, 156–162.

Kimbro, C. D. (1978). The relationship between nurses and nurse-midwives. *Journal of Nurse-Midwifery, 22*, 28–31.

Kinsley, M. (2005). You've come a long way! *Nursing Spectrum (New York/New Jersey), 17*, 4–5.

Klaich, K. (1990). Transitions in professional identity of nurses enrolled in graduate educational programs. *Holistic Nursing Practice, 4*, 17–24.

Kleinpell, R. (2001). Nurse anesthetists hold fast under physicians' blast of supervision ruling. *The Nursing Spectrum, 11*, 26–27.

Kleinpell, R. (2005). Acute care nurse practitioner practice: Results of a 5-year longitudinal study. *American Journal of Critical Care, 14*, 211–221.

Kleinpell-Nowell, R. (1999). Longitudinal survey of acute care nurse practitioner practice: Year 1. *AACN Clinical Issues, 10*, 515–520.

Kleinpell-Nowell, R. (2001). Longitudinal survey of acute care nurse practitioner practice: Year 2. *AACN Clinical Issues, 12*, 447–452.

Kramer, M. (1974). *Reality shock*. St. Louis: Mosby.

Leininger, M. M. (1994). The tribes of nursing in the United States. *Journal of Transcultural Nursing, 6*, 18–22.

Levy, J. (1968). The maternal and infant mortality in midwifery practice in Newark, NJ. *American Journal of Obstetrics and Gynecology, 77*, 42.

Llahana, S. V., & Hamric, A. B. (2011). Developmental phases and factors influencing role development in diabetes specialist nurses: A UK study. *European Diabetes Nursing, 8*, 18–23a.

Lindblad, E., Hallman, E., Gillsjo, C., Lindblad, U., & Fagerstrom, L. (2010). Experiences of the new role of advanced practice nurse in Swedish primary health care—A qualitative study. *International Journal of Nursing Practice, 16*, 69–74.

Lurie, E. E. (1981). Nurse practitioners: Issues in professional socialization. *Journal of Health and Social Behavior, 22*, 31–48.

Martin-Misener, R., Bryant-Lukosius, D., Harbman, P., Donald, F., Kaasalainen, S., Carter, N., et al. (2010). Education of advanced practice nurses in Canada. *Canadian Journal of Nursing Leadership, 23*, 60–84.

McAiney, C. A., Haughton, D., Jennings, J., Farr, D., Hillier, L., & Morden, P. (2008). A unique practice model for nurse practitioners in long-term care homes. *Journal of Advanced Nursing, 62*, 562–571.

McFadden, E. A., & Miller, M. A. (1994). Clinical nurse specialist practice: Facilitators and barriers. *Clinical Nurse Specialist, 8*, 27–33.

McMyler, E. T., & Miller, D. J. (1997). Two graduating master's students struggle to find meaning. *Clinical Nurse Specialist, 11*, 169–173.

McNamara, S. Giguere, V., St.-Louis, L., & Bioleau, J. (2009). Development and implementation of the specialized nurse practitioner role: Use of the PEPPA framework to achieve success. *Nursing and Health Sciences, 11*, 318–325.

Murphy-Ende, K. (2002). Advanced practice nursing: Reflections on the past, issues for the future. *Oncology Nursing Forum, 29*, 106–112.

National Association of Clinical Nurse Specialists (NACNS). (1998). *Statement on clinical nurse specialists practice and education.* Harrisburg, PA: Author.

National Commission on Nurse Anesthesia Education. (1990). Summary of commission findings: Issues and review of supporting documents. *Journal of the American Association of Nurse Anesthetists, 58*, 394–398.

Neale, J. (1999). Nurse practitioners and physicians: A collaborative practice. *Clinical Nurse Specialist, 13*, 252–258.

Nevidjon, B. M., & Simonson, C. J. (2009). Strengthening advanced practice nursing in organizational structures: administrative considerations. In A. B. Hamric, J. A. Spross, & C. M. Hanson (Eds), *Advanced Practice Nursing: An Integrative Approach* (pp. 657–680, 4th ed.). St. Louis: Saunders Elsevier.

Ormond, C., & Kish, C. P. (2001). Role acquisition. In D. Robinson & C. P. Kish (Eds.), *Core concepts in advanced practice nursing* (pp. 269–285). St. Louis: Mosby.

Page, N. E., & Arena, D. M. (1991). Practical strategies for CNS role implementation. *Clinical Nurse Specialist, 5*, 43–48.

Parle, M., Maguire, P., & Heaven, C. (1997). The development of a training model to improve health professionals skills, self-efficacy, and outcome expectancies when communicating with cancer patients. *Social Science & Medicine, 44*, 231–240.

Peplau, H. (1997). *Keynote address.* Presented at the International Congress of Nurses, Vancouver, British Columbia, Canada, June 1997.

Quinn, R. E. (1996). *Deep change: Discovering the leader within.* San Francisco: Jossey-Bass.

Rashotte, J. (2005). Knowing the nurse practitioner: Dominant discourses shaping our horizons. *Nursing Philosophy, 6*, 51–62.

Rich, E. R. (2005). Does RN experience relate to NP clinical skills? *The Nurse Practitioner, 30*, 53–56.

Rich, E. R., & Rodriquez, L. (2002). A qualitative study of perceptions regarding the non-nurse college graduate nurse practitioner. *The Journal of the New York State Nurses' Association, 33*, 31–35.

Roberts, S. J. (1983). Oppressed group behavior: Implications for nursing. *Advances in Nursing Science, 5*, 21–30.

Roberts, S. J. (1996). Breaking the cycle of oppression: Lessons for nurse practitioners? *Journal of the Academy of Nurse Practitioners, 8*, 209–214.

Roberts, S. J., Tabloski, P., & Bova, C. (1997). Epigenesis of the nurse practitioner role revisited. *Journal of Nursing Education, 36*, 67–73.

Rosenfeld, P. (2001). Acute care nurse practitioners: Standard in ambulatory care, they're also useful in hospitals. *American Journal of Nursing, 101*, 61–62.

Rounds, L. R. (1997). The nurse practitioner: A healing role for the nurse. In P. B. Kritek (Ed.), *Reflections on healing: A central nursing construct* (pp. 209–223). New York: National League for Nursing.

Russell, D., VorderBruegge, M., & Burns, S. M. (2002). Effect of an outcomes-managed approach to care of neuroscience patients by acute care nurse practitioners. *American Journal of Critical Care, 11*, 353–364.

Ryden, M. B., Snyder, M., Gross, C. R., Savik, K., Pearson, V., Krichbaum, K., et al. (2000). Value-added outcomes: The use of advanced practice nurses in long-term care facilities. *The Gerontologist, 40*, 654–662.

Safriet, B. J. (1992). Health care dollars and regulatory sense: The role of advanced practice nursing. *Yale Journal on Regulation, 9*, 417–488.

Sangster-Gormley, E., Martin-Misener, R., Downe-Wamboldt, B., & DiCenso, A. (2011). Factors affecting nurse practitioner role implementation in Canadian practice settings: An integrative review. *Journal of Advanced Nursing, 67*, 1178–1190.

Schumacher, K. L., & Meleis, A. I. (1994). Transitions: A central concept in nursing. *Image: The Journal of Nursing Scholarship, 26*, 119–127.

Sechrist, K. R., & Berlin, L. E. (1998). Role of the clinical nurse specialist: An integrative review of the literature. *AACN Clinical Issues, 9*, 306–324.

Stahl, M. A., & Myers, J. (2002). The advanced practice nursing role with multisite responsibilities. *Critical Care Nursing Clinics of North America, 14*, 299–305.

Stein, T. (2000). Struggling for autonomy: Dispute between CRNAs and anesthesiologists continues. *Nurseweek (California Statewide Edition), 13*, 31.

Steiner, S. H., McLaughlin, D. G., Hyde, R. S., Brown, R. H., & Burman, M. E. (2008). Role transition during RN to FNP education. *Journal of Nursing Education, 47*(10), 441–447.

Thomas, S. P. (2003). "Horizontal hostility": Nurses against themselves: How to resolve this threat to retention. *American Journal of Nursing, 103*, 87–91.

Varney, H. (1987). *Nurse-midwifery* (2nd ed.). Boston: Blackwell Scientific.

Waters, R. (March 2007). Scope of practice legislative fights expected to return in 2007. *JNP The Journal for Nurse Practitioners, 3*, 195.

Waugaman, W. R., & Lu, J. (1999). From nurse to nurse anesthetist: The relationship of culture, race, and ethnicity to professional socialization and career commitment of advanced practice nurses. *Journal of Transcultural Nursing, 10*, 237–247.

Evolving and Innovative Opportunities for Advanced Practice Nursing

Jeanne Salyer • Michelle R. Frazelle

Technologic advances and economic and sociocultural conditions have sustained a climate of change in the health care environment, and opportunities for advanced practice nursing continue to emerge in the wake of these changes. As specialties have emerged, many new roles have evolved from specialty nursing practice and have expanded to incorporate some or all of the core attributes of advanced practice nursing (see Chapters 2 and 3). Some of these roles have clearly evolved as advanced practice roles, whereas others are in various stages of evolution. Not all specialties, however, will evolve into advanced practice roles, for a variety of reasons. For example, some specialties evolve away from the core definition of advanced practice nursing, which encompasses direct clinical practice and clinical expertise as essential ingredients. Other specialties, such as informatics and nursing administration, arise as specialties and remain as specialties because direct clinical practice is not a requisite role component.

The purpose of this chapter is to examine some currently evolving specialties and characterize stages in their continuing evolution from specialty nursing practice to advanced practice nursing. Some of these specialties have not yet fully evolved to an advanced level; however, movement within the specialty toward advanced practice may be accelerated as Doctor of Nursing Practice (DNP) programs target these specialties for development. The focus of the discussion is on the various specialties—not on particular advanced practice nursing roles, such as clinical nurse specialist (CNS), nurse practitioner (NP), certified nurse-midwife (CNM), or certified registered nurse anesthetist (CRNA). Specialties selected for inclusion in this discussion were chosen for one or more of the following reasons:

- The specialty has the potential to transition (or is transitioning) to the DNP.
- The specialty has the potential to evolve to advanced practice nursing, given the complexity of care required by the patient population, and direct care is likely to be a defining factor.
- The specialty has arisen as a result of scientific and/ or technologic advances and the influence of these advances on the delivery of health care.
- The specialty is growing because of the rising incidence of health problems in the population.
- The specialty's patient population needs sophisticated care across settings in the complex health care environment.

Opportunities in these evolving specialties for advanced practice nurses (APNs) are discussed and a framework for evaluating progress toward advanced practice status is presented. Exemplars provided by APNs in the specialty were deliberately chosen to illuminate the added value of advanced practice competencies to these evolving specialties.

Patterns in the Evolution of Specialty to Advanced Practice Nursing

Before discussing the evolution of specialty nursing practice into advanced practice nursing, it is important to make a distinction between the two, as well as to clarify the use of the term *subspecialty* in this chapter. Specialization involves focusing on practice in a specific area derived from the field of professional nursing. Specialties can be further characterized as nursing practice that intersects with another body of knowledge, has a direct impact on nursing practice, and is supportive of the direct care provided to patients by other registered nurses (American

Nurses Association [ANA], 2010a). As the profession of nursing has responded to changes in health care, the need for specialty knowledge has increased. For example, in the wake of the National Cancer Act of 1971, which was enacted as a consequence of the increasing incidence of cancer in the population and the need to advance national efforts in prevention and treatment, the oncology specialty became more widely recognized (Oncology Nursing Society [ONS], 2012). The ONS traces its origin to the first National Cancer Nursing Research Conference, supported by the ANA and American Cancer Society, in 1973, after which a small group met to discuss the need for a national organization to support their professional development. From these early efforts, this organization, which was incorporated in 1975, has become a leader in cancer care in the United States and around the world (ONS, 2012).

The classic specialties in nursing have been pediatric, psychiatric and mental health, obstetrics (now termed *women's health*), community and public health, and medical-surgical nursing (now termed *adult health*). Specialties that have emerged include, for example, concentrations in critical care, emergency, and oncology nursing. As a given specialty coalesces, nurses often form specialty nursing organizations out of clinicians' needs to share practice experiences and specialty knowledge. Some examples include the American Association of Critical-Care Nurses, Oncology Nursing Society, and Association of Women's Health, Obstetric, and Neonatal Nurses (AWHONN). Scope and standards of practice statements legitimize specialty designation and prompt efforts to provide opportunities for specialty education and certification. The efforts of the International Transplant Nurses Society (ITNS) to develop and approve a scope of practice statement, a core curriculum, and specialty certification for registered nurses is just one example (ITNS, 2007).

Advanced practice nursing includes specialization but goes beyond it; it involves expansion, which legitimizes role autonomy, and advancement, characterized by the integration of a broad range of theoretical, research-based, and practical knowledge (ANA, 2010; see Chapter 2). Thus, advanced practice nursing reflects concentrated knowledge in a specialty that offers the opportunity for expanded and autonomous practice based on a broader practical and theoretical knowledge base.

The term *specialty* suggests that the focus of practice is limited to parts of the whole (ANA, 2010b). For example, family NPs, who typically see themselves as generalists, have in fact specialized in one of the many facets of health care—namely, primary care. Subspecialization further delineates the focus of practice. In subspecialty practice, knowledge and skill in a delimited clinical area is expanded further. With this expanded knowledge and skill, there is

potentially further advancement of theoretical, evidence-based, and practical knowledge in caring for a specific patient population base. Examples of subspecialty practices within the specialty of adult health nursing include diabetes, transplant, and palliative care nursing. Notably, most of the practice opportunities chosen for discussion in this chapter are subspecialty practices. This distinction between specialty and subspecialty is important, particularly for certification and regulatory reasons, and was recently codified when the National Council of State Boards of Nursing (NCSBN) proposed the regulation of advanced practice nursing in terms of certification requirements at the broad population foci level (e.g., psychiatric and mental health, pediatrics, adult and gerontology), with specialty or subspecialty certification being voluntary (NCSBN, 2008). Regulatory considerations aside, the expansion of advanced practice nursing is increasingly occurring in specialty and subspecialty practice. Expanding these boundaries places APNs on the cutting edge of clinical care delivery in a complex, ever-changing, health care environment. However, for the sake of consistency with the Consensus Model for APRN Regulation (2008), in the remainder of this chapter, we refer to specialty and subspecialty practice as specialties.

The evolution of specialty nursing practice to advanced practice nursing follows a trajectory that has been described by several authors (Beitz, 2000; Bigbee & Amidii-Nouri, 2000; Hamric, 2000; Lewis, 2000; see Chapter 1). Hanson and Hamric (2003) synthesized these observations and characterized this evolution as having distinct stages (Table 5-1). Initially, in stage I, the specialty develops in response to changing patient needs, needs that are usually a result of new technology, new medical specialties, and/or changes in the health care workforce. For example, a lack of pediatric residents created an opportunity for the development of the neonatal NP role (DeNicola, Klied, & Brink, 1994).

A second stage of development is characterized by progress to the point that organized training begins. This training is often institution-specific, on the job training that develops experts in the specialty. Some of these institution-specific programs develop into certificate programs; however, the content may not be standardized, and the quality of these specialty programs may vary. One example is the early transplant coordination role in major transplant centers (see later, "Clinical Transplant Coordination").

In the third stage, the knowledge base required for specialty practice becomes more extensive and the scope of practice of the nurse with specialty training expands. There is growing recognition of the additional knowledge and skill needed for increasingly complex practice. It is not unusual at this stage to see APNs migrate into an

TABLE 5-1	Four Stages in the Evolution of Advanced Practice Nursing	
Stage	Description	Characteristics
I	Specialty begins	Specialty develops in practice settings; development driven by increasing complexity in care demands, new technology, changing workforce opportunities; on the job training, expansion of practice; not exclusively nursing
II	Specialty organizes	Organized training for specialty practice begins; institution-specific training develops; initially uses apprenticeship model; progresses to certificate training; specialty organization forms; certification examination develops but may not be nursing-specific; reports appear on role of nurse in specialty
III	Pressures mount for standardization	Knowledge base grows; pressures mount for standardization, graduate education; knowledge base keeps growing, scope of practice expands for practitioners in the specialty; expanded practice leads to expanded regulatory oversight; leaders call for transition to graduate education and differentiated practice to standardize practice in the specialty; APNs migrate to specialty or specialty nurses return to school; reports appear differentiating APN role in the specialty
IV	Maturity and growing interdisciplinarity	APN practice in the specialty is well articulated, recognized by other providers; APNs practice collaboratively with other practitioners in the specialty; APNs are experts in the specialty or subspecialty; shared knowledge base with other health care professionals recognized; interdisciplinary certification examinations developed

Adapted from Hanson, C.M., & Hamric, A.B. (2003). Reflections on the continuing evolution of advanced practice nursing. *Nursing Outlook, 51,* 203–211.

evolving specialty and further expand practice by infusing it with advanced practice core competencies, making the specialty resemble advanced practice and creating new calls for evolution to this higher level. This transition is clearly evident in wound, ostomy, and continence nursing (see later, "Wound, Ostomy, and Continence Nursing"), as well as in palliative care nursing. Over time, pressure for the standardization of education and skills involved in the specialty arise from clinicians, the profession, and regulators. Certificate-level training programs move into graduate schools that assume responsibility for preparing nurses for these evolving specialties, improving standardization, elevating the status of the specialty, and fostering its emergence as an advanced practice role. In this third stage of the trajectory, graduate education becomes an expected level of preparation (Hanson & Hamric, 2003).

Stage IV, initially described by Salyer and Hamric (2009), is characterized by mature and recognized APN practice in the specialty, along with an emerging understanding of a shared interdisciplinary component. Nurse practitioners in human immunodeficiency virus (HIV) practice who have attained certification as an HIV specialist, awarded by the American Academy of HIV Medicine, are an example of mature expert practitioners who share an interdisciplinary clinical knowledge base with physicians in this specialty.

It is important to note that these stages are dynamic and not mutually exclusive. It is not unusual for specialties to show characteristics of more than one stage simultaneously (e.g., graduate programs began to develop at the same time that most practitioners in the specialty were prepared in certificate programs). In addition, the duration of each stage may vary significantly by specialty. We contend that the evolution from specialty to advanced practice nursing can represent a natural maturation that should result from deliberate logical planning to strengthen the education and broaden the scope of practice of specialty nurses. Some of these roles evolve to fulfill needs of specific patient populations or the needs of organizations. In some cases, changes in the legal recognition and regulation of practice also influence the movement toward advanced practice nursing. For example, nurse midwifery moved toward requiring graduate-level educational preparation for their specialty in response to the national movement among state boards of nursing to require this level of education for all APNs. Complex and often controversial issues must be addressed before and during this evolutionary process (Box 5-1). In the following sections, the evolution of particular specialties to advanced practice nursing is described and these issues are discussed. Some of these specialties are struggling to evolve and change is haphazard. Others are following a planned course of action and have emerged (or will soon do so) at the advanced practice level. All evolving specialties share two challenges—the need to gain support within and external to nursing for these roles, and the need to delineate their potential contributions clearly in the health care environment.

BOX 5-1   Issues in the Evolution of Specialty to Advanced Practice Nursing

- Defining the attributes of advanced practice in the specialty
- Delineating the core competencies of the specialty as encompassing the core competencies of advanced practice
- Delineating a vision of advanced practice that may step outside of nursing's traditional vision of what constitutes an advanced practice role and gaining support within the nursing and health care community for the role
- Standardizing curricula for achieving competency at the advanced practice level
- Clarifying certification and credentialing requirements
- Overcoming legal and regulatory issues that are barriers to patient and/or consumer access to APNs
- Promoting recognition of APNs and nursing as a profession
- Clarifying APN role titles to be consistent and decrease confusion

Adapted from Hanson, C.M., & Hamric, A.B. (2003). Reflections on the continuing evolution of advanced practice nursing, *Nursing Outlook*, 51, 203–211.

Innovative Practice Opportunities: Stage I

The initial stage of the evolution from specialty practice to advanced practice is characterized by the development of a specialty focus. Numerous examples are apparent in the history of nursing, which is replete with accounts of nursing's response to unmet patient needs. As a consequence, definable specialties emerge as nurses expand their practice to include the knowledge and skills necessary to meet the needs of patients requiring specialty care. Examples from our history include the specialty of enterostomal therapy (ET) nursing, now known as wound, ostomy, and continence (WOC) nursing, and forensic nursing, which has historically encompassed care provision in correctional facilities, psychiatric settings, and emergency departments as nurse examiners care for sexual assault and child abuse victims (Burgess, Berger, & Boersma, 2004; Doyle, 2001; Hutson, 2002; Maeve & Vaughn, 2001; McCrone & Shelton, 2001). As specialties begin to coalesce, the practice may not be viewed as a nursing role. For example, early enterostomal therapists were laypersons with ostomies. However, as the specialty evolved, the valuable contributions of nurses began to distinguish them from other care providers.

Several evolving roles in nursing are characterized as being innovative. Some of these roles do not reflect the core competencies of advanced practice nursing and the role components differ significantly, in some cases, from those of an APN. For example, if the focus of practice in forensic nursing had remained on the gathering of legal evidence, not sustained clinical practice using advanced practice core competency elements, the role would not be evolving to an advanced practice level. Regardless, nurses functioning in these subspecialties, some of whom are APNs, make unique contributions to the health of specific populations of patients. One such role to be explored as a stage I specialty is that of the hospitalist.

Hospitalist Practice

The development of the hospitalist movement over the past 15 years represents a break in the tradition of primary care physicians (PCPs) managing patients in inpatient and outpatient settings. In this model, inpatients are cared for by what is termed a *hospitalist physician*—a term coined by Wachter and Goldman (1996)—whose primary professional focus is the general medical care of hospitalized patients (Coffman & Rundall, 2005). The hospitalist model is growing rapidly as a result of the role of managed care in organizations, increasing complexity of inpatient care, fragmentation of care, and pressures experienced by physicians in busy outpatient practices (Freed, 2004; Lee, 2008; Wachter, 2004). In this model, inpatient management is voluntarily transferred by the PCP to the hospitalist during the hospital admission and, on discharge, care is resumed by the PCP. More recently, an opportunity for APNs to practice in this relatively new innovative specialty has evolved out of the physician hospitalist model of care (Nyberg, 2006, Sullivan, 2009).

Although there are limited definitions of the APN hospitalist in the literature, Sullivan (2009) reported the following, which serves as a guide for the role description of the hospitalist APN in the state of Mississippi. This definition states that an APN hospitalist is a nationally certified nurse practitioner whose practice site is the hospital and who has no outside primary or tertiary practice site. As part of a hospitalist team, this APN does the following: (1) admits and discharges patients; (2) diagnoses and manages common health problems in hospitalized patients in collaboration with a physician hospitalist; (3) performs procedures that are within their scope of practice; (4) interprets laboratory and diagnostic tests; and (5) plans and coordinates the discharge, rehabilitation, home health care, and follow-up of patients with acute health problems. This definition, and the specific functions it delineates, illuminates the centrality of direct care practice of APNs in this specialty. As the APN hospitalist specialty continues to evolve, the added value of practice guided by acute care competencies has the potential to improve the quality of care received by hospitalized patients.

EXEMPLAR 5-1   **APN Hospitalist***

The Hospital Medicine Nurse Practitioner Service at Strong Memorial Hospital, University of Rochester Medical Center, was started in 1995 as an initiative to reduce length of stay. Four NPs were hired, along with a hospitalist, to start a short-stay unit. Patients included those with myocardial infarction rule-outs, new-onset atrial fibrillation, and simple cellulitis, as well as those needing observation after procedures. The NPs covered the unit 10 hours/day, 5 days/week, with fellows and other house staff covering the remaining hours (Terboss, 2007).

Since its inception, the service has grown exponentially, primarily in response to the reduced number of medical resident positions and tighter restrictions on resident work hours by the Accreditation Council on Graduate Medical Education (ACGME). In addition, the team's census grew along with the hospital census when two hospitals in the city closed. Other changes included an increase in patients, the addition of physician assistants (PAs) to the team, and orthopedic surgery patients attended to by the Hospital Medicine Service. The service has expanded to cover patients on 15 patient care units, 24 hours/day, 7 days/week, including holidays.

The specialty of hospital medicine is relatively new, and therefore the role of the acute care nurse practitioner (ACNP) in a hospitalist role varies from hospital to hospital. At Strong Memorial, ACNPs have a variety of roles and responsibilities. They collaborate with the Hospital Medicine Division physicians and community-based primary care providers and share responsibility for examinations, documentation, order writing, and discharge planning. The ACNPs also follow patients admitted to subspecialty services, such as gastroenterology, nephrology, cardiology, and infectious diseases. Whereas the subspecialist attending physician or fellow may focus on the organ of interest, the ACNP independently manages comorbidities, updates families, and coordinates care, all of which provide a more holistic perspective to the patient's hospital stay.

Concrete defined tasks include admitting histories, physical examinations, orders, discharge instructions and summaries, and a daily visit with a progress note. ACNPs order and interpret diagnostic and laboratory tests, participate in multidisciplinary unit rounds, and update an electronic sign-out system for safer handoffs. Procedures such as line placement are usually provided by residents as part of their educational experience.

Many of the ACNP's responsibilities are less easily defined or measured. However, in these functions, the ACNP adds value to the care provided by the Hospital Medicine Service. They include coordination of care among the variety of consultants, other health professionals (e.g., physical therapists, nutritionists, social workers), and unit management. In addition, ACNPs update patients and families to maintain open communication and keep them informed of the care plan. They also orient new ACNPs to their role and mentor ACNP students. Most importantly, ACNPs collaborate with the bedside nurses and unit staff. Communication of updates, orders, and plans is essential to ensuring safe, timely, and quality care. The accessibility of the ACNP promotes collaboration and many opportunities for informal teaching. As APNs, ACNPs are often the most knowledgeable about medication information, technology management, or even basic nursing care and can serve as resources for newer, less experienced nurses. Teaching and mentoring are important to ensure staff development and retention as well as safe patient care. The importance of these activities has been difficult to quantify. It has been and continues to be a challenge to the Hospital Medicine Service to measure these contributions and illustrate their value.

The future for ACNPs on Hospital Medicine teams is promising. The specialty is growing, along with the acuity of inpatients and the complexities of discharge planning, both of which ACNPs are well-suited to manage. ACNP programs are incorporating hospital medicine into their curricula and into clinical rotations. The ACNPs on the Hospital Medicine Service have precepted many of these students, some of whom have gone on to join our team. Many challenges are ahead, including finding ways to quantify our contribution in terms of quality of care, length of stay, and patient and staff satisfaction. Orienting new ACNPs to handle the complexity of these inpatients and recruiting for 24-hour, 7-days/week positions is also a challenge.

I find my role as an ACNP on the Hospital Medicine Service to be highly satisfying because I care for patients with a wide variety of health problems. I also have the opportunity every day to teach, learn, and make a difference for a patient or another nurse. Finally, it is very rewarding to work on a team of APNs who are so dedicated to hospital medicine, providing excellent patient care and supporting and helping each other. I am proud to be an ACNP in hospitalist practice.

*We gratefully acknowledge Elizabeth Palermo, MS, RN, APRN-BC, Rochester, NY, for assistance with this exemplar.

The Society of Hospital Medicine (SHM), with over 6000 members, is a multidisciplinary organization (physicians, PAs, NPs) with the following goals (SHM, 2010a):

- Promote high quality care for all hospitalized patients.
- Promote education and research in hospital medicine.
- Promote teamwork to achieve the best possible care for hospitalized patients.
- Advocate a career path that will attract and retain the highest quality hospitalists.
- Define the competencies, activities, and needs of the hospitalist community.
- Support, propose, and promote changes to the health care system that lead to higher quality and more efficient care for all hospitalized patients.

This organization recognizes the contributions of nonphysician providers and has a standing committee within the organizational structure to develop initiatives and programs to promote and define the role of NPs and PAs in hospital medicine (SHM, 2010b). As the role of nonphysician providers continues to evolve, hospitalist practice will become interdisciplinary, and APNs and PAs will continue to be members of collaborative hospitalist teams to provide differentiated levels of care in the inpatient setting.

Commentary: Stage I

Hospitalist practice is a quickly emerging specialty in medicine. Although NPs, particularly and most appropriately ACNPs, are beginning to practice in this specialty, we see this as a stage I specialty for two reasons. First, the specialty is not yet recognized as a nursing specialty, and, although hospitalist practice for nurse practitioners has been defined by at least one state (Sullivan, 2009), describing unique distinctions between an APN hospitalist and physician hospitalist has not yet been attempted. Second, APN preparation for hospitalist practice is continuing to evolve as programs develop competency-based curricula more fully, with practica aimed at the development and refinement of knowledge and skills required for acute care, inpatient practice. One challenge for this stage I specialty is to articulate clearly the unique contributions that APNs can bring to the care of hospitalized patients, which may decrease fragmentation of care and improve interdisciplinary collaboration and overall patient outcomes. In addition, graduate nursing programs offering acute care education can ensure that hospital practice, based on the identified competencies in hospital medicine (Dressler, Pistoria, Budnitz, et al., 2006) and acute care competencies (National Panel for Acute Care Nurse Practitioner Competencies, 2004), are incorporated into required clinical practica. The challenge to any APN moving into this specialty is to maintain APN competencies and avoid a practice that is strictly an extension of medical practice. This transition may be facilitated if acute care nursing organizations promote and support establishment of special interest groups in these organizations to facilitate these transitions.

Specialties in Transition: Stage II

Stage II roles are characterized by progress in the evolution of the specialty to the point that organized training in the specialty begins. This training is often institution-specific, on the job training that develops experts in the specialty. The two roles discussed as demonstrating predominantly stage II characteristics but may exhibit some characteristics of stage III are those of the clinical transplant coordinator (CTC) and forensic nurse. The CTC role is clearly a stage II specialty practice, whereas the forensic nursing role can best be characterized as having several attributes of a stage III specialty (see Box 5-1).

Clinical Transplant Coordination

There is mounting evidence that the role of the CTC is evolving to the level of advanced practice nursing in response to patient care requirements in the referral and evaluation phase for patients, their families, and living donors, and in the pretransplant and post-transplant management phases of candidates and recipients. Specialty nurses with expertise in transplant nursing recognize the complex needs of these patients and many obtain graduate education to prepare them better to deal with the realities of transplant nursing. To the benefit of their patients, these coordinators have expanded the specialty by incorporating advanced practice core competencies.

Two organizations provide opportunities for ongoing education and preparation for certification for nurses who provide care for transplant patients, the North Atlantic Transplant Coordinators Organization (NATCO) and the International Transplant Nurses Society (ITNS). NATCO provides organized education in the specialty in the form of an introductory course for new clinical and procurement transplant coordinators (NATCO, 2009) in preparation for certification by the American Board for Transplant Certification (ABTC, 2007). ITNS, an organization focusing on the professional growth and development of the transplant clinician (ITNS, 2012), provides education on advances in transplantation and transplant patient care. ITNS has published a core curriculum (Ohler & Cupples, 2007) and scope and standards of a practice statement (ANA & ITNS, 2009) for the specialty that incorporates core competencies. Unlike the NATCO core competencies for the advanced practice transplant professional (APTP), which define the APTP as a provider who is not a physician but is licensed to diagnose and treat patients in collaboration with a physician (NATCO, 2010), the scope and standards of practice document developed by ITNS (2012) clearly address the scope of practice for transplant nurses, clinical and procurement transplant coordinators, and advanced practice transplant nurses, both NPs and CNSs. Building on the practice of the registered nurse generalist in transplant care and transplant nurse coordinator by demonstrating a greater depth and breadth of knowledge, greater synthesis of data and interventions, and significant role autonomy, which may include medical diagnosis and prescriptive authority, APNs working in transplant centers integrate and apply a broad range of theoretical and evidence-based knowledge using specialized and expanded knowledge and skills (ITNS, 2007).

It can be argued that the complex needs of patients with end-stage organ disease require higher levels of clinical reasoning and analytic skills, such as those possessed by APNs; however, to advance the CTC role (not just individuals in the role) to this higher level, attention to several issues is necessary. First and foremost, leaders in this specialty must systematically determine whether advanced practice core competencies (see Chapter 3) are required to enact the role fully or whether two levels of differentiated practice-generalist professional and APN—should be defined. Second, the specialty's leadership must agree that the role is a nursing role. Because some CTCs are not nurses, making these decisions may disenfranchise many committed and experienced transplant professionals who are essential care providers. Similar to the different certifications in place for diabetes educators and advanced diabetes managers, a similar method of differentiation, which would recognize the added value that advanced practice knowledge and skill brings to the CTC role, might serve to acknowledge the contributions of APNs and other transplant professionals. Both ITNS and NATCO are moving in this direction by doing the following: (1) delineating the core competencies required for clinical and procurement transplant coordinators (NATCO, 2009; ITNS, 2007), (2) developing a core curriculum for transplant nursing at the generalist level (Ohler & Cupples, 2007); and (3) as of 2004, initiating a certification examination for the clinical transplant nurse (certified clinical transplant nurse, CCTN; American Board for Transplant Certification [ABTC], 2007). Institution-specific, on the job education and experience, attributes that characterize a stage II specialty, continue to be widely embraced in the specialty; however, efforts to provide more formalized education are now the standard.

The issue of specialty certification is an issue for all evolving advanced practice nursing specialties. Educational institutions that prepare APNs must consider the certification requirements and ensure that their graduates are eligible to sit for APN certification examinations approved for legal recognition of an APN role. Specialty certification offered by specialty organizations, although optional, demonstrates a knowledge base shared among clinicians in the specialty and improves clinical credibility.

The evolution toward advanced practice nursing has been haphazard as a result of inattention to several issues. Most notably, the lack of recognition that the role requires advanced practice competencies and the lack of opportunities for advanced practice specialty certification may impede expansion into advanced practice nursing as an expectation of coordinator roles. The issue of specialty certification (at the generalist level) has been addressed, but no plans for advanced practice certification have been proposed, except for the APTP. Clearly, however, there is a commitment to advanced practice nursing in transplantation and, given that commitment, more attention to these issues will be necessary for the CTC role to evolve to stage III.

Exemplar 5-2 demonstrates the complexity of care required for transplant candidates, recipients, and their families. In addition to expertise in advanced practice core competencies, the exemplar also highlights the skill of the CNS in dealing with systems issues—in the hospital and community—and staff education and coaching, both of which are important components of providing care to this challenging patient population. As a member of a team of care providers, collaboration provides the opportunity to advocate for patients and their family members and influence quality of care. It is our view that the knowledge and expertise of advanced practice nurses could fully enable the potential of the CTC position.

Forensic Nursing

Forensic nursing has emerged as a specialty as a result of the severity of the national public health problems associated with violence. Recognition of the severity of the problem was first addressed in 1985 at the Surgeon General's Workshop on Violence and Public Health. In opening remarks, Dr. C. Everett Koop championed a multidisciplinary approach that addressed the prevention of violence and provision of better care for victims of violence. The severity of the problem was again addressed by the World Health Organization (WHO) in the *World Report on Violence and Health* (WHO, 2002). As the first comprehensive summary on the global impact of violence, it stated that more than 1.6 million people die from violence every year and more are injured and suffer mental health consequences.

In 1991, the ANA published a position statement on violence as a nursing practice issue and, in 1995, at the request of the International Association of Forensic Nurses

EXEMPLAR 5-2   Heart Transplant Coordinator*

Given the complexity of care associated with solid organ transplant patients, most transplant programs have multidisciplinary teams that care for candidates and recipients (Donaldson, 2003). The clinical transplant coordinator's role is to facilitate the care of the patient, in collaboration with the multidisciplinary team, throughout the transplantation process. This process begins with the patient's initial referral to the transplant program and often continues for the rest of the patient's life.

As a CNS, my clinical transplant coordinator position affords me the opportunity to incorporate the core competencies of advanced practice nursing. My clinical practice role includes direct and indirect care activities. For example, key direct care activities involve coordinating detailed discharge planning, seeing patients in the transplant clinic, and triaging telephone calls from candidates, recipients, and family members. Indirect care activities include participating in interdisciplinary clinical rounds (e.g., transfer conferences as patients transition from the intensive care unit to the intermediate care unit), developing protocols and patient education materials, participating in performance evaluation and improvement activities, initiating referrals to other health care specialists, and facilitating staff support groups. One example of staff support involved a transplant candidate with biventricular mechanical support who remained hospitalized for over 12 months until a suitable donor organ became available.

Over the course of this prolonged hospitalization, the nursing staff encountered several challenging problems. Many of the patient-staff conflicts revolved around the patient's desire for autonomy and the staff's need to provide care in a timely manner (e.g., dressing changes, physical therapy). To provide support for the staff as they worked toward resolving these problems, I organized consultative sessions with the transplant team's neuropsychologist and social worker that were held biweekly. The neuropsychologist enhanced the staff's understanding of the patient's cognitive status and the social worker helped the staff articulate their frustrations. Over time, in collaboration with the patient, mutually acceptable strategies were devised and implemented. For example, I coached the staff members in how to negotiate with the patient to develop a daily schedule that permitted him to sleep in on weekends when the census was typically low and the staff had more flexibility in providing care. In turn, the patient agreed to follow a more rigid schedule on weekdays.

My role affords many opportunities for staff and patient education. Staff education is formal (e.g., teaching in the critical care nurse internship program) and informal (e.g., answering staff nurses questions during rounds). I provide patient education, which involves extensive teaching sessions with prospective transplant candidates and their family members. The purpose of these sessions is to provide patients with information so they can make informed decisions about whether they wish to proceed with transplantation. Once a patient decides to proceed and is placed on the waiting list, additional education is provided during monthly support group meetings, which I lead. After the transplant procedure, recipients and family members attend comprehensive discharge education sessions. Post-discharge education is provided through newsletters, support group meetings, and individual counseling sessions during clinic visits.

One example of my role as collaborator is my participation with the interdisciplinary team that discusses, plans, implements, and evaluates the ongoing care of transplant candidates and recipients. One of our major responsibilities, as members of the transplant team, is to collaborate with other team members regarding whether a particular patient meets the heart transplant program's physiological and psychosocial eligibility criteria for placement on the waiting list. A second example concerns technology transfer, more specifically, the transfer of scientific advances of mechanical assist device technology into clinical practice. When the heart transplant team was about to discharge our first patient with a left ventricular assist device (LVAD), I coordinated this process working with the heart transplant research nurse, social worker, NP, physicians, hospital administrators, MedStar flight crew members, and community resource providers (e.g., the local power companies). The purpose of this collaborative effort was to establish physiologic and psychosocial criteria for discharge and develop policies and procedures regarding emergent and routine follow-up care.

Last, I have had the opportunity to collaborate with an international, multidisciplinary task force in reviewing the literature pertaining to the biopsychosocial outcomes of cardiothoracic transplantation, evaluating the strength of the evidence, and developing specific recommendations for future research designed to improve psychosocial and clinical outcomes.

*We gratefully acknowledge Sandra A. Cupples, DNSc, RN, Washington, DC, for assistance with this exemplar.

(IAFN), they officially recognized forensic nursing as a specialty. In the wake of the ANA position statement, the American College of Nurse Midwives (in 1995) and the Emergency.Nurses Association (in 1996) issued similar statements (Burgess et al., 2004). The scope and standards of forensic nursing practice was initially published in 1997 (ANA, 1997). These standards were updated in 2009 in collaboration with the IAFN (ANA, 2009).

Since the 1970s, nurses have been formally recognized providers of health care services to victims of violence. Nurses have volunteered at rape crisis centers and, by the mid-1980s, were widely acknowledged for the expertise they had developed. In addition, nurses were also being recognized for their research competence. This combination of factors opened doors for nurses to collaborate with other health care providers, initiate courses and programs of research on victimology and traumatology, influence legislation and health care policy, and ultimately create a new specialty (Burgess et al., 2004). One organization, the Academy on Violence and Abuse (AVA), established in 2005 in response to the challenge issued by the Institute of Medicine (IOM, 2011; Cohn, Salmon, & Stobo, 2002) to educate and train health professionals better about the often unrecognized health effects of violence and abuse, has worked extensively with interdisciplinary experts in violence and abuse prevention (e.g., nurses, dentists, social workers, psychologists, counselors, physicians). Their goal was to develop competencies at the level of the health care system, educational institution, and individuals to be a common starting point for profession-specific criteria regarding the skills, knowledge, and attitudes required for prevention (Ambuel et al., 2011). These efforts broaden the scope of influence of forensic nurses and offer opportunities to advance the specialty.

According to the IAFN (2007), forensic nursing practice is the application of nursing science to public or legal proceedings and often involves work with perpetrators and victims of interpersonal violence (sexual assault, abuse, domestic violence), death investigations, and legal and ethical issues. Forensic nurses interact with forensic psychiatric nurses, correctional nurses, emergency nurses, and trauma nurses, as well as a variety of other medical and law enforcement personnel. Forensic nurses may work for specialized hospital units, in medical examiners' offices, for law enforcement, as legal consultants, and for social services agencies (IAFN, 2012). In addition, in collaboration with school nurses, as a consequence of the increasing incidence of school violence, forensic nurses are becoming a significant line of defense for at-risk individuals, groups, agencies, and communities in efforts to reduce school violence (Jones, Waite, & Clements, 2012).

Like most stage II specialties, forensic nursing has traditionally been taught outside of formal educational programs. Some of the earliest programs were institution-based programs preparing nurses as sexual assault nurse examiners (SANEs). Certification is obtained through the Forensic Nursing Certification Board (FNCB), established in 2002 to promote the highest standards of forensic nursing practice. The FNCB offers adult-adolescent (SANE-A) certification to the sexual assault nurse examiner, as well as a sexual assault nurse examiner–pediatric (SANE-P) certification. Newer educational programs, such as those that prepare sexual assault forensic examiners (SAFEs) or forensic nurse examiners (FNEs), have expanded the scope of forensic nursing practice to include not only sexual assault incidents but also the gathering of forensic evidence in cases of domestic abuse or vehicular accident (IAFN, 2012).

The trend of educating forensic nurses in certificate programs is changing as graduate nursing programs are established; thus, forensic nursing is a specialty in transition. Similar to previous efforts to move wound, ostomy, and continence (WOC) nursing into graduate nursing education programs (Gray et al., 2000), forensic nursing has been taught at the graduate level in a few institutions for several years. Although certificate programs are sometimes the route to preparation, there are now ten master's programs offering this specialty preparation, and one of these programs recently transitioned to offer a DNP in forensic nursing (IAFN, 2012).

Commentary: Stage II

Forensic nursing provides a different perspective on evolving specialties and is used here to illustrate a stage II practice that may become advanced practice, integrating multiple other specialties such as the family NP, psychiatric and mental health NP and CNS, and women's health NP. In stage II, the specialty becomes more organized and visible. Formal training programs develop, specialty organizations form, and certification moves beyond individual institution-based certificates for completion of training to national certification examinations. All these developments lend strength and credibility to the specialty and its practitioners. Although many forensic nurses are prepared in certificate programs, being a specialty in transition to advanced practice nursing presents some opportunities for this particular specialty to evolve.

One of the major challenges in stage II is demonstrating that the specialty is a nursing specialty. There are a number of evolving specialties, such as clinical research coordinators and clinical transplant coordinators, whose practitioners include non-nurses and nurses. Clearly, these roles cannot emerge as advanced practice nursing roles without clear distinctions being drawn between non-nursing practice and nursing practice in the specialty. Specialty organizations with members who are non–health care providers, such as NATCO, must face this challenge. In the case of transplantation, for example, recognition of an APN level of practice or a sanctioning of practice at the APN level for all specialty providers is evolving. For CTCs or other advanced practice nurses working with transplant candidates or recipients, a mechanism for certifying advanced practice transplant nurses (e.g., through the ITNS) is necessary to recognize nursing's essential role in transplantation, without diminishing the contributions of others who also provide essential care and services.

Emerging Advanced Practice Nursing Specialties: Stage III

In the third stage of evolution to advanced practice, a specialty's knowledge base is growing and the scope of practice of nurses with specialty education is expanding. There is growing recognition of the additional knowledge and skills needed for increasingly complex practice in the specialty (Hamric, 2000). Pressures for standardization of education and skills required for specialty practice create incentives to move certificate-level training programs into graduate-level educational settings to increase standardization and raise the status of the specialty to an advanced practice level (Hanson & Hamric, 2003). According to Hanson and Hamric (2003), antecedents to legitimizing advanced practice must be addressed for a given specialty to evolve to advanced levels of practice (see Box 5-1). Two organizations that are addressing the issues necessary to legitimize advanced practice in their specialties are the Wound, Ostomy and Continence Nurses Society (WOCN) and interventional pain practice by the American Association of Nurse Anesthetists (AANA). Although these organizations have adopted differing approaches to advancing practice in their respective specialties, in each case the process was unified and proactive and depicts a framework that can guide other specialty organizations as they chart a course to advanced levels of practice.

Interventional Pain Practice

Millions of individuals suffer from acute or chronic pain every year and the effects of pain exact a tremendous cost on our country in health care costs, rehabilitation and lost worker productivity, and the emotional and financial burden it places on patients and their families (American Academy of Pain Medicine [AAPM], 2012). According to the AAPM (2012), pain affects more Americans than diabetes, heart disease, and cancer combined. Patients' unrelieved chronic pain problems often result in an inability to work and maintain health insurance. According to a recent IOM report, *Relieving Pain in America: A Blueprint for Transforming Prevention, Care, Education, and Research*

(2011), pain is a significant public health problem that costs society at least $560 to $635 billion annually, an amount equal to about $2,000 for everyone living in the United States. Much more needs to be done to meet the challenges of chronic pain management.

Because it is underrecognized and undertreated, the overall quality of pain management is and has been unacceptable to millions of patients with chronic pain. Pain management, particularly acute pain management, has been widely embraced in the inpatient and outpatient settings and is provided by a variety of health care professionals, including physicians, PAs, CRNAs, CNSs, and NPs. Interventional pain management, however, has emerged as the need to treat chronic pain has grown. APNs as interventional pain practitioners face complex and often controversial issues that challenge the legitimacy of this practice.

One example is that of CRNAs who have expanded their scope of practice to incorporate pain management specifically (AANA, 1994). In the wake of the 2001 Centers for Medicare and Medicaid Services (CMS) policy, which allowed states to opt out of the reimbursement requirement that a surgeon or anesthesiologist oversee the provision of anesthesia by CRNAs, several challenges to this option have been levied in several states to restrict more autonomous practice by these APNs. It is the position of the American Society of Interventional Pain Management Physicians (Douglas, 2008) and the American Society of Anesthesiologists (2009) that interventional pain management is the practice of medicine. Thus, actions have been taken in several states to restrict CRNAs scope of practice in chronic pain management. Although the outcomes of these actions have been equivocal, in one response by the Federal Trade Commission (FTC), Office of Policy Planning, Bureaus of Economics and Competition, AANA directors replied to an invitation to comment on legislation that would regulate (restrict) providers of interventional pain management services. Insightful comments in this reply addressed the recent IOM report (IOM, 2011) that identified a key role for APNs in improving access to health care and cautioned that restrictions on scope of practice have undermined nurses' ability to provide and improve general and advanced care (IOM, 2011). Furthermore, directors expressed concerns that access problems to these services may be especially acute for older patients with chronic pain, as well as rural and low-income individuals. Because a major component of the legislation addressed consumer protection, legislators were advised to investigate the need for the bill and its potential negative effects on cost, access, consumer choice and, in the absence of safety concerns, reject the legislation (FTC, 2011). Notably, research has demonstrated no increase in adverse outcomes in opt-out or non–opt-out states as a

EXEMPLAR 5-3 Interventional Pain Practice*

The inception of PainCare in 1992 marked the beginning of multidisciplinary interventional pain management in the northern New England regions of Maine, New Hampshire, and Vermont. This organization began to address a growing need for management of untreated chronic pain in underserved and remote regions of the northeast. Five CRNAs work as fully autonomous clinicians within this highly specialized practice setting; they provide comprehensive pain management services to those suffering from a wide variety of chronic pain conditions, many of whom have suffered for years without relief as the result of lack of access to specialized pain care.

In our pain management facility, the process of treating chronic painful conditions begins with meeting the patient during an initial office visit. The referral base for our patients includes specialty physicians (neurosurgical and orthopedic surgeons), primary care physicians, and nurse practitioners. This initial consultation entails taking a comprehensive and detailed medical and surgical history and performing a focused physical examination. At the conclusion of the initial office visit, we order the appropriate laboratory and imaging studies based on best evidence. Diagnostic studies may include electromyelography, ultrasound scanning, angiography, and/or bone scans. Because pain management is often interdisciplinary, we may make referrals to specialists such as neurologists, physiatrists, endocrinologists, oncologists, or orthopedic surgeons.

One of our roles as a CRNA pain practitioner is to assimilate the findings from the patient's detailed medical history, extensively focused physical examination and diagnostic testing. This is essential in identifying the causative pain generator and engaging an accurate treatment plan. Chronic pain can be difficult to treat and standard, conservative, and surgical treatments may prove unsuccessful. Prior surgical interventions often contribute to a patient's suffering. Furthermore, most patients who seek care at the pain center are currently taking prescription narcotics. Large doses of narcotics contribute significantly to tolerance issues. Side effects and systemic complications related to these potent medications are evident during the initial consultation with the patient. In these cases, pain relief is no longer forthcoming. The patient in chronic pain may experience many years of treatment and mistreatment prior to seeking care at our pain center.

Management of chronic pain requires a multimodal treatment plan. Once the process of patient counseling is initiated, it is our responsibility to initiate the discussion about realistic pain management expectations through patient education. Educating patients with regard to their pathology and treatment plan helps them gain a sense of control and understanding and places them as the central change agent. These chronic pain management patients are expected to attend all scheduled appointments and be an active participant in the treatment plan. The patient must know that management of his or her pain will take time and that improving quality of life is a major goal of treatment.

As pain managers, we regularly make referrals as an integral component of clinical practice. Referrals may be made for one or a combination of the following: physical therapy, occupational therapy, chiropractic sessions, acupuncture, craniosacral therapy, and/or message therapy. We may refer obese or diabetic patients to nutritionists for counseling if it is thought that these conditions may be contributing to their pain. Additionally, therapeutic devices such as lumbar, thoracic, and cervical support braces, transcutaneous electrical nerve stimulation (TENS) units, or orthotics may be incorporated into the treatment plan for spine and extremity pain. Smoking cessation, biofeedback, and hypnosis may also play a role in effective pain management treatment plans.

Frequently, we see patients with coexisting psychiatric issues such as anxiety, depression, bipolar disease, substance abuse, and post-traumatic stress disorder. Psychiatric professionals provide treatment and counseling as an essential part of an effective treatment plan. If a question of substance abuse arises, referrals for substance abuse evaluation and treatment are initiated. Our practice environment includes a comprehensive substance abuse program that plays an integral role in our multidisciplinary treatment facility.

An essential part of the practice includes medication management. Prescribing and selecting from a wide array of medications with various mechanisms of action contribute to the goal of relieving the patient's suffering. For example, opioids are prescribed for severe persistent pain and offer significant relief when other pharmacologic agents are not effective. On the other hand, more invasive procedures such as interventional injections may be used, which directly address causative pain generators. For example, during any given week, I may administer 40 to 50 cervical, thoracic, and lumbar epidural steroid injections, transforaminal injections, facet joint and medial branch nerve blocks to the cervical,

Interventional Pain Practice*—*cont'd*

thoracic, and lumbar regions, stellate ganglion blocks, lumbar sympathetic blocks, hypogastric plexus blocks, occipital nerve blocks, intra-articular joint injections, and peripheral nerve blocks.

To improve accuracy and maximize safety, all invasive procedures are performed under direct fluoroscopic guidance to ensure accurate needle placement. Every interventional injectionist must be an expert with regard to imaging analysis and interpretation. CRNAs involved in pain management recognize the potential for serious and sometimes fatal complications related to these procedures. Profound and lasting pain relief, and quality and safety in practice, mandate that the pain practitioner be well trained in invasive and noninvasive pain management techniques as well as radiation safety.

Prior to independent practice, I was trained under the direct supervision of an anesthesiologist–interventional pain physician. Successful completion of interventional injection procedures under direct supervision and documentation of hundreds of procedures was required to be involved in this type of advanced practice. My clinical privileges were granted on written request and approved by the medical director and clinical board members. In 2009, I earned a Doctor of Nurse Anesthesia Practice (DNAP) degree that has further prepared me to incorporate best evidence into my clinical practice, contribute to nurse anesthesia scholarship, and assume various leadership roles. Additionally, I am certified with the American Academy of Pain Management as a Diplomate. This certification requires a doctoral degree, a 2-year practice in a pain management setting, recommendations from colleagues, and successful completion of a written certification examination. Additional study and training include participation in interventional pain cadaver conferences and completion of continuing education via the American Academy of Pain Management and the International Association for the Study of Pain (IASP).

The nurse anesthesia subspecialty of pain management is evolving in many exciting and innovative ways. For example, Excel Anesthesia and Pain Management Associates (EAPMA) is a group of CRNAs who provide training for university-based student registered nurse anesthetists (SRNAs) and other CRNA populations. Under Medicare guidelines, EAPMA CRNAs are able to bill for direct supervision and training of resident SRNAs. This unique billing arrangement is expected to enhance and expand CRNA pain practice. One U.S. university has developed a specialized pain track for nurse anesthetists earning a clinical doctoral degree. Graduates of this program will qualify to sit for the AAPM certification examination. Members of EAPMA are also developing a separate certification examination for subspecialty pain management practice.

I believe the training and certification of CRNA pain managers is at an exciting turning point and will continue to establish itself. These well-trained and qualified pain practitioners will be a new generation of clinicians able to provide access to pain management services to underserved, critical access, and remote regions of the United States in which these services are currently unavailable. With over 400 patients under my care, I function autonomously in the role of pain manager. It is a true joy to practice in a setting where I am respected as an equal among interventional pain physicians, physiatrists, anesthesiologists, nurse practitioners, physician assistants, and primary care physicians. Almost all patients make significant progress in managing their chronic pain using a multidisciplinary treatment plan. Patients too often arrive at a pain center misunderstood and misdiagnosed, and their complaints deemed questionable. My role as pain manager at our facility is vital and serves an important public health function. The most gratifying part of my work is to witness patients who obtain pain relief for the first time in their lives.

*We gratefully acknowledge Russell Plewinski, DNAP, CRNA, DAAPM, Somersworth, New Hampshire, and Suzanne M. Wright, PhD, CRNA, Richmond, Virginia, for assistance with this exemplar.

consequence of CRNAs practicing without supervision (Dulisse & Cromwell, 2010).

Although these scope of practice issues are unresolved, attention to opportunities for multidisciplinary collaboration are essential for the pain interventionist role to grow and for APNs to be recognized as competent providers. To be recognized for their role in chronic pain management, APNs must be more visible in organizations

such as the American Academy of Pain Management and the American Pain Society (APS). Both these organizations welcome providers from multiple disciplines, but nursing is underrepresented. The APS has reported that approximately 50% of its members are physicians and only 7.4% are nurses. Membership and participation in this organization would improve visibility, recognition, and colleagueship with others providing chronic pain management services. The American Academy of Pain Management (2011) endorses the collective benefits that professionals from a variety of disciplines can make to the specialty of pain management. Unlike the APS, the American Academy of Pain Management does offer a credentialing examination. This examination is designed to ensure a minimum level of competency as an interdisciplinary pain practitioner. There are three levels of credentialing, which all require 2 years of pain management practice prior to examination application—diplomate, fellow, and clinical associate. The diplomate credential requires a doctoral degree in a related health care field, the fellow credential requires a master's degree, also in a related health care field, and the clinical associate credential requires a bachelor's degree (or its equivalent) in a related health care field. A credentialing review committee determines eligibility to sit for the examination; administration, scoring, psychometric consultation, and analysis of the examination are conducted by an external agency. Although this credential would not be required for specialty practice in chronic pain management, obtaining this certification would ensure a common knowledge base and competencies among all disciplines. Because knowledge and competency have been addressed in challenges to scope of practice, which incorporates chronic pain management, this credential would ensure continuing education and upholding the standards of care in pain management practice. In an emerging APN specialty, interdisciplinary certification encompassing the core competencies of the specialty and certification as an APN demonstrate credibility in the specialty in addition to the core competencies of advanced practice, and promotes recognition of advanced practice nursing and nursing as a profession.

Wound, Ostomy, and Continence Nursing

WOC nursing, a specialty that developed in response to unmet patient needs after fecal or urinary diversion surgery, has evolved significantly since its inception in the 1960s. Historically, lay persons developed the subspecialty, dedicated exclusively to the care of ostomy patients (WOCN, 1998). As health care changed and new patient needs arose, the original ET role evolved into a nursing specialty whose scope of practice expanded to include wound, skin, and continence care, in addition to ostomy care. The WOCN now recognizes three levels of care providers: WOC advanced practice registered nurses, WOC specialty nurse, and wound treatment associate. Thus, the WOCN and Wound Ostomy Continence Nursing Certification Board (WOCNCB) differentiate among levels of care providers based on certification. The appropriate use of each level of wound care provider is endorsed (WOCNS, 2012).

The educational preparation for WOC nurses, which began as clinical training programs based heavily on experiential knowledge about ostomy management, has been provided in post–baccalaureate educational programs. Some of these programs have begun to offer graduate-level course work in the specialty. Thus, the content has been integrated to a limited extent into graduate curricula of some U.S. universities (Gray et al., 2000; WOCN, 2012).

To be eligible for advanced practice certification in WOC nursing requires a registered nurse (RN) license and/or a license to practice as an APN and a master's degree in nursing in an advanced practice role (WOCNCB, 2012). These recent decisions by the WOCNCB to differentiate certification based on education clearly represent progress in addressing the added value of APNs in this specialty. This is a critical decision point for this stage III specialty. Similar to the work done by the International Society of Nurses in Genetics (ISONG; see later, stage IV, "Genetics Advanced Practice Nursing"), who established levels of genetics knowledge, practice, and certification, WOC nursing has advocated for APNs as having unique characteristics and contributions to make. These contributions reflect advanced practice core competencies obtained in graduate nursing education in addition to competencies attained in a specialty program aimed at preparing WOC nurses. The advanced practice certification builds on the entry-level certification and offers an incentive to entry-level WOC nurses to complete graduate nursing education as an APN; it also further legitimizes the advanced practice of WOC nursing.

APNs in the specialty may also wish to pursue additional recognition for advanced practice competency. Some nurses with graduate education in wound, ostomy, and/or continence nursing may seek certification as a wound management specialist (certified wound specialist [CWS]) awarded to qualified clinicians by the American Academy of Wound Management, a multidisciplinary organization, or as a urologic specialist, for CNSs or NPs, by the certification board of the Society of Urologic Nurses and Associates. In particular, the CWS certification recognizes a shared clinical knowledge base among professionals providing care to patients with complex wounds and may foster collaborative relationships that would further advance this specialty.

Commentary: Stage III

The stage III specialties discussed here are characterized by a growing knowledge base and an expanded scope of practice. For example, APNs practicing as pain interventionists, most notably CRNAs, have expanded their scope of practice to incorporate advanced diagnostic and treatment knowledge and skills to make pain intervention more accessible. As a consequence, questions

BOX 5-2   Questions to Address in Charting Specialty Evolution

- Are advanced practice nursing competencies required to enact specialty practice fully, or are they an added value?
- What are the distinct advanced practice nursing roles within the specialty?
- How can the organization best recognize and value existing providers while moving to new expectations?
- How should certification and educational expectations be structured, especially if differentiating practice between non-APNs and APNs continues within the specialty?
- How should subspecialty certification within the context of advanced practice nursing regulation be addressed?
- How can the centrality of direct clinical practice be maintained?

regarding their qualifications to provide these services have led to legal challenges. Some APNs in this specialty, in addition to advanced practice certification, have responded to these challenges by seeking credentialing by multidisciplinary specialty organizations, a strategy that lends credibility to their practice. This barrier to evolution to a stage IV specialty is likely to be overcome as more APNs transition to this specialty and demonstrate practice competencies. Exemplar 5-3 (see earlier) depicts a multidisciplinary collaborative practice and the CRNA's knowledge and expertise to deliver patient-centered, evidence-based care. To increase awareness of what can safely and competently be provided by CRNAs in pain management practice, these APNs need to increase their visibility through membership in pain management specialty organizations and credentialing as pain practitioners, better positioning the specialty to emerge as a stage IV role.

WOC nurses have clearly differentiated basic professional practice from advanced practice in the specialty. However, attention to several issues is still necessary for the specialty to emerge fully at the advanced (stage IV) level (Box 5-2). For example, WOC nurses are often educated in certification programs. Some programs offer graduate credit for coursework. Preparation in graduate or post–master's programs would standardize education and advance practice in the specialty. There are levels of practice in place that differentiate advanced practice nursing through their certification process. Thus, this specialty is poised to emerge as a stage IV specialty as a result of efforts clarifying certification and credentialing

requirements and the initiation of advanced practice certification.

Established Advanced Practice Nursing Roles: Stage IV

The fourth stage in the evolution of specialty practice to advanced practice is characterized by mature specialties. APNs practicing in these specialties are experts in the specialty, secure in understanding the unique contributions that they make in the direct care of patients. However, they embrace the notion that aspects of their practice are shared by experts from other disciplines essential to the care of their patients. Because of its origins in interdisciplinary practice, the advanced diabetes manager characterizes an established APN role. APNs in genetics have overcome obstacles to interdisciplinary practice through the development of multidisciplinary collaborative relationships and have also emerged as a stage IV APN role.

Advanced Diabetes Manager

The rising incidence of diabetes mellitus (DM) has created new opportunities for APNs. Advances in the science and technology of diabetes care and findings from two clinical research trials have redefined the roles of health care providers in diabetes care. Two classic studies, the Diabetes Control and Complications Trial (DCCT; 1993) and the United Kingdom Prospective Diabetes Study (UKPDS; 1998) have demonstrated the value of multidisciplinary teams consisting of dietitians, nurses, and pharmacists in the clinical management of those with DM. Before the results of these clinical trials were released, however, the American Association of Diabetes Educators (AADE; 2004) published multidisciplinary scope and standards of practice guidelines, which were revised as recently as 2005 (Martin, Daly, McWhorter, et al., 2005). An advanced practice task force was established in 1993 and the dialogue among the three major disciplines constituting the membership of the association—nurses, dietitians, and pharmacists—and their credentialing bodies was initiated (Hentzen, 1994; Tobin, 2000). These collaborative efforts resulted in a definition of advanced practice in diabetes as the highest of various levels of practice used along the full continuum of diabetes care (Hentzen,1994; Tobin, 2000). These levels are identified as the certified diabetes educator (CDE) and the board-certified advanced diabetes manager (BC-ADM; Martin et al., 2005).

The CDE is a health care provider who meets educational and practice requirements, successfully completes the certification examination for diabetes educators, and is credentialed by the National Certification Board for Diabetes Educators (NCBDE). The CDE can provide the following: case management; diabetes education program development, coordination, and implementation; and referral to advanced practitioners, other health care team members, or community resources.

The BC-ADM, launched in 2000 as a result of unprecedented multiorganizational collaboration and initially credentialed by the ANCC, is now credentialed by the AADE (AADE, 2011). This advanced practice credential focuses the on management of diabetes, including prescribing medications, rather than on diabetes education. Thus, this credential distinguishes between two sets of skills (Daly et al., 2001; Valentine, Kulkarni, & Hinnen, 2003). This level of credentialing is designed for licensed health care professionals, including registered dietitians, registered nurses, and registered pharmacists, who hold graduate degrees and have recent clinical diabetes management experiences after they have been licensed. Credentialing as a CDE is not required to take the advanced management examination.

Notably, the BC-ADM designation is unique. Although each discipline eligible for certification takes a different examination (Valentine et al., 2003), it was the first multidisciplinary approach to the certification of nurses, dietitians, and pharmacists ever developed by the ANCC (Daly et al., 2001; Valentine et al., 2003). The fact that the ANCC agreed with the AADE's request to support the advanced-level examination for disciplines other than nursing to promote team collaboration and improve quality of care for individuals with diabetes represented the emergence of a new model of collaboration among practitioners who formerly may have competed for recognition by patient and consumer groups. The potential benefits of multidisciplinary certification include increased credibility with colleagues, patients and consumers, employers, and other health care professionals as a result of a shared knowledge base, differentiation of these providers as having advanced-level expertise in diabetes management, greater autonomy in the delivery of care and services, and improved reimbursement (Daly et al., 2001). In this multidisciplinary model, APNs fill a niche in the care of these patients that facilitates self-care and achievement of treatment goals. Nurses constitute the largest group of health care professionals who deliver care to individuals with DM across the life span and in a variety of settings; therefore, graduate-level preparation for APNs in diabetes management, consistent with American Diabetes Association standards, would fulfill the need for care providers in acute and primary care settings.

Genetics Advanced Practice Nursing

Mapping the human genome and the relevance of the Human Genome Project to health and disease have been revolutionizing the provision of genetics services specifically and health care generally. New genetic discoveries have made available an increasing number of genetic technologies for carrier, prenatal, diagnostic, and presymptomatic testing for genetic conditions. These discoveries are creating changes in the delivery of genetic services, the most immediate being the integration of genetics into the prevention and treatment, for example, of cardiovascular disease (Arnett et al., 2007), obesity (Yang, Kelly, & He, 2007), and cancer (Balmain, Gray, & Ponder, 2003). Although brought to the forefront of public awareness by the mapping of the human genome, genetics services initially emerged out of a need for professionals who could provide genetic information, education, and support to patients and families with current and future genetic health concerns. Genetics experts in academic, medical, public health, and community-based settings have tradionally provided these services. In each setting, genetics professionals, including medical geneticists, genetics counselors, and genetics APNs, provide genetics services to patients and families. Working with other team members, genetics specialists obtain and interpret complex family history information, evaluate and diagnose genetic conditions, interpret and discuss complicated genetic test results, support patients throughout the genetics counseling process, and offer resources for additional individual and family support. Over time, through interaction with these specialists, patients and family members come to learn and understand relevant aspects of genetics to make informed health decisions and receive support in integrating personal and family genetics information into their daily lives (Lea, Jenkins, & Francomano, 1998).

According to ISONG, the scope of genetics nursing practice is basic and advanced. At the basic level, genetics nurses are prepared to perform assessments to identify risk factors, plan care, provide interventions such as information, and evaluate for referral to genetic services. At the advanced level, master's-prepared nurses provide genetics counseling, case management, consultation, and evaluation of patients, families, resources, and/or programs (ANA-ISONG, 2007). Nurses in genetics clinical practice are certified by the Genetic Nursing Credentialing Commission (GNCC), established in 2001 in cooperation with the ISONG. Two levels of practice and recognition, which correspond to the scope of genetics nursing practice, currently exist, the genetics clinical nurse (GCN) and APN in genetics (APNG). The credentials conferred by the GNCC mandate that specific educational, practice, and professional service requirements are met. The process is accomplished using a portfolio review. Eligibility for the APNG certification requires the following: (1) proof of RN licensure in good standing; (2) completion of 300 hours of genetics practicum experiences as a clinical genetics nurse, with more than 50% genetics practice component; (3) a log of 50 cases within 5 years of the application; (4)

four written case studies reflecting ISONG Standards of Clinical Genetics Nursing Practice; (5) graduation from an accredited graduate program in nursing; and (6) 50 hours of genetics content in the past 5 years through academic courses or continuing education (ISONG, 2012).

Only four programs offer graduate-level genetics programs for nurses. Currently, educational preparation for APNs occurs in master's programs in nursing. Although an increased focus on genetics has been occurring in graduate nursing programs as a result of recent revisions in the *Essentials of Master's Education in Nursing* (American Association of Colleges of Nursing [AACN], 2011), genetics content is usually obtained later in post–baccalaureate educational programs or through continuing education courses. Regardless of the type of program or course, the course content must reflect the following: information in human genetics; molecular and biochemical genetics; ethical, legal, and social issues in genetics; genetic variations in populations; and clinical application of genetics, including genetics counseling to meet requirements for certification. Expectations for evidence-based practice, an advanced practice competency, which has the potential to transform health care because of integration of genetics knowledge, requires the knowledge acquired in graduate nursing education. In addition, the ethical decision making skills of APNs are important to this specialty. Because graduate nursing educational preparation required for the APNG credential places these nurses at the same level as other genetics services providers, such as genetics counselors, professional diversity and interdisciplinary collaboration are fostered.

The American Board of Genetics Counselors (ABGC) certifies some nurses; however, this avenue is not open to nurses unless they complete graduate education and clinical practice requirements in genetics medicine, human genetics, and/or genetic counseling. Nurses who wish to pursue graduate education solely in nursing are not eligible for this certification. Because the scope of practice for the APNG is much broader than that of a genetics counselor, differentiation based on credentials is appropriate. In addition to counseling, the APNG diagnoses and treats patients with a variety of clinical disorders (e.g., birth defects, chromosomal abnormalities, genetic disorders presenting in newborn, child, and adult muscular disorders, and intrauterine teratogen exposure) and inherited conditions. Because of the complexity of care required, collaboration among these professionals is necessary for appropriate genetics services delivery. Toward this end, the National Society of Genetics Counselors (NSGC) and ISONG jointly developed a position statement advocating a multidisciplinary collaborative approach to enhance the quality of genetic services and care (ISONG, 2006). These efforts by the ISONG have positioned the specialty to transition to a stage IV specialty as a result of collaborative efforts with genetics counselors who are master's-prepared for their role.

EXEMPLAR 5-4   **Insights from Leaders in the Genetics Specialty***

In 1976, the Genetic Diseases Act was passed by Congress and the Genetic Diseases Services Branch of the Office of Maternal Child Health, Health Services Administration, Department of Health and Human Services, was established. At that time, a small and academically diverse group of nurses was working with genetics programs in tertiary health care settings. They tended to come from practice backgrounds in pediatrics or obstetrics, which made sense because genetic services at that time were centered primarily on the delivery of prenatal diagnostic procedures and the evaluation of the dysmorphic child or the child with developmental delays. A relatively small number of master's-prepared genetics counselors also were working in settings similar to those of the nurses. In the 1980s, however, medical geneticists started to employ nurses rather than counselors for a variety of reasons, including the limited number of counselors available and the broader scope of practice of nurses.

Differing perspectives emerged regarding basic requirements for certification and the appropriate credentialing body for awarding certification. Genetics counselors required a degree from an approved master of science in genetics counseling program and were credentialed through the American Board of Medical Genetics (ABMG). In contrast, nurses advocated for a professional nursing organization as an appropriate credentialing body and graduate education in nursing as an acceptable educational route.

The number of genetics counselors increased faster than the number of genetics nurses in the 1980s. This led to the educational meetings of the NSGC becoming focused on the learning needs of genetics counselors, not consistently and sufficiently addressing the issues that confronted genetics nurses. After the initial NSGC educational meetings, a bond was formed among those nurses working in genetics and monies were found to form the Genetics Nurse Network. In 1987, there was significant discussion among the members of the network regarding the benefits of establishing a formal professional organization for genetics nurses. The lack of a professional group and the inability to obtain

EXEMPLAR 5-4   **Insights from Leaders in the Genetics Specialty***—*cont'd*

certification that would be recognized by the nursing profession led to the development of ISONG. Membership in the organization has continued to grow since 1987, but the issue of certification remained unresolved. Nurses working in genetics had academic preparation ranging from diplomas to doctoral degrees. Some were already certified as genetics counselors and others were certified as nurse practitioners in their specialty area. After significant discussion by the membership of the ISONG, it was thought that the core knowledge required by genetics nurses was broader, but there was also the issue of recognition of a credential provided by a non-nursing organization being accepted by the nursing community. Also, it was understood that at that time there were not enough nurses to sit for a written examination to provide for test item validation. Therefore, the GNCC was established to investigate alternatives that would address these issues. After extensive work, the GNCC announced the establishment of the APNG credential and awarded the first credentials in 2001.

As genetics knowledge continues to develop, genetics will become an integral part of the clinical practice of all nurses. The ISONG has worked with the National Coalition for Health Professional Education in Genetics (NCHPEG) to develop competencies for health care professionals at the generalist and specialty levels and has collaborated with the ANA to publish competencies specific to nurses. ISONG continues to grow and develop to meet the needs of nurses who are at any point on the novice to expert continuum and who focus on clinical practice, professional or consumer education, or research.

*We gratefully acknowledge Shirley Jones, PhD, RN, Louisville, KY, and Judith Lewis, PhD, RN, Richmond, VA, for their assistance with this exemplar.

Commentary: Stage IV

Caring for persons with diabetes has become complex, requiring the expertise and efforts of interdisciplinary teams. Because the nature of caring for patients with diabetes has historically required interdisciplinary collaboration, health care providers from these disciplines are secure in understanding the unique contributions that they make in patient management. They are experts—secure in their individual and shared clinical knowledge base—and embrace the challenges and opportunities inherent in multidisciplinary collaboration. This model of collaboration is somewhat unique and has been expertly developed by leaders in the AADE. The trajectory of change that was initiated in the early 1990s exemplifies the natural maturation of the specialty resulting from deliberate logical planning to strengthen the education and broaden the scope of practice of practitioners in this specialty. Similarly, and strategically, ISONG has made tremendous progress in defining roles for health care providers, including APNs who are experts in genetics, fostering a collaborative relationship with genetic counselors, and differentiating levels of practice within multidisciplinary teams.

Conclusion

As can be seen from Chapter 1, the evolution of specialties in nursing has a long and rich history that continues in the present. The progress made by members of specialty organizations that have evolved their specialties to advanced levels of practice (stages III and IV) can serve as examples for others that are struggling to evolve (stage II) or are newly emerging (stage I).

In this chapter, we have examined each of these stages in the context of selected specialty groups and the evolving and innovative roles that characterize progression toward advanced practice nursing. Clearly, the ability to be deliberate in efforts to evolve the specialty speeds progress, as demonstrated by organizations such as the WOCN, AADE, and ISONG. Some specialties have evolved haphazardly. Others may not evolve into advanced practice nursing; without commitment from the nursing community and attention to the issues noted in Boxes 5-1 and 5-2, the move toward advanced practice nursing may be an unrealistic goal. It is important to recognize that progression to advanced levels of practice is neither inevitable nor necessary. For example, staff development educators are a respected specialty group within the nursing profession, yet their competencies are not consistent with those of advanced practice nursing (Hanson & Hamric, 2003). As specialties move through the stages described here, one important question for the specialty's leadership is whether the specialty is best advanced by deliberate evolution to the advanced level of practice, development of differentiated levels of practice with distinct expectations and certifications, or continued development as a specialty (see Box 5-2). In these decisions, it is critically important to affirm the roles and value of all providers in the specialty, even as differentiation occurs for advancement and strengthening of specialty roles.

⊙ TABLE 5-2 **Specialty Organizations Offering Advanced-Level Certification**

Specialty Organization	Credentialing Organization; Credential Awarded	Graduate Nursing Education Required?
American Academy of HIV Medicine*	American Academy of HIV Medicine; HIV specialist	Implied (must be licensed as an NP)
American Academy of Pain Management*	American Academy of Pain Management; credentialed pain practitioner	Yes (for diplomate or fellow status)
American Academy of Wound Management*	American Academy of Wound Management; CWS	Yes (for diplomate or fellow status)
American Association of Critical-Care Nurses	AACN Certification Corporation; CCNS, ACNPC	Yes
American Association of Diabetes Educators*	American Association of Diabetes Educators; BC-ADM	No (master's in nursing or related field)
Association of Nurses in AIDS Care	HIV/AIDS Nursing Certification Board; AACRN	Yes
Hospice and Palliative Care Nurses Association	National Board for Certification of Hospice and Palliative Care Nurses; ACHPN	Yes
International Society of Nurses in Genetics	Genetic Nursing Credentialing Commission; APNG	Yes
International Nurses Society on Addictions	Addictions Nursing Certification Board; CARN-AP	No (master's in nursing or related field)
Oncology Nursing Society	Oncology Nursing Certification Corporation; AOCNS, AOCNP	Yes
Wound, Ostomy, and Continence Nursing Society	Wound Ostomy Continence Nursing Certification Board; CWOCN-AP, CWON-AP, CWCN-AP, CCCN-AP	Yes
Society of Urologic Nurses and Associates*	Certification Board of Urologic Nurses and Associates; CUNP, CUCNS	Yes (must already be NP or CNS)

*Multidisciplinary membership.
AACRN, Advanced AIDS Care Registered Nurse; *ACHPN,* Advanced Certification in Hospice and Palliative Care Nursing; *ACNPC,* Acute Care Nurse Practitioner Certification; *AOCNP,* Advanced Oncology Certified Nurse Practitioner; *AOCNS,* Advanced Oncology Clinical Nurse Specialist; *APNG,* Advanced Practice Nurse in Genetics ; *CARN-AP,* Certified Addiction Registered Nurse Advanced Practice; *CCNS,* Critical Care Clinical Nurse Specialist; *CWOCN-AP,* Certified Wound Ostomy Continence Nursing Advanced Practice.

Concern over whether a role is a nursing role (versus exclusively a nursing role) is an issue that will need to be examined in particular specialties. In the history of nursing, some roles have been characterized as sharing attributes with other types of health care providers. For example, some psychiatric CNSs attained their credentials to practice as licensed professional counselors. Other health care providers (e.g., counselors, psychologists) also receive this same credential, despite educational differences. Failure to acknowledge the value of multidisciplinary teams, shared knowledge, and overlapping expertise may limit opportunities for APNs in the current health care environment and impede the advancement of specialties in the discipline. As a profession, nursing must embrace the notion that some roles are not exclusively nursing and must endorse differentiated practice models.

At the same time, the profession must define the advanced level of practice within the interdisciplinary model. This is critical for regulatory purposes, standardization of APN competencies in the practice, and recognition by the public and insurers. In addition to the AADE, other specialty organizations (Table 5-2) certify health care providers who share a common knowledge base. These organizations are models of collaboration that communicate to consumers, other providers, third-party payers, and other stakeholders that there are national standards in the specialty that are upheld by these specialty care providers. These multidisciplinary collaborative models represent a trend in health care that has given rise to a fourth stage in the evolution of advanced practice nursing. This stage is characterized by APNs who are mature expert practitioners in a specialty, secure in understanding the unique contributions that they make in the direct care of patients, yet embracing the notion that some aspects of their practice are shared by experts from other disciplines essential to the care of their patients.

The proliferation of role titles seen in evolving specialties requires special attention as APNs begin practicing in the specialty. For example, within the transplant specialty, role titles such as clinical transplant coordinator, transplant coordinator, transplant nurse, transplant NP, and transplant CNS have been used in practice settings. The advanced practice role titles of CNS, NP, CRNA, and CNM need to be consistently applied to APNs who are practicing in particular specialties to decrease role confusion. In addition, this consistency is important for promoting the recognition of advanced practice nursing

within evolving specialties and the profession as a whole. For specialties that develop nonadvanced and advanced levels of practice, consistent titles are necessary to avoid confusion among providers and patients.

This is an extraordinarily interesting time in the history of the nursing profession. Opportunities and challenges for advanced practice nursing abound. What will the history books say about this period in the evolution and expansion of the nursing profession? As Hamric (2000) wrote in addressing the WOC specialty group, "[Our] hope is that they will say [we] clearly saw patients' needs and developed [our] skills to meet those needs; that [we] grasped the role opportunities that were possible and created new ones; and, most importantly, that [we] moved forward together" (p. 47).

References

Ambuel, B., Trent, K., Lenahan, P., Cronholm, P., Downing, D., Jelley, M., et al. (2011). *Competencies needed by health professionals for addressing exposure to violence and abuse in patient care, academy on violence and abuse.* Eden Prairie, MN: Academy on Violence and Abuse.

American Association of Pain Management. (2011). Credentialing brochure. (http://www.aapainmanage.org).

American Academy of Pain Medicine. (2012).Facts and figures on pain. (http://painmed.org/patientcenter/facts_on_pain.aspx#refer).

American Association of Colleges of Nursing. (2011). *Essentials of Master's Education in Nursing.* Washington, DC: Author.

American Association of Diabetes Educators (AADE). (2004). The scope of practice, standards of practice,, and standards of professional performance for diabetes educators. *Diabetes Educator, 31,* 487–512.

American Association of Diabetes Educators. (2011). AADE re-launches the BC-ADM credential: Are you ready to take the exam? (http://www.diabeteseducator.org/Professional Resources/Periodicals/eFYI/eFYI2011.04_April/articles.html).

American Association of Nurse Anesthetists (AANA), Board of Directors. (1994). *Position statement: Pain management.* Ridge Park, IL: Author.

American Board for Transplant Certification (ABTC). (2007). *Candidate handbook: Clinical transplant coordinators, procurement transplant coordinators, clinical transplant nurses.* Lanexa, KS: Author.

American Nurses Association (ANA). (2009). *Scope and standards of forensic nursing practice.* Washington, DC: Author.

American Nurses Association (ANA). American Nurses Association. (2010a). *Nursing: Scope and standards of practice* (2nd ed.). Silver Spring, MD: American Nurses Association.

American Nurses Association (ANA). (2010b). *Nursing's social policy statement: The Essence of the profession.* Silver Spring, MD: American Nurses Association.

American Nurses Association (ANA)/International Society of Nurses in Genetics (ISONG). (2007). *Genetics/genomics*

nursing: Scope and standards of practice. Washington DC: Author.

American Nurses Association (ANA)/International Transplant Nurses Society (ITNS). (2009). *Transplant nursing: Scope and standards of practice.* Silver Spring, MD: Nursesbooks.org.

American Society of Anesthesiologists. (2009). Position paper: Interventional pain management is the practice of medicine (http://www.asahq.org/For-Members/Advocacy/Federal-Legislative-and-Regulatory-Archive/Positionpaper).

Arnet, D. K., Baird, A. K., Barkley, R. A., Basson, C. T., Boerwinkle, E., Ganesh, S. K., et al. (2007). Relevance of genetics and genomics for prevention and treatment of cardiovascular disease: A scientific statement from the American Heart Association Council of Epidemiology and Prevention, the Stroke Council, and the Functional Genomics and Translational Biology Interdisciplinary Working Group. *Circulation, 155,* 2878–2901.

Balamin, A., Gray, J., & Ponder, B. (2003). The genetics and genomics of cancer. *Nature Genetics, 33*(Suppl), 238–244.

Beitz, J. M. (2000). Specialty practice, advanced practice, and WOC nursing: Current professional issues and future opportunities. *Journal of Wound, Ostomy and Continence Nursing, 27,* 55–64.

Bigbee, J. L., & Amidii-Nouri, A. (2000). History and evolution of advanced nursing practice. In A. B. Hamric, J. A. Spross, & C. M. Hanson (Eds.), *Advanced nursing practice: An integrated approach* (pp. 3–32, 2nd ed.). Philadelphia: Saunders.

Burgess, A. W., Berger, A. D., & Boersma, R. R. (2004). Forensic nursing: Investigating the career potential in this emerging graduate specialty. *American Journal of Nursing, 104,* 58–64.

Coffman, J., & Rundall, T. G. (2005). The impact of hospitalists on cost and quality of inpatient care in the United States: A research synthesis. *Medical Care Research Review, 62,* 379–406.

Cohn, F., Salmon, M. E., Stobo, J. D. (2002). *Confronting chronic neglect: The education and training of health professionals on family violence.* Washington, D.C.: National Academy Press.

Daly, A., Kulkarni, K., & Boucher, J. (2001). The new credential: Advanced diabetes management. *Journal of the American Dietetic Association, 101,* 940–943.

DeNicola, L., Klied, D., & Brink, L. (1994). Use of pediatric physician extenders in pediatric and neonatal intensive care units. *Critical Care Medicine, 22,* 105–106.

Diabetes Control and Complications Trial (DCCT) Research Group. (1993). The effect of intensive treatment of diabetes on the development and progression of long-term complications in insulin-dependent diabetes mellitus. *New England Journal of Medicine, 329,* 977–988.

Donaldson, T. A. (2003). The role of the transplant coordinator. In S. A. Cupples & L. Ohler (Eds.), *Transplantation nursing secrets* (pp. 17–26). Philadelphia: Hanley & Belfus.

Douglas, E. (2008). State initiatives aim to expand role of nurse anesthetists. *Anesthesiology News. 34,* 9.

Doyle, J. (2001). Forensic nursing: A review of the literature. *Australian Journal of Advanced Nursing, 18,* 32–39.

Dressler, D. B., Pistoria, M. J., Budnitz, T. L., McKean, S. C. W., & Amin, A. N. (2006). Core competencies in hospital medicine: Development and methodology. *Journal of Hospital Medicine, 1,* 48–56.

Dulisse, B. & Cromwell, J. (2010) No harm found when nurse anesthetists work without supervision by physicians. *Health Affairs 29,* 1469–1475.

Federal Trade Commission (2011). *Response to invitation for comments on Tennessee House Bill 1896 (H.B. 1896).* Washington DC: Federal Trade Commission.

Freed , D. H. (2004). Hospit6alists: Evolution, evidence, and eventualities. *Health Care Management, 23,* 238–256.

Gray, M., Ratliff, C., & Mawyer, R. (2000). A brief history of advanced practice nursing and its implications for WOC advanced nursing practice. *Journal of Wound, Ostomy and Continence Nursing, 27,* 48–54.

Hamric, A. B. (2000). WOC nursing and the evolution to advanced practice nursing. *Journal of Wound, Ostomy and Continence Nursing, 27,* 46–47.

Hanson, C. M., & Hamric, A. B. (2003). Reflections on the continuing evolution of advanced practice nursing. *Nursing Outlook, 51,* 203–211.

Hentzen, D. (1994). AADE moves to advanced practice model for diabetes education and care. *Diabetes Educator, 20,* 190.

Hutson, L. A. (2002). Development of sexual assault nurse examiner programs. *Nursing Clinics of North America, 37,* 79–88.

Institute of Medicine (IOM) Report, (2002). *Confronting chronic neglect: The education and training of health professionals on family violence.* Washington: National Academies Press.

Institute of Medicine (IOM) Committee on the Robert Wood Johnson Initiative on the Future of Nursing. 2011. *The future of nursing: Leading change, advancing health.* Washington DC: National Academies Press, Institute of Medicine.

Institute of Medicine Report from the Committee on Advancing Pain Research, Care, and Education. *Relieving pain in America: A blueprint for transforming prevention, care, education and research* (2011). Washington: National Academies Press.

International Association of Forensic Nurses (IAFN). (2007). IAFN mission (www.iafn.org/ about/aboutHome.cfm).

International Association of Forensic Nurses (IAFN). (2012). Forensic nursing degree programs (http://www.iafn.org/displaycommon.cfm?an=1&subarticlenbr=542).

International Society of Nurses in Genetics (ISONG). (2006). Provision of quality genetic services and care: Building a multidisciplinary collaborative approach among genetic nurses and genetic counselors (www.isong.org/ISONG_PS_quality_genetic_services.php).

International Society of Nurses in Genetics. (2012). Credentialing requirements (http://www.geneticnurse.org/advancedpracticeapng.html).

International Transplant Nursing Society (ITNS). (2007) Scope and standards of transplant nursing (http://itns.org/scope-and-standards-of-transplant-nursing).

International Transplant Nurses Society. (2012). About ITNS (http://www.itns.org/About/About//aboutitne.html).

Jones, S. N., Waite, R. & Clements, P. T. (2012). An evolutionary concept analysis of school violence: From bullying to death. *Journal of Forensic Nursing,* 4–12. doi: 10.1111/j.1939-3938.2011.x.

Lea, D. H., Jenkins, J., & Francomano, C. A. (1998). *Genetics in clinical practice: New directions for nursing and health care.* Sudbury, MA: Jones & Bartlett.

Lee, K. H. (2008). The hospitalist movement—a complex adaptive response to fragmentation of care in hospitals. *Annals of Academic Medicine in Singapore, 37,* 45–50.

Lewis, J. A. (2000). Advanced practice in maternal/child nursing: History, current status, and thoughts about the future. *Maternal Child Nursing, 25,* 327–330.

Maeve, M. K., & Vaughn, M. S. (2001). Nursing with prisoners: The practice of caring, forensic nursing or penal harm? *Advances in Nursing Science, 24,* 47–64.

Martin, C., Daly, A., McWhorter, L. S., Shwide-Slavin, C., Kushion, W., & 2004-2005 American Association of Diabetes Educators Professional Practices Committee. (2005). The scope of practice, standards of practice, and standards of professional performance for diabetes educators. *Diabetes Educator, 31,* 487–512.

McCrone, S., & Shelton, D. (2001). An overview of forensic psychiatric care of the adolescent. *Issues in Mental Health Nursing, 22,* 125–135.

National Council of State Boards of Nursing (NCSBN), Advanced Practice Registered Nurse Joint Dialogue Group. (2008). *Consensus statement on advanced practice registered nursing: Report of the APRN Consensus Work Group.* Chicago, IL: Author.

National Panel for Acute Care Nurse Practitioner Competencies. (2004). *Acute care nurse practitioner competencies.* Washington, DC: National Organization of Nurse Practitioner Faculty.

North American Transplant Coordinators Organization (NATCO). (2009). *Core competencies for the clinical transplant coordinator.* Lanexa, KS: Author.

North American Transplant Coordinators Organization (NATCO). (2010). *Core competencies for the advanced practice transplant professional.* Lanexa, KS: Author.

Nyberg, D. (2006). Innovations in the management of hospitalized patients. *Nurse Practitioner, Spring* (Suppl), 2–3.

Ohler, L., & Cupples, S. (Eds.). (2007). *Core curriculum for transplant nurses,* St. Louis: Mosby.

Oncology Nursing Society (ONS). (2012). About ONS. (www. ons.org/about).

Salyer, J. & Hamric, A. B. (2009). Evolving and innovative opportunities for advanced practice nursing. In Hamric, A. B., Spross, J. A. & Hansom, C. M. (Eds.), *Advanced practice nursing: An integrative approach* (pp. 520–540, 4th ed.). St. Louis: Elsevier.

Society of Hospital Medicine (SHM). (2010a). Mission statement and goals. (http://www.hospitalmedicine.org/AM/Template. cfm?Section=General_Information&Template=/CM/HTMLDisplay.cfm&ContentID=14047).

Society of Hospital Medicine (SHM). (2010b). Non-physician provider committee (http://www.hospitalmedicine.org/AM/Template.cfm?Section=General_Information&TEMPLATE=/CM/ContentDisplay.cfm&CONTENTID=30050).

Sullivan, D. (February, 2009). A new role for advanced practice nurses—the hospitalist. (www.StuNurse.com. http://stunurse.com/files/ne_ed11.pdf).

Terboss, M.A. (2007). Personal communication.

Tobin, C. T. (2000). A rainbow of opportunities: Advanced practice. *Diabetes Educator, 26,* 216, 326–327.

United Kingdom Prospective Diabetes Study (UKPDS) Group. (1998). Intensive blood glucose control with sulfonylurea or insulin compared with conventional treatment and risk of complications in patients with type 2 diabetes. *Lancet, 352,* 837–853.

Valentine, V., Kulkarni, K., & Hinnen, J. (2003). Evolving roles: Diabetes educator to advanced diabetes manager. *Diabetes Educator, 29,* 598–610.

Wachter, R. M. (2004). Hospitalists in the United States: Mission accomplished or work in progress? *New England Journal of Medicine, 350,* 1935–1936.

Wachter, R. M., & Goldman, L. (1996). The emerging role of "hospitalists" in the American health care system. *New England Journal of Medicine, 335,* 514–517.

World Health Organization (WHO). (2002). *World report on violence and health: summary.* Geneva: Author.

Wound Ostomy and Continence Nursing Certification Board (WOCNCB). (2012). Eligibility for advanced practice certification exam (http://www.wocncb.org/become-certified/advanced-practice/eligibility.php).

Wound Ostomy and Continence Nurses Society (WOCNS). (1998). *Commemorative program for opening session: 30th anniversary conference.* Laguna Beach, CA: Author.

Wound Treatment Associate Task Force. (2012). Position statement about the role and scope of practice for wound care providers. *Journal of Wound, Ostomy and Continence Nursing, 39,* 52–54.

Yang, W., Kelly, T., & He, J. (2007). Genetic epidemiology of obesity. Epidemiologic reviews advance access. (http://epirev.oxfordjournals.org/cgi/content/abstract/mxm004v1).

International Development of Advanced Practice Nursing

Joyce Pulcini

CHAPTER CONTENTS

Advanced practice nursing has evolved in the international arena over the last half-century. With an initial focus in the United States, advanced practice nurse (APN) roles are now becoming more visible as a response to improving health care for people in all parts of the world. Internationally, health care problems have rapidly evolved from a major focus on deadly diseases, high infant mortality, and maternal morbidity to a new focus on chronic or noncommunicable diseases, an aging population, and lifestyle choices that promote health (Skolnik, 2008). Many areas of the world, such as sub-Saharan Africa, continue to have dire health care problems with communicable diseases and mortality, but managing chronic diseases and promoting healthy lifestyles have eclipsed infectious diseases worldwide as infant and child mortality rates have begun to drop globally (Liu, Johnson, Cousens, et al., 2012; World Health Organization [WHO], 2011). Child mortality has decreased to a point that some of the poorest countries are projected to meet Millennium Development Goal 4 for reducing child mortality (Demombynes & Trommlerova, 2012). Many countries are realizing that their aging population will have very different needs in the future and are gearing up to meet the chronic health care problems that accompany aging. Maternal mortality which was a huge problem in parts of South America and Africa, has begun to resolve itself with a greater emphasis on population control and women's health (Grady, 2010;

Hogan, Foreman, Mohsen, et al., 2010). Nurses have played a key and relatively independent role in providing health care in rural areas, particularly in parts of Africa and Australia, where major physician shortages exist. Increasingly, these nurses are entering programs that educate them for role expansion. As the incidence of chronic diseases increases, nurses and APNs will have an even greater role to play in managing these problems and educating the public on lifestyle issues.

Other issues, such as the global health worker shortage and mass migration of health care workers to more developed countries, are important drivers of continued gaps in care. Along with these shortages are huge inequities of care across the globe, with some urban areas having an acute oversupply of providers and excellent health care facilities and others with desperate inequities and shortages of care. Economic disparities have increased over the last 30 years and this rate has accelerated with the recent worldwide recession, starting in 2008 (Leach-Kemmon, Chou, Schneider, et al., 2012). APN educational programs have also been developing in many areas of the world and, as these programs increase, the nursing workforce will be better prepared to function with advanced nursing knowledge. Recently, the World Health Organization (WHO) (2010) issued an important report underscoring the need to enhance the global nursing and midwifery workforce.

EXEMPLAR 6-1   **Evolution of the Nurse Practitioner Role in the Netherlands***

Lillian Garcia Maas, RN, MS

The first NP program was created in collaboration between the Hanze University of Applied Sciences and Groningen University Hospital in Groningen, the Netherlands. Petrie Roodbol, RN, PhD, developed the first program in 1997, with six students in the inaugural class. The NP role originated because of the lack of medical specialists in the hospitals; as a result, so-called supernurses, initially called NPs and now called nurse specialists, were trained to take over medical tasks. This need for medically oriented nurses led to the development of a master's program for NPs, which was the first master's degree for clinically focused nursing at a university of applied sciences. Prior to this graduate degree, a Master of Science degree was available for nursing researchers. Keeping nurses at the bedside is the focus of the master's in advanced nursing practice programs at universities of applied sciences in the Netherlands. Since 1997, NP education has expanded to a total of nine universities of applied sciences across the Netherlands. The Dutch Minister of Health designates and subsidizes approximately 300 NP student placements per year; the trend is to increase the number of NP students in the near future. The full-time Master's in Advanced Nursing Practice (MANP) program is a 2-year work study program. The students work 3 or 4 days in their clinical work setting while attending class one day per week. The students are paid as NPs in training during the program. The MANP faculty works closely with the medical and nursing preceptors to ensure that the competencies are being met within their clinical practice. The final project in the MANP is completion of a master's thesis on a clinical topic. The focus of NP education is to bridge care and cure while providing holistic healthcare.

The roles of the Dutch NP are based on the CanMEDS model for medical specialist, which is based on a medical model developed by the Royal College of Physicians and Surgeons of Canada (2011). This is the current model for medical education in the Netherlands and has been translated to advanced nursing practice. The roles of the model are further adapted to meet the competencies of advanced nursing practice. The core role of advanced practice nurses is the clinical expert. The six complementary roles to support the clinical expert are as follows: (1) professional; (2) communicator; (3) collaborator; (4) manager; (5) health advocate; and (6) scholar. These roles have been adapted to advanced practice nursing competencies.

NP specialty practices include the following:
1. Preventive care (e.g., pediatric screening clinics, travel health, family care)
2. Acute care (e.g., prehospital, emergency room)
3. Intensive care (e.g., transplantation, cardiology)
4. Chronic care (e.g., nursing homes, rehabilitation facilities)
5. Mental health care (e.g., health care clinics, hospitals)

NP students must meet the competencies of their specific practice focus to graduate and legally practice in their role. Following successful completion of the required competencies from an accredited MANP program, the students can register to practice as a nurse specialist (Verpleegkundig Specialisten Register, 2012). The title of NP–nurse specialist is legally protected and recognized. To maintain their license, NPs–nurse specialists are required to become recertified every 5 years by meeting a set of requirements, such as the number of clinical hours at the bedside and certified continuing education courses. NPs–nurse specialists in the Netherlands are legally able to diagnose autonomously, perform a set of delegated medical procedures, and prescribe within their specialty domain.

As of January 2012, there were 1373 registered NPs–nurse specialists. The following are the totals of registered NPs in the five specialties (Verpleegkundig Specialisten Register, 2012): preventive care, 34; acute care, 80; intensive care, 691; chronic care, 271; and mental health care, 297.

Trends in Education: Internationalization of the Nurse Practitioner Curriculum

An international experience has become increasingly common for many MANP programs in the Netherlands. Because of the limited number of NP role models, many MANP programs have developed international experiences in the United States. The NP role originated in the United States, so many students are interested in spending time with their American counterparts. The international experience is used as an educational tool to develop the role further by benchmarking one's own health care and nursing system and exchanging ideas with her or his international NP colleagues, an idea that can be a model for student experiences (Maas, 2011).

One unique example of organizing short-term international group immersion trips to the United States is the Rotterdam University (RU) of Applied Sciences. RU requires an international experience prior to graduation

---

EXEMPLAR 6-1   **Evolution of the Nurse Practitioner Role in the Netherlands—*cont'd***

and is the first of its type in Europe. In addition, internationalization is emphasized in the curriculum to create borderless NPs who are open to other philosophies, cultures, and possibilities (Maas & ter Maten, 2009). The global village is at our doorstep, and RU wants to support its students in looking across borders for solutions and opportunities.

As of March 2012, 161 NP–nurse specialist students have been to the United States and participated in clinical observations. The international experience allows students to witness well-established NP environments. Seeing the NP role accepted has empowered Dutch NP–nurse specialist students to create a vision for themselves and lays the foundation for role development. The challenge of distinguishing advanced nursing practice as an autonomous level of practice becomes clearer (ter Maten & Maas, 2009). The international experience fosters a new sense of nursing pride for the students. For many years, RU has collaborated with the NP program at Texas Woman's University. Eight weeks prior to the international experience, the NP–nurse specialist students work on collaborative keypal assignments with their U.S. counterparts. The keypal exchange is an effective acculturation tool for an international experience (Maas, 2009). The assignment consists of seven weekly topics of health care, nursing system, and professional issues. In addition, the students work on joint clinical case studies. When the Dutch and U.S. students meet, they are able to meet their keypal and discuss the differences and similarities of their clinical case studies and health care and nursing systems. Ultimately, an international experience can instill new vision and confidence to help support leadership skills for future Dutch NPs–nurse specialists.

*The author thanks Lillian Garcia Maas, RN, MS, International Coordinator and Faculty Member, Institute of Healthcare, Rotterdam University of Applied Sciences, Rotterdam, The Netherlands, for authoring this exemplar.

TABLE 6-1 Specialties (Types) of NPs and APNs*

Specialty	Percent of Countries
Community health	76
Mental health	76
Hospital, acute care	71
Specialty	
Disease-specific	67
Age- or population-specific	57
FNP	52
GNP	62
PNP	71
ANP	62
Women's health, midwifery	71
Other	38

*Survey of NPs and APNs educated in 21 countries.
ANP, Adult nurse practitioner; *FNP,* family nurse practitioner; *GNP,* geriatric nurse practitioner; *PNP,* pediatric nurse practitioner.
Adapted from Pulcini, J., Jelic, M., Gul, R., & Loke, A.Y. (2010). An international survey on advanced practice nursing education, practice and regulation. *Journal of Nursing Scholarship, 42,* 31–39.

TABLE 6-2 Most Common Types of Positions Held by NPs and APNs*

Specialty	Percent of Countries
Hospital	96
Hospital-based clinic	80
Community-based clinic	80
Mental health	80
Specialty practice (disease-based)	76
Public health or Ministry of Health agency	72
Faculty position	68
Administration	64
Research	52
Home health care facility	52
Independent nursing practice	44
Long-term care facility	44
School health	44
Occupational health	40
Physician's office	40
Other	12

*Survey of NPs and APNs in 25 countries.
Adapted from Pulcini, J., Jelic, M., Gul, R. & Loke, A.Y. (2010). An international survey on advanced practice nursing education, practice and regulation. *Journal of Nursing Scholarship, 42,* 31–39.

The purpose of this chapter is to provide an overview of international developments related to advanced practice nursing. A key premise is that APNs are part of the solution to global health care problems and, if used appropriately, can partner with other health care providers to improve global health.

Definitions

There are several definitions of advanced practice nursing. The definition used in this text (see Chapter 3) states that "Advanced practice nursing is the patient-focused application of an expanded range of competencies to improve health outcomes for patients and populations within a specialized clinical area of the larger discipline of nursing" (see p. 71). Key elements of the definition are required graduate education and APN certification and the identification of seven core competencies, which distinguish APN-level practice regardless of role. The four specific APN roles used in this book are those used in the United States—nurse practitioner (NP), certified nurse midwife (CNM), certified registered nurse anesthetist (CRNA), and clinical nurse specialist (CNS). These different roles, as they are being developed in a global context, will be discussed later in the chapter.

The International Council of Nurses (ICN)–International Nurse Practitioner/Advanced Practice Nursing Network (INP/APNN) definition states that "A nurse practitioner/advanced practice nurse is a registered nurse who has acquired the expert knowledge base, complex decision-making skills and clinical competencies for expanded practice, the characteristics of which are shaped by the context and/or country in which s/he is credentialed to practice. A master's degree is recommended for entry level" (ICN–INP/APNN, 2012). Although some notable similarities exist among definitions, particularly in acknowledging competencies, expanded practice, and recommending graduate education, the ICN definition is general and recognizes that the terms *nurse practitioner* and *advanced practice nurse* are used interchangeably in some parts of the world. This definition incorporates nurse practitioner and advanced practice nurse into one definition to reflect a broad interpretation of APN roles as they are applied in different countries. This definition advances educational expectations by recommending a master's level education, an important milestone for achieving advanced-level practice.

International Evolution of the Advanced Practice Nurse

When looking at the four APN roles from an international perspective, it is apparent that each of the roles is evolving with country- or region-specific differences. More time is needed to move to the standardization of roles, titles, and responsibilities for the various APN roles internationally, but this work is clearly beginning with a focus on competencies and scope of practice rather than on specific titles (ICN, 2009; ICN–INP/APNN, 2012). All these roles are discussed in detail in other chapters; this section will emphasize the international evolution of APNs.

Nurse Practitioner

The NP had its origins in the United States and has had more than 45 years to develop as a primary care specialty, with additional foci on specialty care and acute care. In other countries, such as the United Kingdom, the NP role is at best 20 years old and is still developing, having evolved from routine well or primary care to the management of more complex specialty conditions in the context of an interdisciplinary team (Sibbald, Laurant, & Reeves, 2006).

The United States and United Kingdom often serve as models for the evolution of the NP role. In Canada, Australia, and New Zealand, the use of a specific nursing title is restricted to those who have met certain requirements to practice. Also, in these countries, national standards for the regulation of and education for the role are becoming well developed and NP prescribing is regulated (Canadian Nurses Association [CNA], 2008; Nursing and Midwifery Board of Australia, 2011; Nurse Practitioner Council of New Zealand, 2012). Although there are also NPs in England, both in primary care and specialty care, variability exists as to the level of education and prescribing abilities; nurses in general who have specific education can prescribe drugs from the British formulary (Kroezen, van Dijk, Groenewegen, & Francke, 2011). To add to the variability, some countries do not use the term *nurse practitioner*. In the Netherlands, the term *nurse specialist* has recently been adopted, replacing the NP title with five recognized specialties—intensive care, acute care, chronic care, mental health care, and preventive care (Frauenfelder, 2012; see Exemplar 6-1). In other countries such as in Singapore, the term *advanced practice nurse* is used instead of NP and is generally preferred. In Singapore, APNs initially function in hospital settings and some outpatient facilities or polyclinics in the community (Mei, 2012; Schober, 2012; see Exemplar 6-2).

The survey by Pulcini and colleagues (2010) also identified the most common types of NP-APN specialties. This survey used the term *NP-APN* but was intended to survey NP roles, listed in Table 6-1. Table 6-2 indicates the most common types of positions held by NP-APNs from the survey.

⊙ EXEMPLAR 6-2   **Advanced Practice Nursing Development in Singapore***

Madrean Schober, RN, ANP, MN, FAANP

Formal and informal discussions among nursing leaders and key decision makers have provided the conceptual beginnings for advanced nursing roles in Singapore. In 1997, a national Nursing Task Force recommended implementation of a nurse clinician role to keep highly skilled nurses in clinical practice (Lim, 2005). A hybrid model based on the clinical nurse specialist and NP roles in the United States provides the foundation for the current Singaporean APN role (Kannusamy, 2006). The Singapore city-state of 5.5 million people has steadily established the APN role in Asia. The initial academic program was introduced at the National University of Singapore (NUS) in January 2003, under the auspices of the Yong Loo Lin School of Medicine. The program is now managed solely under the direction of the Head of Department for the Alice Lee Centre of Nursing Studies. The Head of Department confers with the Dean of School of the Medicine when there are major changes, such as the addition of a new specialty to the program.

The use of the title *advanced practice nurse* is protected under the Amendment to the Singapore Nurses' and Midwives' Act, passed in 2005 (Nurses and Midwives Act, amended by Act 15 of 2005). These regulations include a role definition, scope of practice, and competencies that delineate the role. From concept to current development, the Ministry of Health (MOH) has been pivotal to the feasibility and sustainability of the APN initiative. Unlike the United States, where candidates for education programs are often self-funded and potential students choose their university or program, all student fees are fully funded by the Singapore MOH and an employer (hospital, polyclinic, or other health care institution) selects the potential candidate from the current nursing staff. In addition, the employing institution pays the full salary during the period that the individual is a student and requires the nurse to agree to fulfill a bonding period for 2 to 3 years following graduation and successful completion of their internship. Upon successful completion of the Master of Nursing (MN) at the National University of Singapore, the aspiring APN must complete a minimum of a one-year internship in order to qualify for certification, registration and licensure as an APN.

Impetus for Role Development

Historically, Singapore had been losing highly skilled nurses to management and education career tracks for promotion and remuneration. Key decision makers envisioned that the creation of a clinical career path would retain nurses in clinical practice (Ang, 2002). The APN initiative is still in its infancy; therefore, it is too early to determine the success of this strategy. However, since the entrance of the first students into the Master's in Nursing program in 2003, the number of APN students has grown from 15 in the initial cohort to annual intakes of 20 to 25. As of July 2012, 138 students have completed the APN program. The program began as an 18-month master's program that has now expanded to a 24-month, 2-year master's.

Impetus for the APN role in Singapore has been attributed to a plea by nursing and nurse leaders for clinical career advancement, along with a view that nurses with advanced skills and knowledge could fill gaps and add quality to the provision of health care services. The Singapore national health care agenda has developed an increased focus on chronic illness and mental health needs, especially as they relate to the aging population. In addition, the MOH has envisioned that more services should be accessible in the community. The anticipation of increased demands on health care systems in the country and a shortage of physicians in certain specialties has provided additional momentum for APNs in various settings. Presently, most APNs are hospital-based, in settings ranging from intensive care units, heart failure clinics, preoperative services, and mental health specialties. In 2012, a decision was made to include pediatrics in the academic curriculum.

As is often the case when launching a new idea, progress has been turbulent at times, with some graduates of the APN program choosing not to complete the compulsory internship. Further attrition is associated with the inability of APN interns to complete the certification process successfully. The path to successful role implementation has also been fraught with confusion over what the APN can do that is different from the generalist nurse or nurse clinicians who already hold positions of advanced responsibility in Singapore health care systems. Nurse clinicians are educated in 8-month advanced diploma programs and function in the capacity of care managers in health care settings throughout Singapore. Physicians and nurse managers continue to be puzzled over the inclusion of APNs in the health care workforce, even though the support for this new nursing role is positive.

Future Directions

To make nursing attractive and competitive as a professional option, a massive infusion of funds for

EXEMPLAR 6-2   **Advanced Practice Nursing Development in Singapore—*cont'd***

scholarships is available in Singapore for those leaving secondary education or wishing to make a career switch into nursing. This financial support extends to APN education, with growth fueled by an MOH mandate to have 200 APNs in place, practicing in a clinical role in Singapore by 2015. As of April 2012, there were 78 certified APNs and 15 APN interns preparing for the certification process (Singapore Nursing Board, 2012). Although the numbers seem small compared with the APNs in the United States and other countries with a longer history of NP or APN roles, the challenges in role

implementation are significant in a context in which the nursing culture is barely emerging from an apprenticeship model of training nurses.

The implementation of APN roles is having a transformative effect on the health care network in Singapore. Government officials, nursing leaders, physicians, and managers share a sense of pride in the anticipated increased status and professional development that has accompanied academic education and advanced nursing roles, even as the country faces the challenges that occur with such a significant change.

*The author thanks Madrean Schober, RN, ANP, MSN, FAANP, Senior Visiting Fellow, Alice Lee Centre for Nursing Studies, National University of Singapore, for authoring this exemplar.

Practice Settings

In the survey by Pulcini and colleagues (2010), a large proportion of NPs and APNs worked in hospitals, community or hospital-based clinics, and mental health. A high proportion of the APNs worked in specialty practices. Also, mental health is emerging as an important area for APN practice (Maas, Ezeobele, & Tettero, 2012; see Exemplar 6-1). In New Zealand, for example, mental health NPs are recognized formally and have prescribing privileges (Lewis, 2012). In Singapore, mental health APNs work with patients with psychosis (Chng, 2012). This shows the variety of roles and range of practice reported and may suggest differing interpretations of how roles are being implemented. Further survey work is needed to track the changes over time.

Nurse Midwifery

Nurse midwifery (CNM in the United States) has had a different history and evolved initially in many countries, such as the United Kingdom, as a basic competency within initial nurse education or as a postgraduate course (Barton, 1998). The more specialized role of the nurse midwife has prevailed, and most midwifery education is now provided in specialized courses or university programs. Some of these changes may have occurred as a result of specialization within the medical profession, as well as with changes in nursing. Complicating the CNM role is the fact that some midwives are not nurses; this is a common development, especially in low-resource countries in which skilled birth attendants have improved maternal and infant mortality rates (WHO, 2010). Differing types and levels of CNM education currently exist internationally and are evolving, along with the other APN roles (McAuliffe, 2012). However, the role is still in great demand and evidence has shown that nurse midwives make a great

difference in maternal-infant outcomes, especially in resource-poor settings (WHO, 2010).

Nurse Anesthetist

The CRNA role is common in the United States and has evolved in other countries, such as France. A survey by the International Congress of Nurse Anesthetists has found that nurse anesthetists are common internationally. Phase I of the survey found that in 107 countries (59% of all WHO member states), nurses administer anesthesia; nine countries reported that nurses assist in anesthesia administration. It is not clear what "assist in" anesthesia is meant in this survey. In a second phase of the study, nurse anesthetists were reported to provide as much as 77% of the anesthesia in urban areas and 75% of anesthetics in rural areas of their countries (International Federation of Nurse Anesthetists [IFNA], 2012; McAuliffe, 2012). IFNA has stated that that nurse anesthetists are participating in more than 80% of all anesthesia provided worldwide and are the sole providers in 60% of the cases. Thus, this role is prevalent globally and is an area of nursing practice that continues to expand, especially with improved health care technologies and more surgeries being performed.

Clinical Nurse Specialist

The CNS had its origins in the United States in hospital settings. Dating back to the 1950s, when the first clinically oriented master's level nursing programs were instituted in the United States (see Chapter 1), this role predates that of the NP. Other countries such as Canada also developed the role of CNS as these programs began to be offered at the master's level (CNA, 2008). Initially, the distinction between the NP and the CNS centered around the following:

1. Primary care practice versus hospital practice
2. Direct care versus indirect care
3. Generalist practice in primary care versus specialty practice based on disease conditions or systems

The CNS role initially was carried out in hospital settings, in psychiatry and oncology nursing, and the NP role first occurred in primary care settings (Hanson & Hamric, 2003; Maas, Ezeobele, & Tettero, 2012; Reasor & Farrell, 2005). The CNS role was more focused on indirect care, such as consultation, leadership, staff education, and management of complex patients with specific diagnoses (e.g., cardiac or respiratory disease, cancer), whereas the NP role had more of a direct care focus. As acute care nurse practitioners (ACNPs) became more common in the United States, some confusion resulted in distinguishing these two roles. This pattern is seen in the international context and in the example of the APN in Singapore. In many countries, most notably in Asia, advanced practice started in the hospital setting with specialized foci such as respiratory or cardiac care, and was not as successful in primary care settings (Schober, 2012). In these countries, lack of clarity around terminology has been common—that is, whether hospital-based APNs function as NPs or as CNSs.

Advanced Practice Nurse Issues Worldwide

When examining the evolution of APN roles internationally, some similar themes emerge, which represent evolutionary issues common to all APNs. These will change as APN roles are incorporated into the mainstream. This evolution may reflect the growth of nursing knowledge as well as the depth and complexity of specialty practice. Great differences between regions, and even in countries within regions or continents, in the level of APN practice are seen in educational preparation and regulatory issues (Schober & Affara, 2006; Sheer & Wong, 2008). The speed of progress is highly variable because of economic, social, or political issues in the country or in the strength of leadership and influence that nurses exhibit in the health care system over time. Some universal APN issues being played out to various degrees worldwide are presented here.

Titling

For the NP and CNS, titling issues have and will continue to have a rather significant effect on the evolution of APN roles because they have yet to be clarified and standardized internationally. In an international survey of INP and APNN members in 32 countries, Pulcini and associates (2010) found at least 14 titles for NP and APN roles (Table 6-3). Language clearly differed from country to country

TABLE 6-3 Titles for Advanced Practice Nurses

Title Given as NP or APN Equivalent*	Frequency (%)
Nurse practitioner	38 (44)
Advanced practice nurse	15 (17)
Advanced nurse practitioner	9 (10)
Clinical nurse specialist	7 (8)
Nurse specialist	4 (4)
Professional nurse	2 (2)
Expert nurse	1 (1)
Certified registered nurse practitioner	1 (1)
Chief professional nurse with postbasic training in primary health care	1 (1)
Nurse consultant	1 (1)
Specialist nurse practitioner	1 (1)
Primary health care nurse	1 (1)
Advanced nurse in a specialty	1 (1)
Staff nurse, registered nurse, basic nurse	4 (5)

*86 respondents.

Adapted from Pulcini, J, Jelic, M., Gul, R. Loke, A.Y. (2010). An international survey on Advanced Practice Nursing education, practice and regulation. *Journal of Nursing Scholarship*, 42, 31–39.

and was inconsistent at best, even within a country. Such titling difficulties can lead to role confusion, not only among the nurses but also among patients and other professions. A survey by Rieck-Buckley and Heale (2012) found that 16 of the 36 countries responding had the NP title, 12 used APN, 18 had the CNS title, and 15 used nurse specialist. The functions performed by nurses considered to be APNs in one country may be different from the practices in another. Differences sometimes have to do with country-level preferences and political factors, having little to do with professional standards (Schober, 2012).

Power Differential Between Nursing and Medicine

One common issue relates to the power base of the APN in relation to the physician. Nurses in different parts of the world possess different levels of power, authority, and influence. Usually, nurses have less authority than physicians, but may be important in influencing change through their positive association with the patient. In most parts of the world, nursing is considered to be a female profession, but in some countries, such as Saudi Arabia, Italy, Israel, and Kenya, the percentage of male nurses is above 20%. In other areas, such as India and

Spain, this percentage is also rising because of higher wages and subsequent status (Regan, 2012). Historically, in the United States, the fact that nursing was a female profession often left it without the same authority and power as physicians, who tended to be male (Ashley, 1976).

The power differential between nurses and physicians continues to be seen internationally, especially when nursing is considered to be a low-status, low-wage profession. In many areas of the world, such as South and Central America and Pakistan, physicians have such high status that women who would be well-qualified nurses tend to gravitate into medicine, leaving a major shortage of qualified nurses (Fooladi, 2008; Siantz & Malvarez, 2008). This low status and lack of high-quality formal education can also translate into a negative public image of the nurse, who can be seen as poorly prepared and not having professional status. This problem reinforces itself and ultimately can lead to a self-fulfilling prophesy, in which less is expected of nurses and thus their performance remains at a relatively low level. Often, these nurses are highly motivated to care for sick people and accept low status and wages. The public image of the nurse is also often damaged by stereotypical images of the handmaiden and the impression that nurses are assistants to physicians. For example, in China, nursing is considered a subdiscipline of medicine and is not considered to be equal to other health care disciplines (Zou, Li, & Arthur, 2012). In this case, the Ministry of Health in China has formulated the Nursing Development Plan to establish and develop nurse specialist roles in China and other parts of Asia, and hopefully APN roles as well. Many countries have a long way to go to raise nursing's (and women's) status so that a natural progression to APN development can occur. In China and many other Asian countries, nursing education is taking the lead by developing strong nursing research programs to support the advancement of the field.

Lack of Physician Support for Advanced Practice Nurse Roles

Another common and related issue is that organized medical groups often fail to support APN roles, even though many individual physicians support their advancement. In the 32-nation study by Pulcini and coworkers (2010), when asked to list opponents to the NP role, 83% of respondents said that organized medical groups opposed their role, whereas 67% said that individual physicians opposed the role. Interestingly, in the more recent international survey by Rieck-Buckley and Heale (2012), the majority of respondents said that they did not experience opposition from other health care providers.

Of those respondents who did experience opposition, opposition from physicians was usually cited. To implement any advanced practice role, physician support is often essential and is granted, at least initially. This support can be withdrawn if the APN is seen as a threat to physician practice. Clearly, in countries in which nursing does not enjoy a high status, this opposition can be a major barrier to implementation of the roles.

Level of Educational Preparation

A key component in the development of APN roles in any country is the level of educational preparation for nursing and advanced practice, especially because graduate-level education is becoming the international standard for APN education. In some areas or countries, such as Africa, basic nursing is just beginning to be provided in universities and graduate education is rare. In other areas, such as Asia, graduate education is quickly advancing and becoming more prevalent for APN education. In the survey by Pulcini and others (2010), the master's degree was the most prevalent credential granted, by 50% of the respondents, the advanced diploma, which is a post–registered nurse (RN) program, at 20%, the bachelor's degree, at 15%, and the certificate at 15%. The 2012 study similarly reported that about 50% of the countries surveyed had the master's degree as the most prevalent credential (Rieck-Buckley & Heale, 2012).

Education for APNs has been evolving rapidly in the United States with the Doctor of Nursing Practice (DNP) degree rapidly increasing. The American Association of Colleges of Nursing (AACN; 2012) stated that the number of schools offering the DNP increased from 20 programs in 2006 to 184 programs in 2011, with another 101 programs in the planning stages. According to the International Network for Doctoral Education in Nursing (INDEN), internationally, doctorate-level programs have emerged primarily in parts of Asia, Europe, and the United Kingdom but other areas still must send their nurses abroad for doctoral education or import nurses with this level of education (INDEN, 2012; Zou, Li, & Arthur 2012). This will change in the future, especially in areas in which nursing education is well established in universities. More data are needed on the current status of APN education internationally because it is still variable across the globe.

Valuing Clinical Practice Expertise

In addition to developing formal educational pathways, an important area for the future of APN education is the degree to which clinical practice is valued and encouraged, not only at the practice level but also in educational institutions in which APNs are being educated. As nursing evolves to higher levels of education, one message is clear—information must emanate from clinical practice, and the best evidence available must guide practice. In some areas, such as parts of Asia, it is still common to sideline practice, especially faculty practice, or to move expert nurses into career ladders or pathways toward management positions rather than to see practice as a long-term goal (Chiang-Hanisko, Ross, Boonyanurak, et al., 2008). The career ladder for APNs is not necessarily to move to administrative positions or even to faculty positions but to become clinical experts who remain engaged in direct practice. If nurses who are clinical experts are rewarded with higher salaries, one may assume that their status will also rise; in the end, what is valued most highly is most highly compensated.

Infusing Evidence into Role Development

Canada is an example of a country that has made significant progress in the last decade in the evolution of the NP and CNS roles but which has had setbacks and uneven growth (CNA, 2008). The CNS role in Canada was initiated in the 1960s and evolved from needs emanating from the complexity of hospital care. The NP role arose from the need for services in underserved and rural areas of Canada (Bryant-Lukosius, Carter, Kilpatrick, et al., 2010; Sangster-Gormley, 2012). Although initiated in 1970s, the NP role was stifled because of a perceived oversupply of physicians by the 1990s. The Canadian NP initiative began in 2004, with a strong push by Canadian nurses to reinitiate the role. Their success is evident in the increasing numbers of NPs practicing in Canada today (Bryant-Lukosius et al., 2010; CNA, 2008; DiCenso & Bryant-Lukosius, 2010).

Their method of reintroducing the role was greatly enhanced by the work of Bryant-Lukosius and DiCenso (2004), who introduced the PEPPA framework (participatory, evidence-based, patient-focused process for advanced practice nursing role development, implementation, and evaluation); this sets forth nine steps to determine whether a particular advanced practice role is needed in an area or country (see Chapter 4 for a diagram of the framework [Fig. 4-2]). The evidence proposed by this framework is a key component for the successful introduction of any new role into a country. Canada has made great strides to make regulatory and educational requirements for APNs more uniform across the different Canadian provinces (CNA, 2008; DiCenso & Bryant-Lukosius, 2010). Thus, APN roles have to fit into the system in which they are introduced and make sense to the policy and regulatory bodies that govern these roles.

Cultural Norms

Other issues that lead to the differences in APN roles seen internationally are language differences and cultural expectations and norms. Most countries with successful APN roles are English-speaking or are bilingual. Although not equitable, the most common language for nursing and medical education is English, so great advantage is gained thru Internet-based sources written in English, as well as direct education and consultation from experts. Throughout most of Europe, Asia, and Africa, for example, English is still one of the most common second languages. Spanish-speaking countries in South and Central America can be disadvantaged simply by being outside of this common language.

Cultural issues are complex and have to do with mores and norms surrounding health and illness, who can provide care, and issues related to the role of women (see earlier). Expectations of what nurses can accomplish, and culture- and gender-based power relationships, are also related to status and professional advancement. Patient expectations also come into play here and cultural norms regarding the use of ethnic healers, who for centuries have provided care in remote areas such as those in China and Australia (Aitken-Sallows, 2012; Jackson Allen, 2012). APNs recognize these cultural factors and see patients more holistically, embracing cultural diversity and teaching students to embrace these concepts (Jackson Allen, 2012).

Health Care Delivery System Values

Health care financing systems create powerful incentives, not only for what care is delivered but also who delivers the care. For example, in Germany, strong incentives exist for physician-delivered care through reimbursement systems that reward physicians to provide chronic care that in other countries would be provided by nurses (Schoen, Osborn, Huynh, et al., 2006). Conflicts can be created if APNs are viewed as taking money out of the pockets of more powerful professionals. Financial incentives are strong drivers for care providers as seen in the United States, with physicians as the major recipients of financing for many health care services. If APN services are not covered and not paid for, they will not be maximally used.

The depth and breadth of the health care system in a particular country is another factor in the development of advanced practice. For example, in poorer countries with few resources, such as Haiti, the health care system may be focused on delivering primary care, with weak and underfunded acute care services (Doctors Without Borders, 2011). Others, such as the United Kingdom, have a strong history of public health and community care and of including nurses at the community level, as well as strong acute care systems. Another health care system difference is the percentage of specialists versus primary care providers. In the United States, this ratio has been about 30% primary care providers and 70% specialists, but in most countries the mix is more equal, 50% and 50%. In contrast to the physician ratio, in the United States, at least 65% of NPs work in primary care practices and the rest are in specialty practice or in an acute care facility (AACN, 2012). If primary care is a focus for a country, there is a better chance that primary care NPs will be used, all else being equal. If the focus is on inpatient care, this may lead to more APNs focused on hospital-based care.

Advanced Practice Nurse Payment

Another important issue involves reimbursement structures that dictate how care is paid for and who gets paid. This is relevant for all APNs but one can see the direct consequences of these policies on CNMs and CRNAs, whose practices can be limited through adverse regulatory and reimbursement strategies. In privatized systems, such as in the United States, reimbursement policies have strongly influenced which APNs can practice. In countries with universal government-sponsored health care, practice and reimbursement are regulated by government policies and will not vary as much as in privatized systems. However, many countries have a combination of fee-for-service and government-sponsored care (Kroezen, van Dijk, Groenewegen, & Francke, 2011). The literature is sparse on reimbursement for APNs outside of the United States; more is needed to clarify the important issues related to this topic and to delineate how reimbursement is related to regulation (Schoen et al., 2006).

Advanced Practice Nurse Regulations and Standards

In the United States, state policy is as important as federal policy in reimbursing and regulating APNs, a key issue in the ability for APNs to practice optimally. Each of the 50 states has the right to create its own specific regulations for APNs, so pressure in this system is often applied through influencing state regulatory boards; there is no central federal oversight of APN practice. The United States has a long way to go to standardize APN practice, but efforts have begun.

National standards are often needed to ensure that roles are relatively uniform within and across countries so that consumers can have clear expectations on scope of practice and regulation for APNs. Attempts over the past 10 years to standardize how U.S. APNs are educated and regulated have culminated in the Consensus Model, or the LACE (licensing, accreditation, certification and educational) model, which sets standards for master's level advanced practice registered nurse (APRN) titling and regulation and for the designation of subspecialty areas (APRN Consensus Work Group et al., 2008). This work represents collaboration among educators, certifiers, accreditors, and boards of nursing who license APRNs (see Chapter 21).

In Canada, efforts have been made to have a coordinated national approach to APN regulation (CNA, 2008, DiCenso & Bryant-Lukosius, 2010), although currently some distinctions still occur at the provincial level. This work is essential as APN roles become more mainstream so that consumers and policy makers understand that a uniform set of regulations and standards is in place, such as in Canada and Australia. The regulatory environment can hold back progress if nurses in general, and APNs in particular, do not have clear and broad enough laws and regulations governing practice to allow for change and advancement of the profession. Title protection is an important regulatory term, and the goal would be to ensure that those who use a particular title are using that title uniformly and are duly authorized through licensure to ensure that title or designation.

High-Quality, Interdisciplinary, Advanced Practice Nurse Education

If APN roles are to develop and flourish, education that leads to an understanding of interdisciplinary practice is essential. Many examples exist in the United States, but more work is needed to integrate interprofessional concepts into education. The APN role will only succeed when it is integrated into the mainstream of education in any country. Many factors will determine whether that education is accepted and flourishes and becomes the mainstream of nursing education in a country, or if it fails to progress. A key component of this education is faculty who are well trained and who continue to practice in an APN role. The clash of the demands of academia and the needs of students in clinically based education programs can lead to an undervaluing of faculty practice, a concept that is at the foundation of the success of APN roles in the United States. Hawkins and colleagues (2012) have discussed the concept of cognitive dissonance, with the competing demands for faculty to engage in practice, teaching, research, and service.

This text fully recognizes that APN roles and educational models are evolving. When trying to establish APN programs or educational policy in a particular country or area, many factors should come into consideration and serve as long term goals, including the following:

1. Standardized educational level—an agreed on level or goal for preparation for each role. Confusion in this area can delay implementation of APN education at the graduate level. Some countries have incorporated certificate or advanced diploma programs that meet some of the requirements for a solid educational program but that confuse nurses and the public as to which level is required for entry into the particular APN role.

2. APN program outcomes and competencies. Educational outcomes and requisite APN competencies can be adapted from internationally recognized groups that govern APN education, such as the. National Organization of Nurse Practitioner Faculties (NONPF) in the United States, which develops and updates curricular and outcome competencies for NP education, or the International Confederation of Midwives (ICM), which produces modules for education of nurse midwives. The International Federation of Nurse Anesthetists (IFNA) is an organization that represents nurse anesthetists worldwide and promotes quality educational standards and practices. The National Association for Clinical Nurse Specialists (NACNS) serves as the U.S. authority on CNS education and develops educational standards for the education of CNSs.

3. Interprofessional competency. The use of interprofessional concepts in APN education serves to stimulate change in practice environments when disciplines are taught and are in practice together (O'Brien, Martin, & Meyer, 2009; Schoen et al., 2006). One example is the Interprofessional Education for Collaborative, Patient-Centered Practice (IECPCP) initiative in Canada, which has been successful in promoting these concepts (Canadian Interprofessional Health Collaborative [CNPI], 2012).

4. Continued APN competency. Another key issue to consider is provision for continued competency once a role has been established through mechanisms such as certification, recertification, licensure, professional portfolios, and/or continuing education programs. Now that APN roles are becoming well established, Canada and England are examples of countries considering processes for ensuring continued competency in addition to the current process of using professional portfolios for continued licensure as a nurse (CNPI, 2006; Inman, Shortland, & East, 2012).

Looking to the Future: What Do We Have To Learn From Each Other?

APN practices will inevitably have a major impact on the world's health. A critical issue here will be the evaluation of outcomes of APN practice as the field moves forward. The question is determining how soon this will occur. WHO (2010) has recognized nursing's potential contribution to the world's health care needs. Models that work in one region or country may not work in others, but APN leaders can learn from each other as each country develops APN practices and related roles. Some principles to be considered when working toward continued international development of advanced practice nursing are the following:

- Although each APN role has unique features in its contribution and application in a country or area, common or similar titling would create more clarity for advancing these roles.
- Cultural differences must be honored and celebrated by all APNs as they create the future.
- The goal of expanding advanced practice nursing worldwide is to improve health outcomes for the neediest populations, and for more affluent ones, as health care needs change and evolve.
- Nurses have special expertise in coordinating care, managing transitions across settings, and focusing on maintaining or improving health status.
- An important goal for APNs internationally is to aim for consistent competencies, common definitions, regulatory clarity, and educational standards so that nurses can move freely around the world and use their knowledge and skills without undue barriers (Lowe, Plummer, O'Brien, & Boyd, 2011).

Nurses are increasingly being seen as part of the solution to many of the world's most significant health care problems. The future is bright for APNs, whose expertise and public image are improving at a rapid rate. Currently, APNs comprise a minority of nurses worldwide but these numbers are expected to grow as the complex needs of patients are met and consumers seek out APN services (Schober, 2012). Much work is needed to achieve the goal of creating a common global understanding of APN roles. If advanced practice nursing is to be moved forward, education and cross fertilization with areas outside of one's own country that are implementing innovations are necessary. Progress will be reflected in better health and health care for the diverse populations across the globe.

References

Aitken-Sallows, R. A. (2012). *Nurse practitioners: An innovation in remote, indigenous health care.* Presented at the International Nurse Practitioner/Advanced Practice Nursing Network Conference, London.

American Association of Colleges of Nursing. (2012). New AACN data show an enrollment surge in Baccalaureate and Graduate Programs amid calls for more highly educated nurses (http://www.aacn.nche.edu/news/articles/2012/enrollment-data).

Ang, B. C. (2002). The quest for nursing excellence. *Singapore Medical Journal, 43,* 493–495.

APRN Consensus Work Group and National Council of State Boards of Nursing APRN Advisory Committee. (2008). Consensus model for APRN regulation (www.aacn.nche.edu/education-resources/APRNReport.pdf).

Ashley, J. (1976). *Hospitals, paternalism and the role of the nurse.* New York: Teachers College.

Barton, T. D. (1998). The integration of nursing and midwifery education within higher education: Implications for teachers—a qualitative research study. *Journal of Advanced Nursing, 27,* 1278–1286.

Bryant-Lukosius, D., & DiCenso, A. (2004). A framework for introduction and evaluation of advanced practice nursing roles. *Journal of Advanced Nursing, 48,* 530–540.

Bryant-Lukosius, D., Carter, N., Kilpatrick, K., Martin-Misener, R., Donald, F., Kaasalainen, S., et al. (2010). The clinical nurse specialist role in Canada. *Nursing Leadership, 23,* 140–166.

Canadian Interprofessional Health Collaborative. (2012). Education for collaborative, patient-centered practice (IECPCP). (http://cihc.wikispaces.com/Interprofessional+Education+for+Collaborative,+Patient-Centred+Practice).

Canadian Nurse Practitioner Initiative (CNPI). (2006). Competence assessment framework for nurse practitioners in Canada (http://www2.cna-aiic.ca/CNA/documents/pdf/publications/cnpi/tech-report/section1/07_Report_Tool2.pdf).

Canadian Nurses Association (CNA). (2008). Advanced nursing practice: A national framework. (http://www.srna.org/images/stories/pdfs/nurse_resources/2009_advanced_NP.pdf).

Chiang-Hanisko, L., Ross, R., Boonyanurak, P., Ozawa, M., & Chiang, L. (2008). Pathways to progress in nursing: understanding career patterns in Japan, Taiwan and Thailand (http://www.nursingworld.org/MainMenuCategories/ANAMarketplace/ANAPeriodicals/OJIN/TableofContents/vol132008/No3Sept08/CareerPatternsinJapanTaiwanandThailand.aspx).

Chng, C. (2012). *The impact of an APN-led clinic on patients with psychosis.* Presented at the International Nurse Practitioner/Advanced Practice Nursing Network Conference, London, August 2012.

Demombynes, G., & Trommlerova, S. K. (2012). What has driven the decline of infant mortality in Kenya? (http://econ.worldbank.org/external/default/main?pagePK=64165259&theSitePK=469372&piPp=64165421&menuPK=64166093&entityID=000158349_20120503152728).

DiCenso, A., & Bryant-Lukocious, D. (2010). Clinical nurse specialists and nurse practitioners in Canada: A decision support synthesis (http://www.chsrf.ca).

Doctors without Borders. (2011). Special report: Haiti one year after: Looking ahead (http://www.doctorswithoutborders.org/publications/article.cfm?id=4963&cat=special-report).

Fooladi, M. (2008). Gender influence on nursing education and practice at Aga Khan University School of Nursing in Karachi Pakistan. *Nurse Education in Practice, 8,* 231–238.

Frauenfelder, O. (2012). *Regulation for ANP and nurse prescribing in the Netherlands.* Presented at the International Nurse Practitioner/Advanced Practice Nursing Network Conference, London, August 2012.

Grady, D. (2010). Maternal deaths decline sharply across the globe (http://www.nytimes.com/2010/04/14/health/14births.html?pagewanted=all).

Hanson, C., & Hamric, A. (2003). Reflections on the continuing evolution of advanced practice nursing. *Nursing Outlook, 51,* 203–211.

Hawkins, J., Fontenot, H., & Weiss, J. (2012). Cognitive dissonance experienced by nurse practitioner faculty. *Journal of the American Academy of Nurse Practitioners, 24,* 507–513. doi: 10.1111/j.1745-7599.2012.00726.

Hogan, M., Foreman, K., Mohsen, N., Ahn, S., Wang, M., Makela, S., et al. (2010). Maternal mortality for 181 countries, 1980–2008: A systematic analysis of progress towards Millennium Development Goal 5. *Lancet, 375,* 1609–1623.

Inman, C., Shortland, S., & East, L. (2012). *Demonstrating advanced practice nursing practice: The professional portfolio.* Presented at the International Nurse Practitioner/Advanced Practice Nursing Network Conference, London, August 2012.

International Council of Nurses. (2009). *ICN framework of competencies for the nurse specialist.* Geneva Switzerland: Author.

International Council of Nurses–International Nurse Practitioner/Advanced Practice Nursing Network. (2012). Definition and characteristics of the role (http://icn-apnetwork.org).

International Federation of Nurse Anesthetists (IFNA). (2012). About INFA (http://ifna-int.org/ifna/page.php?16).

International Network for Doctoral Education in Nursing (INDEN). (2012). Directory of international doctoral programs. http://nursing.jhu.edu/academics/programs/doctoral/phd/inden/programs.html

Jackson Allen, P. (2012). *Educating western nurse practitioners in traditional Chinese medicine.* Paper presented at the International Nurse Practitioner/Advanced Practice Nursing Network Conference, London, August 2012.

Kannusamy, P. (2006). A longitudinal study of advanced practice nursing in Singapore. *Critical Care Nursing Clinics of North America, 18,* 545–551.

Kroezen, M. van Dijk, L., Groenewegen, P. P., & Francke, A. (2011). Nurse prescribing of medicines in Western European and Anglo-Saxon countries: A systematic review of the literature (http://www.biomedcentral.com/1472-6963/11/127).

Leach-Kemmon, K., Chou, D., Schneider, M., Tardif, A., Dieleman, J., Brooks, B., et al. (2012). Slowdown of growth of funding to improve health in many developing countries. *Health Affairs, 31,* 228–235. doi: 10.1377/hlthaff.2011.1154.

Lewis, S. (2012). *The mental health nurse practitioner role in rural Queensland, Australia.* Paper presented at the

International Nurse Practitioner/Advanced Practice Nursing Network Conference, London, August 2012.

Lim, D. (2005). Developing professional nursing in Singapore: A case for change. *Singapore Nursing Journal, 32,* 34–47.

Liu, L., Johnson, H. L., Cousens, S., Perin, J., Scott, S., Lawn, J. E., et al. (2012). Global, regional, and national causes of child mortality: an updated systematic analysis for 2010 with time trends since 2000. *Lancet, 379,* 2151–2161.

Lowe, G., Plummer, V., O'Brien, A. P., & Boyd, L. (2011). Time to clarify: The value of advanced practice nursing roles in health care. *Journal of Advanced Nursing, 68,* 677–685. doi: 10.1111/j.1365-2648.2011.05790.x.

Maas, L., Ezeobele, I. E., & Tettero, M. (2012). An American and Dutch partnership for psychiatric mental health advanced nursing practice: Nurturing a relationship across the ocean. *Perspectives in Psychiatric Care, 48,* 165–169. doi: 10.1111/j.1744-6163.2011.00319.x.

Maas, L. G. (2011). Benchmarking one's own healthcare system: professional development through an international experience. *Nurse Education in Practice, 11,* 293–297. doi: 10.1016/j.npr.2011.01.005.

Maas, L. G. (2009). Nursing keypal exchange: An effective acculturation strategy to prepare for an international experience. *International Nursing Review, 56,* 142–144.

Maas, L. G., & ter Maten, A. (2009). The Bologna Agreement and its impact on the Master's In Advanced Nursing (MANP) program at Rotterdam University of Applied Science: Incorporating mandatory internationalization in the curriculum. *International Nursing Review, 56,* 393–395.

McAuliffe, M. (2012). Nurse anesthesia worldwide: Practice, education and regulation (http://ifna-int.org/ifna/e107_files/downloads/Practice.pdf).

Mei, S. L. (2012). *Journey towards certification as an advanced practice nurse (APN) in Singapore.* Paper presented at the International Nurse Practitioner/Advanced Practice Nursing Network Conference, London, August 2012.

Nurse and Midwives ACT. (1999). Amended by Act 15 of 2005 (http://statutes.agc.gov.sg).

Nursing and Midwifery Board of Australia. (2011). Scope of practice of nurse practitioners (http://www.nursingmidwiferyboard.gov.au/documents/default.aspx?record=WD11%2F6875&dbid=AP&chksum=eD0zXENVNtaQrYfktmge%2FA%3D%3D).

Nursing Council of New Zealand. (2012). *Nurse practitioner—scope of practice* (http://www.nursingcouncil.org.nz/index.cfm/1,41,0,0,html/Nurse-Practitioner).

O'Brien, J., Martin, D., Heyworth, J., & Meyer, N. (2009). A phenomenological perspective on advanced practice nurse-collaboration within an interdisciplinary healthcare team. *Journal of the American Academy of Nurse Practitioners, 21,* 444–453.

Pulcini, J., Jelic, M., Gul, R., & Loke, A. Y. (2010). An international survey on advanced practice nursing education, practice and regulation. *Journal of Nursing Scholarship, 42,* 31–39.

Reasor, J., & Farrell, S. (2005). The effectiveness of advanced practice registered nurses as psychotherapists. *Archives of Psychiatric Nursing, 19,* 81–92.

Regan, H. (2012). Male nurses worldwide (http://realmanswork.com/2012/05/05/male-nurses-worldwide).

Rieck-Buckley, C., & Heale, R. (2012). *Regulation of advanced nursing practice roles: A global update.* Presented at the International Nurse Practitioner/Advanced Practice Nursing Network Conference, London, August 2012.

Royal College of Physicians and Surgeons. (2011). The CanMEDS framework (http://www.collaborativecurriculum.ca/en/modules/CanMEDS/CanMEDS-intro-background-01.jsp).

Sangster-Gormley, E. (2012). *Understanding factors that influence nurse practitioner role implementation.* Presented at the International Nurse Practitioner/Advanced Practice Nursing Network Conference, London, August 2012.

Schober, M., & Affara, F. (2006). *Advanced nursing practice.* Geneva Switzerland: International Council of Nurses.

Schober, M. (2012). Globalisation of advanced practice, global vision, global reality. Presented at the International Nurse Practitioner/Advanced Practice Nursing Network Conference, London, August 2012.

Schoen, C., Osborn, R., Huynh, P. T., Doty, M., & Peugh, J., Zapert, K. (2006). On the front lines of care: Primary care doctors' office systems, experiences, and views in seven countries. *Health Affairs (Millwood), 25,* 555–571.

Sheer, B. Wong, F. (2008). The development of advanced nursing practice globally. *Journal of Nursing Scholarship, 40,* 204–211. doi: 10.1111/j.1547-5069.2008.00242.x.

Siantz, S., & Malvarez, S. (2008). Migration of nurses: A Latin American perspective (http://www.nursingworld.org/MainMenuCategories/ANAMarketplace/ANAPeriodicals/OJIN/TableofContents/vol132008/No2May08/LatinAmericanPerspective.html).

Sibbald, B., Laurant, M. G., & Reeves, D. (2006). Advanced nurse roles in UK primary care. *Medical Journal of Australia, 185,* 10–12.

Singapore Nursing Board. (2012). Personal communication.

Skolnik, R. (2008). *Essentials of global health.* Boston: Jones and Bartlett.

Ter Maten, A., & Maas, L. G. (2009). Nurse practitioner leadership development through a short-term international immersion. *International Journal of Nursing Education, 48,* 226–231.

Verpleegkundig Specialisten Register. (2012). (http://www.verpleegkundigspecialismen.nl/Registratiecommissie.aspx).

World Health Organization. (2010). *Strategic directions for strengthening nursing and midwifery services: 2011-2015.* Geneva: WHO.

World Health Organization. (2011). New WHO report: Deaths from non communicable diseases on the rise, with developing world hit hardest (http://www.who.int/mediacentre/news/releases/2011/ncds_20110427/en/index.html).

Zou, H., Li, Z., & Arthur, D. (2012). Graduate nursing education in China. *Nursing Outlook, 60,* 116–120.

Direct Clinical Practice

Mary Fran Tracy

CHAPTER CONTENTS

irect care is the central competency of advanced
practice nursing. This competency informs and
shapes the execution of the other six competencies. Direct
care is essential for a number of reasons. To consult, collaborate, and lead clinical staff and programs effectively,
an advanced practice nurse (APN) must have clinical
credibility. With the deep clinical and systems understanding that APNs possess, they facilitate the care processes that ensure achievement of outcomes for individuals
and groups of patients. Advanced practice occurs within
a health care system that is constantly changing—changing
delivery models, reimbursement structures, regulatory
requirements, population-based management, and even
proposed changes in the basic educational requirements
for advanced practice nurses through the Doctor of
Nursing Practice (DNP) degree. The challenge that many

APNs face is how to maintain the characteristics of care
that have helped patients achieve positive health outcomes
and afforded APN care a unique niche in the health care
marketplace. Characteristics such as the use of a holistic
perspective and formation of therapeutic partnerships
with patients to coproduce individualized health care are
challenged by cost containment strategies that emphasize
standardization of care to achieve population-based
outcome targets. Conversely, characteristics of APN care
such as health promotion, fostering self-care, and patient
education are valued by practices offering care to patients
because they result in an appropriate use of health care
resources and sustain quality. This chapter describes the
direct clinical practice of APNs and helps readers understand how it differs from the practice of experts by experience, describes strategies for balancing direct care with

other competencies, and describes strategies for retaining a direct care focus. The six characteristics of APN practice are identified.

Direct Care Activities

Direct Care and Indirect Care

Direct care is the central APN competency (see Chapter 3). The APN is using advanced clinical judgment, systems thinking, and accountability in providing evidence-based care at a more advanced level than the care provided by the expert registered nurse. The APN is prepared to assist individuals through complex health care situations by the use of education, counseling, and coordination of care (American Association of Colleges of Nursing [AACN], 2006). Although an expert registered nurse may, at times, demonstrate components of care that are at an advanced level, it is care that is gained through experience and is exemplary (not expected) at that level. Essentials I and II of practice doctorate education for APNs delineate that APN-level care is demonstrated through advanced, refined assessment skills and implementation and evaluation of practice interventions based on integrated knowledge from a number of sciences, such as biophysical, psychosocial, behavioral, cultural, economic, and nursing science (AACN, 2006). Graduate-level APN education provides a foundation for the evolution of practice over time as necessitated by health care and patients. This advanced level of practice is an expected competency of all APNs, not an exemplary skill that is intermittently or inconsistently displayed by staff or expert nurses.

For the purposes of this chapter, the terms *direct care* and *direct clinical practice* refer to the activities and functions that APNs perform within the patient-nurse interface. Depending on the focus of an APN's practice, the patient may, and often does, include family members and significant others. The activities that occur in this interface or as direct follow-up are unique because they are interpersonally and physically coenacted with a particular patient for the purpose of promoting that patient's health or well-being. Many important processes transpire at this point of care, including the following:

- The patient-provider therapeutic partnership is established.
- Health problems become mutually understood through information gathering and effective communication.
- Health, recovery, or palliative goals are expressed by the patient.
- Management and treatment options are explored.
- Physical acts of diagnosis, monitoring, treatment, and pharmacologic and non-pharmacologic therapy are performed.

 BOX 7-1   Examples of Advanced Practice Nurse Indirect Care Activities

- Consultation with other health care providers (e.g., physicians, nurses, pharmacists)
- Discharge planning
- Care coordination
- Communication with insurance organizations
- Guidance of bedside nurses
- Unit rounds
- Researching care guidelines
- Leading quality of care initiatives

- Education, support, coaching, counseling, and comfort are provided.
- Decisions regarding future actions to be taken by each party are made.
- Future contact is planned.

Advanced practice nursing activities occurring before and adjacent to the patient-nurse interface have a great influence on the direct care that occurs; however, they are not performed with an individual patient or their main purpose is tangential to the direct care of the patient. Activities such as collaboration, consultation, and mentoring of staff may all be occurring in relation to the direct care interface. It is often difficult to separate out these indirect care interventions, which are equally necessary for adequate fulfillment of the APN role and care of the patient (Box 7-1). For example, when an APN consults with another provider regarding the nature of a patient's condition or the care that should be recommended to a patient, the APN is engaging in advanced clinical practice, but it is not direct care. Even though the APN is accountable for the consultation, the primary purpose of that contact is to acquire information and understanding to use in formulating recommendations for the patient's direct care provider (see Chapter 9). Thus, according to the definition of direct care used in this chapter, the APN is engaged in clinical practice but he or she is not providing direct care to the patient. The direct care role of the clinical nurse specialist (CNS) may not be as apparent to observers as it is for a nurse practitioner (NP), certified registered nurse anesthetist (CRNA), and certified nurse-midwife (CNM) because the CNS frequently shifts from direct to indirect activities depending on the situation and the providers involved. See Exemplar 7-1. For the CNS, these shifts may occur during one patient encounter, and certainly across a day. Most APNs will have a role in ensuring that others are providing quality and safe care through indirect practice.

○ EXEMPLAR 7-1 **Examples of Direct and Indirect Care Provided by Advanced Practice Nurses**

Direct Care

The medical intensive care unit (MICU) acute care nurse practitioner (ACNP) was called into a patient's room by a novice staff nurse. On quick visual assessment of the patient and room, and a verbal update by the nurse, the ACNP ascertained that this was a 65-year-old man with acute respiratory distress syndrome who was intubated and on a ventilator, with an FiO_2 at 60%. His current SaO_2 reading was 84%, blood pressure was 88/60 mm Hg and dropping, and heart rate was 110 beats/min. The patient was sedated and his skin was pale. The alarm on the ventilator was sounding with high peak inspiratory pressures. The staff nurse appeared anxious and stated that she had been unable to determine why the alarm was sounding. When the nurse noticed that that the patient's status was deteriorating, she called for the ACNP to help.

Recognizing that it was not an appropriate time to talk the staff nurse through troubleshooting the ventilator, the ACNP assumed responsibility for the nursing interventions by increasing the FiO_2 on the ventilator and hyperventilating the patient. However, she explained each action she was taking to the staff nurse. The ACNP suctioned the patient and removed a large mucus plug. The patient's color slowly returned to pink, blood pressure started to increase, heart rate started to decrease, and SaO_2 rose to 92%.

After ensuring that the patient was stable, the ventilator was functioning, and returning the ventilator to the original settings, the ACNP reviewed the situation with the staff nurse. She reviewed each step, describing indicators and appropriate actions to take, and answered the staff nurse's questions. In this case, the ACNP assumed direct care activities for the patient to address an urgent situation.

Indirect Care

The MICU clinical nurse specialist (CNS) was approached by an experienced staff nurse who was struggling to develop an interpersonal relationship with the family of a complex critically ill patient. The family was very anxious and was having difficulty synthesizing the information that the staff nurse was trying to provide to them.

Rather than intervene directly with the family, the CNS recognized that this would be a good opportunity for the staff nurse to develop and expand her skills at interpersonal relationship building. The CNS explored the interventions she had already attempted with the nurse and reviewed with her the literature regarding family stressors in critical care, family needs, and the goal of assessing and addressing what the family perceives as their educational and care needs. Armed with this information, the nurse felt comfortable in working with the family to assess their priority educational and psychosocial needs to obtain the resources and information they needed.

The CNS could have intervened by establishing a direct relationship with the family, which would have been providing direct care. In this case, however, she determined that it was more important to assist the staff nurse in the development of the relationship as a growth opportunity and to help the nurse form an ongoing partnership with the family, with whom she would be interacting on a continuing basis.

APN roles tend to diverge when comparing the amount of time spent in each of the direct care activities (Becker et al., 2006; Verger, Marcoux, Madden, et al., 2005). A research study by Oddsdottir and Sveinsdottir (2011) has demonstrated that CNSs spend most of their time in education and expert practice in the institutional domain; the authors recommended that the focus for CNSs needs to be spent on direct practice in the client-family domain. Critical care CNSs reported spending 36% of their time with nursing personnel, 21% with patient population work, and 17% on organizational and system work. Only 26% of their time was spent with individual patients, whereas ACNPs spent 74% of their time with individual patients (Becker et al., 2006). This finding is consistent with other studies reporting that NPs spend more time on individual patient care and less time on indirect and service-related care (ANCC, 2004; Gardner et al., 2010). Other studies have supported the finding that NPs and CNMs are spending most of their time in direct care with patients (Holland & Holland, 2007; McCloskey, Grey, Deshefy-Longhi, et al., 2003; Rosenfeld, McEvoy, & Glassman 2003; Swartz et al., 2003).

This delineation of direct and indirect practice is not intended to denigrate clinical activities that occur outside the patient-nurse interface—quite the contrary. These clinical activities and functions should be recognized as influencing what happens in the interface and as having a significant impact on patient outcomes. Because these other clinical activities significantly affect patient outcomes, they must be valued by the nursing community and health care systems. In the current environment of cost containment and technologic development, all activities that enhance patients' health, recovery, and adjustment are critical components of care delivered by APNs. Ball and Cox (2003), based on a study of CNSs and NPs, found that APNs engage in a range of strategic activities, an excellent characterization of the direct and indirect but adjacent actions that make up the clinical practice of APNs as depicted in exemplars below.

Researchers are beginning to understand the specific activities that constitute the direct care component of various advanced practice nursing roles. However, it is difficult to make generalizations about these activities because the APNs studied had different roles and worked in different settings, with different populations. Different classification schemas were used to categorize APN actions. For example, in some studies, investigators used the term *activities* to classify APN actions; in others, the term *interventions* was used. The variability in terminology and definitions makes it difficult to compare results across APN roles, settings, and populations. Nevertheless, a review of these studies yields some insights into the extent and nature of direct care activities in APN roles.

Many direct care activities performed are similar across APN roles, and preparation of all APNs must include the 3 Ps—pathophysiology, advanced physical assessment, and pharmacology (AACN, 2011). Additional direct care activities that are similar across roles include patient and family education and counseling, ordering laboratory tests and medications, and performing procedures (Becker et al., 2006; Verger et al., 2005). Verger and colleagues (2005) surveyed pediatric critical care NPs regarding their direct care activities, which included physical assessments, patient and family teaching, and performing procedures such as venipuncture, IV insertions, lumbar punctures, feeding tube placements, endotracheal intubations, and central line placements. CNMs reported expansion of their direct care procedures to include first assisting during cesarean sections and performing endometrial biopsies (Holland & Holland, 2007). CNSs and administrators need to have ongoing monitoring of the direct care components of the CNS role. With increasing complexity and diversity of the role, there is a propensity to have CNSs perform less and less expert direct care of patients, which is the main characteristic of APN practice (Lewandowski & Adamle, 2009).

Regardless of the population being cared for, surveillance was a key direct care activity of APNs identified in studies (Brooten, Youngblut, Deatrick, et al., 2003; Brooten, Youngblut, Donahue, et al., 2007; Hughes et al., 2002). Surveillance is described as watching for physical and emotional signs and symptoms and monitoring dressing and wound care, laboratory results, medications, nutrition, response to treatment, and caretaking and parenting. Thus, surveillance refers to an APN's vigilant

assessment of patient status, the rapid diagnosis of subtle or emergent conditions, and quick intervention to prevent or reverse a potentially negative outcome. APNs in these studies also used extensive teaching, guidance, and counseling in many of the same areas in which they were using surveillance. The extent of surveillance and teaching may fluctuate depending on the phase of care and the particular population being cared for. Nursing surveillance can have a particularly important impact on the patient safety indicator of failure to rescue—situations in which providers fail to notice symptoms or respond adequately or swiftly to clinical signs, resulting in patient death from preventable complications. Failure to rescue has been linked to nursing surveillance; for example, the higher the nursing surveillance, as defined by staffing ratios, the lower the number of cases of failure to rescue (Aiken et al., 2002; Clarke & Aiken, 2003). A study by Shever (2011) has also supported the concept that patients who receive higher surveillance, as documented by nursing in the electronic health record, are less likely to be involved in a failure to rescue situation.

In summary, direct care activities make up a large part of what most APNs do, although there is considerable variation in which activities are performed and how much time is devoted to the direct care function across roles, settings, and patient populations.

Six Characteristics of Direct Clinical Care Provided by Advanced Practice Nurses

APNs function in many roles and settings, and with different populations. Despite such variability in role implementation, there is a similarity in the components of direct care provided. Characteristics of advanced practice nursing care extend across advanced practice roles, health care settings, and populations of patients. These characteristics include the following:

- Use of a holistic perspective
- Formation of therapeutic partnerships with patients
- Expert clinical performance
- Use of reflective practice
- Use of evidence as a guide to practice
- Use of diverse approaches to health and illness management

Accumulating evidence supports these features of APN practice as having positive influences on patient outcomes. Throughout this chapter, the empirical evidence cited regarding claims about APN practice is illustrative and not based on a systematic review of research. The research regarding outcomes of APN practice is addressed comprehensively in Chapter 24.

The six characteristics of advanced direct care practice have their roots in the traditional values of the nursing profession. These values are defined in nursing's social contract with society, as outlined by the American Nurses Association (ANA; 2010, p. 6):

- People manifest an essential unity of mind, body, and spirit.
- People's experiences are contextually and culturally defined.
- Health and illness are human experiences. The presence of illness does not preclude health, nor does optimal health preclude illness.
- The relationship between the nurse and patient occurs within the context of the values and beliefs of the patient and nurse.
- Public policy and the health care delivery system influence the health and well-being of society and professional nursing.
- Individual responsibility and interprofessional involvement are essential.

Nurses in advanced practice roles often have a deep commitment to the values on which these characteristics rest and are able to advocate persuasively and incorporate these values in daily practice. The expanded scope of practice of APN roles often enables APNs to fully enact these characteristics in their daily interactions with patients. An overview of strategies for enacting these characteristics is provided in Box 7-2.

Use of a Holistic Perspective

Holism Described

Holism has a variety of meanings. A broad view is that holism involves a deep understanding of each patient as a complex and unique person who is embedded in a temporally unfolding life. The holistic perspective recognizes the multiple dimensions of each person—physiologic, social, emotional, cognitive, and spiritual—and that the relationships among these dimensions result in a whole that is greater than the sum of the parts. The broad perspective also recognizes that the individual is "a unitary whole in mutual process with the environment"(American Holistic Nurses Association, 2007). People are in constant interaction with themselves, others, and the environment and universe and exhibit maximum well-being when all parts are balanced and in harmony (Erickson, 2007); this state of well-being can exist whether there are physical disorders or not. This comprehensive and integrated view of human life and health is considered in the health care encounter in context of the full range of factors influencing patients' experiences (Box 7-3) Clearly, high-tech care environments with many health care providers, each focused on a particular aspect of a patient's condition and treatment, require designated coordinators who have a comprehensive and integrated appreciation of the patient and his or her experience of care as a whole.

APNs' capacity to keep the pieces together and promote continuity of care in a way that focuses care on the unique individual is undoubtedly why many clinical programs have an APN member or coordinator (see later, "Management of Complex Situations" on p. 172). The Shuler nurse practitioner practice model is based on a holistic understanding of human health and illness in older adults that integrates medical and nursing perspectives (Shuler, Huebscher, & Hallock, 2001; see Chapter 2).

Holism and Health Assessment

When working with a relatively healthy person, the APN seeks to understand the person's life goals, functional interests, and health risks to preserve quality of life in the future. In contrast, when working with an ill patient, the APN is interested in what the person views as problems, how he or she is responding to problems, and what the problems and responses mean to the individual in terms of daily living and life goals. In a study of 199 primary care clinical situations (Burman, Stepans, Jansa, et al., 2002), NPs were found to engage in holistic assessment and ground their decision making within the context of the patient's life.

The ability to function in daily activities and relationships is an important consideration for patients when they evaluate their health, so it is an appropriate and essential focus for holistic, person-centered assessment. Most functional assessment formats focus on the following: (1) how patients view their health or quality of life; (2) how they accomplish self-care and household or job responsibilities; (3) the social, physical, financial, environmental, and spiritual factors that augment or tax their functioning; and (4) the strategies that they and their families use to cope with the stresses and problems in their lives.

In pediatrics, measures of functional status such as one for children with asthma (Centers for Disease Control and Prevention [CDC], 2012) have been developed. In adults, APNs may choose to use a disease- or problem-focused tool such as measurement of functional status in heart failure patients (Rector, Anand, & Cohn, 2006), of symptom distress in cancer patients (Cleeland et al., 2000; Chen & Lin, 2007), or of function and disability in geriatric patients (Denkinger et al., 2009), or a widely used general measure such as the Short Form-36 Health Survey (SF-36), which measures overall health, functional status, and well-being in adults and is available in several languages (Ware & Sherbourne, 1992).

Nursing Model or Medical Model

As APNs have taken on responsibilities that were formerly in the purview of physicians, some have expressed concern that APNs are being asked to function within a medical

BOX 7-2   Characteristics of Advanced Direct Care Practice and Strategies for Enacting Them

Use of a Holistic Perspective

- Take into account the complexity of human life.
- Recognize and address how social, organizational, and physical environments affect people.
- Consider the profound effects of illness, aging, hospitalization, and stress.
- Consider how symptoms, illness, and treatment affect quality of life.
- Focus on functional abilities and requirements.

Formation of Therapeutic Partnerships with Patients

- Use a conversational style to conduct health care encounters.
- Optimize therapeutic use of self.
- Encourage the patient to participate actively in decision making.
- Look for cultural influences on health care discourse.
- Listen to the indirect voices of patients who are noncommunicative.
- Advocate the patient's perspective and concerns to others.

Expert Clinical Performance

- Acquire specialized knowledge.
- Seek out supervision when performing a new skill.
- Invest in deeply understanding the patient situations in which you are involved.
- Generate and test alternative lines of reasoning.
- Trust your hunches—check them out.
- Be aware of when you are time-pressured and likely to make thinking errors.
- Consider multiple aspects of the patient's situation when you are deciding how to treat.
- Make sure that you know how to use technical equipment safely.
- Make sure that you know how to interpret data produced by monitoring devices.
- Pay attention to how you move and touch patients during care.
- Anticipate ethical conflicts.

- Acquire computer-related skills for accessing and managing patient data and practice information.

Use of Reflective Practice

- Explore your personal values, belief systems, and behaviors.
- Identify your basic assumptions about health care, the APN role, and the rights and responsibilities of patients.
- Consider how your assumptions affect your judgments.
- Talk to colleagues and your teachers about your clinical experiences.
- Consider use of a journal to document experiences.
- Assess your current skill and comfort in reflection.

Use of Evidence as a Guide For Practice

- Learn how to search health care databases for studies related to specific clinical topics.
- Read research reports related to your field of practice.
- Seek out systematic revision of research and research-based clinical guidelines.
- Acquire skills in appraising the various forms of evidence.
- Work with colleagues to consider evidence-based improvements in care.

Diverse Approaches and Interventions to Health and Illness Management

- Use interpersonal interventions to influence patients.
- Acquire proficiency in new ways of treating and helping patients.
- Help patients maintain health and capitalize on their strengths and resources.
- Provide preventive services appropriate to your field of practice.
- Coordinate services among care sites and multiple providers.
- Acquire knowledge about complementary and alternative therapies.

model of practice rather than within a holistic nursing model. This concern is raised when APNs substitute for physicians. However, there is evidence that a nursing orientation is an enduring component of APN practice, even when medical management is part of the role (Blasdell, Klunick, & Purseglove, 2002; Hoffman, Tasota, Scharfenberg, et al., 2003; Hoffman, Happ, Scharfenberg, et al., 2004; Lambing, Adams, Fox, et al., 2004; Sidani et al., 2006; Watts et al., 2009; Box 7-4). Activities described in these studies clearly reflect a nursing-focused practice.

Statements from professional organizations indicate that APNs value their nursing orientation and their medical functions. For example, the description of APNs in the ANA's nursing social policy statement includes strong endorsement of specialized and expanded knowledge and skills within the context of holistic values (ANA, 2010). On the theoretical front, several models of advanced practice blend nursing and medical orientations (see the Shuler nurse practitioner practice model and the Dunphy-Winland models in Chapter 2).

BOX 7-3   Factors to Consider When Helping the Patient Holistically

- Patient's view of his or her health or illness
- Patterns of physical symptoms and amount of distress they cause
- The effect of physical symptoms on the patient's daily functioning and quality of life
- Symptom management approaches that are acceptable to the patient
- Life changes that could affect the patient's physical or psychological well-being (e.g., relationship break-up, job change, intrafamily conflict, retirement, death of a loved one)
- Context of the patient's life, including the nuclear family unit, social support, job responsibilities, financial situation, health insurance coverage, responsibilities for the care of others (e.g., children, chronically ill spouse or partner, older parents)
- Spiritual and life values (e.g., independence, religion, beliefs about life, acceptance of fate)

 BOX 7-4   Nursing-Focused Advanced Practice Interventions

- Engagement of patients in their own care
- Patient education
- Care planning
- Physical and occupational therapy referrals
- Use of communication skills
- Promotion of continuity of care
- Teaching of nursing staff
- Advance directive discussions
- Wellness and health promotion model

Formation of Therapeutic Partnerships with Patients

The Institute of Medicine (IOM) has recommended patient-centered care as the foundation of safe, effective, and efficient health care (IOM, 2001). The person-centered, holistic perspective of APNs serves as the foundation for the types of relationships that they cocreate with patients. APNs are well prepared to develop therapeutic relationships as the cornerstone of patient-centered care (Badger & McArthur, 2003; Coddington & Sands, 2008). The Gallup Poll has consistently reported that the public views nurses as the most trusted professionals (ANA, 2011). The skill of APNs to develop therapeutic relationships with individual patients can influence broader public perceptions.

The development and maintenance of therapeutic relationships with patients and families is one of the key criteria in *The Essentials of Doctoral Education for Advanced Nursing Practice,* which is specific and foundational to advanced practice nursing (AACN, 2006). Studies have shown that APNs form collaborative relationships with patients. Dontje and colleagues (2004) have described the primary care environment as particularly conducive to developing sustained partnerships with patients. In a synthesis of the literature, a review of qualitative data, and reflection on their own clinical experiences, the authors identified the following as goals of therapeutic partnerships in primary care: self-management of care, promotion of shared decision making, and a holistic approach to care that promotes continuity. The authors posited that these characteristics of APN partnerships may contribute to high-quality care through the adoption of preventive care practices, improved patient satisfaction, appropriate use of resources, and overall better patient outcomes, although more research is needed in this area. In addition, Drennan and colleagues (2011) found that patients were satisfied with their relationships with nurses and midwives, including the consultation process, patient education, medication advice, and the patient's intent to comply with provider advice.

APNs' therapeutic use of self contributes to the optimization of a therapeutic relationship with patient and family. Therapeutic use of self involves APN awareness of personal feelings, attitudes, and values and how that awareness influences the patient-provider relationship (Warner, 2006). This increased awareness on the part of the APN helps increase empathy, allowing the APN to engage more deeply with patients while maintaining appropriate boundaries to maintain objectivity (Warner, 2006).

Shared Decision Making

In addition to eliciting information that increases understanding of the patient's illness experience, APNs, in the studies cited, encourage patients to participate in decisions regarding how their diseases and illnesses should be managed. There is a continuum of patient involvement in making decisions for her or his own health care. At one end of the continuum are patients who want to be fully engaged in a partnership with providers in making decisions, whereas at the other end of the continuum are patients who want to rely on family members or care providers to make all treatment decisions. This may include patients who are older, sicker, or cognitively impaired, or who have cultural beliefs that lead them to defer decisions to others. Regardless of where the patient falls on this continuum, it is still incumbent on the provider to establish a collaborative partnership to ensure that regardless of whom the patient wants to make decisions, it is done in congruence with the patient's beliefs and values.

APNs should individually determine each patient's preference for participation in decision making and be sensitive to the fact that patients' preferences may change over time as they get to know the provider better and as different types of health problems arise. Once the patient's preference has been elicited, the provider should tailor his or her communication and decision making style to the patient's preference. Many patients have not had prior health care experiences in which shared decision making was even a possibility but, when offered the opportunity, many choose it—tentatively in some cases, enthusiastically in others. Trying on a more active role may require some help from the provider, such as explaining how it would work and which responsibilities are the patient's and which are the provider's. Providers can encourage patients to bring up issues by asking open-ended questions such as "So, how have you been?" and focused but open questions such as "So, how are things going at home?" Patients can be encouraged to participate in decision making by offering them explicit opportunities in the form of questions such as "Does one of those approaches sound better to you than the other?" Gradually, patients approached in this way will learn that health care encounters will be organized around their concerns, not around a series of questions asked by the provider, and that they should feel safe to express their concerns and preferences.

Open and honest communication is foundational to a shared decision making philosophy. APNs have reported more advanced communication skills than those reported by basic RNs (Sivesind et al., 2003). The ability to adapt communication styles is a needed skill of APNs (Lawson, 2002; McCourt, 2006) and can result in patients who report that they have more knowledge and control of their own care. It is a skill that is necessary for an APN to maintain a therapeutic relationship with a patient while also supporting her or him in effective decision making . The APN needs to use an approach that incorporates verbal and nonverbal behaviors exhibited by the patient while being careful to maintain professional boundaries (Elliott, 2010).

APNs must be cognizant of their own personal beliefs and value systems in a partnership in which they are coaching patients in decision making (see Chapter 8). Although they are uniquely prepared to facilitate the holistic management of the physical, psychosocial, and spiritual aspects of care in these particular situations, APNs may be involved in interactions in which it is difficult for them to help patients make decisions. If the APN

is unaware or has unresolved issues of his or her own, he or she may risk exercising undue or unintentional influence on a patient's decision in emotionally charged situations (Bialk, 2004). Bringing one's own beliefs and values to consciousness prior to a discussion focused on patient decision making, reflecting on one's own cognitive and affective responses to such discussions, and debriefing with a colleague can help APNs maintain a therapeutic approach (or determine when it is appropriate for another clinician to become involved).

Cultural Influences on Partnerships

Another important factor affecting whether and how persons want to participate in health care decision making is their cultural background. It is easy to forget that not all cultures value individual autonomy as much as North Americans of Anglo-Saxon ancestry. Increasingly, recognizing and respecting the cultural identification of patients is being viewed as essential to building meaningful partnerships. Cultural groups form along lines of racial, national origin, religious, professional, organizational, sexual orientation, or age group identification. Some cultural groups are easier to identify than others. Physical differences in appearance often indicate to the provider that he or she is dealing with a person of a different cultural orientation. Other cultural identifications are less obvious—for example, people with religious beliefs about fate, God as healer, or treatment taboos. However, it is important to avoid making assumptions about cultural beliefs simply based on physical appearance or dress. In today's increasingly diverse society, many families have blended traditional beliefs and practices from a number of cultures. These beliefs are learned by asking the patient open-ended questions and responding in a way that makes the patient feel understood.

The DNP *Essentials* identifies the need for APNs to synthesize and incorporate principles of cultural diversity into preventive and therapeutic interventions for individuals and populations (AACN, 2006). The preparation of APNs in the area of cultural competence and culturally appropriate care is key, because the demographics of nurses and APNs do not match the overall demographics of the United States population (McNeal & Walker, 2006; Ndiwane et al., 2004). Interactions that are complicated by cultural misunderstandings can result in incomplete or inaccurate assessments and even in misdiagnoses and suboptimal outcomes (Barakzai, Gregory, & Fraser, 2007; Sobralske & Katz, 2005). The APN needs to individualize care based on an assessment of the cultural influences on the perception of illness and reporting of symptoms. Otherwise, differences in perceptions can cause confusion, misunderstandings, and even conflicts that disrupt the patient-provider relationship and discourse. Moreover, they often complicate attempts to resolve misunderstandings because different cultural groups approach conflict negotiation differently. Studies have shown that NPs can engender trust in a population such as African Americans to a greater extent than physicians (Benkert, Peters, Tate, et al., 2008). In every encounter, the provider should expect that the patient may have values that are different in some ways from his or her own and must make a special effort to ensure that the care being given meets the patient's needs and is acceptable to him or her (Escallier & Fullerton, 2009). APNs must always remain nonjudgmental and not impose their own beliefs or biases onto the patient.

Communication with Patients

A foundation of good communication with patients is essential to developing a therapeutic relationship. Research has shown that good communication between the APN and patient can increase patient satisfaction, establish trust, increase adherence to a treatment plan, and improve patient outcomes (Burley, 2011; Charlton, Dearing, Berry, et al., 2008; Gilbert & Hayes, 2009; Persson, Hornsten, Wirkvist, et al., 2011; Sandhu, Dale, Stallard, et al., 2009). Learning good communication skills takes ongoing practice throughout the APN's career. Simulation laboratories have been shown to be helpful in assisting APN students to learn communication techniques in situations such as working with angry patients, delivering bad news to patients and families, providing empathy, and optimal motivational interviewing (Rosenzweig, Hravnak, Magdic, et al., 2008).

One aspect of optimal communication is listening. Listening has been described as being fully present with the patient to garner patient details, increase the level of trust in the relationship, and improve patient compliance (Browning & Waite, 2010). Listening takes as much concerted effort to perform optimally as verbal communication. Key to good listening is the ability on the APN's part to avoid being distracted by personal thoughts, forming instant judgments, and formulating a reply while the patient is still speaking and telling her or his story. In addition, the APN must become aware of how individual expectations, experiences, and cultural paradigms can result in biases and misperceptions when working with patients (Browning & Waite, 2010). Reflective listening techniques can be useful when APNs convey to patients that they have been heard and understood without judgment and can assist patients to explore their personal situations more fully (Resnicow & McMaster, 2012). These techniques include taking patient statements and restating, rephrasing, reframing, and reflecting thoughts, feelings, and emotional undertones back to the patient (Miller, 2010). APN use of reflective listening has been shown to assist in behavioral change and self-care decision making in heart failure patients (Riegel et al., 2006).

Therapeutic Partnerships with Noncommunicative Patients

Some patients are not able to enter fully into partnership with APNs because they are too young, have compromised cognitive capacity, or are unconscious. Clinical populations who may be unable to participate fully in shared decision making are listed in Box 7-5. Unfortunately, staff nurses working with noncommunicative patients can become so focused on providing care that they forget about having meaningful interactions with the patient (Alasad & Ahmad, 2005). APNs can role-model alternative forms of communication so that noncommunicative patients can receive optimal care.

Although these patients may have limited ability to speak for themselves, they are not entirely without opinion or voice. Situations in which patients will experience temporary alterations in cognition or verbal ability can often be anticipated. For example, in planned perioperative situations in which general anesthesia and intubation will be used, the CRNA has the opportunity to dialogue with the patient prior to the procedure. This creates a shared relationship in which the patient can feel comforted and confident about the upcoming procedure (Rudolfsson, von Post, & Eriksson, 2007). The CRNA can prepare patients for the period when communication will

---

BOX 7-5 Patient Populations Unable to Participate Fully in Partnership

- Infants and preverbal children
- Anesthetized patients
- Unconscious or comatose patients
- People in severe pain
- Patients receiving medications that impair cognition
- People with dementia
- People with psychiatric conditions that seriously impair rational thought
- People with conditions that render them incapable of speech and conversation
- People with congenital or acquired cognitive limitations
- People whose primary language is different from the provider's

be a challenge and propose alternative methods for communication. In addition, the CRNA can discuss patients' preferences for handling possible events beforehand to elicit their wishes.

In the absence of this type of prior dialogue, experts who work with patients who cannot verbalize their concerns and preferences learn to pay close attention to how patients are responding to what happens to them; facial expressions, body movement, and physiologic parameters are used to ascertain what causes the patient discomfort and what helps alleviate it. In a study of persons who had experienced and recovered from unconsciousness (Lawrence, 1995), 27% of the patients reported being able to hear, understand, and respond emotionally while they were unconscious. These findings suggest that nurses should communicate with unconscious patients by providing them with interventions such as reassurance, bodily care, pain relief, explanations, and comforting touch. APNs should view these interactions as not merely one-way imparting of information but also as providing key emotional support (Alasad & Ahmad, 2005; Geraghty, 2005).

There are tools that can be used for patients who are conscious but unable to communicate. Unfortunately, many nurses are not adequately educated in using alternative methods of communication and, if they are, may not be familiar or comfortable with the particular method required for an individual patient (Finke, Light, & Kitko, 2008). Other barriers include not having access to communication devices and time pressures that may not allow providers to engage adequately in a process that could take more time.

Other sources of information about patients who are unable to respond physically or to communicate should also be identified. For example, siblings visiting an adolescent male with a major head injury would be able to tell you what type of music he likes to listen to and would probably even bring you a CD to play for the patient. His mother would know what has caused him to have skin reactions in the past. Responding to his father's offhand comment that he cannot stand to be without his glasses when he is not wearing his contact lenses would most likely help father and son. All these are ways of building a partnership with an unconscious teenager in an intensive care unit (ICU). In adults and adolescents, advance directives, heath care proxy documents, and organ donation cards are other sources of information regarding patients' wishes. Thus, noncommunicative patients are not without voices, but hearing their voices does require presence and attentiveness, and establishing a relationship. Box 7-6 summarizes options for the APN when engaging with noncommunicative patients.

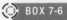 **BOX 7-6   Techniques for Communicating with Noncommunicative Patients**

- Maintain verbal interactions and eye contact with patient throughout care.
- Explain procedures.
- Monitor tone of voice so you are not inadvertently relaying emotional subcontext to the actual words used.
- Use appropriate touch for reassurance.
- Use other communication devices such as alphabet and word boards, writing, computers, electronic communication devices.
- Use interpreters for foreign languages and sign language.
- Use other sources of information for patient's likes and dislikes—family, primary care providers, friends.
- Use physiologic cues as appropriate to evaluate patient responses to care and treatments—grimacing, frowning, turning away from touch, relaxing facial muscles, blood pressure and heart rate responses.

Expert Clinical Performance

Few studies have clearly differentiated between the expert skills of the APN and the practice of the basic RN. The expert performance of an APN encompasses clinical thinking and skills. An expert's clinical judgment is characterized by the ability to make fine distinctions among features of a particular condition that were not possible during beginning practice. Benner's studies of expert clinical judgment, although not with APN participants, inform this discussion of APNs' clinical expertise (1984). Tanner (2006) has reviewed the literature regarding clinical judgment and found that it requires three main categories of knowledge. The first is scientific and theoretical knowledge that is widely applicable. The second is knowledge based on experience that fills in gaps and assists in the prompt identification of clinical issues. The final category is knowledge that is individualized to the patient, based on an interpersonal connection.

Clinical Thinking

APNs' specialized knowledge accrues from a variety of sources, including graduate and continuing education, clinical experience, professional reading, reflection, mentoring, and exchange of information and ideas with colleagues within and outside nursing. The integration of knowledge from these sources provides a foundation for the expert clinical thinking that is associated with advanced direct care practice. Once an APN has been in practice for a while, formalized knowledge and experiential knowledge become so mixed together that they may not be distinguishable to the outside observer. Illness trajectories and presentations of prior patients make an impression and come to mind when a patient with a similar problem is seen later (Benner, 1984). The expert also remembers which interventions worked and did not work in certain situations. Eventually, the expert's clinical knowledge consists of a complex network of memorable cases, prototypic images, research findings, thinking strategies, moral values, maxims, probabilities, behavioral responses, associations, illness trajectories and timetables, and therapeutic information. Thus, experts have extensive, varied, and complex knowledge networks that can be activated to help them understand clinical situations and events. These networks are comprised of internal and external resources. The APN may mentally review internal resources such as educational knowledge, typical cases, and previously experienced cases when confronted with a complex or challenging case. However, the APN is also cognizant of when internal resources are no longer adequate and knows when to refer to external resources for consultation, more data, or guidance.

Clinical reasoning brings together the clinical knowledge of the provider with specific observations, perceptions, events, and facts from the situation at hand to produce an understanding of what is occurring (O'Neill, 1995). Sometimes, the understanding is arrived at by using cognitive processes to consider evidence and alternative explanations logically. At other times, the insight or understanding arrives intuitively—that is, through direct apprehension without recourse to deliberate reasoning (Benner et al., 1996; Tanner, 2006). In these situations, APNs can use reflective practice to sort through the intuition to understand the components better and identify new insights. With experience, they can then repackage these insights and incorporate them into their experiential learning to use the information in the next relevant case prospectively and deliberately.

APN experts have the ability to scan a situation rapidly (e.g., past records, patient's appearance, the patient's unexpressed concern or discomfort) and identify salient and relevant information. The APN is able to suspend judgment purposefully about personal strongly held beliefs that may be proposed by others, such as "he's a difficult patient" or "she's just drug seeking." The ability to do this ensures as much objectivity as possible when caring for patients. For example, research has shown that expert

CNSs are able to transcend the labeling of a "difficult patient" to problem resolution through the use of patient respect, communication skills, and increased self-efficacy (Wolf & Robinson-Smith, 2007). Relying heavily on their perceptions, observations, and assessment skills, APNs quickly activate one or several lines of reasoning regarding what might be occurring. They then conduct a more focused assessment to determine which one best explains the situation at hand. These lines of reasoning can be informal personal theories about the specific patient situation; this formulation draws from personal knowledge of the particular patient, personal knowledge acquired from previous experiences, and formalized domain-specific knowledge (Tanner, 2006). In implementing the solutions, these lines of reasoning can be tested by performing a clinical intervention and noting how the patient responds. Throughout this process, the APN may be teaching and role modeling with staff to assist in staff nurse self-awareness and reflection. A novice APN may need to work through the situation in a formal logical way and be more deliberate about the use of formal educational knowledge, enriching it over time with experiential knowledge (Tanner, 2006).

It has been shown that the values and underlying knowledge a nurse brings to a situation also has a profound influence on his or her assessment of the patient. Results of one study demonstrated that a nurse's beliefs about older adults can affect how a nurse assesses the older confused patient and can affect prioritization of that patient's needs (Dahlke & Phinney, 2008). Another example is when a nurse's moral opinion of drug addiction and the interpretation of behavior as drug seeking may have more influence on the treatment of a patient's pain, rather than the actual assessment of the pain.

Most patient accounts unfold in a fairly predictable way and the APN arrives at a diagnosis and/or intervention with considerable confidence in her or his clinical inferences. At other times, however, there is uncertainty and lack of understanding regarding the situation. The uncertainty may pertain to information the patient provides, the diagnosis, the best approach to management, or to how the patient is responding (Brykczynski, 1991). When there is ambiguity, experts often break into conscious problem solving or "detective-like thinking and questioning" (Benner et al., 1996; Benner, Hooper-Kyriakidis, & Stannard, 1999) to try to determine what is going on.

Knowing the patient may be critical to perceptive and accurate clinical reasoning. Knowing the patient as an individual with certain patterns of responses enables experienced nurses to detect subtle changes in a patient's condition over time (Tanner, 2006; Tanner, Benner,

Chesla, et al., 1993). The extent to which any nurse knows a patient may be associated with that nurse's ability to do the following:

- Recognize that risk factors are present.
- Detect early indicators of a problem (e.g., a subtle change in pattern).
- Take timely preventive action.
- Recognize nonfitting and atypical data.

Nonfitting data suggest to experts that they need to generate new or additional hypotheses because the current observations and parameters do not fully explain the clinical picture as it has been or as it should be. For example, when faced with a nonfitting sign or symptom, the nurse may generate alternative hypotheses pertaining to the onset of a complication or worsening of the disease process (Burman et al., 2002).

Thinking Errors

The clinical acumen of APNs and the inferences, hypotheses, and lines of reasoning that they generate are highly dependable. However, as practice becomes repetitive, APNs may develop routine responses and then run the risk of making certain types of thinking errors (Schön, 1992). Errors of expectancy occur when the correct diagnosis is not generated as a hypothesis because a set of circumstances, in the clinician's experience or patient's circumstances, predisposes the clinician to disregard it. For example, the NP who over several years has seen an older woman for problems associated with chronic pulmonary disease may fail to consider that the most recent onset of shortness of breath and fatigue could be related to worsening aortic stenosis; the NP has come to expect pulmonary disease, not cardiac disease.

Erroneous conclusions are also more likely when the situation is ambiguous—that is, when the meaning or reliability of the data is unclear, the interpretation of the data is not clear-cut, the best approach to treatment is debatable, or one cannot say for sure whether the patient is responding well to treatment (Brykczynski, 1991). To avoid errors in these types of situations, experts often revert to the use of maxims (a succinct metaphor for a general truth) to guide their thinking (Brykczynski, 1989). One of the maxims that NPs use to deal with uncertain diagnoses is "When you hear hoof beats in Kansas, think horses, not zebras." This reminds clinicians who are about to make a diagnosis that occurs infrequently to consider the incidence of the condition in the population. Thus, an older adult with respiratory problems seen in a suburban office is unlikely to have tuberculosis; pneumonia is a more likely diagnosis. Because tuberculosis is rare in the older adult population, the clinical data for tuberculosis should be convincing if that diagnosis is proposed.

Poor judgment can also result from the following: tunnel vision; overgeneralization; influence by a recent dramatic experience; premature closure (Croskerry, 2003); and fixation on certain problems to the exclusion of others (Benner et al., 1999). Faulty thinking is not the only source of error in clinical decision making. Others include inaccurate observations, misinterpretation of the meaning of data, a sketchy knowledge of the particular situation, and a faulty or outdated model of the disease, condition, or response.

It is important that APNs recognize the potential for and avoid leaping to conclusions and making snap judgments. It can become easy to allow biases to lead to premature diagnoses without fully listening to or assessing patients. The expert APN has learned to scan data constantly and look for deviations. The ability to differentiate effectively between significant and insignificant data is needed to have safe practice. See Box 7-7 for actions that APNs can take to prevent thinking errors.

Time Pressures

Regardless of setting, practitioners worry about the effect that time pressures have on the accuracy and completeness of their clinical thinking and decision making. The IOM's galvanizing report on errors and patient safety cited studies in which between 3% and 46% of hospitalized patients in the United States were harmed by error or negligence (IOM, 2000). It is estimated that more than 100,000 patients die from medical errors and a more recent study, in 2009, suggested that little progress has been made in the decade since it was published (see http://content.healthaffairs.org/content/29/1/165.abstract). The committee called for transformation and

 BOX 7-7   Actions to Use to Avoid Thinking Errors

- Listen fully to patients' concerns and descriptions of their problems.
- Listen to input from other providers as to their assessments and perspectives.
- Pay attention to intuition that points to an incongruence in data.
- Avoid reliance on knowledge derived solely from rote memorization or repetition, but critically think through the source of knowing and how it relates to the individual patient.
- Remain constantly open to reevaluation of working diagnoses and treatments.
- Be aware of personal biases and assumptions.
- Continually evaluate what is "critical" data in each patient case.

redesign of the health care system. The wide variation is the result of varying definitions of what constitutes adverse events and various methods of detecting their occurrence. A heavy workload is associated with feelings of pressure, being rushed, cognitive overload, and fatigue adding to already burdened clinicians; these feelings clearly contribute to unsafe acts and omissions in care (IOM, 2000). Evidence in support of this inference comes from studies of nurse staffing in hospitals in which fewer hours of nursing care per patient per day and less care provided by registered nurses were associated with poorer patient outcomes (Aiken, Cimiotti, Sloane, et al., 2011; Blegen, Goode, Spetz, et al., 2011; Kaen, Shamliyan, Mueller, et al., 2007; Needleman, Beurhaus, Pankratz, et al., 2011; Van den Heede, Lesaffre, Diya, et al., 2009). Effectively addressing the issues of time pressures and insufficient hours of nursing care requires culture change, process redesign, and appropriate use of technology. The patient safety movement has led to a variety of efforts aimed at preventing errors—root cause analysis of sentinel events, improved work processes, redesign of delivery systems, use of technologic aids, communication training, human factors analysis, and team building. All these factors can have significant direct and indirect effects on workload, fatigue, and time available for direct patient care.

The effects of a heavy workload on patient outcomes in nonhospital settings are less well understood; thus, actions to address this issue have received less attention. However, as lengths of visits or contact times are decreased or the number of patients whom practitioners are expected to see in a day is increased, it is logical to assume that the number of errors in clinical thinking will increase. Each contact requires the practitioner to reset his or her clinical reasoning process by closing out one thinking project and starting on an entirely new one. This resetting, which is done back to back often during a day, is cognitively and physically demanding. How these performance expectations affect clinical reasoning accuracy is unknown.

Moreover, time pressures often get compounded by hassles, which come in the form of interruptions, noise in the environment, missing supplies, and system glitches that make clinical data or even whole charts unavailable to providers. These hassles likely interfere with providers' ability to concentrate on what the patient is saying and disrupt their efforts to make clinical sense of a patient's account. In many settings, providers are required to multitask. They start a task but must attend to another before completing the original one. This clearly increases the risks of failure to obtain needed information, broken lines of thought, technologic missteps, omissions in care, and failure to respond to patients' requests for service (Cornell, Riordan, Townsend-Gervis, et al., 2011; Ebright, Patterson, Chalko, et al., 2003).

Studies of emergency physicians and emergency NPs have demonstrated that their workflow patterns have frequent interruptions, which can result in short cuts, failure to return to the original task, increased perceptions of stress, and a potential for commission of errors (Burley, 2011; Chisholm, Weaver, Whenmouth, et al., 2011; Westbrook, Woods, Rob, et al., 2010). Emergency physicians are what is referred to as interrupt-driven. Admittedly, the emergency department may be an extreme example of a multitasking environment, but other settings also impose interruptions at a very high rate. An experienced APN may be more skilled at focusing on and prioritizing tasks and quickly dismissing interruptions and extraneous information. The novice APN, conversely, may take longer to perform tasks (allowing for more interruptions) and may need more assistance with consultations or accessing resources (Phillips, 2005). As time pressures for clinicians increase, organizational efforts to monitor for errors and potential errors and seek correction when there are system weaknesses are actions that APNs owe patients and themselves as providers functioning in busy environments.

Many patients are sensitive to the pace with which staff and providers greet them, talk with them, and do things, particularly those activities that involve verbal interaction and physical contact. Some patients respond to the fast-paced talk and hurried movements of providers by not bringing up some of the questions that they had intended to ask. Others may just get flustered and forget to mention important information; still others may become hostile and withhold information. Thus, errors in the form of information omission by the patient enter the clinical reasoning and decision making process.

In summary, clinical thinking is a complex task. It involves drawing on knowledge in memory and attending to multiple sources of situational input, some of which are difficult to interpret. Often, multiple clinical issues must be addressed during a patient encounter. These complexities make clinical thinking a challenging task, even under the best of circumstances. Situational awareness—perceptions of the current environment in which the APN is functioning—can make the APN more cognizant of the potential for error and improve diligence to the thought process at critical junctures, such as when writing orders or performing procedures, or during handoffs (Phillips, 2005).

Ethical Reasoning

Clinical reasoning is inextricably linked to ethical reasoning. Clinical reasoning generates possibilities of what could be done in a situation, whereas ethical reasoning adds the dimension of what should be done in the situation (see Chapter 13). Advances in health care and medical technology have increasingly resulted in gaps between care that is medically possible and care that is in the best interest of the patient. These gaps may be most notable when making decisions regarding withdrawing or withholding nutrition, hydration, or a treatment, when dealing with reproductive technology or human genetics, and when cost must figure into clinical treatment decisions. These situations are at high risk for becoming ethically problematic.

The literature regarding how to resolve ethical issues is extensive. One approach, incorporating preventive or prospective ethical considerations into clinical thinking and decision making, makes a great deal of sense (Epstein, 2012). This approach places an emphasis on preventing ethical conflicts from developing rather than waiting until a conflict arises by shaping the process of clinical care so that potential value conflicts are anticipated and discussed before outright conflict occurs. APNs can use this approach with routine encounters with patients. For example, during an encounter with a healthy patient, an APN may be able to say, "I'd like to discuss an important issue with you while you're well so I will know how to best help you." Such issues could include pain management, advance directives, or organ donation. In addition to emphasizing early communication among the patient, significant others, and the health care provider(s) about values, preventive ethics requires explicit critical reflection on the institutional factors that lead to conflict (Epstein, 2012). A third aspect of preventive ethics is an effort to create and preserve trust and understanding among providers, as well as between providers and patients (and their families). Thus, the use of preventive ethics can be considered proactive in that it requires providers to consider how the routine processes of care foster or prevent conflicts from occurring or, at the very least, ensure that such issues are identified at an early stage. The preventive approach has the potential to avoid conflicts because clinicians integrate ethical reasoning into clinical reasoning at an earlier point in time than when a traditional, conflict-based ethics approach is used.

The concept of moral distress is being recognized increasingly as an issue for all nurses, including APNs. Moral distress is defined as knowing what the ethically appropriate action should be but encountering barriers that discourage the provider from carrying out the action (American Association of Critical-Care Nurses, 2004; Rushton, 2006). This results in internal conflict that is not resolved (see Chapter 13).

Laabs (2005) has found that among primary care NPs, distress is most frequently caused by patient refusal of appropriate treatment. This creates a conflict for the NPs between promoting patient autonomy and beneficence on the part of the NP, resulting in feelings of frustration and powerlessness. Some NPs changed jobs and others considered leaving advanced practice altogether.

The American Association of Critical-Care Nurses (2004) has developed a model to address moral distress. APNs can use this four As model to understand and work toward the resolution of distressing situations; the four As include the following (American Association of Critical-Care Nurses, 2004; Rushton, 2006):

- Ask—explore and understand where the distress is coming from.
- Affirm—confirm the distress and consider one's professional obligations.
- Assess—use self-awareness, reflection, and evaluation to assess barriers, opportunities, and potential consequences in preparation for action.
- Action—put into place actions that will initiate resolving the distress, anticipating setbacks and ways to cope with them.

Encountering these situations can feel overwhelming but can also be opportunities for an APN to reassess her or his current beliefs and values. The APN can use concurrent and retrospective reflection on these situations as a growth and development experience that can be used in positive proactive interventions with future patient encounters (Rushton, 2006).

Skillful Performance

Although the health care professions place high value on knowledge and expert clinical reasoning, it is important to keep in mind that the public values skillful performance in physical examinations, delivery of treatments, diagnostic procedures, and comfort care. Most graduate schools require students to perform a specific set of procedural skills recommended by a national specialty organization before they complete their program. However, little is known about how APNs acquire competency in new or expanded procedural skills once they are in practice. Presumably, competency of APNs to perform specific procedures and treatments is initially ensured through the processes that agencies use to credential and grant privileges to APNs. After that, the responsibility for acquiring new competencies lies with the individual APN and employing agency. When an APN or agency recognizes that patients would receive better care if the APN would perform a new procedure, an agreement should be reached regarding exactly which new procedure the APN will perform, the conditions under which the procedure will be done, how the APN will acquire the necessary skill, and how supervision will be provided during the learning period. The APN must also be aware that refinement of the technical component is only a piece of the procedure. He or she must also understand indications, contraindications, complications, and consequences of performing the procedures (Hravnak, Tuite, & Baldisseri, 2005). Documented evidence that formal training has occurred is required for regulatory purposes.

The types of skills nurses have performed have evolved over time. For example, it used to be within the physician's scope of practice (and outside the nurse's) to measure blood pressure and administer chemotherapy. With the advent of the APN role, APNs have acquired new performance skills when it made sense within their role and for the comfort, convenience, and satisfaction of patients. It is key for APNs to be cognizant of the scope of their role, regulatory requirements of the states, and the reasonableness of acquiring the skill.

Advanced Physical Assessment

Discussion continues about what actually constitutes advanced physical assessment in the differentiation between the basic RN and APN practice. In one survey, 99 APNs, physician assistants (PAs), and their corresponding preceptor physicians were asked to rank the importance of 87 competencies as an advanced skill (Davidson, Bennett, Hamera, et al., 2004). All skills were ranked fairly high as being necessary for advanced practice care. Skills ranked highest as advanced skills were cardiac assessments, such as rhythm interpretation, and women's health skills, such as gynecologic and breast examinations. Competencies such as head, neck, and throat and skin assessment skills were rated lower on the advanced skill priority scale. The authors reported that higher rated skills appeared to need more use of clinical judgment to interpret or differentially diagnose when compared with lower rated skills, which tended to be more demonstration or technical skills.

Another component of advanced assessment is the use of evidence in assessing and formatting a diagnosis (Munro, 2004). APNs should be skilled at understanding and using the concepts of sensitivity, specificity, and the kappa statistic to differentiate the likelihood of presence or absence of disease based on physical signs and the reliability of that finding. The increased use of technology does not preclude the importance of the physical assessment in reaching an accurate diagnosis (Munro, 2004).

Patient Education

Patient education is a central and well-documented function of all nurses in any setting, and evidence of its effectiveness has been well established (Redman, 2004). Teaching and counseling are significant clinical activities in nurse-midwifery (Holland & Holland, 2007) and CNS practice (Parry et al., 2006). There are several examples of the role of nurse practitioners in patient education to promote adherence to treatment regimens and provide health care information (Lerret & Stendahl, 2011; Madsen, Craig, & Kuban, 2009; Mao & Anastasi, 2010; McAfee, 2012). A study of NP students revealed that many of their interventions were also directed toward education. Of 3733 patient visits, Knowledge Deficit was one of the top four nursing diagnoses made by NP students (O'Connor, Hameister, & Kershaw, 2000). Using the Nursing Interventions Classification (NIC) system, O'Connor and colleagues (2000) also found that patient education was one of the top four intervention classifications used by NP students. APNs must understand the basic principles of patient education and the specific educational needs of their clinical populations. APNs must be aware of the research in their specialties and be responsible for knowing the theoretical and scientific bases for patient teaching and coaching in their specialties and practice settings.

Students can develop competence by developing and implementing patient education. For example, a student could negotiate with a preceptor to colead a self-management group for patients with a chronic condition, using motivational interviewing and other chronic disease management strategies. Other activities could include the following: developing limited literacy tools or evaluating existing patient education materials with regard to the appropriateness of content and health literacy level (Quirk, 2000); assessing the cost-effectiveness of a patient education initiative (Welch, Fisher, & Dayhoff, 2002); and evaluating the reliability and appropriateness of health information on the Internet (Clark & Gomez, 2001). The Internet is a resource used by many health care consumers. Students should know the health information resources likely to be used by their patient populations and be able to advise patients on those that are reliable and regularly updated.

Assessment of functional health literacy must be done sensitively. Years of education completed may not be an adequate indicator of reading and computational literacy. In addition, people with higher levels of education who experience a new diagnosis or other stresses may be unable to process complex information and consequently may benefit from the use of limited literacy materials (Stableford & Mettger, 2007). A variety of tools are available to assist clinicians in assessing patient literacy (Pawlak, 2005; Quirk, 2000). APNs involved in developing programmatic approaches to patient education must ascertain that materials are appropriate to the literacy level of participants in educational programs. Educational materials should use plain language—that is, text that exemplifies clear communication (National Institutes of Health, 2012; Stableford & Mettger, 2007). The term *plain language* is also used to describe the approach to developing such materials: "evidence-based standards are used in structuring, writing and designing [materials] to create reading ease" (Stableford & Mettger, 2007, p. 75). Plain language text is accessible, engaging, and reader-friendly. Stableford and Mettger noted that reading levels alone are insufficient to determine whether text was prepared using plain language principles. They also asserted that addressing health literacy effectively will mitigate many of the problems that are the focus of national initiatives, including reducing health disparities and improving quality and safety. Readers are encouraged to read the Stableford and Mettger article (2007) to gain an understanding of the clinical and policy issues associated with health illiteracy, and to learn more about barriers to and strategies for improving the quality and usefulness of patient educational materials.

Numerous resources exist to help APNs improve their abilities to assess health literacy and prepare useful, readable instructional materials. The Harvard School of Public Health (2010) site is particularly useful; it includes slides documenting the problem of health literacy and its effects on health, as well as links to numerous resources. As APNs work to improve the quality of educational materials for patients with limited literacy, they may encounter resistance to simplifying language and educational tools (Stableford & Mettger, 2007); therefore, slides and other resources that document the extent and impact of health illiteracy may be useful.

Adverse Events and Performance Errors

Since the publication of the IOM's report "To Err is Human," medical errors have been prominent in the public eye, as well as a focus of reform for health care institutions (IOM, 2000). Ideally, institutions and care providers should focus on improving the reliability of complicated systems to prevent failures or quickly identify, redesign, and rectify failures that do occur. Improving reliability ensures that care is consistently and appropriately provided. Traditionally, institutions and providers have been reluctant to be forthcoming with patients when errors or near misses have occurred. That stance is slowly changing with the movement toward increasing transparency in care and a focus on addressing system dysfunction to improve patient safety. In 2002, the National Quality Forum (NQF) first identified a list of adverse medical events that health care systems should work to prevent and publicly report when they occur to encourage public access to information about health care performance (NQF, 2008). This list was updated in 2006 and 2011. The following are categorized (29 total events): surgical or invasive procedure events, product or device events, patient protection events, care management events, environmental events, radiologic events, and potential criminal events (NQF, 2011). The Centers for Medicare and Medicaid Services (CMS) is now

denying payment for some of these publicly reported events and it is anticipated that additional events will continue to be identified for denial of payment. There are increasing resources available in clinics and health care settings to try to prevent adverse events, including computer-generated alerts for ordering medications and laboratory tests, interdisciplinary colleagues, such as pharmacists and dietitians, electronic resources to access and verify recommendations and practice guidelines, appropriate steps in patient identification, and optimal team communication techniques (White, 2012). It is critical that APNs consistently use them and be involved in decisions related to their development.

These changes are relevant to APNs as it relates to their direct care role and the potential to be involved in "never," near miss, or medical error situations. It would be to the APN's advantage to be cognizant of the institution's or practice group's policies related to appropriate actions when errors occur and what is required to be reported publicly based on federal and state regulations. APNs may find themselves involved in these situations as a result of the many issues discussed, such as thinking errors and time pressures. APNs involved as caregivers in these types of events should anticipate the need to inform the patient and family readily of the event. Honest open communication and sensitivity will help preserve trust and support ongoing care, and may reduce emotional trauma (Gallagher, Waterman, Ebers, et al., 2003; Vincent, 2003). Medical research has shown that patients expect to be told of medical errors and are more likely to consider legal recourse if the physician has withheld information about the error (Witman, Park, & Hardin, 1996).

A consensus group of Harvard hospitals (Massachusetts Coalition for the Prevention of Medical Errors, 2006) has recommended four steps for communicating about adverse events:

1. Tell the patient what happened immediately, but leave details of how and why for later when a thorough review has occurred.
2. Take responsibility for the incident.
3. Apologize and communicate remorse.
4. Inform the patient and family what will be done to prevent similar events.

APNs should take advantage of training and educational opportunities on how to communicate bad news and ways to promote safety. In addition, APNs involved in incidents should anticipate the need for their own emotional support during this time.

Use of Reflective Practice

To continually grow and develop, APNs must be reflective practitioners. APNs may be familiar with multiple methods of learning—didactic, small group projects, clinical experiences with preceptors—but may be less familiar with this method of learning, which will be useful to them throughout their careers. Reflective practice is a way to take the experiences a practitioner has (positive or negative) and explore them for the purpose of eliciting meaning, critically analyzing, and synthesizing and using learning to improve practice (Atkins & Murphy, 1995; Kumar, 2011; Schön, 1992). The goal is to turn experience into personal knowledge by seeking insights that are not available with superficial recall (Atkins & Murphy, 1995; Kumar, 2011; Rolfe, 1997; Schön, 1992). Research findings have shown that reflective practice by nurses is a valuable learning method, may increase self-confidence as a practitioner, and may promote accountability (Astor, Jefferson, & Humphrys, 1998; Davies, 1995; Wong et al., 1997).

Forms of clinical supervision are frequently used in mental health nursing. Barron and White (2009) have described clinical supervision in this realm as a relationship between a more experienced and more novice nurse in which the expected outcome is to assist the less-experienced nurse in the professional development of knowledge, skills, and autonomy. In these cases, clinical supervision may be used as a debriefing with a trusted and more experienced colleague of a situation that has been complex, intense, or characterized by uncertainty.

Reflection is not just a retrospective activity; it may occur prospectively or concurrently (Atkins & Murphy, 1995) while providing care. Retrospective reflection occurs when an APN takes the opportunity to consider how a situation could have been handled differently. Prospective reflection may occur when an APN prepares to enter a difficult or uncertain clinical situation; one draws on experience and scientific knowledge to plan an approach and anticipates possible reactions or outcomes. Reflection can also occur concurrently. Concurrent reflection is termed *reflection-in-action* and can promote flexibility and adaptation of interventions to suit the situation. Reflection-in-action may be the goal of a more expert practitioner who has honed the skill of reflection (Benner et al., 1999). Although Benner's work was done with bedside staff nurses, it may be applicable to APNs as well, as research by Bryzycznski and Fenton suggested (see Chapter 2). Several models have been proposed to gain expertise in reflective practice (Atkins & Murphy, 1995; Brubakken, Grant, Johnson, et al., 2011; Johns, 2000; Kim, 1999) although they use similar processes to guide the practitioner through the reflective process. The model Spross proposed (see Chapter 8) explains expert coaching as a process that relies on self-reflection to integrate technical competencies, clinical competencies, and interpersonal competencies fully; it may apply equally to the direct care competency. Deliberate self-reflection allows the APN to anticipate alternative possibilities, remain flexible in challenging and changing situations, and strategically integrate the results of self-reflection with best practices to match interventions to patient and family needs.

Strengthening skills in self-reflection can be done in a number of ways for the APN—through solitary self-evaluation, with a supervisor or teacher, or in small groups of supportive colleagues. With experience, the APN may be asked to be the mentor in guiding others through a self-reflective process. Regardless of which model is used for reflection, the following guidelines can be considered:

- If reflection occurs in a small group, participants must feel safe to express thoughts, emotions, and thinking processes without fear of judgment.
- Practitioners need to gain self-awareness of personal values, beliefs, and behaviors.
- Practitioners need to develop the skills to articulate a situation with objective and subjective details.
- Critical debriefing and analysis are used to identify practitioner goals in the situation, extent of knowledge that was present or missing, feelings on the part of the practitioner and patient, consequences of actions, and which alternative options existed.
- Knowledge gained through this process can be integrated with current knowledge to change interventions in a current situation or improve approaches in future situations.
- Evaluation of this reflective process supports masterful practice and creates lasting improvements in practice.

There are several barriers to using reflection in daily practice. Lack of time may result in care and interventions becoming routine. The use of a reflective practice process will require dedicated time. If not thoughtfully arranged, it may seem to be extraneous and a "nice thing to do" rather than a necessary component to the APN role. Acknowledging that we do not always know the right answer can be difficult for an APN who is trying to establish a practice and role. In addition, reflection may elicit emotions that may be painful or difficult to deal with. It takes experience and skill to use reflection, which is particularly important when an APN is very involved in a situation. Novice APNs may need guidance in performing reflection to assist in ascertaining meaning and making connections that otherwise might be missed (Johns, 2000). Finally, some may see reflective practice discussions as official surveillance when supervisors are involved, and depending on the context (Clouder & Sellars, 2004). However, when reflective thinking is developed and incorporated into one's practice, it can be a means to demonstrate professional accountability for practice and a source of lifelong learning (Clouder & Sellars, 2004). Knowledge from reflection informs future clinical decision making, especially in those situations for which no benchmarks or best practice guidelines exist.

Use of Evidence as a Guide to Practice

An important form of knowledge that must be brought to bear on clinical decision making, for individuals and for populations, is the ever-increasing volume of evidence. For the nursing profession, the use of evidence as a basis for practice is more than the latest trend. The profession has been intensively exploring and considering issues regarding the use of research since the early 1970s. Historically, CNSs have led efforts in many agencies to move toward research-based practice (DePalma, 2004; Hanson & Ashley, 1994; Hickey, 1990; Mackay, 1998; Stetler, Batista, Vernale-Hannon, et al., 1995). They have brought research findings to the attention of the nursing staff and interdisciplinary teams and worked to develop the research appraisal skills of nursing staffs. The profession, agencies, and APNs themselves view evidence-based practice skills as central to APNs' research competency and as a more appropriate expectation of APNs than the conduct of the research itself (see Chapter 10).

Identifying and locating research findings is becoming easier with improved technology and categorization. However, clinicians often do not have sufficient experience in the use of various search engines available to retrieve information from databases. Research has shown that clinicians are not skilled in writing a researchable question that is clearly articulated or in searching for evidence (Meats, Brassey, Heneghan, et al., 2007). APNs could benefit from education on simple tools that could greatly increase the efficiency of their searches. APNs in all settings engaging in an evidence-based practice project would be well served by developing a relationship with a health care librarian who can assist with searches, save time, and prevent the omission of relevant evidence.

Evidence can be used in a variety of ways. Differentiating between research-sensitive practice, research-based practice, and evidence-based practice provides a useful way of thinking about how APNs can incorporate evidence into their practices.

Evidence-Based Practice

It would be ideal to have all health care delivery based on research. However, in reality, there frequently may be no research on which to base decisions. Sackett (1998) has defined evidence-based practice as the explicit and judicious integration of best evidence with clinical expertise and patient values. Using only external evidence to make practice decisions is as unacceptable as using only individual clinical expertise.

Usually, when APNs are involved in designing care for a population of patients, all forms of objective evidence should be used, including quality improvement data, data from internal databases, expert opinion panels, consensus statements, national guidelines data from benchmarking partners, and data from state and national databases (e.g., the CDC). Agency-specific information, collected to pinpoint the nature of a problem, is particularly useful evidence that should be combined with the more general knowledge gained from research evidence (Brown, 2001; see Chapter 10).

The process and extent of quality improvement (QI) has advanced significantly in the past few years with APNs as QI leaders in their health care settings. Use of improved QI methods and tools and a national focus on the need to make significant changes in the care of patients provides nurses with the opportunity to identify patient care issues, evaluate the problem, and implement potential solutions in a more rapid fashion than ever before. APNs can use QI methods such as the plan-do-study-act (PDSA) process and tools (Institute for Health care Improvement [IHI], 2011b) and lean principles (IHI, 2011a) to lead and facilitate teams in improving care. Although QI data does not have broad generalizability and the rigor of official research, it can provide evidence for significant improvements that the APN can implement on a daily local basis.

Research-sensitive practice is practice in which the individual clinician brings research findings to bear on practice in an unstructured way. To do this, an APN would do the following: (1) read primary research reports and summaries of research findings on a regular basis; (2) informally evaluate the soundness of the methods; and (3) adjust or fine-tune his or her own practice on the basis of credible findings. This is the form of research use in which every professional nurse should engage. It is part of staying abreast of new knowledge in one's area of clinical practice.

Research-sensitive practice could take the form of setting time aside to scan clinical journals systematically for reports relevant to one's clinical specialty. APNs can subscribe to list serves, such as those from the Agency for Healthcare Research and Quality (AHRQ), which send timely summaries of emerging evidence and new national guidelines. Alternatively, an APN could join or form a multidisciplinary group that meets monthly to discuss several research reports on topics of mutual interest. Some APNs keep a small notebook in which to jot down clinical issues and questions about which they are uncertain.

Then they can make the most efficient use of library time to explore the evidence related to the questions of interest.

Evidence-based practice is a more systematic, rigorous, and precise way of translating research findings into practice. The evidence based practice process is used in an organization to design a standard of care for a population of patients. This process is more formal because evidence-based care will be widely used as a guide to care; therefore, the scientific conclusions on which it is based must be as free of bias and error as possible. In general terms, the process involves four steps: (1) locating, evaluating, and summarizing the science; (2) translating the science into clinical recommendations; (3) strategically implementing the recommendations; and (4) measuring and reporting its impact. The recommendations may take the form of a clinical practice guideline, decision algorithm, clinical protocol, the components of a clinical program, or change in policies or procedures.

Clinical Guidelines

Evidence-based clinical practice guidelines can be useful decision making and planning aids for clinicians. Many guidelines have been developed in close association with providers, are based on systematic and thorough reviews of research evidence, and have attained a balance between optimal care and economic reality. However, contractors also use clinical guidelines to ensure quality, limit variation of care, and control resource use. Guidelines should be based on research evidence that is evaluated and summarized by a credible panel, inside or outside the system, to ensure that the guidelines serve to incorporate science into practice and contain costs. Providers involved in the care of patients with the condition that the guideline addresses should have the opportunity to adapt guidelines produced by others. Ideally, clinicians should review proposed guidelines and negotiate problematic recommendations in advance to avoid situations in which the care of the individual becomes the focus of negotiation. In addition, clinicians should acknowledge that although the guidelines may serve most patients well, some patients will require treatment and interventions not recommended in the guidelines. An explicit method for advocating for individual needs should be available to clinicians. Several national groups have evaluated evidence and posted their recommendations for population use. Guidelines can be found through organizations such as the National Guideline Clearinghouse (www.guideline.gov), AHRQ (www.ahrq.gov), and professional organizations such as the American Heart Association. Clinicians should review published guidelines carefully and be familiar with the grading criteria each organization uses to grade the strength of the evidence used to make care recommendations. It is important that APNs be part of the teams that are developing new guidelines for practice.

Theory-Based Practice

The preceding discussion of research-based practice recognizes how research evidence informs practice but ignores the role of theory. APNs are becoming comfortable with the idea of research evidence as a guide to practice, yet the idea of theory-based practice is less familiar. It should not be because, contrary to common perception, theory can be a practical tool. Theory often brings together research findings in a way that helps practice be more purposeful, systematic, and comprehensive.

In the past, most discussions of theory-based practice addressed the use of conceptual models of nursing to guide care (Bonamy, Schultz, Graham, et al., 1995; Hawkins, Thibodeau, Utley-Smith, et al., 1993; Laschinger & Duff, 1991; Sappington & Kelley, 1996). However, more recently, emphasis has shifted to middle-range theories, which guide practice more specifically. Middle-range theories typically address a particular patient experience (e.g., living with rheumatoid arthritis) or problem (e.g., managing chronic pain); thus, their range of applicability is relatively narrow. However, this narrow range allows them to be developed to address specific issues encountered in clinical practice. Schwartz-Barcott and associates (2002) have made a strong case for developing theories by using fieldwork so that the theories will be more closely aligned to the realities that practicing nurses encounter. Another approach to developing theories that are more specific to clinical situations is to generate a middle-range theory from one of the broader conceptual models. For example, Whittemore and Roy (2002) developed a middle-range theory describing adaptation to diabetes mellitus based on the concepts and theoretical statements of the broader Roy Adaptation Model. Middle-range theories have a structure of ideas and concepts that are more focused than general nursing theories and are more directly applicable to nursing practice (Smith, 2008).

Smith and Liehr (2008) have delineated middle-range theories that have the potential for impact on clinical nursing practice. The list in Box 7-8 provides a sampling of the middle-range theories currently available to practicing nurses and the reader can see that the topics of the theories are substantively specific, although some are more specific than others. An APN in a particular field may find that only one or two of these theories are applicable to her or his area of practice. However, as middle-range theories are developed for other topics, APNs will be able to use several of these types of theories to guide different aspects of practice.

Diverse Approaches to Health and Illness Management

APNs' holistic approach to care and their commitment to using evidence as a basis for care contribute to how they help patients. Generally, APNs use a variety of interventions to effect change in the health status or quality of life of an individual or family and tailor their recommendations, approaches, and treatment to individual patients. Interpersonal interventions that are psychosocial in nature are frequently termed *support interventions*. Support interventions are somewhat distinct from educational interventions, which are informational in nature. Coaching uses a combination of support and educational strategies (see Chapter 8). There are also discrete physical actions, which are frequently categorized as nonpharmacologic and pharmacological interventions. These distinctions are arbitrary because good clinicians probably craft interventions that are a combination of the various types as they seek to alleviate, prevent, or manage specific physical symptoms, conditions, or problems.

Interpersonal Interventions

Support is not a discrete intervention; it is a composite of interpersonal interventions based on the patient's unique psychological and informational needs. Supportive interpersonal interventions include providing reassurance, giving information, coaching, affirming, providing anticipatory guidance, guiding decision making, listening actively, expressing understanding, and being fully present. Each of these interventions can be described in terms of the circumstances for which it is indicated. For example, reassurance is indicated when a patient is experiencing uncertainty, distress, or lack of confidence; active listening is indicated when a patient has a strong need to tell his or her story. The actions that constitute these interventions are not mutually exclusive. For example, giving factual information can be reassuring, instructional, guiding, or all of these things at the same time.

In practice, these interpersonal interventions are blended and APNs may not be consciously aware of when they are doing one and when they are doing another. This is as it should be. APNs have no need to think "Now I'm doing active listening; now I'm going to do anticipatory guidance." Instead, APNs interact with patients in ways that intermingle the conceptually separate interventions. This crafting of support evolves as the APN talks with patients, infers their worries, fears, and concerns and, without a great deal of conscious thought, acts to alleviate their distress. A patient may experience the interaction as just a good talk with the APN or as a feeling of being understood. However, support is a complex nursing intervention that is strategically crafted and purposefully administered, and that often makes a difference in how the patient feels and acts. See Exemplar 7-2.

Therapeutic Interventions

The decision about whether to treat can be difficult because the practitioner is faced with several probabilities that do not all lead to the same decision. Moreover, there is often pressure from patients to do something. When deciding whether and how to treat patients, clinicians consider the following five types of information:

- The degree of certainty about the diagnosis, condition, or symptom
- What is known about the effectiveness of the various treatment alternatives
- What is known about the risks of the treatment alternatives
- The clinician's comfort with a particular treatment or intervention
- The patient's preference for a certain type of treatment or management

The most clear-cut situation is when the condition is definitely present, a particular treatment is known to be highly effective, the treatment can be expected to be low in risk for the particular patient, and the clinician and patient are comfortable with the treatment. Unfortunately, many (probably most) therapeutic decisions are not so clear-cut. In these cases, the weight of factors in support of a particular treatment and the weight of those against treatment or in support of another treatment are almost equal.

The treatment and management interventions that APNs perform include a wide variety of self-care modalities and low-tech, nonpharmacologic modalities (Day & Horton-Deutsch, 2004; Fowler, 2006; Hiltunen et al., 2005; Riegel et al., 2006). In a study of 10 collaborative pairs of physicians and NPs, NPs and physicians were

EXEMPLAR 7-2   **An Interpersonal Intervention***

JE is a certified nurse midwife in a joint CNM-OB/GYN practice model. The seven CNMs have an independent nurse-midwife patient panel. Consultants for the CNM practice are with the seven OB/GYNs in the shared clinical office space. Patients have access to both services at the initiation of care.

Patient care is coordinated and maintained in the respective patient panels. There is a formal process for patients to be seen by the alternative groups in the practice because patients are not allowed to alternate between CNM and OB/GYN provider patient panels. Transfers of care for patients who wish to have CNM care and are considered low risk are accepted in the same manner as transfers to the OB/GYNs of patients who develop high-risk complications outside the scope of the CNM practice.

JE has an appointment to see a couple in their early 30s who are expecting their first child. In this group CNM practice, he has met Jan and Steve once previously in this pregnancy. They are very excited about the upcoming birth because they are now 37 weeks and 5 days pregnant. Jan and Steve have prepared themselves with childbirth education classes and have hired a doula to assist them in the birthing process.

JE reviews the record and notes that Jan has had no complications during this pregnancy. Accurate dating has been established by the use of an early ultrasound (US), which corresponds with Jan's last menstrual period and estimated due date. Vital signs today are normal and the patient voiced no concerns to the medical assistant who did the initial intake for this routine, scheduled prenatal visit.

JE interviews Jan, who reports she feels well and has no concerns. Jan states that she has had more issues becoming comfortable—at night with increased hip pain, having to get up and urinate frequently, with the baby moving, and with itching. JE asks more about the itching and Jan relates that she has been noticing it more in the last few weeks but hadn't mentioned it before. She had looked up itching in pregnancy on the Internet and discussed it with her doula, who told her that this itching (pruritic urticarial papules and plaques of pregnancy [PUPPs]) seems pretty common in pregnancy. JE asked Jan more questions about the itching, who states that it is primarily on the palms of her hands and soles of her feet and only scratching seems to help. Steve relates it is getting so bad lately it's like "watching a dog with an unrelenting scratch." Jan states that she has tried Benadryl a couple of times but it didn't help.

JE performs a physical examination, which reveals some minor stretch marks but no notable trunk rash, as would be expected with PUPPs. There are some excoriated marks on Jan's palms because she has been rubbing her hands during the interview.

JE recognizes that this does not appear to be a typical PUPP presentation and believes that the itching may be a symptom of intrahepatic cholestasis of pregnancy (ICP), a potentially serious complication. JE relays his thoughts to Jan and Steve and tells them that his is going to order additional blood tests. He orders a complete blood count (CBC), liver function tests (LFTs) and total bile acid tests.

The laboratory results reveal a normal CBC but an elevated total bile acid level of 27.6 μmol/liter (normal range, 0 to 7.0 μmol/liter) and alanine aminotransferase (ALT) level of 104 IU/liter (normal range, 0 to 50 IU/liter). These results confirm that the itching is related to ICP, which puts Jan at an increased risk of intrauterine fetal demise (IUFD). With confirmation laboratory data and a term pregnancy, JE calls Jan and informs her of the diagnosis and the need for induction of labor because of the increased risk of IUFD. She is upset and wants to have a direct conversation in the clinic to discuss if induction is really necessary.

JE sees Jan and Steve in the clinic and provides answers to their many questions about ICP. They want to discuss alternatives to induction because they had planned for a low-intervention, spontaneous labor and delivery. JE reviews with the couple that ICP is associated with a substantial risk of IUFD. This risk increases as a pregnancy approaches term. He explains that induction is considered the best option with a term pregnancy because routine antepartum testing such as US or electronic fetal monitoring (EFM) are used to evaluate for a placental insufficiency disease process and do not have the specificity to predict an increased risk of IUFD in ICP. JE also explains that the elevated bile acids in the amniotic fluid can cause the fetus to experience a sudden cardiac death because of effects on the umbilical artery and/or the electrical activity in the fetal heart. JE reviews other treatment options with the couple. Using ursodiol has been effective at decreasing the level of bile acids in the maternal system in preterm pregnancies, but its use to extend pregnancies to spontaneous labor is not recommended because the risk for IUFD still remains, even with decreased maternal bile acids at or beyond term. JE also informs Jan that the elevated levels of bile acid are caused by a genetic enzyme deficiency that she has and is not related to anything she did or did not do during her pregnancy.

Jan is crying out of fear and disappointment. JE reviews the couple's birth plan with them, pointing out that the desires they had expressed in their birth plan do not have to be revised at this time because of the need for induction. Although constant EFM with induction is required, the use of telemetry will not affect Jan's movement while she is in labor, nor will the use of hydrotherapy as an alternative to pharmaceutical pain management.

Jan and Steve agree with the plan of induction after this consultation and arrive at the hospital with their doula, Rita. After the initiation of induction, JE uses this early labor period to discuss and educate Rita privately on the rationale for induction and the pathophysiology of ICP. JE recognizes that educating Rita is important

so she can use this information with her future clients. JE also knows that as a member of a childbirth cooperative group, Rita is in a place to inform and instruct her doula peers that the subjective signs of increased itching of the palms of the hands and soles of the feet can be indicative of ICP, and they can advise future clients of doulas to notify their health care providers about these findings.

Emily is born to Jan and Steve at 7 pounds, 5 ounces, with an 8/9 Apgar score via normal spontaneous vaginal delivery after a 16-hour labor and delivery hospitalization for induction with prostaglandins and pitocin. Jan's maternal itching is resolved and total bile acid and liver function test results are returning to normal 48 hours postpartum. Baby and mother are discharged, with no additional follow-up needed for ICP, except for the increased risk of recurrence in future pregnancies.

*The author gratefully acknowledges John Eads, CNM, for use of his exemplar.

---

identical in their final recommendations related to medication management, although the processes used to reach decisions were different (Flesner & Clawson, 1998). The NPs elicited more information about the context of the patients' lives and available resources and collaborated with patients more frequently to work out the details of implementing the management plans.

When prescribing or recommending medications, APNs consider the patient's financial status, patient's previous experience with similar medications, ease of taking the medication, how many other medications the person is taking, how often the medications must be taken, the side effect profiles of the drugs being considered, and potential drug and disease interactions. A systematic review of nurses as prescribers has shown that APNs tend to prescribe similar or lower total numbers of medications overall compared with physicians, clinical parameters are the same or better for patients treated by prescribing APNs, and quality of care is similar or better, with similar or improved patient satisfaction (Van Ruth, Mistiaen, & Francke, 2008).

As noted, considerable evidence indicates that APNs use a broad range of interventions, with substantial reliance on self-care and low-tech interventions. Surveillance, teaching, guidance, counseling, and case management are interventions used more often than procedural interventions (Brooten et al., 2003). The frequency with which the various categories of interventions are used varies moderately with patient populations. Several models have been developed for classifying nursing interventions, including

the nursing interventions classification–nursing outcomes classification (NIC-NOC), nursing interventions classification project (Bulechek & McCloskey, 1999), Omaha classification system, and home health care classification, which are on the way to capturing the full range of treatments and interventions that nurses use (Henry, Holzemer, Randell, et al., 1997). The repertoire of interventions used by individual APNs clearly depends on the problems experienced by the population of patients with whom they work. ACNPs, CNMs, CRNAs, and CNSs use repertoires of therapeutic interventions different from those used by APNs who provide primary care. The methods of practice that an individual APN uses also depend on the customs of colleagues, practice setting, and reimbursement system. Nevertheless, APNs must make an effort to extend and refine their repertoire constantly beyond the interventions learned during graduate education.

Individualized Interventions

One goal of treatment decision making is to choose from among several possible interventions and to use the one that will have the highest probability of achieving the outcomes the patient most desires. Usually, that probability is increased by particularizing the treatment or action to the individual patient (Benner et al., 1996, p. 24). Particularizing requires that the recommendation or action take the following into account:

- Acceptability of the treatment to the patient
- What has worked for the patient in the past
- Patient's motivation and ability to use or follow the treatment (self-care)
- Likelihood that the patient will continue to use the treatment, even if side effects are experienced
- Financial burden of the treatment
- Health literacy of the patient

Nursing has always believed that individualizing nursing care—that is, tailoring care to the unique characteristics of the person and his or her situation—produces the best patient outcomes. In contrast, standardization of care and control of wide variation are important to quality control and cost containment. Clearly, a blending of the two perspectives is required to produce care that is effective for an individual and congruent with available resources. This can be accomplished by adopting evidence-based standards and guidelines to provide a framework for care while acknowledging that at the point of care (i.e., in the patient-provider interface), interventions and management may need to be tailored to reflect the patient's unique situation and needs (Brown, 2001).

Unfortunately, research support for the effectiveness of individualized interventions in general is not as strong as most APNs would like. The extent to which the equivocal nature of the evidence is a function of methodologic difficulties in studying individualized interventions is unknown. Part of the difficulty stems from the various ways in which health messages may be customized—personalized, targeted, tailored, and individualized (Ryan & Lauver, 2002). An integrative research review of 20 studies in which interventions with varying degrees of customization to the individual were delivered has revealed that better patient outcomes were achieved with tailored interventions in only 50% of the studies as compared with standard interventions (Ryan & Lauver, 2002). The authors of the review proposed that another reason for the modest support for the efficacy of customized interventions is that patients with certain characteristics are more affected by these interventions than others; such uneven effects across subgroups would offset each other and present an appearance of little or no benefit. Even when a tailored intervention does not result in changed behavior or produce better patient outcomes, it may have other benefits. An example of this collateral gain was found in a study of 43 women with gynecologic cancer (Ward, Donovan, Owen, et al., 2000). The individualized sensory and coping message for pain management intervention had no demonstrable effect on analgesic use, pain intensity scores, or pain interference with life, but the women who received the individualized intervention reported that it contained useful information that helped them to feel more comfortable taking pain medication and to discuss pain more openly with a physician or nurse.

Many patients use computers to access information and educate themselves about their health and diseases. Patients may actually come to appointments knowing more about their disease than the APN does (McMullan, 2006). Although this can be disconcerting, it is important to recognize this as information-seeking behavior and capitalize on the opportunity to work with the patients to help them gain the information they need (Cutilli, 2006). Patients vary widely in terms of how much information they want and how they want it presented. Allowing them to make choices about how and what they learn should help prevent content overload and enhance the relevancy of the information given, resulting in better retention and application. Along similar lines, computer-based programs have been developed to counsel patients faced with major treatment decisions (Cherkin et al., 2002; Frosch, Kaplan, & Felitti, 2001; Morgan et al., 2000). Programs can be designed to allow patients to acquire information that is most important to them and to help them sort out their values, priorities, and preferences in their specific situation. It is apparent that computer-based learning and decision making tools will be more acceptable to some groups of patients than others.

It will be important for APNs to help consumers differentiate among websites that are reputable and offer valid information and those that may not have solid evidence. The Internet is now used for patients with similar or rare diseases to connect with each other as support in a way that might never have been possible before the advent and ease of use of the Internet. APNs can also direct patients to state health department websites as excellent sites for accessing helpful information, such as immunization schedules, tobacco cessation tools, and information on diabetes care, sexually transmitted diseases, tuberculosis, and newborn screening (Alpi, 2005).

Complementary and Alternative Medicine

The extent of public use of complementary and alternative medicine (CAM) was well documented in the 1990s by Eisenberg and colleagues when they reported that approximately 33% of Americans were using at least one unconventional therapy; this was supported in further studies (Eisenberg et al., 1993, 1998; Ni, Simile, & Hardy, 2002). This use has resulted in the establishment of the National Center for Complementary and Alternative Medicine in the National Institutes of Health (NIH). Its use in certain ethnic groups is often higher than the national average. Many patients use alternative therapies in conjunction with conventional medical services; hence, these are also termed *integrative therapies*.

The effectiveness and safety of alternative and complementary therapies vary widely. Some have been scientifically studied (e.g., relaxation, guided imagery, glucosamine and chondroitin for osteoarthritis), whereas others have not been studied at all. Of concern is that some may interact with other medications that the patient is receiving (Norred, 2002; Scott & Elmer, 2002). Another issue specific to dietary supplements and herb therapy is the lack of control over ingredients (Barnes, 2003; Tesch, 2002). Providers are caught between the desire of patients to use alternative therapies and reservations about their safety, often in the face of insufficient scientific evidence.

APNs are incorporating complementary and alternative treatments into their practices in a variety of ways, albeit with some caution (Allaire, Moos, & Wells, 2000; Hayes & Alexander, 2000; Sohn & Loveland Cook, 2002; Thomas, 2003). APNs have expressed interest in being able to provide CAM for patients, even if it means expanding their scope of practice (Patterson, Kaczorowski, Arthur, et al., 2003). They are increasing their engagement in these therapies, are more willing to ask patients about CAM practices, and are counseling patients on appropriate use. Many APNs report a need to increase their own knowledge about CAM to incorporate it fully into care. An interim solution to this situation may be for an APN to consider developing a collaborative relationship with an expert CAM provider. In summary, because patients are using CAM, APNs seem to believe it is better that they do so with provider guidance and awareness.

Clinical Prevention

Population-Based Data to Inform Practice

The hallmark of the APN role that differentiates it from other advanced nursing roles is the direct care that the APN provides in the patient interface. Although this is a key component of the role, it is expected that APNs also use a clinical prevention and population health focus (AACN, 2006). Clinical prevention refers to the health promotion and risk reduction components of individual health care that are learned as a result of population data. APNs are considered to be nursing leaders in achieving national health goals for individuals and populations. Interventions outlined in the Healthy People 2020 campaign (U.S. Department of Health and Human Services, 2010) can frequently be instituted or recommended by APNs, regardless of their roles or settings. Monitoring for current vaccinations, advocating for tobacco cessation with patients, assisting in healthy diets, and identifying opportunities for increasing physical activity are all population-identified behaviors that can be implemented at the individual level. These interventions are key to addressing the increasing disease rates of diabetes, obesity,

lung cancer, and asthma. The Healthy People 2020 website (http://www.healthypeople.gov/2020) is a great resource for APNs and patients to access basic health care information. In addition, APNs should be cognizant of the ever-changing information related to infectious diseases and emergency preparedness based on today's global health care environment.

APNs can use population trends to inform direct care and improve the assessments and interventions used at the direct care interface. Population data are frequently based on the diseases and conditions prevalent in the geographic setting in which the APN practices, such as the following:

- Monitoring for metabolic syndrome in the southeast United States
- Assessing for asthma in Virginia
- Surveillance for neurologic disorders in Minnesota
- Cognizance of altitude-based disorders in mountain states
- High suspicion for tuberculosis in homeless patients with pulmonary symptoms who live in densely populated urban settings

Aggregated, individual clinical outcomes are also useful for the evaluation of program and practice effectiveness. By requiring that care be administered and individual outcomes be documented in standardized ways, the health care system can conduct programmatic evaluations of clinical outcomes. Population-based evaluations can also be used by APNs to evaluate and improve the care they provide. Such evaluations can help answer questions such as the following:

- "Is the specific care I (we) provide patients the best way of managing their health or illness?"
- "Are my (our) patients doing as well as similar patients who are cared for by other providers?"

Conducting such an evaluation involves the following: (1) identifying groups of patients (i.e., populations) who have high costs of care, less than optimal outcomes, or both; (2) monitoring and analyzing variances in outcomes and costs; (3) examining processes of care to determine how management of the condition could be improved; and (4) incorporating management methods found to be effective in research or best practice networks. For example, population data in New Mexico have revealed a high mortality rate from alcoholism, prompting the state to invest more in alcoholism prevention programs and emphasize a sharper clinical focus on substance abuse.

Evaluation of the degree to which desirable outcomes are attained enables health care systems to compare their effectiveness with that of a comparable system or to evaluate the relative effectiveness of a new program or process of care. These types of evaluations and comparisons can lead to the identification of best practice methods at the health care system level. Use of services, readmission rates, complication rates, average total cost per case, and mortality rates are examples of population outcomes used in these types of evaluations and comparisons.

Preventive Services in Primary Care

Health promotion and disease prevention interventions are tools that APNs in primary care regularly use to help people achieve and maintain a high quality of life. These preventive services include the following:

- Counseling regarding personal health practices that can protect a person from disease or promote screening for the presence of disease
- Immunization to prevent specific diseases
- Chemoprevention (e.g., use of aspirin for prevention of cardiovascular events)

Discernment is needed in the use of these interventions because time and effort can be wasted if their use is not based on current scientific knowledge and tailored to the individual person or community. Also, the public is confused regarding many of the preventive recommendations because new research evidence has been unseating long-established recommendations, such as the value of breast self-examination. The U.S. Preventive Services Task Force's "Guide to Clinical Preventive Services" (2010) and the Canadian Task Force on Preventive Health Care (2012) provide specific preventive guidelines for many health conditions. These include valuable summaries of the state of the science for each recommendation; the U.S. guidelines provide cost-effectiveness analyses, which summarize the benefits, harms, and costs of alternative strategies.

An important point made in an earlier version of the "Guide to Clinical Preventive Services" (U.S. Preventive Services Task Force, 1996) is that primary prevention in the form of counseling aimed at changing health-related behavior may be more effective than diagnostic screening and testing. Many healthy people, as well as those who have had a recent health scare, are receptive to—even eager for—information and guidance about how to stay healthy and avoid age-related disabilities. However, other people who engage in one or several unhealthy behaviors can be defensive and resistant to talking about their risks and how behavior changes could reduce risks. Introducing behavior change issues with unreceptive people requires a high level of interpersonal skill and a good sense of timing. An APN must consider that it is possible that no health care provider has previously attempted to discuss the problem (e.g., smoking, lack of exercise, alcohol abuse) with the person, even though signs of a problem have existed for a long time.

Talking about the risks of the current behavior and benefits of the behavior change is not enough. To be effective, counseling regarding these issues should also include a discussion of how the person perceives the burden of changing a personal behavior—that is, what would be lost and what would be required to make the change? The provider must first make the patient feel understood and must elicit how much effort will be required, what would give the individual the confidence to change, and which forms of self-help assistance are acceptable to the individual. Then and only then can a specific recommendation about a strategy or program be made. Theoretical models that can be useful in planning a behavior change program or protocol include the Transtheoretical Model (www.uri.edu/research/cprc/transtheoretical.htm) and the Health Belief Model (www.etr.org/recapp/theories/hbm/index.htm#majorconcepts). Both models include provider strategies for building a person's self-efficacy—confidence in one's ability to take action; see Chapter 8).

Clinicians also have at their disposal a wide array of screening tools, some of which are better with certain populations or age-groups than others. For example, the U.S. Preventive Services Task Force (2010) recommends against routinely screening women older than age 65 for cervical cancer if they have had an adequate recent screening with normal Papanicolaou (Pap) test results and are not otherwise at risk; they also recommend against performing routine Pap tests for women who have had a total hysterectomy as treatment for benign disease. Staying current with the latest screening recommendations in one's area of practice ensures that care is provided in a way that is scientific and cost-effective.

Preventive Services in Hospitals and Home Care

The preventive services provided in inpatient and home care settings are somewhat different from those provided in primary care. Many of the actions and assessments performed on behalf of acutely ill patients are aimed at early detection and prevention of problems related to treatment, disease progression, self-care deficits, or the hospital environment itself. Complications typically result from a complex set of factors, such as inadequate delivery systems or failure to assess patients for risk of complications common to their condition. Nurses assist patients by preventing adverse events and complications, including adverse medication reactions, unexpected physiologic decline, poor communication, pressure ulcers, and death. This function is also termed *surveillance* or *rescuing* (as in rescuing from a bad course of events or death; Aiken, Sochalski, & Lake, 1997). As noted, in five studies of APN interventions with diverse patient groups, surveillance was the predominant APN function (Brooten et al., 2003).

In the home setting, APNs serve as advisors and partners. In addition to assessment and surveillance, coaching and guidance are particularly important. The patient may be new to the role of partner in this setting (Holman & Lorig, 2004). APNs work with patients to prioritize measures that might prevent rehospitalizations. Interventions may include teaching about reportable signs and symptoms, guidance on how to communicate with their providers, and assistance in making connections between behaviors and situations in the home that directly affect health status.

Management of Complex Situations

APNs' direct care often involves the management and coordination of complex situations. Many illustrations of this advanced practice nursing feature may be found in the chapters on specific advanced practice nursing roles (see Chapters 14 through 18). In some settings, APNs have been designated as the providers responsible for coordination of complex follow-up care (Dellasega & Zerbe, 2002) or for education of patients at high risk for complications (Brooten et al., 2007; Naylor et al., 1999). APNs manage diverse patient conditions and care requirements, which include the following:

- Confusion in older hospitalized patients and acute care of the elderly (ACE) units
- Frail older adults (Barton & Mashlan, 2011)
- Pain in patients who are chronically or terminally ill
- Acute pain
- High-risk pregnant women (Brooten et al., 2007)
- Long-term mechanical ventilation (Burns & Earven, 2002)
- Heart failure patients (Albert et al., 2010; Case, Haynes, Holaday, et al., 2010))
- Neurosurgical patients (Yeager, Shaw, Casavant, et al., 2006)
- Pediatric palliative care (Mauricio & Okhuysen-Cawley, 2010)
- Critically ill neonates

Many CNSs have been called in for consultation when there is a need for skilled communication, advocacy, or coordination of the various providers' plans—or some combination thereof (see Exemplar 7-3). The patient's condition may not be improving because wound care, pain management, and physical therapy have not been well thought out and coordinated. Family members may be angry because plans keep changing and they are receiving conflicting information from various providers. Typically, the CNS talks with the patient and family to become familiar with their concerns and objectives and then brokers a new plan of care that reflects the patient's and family's needs and preferences, as well as the clinical objectives of the involved providers. The agreed on plan

must also be consistent with the care authorized by the third-party payers for the patient, or a special agreement must be negotiated. This brokering requires broad clinical knowledge regarding the objectives of various providers, interpersonal skill in dealing with the results of misunderstandings, diplomacy to encourage stakeholders to see each other's points of view, and a commitment to keeping the patient's needs at the center of what is being done.

Helping Patients Manage Chronic Illnesses

Another type of complex situation that APNs manage effectively is chronic illness. Chronic diseases such as multiple sclerosis, cognitive degeneration, psoriasis, heart failure, chronic lung disease, cancer, acquired immunodeficiency syndrome (AIDS), and organ failure with subsequent transplantation affect individuals and families in profound ways. Most chronic illnesses are characterized by a great deal of uncertainty—uncertainty about the future life course, effectiveness of treatment, chances of leading a happy life, bodily functions, medical bills, and intimate relationships (Mast, 1995). Spouses and significant others of those with a chronic illness often bear considerable emotional and caregiving burdens. For a variety of reasons related to the characteristics of advanced practice nursing, APNs are successful in providing care to persons with chronic conditions and their families.

The U.S. Department of Health and Human Services (DHS) has issued proposed rules for health care providers and systems based on the Affordable Care Act to improve the coordination of patient care through the establishment of an accountable care organization (ACO; DHS, 2011). It is believed that through the use of incentives, these voluntary ACO providers of care will coordinate care of patients across health care settings—clinics, hospitals, and long-term care facilities. The goal of this program is to place patients at the center of their care, maintain quality standards of care, and lower health care costs (see Chapter 22).

APNs who see chronically ill patients in a primary care or specialty setting improve care by coordinating the services patients receive from multiple providers. Chronic illnesses often affect several body systems or have numerous sequelae. Thus, persons who are chronically ill often receive care from a primary care provider and several other clinicians, including physicians and APN specialists, social workers, physical therapists, and dietitians. Without coordination, families coping with chronic illness can find themselves in an "agency maze" (Burton, 1995, p. 457). This vivid phrase captures the confusing experiences that ensue when the agencies and providers rendering care to a family do not communicate with one another. Families do not know where to go for help and, as a result, many resort to a trial and error approach to getting what they

⊙ EXEMPLAR 7-3   Management of Complex Patient Situations*

CM is a diabetes clinical nurse specialist with 20 years of experience. She works in an 800-bed academic medical center, where she is accountable for overall outcomes of glycemic control in the inpatient setting. She is also responsible for evaluating, treating, and educating patients with complex diabetes needs.

CM has been asked to consult on and write treatment recommendations for a 30-year-old Somali woman. Before seeing the patient, CM reviewed the chart to ascertain patient history and information. The patient was diagnosed with type 2 diabetes mellitus (DM) 11 years ago and had been on oral hypoglycemic agents, although not well controlled. She has been managed by multiple providers over the years. The patient was not married and had two sons, 13 and 17 years of age; both have been diagnosed with type 1 DM.

Documentation in the chart indicated that the patient had been admitted to the hospital in ketoacidosis caused by presumed nonadherence to her regimen. The health care team had initiated an insulin infusion but had not initiated the diabetic ketoacidosis (DKA) protocol and had been having difficulty getting the patient's glucose level in the target range.

When CM entered the patient's room, she saw an African woman with truncal obesity, a puffy face, acne, and facial hair. The patient did not make eye contact and appeared standoffish. The patient was reluctant to answer questions. CM recognized the need to proceed thoughtfully in developing a relationship with the patient to establish trust. CM also realized that multiple visits would be required to fully ascertain the extent of needs for this complex patient. From CM's experience and knowledge base, she knew that the symptomatology of DM in the African population is different from the typical presentation of DM in Caucasions. Type 1 DM symptoms in the African population may not be as severe on initial presentation and may not reflect ketosis; therefore, this population can be misdiagnosed with type 2 DM and started on oral agents when they actually have type 1 DM and should be treated with insulin. CM suspected that this might have been the case with this patient. In addition, on first glance, CM immediately suspected that the patient had other endocrine issues (e.g., adrenal dysfunction or polycystic ovary syndrome [PCOS]) because of the presence of puffy face, acne, and facial hair.

CM decided the priority for this initial visit was to focus on the physical care aspects while clarifying the diagnosis and prescribing appropriate treatment to control the patient's glucose. She performed a physical examination and ordered the following diagnostic tests:

- C-peptide and antibodies (to differentiate between types 1 and 2 DM)
- Fasting cortisol
- ACTH stimulation test
- Estradiol-androgen panel
- 24-hour urine
- Endocrinologist consult
- Initiation of standardized DKA protocol

CM returned the following day with the intent to explore knowledge and psychosocial areas with the patient. Again, the patient was wary in her interaction but started to have better eye contact. CM started by asking about the patient's psychosocial situation and determined that the patient was making ends meet financially. However, there were income issues, and CM determined that a social work referral was in order. The patient described having a good relationship with her sons and acknowledged an extensive family support system in the community. She identified herself as a Christian, not a Muslim, as most people assumed.

CM then started to inquire about the physical signs she had noticed on the previous visit by asking how long the patient had had acne and facial hair. At that point, the patient started to cry and stated that CM was the first person to have ever asked her about it. They were clearly distressing symptoms for the patient, and she relayed that she had tried multiple over-the-counter products to try to resolve the acne, but without success. CM shared with the patient what she suspected might be happening with other endocrine issues and reassured her that if that were the case, prescription dermatology creams and hormone therapies would help resolve the symptoms. It was at this point that the patient realized that CM was committed to helping her and a therapeutic relationship began to develop. The patient was now more receptive to allowing a full knowledge assessment.

CM discovered that the patient understood DM well and knew how to count carbohydrates and how to use that information when planning meals. Although the patient spoke English well, CM discovered that the patient could not read English and had some visual disturbances. What had been labeled as nonadherence was actually an inability to read and see health care instructions. When CM reviewed the diagnostic test results, it was determined that the patient had Cushing's syndrome, PCOS, and type 1 DM, rather than type 2. Over the following days, in educational sessions with CM, the patient quickly gained knowledge about insulin and how to administer it, and became proficient at using a magnifier to read the insulin syringe. CM developed instructional tools that did not require the ability to read

EXEMPLAR 7-3   **Management of Complex Patient Situations—*cont'd***

complicated English. Whenever the patient's sons were present, they were included in the teaching.

The patient was eventually discharged to home with new knowledge of insulin and type 1 DM management, as well as information about her new diagnoses and medications, ongoing support from external social services, and referral to a physician group that could manage the health needs of the entire family and provide continuity of care over time.

Highlights of Advanced Practice Nursing Care of a Complex Patient

This case exemplifies the role that an APN can play in making accurate diagnoses and optimizing care for a complex patient. CM exhibited the following:

- Use of evidence and knowledge of unique population-based data applied to an individual

patient, which resulted in prompt correction of a diabetes misdiagnosis
- Expert clinical assessment and intervention skills that identified new endocrine diagnoses and assisted in rapid correction of glycemic control
- Holistic approach to care, incorporating cultural assessment, psychosocial needs, and barriers to knowledge
- Individualized interventions to meet patient needs
- Interpersonal approach that allowed for rapid development of a trusting therapeutic relationship with a patient who was traditionally wary of health care providers who had consistently misidentified her as noncompliant

*The author gratefully acknowledges Carol Manchester, CNS, for the use of her exemplar.

need. They often suffer the negative effects of misinformation, repetitive intake interviews, denial of service, conflicting approaches, and unsolved problems. A resource-savvy APN can often assess these situations and intervene to reduce stress, improve communications, and benefit patients and families. By contacting other providers to develop a coordinated management plan and by linking patients with suitable agencies, the APN can do much to relieve the burdens of chronic illness on a family.

Among the reasons that APNs are successful in providing care to persons with chronic illness is their advocacy of patient self-care. It has been proposed that the key to self-care by patients with chronic illness is to provide self-management education in conjunction with traditional patient education (Bodenheimer, Lorig, Holman, et al., 2002). Self-management education is aimed at promoting confidence to carry out new behaviors, teaching the identification and solving of problems and setting patient-directed short-term goals (Bodenheimer et al., 2002; Lorig, Ritter, & Gonzalez, 2003).

Partnership in the management of a chronic illness requires a change in roles for patients and providers. Patients develop daily management skills, changes in behaviors, and accurate reporting of symptoms. Although providers continue as advisers and partners, they now also become teachers, a role that many are not adequately prepared to fulfill (Holman & Lorig, 2004). In this new partnership, patients develop more knowledge and experience over time and they know the most about the real consequences of chronic disease and their behaviors.

The benefits of emphasizing self-care are supported by research showing that when patients are given information about illnesses and helped to manage their illness, such as heart failure, asthma, and arthritis, their courses of illness and quality of life are improved (Bodenheimer et al., 2002; Lorig, 2003; Riegel et al., 2006). Moreover, the evidence suggests that health education for self-management works in part by building patients' self-confidence about controlling their lives, in spite of the presence of disease (Bodenheimer et al., 2002). Hence, many self-management educational interventions for those with chronic conditions are designed to bolster patients' sense of self-efficacy related to coping with their associated disability and gaining control over the impact of the disease on their lives. Also, APNs can help patients make good decisions specific to the context of their disease and their home situation (Riegel et al., 2006).

However, there are barriers to using a self-management education program in today's health care environment. These include lack of trained personnel in this intervention, patient dependence on the medical model that has been facilitated by paternalistic health care providers, and lack of reimbursement for these services (Bodenheimer & Grumbach, 2007). Regardless, results of this model are compelling and need to be promoted because the aging of the U.S. population will only result in increasing numbers of patients living with chronic illness.

Through the use of diverse approaches and individualized, interpersonal, and therapeutic interventions, APNs have the skills and resources to partner in managing populations throughout the care continuum, from preventive care to the most complex care required by patients with a chronic condition. This is important in view of the increasing complexity of patients' health problems in today's society.

Direct Care and Information Management

Health care is an information-rich environment. It has been said that health care encounters occur essentially for the exchange of information—between the patient and care provider and among care providers themselves (IOM, 2001). With the adoption of information technology, health care information management has become increasingly complex. Inadequate resources and difficulty in accessing information at the time it is needed complicate the situation further (IOM, 2001). The IOM report recommended that government, health care leaders, and vendors work collaboratively to build an information infrastructure quickly to eliminate handwritten clinical data by the end of 2010. With the implementation of the Affordable Care Act, the DHS has made recommendations to encourage widespread implementation of electronic systems and databases to facilitate access to seamless and accessible health care information for everyone (DHS, 2010). It is believed that appropriate use of these systems will decrease errors in prescribing and dosing, increase appropriate use of best practice guidelines, reduce redundancy, improve access to information for patients and providers, and improve quality of care. The direct care practice of APNs is directly influenced by these changes as more and more health care systems and clinics implement electronic health records and databases.

The DNP *Essentials* task force recognized the increasing importance of information systems for APN practice and education. Essential IV of the DNP *Essentials* requires that APNs be prepared to participate in design, selection, and evaluation of systems used for outcomes and quality improvement, exhibit leadership in the area of legal and ethical issues related to information systems, and be knowledgeable about how to evaluate consumer sources of information available through technology (AACN, 2006). With rapid changes in technology, it will be an ongoing challenge throughout an APN's career to remain current in this area.

Even basic competence in the use of computers can be a challenge for some APNs. Wilbright and colleagues (2006) surveyed 454 nursing staff at all role levels in their self-reported skill in 11 key areas of computer use. Although the APNs reported excellent to good skills at entering orders and accessing laboratory results, they rated their skills as fair or poor in 5 of 11 areas that were deemed essential to their role. The skills included

bookmarking websites, copying and pasting files, entering data into spreadsheets, searching MEDLINE or CINAHL, and setting patients up for return clinic appointments. If APNs struggle with these basic skills, it will be difficult for them to use tools and their time optimally to care for their patients.

Well-functioning information systems can ease the workload of the APN by optimizing the management of extensive data. However, meaningful information technology needs more development to overcome challenges that APNs may face on a daily basis in their use, such as workflow disruptions, lack of interfaces between systems, work-arounds, in which providers subvert the information technology (IT) to get the job done, and inappropriate use of order entry warning alerts (DePhillips, 2007; Feldstein et al., 2004; Staggers, Thompson, & Snyder-Halpern, 2001). Computer technology may actually require increased staff time when used for complex order entry and clinical documentation.

Health care institutions and private practices are rapidly implementing information systems across the country, so it is likely that APNs will work in an environment in which a system is being implemented or upgraded. In a survey of primary care pediatric practices, it was reported that the larger the size of the practice, the more likely it was that they had an information system. Smaller practices reported difficulty in implementing them, chiefly because of system expense. Even with systems in place, only one third of practices had decision support components available, such as prompts for immunizations or alerts for abnormal laboratory values (Kemper, Uren, & Clark, 2006). APNs can have an impact on how these systems function to make them user-friendly and efficient at the direct care interface. Although APNs may feel they have neither the time, inclination, nor expertise to participate in these implementations, user input is imperative and ultimately affects direct care.

As information systems are implemented, APNs need to be cognizant of the potential for at least a temporary increase in errors, reduced charge capture, incomplete or difficult to access information, and increased time for routine tasks. Implementation of these systems is a major undertaking because it takes time to re-equilibrate workflow and organizational skills, regardless of APN experience. When information systems are well-implemented and used, the APN will be able to use and view data in new ways to improve patient care.

To obtain the information that they need to take care of patients, APNs need to be able to use handheld devices (e.g., smartphones, personal digital assistants [PDAs]) (Krauskopf & Farrell, 2011; Stroud, Smith, & Erkel, 2009), tablets, portable laptops, and desktop computers to access essential information. This technology improves services at the point of care by decreasing time to access information, decreasing the potential for error through access to current information, and increasing opportunities for care planning (Krauskopf & Wyatt, 2006). APNs can feel overwhelmed with these devices if they are not familiar with them because of fear of loss of data, multiple options in devices, cost, and intimidation related to their use. There are numerous resources available, such as free software, web-based purchasing advice, and resources for learning about PDAs and increasing one's expertise in using PDAs clinically (Krauskopf & Wyatt, 2006).

Although information systems and electronic resources can be great tools in the APN's repertoire, the APN must be constantly aware that these technologies bring with them their own pitfalls and unique potential for errors. APNs can play important roles in evaluating proposed technology and information management systems and the impact they have on APN practice and patient care.

Conclusion

The central competency of advanced practice nursing is direct care, regardless of the specific role of the CNS, NP, CRNA, or CNM. APNs are currently providing direct health care services that affect patients' health care outcomes positively and that are qualitatively different from those provided by other health care professionals. Of importance, these services are valued by the public and are cost-effective. APNs can offer this essential care through the use of the six characteristics that comprise APN direct care: use of a holistic perspective, formation of therapeutic partnerships with patients, expert clinical performance, use of reflective practice, use of evidence as a guide to practice, and use of diverse approaches to health and illness management. Their mastery accomplishes several goals, including differentiation of practice at an advanced level and context for the development of other competencies, such as reflective practice, coaching, counseling, and collaboration. Together, these characteristics form a solid foundation for providing scientifically based, person-centered, and outcome-validated health care. Research evidence supports each of these claims and hence substantiates the nursing profession's and public's confidence in the care provided by APNs. As APNs continue to expand the scope and settings of their practice, it will be imperative that these six characteristics continue to be substantiated by solid research in each of the roles. In addition, research will be important in documenting the optimal so-called nurse dose of APN intervention as we continue to face challenges in caring for culturally diverse, aging, and chronically ill populations.

References

Aiken, L., Sochalski, J., & Lake, E. (1997). Studying outcomes of organizational change in health services. *Medical Care, 35*(Suppl), NS6–NS18.

Aiken, L. H., Clarke, S. P., Sloane, D. M., Sochalski, J., & Silber, J. H. (2002). Hospital nurse staffing and patient mortality, nurse burnout, and job dissatisfaction. *Journal of the American Medical Association, 288*, 1987–1993.

Aiken, L. H., Cimiotti, J. P., Sloane, D. M., Smith, H. L., Flynn, L., & Neff, D. F. (2011). Effects of nurse staffing and nurse education on patient deaths in hospitals with different nurse work environments. *Medical Care, 49*, 1047–1053.

Alasad, J., & Ahmad, M. (2005). Communication with critically ill patients. *Journal of Advanced Nursing, 50*, 356–362.

Albert, N. M., Fonarow, G. C., Yancy, C. W., Curtis, A. B., Stough, W. G., Gheorghiade, M., et al. (2010). Outpatient cardiology practices with advanced practice nurses and physician assistants provide similar delivery of recommended therapies. *American Journal of Cardiology, 105*, 1773–1779.

Allaire, A. D., Moos, M. K., & Wells, S. R. (2000). Complementary and alternative medicine in pregnancy: A survey of North Carolina certified nurse-midwives. *Obstetrics and Gynecology, 95*, 19–23.

Alpi, K. M. (2005). State health department websites: Rich resources for consumer health information. *Journal of Consumer Health on the Internet, 9*, 33–44.

American Association of Colleges of Nursing (AACN). (2006). The essentials of doctoral education for advanced nursing practice (www.aacn.nche.edu/DNP/pdf/Essentials.pdf).

American Association of Colleges of Nursing. (2011). The Essentials of Master's Education in Nursing. www.aacn.nche.edu/education-resources/MastersEssentials11.pdf).

American Association of Critical-Care Nurses. (2004). The 4A's to rise above moral distress (http://www.aacn.org/wd/practice/docs/4as_to_rise_above_moral_distress.pdf).

American Holistic Nurses Association. (2007). What is holistic nursing? (www.ahna.org/AboutUs/WhatisHolisticNursing/tabid/Default.aspx).

American Nurses Association. (2011). Nurses keep top spot for honesty and ethics in poll ranking professions (http://nursingworld.org/HomepageCategory/NursingInsider/Archive_1/2011-NI/Dec2011-NI/Nurses-Keep-Top-Spot-for-Honesty-Ethics.html).

American Nurses Association (ANA). (2010). *Nursing's social policy statement.* (3rd ed.). Silver Springs, MD: American Nurses Association.

American Nurses Credentialing Center. (2004). *A role delineation study of seven nurse practitioner specialties.* Silver Spring, MD: American Nurses Credentialing Center.

Astor, R., Jefferson, H., & Humphrys, K. (1998). Incorporating the service accomplishments into pre-registration curriculum to enhance reflective practice. *Nurse Education Today, 18,* 667 675.

Atkins, S., & Murphy, K. (1995). Reflective practice. *Nursing Standard, 9,* 31–37.

Badger, T. A., & McArthur, D. B. (2003). Academic nurse clinics: Impact of health and cost outcomes for vulnerable populations. *Applied Nursing Research, 16,* 60–64.

Ball, C., & Cox, C. L. (2003). Restoring patients to health: Outcomes and indicators of advanced nursing practice in adult critical care. Part 1. *International Journal of Nursing Practice, 9,* 356–367.

Barakzai, M. D., Gregory, J., & Fraser, D. (2007). The effect of culture on symptom reporting: Hispanics and irritable bowel syndrome. *Journal of the American Academy of Nurse Practitioners, 19,* 261–267.

Barnes, J. (2003). Quality, efficacy, and safety of complementary medicines: Fashions, facts and the future. Part I. Regulation and quality. *British Journal of Clinical Pharmacology, 55,* 226–233.

Barron, A. M., & White, P. A. (2009). Consultation. In A. B. Hamric, J. A. Spross, & C. M. Hanson (Eds.), *Advanced practice nursing. An integrative approach.* (pp. 191–216, 4th ed.). St. Louis: Elsevier.

Barton, D., & Mashlan, W. (2011). An advanced practice nurse-led service—consequences of service redesign for managers and organizational structure. *Journal of Nursing Management, 19,* 943–949.

Becker, D., Kaplow, R., Muenzen, P. M., & Hartigan, C. (2006). Activities performed by acute and critical care advanced practitioners: American Association of Critical Care Nurses study of practice. *American Journal of Critical Care, 15,* 130–148.

Benkert, R., Peters, R., Tate, N., & Dinando, E. (2008). Trust of nurse practitioners and physicians among African Americans with hypertension. *Journal of the American Academy of Nurse Practitioners, 20,* 273–280.

Benner, P. A. (1984). *From novice to expert: Excellence and power in clinical practice.* Menlo Park, CA: Addison-Wesley.

Benner, P. A., Hooper-Kyriakidis, P., & Stannard, D. (1999). *Clinical wisdom and interventions in critical care: A thinking-in-action approach.* Philadelphia: WB Saunders.

Benner, P. A., Tanner, C. A., & Chesla, C. A. (1996). *Expertise in nursing practice: Caring, clinical judgment, and ethics.* New York: Springer-Verlag.

Bialk, J. L. (2004). Ethical guidelines for assisting patients with end-of-life decision making. *MedSurg Nursing, 13,* 87–90.

Blasdell, A. L., Klunick, V., & Purseglove, T. (2002). The use of nursing and medical models in advanced practice: Does education affect the nurse practitioner's practice model? *Journal of Nursing Education, 41,* 231–233.

Bodenheimer, T., & Grumbach, K. (2007). *Improving primary care.* New York: McGraw-Hill/Lange.

Blegen, M. A., Goode, C. J., Spetz, J., Vaughn, T., & Park, S. H. (2011). Nurse staffing effects on patients: Safety-net and non–safety-net hospitals. *Medical Care, 49,* 406–414.

Bodenheimer, T., Lorig, K., Holman, H., & Grumbach, K. (2002). Patient self-management of chronic disease in primary care. *Journal of the American Medical Association, 288,* 2469–2475.

Bonamy, C., Schultz, P., Graham, K., & Hampton, M. (1995). The use of theory-based practice in the Department of Veterans' Affairs Medical Centers. *Journal of Nursing Staff Development, 11,* 27–30.

Brooten, D., Youngblut, J. M., Deatrick, J., Naylor, M., & York, R. (2003). Patient problems, advanced practice nurse (APN) interventions, time and contacts among five patient groups. *Journal of Nursing Scholarship, 35,* 73–79.

Brooten, D., Youngblut, J. M., Donahue, D., Hamilton, M., Hannan, J., & Neff, D. F. (2007). Women with high-risk pregnancies: Problems and APN interventions. *Journal of Nursing Scholarship, 39,* 349–357.

Brown, S. J. (2001). Managing the complexity of best practice health care. *Journal of Nursing Care Quality, 15,* 1–8.

Browning, S., & Waite, R. (2010). The gift of listening: JUST listening strategies. *Nursing Forum, 45,* 150–158.

Brubakken, K., Grant, S., Johnson, M. K., & Kollauf, C. (2011). Reflective practice: A framework for case manager development. *Professional CaseManagement, 16,* 170–179.

Brykczynski, K. A. (1989). An interpretive study describing the clinical judgment of nurse practitioners. *Scholarly Inquiry for Nursing Practice 3,* 75–104.

Brykczynski, K. A. (1991). Judgment strategies for coping with ambiguous clinical situations encountered in primary family care. *Journal of the American Academy of Nurse Practitioners, 3,* 79–84.

Bulechek, G. M., & McCloskey, J. C. (Eds.). (1999). *Nursing interventions classification: Effective nursing treatments* (3rd ed.). Philadelphia: Saunders.

Burley, D. (2011). Better communication in the emergency department. *Emergency Nurse, 19,* 32–36.

Burman, M. E., Stepans, M. B., Jansa, N., & Steiner, S. (2002). How do NPs make clinical decisions? *Nurse Practitioner, 27,* 57–64.

Burns, S. M., & Earven, S. (2002). Improving outcomes for mechanically ventilated medical intensive care unit patients using advanced practice nurses: A 6-year experience. *Critical Care Nursing Clinics of North America, 14,* 231–243.

Burton, D. (1995). Agency maze. In I. M. Lubkin (Ed.), *Chronic illness: Impact and interventions* (pp. 457–480, 3rd ed.). Boston: Jones & Bartlett.

Canadian Task Force on Preventive Health Care. (2012). Current recommendations 2011 (www.canadiantaskforce.ca/recommendations_current_eng.html).

Case, R., Haynes, D., Holaday, B., & Parker, V. G. (2010). Evidence-based nursing: The role of the advanced practice registered nurse in the management of heart failure patients in the outpatient setting. *Dimensions of Critical Care Nursing, 29,* 57–62.

Centers for Disease Control and Prevention. (2011-2012). National Survey of Children's Health (http://www.cdc.gov/nchs/slaits/nsch.htm).

Charlton, C. R., Dearing, K. S., Berry, J. A., & Johnson, M. J. (2008). Nurse practitioners' communication styles and their impact on patient outcome: an integrated literature review.

Journal of the American Academy of Nurse Practitioners, 20, 382–388.

Chen, M. L., & Lin, C. C. (2007). Cancer symptom clusters: A validation study. *Journal of Pain and Symptom Management, 34,* 590–599.

Cherkin, D. C., Deyo, R. A., Sherman, K. J., Hart, L. G., Street, J. H., Hrbek, A., et al. (2002). Characteristics of visits to licensed acupuncturists, chiropractors, massage therapists, and naturopathic physicians. *Journal of the American Board of Family Practice, 16,* 463–472.

Chisholm, C. D., Weaver, C. S., Whenmouth, L., & Giles, B. (2011). A task analysis of emergency physicians activities in academic and community settings. *Annals of Emergency Medicine, 58,* 117–122.

Clark, P., & Gomez, E. (2001). Details on demand: Consumers, cancer information, and the Internet. *Clinical Journal of Oncology Nursing, 5,* 19–24.

Clarke, S. P., & Aiken, L. H. (2003). Failure to rescue. *American Journal of Nursing, 103,* 42–47.

Cleeland, C. S., Mendoza, T. R., Wang, X. S., Chou, C., Harle, M. T., Morrissey, M. et al. (2000). Assessing symptom distress in cancer patients: The M.D. Anderson Symptom Inventory. *Cancer, 89,* 1634–1646.

Clouder, L., & Sellars, J. (2004). Reflective practice and clinical supervision: An interprofessional perspective. *Journal of Advanced Nursing, 46,* 262–269.

Coddington, J. A., & Sands, L. P. (2008). Cost of health care and quality outcomes of patients at nurse-managed clinics. *Nursing Economics, 26,* 75–83.

Committee on Quality of Health Care in America, Institute of Medicine (IOM); Kohn, L. T., Corrigan, J. M., & Donaldson, M. S. (Eds.). (2000). *To err is human: Building a safer health system.* Washington DC: National Academy Press.

Committee on Quality of Health Care in America, Institute of Medicine (IOM). (2001). *Crossing the quality chasm: A new health system for the 21st century.* Washington DC: National Academy Press.

Cornell, P., Riordan, M., Townsend-Gervis, M., & Mobley, R. (2011). Barriers to critical thinking: Workflow interruptions and task switching among nurses. *Journal of Nursing Administration, 41,* 407–414.

Croskerry, P. (2003). Cognitive forcing strategies in clinical decision-making. *Annals of Emergency Medicine, 41,* 110–121.

Cutilli, C. C. (2006). Accessing and evaluating the Internet for patient and family education. *Orthopaedic Nursing, 25,* 333–338.

Dahlke, S., & Phinney, A. (2008). Caring for hospitalized older adults at risk for delirium. *Journal of Gerontological Nursing, 34,* 41–47.

Davidson, L. J., Bennett, S. E., Hamera, E. K., & Raines, B. K. (2004). What constitutes advanced assessment? *Journal of Nursing Education, 43,* 421–425.

Davies, E. (1995). Reflective practice: A focus for caring. *Journal of Nursing Education, 34,* 167–174.

Day, P. O., & Horton-Deutsch, S. (2004). Using mindfulness-based therapeutic interventions in psychiatric nursing practice. Part 1. Description and empirical support for mindfulness-based interventions. *Archives of Psychiatric Nursing, 18,* 164–169.

Dellasega, C., & Zerbe, T. M. (2002). Caregivers of frail rural older adults: Effects of an advanced practice nursing intervention. *Journal of Gerontological Nursing, 28,* 40–49.

Denkinger, M. D., Igl, W., Coll-Planas, L., Bleicher, J., Nikolaus, T., & Jamour, M. (2009). Evaluation of the short form of the late-life function and disability instrument in geriatric inpatients—validity, responsiveness, and sensitivity to change. *Journal of the American Geriatrics Society, 57,* 309–314.

DePalma, J. A. (2004). Advanced practice nurses' research competencies: Competency I—using evidence in practice. *Home Health Care Management and Practice, 16,* 124–126.

DePhillips, H. A. III. (2007). Initiatives and barriers to adopting health information technology. *Disease Management and Health Outcomes, 15,* 1–6.

Dontje, K., Corser, W., Kreulen, G., & Teitelman, A. (2004). A unique set of interactions: The MSU sustained partnership model of nurse practitioner primary care. *Journal of the American Academy of Nurse Practitioners, 16,* 63–69.

Drennan, J., Naughton, C., Allen, D., Hyde, A., O'Boyle, K., Felle, P., et al. (2011). Patients' level of satisfaction and self reports of intention to comply following consultation with nurses and midwives with prescriptive authority: A cross-sectional survey. *International Journal of Nursing Studies, 48,* 808–817.

Ebright, P. R., Patterson, E. S., Chalko, B. A., & Render, M. L. (2003). Understanding the complexity of registered nurse work in acute care settings. *Journal of Nursing Administration, 33,* 630–638.

Eisenberg, D., Kessler, R., Foster, C., Norlock, F., Calkings, D., & Delbanco, T. (1993). Unconventional medicine in the United States. *New England Journal of Medicine, 328,* 246–252.

Eisenberg, D. M., Davis, R. B., Ettner, S. L., Appel, S., Von Rampay, M., & Kessler, R. C. (1998). Trends in alternative medicine in the United States, 1990–1997: Results of a follow-up national survey. *JAMA, 280,* 1569–1575.

Elliott, N. (2010). "Mutual intacting": A grounded theory study of clinical judgment practice issues. *Journal of Advanced Nursing, 66,* 2711–2721.

Epstein, E. G. (2012). Preventive ethics in the intensive care unit. *AACN Advanced Critical Care, 23,* 217–224.

Erickson, H. L. (2007). Philosophy and theory of holism. *Nursing Clinics of North America, 42,* 139–163.

Escallier, L. A., & Fullerton, J. T. (2009). Process and outcomes evaluation of retention strategies within a nursing workforce diversity project. *Journal of Nursing Education, 48,* 488–494.

Feldstein, A., Simon, S. R., Schneider, J., Krall, M., Laferriere, D., Smith, D. H., et al. (2004). How to design computerized alerts to ensure safe prescribing practices. *Joint Commission Journal on Quality and Safety, 30,* 602–613.

Flesner, M., & Clawson, J. (1998). Clinical management by family nurse practitioners and physicians in collaborative practice: A comparative analysis. In T. J. Sullivan (Ed.), *Collaboration: A health care imperative* (pp. 207–224). New York: McGraw-Hill.

Fowler, T. L. (2006). Alcohol dependence and depression: Advanced practice nurse interventions. *Journal of the American Academy of Nurse Practitioners, 18,* 303–308.

Frosch, D. L., Kaplan, R. M., & Felitti, V. (2001). The evaluation of two methods to facilitate shared decision making for men considering the prostate-specific antigen test. *Journal of General Internal Medicine, 16*, 391–398.

Finke, E. H., Light, J., & Kitko, L. (2008). A systematic review of the effectiveness of nurse communication with patients with complex communication needs with a focus on the use of augmentative and alternative communication. *Journal of Clinical Nursing, 17*, 2102–2115.

Gallagher, T. H., Waterman, A. D., Ebers, A. G., Fraser, V. J., & Levinson, W. (2003). Patients' and physicians' attitudes regarding the disclosure of medical errors. *Journal of the American Medical Association, 289*, 1001–1007.

Gardner, G., Gardner, A., Middleton, S., Della, P., Kain, V., & Doubrovsky, A. (2010). The work of nurse practitioners. *Journal of Advanced Nursing, 66*, 2160–2169.

Geraghty, M. (2005). Nursing the unconscious patient. *Nursing Standard, 20*, 54–64.

Gilbert, D. A., & Hayes, E. (2009). Communication and outcomes of visits between older patients and nurse practitioners. *Nursing Research, 58*, 283–293.

Hanson, J. L., & Ashley, B. (1994). Advanced practice nurses' application of the Stetler Model for research utilization: Improving bereavement care. *Oncology Nursing Forum, 21*, 720–724.

Harvard School of Public Health. (2010). Health literacy studies (www.hsph.harvard.edu/healthliteracy/index.html).

Hawkins, J. W., Thibodeau, J. A., Utley-Smith, Q. E., Igou, J. F., & Johnson, E. E. (1993). Using a conceptual model for practice in a nursing wellness centre for seniors. *Perspectives, 17*, 11–16.

Hayes, K. M., & Alexander, I. M. (2000). Alternative therapies and nurse practitioners: Knowledge, professional experience, and personal use. *Holistic Nursing Practice, 14*, 49–58.

Henry, S. B., Holzemer, W. L., Randell, C., Hsieh, S. F., & Miller, T. J. (1997). Comparison of nursing interventions classification and current procedural terminology codes for categorizing nursing activities. *Image: The Journal of Nursing Scholarship, 29*, 133–138.

Hickey, M. (1990). The role of the clinical nurse specialist in the research utilization process. *Clinical Nurse Specialist, 4*, 93–96.

Hiltunen, E. F., Winder, P. A., Rait, M. A., Buselli, E. F., Carroll, D. L., & Rankin, S. H. (2005). Implementation of efficacy enhancement nursing interventions with cardiac elders. *Rehabilitation Nursing, 30*, 221–229.

Hoffman, L. A., Happ, M. B., Scharfenberg, C., DiVirgilio-Thomas, D., & Tasota, F. J. (2004). Perceptions of physicians, nurses, and respiratory therapists about the role of acute care nurse practitioners. *American Journal of Critical Care, 13*, 480–488.

Hoffman, L. A., Tasota, F. J., Scharfenberg, C., Zullo, T. G., & Donahoe, M. P. (2003). Management of patients in the intensive care unit: Comparison via work sampling analysis of an acute care nurse practitioner and physicians in training. *American Journal of Critical Care, 12*, 436–443.

Holland, M. L., & Holland, E. S. (2007). Survey of Connecticut nurse-midwives. *Journal of Midwifery & Women's Health, 52*, 106–115.

Holman, H., & Lorig, K. (2004). Patient self-management: A key to effectiveness and efficiency in care of chronic disease. *Public Health Reports, 119*, 239–243.

Hravnak, M., Tuite, P., & Baldisseri, M. (2005). Expanding acute care nurse practitioner and clinical nurse specialist education: Invasive procedure training and human simulation in critical care. *AACN Clinical Issues, 16*, 89–104.

Hughes, L. C., Robinson, L., Cooley, M. E., Nuamah, I., Grobe, S. J., & McCorkle, R. (2002). Describing an episode of home nursing care for elderly postsurgical cancer patients. *Nursing Research, 51*, 110–118.

Institute for Healthcare Improvement. (2011a). Going lean in health care (www.ihi.org/knowledge/Pages/IHIWhitePapers/GoingLeaninHealth care.aspx).

Institute for Healthcare Improvement. (2011b). Plan-do-study-act worksheet (www.ihi.org/knowledge/Pages/Tools/PlanDoStudyActWorksheet.aspx).

Johns, C. (2000). *Becoming a reflective practitioner.* London: Blackwell Science.

Kane, R. L., Shamliyan, T. A., Mueller, C., Duval, S., & Wilt, T. J. (2007). The association of registered nurse staffing levels and patient outcomes: Systematic review and meta analysis. *Medical Care, 45*, 1195–1204.

Kemper, A. R., Uren, R. L., & Clark, S. J. (2006). Adoption of electronic health records in primary care pediatric practices. *Pediatrics, 118*, e20–e24.

Kim, H. S. (1999). Critical reflective inquiry for knowledge development in nursing practice. *Journal of Advanced Nursing, 29*, 1205–1212.

Krauskopf, P. B., & Farrell, S. (2011). Accuracy and efficiency of novice nurse practitioners using personal digital assistants. *Journal of Nursing Scholarship, 43*, 117–124.

Krauskopf, P. B., & Wyatt, T. H. (2006). Even technophobic NPs can use PDAs. *Nurse Practitioner, 31*, 48–52.

Kumar, K. (2011). Living out reflective practice. *Journal of Christian Nursing, 28*, 139–143.

Laabs, C. A. (2005). Moral problems and distress among nurse practitioners in primary care. *Journal of the American Academy of Nurse Practitioners, 17*, 76–83.

Lambing, A. Y., Adams, D. L. C., Fox, D. H., & Divine, G. (2004). Nurse practitioners' and physicians' care activities and clinical outcomes with an inpatient geriatric population. *Journal of the American Academy of Nurse Practitioners, 16*, 343–352.

Laschinger, H. K., & Duff, V. (1991). Attitudes of practicing nurses towards theory-based nursing practice. *Canadian Journal of Nursing Administration, 4*, 6–10.

Lawrence, M. (1995). The unconscious experience. *American Journal of Critical Care, 4*, 227–232.

Lawson, M. T. (2002). Nurse practitioner and physician communication styles. *Applied Nursing Research, 15*, 60–66.

Lerret, S. M., & Stendahl, G. (2011). Working together as a team: Adolescent transplant recipients and nurse practitioners. *Progress in Transplantation, 21*, 288–298.

Lewandowski, W., & Adamle, K. (2009). Substantive areas of clinical nurse specialist practice. A comprehensive review of the literature. *Clinical Nurse Specialist, 23*, 73–90.

Lorig, K. (2003). Self-management education: More than a nice extra. *Medical Care, 41*, 699–701.

Lorig, K., Ritter, P. L., & Gonzalez, V. (2003). Hispanic chronic disease self-management: A randomized community-based outcome trial. *Nursing Research, 52,* 361–369.

Mackay, M. H. (1998). Research utilization and the CNS: Confronting the issues. *Clinical Nurse Specialist, 12,* 232–237.

Madsen, L. T., Craig, C., & Kuban, D. (2009). A multidisciplinary prostate cancer clinic for newly diagnosed patients: Developing the role of the advanced practice nurse. *Clinical Journal of Oncology Nursing, 13,* 305–309.

Mao, A. J., & Anastasi, J. K. (2010). Diagnosis and management of endometriosis: The role of the advanced practice nurse in primary care. *Journal of the American Academy of Nurse Practitioners, 22,* 109–116.

Massachusetts Coalition for the Prevention of Medical Errors. (2006). When things go wrong: Responding to adverse events (http://www.macoalition.org/documents/respondingTo AdverseEvents.pdf).

Mast, M. E. (1995). Adult uncertainty in illness: A critical review of research. *Scholarly Inquiry for Nursing Practice, 9,* 3–24.

Mauricio, R. V., & Ohuysen-Cawley, R. (2010). The caring continuum: Role of the pediatric critical care advanced practice nurse in palliative care program development. *Critical Care Nurse Quarterly, 33,* 292–297.

McAfee, J. L. (2012). Developing an advanced practice nurse-led liver clinic. *Gastroenterology Nursing, 35,* 215–224.

McCloskey, B., Grey, M., Deshefy-Longhi, T., & Grey, L. J. (2003). APRN practice patterns in primary care. *Nurse Practitioner, 28,* 39–44.

McCourt, C. (2006). Supporting choice and control? Communication and interaction between midwives and women at the antenatal booking visit. *Social Science and Medicine, 62,* 1307–1318.

McMullan, M. (2006). Patients using the Internet to obtain health information: How this affects the patient-health professional relationship. *Patient Education and Counseling, 63,* 24–28.

McNeal, G. J., & Walker, D. (2006). Enhancing success in advanced practice nursing: A grant-funded project. *Journal of Cultural Diversity, 13,* 10–19.

Meats, E., Brassey, J., Heneghan, C., & Glasziou, P. (2007). Using the Turning Research into Practice (TRIP) database: How do clinicians really search? *Journal of the Medical Library Association, 95,* 156–163.

Miller, N. H. (2010). Motivational interviewing as a prelude to coaching in health care settings. *Journal of Cardiovascular Nursing, 25,* 247–251.

Morgan, M. W., Deber, R. B., Llewellyn-Thomas, H. A., Gladstone, P., Cusimano, R. J., O'Rourke, K., et al. (2000). Randomized, controlled trial of an interactive videodisc decision aid for patients with ischemic heart disease. *Journal of General Internal Medicine, 15,* 685–693.

Munro, N. (2004). Evidence-based assessment: No more pride or prejudice. *AACN Clinical Issues, 15,* 501–505.

National Institutes of Health. (2012). Plain language (www.nih.gov/clearcommunication/plainlanguage.htm).

National Quality Forum. (2008). Serious reportable events (www.qualityforum.org/Publications/2008/10/Serious_Reportable_Events.aspx).

National Quality Forum. (2011). Serious reportable events in health care—2011 update. A consensus report (www. qualityforum.org/Publications/2011/12/Serious_Reportable_ Events _in_Health care_2011.aspx).

Naylor, M. D., Brooten, D., Campbell, R., Jacobsen, B. S., Mezey, M. D., Pauly, M. V., et al. (1999). Comprehensive discharge planning and home follow-up of hospitalized elders: A randomized clinical trial. *JAMA, 281,* 613–620.

Ndiwane, A., Miller, K. H., Bonner, A., Imperio, K., Matzo, M., McNeal, G., et al. (2004). Enhancing cultural competencies of advanced practice nurses: Health care challenges in the twenty-first century. *Journal of Cultural Diversity, 11,* 118–121.

Needleman, J., Buerhaus, P., Pankratz, V. S. Leibsno, C. L., Stevens, S. R., & Harris., M. (2011). Nurse staffing and inpatient hospital mortality. *New England Journal of Medicine, 364,* 1037–1045.

Ni, H., Simile, C., & Hardy, A. M. (2002). Utilization of complementary and alternative medicine by United States adults: Results from the 1999 National Health Interview Survey. *Medical Care, 40,* 353–358.

Norred, C. L. (2002). Complementary and alternative medicine use by surgical patients. *Journal of American Operating Room Nurses, 76,* 1013–1021.

O'Connor, N. A., Hameister, A. D., & Kershaw, T. (2000). Developing a database to describe the practice patterns of adult nurse practitioner students. *Journal of Nursing Scholarship, 32,* 57–63.

Oddsdottir, E. J., & Sveinsdottir, H. (2011). Content of the work of clinical nurse specialists described by use of daily activity diaries. *Journal of Clinical Nursing, 20,* 1393–1404.

O'Neill, E. S. (1995). Heuristics reasoning in diagnostic judgment. *Journal of Professional Nursing, 11,* 239–245.

Parry, C., Kramer, H. M., & Coleman, E. A. (2006). A qualitative exploration of a patient-centered coaching intervention to improve care transitions in chronically ill older adults. *Home Health Care Services Quarterly, 25,* 39–53.

Patterson, C., Kaczorowski, J., Arthur, H., Smith, K., & Mills, D. A. (2003). Complementary therapy practice: Defining the role of advanced nurse practitioners. *Journal of Clinical Nursing, 12,* 816–823.

Pawlak, R. (2005). Economic considerations of heath literacy. *Nursing Economics, 23,* 173–180.

Persson, M., Hornsten, A., Wirkvist, A., & Mogren, I. (2011). "Mission impossible?" Midwives' experiences counseling pregnant women with gestational diabetes mellitus. *Patient Education and Counseling, 84,* 78–83.

Phillips, J. (2005). Neuroscience critical care: The role of the advanced practice nurse in patient safety. *AACN Clinical Issues, 16,* 581–592.

Quirk, P. (2000). Screening for literacy and readability: Implications for the advanced practice nurse. *Clinical Nurse Specialist, 14,* 26–43.

Rector, T. S., Anand, I. S., & Cohn, J. N. (2006). Relationships between clinical assessments and patients' perceptions of the effects of heart failure on their quality of life. *Journal of Cardiac Failure, 12,* 87–92.

Redman, B. K., (2004). *Advances in patient education.* New York: Springer.

Resnicow, K., & McMaster, F. (2012). Motivational interviewing: Moving from why to how with autonomy support. *International Journal of Behavioral Nutrition and Physical Activity, 9,* 19.

Riegel, B., Dickson, V. V., Hoke, L., McMahon, J. P., Reis, B. F., & Sayers, S. (2006). A motivational counseling approach to improving heart failure self-care: Mechanisms of effectiveness. *Journal of Cardiovascular Nursing, 21,* 232–241.

Rolfe, G. (1997). Beyond expertise: Theory, practice, and the reflexive practitioner. *Journal of Clinical Nursing, 6,* 93–97.

Rosenfeld, P., McEvoy, M. D., & Glassman, K. (2003). Measuring practice patterns among acute care nurse practitioners. *Journal of Nursing Administration, 33,* 159–165.

Rosenzweig, M., Hravnak, M., Magdic, K., Beach, M., Clifton, M., & Arnold, R. (2008). A communication simulation laboratory for students in an acute care nurse practitioner program. *American Journal of Critical Care, 17,* 364–372.

Rudolfsson, G., von Post, I., & Eriksson, K. (2007. The perioperative dialogue. Holistic nursing in practice. *Holistic Nursing Practice, 21,* 292–298.

Rushton, C. H. (2006). Defining and addressing moral distress: Tools for critical care nursing leaders. *AACN Advanced Critical Care, 17,* 161–168.

Ryan, P., & Lauver, D. R. (2002). The efficacy of tailored interventions. *Journal of Nursing Scholarship, 34,* 331–337.

Sackett, D. L. (1998). Evidence-based medicine. *Spine, 23,* 1085–1086.

Sandhu, H., Dale, J., Stallard, N., Crouch, R., & Glucksman, E. (2009). Emergency nurse practitioners and doctors consulting with patients in an emergency department: A comparison of communication skills and satisfaction. *Emergency Medicine Journal, 26,* 400–404.

Sappington, J., & Kelley, J. H. (1996). Modeling and role-modeling theory: A case of holistic care. *Journal of Holistic Nursing, 14,* 130–141.

Schön, D. A. (1992). *The reflective practitioner: How professionals think in action* (2nd ed.). San Francisco: Jossey-Bass.

Schwartz-Barcott, D., Patterson, B. J., Lusardi, P., & Farmer, B. C. (2002). From practice to theory: Tightening the link via three fieldwork strategies. *Journal of Advanced Nursing, 39,* 281–289.

Scott, G. N., & Elmer, G. W. (2002). Update on natural product–drug interactions. *American Journal of Health-System Pharmacy, 59,* 339–347.

Shever, L. L. (2011). The impact of nursing surveillance on failure to rescue. *Research and Theory for Nursing Practice, 25,* 107–126.

Shuler, P. A., Huebscher, R., & Hallock, J. (2001). Providing wholistic health care for the elderly: Utilization of the Shuler Nurse Practitioner Practice Model. *Journal of the American Academy of Nurse Practitioners, 13,* 297–303.

Sidani, S., Doran, D., Porter, H., LeFort, S., O'Brien-Pallas, L. L., Zahn, C., et al. (2006). Processes of care: Comparison between nurse practitioners and physician residents in acute care. *Canadian Journal of Nursing Leadership, 19,* 69–85.

Sivesind, D., Parker, P. A., Cohen, L., Demoor, C., Bumbaugh, M., Throckmorton, T., et al. (2003). Communicating with patients in cancer care. *Journal of Cancer Education, 18,* 202–209.

Smith, M. C. (2008). Disciplinary perspectives linked to middle range theory. In Smith, M. J., & Lierh, P. R. (Eds). *Middle range theory for nursing.* (pp. 1–31). New York: Springer.

Smith, M. J., & Liehr, P. R. (Eds). (2008). *Middle range theory for nursing* (2nd ed.). New York: Springer.

Sobralske, M., & Katz., J. (2005). Culturally competent care of patients with acute chest pain. *Journal of the American Academy of Nurse Practitioners, 17,* 342–349.

Sohn, P. M., & Loveland Cook, C. A. (2002). Nurse practitioner knowledge of complementary alternative health care: Foundation for practice. *Journal of Advanced Nursing, 39,* 9–16.

Stableford, S., & Metter, W. (2007). Plain language: A strategic response to the health literacy challenge. *Journal of Public Health Policy, 28,* 71–93.

Staggers, N., Thompson, C. B., & Snyder-Halpern, R. (2001). History and trends in clinical information systems in the United States. *Journal of Nursing Scholarship, 33,* 75–81.

Stetler, C. B., Bautista, C., Vernale-Hannon, C., & Foster, J. (1995). Enhancing research utilization by clinical nurse specialists. *Nursing Clinics of North America, 30,* 457–473.

Stroud, S. D., Smith, C. A., & Erkel, E. A. (2009). Personal digital assistant use by nurse practitioners: A descriptive study. *Journal of the American Academy of Nurse Practitioners, 21,* 31–38.

Swartz, M. K., Grey, M., Allan, J. D., Ridenour, N., Kovern, C., Walker, P. H., et al. (2003). A day in the lives of APNs in the U.S. *Nurse Practitioner, 28,* 32–39.

Tanner, C. A. (2006). Thinking like a nurse: A research-based model of clinical judgment in nursing. *Journal of Nursing Education, 45,* 204–211.

Tanner, C. A., Benner, P., Chesla, C., & Gordon, D. R. (1993). The phenomenology of knowing a patient. *Image: The Journal of Nursing Scholarship, 25,* 273–280.

Tesch, B. J. (2002). Herbs commonly used by women: An evidence-based review. *Disease-A-Month: DM, 48,* 671–696.

Thomas, L. A. (2003). Clinical management of stressors perceived by patients on mechanical ventilation. *AACN Clinical Issues, 14,* 73–81.

U.S. Department of Health and Human Services. (2010). Healthy people 2020 (http://www.healthypeople.gov/2020).

U.S. Department of Health and Human Services. (2011). Affordable Care Act to improve quality of care for people with Medicare (www.hhs.gov/news/press/2011pres/03/20110331a.html).

U.S. Department of Health and Human Services, Office of the National Coordination for Health Information Technnology. (2010). Electronic eligibility and enrollment (http://healthit.hhs.gov/portal/server.pt?open=512&mode=2&objID=316).

U.S. Preventive Services Task Force. (1996). *Guide to clinical preventive services: Report of the U.S. Preventive Services Task Force* (2nd ed.). Baltimore: Williams & Wilkins.

U.S. Preventive Services Task Force. (2010). Guide to clinical preventive services 2011: Recommendations of the U.S. Preventive Services Task Force (www.ahrq.gov/clinic/pocketgd1011).

Van den Heede, K., Lesaffre, R., Diya, L., Vieugels, A., Clarke, S. P. Aiken, L. H., et al. (2009). The relationship between inpatient cardiac surgery mortality and nurse numbers and educational level: analyzing administrative data. *International Journal of Nursing Scholarship, 46,* 796–803.

Van Ruth, L. M., Mistiaen, P., & Francke, A. L. (2008). Effects of nurse prescribing of medications: A systematic review (http://www.ispub.com/journal/the-internet-journal-of-healthcare-administration/volume-5-number-2/effects-of-nurse-prescribing-of-medication-a-systematic-review.html).

Verger, J. T., Marcoux, K. K., Madden, M. A., Bojko, T., & Barnsteiner, J. H. (2005). Nurse practitioners in pediatric critical care: Results of a national survey. *AACN Clinical Issues, 16,* 396–408.

Vincent, C. (2003). Understanding and responding to adverse events. *New England Journal of Medicine, 348,* 1051–1056.

Ward, S., Donovan, H. S., Owen, B., Grosen, E., & Serlin, R. (2000). An individualized intervention to overcome patient-related barriers to pain management in women with gynecologic cancers. *Research in Nursing and Health, 23,* 393–405.

Ware, J. E., & Sherbourne, C. D. (1992). The MOS 36-item short form health survey (SF-36): I. Conceptual framework and item selection. *Medical Care, 30,* 473–483.

Warner, H. (2006). Caring for a child with disabilities: Part 2. The child/family/nurse relationship. *Paediatric Nursing, 18,* 38–43.

Watts, S. A., Gee, J., O'Day, M. E., Schaub, K., Lawrence, R., Aron, D., et al. (2009). Nurse practitioner-led multidisciplinary teams to improve chronic illness care: The unique strengths of nurse practitioners applied to shared medical appointments/medical visits. *Journal of American Academy of Nurse Practitioners, 21,* 167–172.

Welch, J., Fisher, M., & Dayhoff, N. (2002). A cost-effectiveness worksheet for patient education programs. *Clinical Nurse Specialist, 16,* 187–192.

Westbrook, J. I., Woods, A., Rob, M. I., Dunsmuir, W. T. M., & Day, R. O. (2010). Association of interruptions with an increased risk and severity of medication administration errors. *Archives of Internal Medicine, 170,* 683–690.

White, C. S. (2012). Advanced practice prescribing: Issues and strategies in preventing medication error. *Journal of Nursing Law, 14,* 120–127.

Whittemore, R., & Roy, C. (2002). Adapting to diabetes mellitus: A theory synthesis. *Nursing Science Quarterly, 15,* 311–317.

Wilbright, W. A., Haun, D. E., Romano, T., Krutzfeldt, T., Fontenot, C. E., & Nolan, T. E. (2006). Computer use in an urban university hospital: Technology ahead of literacy. *Computers, Informatics, Nursing: CIN, 24,* 37–43.

Witman, A. B., Park, D. M., & Hardin, S. B. (1996). How do patients want physicians to handle mistakes? A survey of internal medicine patients in an academic setting. *Archives of Internal Medicine, 156,* 2565–2569.

Wolf, Z. R., & Robinson-Smith, G. (2007). Strategies used by clinical nurse specialists in "difficult" clinician-patient situations. *Clinical Nurse Specialist, 21,* 74–84.

Wong, F. K. Y., Loke, A. Y., Wong, M., Tse, H., Kan, E., & Kember, D. (1997). An action research study into the development of nurses as reflective practitioners. *Journal of Nursing Education, 36,* 476–481.

Yeager, S., Shaw, K. D., Casavant, J., & Burns, S. M. (2006). An acute care nurse practitioner model of care for neurosurgical patients. *Critical Care Nurse, 26,* 57–64.

Guidance and Coaching

Judith A. Spross • Rhonda L. Babine

CHAPTER CONTENTS

The competency of guidance and coaching is a well-established expectation of the advanced practice nurse (APN). For example, the ability to establish therapeutic relationships and guide patients through transitions is incorporated into the *DNP Essentials* (American Association of Colleges of Nursing [AACN], 2006). Although there is variability in how this aspect of APN practice is described, standards that specifically address therapeutic relationships and partnerships, coaching, communication, patient-family–centered care, guidance, and/or counseling can be found in competency statements for most APN roles (American College of Nurse Midwives [ACNM], 2012; National Association of Clinical Nurse Specialists [NACNS], 2013; National Organization of Nurse Practitioner Faculties [NONPF], 2012).

Since the last edition, developments in public health and health policy within nursing and across disciplines have influenced the conceptualization of the APN guidance and coaching competency. Professional coaching now is recognized within and outside of nursing as a particular intervention, distinct from guidance, mentoring and counseling. This practice, by nurses and other disciplines,

focuses on health, healing, and wellness; as the broad understanding of professional coaching evolves, it will influence the evolution of the APN guidance and coaching competency. This edition draws from literature on professional coaching by nurses and others to inform and build on the model of APN guidance and coaching presented in previous editions. It is important to understand that APN guidance and coaching are not synonymous with professional coaching. There are several reasons for this:

- The foundational importance of the *therapeutic* APN-patient (client) relationship is not consistent with professional coaching principles.
- The evolving criteria and requirements for certification of professional coaches are not premised on APN coaching skills.
- Empirical research findings that predate contemporary professional coaching have affirmed that guidance and coaching are characteristics of APN-patient relationships.

This chapter considers the core competency of APN guidance and coaching within the context of the nursing profession's efforts to extend and advance the coaching functions of nurses. Some form of coaching is inherent in nursing practice, and developing professional nurse coaching certifications should build on these skills. Foundations of the APN competency are established when nurses learn about therapeutic relationships and communication in their undergraduate and graduate programs, together with growing technical and clinical expertise. Graduate programs deepen students' inherent coaching skills by incorporating evidence-based coaching practices into curricula.

The purposes of this chapter are to do the following: offer a conceptualization of APN guidance and coaching that can be applied across settings and patients' health states and transitions; integrate findings from the nursing literature and the field of professional coaching into this conceptualization; offer strategies for developing this competency; and differentiate professional coaching from APN guidance and coaching. Although the primary focus of this chapter is on guiding and coaching patients and families, applications of the coaching model to students and staff are discussed.

Imperatives for Advanced Practice Nurse Guidance and Coaching

Burden of Chronic Illness

Nationally and internationally, chronic illnesses are leading causes of morbidity and mortality. In 2008, worldwide, over 36 million people died from conditions such as heart disease, cancers, and diabetes (World Health Organization [WHO], 2011, 2012). Similarly, in the United States, chronic diseases caused by heart disease result in 7 out of 10 deaths/year; cancer and stroke account for more than 50% of all deaths (Heron, Hoyert, Murphy, et al., 2009). In 2008, 107 million Americans had at least one of six chronic illnesses—cardiovascular disease, arthritis, diabetes, asthma, cancer, and chronic obstructive pulmonary disease (U.S. Department of Health and Human Services [HSS], 2012); this number is expected to grow to 157 million by 2020 (Bodenheimer, Chen, & Bennett, 2009). These diseases share four common risk factors that lend themselves to APN guidance and coaching—tobacco use, physical inactivity, the harmful use of alcohol, and poor diet. There is evidence that psychosocial problems, such as adverse childhood experiences, contribute to the initiation of risk factors for the development of poor health and chronic illnesses in Americans (Centers for Disease Control and Prevention [CDC], 2010; Felitti, 2002). The physical, emotional, social, and economic burdens of chronic illness are enormous but, until recently, investing in resources to promote healthy lifestyles and prevent chronic illnesses has not been a policy priority. Registered nurses, including APNs, are central to a redesigned health system that emphasizes prevention and early intervention to promote healthy lifestyles, prevent chronic diseases, and reduce the personal, community, organizational, and economic burdens of chronic illness (Hess, Dossey, Southard, et al., 2012; Institute of Medicine [IOM], 2010; Thorne, 2005).

Health Care Policy Initiatives

Accountable Care Organizations and Patient-Centered Medical Homes

The Patient Protection and Affordable Care Act (PPACA; HHS, 2011) in the United States and other policy initiatives nationally and internationally are aimed at lowering health costs and making health care more effective. The PPACA has led payers to adopt innovative approaches to financing health care, including accountable care organizations (ACOs) and patient-centered medical homes (PCMHs; see Chapter 22). To qualify as a medical or health care home or ACO, practices must engage patients and develop communication strategies. Thorne (2005) has analyzed findings from a decade of qualitative research on nurse-patient relationships and communication in chronic illness care in the context of the health policy emphasis on accountable care; many findings were associated with better outcomes. Accountable care initiatives are an opportunity to implement these findings and evaluate and strengthen the guidance and coaching competency of APNs.

Patient-Centered Care, Culturally Competent and Safe Health Care, and Meaningful Provider-Patient Communication

The aging population, increases in chronic illness, and the emphasis on preventing medical errors has led to calls for care that is more patient-centered (Devore & Champion, 2011; IOM, 2001; National Center for Quality Assurance [NCQA], 2011). The Institute for Healthcare Improvement [IHI] has asserted that patient-centered care is central to driving improvement in health care Johnson, Abraham, Conway, et al., 2008). The Joint Commission (TJC) published the *Roadmap for Hospitals* in 2010. Its purpose was "to inspire hospitals to integrate concepts from the communication, cultural competence, and patient- and family-centered care fields into their organizations" (TJC, 2010, p. 11). Similarly, two of ten criteria that primary care PCMHs are expected to meet are "written standards for patient access and communication" and "active support of patient self-management" (NCQA, 2011). In addition, patient-centered communication and interprofessional team communication are important quality and safety education for nurses (QSEN) competencies for APNs

(Cronenwett, Sherwood, Pohl, et al., 2009; http://qsen.org/competencies/graduate-ksas/).

These initiatives signal increasing recognition by all stakeholders that improving health care depends on a patient-centered orientation in which providers communicate meaningfully and effectively and provide culturally competent and safe care (IOM, 2010; Hobbs, 2009; TJC, 2010; Woods, 2010). The provision of patient-centered care and meaningful patient-provider communication activates and empowers patients and their families to assume responsibility for initiating and maintaining healthy lifestyles and/or adopting effective chronic illness management skills. When patient-centered approaches are integrated into the mission, values, and activities of organizations, better outcomes for patients and institutions, including safer care, fewer errors, improved patient satisfaction, and reduced costs, should ensue. APNs have the knowledge and skills to help institutions and practices meet the standards for meaningful provider-patient communication and team-based, patient-centered care.

Interprofessional Teams

Over the last decade, the importance of interprofessional teamwork to achieve high-quality, patient-centered care has been increasingly recognized. The Interprofessional Collaborative Expert Panel (ICEP) has proposed four core competency domains that health professionals need to demonstrate if interprofessional collaborative practice is to be realized (ICEP, 2011; http://www.aacn.nche.edu/education-resources/ipecreport.pdf). These core competency domains are as follows: values and ethics for interprofessional practice; roles and responsibilities; interprofessional communication; and teams and teamwork. The competency related to teams and teamwork emphasizes relationship building as an important element of patient-centered care (see Chapter 12). As interprofessional teamwork becomes more integrated into health care, guidance and coaching will likely be seen as a transdisciplinary, patient-centered approach to helping patients but will be expressed differently, based on the discipline and experience of the provider.

The publication of these competencies, together with research on interprofessional work in the health professions (e.g., Reeves, Zwarenstein, Goldman, et al., 2010), are helping educators determine how best to incorporate interprofessional competencies into APN education. Skill in establishing therapeutic relationships and being able to coach patients based on discipline-related content and skills will be important in achieving interprofessional, patient-centered care. APNs must be able to explain their nursing contributions, including their relational, communication, and coaching skills, to team members.

Furthermore, many APNs will have responsibilities for coaching teams to deliver patient-centered care.

Definitions: Teaching, Guidance, and Coaching

Guidance and coaching by APNs have been conceptualized as a complex, dynamic, collaborative, and holistic interpersonal process mediated by the APN-patient relationship and the APN's self-reflective skills (Clarke & Spross, 1996; Spross, Clarke, & Beauregard, 2000; Spross, 2009). To help the reader begin to discern the subtle differences among coaching actions, the terms that inform this model are defined here, in particular, patient education, APN guidance, including anticipatory guidance, and a revised definition of APN coaching (to distinguish it from professional coaching).

Parry and Coleman (2010) have offered useful distinctions among different strategies for helping patients: coaching, doing for patients, educating, and guiding along five dimensions (Table 8-1). These distinctions are reflected in the definitions that follow.

Patient Education

Patient teaching and education (see Chapter 7) directly relates to APN coaching. Teaching is an important intervention in the self-management of chronic illness and is often incorporated into guidance and coaching. "Patient education involves helping patients become better informed about their condition, medical procedures, and choices they have regarding treatment. Nurses typically have opportunities to educate patients during bedside conversations or by providing prepared pamphlets or handouts. Patient education is important to enable individuals to better care for themselves and make informed decisions regarding medical care" (Martin, eNotes, 2002, http://www.enotes.com/patient-education-reference/patient-education). This definition is necessarily broad and can inform standards for patient education materials and programs targeting common health and illness topics. Patient education may include information about cognitive and behavioral changes but these changes cannot occur by teaching alone. All nurses and APNs should be familiar with the patient education resources in their specialty because these resources can facilitate guidance and coaching.

Guidance

Guidance can be seen as a preliminary, less comprehensive form of coaching. A subtle distinction is that guidance is done by the nurse, whereas coaching's focus is on

TABLE 8-1   Distinctions Among Coaching and Other Processes

	PARADIGM			
Dimension	Do-er and Do-ing	Teacher and Teaching	Coach and Facilitating	Guide and Encourage
Goal	Task completion	Information and skill transfer	Patient engagement and empowerment Information and skill transfer	Information transfer and assistance in choosing direction
Primary focus	Content • Task completion	Content • Assessment • Information and skill transfer	Process of coaching • Patient-centeredness of the interaction (built around patient's goals) • Modeling patient engagement in the coach-patient interaction • Content Information and skill transfer	Content • Practitioner provides information and possible outcomes • Patient receives assistance in choosing direction that best suits her or him • Patient ultimately makes decision
Ownership of the agenda	The doer	The teacher	The patient	The patient and guide
Level of patient engagement	Low	Medium	High	High

Adapted from Parry, C. & Coleman, E. A. (2010). Active roles for older adults in navigating care transitions: Lessons learned from the care transitions intervention. *Open Longevity Science, 4,* 43–50.

empowering patients to manage their care needs. This definition of guidance draws on dictionary definitions of the word and the use of the term in motivational interviewing (MI). To guide is to advise or show the way to others, so guidance can be considered the act of providing counsel by leading, directing, or advising. To guide also means to assist a person to travel through, or reach a destination in, an unfamiliar area, such as by accompanying or giving directions to the person. The term is also used to refer to advising others, especially in matters of behavior or belief. Rollnick and colleagues (2008) have described guiding as one of three styles of doing MI. They compare a guiding style of communication to tutoring; the emphasis is on being a resource to support a person's autonomy and self-directed learning and action.

APN guidance is a style and form of communication informed by assessments, experiences, and information that is used by APNs to help patients and families explore their own resources, motivations, and possibilities. The goals of APN guidance are to raise awareness, contemplate, implement, and sustain a behavior change, manage a health or illness situation, or prepare for transitions, including birth and end of life. The deliberate use of guidance in situations that are acute, uncertain, or time-constrained, offers patients and families ideas for examining alternatives or identifying likely responses. Guidance may also occur in situations in which there may

be insufficient information for a patient to make an informed choice related to a desired outcome.

Anticipatory guidance is a particular type of guidance aimed at helping patients and families know what to expect. Such guidance needs to be wisely crafted to avoid "leading the witness" or creating self-fulfilling prophecies (see Exemplar 8-1). With experience, APNs develop their own strategies for integrating specialty-related anticipatory guidance into their coaching activities. APNs are likely to move between guidance and coaching in response to their assessments of patients. Although we believe that guidance is distinct from coaching, more work is needed to illuminate the differences and relationships between the two.

APN coaching is defined as a purposeful, complex, dynamic, collaborative, and holistic interpersonal process aimed at supporting and facilitating patients and families through health-related experiences and transitions to achieve health-related goals, mutually determined, whenever possible. These goals may include higher levels of wellness, risk reduction, reduced morbidity and suffering from chronic illness, and improved quality of life, including palliative care. The APN coaching process can best be understood as an intervention. It is mediated by the APN-patient relationship and the APN's self-reflective skills and interpersonal, clinical, and technical skills. APNs can usually coach patients independent of setting, cognitive

EXEMPLAR 8-1   Anticipatory Guidance in Primary and Acute Care

Primary Care

A nurse practitioner (NP), doing a health history on a young woman, elicited information about binge drinking that was a concern. Rather than directing or lecturing, she asked the woman if she knew about the effects of alcohol on the body; the woman said "no." The NP then asked if the woman would like to learn about the effects, to which the patient replied "yes." The visit proceeded with a brief overview of the effects of alcohol and provision of more resources.

Acute Care

After multiple experiences with cancer patients, one of the authors (JS) incorporated anticipatory guidance at the start of cancer chemotherapy, using the following approach.

Noting that everyone responds to this type of chemotherapy differently, JS would ask what they had heard about the drugs they would be taking. JS would review the common side effects, what could be done pharmacologically and nonpharmacologically to minimize the effects, and what other patients had done to manage their time and activities during the period receiving chemotherapy. JS pointed out that the first treatment was the hardest because of unknown factors and that if the patient paid attention to his or her own experience—if and when side effects occurred—they would be in a position to work together to make subsequent treatments more tolerable. An important assessment prior to the next chemotherapy cycle focused on the patient's responses to treatment, and what worked and what didn't work, so that a more appropriate side effect management program could be developed.

---

capacity, and stage of illness; it can be done at a distance or face to face.

Advanced Practice Nurse Guidance and Coaching Competency: Theoretical and Empirical Perspectives

This section reviews selected literature reports, including the following: (1) conceptual and empirical work on transitions as a major focus of APN guidance and coaching; (2) the transtheoretical model of behavior change (also known as the stages of change theory) and its associated interventions; and (3) evidence that APNs incorporate expert guidance and coaching as they deliver care.

Transitions in Health and Illness

The notion of transitions and the concept of transitional care have become central to policies aimed at reducing health care costs and increasing quality of care (Naylor, Aiken, Kurtzman, et al., 2011). Early work by Schumacher and Meleis (1994) remains relevant to the APN coaching competency and contemporary interventions, often delivered by APNs, designed to ensure smooth transitions for patients as they move across settings (e.g., Coleman & Boult, 2003; Coleman & Berenson, 2004; U.S. Aging and Disability Resource Center, 2011; Administration on Aging, 2012).

Schumacher and Meleis (1994) have defined the term *transition* as a passage from one life phase, condition, or status to another: "Transition refers to both the process and outcome of complex person-environment interactions. It may involve more than one person and is embedded in the context and the situation" (Chick & Meleis, 1986, pp. 239-240). The definition speaks to the fact that others are affected by, or can influence, transitions. Transitions are paradigms for life and living. Becoming a parent, giving up cigarettes, learning how to cope with chronic illness, and dying in comfort and dignity are just a few examples of transitions. Similar to life, they may be predictable or unpredictable, joyous or painful, obvious or barely perceptible, chosen and welcomed, or unexpected and feared. Understanding patients' perceptions of transition experiences is essential to effective coaching. Chick and Meleis (1986) have characterized the process of transition as having phases during which individuals experience the following: (1) disconnectedness from their usual social supports; (2) loss of familiar reference points; (3) old needs that remain unmet; (4) new needs; and (5) old expectations that are no longer congruent with the changing situation.

Transitions can also be characterized according to type, conditions, and universal properties. Schumacher and Meleis (1994) have proposed four types of transitions—developmental, health and illness, situational, and organizational.

Developmental transitions are those that reflect life cycle transitions, such as adolescence, parenthood, and aging. For the purposes of discussing coaching by APNs, developmental transitions are considered to include any transition with an intrapersonal focus, including changes in life cycle, self-perception, motivation, expectations, or meanings.

Health and illness transitions were primarily viewed as illness-related and ranged from adapting to a chronic illness to returning home after a stay in the hospital (Schumacher and Meleis, 1994). In today's health care system, transitions are not just about illness. They include adapting to the physiologic and psychological demands of pregnancy, reducing risk factors to prevent illness, changing unhealthy lifestyle behaviors, and numerous other clinical phenomena. Some health and illness changes are self-limiting (e.g., the physiologic changes of pregnancy), whereas others are long term and may be reversible or irreversible. In this chapter, health and illness transitions are defined as transitions driven by an individual's experience of the body in a holistic sense.

Studies have suggested that prior embodied experiences may play a role in the expression or the trajectory of a patient's health/illness experience. For example, in the Adverse Childhood Experiences (ACE) Study (Centers for Disease Control and Prevention, 2010), adverse experiences in childhood, such as abuse and trauma, had strong relationships with health concerns, such as smoking and obesity. In a clinical case study, Felitti (2002) proposed that, although diabetes and hypertension were the "presenting concerns" in a 70-year-old woman, the first priority on her problem list should be the childhood sexual abuse she had experienced; effective treatment of the presenting illnesses would depend on acknowledging the abuse and referring the patient to appropriate therapy.

Situational transitions are most likely to include changes in educational, work, and family roles. These can also result from changes in intangible or tangible structures or resources (e.g., loss of a relationship or financial reversals; Schumacher & Meleis, 1994). Developmental, health and illness, and situational transitions are the most likely to lead to clinical encounters requiring guidance and coaching. In practice, APNs remain aware of the possibility of multiple transitions occurring as a result of one salient transition. While eliciting information on the primary transition that led the patient to seek care, the APN attends to verbal, nonverbal, and intuitive cues to identify other transitions and meanings associated with the primary transition. Attending to the possibility of multiple transitions enables the APN to tailor coaching to the individual's particular needs and concerns.

Organizational transitions are those that occur in the environment; within agencies, between agencies, or in society. They reflect changes in structures and resources at a system level. Clinical nurse specialists (CNSs) typically have more involvement in planning and implementing organizational transitions. However, all APNs must be skilled in dealing with organizational transitions, because they tend to affect structural and contextual aspects of providing care. Table 8-2 lists some transitions, based on this typology, that might require APN coaching. Wise APNs pay attention to all four types of transitions in their personal and professional lives.

Outcomes of successful transitions include subjective well-being, role mastery, and well-being of relationships (Schumacher and Meleis, 1994), all components of quality of life. This description of transitions as a focus for APN coaching underscores the need for and the importance of a holistic orientation to caring for patients.

Transtheoretical Model of Behavior Change

The transtheoretical model (TTM; also called the Stages of Change theory), is a model derived from several hundred psychotherapy and behavior change theories

---

TABLE 8-2   **Transition Situations That Require Coaching**

Health/Illness	Developmental	Situational	Organizational
Pregnancy, labor	Parenting	Job loss or change	Mergers
Hospitalization	Adverse childhood experiences	Divorce	Policy changes
Risk reduction	Puberty	Natural or national disasters	Change in leadership
Lifestyle changes	Suffering	Quality of life	Change in organizational structure
Chronic condition	Loss of significant others	Change in social supports	
Disability	Caregiving for older relatives	Social isolation	
Weight loss or gain	Changes in sexual function or activity	Financial reversals or windfalls	
Symptoms		Change in living situations	
Violence		Community trauma	

NOTE: The situations are categorized according to the initiating change. Many of these transitions have reciprocal impacts across categories.

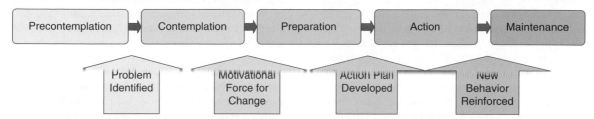

FIG 8-1 Prochaska's stages of change: The five stages of change. *(From R. W. Scholl. [2012]. Personal communication.* Adapted from Prochaska, J.O., DiClemente, C.C., & Norcross, J.C. [1992]. In search of how people change. Applications to addictive behaviours. *American Psychologist, 47,* 1102.)

(Norcross, Krebs & Prochaska, 2011; Prochaska, Redding, & Evers, 2008). Based on studies of smokers, Prochaska and associates (2008) learned that behavior change unfolds through stages. TTM has been used successfully to increase medication adherence and to modify high-risk lifestyle behaviors, such as substance abuse, eating disorders, sedentary lifestyles, and unsafe sexual practices. Change is conceptualized as a five-stage process (Fig. 8-1), in which change can be hastened with skillful guidance and coaching. APNs can use the TTM model to tailor interactions and interventions to the patient's specific stage of change to maximize the likelihood that they will progress through the stages of behavioral change.

Stages of Change

Precontemplation

This is the stage in which people are not yet contemplating change; specifically, they do not intend to take any action within the next 6 months. Precontemplators are not interested in learning more, thinking about, or discussing their high-risk behaviors. Offering specific advice in this stage is counterproductive and can increase resistance and hamper progression through the stages of change. In this stage, the focus of APN coaching is to make the patient feel understood, avoid giving advice, keep lines of communication open, and convey a willingness to be available when the patient is ready to make a change. APNs should also be alert to expressions of emotions about the unhealthy behavior because these are often opportunities to raise a patient's awareness of the impact of the unhealthy behavior, an important precursor to committing to change.

Contemplation

In this stage, people intend to make a change within the next 6 months. They are acutely aware of the hazards of the behavior and are also more aware of the advantages of changing the behavior. Contemplation is not a commitment, and the patient is often uncertain. When the risks of not changing the behavior are approximately equivalent to the advantages of changing, people can become stuck in ambivalence. Offering advice or education at this stage can also impede progress toward successful behavior change. With contemplators, the focus of APN coaching is to try to tip the decisional balance. Evocation requires close attention to the patients' statements and emotions to uncover possible motivations that will move the patient forward; so, interventions in this stage are not directed toward overcoming resistance or increasing adherence or compliance to treatment.

Preparation

This is the stage in which people are ready to take action within 1 month. They have a detailed action plan and may have already taken some action in the past year. Actions may be small (e.g., walking 15 minutes/day) but are clearly stated and oriented toward change; individuals are more open to the APN's advice. In this stage, because ambivalence is not yet completely resolved, the focus of APN coaching is to offer support related to the patient's action plan and to determine the strength of the commitment. This assessment enables the APN to work with the patient on identifying and anticipating difficulties and devising specific strategies to overcome them, a critical intervention in this stage.

Action

This is the stage in which people have already made lifestyle changes within the last 6 months that are leading to a measurable outcome (e.g., number of pounds lost, lower hemoglobin A1c [HbA1C] level). To be categorized as being in the action stage, a measurable marker must be met as a result of an action the patient took that reduced the risk for disease or complications. In this stage, the focus of APN coaching is to support and strengthen the person's commitment to the changes that he or she has made. APNs do this by reinforcing the health benefits of the change, and acknowledging the personal qualities and resources that the patient has tapped to make and sustain this change.

Maintenance

This is the stage in which patients have changed a behavior for longer than 6 months and strive to avoid relapse; they have more confidence in their ability to sustain the change and are less likely to relapse. Even so, relapse is always possible in the action or maintenance stage and may be a response to stressful situations. Relapse can occur over time (e.g., several "just this once, I can…" occasions), but even one slip can initiate a return to the old behavior. The focus of APN coaching is to work with the patient to avoid relapse by reviewing the stages of change, assessing the stability of the change, assessing for new stressors or reduced capacity to cope with stress, reviewing the patient's plans to overcome barriers to change, reminding the patient that vigilance is required, and identifying resources for dealing with new stressors. Regardless of how difficult life becomes, patients are confident that they can sustain the changes they have achieved and will not return to unhealthy coping mechanisms.

Earlier work on transitions by Meleis and others is consistent with and affirms the concepts of the TTM. For example, Chick and Meleis (1986) have characterized the process of transition as having phases during which individuals go through five phases (see earlier). These ideas are consistent with elements of the TTM and offer useful ideas for assessment. Making lifestyle or behavior changes are transitions; the stages of change are consistent with the characteristics of transition phases (Chick and Meleis, 1986). APNs can use nurses' theoretical work on transitions to inform assessments and interventions during each of the TTM stages of change and tailor their guiding and coaching interventions to the stage of readiness. When clinicians adopt the language of change, it prevents labeling and prejudging patients, helps maintain positive regard for the patient, and creates a climate of safety and hope. Patients know that, if and when they are ready to change, the APN will collaborate with them.

Evidence That Advanced Practice Nurses Guide and Coach

Quantitative studies, qualitative studies, and anecdotal reports have suggested that coaching patients and staff through transitions is embedded in the practices of nurses (Benner, Hooper-Kyriakidis, et al., 1999), and particularly APNs (Bowles, 2010; Cooke, Gemmill, & Grant, 2008; Dick & Frazier, 2006; Hayes & Kalmakis, 2007; Hayes, McCahon, Panahi, et al., 2008; Link, 2009; Mathews, Secrest, & Muirhead, 2008; Parry & Coleman, 2010). APN-led patient education and monitoring programs for specific clinical populations have demonstrated that coaching is central to their effectiveness (Crowther, 2003; Brooten, Naylor, York, et al., 2002; Marineau, 2007).

Teaching and counseling are significant clinical activities in nurse-midwifery (Holland & Holland, 2007) and CNS practice (Lewandoski & Adamle, 2009). Studies of NPs and NP students have indicated that they spend a significant proportion of their direct care time teaching and counseling (Lincoln, 2000; O'Connor, Hameister, & Kershaw, 2000). Early studies documented the nature, focus, content, and amount of time that APNs spent in teaching, guiding and coaching, and counseling, as well as the outcomes of these interventions (Brooten, Youngblut, Deatrick, et al., 2003; see Chapter 23). Furthermore, Hayes and colleagues (2008) have affirmed the importance of the therapeutic APN-patient alliance and have proposed that NPs who manage patients with chronic illness apply TTM in their practice, including the use of coaching strategies.

Advanced Practice Nurses and Models of Transitional Care

Among the studies of APN care are those in which APNs provide care coordination for patients as they move from one setting to the other, such as hospital to home. Transitional care has been defined as "a set of actions designed to ensure the coordination and continuity of health care as patients transfer between different locations or different levels of care within the same location" (Coleman & Boult, 2003, p. 556). There are at least three types of evidence-based transitional care programs that have used APNs to support transitions from hospital to home (U.S. Agency on Aging and Disability Resource Center, 2011). Studies of the transitional care model (TCM) and care transitions intervention (CTI) have used APNs as the primary intervener. There is also a model of practice-based care coordination that used an NP and social worker, the Geriatric Resources for Assessment and Care of Elders (GRACE) model (Counsell, Callahan, Buttar, et al., 2006). Based on transitional care research, the provision of transitional care is now regarded as essential to preventing error and costly readmissions to hospitals and is recognized and recommended in current U.S. health care policies (Naylor et al., 2011). Table 8-3 compares the three models of care transitions that used APNs. Because the GRACE model is similar to the TCM and CTI models, it will not be discussed further here.

Transitional Care Model

Extensive research on the TCM has documented improved patient and institutional outcomes and led to better understanding of the nature of APN interventions. Currently, the TCM is a set of activities aimed at providing "comprehensive in-hospital planning and home follow-up for chronically ill high risk older adults hospitalized for common medical and surgical conditions" (Transitional

TABLE 8-3 Care Transition Models Using Advanced Practice Nurses

	MODEL		
	Care Transitions Intervention (CTI)*	Transitional Care Model (TCM)†	Geriatric Resources for Assessment and Care of Elders (GRACE)‡
Short description	Transition coach: • Helps patients and families learn transition-specific self-management skills • Conducts hospital visit to introduce the program and tools (e.g., personal health record [PHR]) • Conducts one home visit 24-72 hr postdischarge • Makes three follow-up phone calls to reinforce coaching offered during the home visit and activation behavior	Transitional care nurse: • Visits patient in the hospital • Conducts home visit within 24 hr of discharge • Accompanies patient on first visit with physician postdischarge and subsequent visits if needed • Facilitates physician-nurse collaboration across episodes of acute care • Conducts weekly home visits for first month • Is on call 7 days/wk • Provides active engagement of patients and family caregivers, with focus on meeting their goals • Provides communication to, between, and among the patient, family caregivers, and health care providers	Resource team: • Conducts in-home initial comprehensive geriatric assessment with patient and family • Meets with larger GRACE team to develop individualized care plan, including protocols • NP and social worker implement care plan and coordinate care between providers and settings through face to face and telephone contacts • Makes contact with other providers for coordination of care
Target population	Individuals ≥ 65 Community-dwelling adults with a working telephone Appropriate for persons with depression or dementia provided they have a willing and able family caregiver	Evaluation includes cognitively intact adults ≥ 65 yr with two or more risk factors, including • Poor self-health ratings • Multiple chronic conditions • History of recent hospitalizations	Individuals ≥ 65 yr Community-dwelling adults with a working telephone Annual household income below 200% of federal poverty level Had one or more primary care visits in past 12 mo
Length of intervention	1 mo	1-3 mo	Research study: 2 yr
Training	1-day training on site or in Colorado	Internet-based training modules	Special training in implementing GRACE protocols and working as an interdisciplinary team during 12 weekly small group seminars
Qualification(s) required	Transition coach needs strong interpersonal and communication skills, ability to make the shift from doing things for patients to facilitating skill transfer so that patients can do more for themselves	Transitional care nurse in published studies was APN Currently evaluating outcomes with baccalaureate-prepared nurses	Resource team includes NP and licensed social worker, both having previous experience in geriatric care; employed by primary care practice Larger GRACE team consists of geriatrician, pharmacist, physical therapist, mental health social worker, and community-based services liaison

Continued

TABLE 8-3   Care Transition Models Using Advanced Practice Nurses—*cont'd*

	MODEL		
	Care Transitions Intervention (CTI)*	Transitional Care Model (TCM)†	Geriatric Resources for Assessment and Care of Elders (GRACE)‡
Estimated costs	From research study: $196/patient	From research study: $982/patient	From research study: $1000/patient/yr
Website	http://www.caretransitions.org	http://www.innovativecaremodels.com/care_models/21/overview	http://medicine.iupui.edu/IUCAR/research/grace.aspx

*Referred to as the Coleman model (Coleman et al., 2004)
†Referred to as the Naylor model (Naylor et al., 2004).
‡Referred to as the GRACE model (Counsell et al., 2006).
Adapted from the U.S. Aging and Disability Resource Center. (2011). Evidence-based care transitions models side-by-side March 2011 (adrc-tae.org/tiki-download_file.php?fileId=30310).

Care Model, 2008-2009; http://www.transitionalcare.info/). Early studies of the model from which TCM evolved have provided substantive evidence of the range and focus of teaching and counseling activities undertaken initially by CNSs, and later NPs, who provided care to varied patient populations. Controlled trials of this model have found that APN coaching, counseling, and other activities demonstrate statistically significant differences in patient outcomes and resource utilization (e.g., Brooten, Roncoli, Finkler, et al., 1994; Naylor, Brooten, Campbell, et al., 1999).

Secondary analyses of data from early transitional care trials have identified the specific interventions that APNs used for five different clinical populations (Naylor, Bowles, & Brooten, 2000): health teaching, guidance, and/or counseling; treatments and procedures; case management; and surveillance (Brooten et al., 2003). The most frequent intervention was surveillance; health teaching was the second or third most frequent intervention, depending on the patient population. APNs used a holistic focus that required clinical expertise, including sufficient patient contact, interpersonal competence, and systems leadership skills to improve outcomes (Brooten, Youngblut, Deatrick, et al., 2003). Currently, the TCM process is focused on older adults and consists of screening, engaging the older adult and caregiver, managing symptoms, educating and promoting self-management, collaborating, ensuring continuity, coordinating care, and maintaining the relationship (http://www.transitionalcare.info/).

Care Transitions Intervention Model

During an illness, patients may transition through multiple sites of care that place them at higher risk for errors and adverse events, contributing to higher costs of care. Building on findings from studies of the TCM, the CTI program supports older adults with complex medical needs as they move throughout the health care system (Parry and Coleman, 2010). Coleman and colleagues have found results similar to those of TCM, a decreased likelihood of being readmitted and an increased likelihood of achieving self-identified personal goals around symptom management and functional recovery (Coleman, Smith, Frank, et al. 2004). Findings were sustained for as long as 6 months after the program ended. Subsequent studies of CTI have demonstrated significant reductions in 30-, 90-, and 180-day hospital readmissions (Coleman, Parry, Chalmers & Min, 2006). Because motivational interviewing (MI) has been part of CTI training, these findings suggest that integration of TTM key principles into APN practice, such as helping patients identify their own goals and having support (coaching) in achieving them, contributes to successful coaching outcomes.

Based on their observations of creating and implementing the CTI with coaches of different backgrounds, Parry and Coleman (2010) have asserted that coaching differs from other health care processes, such as teaching and coordination. Instead of providing the patient with the answers, the coach supports the patient and provides the tools needed to manage the illness and navigate the health care system. According to these authors, a commitment and ability to adopt a coaching role and foster empowerment and confidence in the patient is more important than a disciplinary background.

As APN-based transitional care programs evolve, researchers are examining whether other, sometimes less expensive providers can offer similar services and achieve the same outcome. For example, TCM programs have begun to use baccalaureate-prepared nurses to provide transitional care; Parry and Coleman (2010) have reported on the use of other providers in CTI interventions, including social workers. These initiatives suggest that APNs, administrators, and researchers need to identify those clinical populations for whom APN coaching is necessary.

In medically complex patients, APNs may be preferred and less expensive coaches, in part because of their competencies and scopes of practice.

Model of Advanced Practice Nurse Guidance and Coaching

Assumptions

Several assumptions underlie this model:

1. APNs involve the patient's significant other or patient's proxy, as appropriate.
2. Although technical competence and clinical competence may be sufficient for teaching a task, they are insufficient for coaching patients through transitions, including chronic illness experiences or behavioral and lifestyle changes. For example, patients with diabetes may be taught how to monitor their blood sugar levels and administer insulin with technical accuracy, but if the lifestyle impacts of the transition from health to chronic illness are not evaluated, guidance and coaching do not occur.
3. Although guidance and coaching skills are an integral part of professional nursing practice, the clinical and didactic content of graduate education extends the APN's repertoire of skills and abilities, enabling the APN to coach in situations that are broader in scope or more complex in nature.
4. APNs also apply their guidance and coaching skills in interactions with colleagues, interprofessional team members, students, and others.
5. Effective guidance and coaching of patients, family members, staff, and colleagues depend on the quality of the therapeutic or collegial relationships that APNs establish with them.
6. As with other APN core competencies, the coaching competency develops over time, during and after graduate education.

Overview of the Model

The APN guidance and coaching competency reflects an integration of the characteristics of the direct clinical practice competency (see Chapter 7) but is particularly dependent on the formation of therapeutic partnerships with patients, use of a holistic perspective and reflective practice, and interpersonal interventions. Individual elements of the model include clinical, technical, and interpersonal competence mediated by self-reflection. In identifying these elements, the model of APN guidance and coaching breaks down what is really a holistic, flexible, and often indescribable process. As APNs assess, diagnose, and treat a patient, they are attending closely to the meanings that patients ascribe to health and illness experiences; APNs take these meanings into account in working with patients. APNs also attend to patterns, consciously and subconsciously, that develop intuition and contribute to their clinical acumen. The aim in offering this model is not only to help APNs understand what coaching is but to give them language by which to explain their interpersonal effectiveness. It is important to note that all elements of the model work synergistically to create this competency; separating them for the sake of discussion is somewhat artificial.

APNs integrate self-reflection and the competencies they have acquired through experience and graduate education with their assessment of the patient's situation—that is, patients' understandings, vulnerabilities, motivations, goals, and experiences. Guidance and coaching require that APNs be self-aware and self-reflective as an interpersonal transaction is unfolding so that they can shape communications and behaviors to maximize the therapeutic goals of the clinical encounter. Thus, guidance and coaching by APNs represent an interaction of four factors: the APN's interpersonal, clinical, and technical competence and the APN's self-reflection (Fig. 8-2). These factors are further influenced by individual and contextual factors. The interaction of self-reflection with these three areas of competence, and clinical experiences with patients, drive the ongoing expansion and refinement of guiding and coaching expertise in advanced practice nursing.

Self-Reflection

Self-reflection is the deliberate internal examination of experience so as to learn from it. The APN uses self-reflection during and after interactions with patients, classically described as reflection-in-action and reflection-on-action (Schön, 1983, 1987). Reflection-in-action is the ability to pay attention to phenomena as they are occurring, giving free rein to one's intuitive understanding of the situation as it is unfolding; individuals respond with a varied repertoire of exploratory and transforming actions best characterized as strategic improvisation. APN coaching is analogous to the flexible and inventive playing of a jazz musician. Reflection-in-action requires astute awareness of context and investing in the present moment with full concentration, capabilities that take time to master and require regular practice.

The ability to self-reflect and focus on the process of coaching as it is occurring implies that APNs are capable of the simultaneous execution of other skills. While interacting with patients, APNs integrate observations and information gleaned from physical examinations and

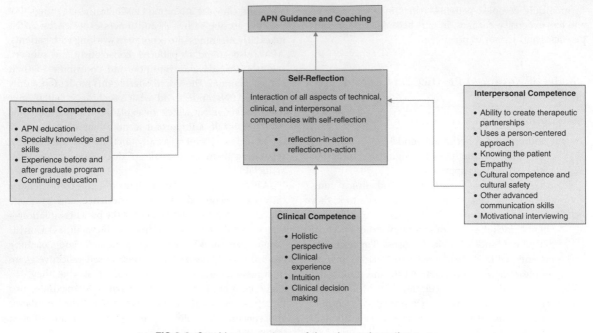

FIG 8-2 Coaching competency of the advanced practice nurse.

interviews with their own theoretical understanding, non-cognitive intuitive reactions, and the observations, intuitions, and theories that they elicit from patients. APNs interpret these multiple sources of information to arrive at possible explanations and interventions. Throughout the process, the APN is aware of the individual and contextual factors that may affect the coaching encounter and these factors also shape interactions—first to elicit and negotiate patient goals and outcomes and then to collaborate with the patient and others to produce those outcomes.

APNs bring their reflections-in-action to their post-encounter reflections on action. Experienced APNs are more likely than inexperienced APNs to pay attention to feelings and intuitions. More often, one is likely to ruminate on negative experiences because the feeling of failure is more uncomfortable than the feeling of satisfaction or success. However, reflecting on satisfying and successful experiences and discerning why they were effective contributes to developing competence and expertise and reveals knowledge about assessments and interventions that will be useful in future interactions. APN students need to be taught that the feelings arising in clinical experiences are often clues to their developing expertise or indicate something that may require personal attention (e.g., a patient who repeatedly comes to clinic intoxicated

elicits memories and feelings of a parent who was alcoholic). Regular self-reflection helps APNs develop skills to describe clinical phenomena and express that which is hard to name.

Clinical and Technical Competence

Clinical and technical competence are well-defined aspects of established advanced practice roles and their importance to coaching cannot be overstated. However, these two factors are not addressed in detail in this chapter. Clinical and technical competence are based on experience with the APN's specialty populations. Pre–graduate school experiences, experiences within graduate clinical practica, and post-graduate clinical experiences provide the grist for analyzing, developing, and revealing the coaching competency of APNs. Over the course of caring for patients, nurses learn the many ways people experience and manage health, birth, illness, pain, suffering, and death (Benner, 1985; Benner et al., 2009). Ongoing development of this competency depends on applying self-reflection to these clinical experiences, including the mastery of technical skills, to acquire new coaching knowledge and skills that cannot be found in any text. For example, novice APNs may experience more difficulty being present with patients because of concern about their technical competence, time pressures, and other sources of anxiety that might interfere with presence in the clinical encounter.

The evolution of APN specialties in nursing has focused on defining and describing the technical and clinical skills required for particular APN roles and clinical populations (see Chapters 1 and 7). The chapters in Part III illustrate the role-specific technical and clinical skills APNs need to enact this competency.

Interpersonal Competence

Interpersonal competence encompasses a set of advanced relational and communication skills that enable APNs to establish therapeutic caring relationships or alliances and communicate effectively, addressing affective and cognitive elements of the patient encounter. Therapeutic relationship skills learned in one's preprofessional nursing education are the basis for developing the advanced relational and communication skills APNs need. Since researchers first identified the teaching-coaching function of expert nurses and APNs (Benner, 1985; Benner et al., 1999; Fenton & Brykczynski, 1993), teaching, guidance, and coaching by APNs have been integrated into research studies, APN competencies, case studies, and other writings about APN practice. There is increasing recognition and evidence that provider-patient relationships and the quality of their communications influence quality, safety, and health outcomes.

The seven elements that comprise interpersonal competence will be discussed in some detail, because they help distinguish APN guidance and coaching from coaching done by staff nurses and other health coaches. Much of the information on the APN-patient relationship as an intervention is found in the psychiatric literature (e.g., Mathews, Secrest, & Muirhead, 2008; Parrish, Peden, & Staten, 2008; Perraud, Delaney, Carlson-Sebelli, et al., 2006). Several common characteristics of therapeutic relationships that inform the concept of interpersonal competence include: creating an alliance or partnership; knowing the patient; a holistic perspective (e.g., Parrish et al., 2008; Mathews et al., 2008); conveying empathy (e.g., Perraud, et al. 2006); presence, trust, and positive regard; and engagement (Elliott, 2010).

Taken together, these findings affirm that APNs use a holistic perspective, establish therapeutic partnerships with patients, and use self-reflection to uncover personal knowledge that can be applied in practice. In addition, it appears that APNs use processes consistent with TTM principles and communication strategies in their coaching. It is apparent that establishing a therapeutic partnership with a patient is a complex process involving a variety of relational and communication skills that are central to an APN's interpersonal effectiveness. These skills are developed and refined through education, experience, and a dialectic process of reflection on experiences with individuals, groups, or populations of patients.

In addition to the complexities cited, several features allow APNs' interpersonal competence to be characterized as advanced. A primary feature is that the interactions are strategic, even when they are spontaneous (Ball & Cox, 2003; Hanley & Fenton, 2007). APNs prepare themselves, however briefly, for an encounter. Aware of possible patient vulnerabilities, APNs strive to create an environment that is interpersonally, physically, psychologically, and culturally safe. APNs collaborate with the patient, family, and other team members to establish goals and use their assessments and guiding and coaching skills to maintain or modify goals and treatments. Another important advanced element is the APN's use of coaching to advocate for patients to their colleagues, thereby helping teams and systems understand patient and family perspectives, working with the whole team (including the patient) to create a safe environment and shape the course of the health and illness, developmental, or situational transition.

Ability to Create Therapeutic Partnerships

Establishing and sustaining a caring therapeutic relationship with a patient demands that the APN be emotionally responsive, not distant; they demonstrate empathy and caring while maintaining professional boundaries. They present authentically, revealing themselves through their eyes, tone of voice, affect, body language, and silences. APNs who rely only on scientific and technical competencies in their relationships with patients are unlikely to appreciate patients' holistic responses or enable patients to express themselves holistically (Gadow, 1980). In a qualitative study of 10 psychiatric APNs, Parrish and associates (2008) found that APNs described this authentic and holistic approach as a primary element of their care of patients with depression. They viewed the therapeutic use of self as a key strategy for involving the patient in their care and engaged with patients as partners in assessment and decision making regarding treatment.

Person-Centered Approach

A patient- and family-centered care approach is now understood as a central component of safe and effective patient care. The TJC (2010) has defined patient- and family-centered care as "An innovative approach to plan, deliver, and evaluate health care that is grounded in mutually beneficial partnerships among health care providers, patients, and families. Patient- and family-centered care applies to patients of all ages, and it may be practiced in any health care setting" (p. 92).

The first QSEN competency for APNs also speaks to the importance of this person-centered stance in noting that APNs "analyze multiple dimensions of patient-centered care [including]: patient/family/community values; coordination and integration of care; information, communication, and education; physical comfort and emotional support; involvement of family and friends; [and] transition and continuity" (Cronenwett, Sherwood, Pohl, et al., 2009, p. 339).

Prior to meeting a patient, APNs do an internal check. This may entail thoroughly looking at the chart, quickly scanning results and notes since the last visit, or simply intending to be present to a patient in the middle of a harried, time-packed day. APNs also attend to relational and communication basics and encourage team members to do the same, such as introducing oneself, explaining her or his role, explaining how the office or unit providers and staff work together to deliver care, and discussing any important principles or policies (e.g., on-call system, late arrivals). APNs are aware of how the environment or behaviors can facilitate or impede communication and ensure that a patient feels safe. For example, an APN might ask permission for a student to be present or to touch the patient prior to conducting an examination. APNs also avoid postures that might convey a power differential, such as standing during an interview while the patient is seated.

APNs must also be able to suspend judgment about a patient's appearance, behavior, background, or other characteristics and transcend difficult or unpleasant clinical presentations, such as a malodorous wound, to convey an unconditional positive regard for the person. APNs also coach team members, through advocacy and mentoring, to develop and convey this quality in their relationships with patients. APNs remain alert to their own emotional and behavioral reactions in clinical situations and develop the resources and skills needed to debrief, process the emotions that arise, and know when to seek support and consultation.

Knowing the Patient

APNs are attentive to the multiple dimensions of being human—physiologic, affective, cognitive, behavioral, social and relational, spiritual, and environmental—knowing that a focus on a particular factor may be the key to a productive therapeutic relationship. This enables APNs not only to know individual patients, but to know populations, acquiring specialized and deep personal knowledge of common features of patients' experiences of health and illness that are integrated into evidence-based assessments and interventions at the point of care. In addition, APNs attend to interaction effects among patients, families, provider systems, and contexts. This specialized personal knowledge of patients, populations, teams, and systems enables APNs to individualize care to the patient. For example, a CNS in diabetes care might find that by understanding the type of work a patient did, she could explain the pathophysiology of the disease in a way that would motivate the patient to begin to make the necessary dietary and lifestyle changes. A pediatric NP might realize that one of the reasons for no-shows of chronically ill children in an urban, academic center clinic was that parents could not manage the time and travel challenges to keep multiple referral appointments. Then, she might work with others to create a one-stop appointment system so that children could be seen by all needed specialists on the same day.

A vital aspect of knowing the patient is what White (2005) has called "sociopolitical knowing." This includes an understanding of the social and political context of the patient, as well as the broader context in which nursing and health care take place. Both the APN's and patient's cultural and political backgrounds powerfully influence their understanding of health, illness, language, identity, social roles, and historical issues. For example, domestic violence, child abuse, and stress-induced illnesses are often responses to political, social, and personal problems. APNs may find that coaching their patients requires that they expose social and political inequities that affect people's health so that they can be addressed, an observation consistent with phase 4 of the ethical decision making competency—that APNs work for social justice (see Chapter 13). Otherwise, the core issues in many patients' transitions will be invisible and unidentified, and the coaching strategies used will be superficial, unfocused, and ineffective.

Bonis' (2009) concept analysis of knowing in nursing, including knowing the patient, clarifies several attributes of knowing relevant to this model of coaching. Personal knowledge is an integration of scientific information with the application of this knowledge in one's practice that becomes refined and synthesized through reflection. Knowing is also shaped through one's personal perspective—not just the nurse's perspective but his or her ability to comprehend the patient's unique perspective and recognize a patient's unique patterns and health-related changes in those patterns. It is this knowing that enables APNs to collaborate with patients to create goals and action plans that take into account a patient's health patterns and experiences. Consequences of knowing for nurses and their patients are understanding, finding meaning, and evoking transformation. Transformation is viewed as "an ongoing process of change involving knowing, understanding, and finding meaning in experience" (Bonis, 2009, p. 1334). This notion of transformation is consistent with our belief that APN coaching can be transformative for patients. Knowing the patient addresses the objective and intuitive elements of care and is a particular aspect of forming partnerships with patients that APNs attend to when guiding and coaching.

Research studies have provided empirical support for the concept of knowing the patient as a central characteristic of nurse-patient (Benner et al., 2009; Morrison, 2011) and APN-patient relationships (Callister & Freeborn, 2007; Parrish et al., 2008).

Empathy

An early study, which has not been reproduced is the work of Squier (1990). Based on an analysis of studies of physicians and APNs, he proposed a model linking a clinician's empathic understanding with a patient's adherence to therapeutic regimens and hypothesized that empathic understanding has two components, cognitive and affective. Clinicians' cognitive ability to take the perspective of the patient accurately enables them to communicate effectively and reflect this understanding back to the patient. Patients are then more likely to elaborate the concerns that brought them to the clinician. Clinicians' sensitivity to patients' emotions and underlying concerns helps reduce the anxiety and stress that often affect the health problems for which patients consult clinicians. This work suggested that a clinician's relational and communication skills work together to create a productive therapeutic relationship.

Findings from later studies have supported Squier's model and show the interaction of the various elements of interpersonal competence. Parry and coworkers (2006), in a qualitative study of 32 of 976 patients who had participated in the CTI program, described patient experiences with the APNs' coaching intervention. First, the APN coach offered continuity and direction at each stage of the transition from one health care setting to the other; patients felt "supported, comforted, and safe" (p. 46). Second, patients identified two crucial components of APNs' coaching in self-management knowledge and skills: (1) during the home visit they were coached in medication management, and (2) they were taught about red flags, signs of disease complications and adverse drug effects that required action. This finding was consistent with Brooten and colleagues' (2003) view that teaching and coaching are related to the health problem under surveillance. In addition, many subjects mentioned that the coach supported their ability to communicate effectively with other providers by helping them generate questions and engage in role playing. This finding seems particularly important in light of Frosch and associates' 2012 study of shared decision making, in which patients reported that they feared being judged as difficult if they spoke up. Third, patients mentioned the importance of caring in the coaching relationship. In addition to feeling cared about, patients mentioned specific behaviors and qualities of the APN coach—meeting the coach prior to discharge, the APN's knowledge, experience, interest, and organizational skills, and the APN's willingness to become more involved in their care. The researchers observed that the patients' perception of feeling cared about may have been related to the APN's accessibility and frequent follow-up activities.

Cultural Competence and Cultural Safety

To coach effectively, APNs must be able to create a sense of cultural safety and demonstrate cultural competence in their communications with patients. Providing culturally safe care means that nurses deliver care that protects individuals' cultural identities, well-being, and practices (Betancourt, Green, & Carrillo, 2002; Nursing Council of New Zealand, 2005; Polaschak, 1998; Woods, 2010). This involves assuming a culturally competent stance that demonstrates an awareness of how persons of a particular group are perceived. Unsafe cultural practices are those that diminish, demean, or disempower the cultural identity and well-being of an individual (Nursing Council of New Zealand, 2005). APNs not only understand how the ways in which patients are different will affect patient care, but how clinicians' perceptions of a particular patient or patient population will affect the team's approach to assessment and care. Patients may avoid seeking care because they are aware of how they are perceived and only seek health care services when a problem is far advanced.

Creating cultural safety requires APNs to reflect deeply on their own experiences, biases, and judgments to understand how they may influence the care that they provide to patients (Woods, 2010). Cultural competence is sometimes regarded as controversial, because, as Wood noted, it requires one to view the patient as different and other and adapt one's practice to the situation, that could, even if inadvertently, disempower the patient. Exemplar 8-2 illustrates a student's recognition of her own biases and what she learned when she set aside her preconceived ideas about a homeless person, enhancing her sensitivity and ability to create cultural safety for future patients. Creating cultural safety should be a focus as APNs establish relationships with patients.

Other Advanced Communication Skills

Effective health communication has the attributes of accuracy, accessibility, balance (e.g., risks and benefits are clearly outlined), consistency, cultural competence, evidence-based care, broad reach (which gets to the largest possible number of people affected by the condition), is credible and reliable, repeated over time, timely, and understandable (Stableford & Mettger, 2007; TJC, 2010). The APN strives to ensure that communications with

EXEMPLAR 8-2   Self-Reflection and Learning Cultural Sensitivity

Reflecting on her experience with a homeless patient, a CNS student noted that when she heard in a report that her patient had a challenging wound care regimen and was homeless, she made a number of (negative) judgments about what this meant. Prior to entering his room, she made the decision to set these judgments aside, to set the intention to be open and respectful, and to learn from this man. She was first surprised by his neat and well-kept appearance. She learned that the man had been so disabled by his chronic illness (the work he used to perform had him on his feet all day, making him vulnerable to foot wounds and infections) that he lost his job and, ultimately, his home. Her patient had negotiated his life creatively—determined to look like he was working while looking for work. He knew in which public places he could find a place to wash and sometimes shower and have his clothes cleaned. He spent his days at the library, when he was not interviewing for a job. This experience forever changed the student—a lesson in suspending judgment to understand and care effectively.

---

patients meet these criteria. APNs also attend to a broader range of verbal and nonverbal cues and quickly determine those that are priorities. They then tailor an interaction to address the important issues embedded in the patient's language, issues that may be more or less relevant to the clinical problem at hand but are central to the patient.

APNs attend to patient communications and nonverbal cues expressed by the patient, significant others, other team members, and the APN's own nonverbal cues, using this information to ask additional questions, to probe for meaning, to reshape the interaction as it is unfolding, and to identify issues that may need to be further assessed at a future encounter. APNs summarize, recap, and interpret as they coach. Verbal and nonverbal skills that characterize advanced, person-centered skills are listed in Box 8-1.

While guiding and coaching, skilled clinicians move easily among various communication styles and skills, informed by the clinical situation, assessments, goals, and cognitive and emotional content of their interactions with patients and families. They are aware of what they are doing and why.

Motivational Interviewing

MI has emerged as one of the most powerful strategies for improving health by helping patients change their thoughts and behaviors (Rollnick, Miller, & Butler, 2008; Rubak, Sandboek, Lauritzen, et al., 2005). In a meta-analysis comparing MI with traditional advice giving, Rubak and colleagues found that MI consistently resulted in better results across a wide range of health outcomes, including body mass index, HbA1C level, total blood cholesterol, and systolic blood pressure.

In brief, MI is an interviewing approach aimed at understanding and resolving a patient's ambivalence about change by raising awareness and building a desire

 BOX 8-1   **Advanced Person-Centered Communication Skills**

- Allow patients to tell their stories using their own language and chronology
- Use a conversational style of interviewing
- Use motivational interviewing techniques and principles
- Elicit patients' thoughts, perspectives, expectations, values, and goals
- Ask about the contexts of patients' lives and the impact of health and illness concerns
- Encourage self-disclosure
- Respond to patients' indirect and nonverbal clues regarding emotions and problems
- Provide patients with self-care information and enable patients' participation in health care decision making
- Create shared understandings with patients
- Develop health care plans collaboratively with patients
- Express concern for patients' well-being
- Respond empathically
- Create social connectedness with patients by means of humor, touch, and appropriate self-disclosure
- Use open-ended questions and paraphrasing to elicit information and validate patients' communications
- Use a tone of voice and pace of speech appropriate to the topic being discussed
- Make eye contact and use a forward-leaning posture

Data from Borrelli (2006), Brown (1999), Montgomery (1993), Phillips-Salimi et al. (2011), and Quirk (2000).

on the part of the patient (motivation) to adopt new behaviors (Borrelli, 2006; Rollnick, Miller, & Butler, 2008). Through MI, patients uncover their own motivations and arguments for change; these become the scaffolding of commitment, self-efficacy, and long-term change. This type of interviewing is consistent with a person-centered style of interaction because it gives the patient an opportunity to air his or her concerns about the impact of changing or not changing. In MI, the APN engages in active and careful listening and poses strategic questions. Questions are asked in ways that engage the patient in self-reflection, aimed at raising awareness and uncovering possible motivations:

- What keeps them from changing?
- What would help them take action?
- Can an intermediate goal be identified?

Rosengren (2009) has noted that MI is not so much a collection of techniques but a set of specific clinician behaviors that are guided by an underlying philosophy, called MI spirit, which is a critical element of MI. MI spirit is defined as "the underlying set of mind and heart within which MI is practiced, including partnership, acceptance, compassion, and evocation" (Miller & Rollnick, 2012, p. 12). Although not unique to MI (e.g., the overlap with skills APNs learn about therapeutic relationships), this philosophy is a key element of MI (Rosengren, 2009).

Rollnick and associates (2008) have identified three communication styles and three communication skills associated with MI. The communication styles are guiding, directing, and following; the communication skills are asking, listening, and informing. It was noted that a directing style, characterized by more use of asking and informing, tends to be overused in practice.

In addition to communication styles and skills (Rollnick, Miller, & Butler, 2008) and MI spirit (Rosengren, 2009), the other key elements of MI include MI principles (RULE), foundational skills (OARS), and change talk or evocation (Rosengren, 2009). The RULE principles and OARS skills are listed in Tables 8-4 and 8-5. Readers are encouraged to consult the MI resources cited here for more information about this important approach.

In a study of the TCM, McCauley and coworkers (2006) have found that APNs use strategies consistent with MI, which helped account for their successful outcomes, and concluded that "identification of the patients' unique goals and connecting achievement of these goals to health-related behaviors.... proved to be a powerful force in gaining patient and caregiver partnership in sustained behavioral change" (McCauley et al., p. 307). Evidence has been accumulating that APNs, whether or not they are educated in the principles and techniques, seem to use MI strategies. However, the consistency with which MI can be implemented by APNs is likely to depend on

TABLE 8-4	Motivational Interviewing Principles: RULE
RULE	Example
Resist the righting reflex	• Refers to the impulse to "fix" the patient by giving advice.
	• Through reflective listening, the APN demonstrates an understanding of the decisional balance that the patient faces and asks questions that invite the patient to voice arguments for change.
Understand the patient's motivation	• The APN asks powerful questions to understand the specific motivators that will enable the patient to persist in changing to reach an identified goal.
Listen to the patient	• The APN uses all the senses to listen intently.
Empower the patient	• The APN identifies and reinforces the patient's best self resources.

Adapted from Rosengren, D. (2009). *Building motivational interviewing skills: A practitioner workbook.* New York: The Guilford Press, p. 9.

the practice setting and patient population in addition to the APN's education in, and experience with, using MI. One of the authors (RB) has been trained in MI and, as a CNS in acute care, she found that she has had to tailor its use in the acute care setting. However, MI has been invaluable in working with the many chronically ill patients she cares for during their acute episodes (see Exemplar 8-3). In addition, she has found this skill to be helpful in working with team members and staff in implementing change.

This review and discussion further speaks to the importance of APNs' therapeutic relationships with patients and the likelihood that they contribute to quality and outcomes of care, and suggests why health coaching has gained traction as a strategy for improving health and outcomes. This discussion of APNs' advanced relational and communication skills demonstrates that there are a number of hard to measure, interpersonal approaches that APNs can use to coach patients, families, teams, and systems to achieve high-quality, patient-centered care.

Conflict Negotiation and Resolution

APN students often express concern about difficult conversations and must be given opportunities to practice these types of communication and debrief their clinical observations and experiences with faculty. Among the many types of difficult conversations are conflicts, bad news, confronting bullying, or reporting an impaired

TABLE 8-5   Motivational Interviewing Technique: OARS

OARS	Techniques	Examples
Open Ended Questions	The patient does most of the talking.	• What would your life be like if you didn't have type 2 diabetes? • How would your life change if you stopped smoking?
Affirmation (with every encounter)	Notice a highly specific action that the patient has taken.	• I see you really invested in yourself by joining a gym. • I notice you have brought a notebook to take notes today.
Reflective listening	Listen for meaning and for incongruities between verbal and nonverbal communication.	• So, you think you are drinking too much but you really like it and don't want to change? • Are you saying that although it is painful for you to go out with friends, you do not want to lose weight?
Summaries	Offer a brief two- or three-sentence summary of the interaction that is easy to understand.	• You came to see me today about your back and leg pain and you have also discussed how concerned you are about your husband's health and your ability to take care of him. When we talked before, you haven't been interested in getting more help at home, which is available from the area Agency on Aging. I know how important it is to you to take care of your husband and we've talked about how you can take care of yourself as well.

Adapted from the Institute for Motivational Change. (2006). About motivational interviewing (http://www. miinstitute.com/index.php?page=about_motivational_interviewing).

EXEMPLAR 8-3   Coaching an End-of-Life Heart Failure Patient

As a CNS student, RB spent one semester with a palliative care team at a tertiary care hospital caring for patients with advanced illness. Within this interprofessional team there was an NP but no practicing CNS or registered nurse (RN). It was enlightening when, only after a few short weeks, RB's preceptor physician could explain what she brought to the team. The physician described the CNS role as a "keeper of the environment," one who connects with the patient and bedside nurse while examining the atmosphere around the patient that might affect care. The APN skills of coaching and motivational interviewing were most apparent with the care of a heart failure patent admitted to the cardiology service. The following referral (story) was sent to the palliative care team by the heart failure CNS, who had worked with the patient for 5 years, requesting that they see this patient.

Summary received from the referring CNS: CB is a 47-year-old man who has been on home dobutamine for the past 10 months for end-stage diastolic heart failure. He is not a transplant candidate by choice because he wants to continue to smoke and drink; maintaining his lifestyle is his priority. He seems at peace with dying; he has a do not resuscitate (DNR) order but wishes to keep his implantable cardiac defibrillator (ICD) activated.

They have discussed the concept of hospice for the past year and he has not felt ready for it. CB has beaten all odds with his disease by continuing to live at home and care for his dad with Alzheimer's; this is incredibly important to him. He drives, despite being advised by us not to. He has a girlfriend but at times their relationship is strained by what she wants (all heroics) and what he wants (DNR and dobutamine). She helps with his care when he allows her. Currently, he is in severe decline with an ICD infection and early kidney failure and is on long-term antibiotics. He is now receptive to my helping him at home and to having me focus on comfort care. CB still has unrealistic expectations about feeling better, and I have worked with him to revise his expectations. I am hoping the palliative care team can help move him forward to a good, final stage in his life. I am concerned that hospice won't accept him with dobutamine and a decision to keep the ICD on. Can you help?"

Palliative Care Team Activities and Interventions: The NP with the palliative care team met with CB and his girlfriend and provided them with information on end-of-life care and hospice options, to which they were receptive. On a follow-up visit, CB had become ambivalent and did not want to talk about end-of-life care. He again thought that his medical condition would improve and he would return home. It was determined that RB would meet with the patient to determine where he was in the decision making process, because she had cared for CB previously on the cardiology unit.

On meeting with the patient, RB reviewed the CNS student role and the purpose of her visit and then allowed the patient to control the conversation. During this initial meeting, RB focused on reflective listening, with open-ended, probing questions. The conversation included CB's disease process, end-of-life care, and current home situation.

CB told his father at the time of his diagnosis of Alzheimer's disease that he would take care of him as long as he could. CB's father can become aggressive at times, so caring for him at home is a challenge. The patient has a supportive brother and girlfriend who are willing to help him, but CB has difficulty asking others for help. During the conversation, RB used affirmations to evoke deeper feelings from the patient: "You know how it feels to take care of someone you love. Your friends and family have the same feelings when they help you." End-of life-decisions were not made during this initial conversation but the existing relationship was strengthened. CB was very appreciative of information regarding end-of-life care, but stated that he wanted to live one day at a time. He described his living situation and how he would continue to sleep upstairs, even if he had to crawl up the stairs, because his bedroom was his sanctuary; the one place where he could be alone. To maintain the momentum of evocation, RB summarized the conversation throughout the coaching session and at the beginning and end of the meeting.

Late on a Friday afternoon, RB met with CB. He was not feeling well, "no fight left in me," and she wanted his father to come to the hospital to visit him. CB wasn't optimistic about this happening because of his father's disease and periods of aggression. CB decided to talk with his brother to see if he would bring his dad into the hospital when he had a "good" day. The conversation turned to his long fight with heart failure, and how he hoped to beat the odds. A few years ago, CB suffered a cardiac arrest, was coded and pronounced dead, but regained a cardiac rhythm and awoke without neurologic deficits. When dobutamine was initiated last year, he was told he would only live a few months, and here he is almost a year later. RB decided not to discuss code status on a Friday afternoon; instead, she coached the nurse assigned to CB over the weekend to explore his feelings with open-ended questions. On Monday morning, CB decided to have his ICD turned off.

The following week, CB felt more short of breath, had increasing abdominal pain, was feeling very tired, and wanted to sleep all the time. He was focused on living one day at a time and hopeful to beat the odds again and to make it home and sleep in his own bed. When prompted about previous conversations about asking for help from friends and family, he believed it was getting easier for him.

CB was discharged home with visiting nurse support later that week, but was only home a few days before returning to the hospital. On readmission, he openly talked about the end of his life and he felt that his time was near. He did not want to be discharged to a hospice house, but wanted to die peacefully in the hospital with the nurses with whom he felt comfortable. He was started on morphine and his dobutamine was weaned off. CB passed away peacefully early one morning, with his brother and girlfriend at his bedside.

---

colleague. Some of these topics are addressed in other chapters of this text and/or professional organization publications. Conflicts are often at the heart of individual and team issues, such as moral distress and workplace bullying, both of which affect the APN's ability to guide and coach effectively. However, conflicts also present opportunities to practice new behaviors. Not all conflicts can be resolved, although skill in negotiating conflict can help APNs manage many difficult interpersonal interactions and coaching situations. The APN's self-awareness and self-reflection with regard to emotions and behavioral responses is no less important in these situations. It is helpful for APNs to identify clinical situations that trigger conflict for them and their usual reactions to conflict in order to recognize conflicts when they occur and evaluate whether their ways of handling conflict could be improved. The first author (JS) has found that APN students acknowledge that their conflict skills are suboptimal and a source of stress and distress; they are eager to learn new tools to handle these situations. There are many resources for assisting APNs to acquire effective skills for managing conflict, such as using the skills described on the Conflict Resolution Network (www.crnhq.org.; Box 8-2).

BOX 8-2   Conflict Resolution Skills: Summary of 12 Skills

1. The win-win approach: How can we solve this as partners rather than opponents?
2. Creative response: Transform problems into creative opportunities.
3. Empathy: Develop communication tools to build rapport. Use listening to clarify understanding.
4. Appropriate assertiveness: Apply strategies to attack the problem not the person.
5. Cooperative power: Eliminate "power over" to build "power with" others.
6. Managing emotions: Express fear, anger, hurt, and frustration wisely to effect change.
7. Willingness to resolve: Name personal issues that cloud the picture.
8. Mapping the conflict: Define the issues needed to chart common needs and concerns.
9. Development of options: Design creative solutions together.
10. Introduction to negotiation: Plan and apply effective strategies to reach agreement.
11. Introduction to mediation: Help conflicting parties move toward solutions.
12. Broadening perspectives: See the three articles on running meetings in conflict-resolving mode (available on the CRN website).

From Conflict Resolution Network. (2012). 12 skills summary (http://www.crnhq.org/pages.php?pID=10). © Conflict Resolution Network, PO Box 1016 Chatswood NSW 2057, Australia; website, www.crnhq.org. Ph +61 2 9419-8500. E-mail: crn@crnhq.org. Fax +61 2 9413-1148. © This CRN material can be freely reproduced provided this copyright notice appears on each page.

Individual and Contextual Factors That Influence Advanced Practice Nurse Guidance and Coaching

Factors that can influence APN guidance and coaching can be grouped in three categories—APN factors, patient factors, and contextual factors.

Advanced Practice Nurse Factors

Individual factors such as demographic characteristics, cultural differences, mood, and years of experience may affect the APN's attention and ability to coach in a particular encounter. Personal factors such as confidence, stress, and competing personal and professional demands can also influence this process. Students and novice APNs, even when they have considerable experience as RNs, indicate that they find it difficult to attend to relational and communication details when they are focused on history taking, performing assessments, and/or learning new technical skills. Skill in implementing APN coaching is a

dialectic process that depends on the APN's ability to reflect in and on practice. Eventually, APNs learn to integrate relational and communication skills with clinical and technical skills so that as they perform these skills, they are also relating and communicating in therapeutic ways with patients.

Patient Factors

As with APNs, demographic and personal characteristics of patients and families can affect their ability to interact with APNs and respond to guiding and coaching interventions. Other factors, such as social support, personal and community resources, motivation, and ambivalence, can also influence patients' readiness to be guided and coached.

Depending as it does on the APN's clinical, technical, interpersonal, and self-reflective abilities, guidance and coaching can be done with patients whose cognition is impaired, even those who are comatose or dying. Effective coaching in these situations is a function of knowing the patient and is often a synthesis of the following: observations of a single patient over time; a single observation of a patient informed by many observations of patients in similar situations (e.g., ventilator weaning or palliative care); information supplied by the family about the patient's personality, interests, and other factors; knowledge of the clinical trajectory of a health concern; and a number of other cognitive, intuitive, and experiential factors. Even if a patient can't communicate, APNs will explain, anticipate, and address common or possible concerns with many of the relational and communication interventions that they use with the cognitively intact patient.

Contextual Factors

There are many contextual factors that facilitate or impede the APN's ability to coach. For example, setting and time pressures are similar to those discussed in Chapter 7 ("Clinical Thinking" and "Skillful Performance" sections). Other influences include agency policies and procedures, reimbursement methods, staffing, availability of resources, and quality of teamwork and team interactions.

Coaching "Difficult" Patients

APNs frequently are asked to care for patients whom other clinicians regard as "difficult." However, situations that others might characterize as difficult, APNs usually see as demanding or challenging. Sometimes, difficulty arises from the setting, patient's emotions (e.g., disappointment, anger, grief), self-sabotaging behavior, family issues, issues not directly related to the health problem, or a combination of factors. Robinson Wolf and Robinson Smith

(2007) have identified a range of patients and situations characterized as difficult—managing physical aspects of an illness, patient attitudes (e.g., never satisfied) and knowledge (knowing too much about medications), and social factors. For persons with chronic illness (or at high risk for it), not everyone is interested in being helped, changing behaviors, improving health, or undertaking any action for the health problem at hand. A person can become stuck or immobilized by the demands of a transition, the underlying nature of the illness (e.g., borderline personality disorder), or personal factors such as limited social support or cognitive ability.

APNs recognize that when colleagues describe patients as difficult, patients can experience stigmatization, marginalization, discrediting, and disconfirmation (Robinson Wolf & Robinson Smith, 2007)—dehumanizing experiences that are not consistent with nursing's values. Thus, APNs frequently bring a "let me roll up my sleeves and try to understand what is going on" perspective to this work; they are tenacious, staying with a patient, family, or situation until some resolution or accommodation has been achieved. This is an area about which little has been written in nursing (there is a literature in medicine on "the hateful patient"), yet APNs frequently find themselves assuming clinical leadership in such situations.

By working effectively with difficult cases, APNs expand their repertoire of coaching interventions. Some patients who are stuck simply need a new coach, someone with a different approach or personality. A smaller population may be help rejecters; in this case, coaching is unlikely to be effective. APNs may find immunity to change analysis helpful for patients who are perceived as difficult and for whom other approaches are not working. This approach delves into underlying assumptions and competing commitments and motivations that may be undermining a person's ability to change (Kegan & Lahey, 2009).

Robinson Wolf and Robinson Smith (2007) have surveyed CNSs to determine which strategies they used with difficult patients. Three of 83 strategies identified centered on the issue of respect. They were priority strategies and the ones most frequently used: respect the patient's dignity; approach the patient and family with respect and openness; and show the patient and family they are respected. Frosch and associates (2012) have found that patients whose physicians were authoritarian are afraid of being perceived as difficult and are less likely to speak up or share in decision making. This finding affirms the importance of a respectful stance and of using a patient-centered style to engage patients in understanding and improving their health.

Liaschenko (1994) has characterized the work of establishing a positive connection with difficult patients as creating a bridge between self and other and viewed this as a moral task. The self-reflective APN may only recognize his or her inability to establish a therapeutic relationship when the repertoire of coaching skills that they have developed in caring for difficult patients has not worked. APNs who can create a moral bridge in these cases can provide important clinical and moral leadership when they and their coworkers are challenged to provide safe, reliable, and quality care under adverse circumstances.

In an effort to look beyond the patient as a source of difficulty, Macdonald (2007) conducted a qualitative study on in-hospital family medicine units and identified four major factors that influenced difficulty in the nurse-patient encounter—context, sources of problems, strategies to manage the problem, and the consequences of using different strategies. These factors ranged from adequacy of staffing, whether staff knew the patients, lack of supplies, and other nurse and system factors. Actions that tended to create harmony were those that involved being inclusive, such as working together. Controlling actions such as enforcing rules and rushing contributed to difficult encounters. Macdonald has noted that although organizations operate based on a linear concept of time, in which things will happen in an orderly and defined manner, nursing values and the nature of nursing care do not always align with this notion of time. These findings can help APNs be aware of the factors in their settings that contribute to difficulty or harmony in creating therapeutic relationships.

Guidance and Coaching Competency and Outcomes

The model of APN guidance and coaching is fundamentally a process. Through guiding and coaching interventions, APNs help patients and families make sense of their experiences of health, illness, and other transitions. These interventions can result in tangible outcomes such as lifestyle changes and better health markers, reduced readmissions and costs, and improved quality of life. Intangible goals are also realized, such as an improved ability to cope with uncertainty, transcending difficulties and limitations, finding resources within themselves or in their communities, and finding new meanings. Even in brief encounters, such as self-limiting illnesses or employee physical examinations, the APN's interpersonal competence can result in efficient care delivery, improved patient satisfaction, and return business, all valued outcomes in primary care practices.

Exemplar 8-4 illustrates the aspects of APN guidance and coaching such as recognizing the need for coaching early in a patient encounter and the risks of not coaching (poor pain management, poor rehabilitation outcome, alienation between staff and patient), identifying the

EXEMPLAR 8-4   **Advanced Practice Nurse Coaching and Complex Pain Management**

A CNS collaborated with a psychologist in the care of a patient named JG who had complex care needs. JG had been admitted to a rehabilitation hospital after a left hip arthroplasty and left tibial traction pin. His immediate postoperative course had been complicated by a staphylococcal infection at the surgical site, for which he was still receiving intravenous antibiotics. JG had a history of substance abuse and had been in a methadone maintenance program. JG was well known to the staff because he had been in the rehabilitation hospital 1 year earlier, after a surgical procedure was performed on his right hip. During both admissions, pain management was a significant problem. He became easily frustrated and impatient and expressed his anger verbally. These characteristics were exacerbated when he was in moderate to severe pain. For example, requests for pain medications were made in demanding and insistent tones. JG currently reports pain in his left hip and left lower leg, as well as some right shoulder and paralumbar pain. According to the nursing assessment, his pain intensity data are as follows: worst pain is 10/10, least pain is 9/10, and average pain is 9/10. He receives Percocet, two tablets every 6 hours PRN, and his pain is never below 9/10. JG did not complete high school and is disabled. His parents are divorced. He has nieces and nephews he adores and has been motivated to stay clean because he is not permitted to see them if he is abusing drugs.

The CNS performed an initial thorough assessment of JG's pain. During this assessment, she initiated coaching by reviewing with him what they had learned during the prior admission about how to manage his pain by using a combination of scheduled opioids and nondrug interventions. JG expressed frustration that he was not as independent as he had been during the prior admission. The CNS explained that during the prior admission, he had had the use of his good leg to compensate for what the treated leg could not do. Although he had made a good recovery, the leg treated last year was not functional enough to support his weight and compensate for the temporary loss of function in the leg being treated during this admission. He acknowledged that this made sense. The CNS knew from having reviewed the admission orders that she would need to talk to the physicians to get the analgesics changed to a more frequent, around the clock schedule so that JG could participate effectively in therapies.

The CNS and psychologist conferred and agreed to share responsibility for coaching, with the CNS having a primary focus on the patient and the psychologist having a primary focus on the staff. The CNS had been

working with the staff for more than a year to improve pain management practices on the unit. However, the staff would need coaching because they were being challenged to apply what they learned about pain management to a patient whose history they believed made his use of opioids for pain risky. The psychologist would help the staff understand this patient and the reasons for treating pain with opioids in an addict who had had surgery and, if needed, help staff see when their attitudes and misconceptions might be interfering with JG's care. JG needed coaching regarding appropriate ways to communicate his pain and his responses to pain management interventions to avoid alienating staff and maximize participation in therapy. In addition, the CNS would work with the nurses and physicians on titrating analgesics to effect. Given JG's history, he was likely to need more analgesic, not less.

The psychologist noticed during the course of working with JG that staff often assumed that JG was drug seeking if he requested medications for pain. Staff had other concerns that needed attention—fear of giving too much pain medication, weaning JG from analgesics as soon as possible (regardless of pain intensity level or impact of unrelieved pain on progress in rehabilitation), and concern that JG would relapse with regard to substance abuse. The psychologist listened to and acknowledged the staff's issues. He offered them new information to encourage them to modify their thinking about how pain in addicts should be managed. Both the psychologist and CNS were able to show staff the effectiveness of their interventions; when JG's pain was well managed, his participation in therapy was better. If someone had withheld or forgotten JG's medication, it showed in a decreased level of activity during physical and occupational therapy.

The CNS coached JG in effective ways to communicate his frustration and explained why angry and blaming communications might make it harder for some staff to help him. The psychologist and CNS used cognitive restructuring strategies to help JG think differently about his problems and learn ways to increase his threshold for frustration. For example, when JG reported that nothing was going right or that he could not do anything, events of the day were reviewed for evidence of some progress. The links between his thinking and behavior were identified. When JG became an outpatient, the psychologist and the CNS praised his self-care and adherence to treatment plans. JG had been discharged 4 weeks after admission with an effective analgesic regimen so that he could continue to make progress

EXEMPLAR 8-4   Advanced Practice Nurse Coaching and Complex Pain
Management—*cont'd*

at home. Before discharge, the psychologist and CNS collaborated with the social worker to find and then coach a primary care physician in the most effective strategies to help JG because he was at high risk of being lost to follow-up. The staff also gained a better

understanding of how to manage pain in a patient with a history of substance abuse. The staff's success with managing JG's pain enabled them to better manage the pain of the occasional future patient who might have a comorbid addiction.

multiple levels of coaching needed (patient, staff, post-discharge caregivers), and using relationships with patients and colleagues to shape a positive outcome in a complex situation.

Development of Advanced Practice Nurses' Coaching Competence

Although scientific and technical knowledge are essential for effective coaching, it is in the integration of the elements of the coaching model that the art of advanced practice nursing is fully expressed. APNs need a highly nuanced range of interpersonal skills to coach people through experiences of health and illness. The strategies used to develop coaching expertise are designed to prepare APNs for reflective practice and a person-oriented interactive style, which are foundational to becoming a skilled coach.

There are at least two types of experiences, during and after graduate education, that can refine and extend one's coaching abilities. Continuous contact with patients over time provides students and APNs with experiences that let them observe how health and illness issues evolve. For example, APNs in acute care may learn the common features of weaning trajectories for patients on ventilators. This knowledge informs their anticipatory guidance of patients' families: "when we first begin weaning we will do this and you can expect this to happen." In primary care, an NP who has coached many patients to increase their exercise by using a pedometer knows which goals might be achievable and which factors will impede or facilitate adopting the new behavior, and uses this information to coach patients.

One-time, episodic encounters are a second experience that can contribute to one's coaching expertise. For example, APNs in the organ donation field may only see a family once or twice, but over a number of one-time encounters they learn the different directions that so-called bad news conversations can take and recognize cues that lead them to use the most appropriate communications and actions for the particular situation. Another example

would be an unusual diagnosis, such as Ludwig's angina; the lessons from one experience with an unusual illness will be available if and when APNs encounter another one. Thus, continuous contact experiences help APNs recognize within-patient patterns that help them coach subsequent patients with similar diagnoses and illness trajectories. The episodic or one-time encounters help APNs recognize across-patient patterns; these lessons can be applied in the next similar encounter. Whether from continuous or episodic encounters, coaching is embedded in a deep knowledge of practice and sound empirical knowledge of the specialty.

Graduate Nursing Education: Influence of Faculty and Preceptors

Graduate faculty and clinical preceptors are highly influential models for APN students seeking to develop coaching skills. Faculty can assist APN students to develop as coaches by being reflective themselves. In particular, faculty need to name and evaluate the processes and pedagogies to which they were exposed, distinguishing between effective, respectful experiences of being taught or coached and ineffective, disrespectful ones. Students who have been effectively coached by teachers and preceptors will know experientially what respectful coaching feels like and be more likely to reproduce these behaviors with patients. Schön (1987) termed this the *hall of mirrors effect*. The teacher, in the very process of supervising and coaching the student, exemplifies the coaching repertoire that the student is attempting to acquire. If disrespectful, ineffective teaching is recognized for what it is, a position-centered style, then students also learn how not to coach.

Clinical preceptors play a particularly salient role in teaching this competency. In effect, there is a double exposure to coaching; the student experiences being coached and observes how patients are coached by the preceptor. Similarly, preceptors need to be able to coach students while coaching patients. A person-centered style of interaction on the part of the preceptor is just as important to developing APN students' coaching skills as it is to helping patients accomplish their health goals.

It is possible to have preceptors who use a person-centered style of interaction with patients, but because of their own student experiences, they adopt a position-centered style of interacting with students. Very experienced APNs can be novice preceptors, so that preceptors themselves may need coaching by faculty and feedback from students to develop in their preceptor roles. Just as APNs tailor their coaching to meet individual patient needs, APN preceptors need to tailor their coaching of students to the level of the student and the situation. Both the NACNS (2013; http://www.nacns.org/docs/GuidelinesForPreceptors.pdf) and ACNM (2010; http://www.midwife.org/Preceptor-Resources) have excellent guidelines for preceptors that APN faculty, students, and preceptors would find helpful.

Faculty and APN preceptors need to make students aware of the range of coaching strategies used in the classroom and clinical area. This is one way students learn how to coach. What was ineffable and undervalued in the process of coaching becomes defined, contextualized, reproducible, and valued (McKinnon & Erickson, 1988). Faculty and APN preceptors need to facilitate student reflection on their experiences and intuitions. APN students should reflect on their previous student experiences, identifying and evaluating effective and ineffective coaching. Bringing these educational moments to full consciousness and naming them is a key first step to envisioning coaching processes that students will want to emulate or discard.

Strategies for Developing and Applying the Coaching Competency

There are now texts on communication and motivational interviewing that can be used to strengthen APN skills in guidance and coaching (Dart, 2011; Miller & Rollnick, 2006; Rollnick, Miller, & Butler, 2008; Rosengren, 2009), including one specifically for APNs (Hart, 2010). These texts can be used to design assignments and inform the teaching strategies to enlarge an APN student's interpersonal repertoire and self-reflective abilities. Expressive writing enables students to recapture important experiences in nursing and reflect on them to arrive at new insights and interpretations. Keeping a journal and writing poetry are other examples of expressive writing.

Journal writing is a helpful strategy for developing coaching and communication skills. Students can document their "thinking about thinking," observations about themselves and demeanor, emotions, and clinical decision making. Such assignments can help students reflect on the experience of being new or uncertain of their skills and can lead to discussions of developmental tasks, such as embracing novicehood or learning to trust one's hands,

heart, gut, and observations. Journaling and online blogs can also be used to help students begin to appreciate the dialectic between reflection-on-action and reflection-in-action. Faculty responses to journals and blogs focus on developmental milestones, offering strategies, noting where clinical intuition may have been operating, identifying situations that would benefit from further exploration between student and preceptor, and helping students elicit feedback from preceptors and patients. Similar to the techniques of MI, faculty respond to student writing with questions, observations, insights, and strategies that can enlarge the students repertoire of thinking strategies, help them recognize developing skill, and encourage and give permission to students to take appropriate communication risks.

In the first author's experience (JS), APN students in their first clinicals tend to reflect on action (after the fact). They need help distinguishing between rumination—for example, revisiting over and over what they should have done and discernment—reflecting sufficiently on a situation to learn from it, but then letting it go. Faculty and preceptors can help students learn to use reflection-on-action to discern developing cognitive and communication skills, attend to what worked, and identify areas for development or improvement. As they advance in their practica, through journaling, faculty can help students recognize when reflection in action has occurred so that students learn how it differs from reflection-on-action-and how the two activities inform each other and contribute to increasing confidence and expertise.

Storytelling is another expressive strategy in which stories, the products of reflection, are relayed orally (Charon, 2006; Mattingly, 2001). Sharing stories about guidance and coaching from practica enables APN students to establish a shared history and provides a means of offering and receiving support while learning about coaching situations and strategies. Done well, the process promotes community, collegiality, critical thinking and risk taking and fosters self-esteem and confidence. Through these expressive methods, cues and strategies for coaching used by different APN students and preceptors become available to a larger group of learners. APNs can encourage storytelling among patients and families. In fact, APNs in palliative care often ask family members, whose loved one is not able to communicate, to tell them about the loved one—for example, memories, personality characteristics, and interests.

Written exemplars of coaching and group debriefing of coaching experiences facilitate self-reflection on coaching and expand one's coaching repertoire. In a study of APNs providing transitional care to cancer patients, Monturo (2003) noted that the APN interveners met regularly to discuss their experiences and support each other.

Aesthetic approaches to developing interpersonal competence can also enhance APNs' coaching skills. Some of the most profound experiences in which nurses are involved can never be known through scientific and transactional writing because of the limitations of these styles of writing. Poetry, literature, and film can be potent triggers for developing reflective practice. They can help students and novice APNs understand what an experience of illness might be for a patient. For example, movies and books with plots involving illness or disability can help students assess needs for coaching, evaluate clinicians' ineffective and effective interpersonal styles, and articulate the gaps in care that might require advanced practice nursing intervention.

Coaching competence can be further strengthened when students develop and implement patient education materials and programs. For example, a student could initiate or colead a self-management group for patients with a chronic condition. Other activities might include developing, implementing, and evaluating limited literacy tools, assessing the cost-effectiveness of a patient education initiative, or evaluating the reliability and appropriateness of health information on the Internet, with particular attention to how these tools facilitate coaching. Students should know the health information resources likely to be used by their patient populations and be able to recommend those that are reliable and regularly updated.

Professional Coaching and Health Care

Given the expansion of professional coaching and the emergence of the professional nurse coach role (Hess, Dossey, Southard, et al., 2012), a brief overview of professional coaching is provided to help readers understand that the APN guidance and coaching competency is different from contemporary professional coaching. Even so, the APN competency and professional coaching have elements in common; the APN model is also informed by professional coaching principles and practices, particularly MI.

The International Coach Federation (ICF) has defined coaching as "partnering with clients in a thought-provoking and creative process that inspires them to maximize their personal and professional potential" (http://www.coachfederation.org/). Through the process of coaching, clients deepen their learning, improve their performance, and enhance their quality of life (ICF, 2011). Although this definition may seem daunting with regard to clinical care, its intent is relevant as health care institutions try to reduce costs and improve outcomes. Goals such as maximizing potential are consistent with the APN guidance and coaching competency.

Box 8-3 lists the competencies of professional coaching promulgated by the ICF (2011) on which ICF-approved certification is based (for professional coaching competencies that are not self-explanatory, ICF definitions are given).

 BOX 8-3   International Coach Federation: Professional Coaching

Competencies

A. Setting the foundation
   1. Meeting ethical guidelines and professional standards
   2. Establishing the coaching agreement
B. Cocreating the relationship
   3. Establishing trust and intimacy with the client
   4. Coaching presence (ability to be fully conscious and create a spontaneous relationship with the client, using a style that is open, flexible, and confident)
C. Communicating effectively
   5. Active listening
   6. Powerful questioning (ability to ask questions that reveal the information needed for maximum benefit to the coaching relationship and the client)
   7. Direct communication (ability to communicate effectively during coaching sessions, and to use language that has the greatest positive impact on the client)
D. Facilitating learning and results
   8. Creating awareness (ability to integrate and accurately evaluate multiple sources of information and to make interpretations that help the client gain awareness and thereby achieve agreed-on results)
   9. Designing actions (ability to create with the client opportunities for ongoing learning, during coaching and in work-life situations, and for taking new actions that will most effectively lead to agreed-on coaching results)
   10. Planning and goal setting
   11. Managing progress and accountability (ability to hold attention on what is important for the client and to leave responsibility with the client to take action)

NOTE: Readers are encouraged to view the website, which contains greater detail.
Adapted from the International Coach Federation. (2011). ICF core competencies (http://www.coachfederation.org/icfcredentials/core-competencies).

Professional health and wellness coaching programs are often informed on the ICF competencies. A review of these programs is beyond the scope of this chapter but readers are encouraged to attend to this rapidly evolving field; it is likely that APNs will work on teams with health coaches or make referrals to these professionals.

The professional coaching process is not usually effective in clients with severe mental illness or compromised mental status, such as intoxication or confusion. Professional coaching can be highly effective in those at risk for chronic illness or those who already have a chronic disease, such as type 2 diabetes mellitus or heart disease, if they are emotionally healthy, cognitively intact, and willing to use the services of a professional coach. Many patients seen by APNs meet these criteria but there are other populations (e.g., infants, persons with dementia) who do not.

Unlike professional coaching, the APN guidance and coaching competency is rooted in nursing's disciplinary perspective and societal mandate to treat and care, and therefore applies across a wide range of patient characteristics and contexts—an important distinction from professional coaching. The reader is invited to consider how theoretical and empirical support for APN guidance and coaching are consistent with, and even overlap, the competencies of professional coaching listed in Box 8-3.

Advanced Practice Nurse Guidance and Coaching and Coach Certification

Given the expansion of professional coaching and the emergence of the professional nurse coach role, APNs need to be able to distinguish the APN guidance and coaching competency from professional or health coaching. The health policy emphasis on care aimed at preventing illness and reducing morbidity, emergence of health and wellness coaching, and call for integrating coaching skills into the health professions have resulted in a number of efforts to advance coaching as a means of improving patient outcomes. Most important is the work of the Professional Nurse Coach Workgroup (PNCW) (Hess, Dossey, Southard, et al., 2012) and the requests for nurses to be health coaches (Luck, 2010).

The PNCW was established to develop standards and competencies for professional nurse coaching (Hess, Dossey, Southard, et al., 2012). They have defined a professional nurse coach as follows: "The Professional nurse coach (PNC) is a registered nurse who integrates coaching competencies into any setting or specialty area of practice to facilitate a process of change or development that assists individuals or groups to realize their potential. Professional nurse coaching is a skilled, purposeful, results-oriented, and structured relationship-centered interaction with clients provided by RNs for the purpose of promoting

achievement of client goals" (Hess, Dossey, Southard, et al., 2012, p. 6). This definition is consistent with that of the ICF (see Box 8-3). The PNCW has asserted that nurse coaching is not a specialty and that coaching builds on traditional nursing theories, values, and processes. They also assert that the nurse coaching process is a reorientation of the nursing process. How this type of coaching would meet the needs of patient populations who cannot establish goals and make choices for themselves is unclear.

It also is not yet clear whether all preprofessional nursing curricula will eventually reflect the professional nurse coach standards and competencies, proposed by Hess and colleagues (2012), and therefore be reflected on National Council Licensure Examination (NCLEX) examinations, or whether all registered nurses should be prepared to sit for professional nurse coaching credentials. The issue of basic and advanced coaching by nurses is also not addressed but is likely to arise as more APNs seek some type of coaching certification to add value to their existing roles. Alternatively, APNs may choose to become certified health or professional coaches; this choice may mean that they do not have the same clinical responsibilities with patients as they had when practicing in an APN role. These issues will need to be clarified, and national APN stakeholder organizations should play a part in this clarification. Nevertheless, it is significant that the profession is actively advocating that coaching be integrated into basic nursing practice. APNs should be involved as the nursing profession defines coaching by nurses.

In addition to this intraprofessional coaching activity, APNs should be aware of other health coaches and their preparation and certification (e.g., see Health Sciences Institute, n.d.; retrieved April 6, 2013, from http://www.healthsciences.org/). Insurers, corporations, and large clinical practices are hiring health coaches to reduce costs. The availability of other types of health coaches has implications for APNs' consultations, referrals, and interprofessional collaboration. The following questions need to be addressed:

- How do the APN's coaching activities with a patient and family interface with those of a certified health coach?
- When should an APN encourage a patient to contact their insurer about having a health coach?
- What are the qualifications of the coach and do the qualifications match the needs of the patient?
- How should the APN best communicate with health coaches?
- Do APNs notice important clinical differences between patients with health coaches for a chronic illness and those who do not have such coaches?

These and other important questions remain to be answered.

Conclusion

This chapter has defined and described the APN competency of guidance and coaching, a core of all APN roles. This is an opportune time to examine the role of APN guidance and coaching in producing favorable clinical and institutional outcomes. Further research is needed on the nature of this competency and its contribution to patient-centered, high-quality care, positive patient outcomes, and reduced health costs. Given the effectiveness of coaching by APNs and others, these studies should be a priority. Such research can inform policy by doing the following: (1) identifying the patient populations for whom APN coaching results in the best outcomes at reasonable costs for patients and delivery systems, measured not only in dollars but provider time, prevention or reduction of morbidity and complications, longer times between health visits or hospital readmissions, and other meaningful patient outcomes; and (2) determining the "nurse dose" (a concept introduced by Brooten and Youngblut, 2006) of coaching needed. Perhaps an APN is the appropriate initial coach for medically complex older patients making the transition from hospital to home, after which a professional nurse coach or certified health coach can assume responsibility. Findings will enable delivery systems and patients to choose coaches for particular situations in order to design the most effective coaching plans.

The term *coaching* has long been used in a variety of disciplines and settings. Even as a broad definition of health coaching is evolving, it is important for APNs and other health professionals who coach patients in areas of health, wellness, and illness to represent the nature of their discipline-specific coaching accurately. Challenges in the coming years will be to continue to clarify the nature of health and chronic illness coaching, distinguish between professional coaching and therapeutic coaching done by APNs as compared with other providers, and determine effective coaching interventions that are interprofessional and those that are discipline-specific. APNs practicing to their full scope must be mindful that theirs is first a therapeutic relationship in which they integrate their additional coaching preparation as they care for patients.

References

Administration on Aging. Department of Health and Human Services. (2012). Retrieved January 2, 2013, from http://www.aoa.gov/AoA_programs/HCLTC/ADRC_CareTransitions/index.aspx

American Association of Colleges of Nursing. (2006). *The essentials of doctoral education for advanced nursing practice.* Washington DC: Author.

American College of Nurse Midwives. (2012). Core competencies for basic midwifery practice (http://www.midwife.org/ACNM/files/ACNMLibraryData/UPLOADFILENAME/000000000050/Core%20Competencies%20June%202012.pdf).

American College of Nurse Midwives. (2010). Preceptor resources. Retrieved January 2, 2013, from http://www.midwife.org/Preceptor-Resources

Ball, C., & Cox, C. I. (2003). Part one: Restoring patients to health—outcomes and indicators of advanced nursing practice in adult critical care. *International Journal of Nursing Practice, 9,* 356–367.

Benner, P. (1985). The oncology clinical nurse specialist as expert coach. *Oncology Nursing Forum, 12,* 40–44.

Benner, P., Hooper-Kyriakidis, P., & Stannard, D. (1999). *Clinical wisdom and interventions in critical care: A thinking-in-action approach.* Philadelphia: WB Saunders.

Benner, P., Tanner, C. A., & Chesla, C. A. (2009). *Expertise in nursing practice: Caring, clinical judgment, and ethics.* New York: Springer.

Betancourt, J., Green, A., & Carrillo, J. (2002). Cultural competence in health care: Emerging frameworks and practical approaches (http://www.cmwf.org/usr_doc/betancourt_culturalcompetence_576.pdf)

Bodenheimer, T., Chen, E., & Bennett, H. (2009). Confronting the growing burden of chronic disease: Can the U.S. health care workforce do the Job? *Health Affairs, 28,* 64–74.

Bonis, S. A. (2009). Knowing in nursing: a concept analysis. *Journal of Advanced Nursing, 65,* 1328–1341. doi: 10.1111/j.1365-2648.2008.04951.x

Borrelli, B. (2006). Using motivational interviewing to promote patient behavior change and enhance health (http://www.medscape.com/viewprogram/5757_pnt).

Bowles, K. H. (2010). Nurse practitioner–provided home telemonitoring and medication management improves glycemic control in primary care patients with type 2 diabetes more than monthly care coordination telephone call. *Evidence-Based Nursing, 13,* 74–75.

Brooten, D., Naylor, M. D., York, R., Brown, L. P., Munro, B. H., Hollingsworth, A. O., et al., (2002). Lessons learned from testing the quality cost model of Advanced Practice Nursing (APN) transitional care. *Journal of Nursing Scholarship, 34,* 369–375.

Brooten, D., Roncoli, M., Finkler, S., Arnold, L., Cohen, A., & Mennutti, M. (1994). A randomized clinical trial of hospital discharge and nurse specialist home follow-up of women with unplanned cesarean birth. *Obstetrics and Gynecology, 84,* 832–838.

Brooten, D., Youngblut, J., Deatrick, J., Naylor, M., & York, R. (2003). Patient problems, advanced practice nurse (APN) interventions, time and contacts among five patient groups. *Journal of Nursing Scholarship, 35,* 73–79.

Brooten, D., & Youngblut, J. (2006). Nurse dose as a concept. *Journal of Nursing Scholarship, 38,* 94–99.

Brown, S. J. (1999). Patient-centered communication. *Annual Review of Nursing Research, 17,* 85–104.

Callister, L. C., & Freeborn, D. (2007). Nurse midwives with women: Ways of knowing in nurse midwives. *International Journal for Human Caring, 11,* 8–15.

Centers for Disease Control and Prevention. (2010). Adverse childhood experiences (ACE) study: Major findings (http://www.cdc.gov/ace/findings.htm).

Charon, R. (2006). The perilous fate of the teller, or what bench? what desolation? *Literature and Medicine, 25,* 412–438.

Chick, N., & Meleis, A. (1986). Transitions: A nursing concern. In P. Chinn (Ed.), *Nursing research methodology: Issues and implementation* (pp. 237–258). Rockville, MD: Aspen.

Clarke, E. B., & Spross, J. A. (1996). Expert coaching and guidance. In A. B. Hamric, J. A. Spross, & C. M. Hanson (Eds.), *Advanced practice nursing: An integrative approach* (pp. 139–164). Philadelphia: WB Saunders.

Coleman, E. A., & Boult, C. (2003). Improving the quality of transitional care for persons with complex care needs: Position statement of The American Geriatrics Society Health Care Systems Committee. *Journal of the American Geriatrics Society, 51,* 556–557.

Coleman, E. A., & Berenson, R. A. (2004). Lost in transition: Challenges and opportunities for improving the quality of transitional care. *Annals of Internal Medicine, 140,* 533–536.

Coleman, E. A., Smith, J. D., Frank, J. C., et al. (2004). Preparing patients and caregivers to participate in care delivered across settings: The care transitions intervention. *Journal of the American Geriatrics Society, 52,* 1817–1825.

Coleman, E. A., Parry, C., Chalmers, S., & Min, S. J. (2006). The care transitions intervention: Results of a randomized control trial. *Archives of Internal Medicine, 166,* 1822–1828.

Conflict Resolution Network. (2012). 12 skills summary (http://www.crnhq.org/pages.php?pID=10). © Conflict Resolution Network, PO Box 1016, Chatswood, NSW 2057, Australia; website, www.crnhq.org.

Cooke, L., Gemmill, R., & Grant, M. (2008). Advanced practice nurses core competencies: A framework for developing and testing an advanced practice nurse discharge intervention. *Clinical Nurse Specialist CNS, 22,* 218–225.

Counsell, S. R., Callahan, C. M., Buttar, A. B., Clark, D. O., & Frank, K. I. (2006). Geriatric resources for assessment and care of elders (GRACE): A new model of primary care for low-income seniors. *Journal of the American Geriatrics Society, 54,* 1136–1141. doi: 10.1111/j.1532-5415.2006.00791.x

Cronenwett, L., Sherwood, G., Pohl, J., Barnsteiner, J., Moore, S., Sullivan, D. T., et al. (2009). Quality and safety education for advanced nursing practice. *Nursing Outlook, 6,* 338–348. (http://www.qsen.org/ksas_graduate.php)

Crowther, M. (2003). Optimal management of outpatients with heart failure using advanced practice nurses in a hospital-based heart failure center. *Journal of the American Academy of Nurse Practitioners, 15,* 260–265.

Dart, M. A. (2011). *Motivational interviewing in nursing practice: Empowering the patient.* Sudbury, MA: Jones and Bartlett.

DeVore, S., & Champion, R. W. (2011). Driving population health through accountable care organizations. *Health Affairs, 30,* 41–50.

Dick, K., & Frazier, S. C. (2006). An exploration of nurse practitioner care to homebound frail elders. *Journal of the American Academy of Nurse Practitioners, 18,* 325–334.

Elliott, N. (2010). 'Mutual intacting': A grounded theory study of clinical judgement practice issues. *Journal of Advanced Nursing, 66,* 2711–2721. doi: 10.1111/j.1365-2648.2010.05412.x.

Felitti, V. (2002). [The relationship between adverse childhood experiences and adult health: Turning gold into lead.] *The Permanente Journal, 6,* 1–7.

Fenton, M., & Brykczynski, K. (1993). Qualitative distinctions and similarities in the practice of clinical nurse specialists and nurse practitioners. *Journal of Professional Nursing, 9,* 313–326.

Frosch, D. L., May, S. G., Rendle, K. A. S., Tietbohl, C., & Elwyn, G. (2012). Authoritarian physicians and patients' fear of being labeled 'difficult' among key obstacles to shared decision making. *Health Affairs, 31,* 1030–1038.

Gadow, S. (1980). Existential advocacy: Philosophical foundations of nursing. In S. Spicker & S. Gadow (Eds.), *Nursing: Images and ideas* (pp. 79–101). New York: Springer-Verlag.

Hanley, M. A., & Fenton, M. V. (2007). Exploring improvisation in nursing. *Journal of Holistic Nursing, 25,* 126–133.

Hart, V. A. (2010). *Patient-provider communications: Caring to listen.* Sudbury, MA: Jones and Bartlett.

Hayes, E., & Kalmakis, K. A. (2007). From the sidelines: coaching as a nurse practitioner strategy for improving health outcomes [review]. *Journal of the American Academy of Nurse Practitioners, 19,* 555–562. doi: 10.1111/j.1745-7599.2007.00264.x.

Hayes, E., McCahon, C., Panahi, M. R., Hamre, T., & Pohlman, K. (2008). Alliance not compliance: Coaching strategies to improve type 2 diabetes outcomes [review]. *Journal of the American Academy of Nurse Practitioners, 20,* 155–162. doi: 10.1111/j.1745-7599.2007. 00297.x.

Health Sciences Institute. (n.d.). Retrieved April 6, 2013, from http://www.healthsciences.org/.

Heron, M., Hoyert, D. L., Murphy, S. L., Xu, J., Kochanek, K. D., Tejada-Vera, B. (2009). Deaths: Final data for 2006. In National Center for Health Statistics (Ed.), *National vital statistics report* (*vol 57*). Hyattsville, MD: National Center for Health Statistics.

Hess, D., Dossey, B., Southard, M. E., Luck, S., Schaub, B. G., Bark, L. (2012). Nurse coach role: Scope and competencies (http://www.ahncc.org/nursecoachrole.html).

Hobbs, J. L. (2009). A dimensional analysis of patient-centered care. *Nursing Research, 58,* 52–62.

Holland, M. L., & Holland, E. S. (2007). Survey of Connecticut nurse-midwives. *Journal of Midwifery & Women's Health, 52,* 106–115.

Institute of Medicine (IOM). (2010). The future of nursing: Leading change, advancing health (http://www.iom.edu/Reports/2010/The-Future-of-Nursing-Leading-Change-Advancing-Health.aspx).

Institute of Medicine, Committee on Quality Health Care in America. (2001). *Crossing the quality chasm: A new health system for the 21st century.* Washington, DC: National Academies Press.

International Coach Federation (ICF). (2011). ICF core coaching competencies (http://www.coachfederation.org/icfcredentials/core-competencies).

International Coach Federation (ICF). (2011). Retrieved January 2, 2013, from http://www.coachfederation.org/

Interprofessional Education Collaborative Expert Panel. (2011). *Core competencies for interprofessional collaborative practice: Report of an expert panel.* Washington, DC: Interprofessional Education Collaborative. Retrieved January 2, 2013, from http://www.aacn.nche.edu/education-resources/ipecreport.pdf

Johnson, B., Abraham, M., Conway, J., Simmons, L., Edgman-Levitan, S., Sodomka, P., et al. (2008). Partnering with patients and families to design a patient- and family-centered health care system: Recommendations and promising practices (http://www.ihi.org/knowledge/Pages/Publications/PartneringwithPatientsandFamiliesRecommendationsPromisingPractices.aspx).

Kegan, R., & Lahey, L. (2009). *Immunity to change: How to overcome it and unlock the potential in yourself and your organizations.* Boston: Harvard Business School Publishing.

Lewandowski, W., & Adamle, K. (2009). Substantive areas of clinical nurse specialist practice: A comprehensive review of the literature. *Clinical Nurse Specialist CNS, 23,* 73–92. doi: 10.1097/NUR.0b013e31819971d0

Liaschenko, J. (1994). Making a bridge: the moral work with patients we do not like. *Journal of Palliative Care, 10,* 83–89.

Lincoln, P. E. (2000). Comparing CNS and NP role activities: A replication. *Clinical Nurse Specialist, 14,* 269–277.

Link, D. G. (2009). The teaching-coaching role of the APN. *Journal of Perinatal & Neonatal Nursing, 23,* 279–283. doi: 10.1097/JPN.0b013e3181b0b8d2.

Luck, S. (2010). Changing the health of our nation—the role of nurse coaches. *Alternative Therapies, 16,* 68–70.

Macdonald, M. (2007). Origins of difficulty in the nurse-patient encounter. *Nursing Ethics, 14,* 510–521.

Marineau, M. L. (2007). Special populations: Telehealth advance practice nursing: The lived experiences of individuals with acute infections transitioning in the home. *Nursing Forum, 42,* 196–208. doi: 10.1111/j.1744-6198.2007.00088.x.

Martin, J. N. (2002). Patient education: Definition. *E-notes: Gale Encyclopedia of nursing and allied health.* http://www.enotes.com/patient-education-reference/patient-education. Accessed January 4, 2012.

Mathews, S. K., Secrest, J., & Muirhead, L. (2008). The interaction model of client health behavior: A model for advanced practice nurses. *Journal of the American Academy of Nurse Practitioners, 20,* 415–422. doi: 10.1111/j.1745-7599.2008.00343.x

Mattingly, C., & Garro, L. C. (2001). *Narrative and the cultural construction of illness and healing.* Berkeley, CA: University of California Press.

McCauley, K. M., Bixby, B., & Naylor, M. D. (2006). Advanced practice nurse strategies to improve outcomes and reduce cost in elders with heart failure. *Disease Management, 9,* 302–310.

McKinnon, A., & Erickson, G. (1988). Taking Schön's ideas to a science teaching practicum. In P. Grimmett & G. Erickson (Eds.), *Reflection in teacher education* (pp. 113–137). New York: Teacher's College Press.

Miller, W., & Rollnick, S. (2012). Glossary of motivational interviewing terms. Retrieved January 2, 2013, from http://www.motivationalinterviewing.org/sites/default/files/elfinder_uploads/ColleenMarshall/Glossary%20of%20MI%20Terms.pdf

Miller, W., & Rollnick, S. (2006). *Motivational interviewing: Preparing people to change.* New York: Gilford Press.

Montgomery, C. L. (1993). *Healing through communication.* Newbury Park, CA: Sage.

Monturo, C. A. (2003). The advanced practice nurse in research: From hospital discharge to home. *Oncol Nurs Forum, 30,* 27–28.

Morrison, S. M. (2011). An integrative review of expert nursing practice. *Journal of Nursing Scholarship, 43,* 163–170.

National Association of Clinical Nurse Specialists (NACNS). (2013). Precepting guidelines for Clinical Nurse Specialists. Retrieved January 2, 2013, from http://www.nacns.org/docs/GuidelinesForPreceptors.pdf

National Committee for Quality Assurance. (2011). *PCMH (patient-centered medical home): Standards and guidelines.* Washington, DC: Author.

National Organization of Nurse Practitioner Faculties (NONPF). (2012). Nurse practitioner entry level competencies (http://www.nonpf.com/associations/10789/files/NPCoreCompetenciesFinal2012.pdf).

Naylor, M. D., Aiken, L. H., Kurtzman, E. T., Olds, D. M., & Hirschman, K. B. (2011). The importance of transitional care in achieving health reform. *Health Affairs, 30,* 746–754.

Naylor, M., Bowles, K., & Brooten, D. (2000). Patient problems and advanced practice nurse interventions during transitional care. *Public Health Nursing, 17,* 94–102.

Naylor, M. D., Brooten, D. A., Maislin, G., McCauley, K. M., & Schwartz, J. S. (2004). Transitional care of older adults hospitalized with heart failure: A randomized, controlled trial. *Journal of the American Geriatrics Society, 52,* 675–684.

Naylor, M. D., Brooten, D., Campbell, R., Jacobsen, B. S., Mezey, M. D., Pauly, M. V., et al. (1999). Comprehensive discharge planning and home follow-up of hospitalized elders. *JAMA: Journal of the American Medical Association, 281,* 613–620.

Norcross, J. C., Krebs, P. M., & Prochaska, J. O. (2011). Stages of change. *Journal of Clinical Psychology, 67,* 143–154.

Nursing Council of New Zealand. (2005). *Guidelines for cultural safety, the Treaty of Waitangi and Maori health in nursing education and practice.* Wellington, New Zealand: Nursing Council of New Zealand.

O'Connor, N. A., Hameister, A. D., & Kershaw, T. (2000). Developing a database to describe the practice patterns of adult nurse practitioner students. *Journal of Nursing Scholarship, 32,* 57–63.

Parrish, E., Peden, A., & Staten, R. (2008). Strategies used by advanced practice psychiatric nurses in treating adults with depression. *Perspectives in Psychiatric Care, 44,* 232–240.

Parry, C., & Coleman, E. A. (2010). Active roles for older adults in navigating care transitions: Lessons learned from the care transitions intervention. *Open Longevity Science, 4,* 43–50.

Parry, C., Kramer, H. M., & Coleman, E. A. (2006). A qualitative exploration of a patient-centered coaching intervention to improve care transitions in chronically ill older adults. *Home Health Care Services Quarterly, 25,* 39–53.

Perraud, S., Delaney, K. R., Carlson-Sabelli, L., Johnson, M. E., Shephard, R., & Paun, O. (2006). Advanced practice psychiatric mental health nursing, finding our core: The therapeutic relationship in 21st century. *Perspectives in Psychiatric Care, 42,* 215–226.

Phillips-Salimi, C. R., Haase, J. E., & Carter Kooken, W. (2011). Connectedness in the context of patient-provider relationships: A concept analysis. *Journal of Advanced Nursing, 68,* 230–245. doi: 10.111/j.1365-2648.2011.05763.x

Polaschak, N. R. (1998). Cultural safety: A new concept in nursing people of different ethnicities. *Journal of Advanced Nursing, 27,* 452–457

Prochaska, J., Redding, C., & Evers, K. (2008). The transtheoretical model and stages of change. In K. Glanz, B. Rimer, & K. Viswanath (Eds.), *Health behavior and health education* (pp. 99–120, 4th ed.). San Francisco: Jossey-Bass.

Quirk, P. (2000). Screening for literacy and readability: Implications for the advanced practice nurse. *Clinical Nurse Specialist CNS, 14,* 26–32.

Reeves, S., Zwarenstein, M., Goldman, J., Barr, H., Freeth, D., Koppel, I., et al. (2010). The effectiveness of interprofessional education: Key findings from a new systematic review. *Journal of Interprofessional Education, 24,* 230–241.

Robinson Wolf, Z., & Robinson Smith, B. (2007). Strategies used by clinical nurse specialists in "difficult" clinician-patient situations. *Clinical Nurse Specialist CNS, 21,* 74–84.

Rollnick, S., Miller, W., & Butler, C. (2008). *Motivational interviewing in health care: helping patients change behavior.* New York: Guilford Press.

Rosengren, D. (2009). *Building motivational interviewing skills: A practitioner workbook.* New York: The Guilford Press.

Rubak, S., Sandboek, A., Lauritzen, T., & Christensen, B. (2005). Motivational interviewing: A systematic review and meta-analysis. *British Journal of General Practice, 55,* 305–312.

Schön, D. (1983). *The reflective practitioner: How professionals think in action.* New York: Basic Books.

Schön, D. (1987). *Educating the reflective practitioner: Toward a new design for teaching and learning in the professions.* San Francisco: Jossey-Bass.

Schumacher, K., & Meleis, A. (1994). Transitions: A central concept in nursing. *Image—The Journal of Nursing Scholarship, 26,* 119–127.

Spross, J. (2009). Expert coaching and guidance. In A. B. Hamric, J. A. Spross, & C. M. Hanson (Eds.), *Advanced nursing practice: An integrative approach* (4th ed., pp. 159–190). St. Louis: Elsevier Saunders.

Spross, J. A., Clarke, E. B., & Beauregard., J. (2000). Expert coaching and guidance. In A. B. Hamric, J. A. Spross, & C. M. Hanson (Eds.), *Advanced nursing practice: An integrative approach* (2nd ed., pp. 183–215). Philadelphia: WB Saunders.

Squier, R. (1990). A model of empathic understanding and adherence to treatment regimens in practitioner-patient relationships. *Social Science and Medicine, 30,* 325–339.

Stableford, S., & Mettger, W. (2007). Plain language: A strategic response to the health literacy challenge. *Journal of Public Health Policy, 28,* 71–93.

The Joint Commission. (2010). *Advancing effective communication, cultural competence, and patient- and family-centered care: A Roadmap for hospitals.* Oakbrook Terrace, IL: Author.

Thorne, S. (2005). Patient-provider communication in chronic illness: A health promotion window of opportunity. *Family & Community Health, 19,* 4S–11S.

Transitional Care Model. (2008-2009). Retrieved January 2, 2013, from http://www.transitionalcare.info/

U.S. Aging and Disability Resource Center. (2011). Evidence-based care transitions models side-by-side March 2011 (adrc-tae.org/tiki-download_file.php?fileId=30310).

U.S. Department of Health and Human Services (HHS). (2011). Patient Protection and Affordable Care Act (http://www.healthcare.gov/law/full/index.html).

U.S. Department of Health and Human Services (HHS). (2012). Healthy people 2020 (http://www.healthypeople.gov/2020/default.aspx).

White, J. (2005). Patterns of knowing: Review, critique, and update. In L. Andrist, P. K. Nicholas, and K. A. Wolf (Eds.), *A history of ideas in nursing* (pp. 139–150). Sudbury, MA: Jones and Bartlett.

Woods, M. (2010). Cultural safety and the socioethical nurse. *Nursing Ethics, 17,* 715–725. doi: 10.1177/0969733010379296.

World Health Organization. (2012). Obesity and overweight: Fact Sheet. Geneva, Switzerland: (http://www.who.int/mediacentre/factsheets/fs311/en/index.html).

World Health Organization. (2011). WHO global status report on non-communicable diseases 2010 Geneva, Switzerland: Author. (http://www.who.int/nmh/publications/ncd_report_full_en.pdf).

Consultation

Julie Vosit-Steller • Allison B. Morse

CHAPTER CONTENTS

Consultation is an important aspect of advanced practice nursing. As advanced practice nursing has evolved over the years, the consultation competency has received increased attention and is now explicitly addressed as a role expectation. The American Association of Colleges of Nursing (AACN, 2006, 2011) has highlighted consultation as an essential component of master's and Doctor of Nursing Practice (DNP) programs. In defining the essentials of DNP education, the AACN emphasizes the need for exquisite skills in the areas of collaboration and consultation for DNP-prepared advanced practice nurses (APNs). Collaboration is considered in depth in Chapter 12. The complexities of today's health care settings require that all APNs offer and receive consultation and understand, clinically and legally, the differences between consultation and collaboration.

This chapter will address APN consultation in the following manner:

- Establishing consultation as an essential component in APN practice
- Defining consultation and distinguishing it from other APN relationships/responsibilities

- Describing consultation in the context of specific APN roles
- Reviewing a model of consultation developed by Barron and White (2009)
- Highlighting the importance of consultation in education
- Evaluating the consultation process
- Exploring consultation in the international arena

Clarity regarding consultation has the potential to increase patient access to APNs' expert nursing care. Skill with consultation will augment the APN's capability to provide quality care by providing patients with key resources to address their needs. Provision of care to patients with complex needs requires continual development of this competency. APNs can also develop their own consultative skills and use their expertise to enhance their colleagues' nursing practice. The sharing of expertise through a consultative relationship is an important way to promote professional development and enhance clinical understanding.

The enduring works of Caplan (1970), Caplan and Caplan (1993), and Lipowski (1974, 1981, 1983) continue to inform our thinking, writing, and practice in the area of consultation. A number of the sources used to prepare this chapter are considered classics or have ongoing relevance, despite their early publication dates.

Consultation and Advanced Practice Nursing

APN consultation requires the building of relationships with health care professionals within nursing and across disciplines; in advanced practice consultation, the APN offers his or her expertise with colleagues to optimize patient care. Barron and White (2009) have made the important point that consultation may be a significant variable that can contribute to the effectiveness of APNs. Opportunities to consult present themselves to APNs on a daily basis. In clinical practice, the APN applies expertise to the clinical situation and consults with other professionals across disciplines—with an APN colleague regarding a difficult clinical problem, with a physician colleague about how to address a specific patient management issue, or with the nursing staff about how to manage a patient's symptoms or how to follow the clinical guidelines required to handle a unique clinical problem (e.g., infectious disease precautions). In the context of consultation across disciplines, the APN has a unique understanding of the clinical situation from a nursing perspective and is therefore viewed as an expert. Even in a situation in which the APN is working with someone with more experience, such as a specialist physician who is also involved in the patient's care, the unique nursing perspective and expertise of the APN can be brought to bear in the discussion, and it is requisite for the APN to offer these specific insights. This supports Barron and White's (2009) position that the ability of the APN to consult effectively directly influences his/her performance and success in the role.

It is important to mention that there are still some state laws and regulations that mandate a consulting or collaborating physician for advanced practice nurses and for prescriptive privileging. The wording of these mandates often directly states or implies a hierarchical relationship between the APN and physician, which is contrary to the description of consultation being put forth here. As far back as 1999, Minarik and Price described the critical importance of conceptual clarity for legislative and regulatory reform and its far-reaching impact on APN practice. At the state and federal levels, medical societies have attempted to limit advanced practice nursing, so the terminology included in the legislation describing the relationship between physicians and APNs is of enormous significance with regard to collaboration and consultation. Minarik and Price (1999) made the compelling argument that the practical effect of the language of legislation related to the financing of health care can be devastating to advanced practice nursing, even though state boards of nursing are clear in their regulations about the appropriateness of the expanded scope of practice for APNs (LeBuhn & Swankia, 2010). The *Future of Nursing* report by the Institute of Medicine (IOM, 2011) highlights the ever-increasing need for all nurses, including APNs, to be able to function at the full capacity of their education to meet the increasing needs of patients. APNs must be sophisticated readers of legislative proposals that include mandated relationships between physicians and APNs. Because legislation is drafted regarding scope of practice and direct reimbursement for practice, APNs need to be clear and articulate about the implications of such terms as *collaboration, supervision, direction,* and *consultation.* Medical societies may propose such terminology with a clear intent to mandate hierarchical relationships with physicians to limit advanced practice nursing. Because mandated relationships between APNs and physicians may constrain advanced practice nursing consultation, APNs should be aware of the statutes and norms that regulate their practices.

The goals and outcomes of consultation are relevant to ongoing efforts to reform health care. APNs can help bring about the national goal of high-quality, cost-effective health care for every American, as outlined in the IOM report (IOM, 2011). Through consultation, APNs create networks with other APNs, physicians, and colleagues, offering and receiving advice and information that can improve patient care and their own clinical knowledge and skills. Interacting with colleagues in other disciplines can enhance interdisciplinary collaboration and subsequently enhance patient outcomes (see Chapter 12). Consultation can also help shape and develop the practices of consultees and protégés, thereby indirectly but significantly improving the quality, depth, and comprehensiveness of care available to patients and families. Consultation offers APNs the opportunity to influence health care outcomes positively, beyond the direct patient care encounter.

Given the importance of consultation for all APNs, it is surprising that so little emphasis is reflected in advanced practice nursing literature. Consultation within advanced practice nursing may be less visible, less common, or just not a major publication emphasis, but consultation activities may be an important variable in explaining the effectiveness of APNs. Given the complexity of care needs addressed in all settings, the wide-ranging needs of an aging population, and significant time constraints in practice, developing and studying consultation as a core competency in APN practice is imperative. All APNs should be mindful to recognize the significance of consultation in their practice and to communicate the issues, concerns, and successes of this aspect of practice. Advanced practice nursing researchers must also study the role played by

| | TABLE 9-1 | Clarifying Definitions of Clinical Consultation, Comanagement, and Referral |

Type of Interaction	Goals	Focus	Responsibility for Clinical Outcomes
Clinical consultation	To enhance patient care and/or improve skills and confidence of consultee	Consultant may or may not see patient directly Degree of focus on consultee's skill is negotiated with consultee	Remains with consultee, who is free to accept or reject the advice of consultant
Comanagement	To enhance patient care through availability of expertise of two (or more) professionals working together to optimize outcomes	Both professionals see patient directly and coordinate their care with one another (e.g. physician may monitor complex medication regimen while APN focuses on adaptation and human response)	Shared
Referral	To enhance patient care by relinquishing care (or aspects of care) to another professional whose expertise is perceived to be more essential to care than that of the professional making the referral.	Establish connection between patient and professional who is accepting referral Negotiate responsibilities for outcomes	Negotiated, but responsibility is often assumed (at least for aspects of care by professional accepting referral)

Adapted from Barron, A. M., & White, P. (2009). Consultation. In A. B. Hamric, J. A. Spross, & C. M. Hanson (Eds.), *Advanced practice nursing: An integrative approach* (3rd ed., pp. 191–216). Philadelphia: WB Saunders.

timely consultations in the high-quality, cost-effective care delivered by APNs. Consultation is a variable that should be considered in health care outcomes research. Looking specifically at APN consultation and its impact on patient and institutional outcomes may illuminate the role APNs play in improving the care delivery processes.

Defining Consultation

The term *consultation* is used in many ways. It is sometimes used to describe direct care—the practitioner is in consultation with the patient. It may be used interchangeably with the terms *referral* and *collaboration*. Thus, how the term is being used in a given situation may be unclear, and it may be difficult to determine exactly what is being requested and what is expected. A lack of clarity about the specific process being used for clinical problem solving leads to confusion about roles and clinical accountability. The more precisely the word *consultation* is defined, the more likely consultation will be used for its intended purposes of enhancing patient care and promoting positive professional relationships that result in true collaboration and optimal patient outcomes. Because consultation is a core competency of advanced practice nursing, this precision is needed for communication within and outside the profession. It is extremely important to understand the differences between consultation and other types of professional interactions. Table 9-1 summarizes these differences, which are further described in the remainder of this section.

Distinguishing Consultation from Comanagement, Referral, and Collaboration*

Four terms with similar meaning are often used interchangeably; each term suggests specific relationships and responsibilities. The subtle differences between the terms *consultation, comanagement, collaboration,* and *referral* are identified when one examines the degree to which an APN assumes responsibility for the direct management of a clinical or administrative problem.

Consultation is an interaction between two professionals in which the consultant is recognized as having specialized expertise (Caplan, 1970; Caplan & Caplan, 1993). The consultee requests the assistance of that expert in handling a problem that he or she recognizes as falling within the expertise of the consultant. Consultation is a role function used by APNs to offer clinical expertise to other colleagues, as a specialty consultant, or to seek additional information to enhance their own practice. Given APNs' advanced knowledge and assessment skills, and in some cases expansion of the APN role into areas of specialization, consultation for peer APN expertise can foster improved accessibility, consultation, and timely and potentially improved care for patients waiting to be seen for patients with unique conditions.

*In this chapter, we use the term *collaboration* to refer to a specific advanced practice nursing competency (see Chapter 10) and the term *comanagement* to refer to a specific type of collaborative interaction (see Table 9-1). Thus, we consider comanagement as one of many collaborative processes used by APNs. In American College of Nurse-Midwives (ACNM) documents, the terms *comanagement* and *collaboration* are used synonymously (ACNM, 2011; Hamric, Spross, & Hanson, 2009).

Comanagement is the process whereby one professional manages some aspects of a patient's care while another professional manages other aspects of the same patient's care. Effective comanagement requires excellent communication, coordination, and collaborative skills. Professionals who work within the same interdisciplinary team often develop systems that facilitate seamless and effective comanagement. In comanagement, both providers retain responsibility for the patient's care (Table 9-1).

APNs are often confused in practice between consultation and collaboration. Chapter 12 provides a thoughtful definition of collaboration that was first offered by Hanson and Spross in 1996: *"Collaboration is a dynamic, interpersonal process in which two or more individuals make a commitment to each other to interact authentically and constructively to solve problems and to learn from each other in order to accomplish identified goals, purposes, or outcomes. The individuals recognize and articulate the shared values that make this commitment possible."* Collaboration is a process that underlies the professional interactions involved in consultation, comanagement, and referral. Whatever the nature of the consulting relationship, the APN keeps the patient at the center of her or his actions; therefore, consultation requires collaboration on some level when two professionals come together to meet patient-centered goals. Recruiting other professionals for collaboration organizes support of an interdisciplinary group, thereby increasing the impact on the patient or problem through the synergy of multiple experts. An example of collaboration may involve a geriatric clinical nurse specialist (CNS) and palliative care nurse practitioner (NP) participating in a family meeting to discuss goals of care with a frail older patient and his or her family regarding end-of-life wishes, including code status and hospice.

A referral describes a situation in which a clinician relinquishes responsibility for care (or aspects of care), temporarily or permanently, to another clinician who is likely a specialist for an opinion or management of part of a patient's care. In most cases, once the care associated with the referral is complete, the patient will return to the full-time care of the referring clinician.

Consultation occurs when the APN requests the advice or opinion of a physician or other health care team member and the APN maintains primary responsibility for the patient's care. The ACNM uses the term *collaboration* to describe the process whereby the CNM and physician jointly manage the care of the woman or newborn. Another frequently encountered term, *referral,* describes a situation in which the clinician making the referral relinquishes responsibility for care (or aspects of care), temporarily or permanently.

Background

Types of Consultation

According to Caplan's classic definition (1970), there are four different types of consultation. Client-centered case consultation is the most common type of consultation. The primary goal of this type of consultation is assisting the consultee to develop an effective plan of care for a patient who has a particularly difficult, complex, or unique problem. In client-centered case consultation, the consultant often sees the patient directly to complete an assessment of the patient and to make recommendations to the consultee for the consultee's management of the case. This is often a one-time evaluation, although follow-up by the consultant is sometimes needed. The primary goal is to assist the consultee in helping the patient. A positive experience when handling that specific case will enhance the consultee's ability so that future patients with similar problems can be treated more effectively. For example, the APN may consult an infectious disease APN to elicit her or his opinion on an ongoing infection in a human immunodeficiency virus (HIV)–positive patient. This consultation would be specific to the clinical problem at hand and result in recommendations for the consultee to manage or comanage a challenging clinical infection with the assistance of an expert infectious disease APN. The recommendations could include information such as which antibiotics are recommended to treat the infection, how to monitor response to the antibiotics, and potential adverse effects of the treatment plan.

In consultee-centered case consultation, improving patient care is important but the emphasis is focused directly on the consultee's ability to handle a challenging situation. Thus, the primary goals are to assess the consultee's needs and address the problem effectively. In consultee-centered case consultation, the task for the consultant is to understand and remedy the problems of the consultee in managing a particular case. A usual problem is lack of knowledge, skill, confidence, or objectivity. Therefore, the consultant may educate the consultee further on the issues presented by the patient or may suggest alternative strategies for dealing with the problem. This is probably the most common type of consultation sought by APNs. The consultant may seek to bolster the confidence of the consultee in handling the problem if, in the opinion of the consultant, the consultee has the ability and potential to do so. If the problem presented by the consultee is a lack of professional objectivity, the consultant can help the consultee identify the factors interfering with the consultee's ability to see the patient realistically. The consultee may hold a stereotyped view of the patient, or perhaps the patient's difficulties in some way mirror or symbolize the consultee's personal difficulties and cloud the consultee's ability to see the reality of the situation.

Effective consultation can foster orderly reflection and extend the frames of reference used by the consultee to solve clinical problems (Caplan & Caplan, 1993). Both client-centered and consultee-centered case consultations have been important activities in traditional CNS practice. For example, the psychiatric CNS is often consulted by the APN in the hospitalist role who has patients with advanced dementia, behavioral disorders, or long-standing psychiatric diagnoses that may need adjustment now that the patient has been hospitalized. Although the APN hospitalist is comfortable with behavioral assessment and continuity of care, he or she may not be adept at treating the changes in behavior that can occur while the patient is hospitalized. The psychiatric CNS can apply specific knowledge, along with the necessary medical treatment, to maximize patient care while she or he is hospitalized and teach the APN these diagnostic and management techniques. In the primary care setting, this type of consultation can be seen when APNs confer with their physician or APN colleagues to confirm their differential diagnoses or individualize a treatment plan.

Program-centered administrative consultation focuses on the planning and administration of clinical services whereby the APN consultant steps in to offer needed clinical expertise in a clinical program focused on a patient population. Consultee-centered administrative consultation focuses on the consultee's (or group of consultees') difficulties as they interface with the organization's objectives. For example, an APN may consult with a group of administrators who want to implement a clinical service, such as wound care or breast health. To assist in the development of these two programs, the APN's consultation can offer perspective on how specific needs—both clinical and psychosocial—of these two patient populations can be met.

APNs may be involved in all four types of consultation at various times. This chapter specifically considers the first two types of consultation, client-centered case consultation and consultee-centered case consultation, because the focus here is the process of interacting with other professionals regarding the care of individual patients. Case consultation can bridge the gap between evidence or knowledge and practice, assisting staff in improving care for patients and families through broadening perspectives, expanding expertise, and generalizing knowledge appropriately (Lewandowski & Adamle, 2009).

Consultation and Specific Advanced Practice Nurse Roles

The consultation competency has received significant attention in the four APN roles and is explicitly addressed as a role expectation (AACN, 2006; 2011; American Association of Nurse Anesthetists [AANA], 2005; ACNM, 2011, 2012; National Association of Clinical Nurse Specialists (NACNS), 2004; National CNS Task Force, 2010; National Organization of Nurse Practitioner Faculties [NONPF], 2011). Although all APNs seek and provide consultation, the literature on consultation in specific APN roles varies. Certified nurse-midwives (CNMs), for example, specifically address consultation as an expectation (ACNM, 2011). In addition, consultation has long been a specific expectation for those in CNS positions. Consultation as a competency is less frequently addressed in the certified registered nurse anesthetist (CRNA) and NP literature, although they are likely to consult and be consulted formally and informally in practice on a regular basis.

Of the four APN roles, the CNS literature contains the largest amount of information regarding consultation. As a CNS, the professional focus remains on clinical nursing, although the CNS also spends time in nursing staff education, evidence-based practice, and system change and innovation. As a clinical expert, a CNS hones consultant-consultee relationships with the nurses who provide bedside care in the acute setting (Dias, 2010). In these consultant-consultee interactions, the CNS can influence patient outcomes by modeling and leading nurses to use evidence in making clinical decisions. For example, a CNS may discuss the chemotherapy care plan or wound care protocol with the staff nurse prior to implementation to ensure that the nurse has a complete understanding of the interventions to be provided.

In the CNM role, managing patient risk and responding to the patient's best interest drives the decision to refer for an obstetric consultation (Skinner & Foureur, 2010). In New Zealand, the obstetric consultation rate is 35%. Although the consultation rate may seem high, the reasons for consultation were significantly justified and the midwives usually continued to provide some midwifery care for the patients, even when risk had been identified. The consultation with the obstetrician did not automatically result in comanagement of the pregnant patient by the physician and CNM; rather, most patients returned to the care of the midwife with the consultant's input (Skinner & Foureur, 2010).

Some examples of NPs as consultants have been described in the literature. The development of mental health NP consultant liaisons who consult on emergency department (ED) patients has been explored in Australia (Wand & Fisher, 2006; Van Der Watt, 2010). These NPs consult with ER colleagues on patients with behavioral issues who present to the ED using therapeutic techniques and medications for acute crises, and making referrals, as needed. These roles have been shown to increase collaboration and improve patient and family satisfaction and are seen as complementary to rather than a replacement for medical psychiatric care (Wand & Fisher, 2006). Other examples of NP consultation have been illustrated—NP-led rapid response teams demonstrate decreases in need for cardiopulmonary resuscitation while providing patient treatment and staff education (Benson et al., 2008), and NPs in interventional radiology provide consultation related to vascular access and diagnostic procedures (Dryer, 2006).

Model of Advanced Practice Nursing Consultation

Barron (1989) proposed a model of consultation for CNSs that was based on the nursing process and incorporated principles from the work of Caplan (1970) and Lipowski (1974, 1981, 1983). This model, expanded by Barron and White (1996), has evolved into the model of advanced practice nurse consultation shown in Figure 9-1. This model is based on the following principles of consultation derived from the field of mental health (Caplan, 1970; Caplan & Caplan, 1993; Lipowski, 1981):

- The consultation is usually initiated by the consultee.
- The relationship between the consultant and consultee is nonhierarchical and collaborative.
- The consultant always considers contextual factors when responding to the request for consultation.
- The consultant has no direct authority for managing patient care.

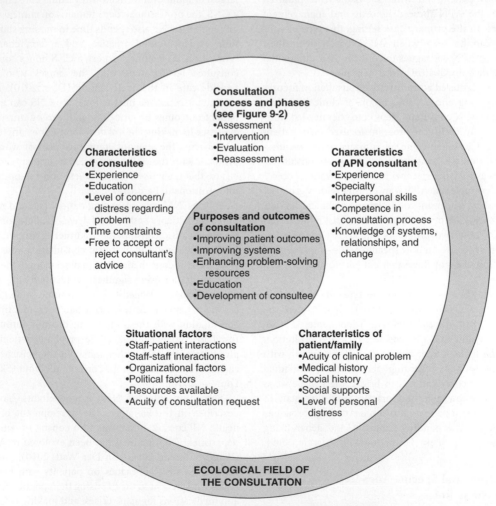

Consultation process and phases (see Figure 9-2)
- Assessment
- Intervention
- Evaluation
- Reassessment

Characteristics of consultee
- Experience
- Education
- Level of concern/ distress regarding problem
- Time constraints
- Free to accept or reject consultant's advice

Characteristics of APN consultant
- Experience
- Specialty
- Interpersonal skills
- Competence in consultation process
- Knowledge of systems, relationships, and change

Purposes and outcomes of consultation
- Improving patient outcomes
- Improving systems
- Enhancing problem-solving resources
- Education
- Development of consultee

Situational factors
- Staff-patient interactions
- Staff-staff interactions
- Organizational factors
- Political factors
- Resources available
- Acuity of consultation request

Characteristics of patient/family
- Acuity of clinical problem
- Medical history
- Social history
- Social supports
- Level of personal distress

ECOLOGICAL FIELD OF THE CONSULTATION

FIG 9-1 Model of Advanced Practice Nurse consultation.

- The consultant does not prescribe, but makes recommendations.
- The consultee is free to accept or reject the recommendations of the consultant.
- The consultation should be documented.

Ecologic Field of the Consultation Process

APNs tend to have a holistic orientation and understanding of systems theory that enables them to apply this consultation model in practice. At the center of Barron and White's (1996) proposed model are the purposes and outcomes of consultation. Surrounding the center is the ecologic field of the consultation. Consultations are embedded in the context of the specific circumstances surrounding the consultation request, so the ecologic field in which the consultation takes place must be understood to provide effective consultation (Caplan & Caplan, 1993). This involves an appreciation of the interconnection and interrelatedness of the systems and contexts influencing the consultation problem and process. Thus, the consultation process is an integral part of the ecologic field. The process—in which the consultant evaluates the request, performs an assessment, determines the skills required

to address the problem, intervenes, and evaluates the outcome—is expanded in Figure 9-2. Other elements of the ecologic field include the characteristics of the consultant, consultee, patient and family, and situational factors. We assume that there are reciprocal influences among the purposes, process, and contextual factors that can affect consultation processes and outcomes. Each component of the model is elaborated in the following sections.

Purposes and Outcomes

The purpose of a consultation may be to improve care delivery processes and patient outcomes, enhance health care delivery systems, extend the knowledge available to solve clinical problems, foster the ongoing professional development of the consultee, or a combination of these goals. Consultants should be aware that the purposes for which they have been consulted may contract or expand during the process of consulting. Often, APN consultants accomplish several purposes at once. If additional purposes and possible outcomes are uncovered during consultation, these should be made clear to the consultee. The consultee may want the consultant's assistance with a patient but does not have the time or interest to focus on

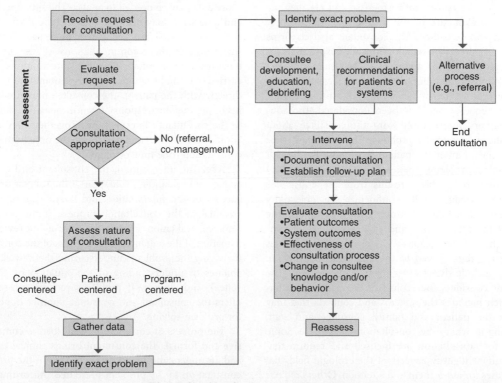

FIG 9-2 Algorithm for the consultation process.

his or her own development. Patients may also reveal information that requires a shift in the consultation's focus, purpose, and outcome. Over the course of the consultation, being explicit about the goal or outcome of the consultation is essential if APNs are to evaluate the impact of consultation on practice.

Consultation Process for Formal Consultation

Figure 9-2 presents an algorithm of the consultation process. With experience and expertise, the process may occur fairly rapidly so that the expert consultant may not be consciously aware of using these steps. In addition, in some situations, the problem for which help is sought is clear-cut and the consultation is brief. These types of consultations are discussed later in the chapter.

Once a request for consultation has been received, assessment of the consultation problem begins with evaluation of the request itself. An important component of assessment is confirming with the consultee that consultation is, in fact, the appropriate strategy for addressing the problem (e.g., rather than a referral). At this stage, the consultant and consultee may decide that an alternative process is needed (e.g., a shift to comanagement or referral). The consultant confirms that the problem has been accurately identified and falls within the realm of the consultant's expertise and clarifies the nonhierarchical nature of the relationship between the consultant and consultee. The consultant also confirms that the consultee will remain clinically responsible for the patient who is the focus of the consultation. The consultant must remember that the consultee is ultimately free to accept or reject her or his recommendations. Once the request itself has been considered, the consultant gathers information from the consultee about the specific nature of the problem. The consultant tries to determine whether the patient has unusually difficult and complex problems (patient-centered consultation) and whether the problem results from the consultee's lack of knowledge, skill, confidence, or objectivity (consultee-centered consultation). Once the request, the nature of the relationship, and appropriateness of consultation have been established, the consultant focuses on gathering data related to the consultation problem. This may include direct assessment of the patient. The consultant considers the ecologic field of the consultation, which includes the systems and contexts that may influence the patient and family, consultee and staff, and setting in which the consultation takes place. Some requests for consultation are focused and require that the consultant identify aspects of the ecologic field that are priorities for assessment and attention. Others require more comprehensive assessment.

The consultant uses available resources such as patient records, direct assessment of the patient, and interviews with staff and family to identify the exact problem(s) that is (are) to be the focus of consultation. This may or may not be the problem for which help has been sought. Some consultation problems are simple and do not require extensive data collection. Others are complex and may require extensive chart review for a long-standing problem or calls to referring clinicians when incomplete data have been provided. The consultant shares the identified problem with the consultee and validates this with the consultee. If part of the problem is the consultee's lack of expertise, the consultant will want to use tact as the problem is identified and discussed. Interpersonal qualities of the consultant are crucial (see later).

Once the specific problem or problems have been identified, the consultant and consultee consider interventions that will address the problem(s). The consultant may intervene directly with the consultee by using approaches such as education, assistance with reinterpretation of the problem, or identification of appropriate resources if the problem is the consultee's lack of experience. If the problem results from a particularly difficult patient situation, the consultant may assist with the process of clinical decision making by providing alternative perspectives on the problem and recommending specific interventions. More data may be needed to analyze the situation further, and a decision may need to be made about whether the consultee or consultant will gather more data. If the consultee accepts the recommendations of the consultant, together they negotiate how the interventions will be carried out, and by whom. If the consultant is to intervene directly with the patient, the consultee must understand his or her ongoing responsibility for the patient and agree to the consultant's interventions. Together, they identify additional resources and determine the time frame for the consultation (one time or ongoing).

After the intervention, the consultant and consultee engage in evaluation. Evaluation of the success or lack of success of the intervention and overall consultation is essential to the consultation process. If the problem is resolved, evaluation offers an opportunity for review, confirmation of the enhanced effectiveness of the consultee in managing the problem (underscoring the new skills and abilities or understanding of the situation by the consultee), and closure. If problems remain, reassessment offers the consultant and consultee another opportunity for problem solving.

The process of consultation described is comprehensive and formal. The consultant brings clinical expertise and an understanding and appreciation of the process of consultation to the problem presented. According to the model, the consultant considers all elements of the nursing process in relation to the consultation problem. However, what about the quick questions to the consultant, when what is needed is a piece of information and a brief description of how to apply the information? Are these brief interactions, sometimes called "corridor consultations," related to circumscribed problems true consultations? They are, absolutely, but the consultant needs to make a conscious decision about responding briefly and simply to the request and needs to consider with the consultee whether the quick response addresses the problem. Sometimes, the problem presented oversimplifies a complex concern, requiring a more comprehensive approach. If the consultant and consultee consider the problem together, they can determine whether the quick response is adequate or whether consultation is needed. Conversely, sometimes what is truly needed is a short answer to a clinical question or validation that the approach to the problem is appropriate.

Staff nurses sometimes equate this brief type of consultation with consultation in general because they have experienced only this type of consultation with physicians, who quickly impart information and are then off to the next patient. The idea of the roving clinical expert dropping by with tidbits of expert advice is the idea that non-APNs can have of a consultant. This is another reason why it is important to make a conscious decision about responding in a brief way to the consultation request. In the informal situation, the consultee may not realize that a more comprehensive and thorough investigation of the problem and solutions with the consultant is possible. Also, some clinical situations require a more formal approach to the consultation problem. APNs should consider the types of problems in practice that require a formal approach and develop a system for integrating nurse-nurse and interdisciplinary consultations, which make advanced practice nursing skills more visible and extend their knowledge and skills.

Characteristics of the Advanced Practice Nurse Consultant

In addition to theoretical understanding, self-awareness and interpersonal skills are essential for the consultant (Barron, 1989; Barron & White, 2009). For a model of consultative practice to be implemented, it is critical that APNs first value themselves and the specialized expertise that they have developed. One must appreciate one's own skills and knowledge before the possibilities for consultation can be envisioned (see Chapters 3 and 7). APNs have developed specialized expertise in the following: direct care of underserved populations, such as the homeless; frail older adults; persons who are chronically mentally ill, home-bound, or institutionalized; and patients with HIV infection. The knowledge and skills acquired

by APNs could serve to inform and expand the practices of staff nurses, other APNs, and health care professionals of various disciplines involved in the care of these populations of patients. However, APNs must first appreciate that they have valuable understanding and knowledge to share.

Ideally, consultants know themselves well—they are aware of their own personal issues, strengths, weaknesses, and motives. A good consultant must be able to suspend judgment and avoid stereotyping. When consultation is sought, a fresh perspective is often needed. Self-understanding allows the consultant to see consultation issues realistically, without prejudice. It is not uncommon for a consultant to step into a highly emotionally charged situation. Self-awareness, understanding, and being able to remain centered and self-possessed are key to remaining objective and clear. It can be meaningful and helpful for the consultant to have a trusted colleague or supervisor with whom to share and review consultation situations. These discussions can offer support and enhance the consultant's understanding of personal and interpersonal responses to the consultation material.

The consultant should also be able to establish warm, respectful, and accepting relationships with consultees (Carter & Berlin, 2007; Perry, 2011). The initiation of a consultation request is often associated with a sense of vulnerability on the part of the consultee, who recognizes that assistance is required to help manage the situation at hand. The consultant must communicate (and sincerely believe) that the problem and consultee are important and worthy of consideration. The consultant must also communicate confidence in the consultee's ability to overcome the difficulties resulting in the consultation request. When the consultant creates a climate of trust and acceptance, the consultee can then be willing to risk vulnerability and genuineness with the consultant. When a respectful trusting connection is made between the consultant and consultee, a deep examination of the problem, implications, and solutions is possible.

An APN is sometimes the consultee, and often the APN requests consultation from a physician. As a consultee, the APN should be able to identify and articulate the nature of the problem for which help is being sought. It may be necessary to clarify the collegial, nonhierarchical nature of the consultation relationship. When consulting with an APN colleague or physician, often an APN has already tried alternative plans or is thinking about possible directions to take based on knowledge of the patient or clinical situation. Consultants find such information useful in planning their approaches to the consultation. Dialogue with APN colleagues and physicians can improve the effectiveness and efficiency of the consultation and can strengthen collaboration among colleagues. In addition to their intrapersonal knowledge and interpersonal skills, APNs must be competent in the consultative process.

To be an effective consultant, an APN must be knowledgeable about systems, relationships, and change (see Chapter 11). Although skill in consultation develops over time, the attributes of the consultant and consultation process described here can help novice APNs who are open to learning approach consultation with confidence (see later, "Developing Consultation Skills in Advance Practice Nurse Students"; Carter & Berlin, 2007).

Characteristics of the Consultee

The consultee identifies a problem that exists in a clinical situation because of uncertainty, complexity, or a lack of knowledge on his or her part and believes that increased knowledge and assistance with clinical decision making would enhance practice. Characteristics of the consultee may need to be considered. Education, experience, the consultee's level of distress regarding the clinical problem for which help is sought, organizational skills, and availability to solve problems with the consultant are factors that can influence the consultation.

Patient and Family Factors

Among factors to consider are the acuity and complexity of the clinical problem, the patient's medical history, social history, and social supports, and other resources. Depending on the nature of the problem, it may be important to consider concurrent stresses being experienced by the patient and family. An acute problem may demand the consultant's immediate assistance, requiring a shift in the consultant's priorities. A complex or unusual problem may take more time to solve.

Situational Factors

In this model, the term situational factors refer to those inherent factors in the organization and staff caring for the patient. Numerous situational factors can affect the consultation process. The quality of relationships and interactions between staff and patients or among staff members themselves may be important issues. For example, a patient perceived as being nonadherent to some therapy may be responding to conflicts among team members that the patient has inferred from clinicians' behaviors. A clinician may seek validation from a consultant as a way of getting support for an unpopular but potentially productive approach to a clinical problem. Time pressures and lack of adequate resources can affect consultation. Organizational factors include legal factors, regulatory considerations, and credentialing mechanisms for a specialty practice. Organizational politics, power imbalances, and rapid or frequent system changes also are to be considered. All these factors can affect the consultee's view of the

importance of the request. For APNs, the status of advanced practice nursing and APNs in a particular agency or state may influence consultation. For example, organizational policies and procedures regarding consultation, statutes regarding APN-physician consulting relationships, protocol agreements, reimbursement policies, and degree of prescriptive authority may affect the consultation process.

Common Advanced Practice Nurse Consultation Situations

Depending on one's particular advanced practice nursing role, certain consultation situations may be more common than others. APNs are most likely to receive requests for patient- and consultee-centered case consultations. These types of consultations are described here. Experienced APNs may extend their consultative skills into other types of consultations, such as program-centered consultations. The exemplars included here vary in the complexity of consultations and the extent to which aspects of the consultation model are made explicit. The reader is encouraged to examine how the proposed model of advanced practice nursing consultation is applied and consider ways in which it can be applied in his or her own practice.

Advanced Practice Nurse Consultation in Practice

Within their specialty or setting, APNs may take for granted the available APN consulting resources. They may not think of their interactions regarding patient care as a consultation because they occur as they are engaged in practice, in the hallway, or over coffee. Consultation among APNs may be more or less formal, depending on the culture of the unit or clinic, relationships among the APNs, and specialty populations seen in the facility. Consultations are likely to involve specific patient issues—for example, "Could you look at this rash?" or "I've done everything I can think of to try to make sure this pregnant teen comes to her prenatal visits, and she still misses them. Here's what I've done. … Can you think of anything else I can try before I get the city department of social services involved?" Exemplar 9-1 illustrates a formal consultee-centered consultation between a primary care NP and a CNS-NP specializing in HIV/AIDS; this consultation also led to a plan to comanage the patient.

Exemplar 9-1 highlights formal consultation and comanagement of a client's needs, which are chronic and complex and require the resources of many professionals. The CNS specialist in HIV/AIDS provided consultee-centered consultation, enhancing the knowledge base of the primary care NP and providing insight into the expected course of adjustment of patients with AIDS and

EXEMPLAR 9-1 Nurse Practitioner–Clinical Nurse Specialist Consultation on Infectious Disease

Ms. L is a 29-year-old woman who has been followed regularly for primary care through her young adulthood in the family practice. She presented 2 years ago with symptoms initially thought consistent with bronchitis. Her symptoms worsened, and she was eventually hospitalized and diagnosed with pneumocystis pneumonia. A diagnosis of acquired immunodeficiency syndrome (AIDS) was then made. Ms. L was subsequently referred to the infectious disease specialists in a tertiary setting for ongoing management of AIDS; she continued to have her general primary care needs met at the family practice. The primary care NP was pleased that her patient wanted to continue to be cared for in the family practice but was challenged by the increasing complexities in management of her new illness and the patient's struggles in coping with this disease. The primary care NP scheduled a telephone consultation with the APN in the infectious disease clinic where Ms. L received her care for AIDS.

The APN was a blended role CNS who had extensive knowledge and experience in the care of clients with HIV/AIDS. She was able to provide the primary care NP with specific knowledge regarding expected and unusual side effects of the medication regimen and commonly encountered drug-drug interactions. Although the CNS would continue to prescribe and oversee the medication regimen, they discussed what they would do to comanage Ms. L's care. The NP agreed that she felt comfortable with managing common side effects and would collaborate to monitor Ms. L for any problems with adherence to the treatment regimen between visits to the specialty clinic. When discussing how the patient was coping, the CNS reassured the NP that her patient's response was appropriate for her stage of illness and suggested communication strategies that might further assist the patient in dealing with the reactions of family, coworkers, and friends. In addition, they acknowledged that the NP was likely to have more opportunities to help Ms. L with coping with the disease, so the CNS agreed to send the NP some recent relevant literature on the unique challenges of integrating the experience of living with AIDS into one's life. The CNS provided information about a support group and other resources that the patient might find helpful.

suggestions for community-based support. The primary care NP continued providing primary care and monitoring the patient's response to treatment and adjustment to the illness, comanaging Ms. L's illness with the HIV/AIDS CNS and her colleagues at the specialty clinic.

As noted, the role of the midwife assumes a large amount of risk. As a result, liability is a significant consideration. Xu and colleagues (2008) conducted a survey of nurse midwives in Michigan in which 69% (*N* = 145) reported that liability concerns negatively affected their clinical decision making. Of the respondents, 35% had been named in a malpractice claim at least once in their careers. This is one example of what CNMs have to navigate in the U.S. health care delivery system. As such, Exemplar 9-2 addresses how peer to peer consultation can play a positive role in patient care.

This case is an example of consultee-centered consultation. Kathy provided clinical support and reassurance to Molly that she was using sound clinical judgment. The team physicians agreed that Molly made a good decision to allow the patient to proceed to natural childbirth delivery on her own; this reassured the patient that her caregivers were listening to her requests and working together to meet her needs.

Advanced Practice Nurse–Physician Consultation

Consultation and collaboration with the physician and patient care team remain integral components of APN interprofessional development. When consulting with other nurses or physicians, an APN is likely to be far along in the problem-solving process. The need for consultation is often related to the consultee's level of diagnostic uncertainty or complex management issues. Experienced APNs often have a clear definition of the problem and a preliminary plan to address it that they wish to validate or reformulate, depending on the consultant's advice. Truly collaborative relationships between physicians and APNs ensure consultation that is bidirectional. Physicians in primary care often consult APNs regarding issues such as assisting patients in making lifestyle changes or in coping with the effects of chronic illness. Many APNs in primary care have special expertise in women's health care and are sought out by physicians for consultation on such issues. Physicians might then choose to comanage patients with APNs so that patients benefit from the expertise of both professionals. APNs, in turn, might consult a physician regarding a patient in a medically unstable condition, which evolves into comanagement by the physician and

EXEMPLAR 9-2   Certified Nurse Midwife–Certified Nurse Midwife Consultation

Molly, a CNM, is an experienced midwife of 5 years; she practices in a large hospital-based, urban, maternal-child health unit. She is in practice with Kathy, a more senior CNM. Molly has a healthy 29-year-old patient, Kim (G1P0), who is very articulate in the prenatal visits about her desire to experience natural childbirth. She is married and in a monogamous relationship. She has no medical problems and no past surgical history. She has not consumed alcohol or smoked cigarettes since she learned of her much desired pregnancy.

At 35 weeks, Kim's blood pressure begins to increase. She is asymptomatic and has no protein in her urine. Molly discusses early stages of pregnancy-induced hypertension (PIH) with Kim and the patient is adamant that she is not going to have an induction; she is insistent on experiencing a natural childbirth. Once she reaches 39 weeks, Kim is diagnosed with PIH. Her urine protein begins to rise slightly and she is started on low-dose labetalol, with good effect; Kim remains committed to a natural birth plan and the fetal heart tracing remains reassuring.

Given the circumstances, Molly approaches her senior CNM colleague, Kathy, for advice about approaching the patient to discuss the possibility of induction because of her PIH. They discuss the risks and benefits of letting the patient continue her pregnancy until she experiences natural labor. They discuss the principles of midwifery and the importance of supporting the patient's wishes if it is safe to do so, and at what point they should consider referral to the collaborating physician. Once Kim reaches 40 weeks, Kathy meets with the patient and Molly to review the clinical situation and the possible need for induction in the setting of PIH and pregnancy after her due date. Together, both midwives and the patient decide to let the pregnancy progress naturally. To do so, Kathy and Molly meet with their collaborating physician to review their clinical decision making. Ultimately, the patient delivers a healthy baby boy at 41 weeks via natural childbirth.

APN, with each assuming responsibility for the outcomes of decision making.

The ACNM (2011) was deliberate in describing the various types of interactions that CNMs have with physicians. Unfortunately, APN-physician consultative relationships have often been structured by laws and regulations that mandate or imply supervisory oversight, which can reinforce stereotypical nurse-physician relationships. Many organizational cultures reinforce traditional nurse-physician relationships and the behavioral norms associated with them. One of the major challenges facing advanced practice nursing educators is to address students explicitly prior to socialization to nurse-physician relationships that might undermine the full expression of autonomous advanced practice nursing. When a hierarchical relationship exists between an APN and physician, the APN who consults may defer to the physician's decisions, downplaying or ignoring first-hand knowledge of the patient. However, there are successful interactions between physicians and APNs and these practices embrace the collaborative relationships that are key to effective consultation (see Chapter 12).

Consultation between APNs and physicians can highlight the strengths of each—that is, the APN's deep appreciation for the human responses related to health and illness and the physician's deep understanding of disease and treatment. When both areas of expertise are available

to patients and their families, truly holistic, comprehensive, and individualized care is offered. As APN knowledge evolves and deepens, an emerging issue in relation to APN-physician consultation is the crossing of traditional nurse-physician boundaries. As APNs become more and more specialized, the knowledge embedded in practice may be more closely related to what is generally thought of as medical practice. For example, a CRNA may have highly developed skills in the area of pain management and the requisite skills to perform procedures to address complex pain issues. In women's health practices, APNs may specialize in using complementary therapies for menopausal symptoms. Physicians often refer interested patients to the collaborating women's health APN in the practice for consultation about using naturopathic medications, herbal remedies, and compounded estrogens. Tact and understanding of the long-standing boundaries that are being crossed can elevate the consultation relationship to a new level.

Advanced Practice Nurse–Staff Nurse Consultation

Early on, as CNSs implemented their consultative roles, it became apparent that the culture of nursing had not adopted consultation as an important strategy in providing patient care (Barron, 1983). Staff nurses were expected to take care of the patients themselves. A novice might consult a head nurse or more senior nurse, but staff members were expected to know how to solve problems and use the policy and procedure manual. An important component of implementing consultation means teaching staff members how and when to consult. During that time, CNSs often engaged in active case finding to identify patients who needed the knowledge and skills they had because CNSs were not actually assigned to patients and staff nurses. By building this type of clinical caseload, they demonstrated to staff how consultation might be helpful. Of note, CNSs tended to carry out direct consultation with patients and to consult with other professionals to assist the staff with problem solving and enhancing patient care. For example, staff nurses might call the medical-surgical CNS regarding a patient with Guillain-Barré syndrome because they had no experience caring for patients with this disorder. The CNS may have had little or no experience as well but could mobilize the resources needed, such as arranging an in service by the neuroscience or rehabilitation CNS, providing articles, being available to staff on all shifts as they implemented unfamiliar assessments, and assisting with care plan development. The APN initiates processes (including additional consultation) and provides knowledge directly.

Once relationships are established and staff perceive that the APN consultant is approachable, respectful, and helpful, staff will initiate contact with the consultant when complex clinical issues arise. See Exemplar 9-3 for an example of staff RN to APN consultation.

This example demonstrates the consultation process. The NP has specific clinical expertise and is called on to support the oncology RN in her care for patient JM. Through this consultation, the NP has provided the oncology RN with evidence-based practice (EBP) knowledge that she will be able to use when caring for future patients with the same issue.

In Exemplar 9-4, intensive care unit (ICU) nurses requested a psychiatric liaison nursing consultation. The staff and consultant had a well-established relationship.

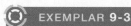 **EXEMPLAR 9-3** **Oncology Registered Nurse–Oncology Nurse Practitioner Consultation**

JM is a 65-year-old man with adenocarcinoma of the tonsils who underwent radical neck surgery and will begin radiation therapy. His nurse is doing radiation therapy teaching with JM and his family. JM already suffers from dry mouth and they are concerned that the radiation therapy could also cause xerostomia. The oncology nurse consults the oncology NP to ask for management and treatment guidance because she has only taken care of one patient with xerostomia who was undergoing radiation therapy. Because JM already has an underlying xerostomia, she would like to strategize about how to prevent JM from experiencing severe symptoms.

The oncology NP who was consulted to manage JM's potential xerostomia during radiation therapy would search the literature, offer clinical pearls based on his or her experience, describe population-based data (e.g., men with adenocarcinoma of the tonsils), and/or strategize about prevention of this specific symptom with oncology patients treated at the same facility with the same drug.

 EXEMPLAR 9-4 **Clinical Nurse Specialist–Intensive Care Unit Staff Consultation**

An 18-year-old man who overdosed on acetaminophen was admitted to the ICU several hours before consultation was sought. His medical condition was grave. The psychiatric CNS was consulted to assess the patient's current suicidal risk and make treatment recommendations. Her initial recommendations focused on support for the nurses as they were managing the grief, fear, and guilt of the young man and his mother. The medical implications of his actions were real and the teaching the nurses provided was very important. The nurses were very concerned about the young man and his family. The patient was expressing regret about the overdose, saying he was no longer suicidal. He was terrified by the potential for liver failure and dying. His mother was beside herself with guilt. The night before admission, the patient had come home intoxicated, telling his mother that he had taken the acetaminophen. She did not believe him; she thought he was looking for sympathy to avoid getting into trouble for drinking. She also reasoned that if he had taken the acetaminophen, it was no big deal; after all, it was a relatively mild and safe drug. When he woke up in the morning very ill, she brought

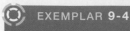

Clinical Nurse Specialist–Intensive Care Unit Staff Consultation—*cont'd*

him to the local emergency department for care. Treatment was initiated and he was transferred by ambulance to the medical center.

The gastroenterologist was not confident that liver failure could be prevented. The psychiatrists assessed that the patient was no longer at risk of suicide. Everyone involved was deeply moved and distressed by the tragedy they were witnessing. The nurses requested that the psychiatric CNS be available for additional supportive care for the patient, support and referral for the family, and assistance in planning nursing care for the patient. The nurses continued to request additional intervention and knowledge about how to care for this young man with liver failure, who was dying following a seemingly innocent gesture. The CNS was available to provide consultation to the nurses who had specific concerns regarding liver failure and death and dying.

After 36 hours, the patient became comatose and his organs began to fail. It was clear that he was dying. His mother accepted referral to her local mental health center, which was arranged by the psychiatric CNS. After her son became comatose, she did not spend much time in the ICU. She said it was just too painful for her to see him deteriorate. Other family members and friends spent a great deal of time in the unit. The psychiatric CNS stopped by the unit frequently, talking with staff and family members. Everyone

(including the CNS) had a great need to talk through the sorrow and sense of impotence in the situation. Everything that could be done was being done, but that was not enough to change the outcome. The presence of the CNS and her skill at facilitating a debriefing were powerful tools in a time of need for the staff and family.

The patient lived for 5 days; on the sixth day, death was not far away. The nursing staff was concerned about how to respond to his mother when he died. The CNS was present with the family and friends to support the patient in the process of dying. His mother did not return to the hospital. After the emotionally tumultuous week with the young patient, there was some sense of satisfaction in knowing that if his death could not be prevented, a peaceful and dignified death could be facilitated. The family and friends expressed their deep gratitude for that facilitation.

This client-centered consultation addressed the needs of the nurses, patient, and family regarding the patient's liver failure and unexpected death. The consultation clarified the goal to promote a peaceful and comfortable death, because cure was no longer possible. The CNS consultation contributed to an active and compassionate nursing presence, which allowed for a peaceful and dignified death for the young patient and a referral for ongoing support for a grieving mother.

Consultation in the International Community

Within the past 10 years, there has been increased success in establishing international consultative relationships in nursing. The role and use of consultation internationally has expanded, especially in the areas of midwifery (Vosit-Steller, Morse, & Mitrea, 2011) and palliative care. Vosit-Steller and coworkers (2011) reported that with the support of agencies such as Sigma Theta Tau International and the International Council of Nurses, cross-cultural consultation has grown to provide more advanced nursing care to many rural areas of the world.

International consultation is challenging and rewarding. The creation of sustainable international collaborations that attend to consultation is congruent with the mission and values of nursing and the philosophy of nursing education (Vosit-Steller et al., 2011). Consultative relationships must initially be built on trust and a common mission, with excitement, and a committed relationship. Once rapport and appreciation for cultural differences have been established, effective communication can be

achieved by personal visits, telecommunication, Skype, and written vehicles for collaboration. Consultation is a dynamic process that benefits both parties when they understand one another's need (see Exemplar 9-5). There is a current need to expand consultation in the areas of training resources in primary care and specialty areas, expand education, transforming support in telecommunications and writing for publication (Vosit-Steller et al., 2011).

Mechanisms to Facilitate Consultation

Mechanisms to facilitate consultation need to be considered by all APNs, regardless of setting. As health care becomes more community-focused and APNs provide care to increasingly diverse and vulnerable populations, the breadth and depth of skill required for these newer roles will be considerable. APN-APN consultation is an important means of developing these evolving skills.

EXEMPLAR 9-5 **American Advanced Practice Nurse–Romanian Registered Nurse International Consultation**

Mrs. P is a 60-year-old widow who has lived all of her life in Romania. She is Christian Orthodox, but does not practice her religion. She receives a modest pension from the government, which meets her financial needs. Her past medical history includes cardiovascular disease. Mrs. P was diagnosed with breast cancer this year and was treated surgically. Following her mastectomy, she refused chemotherapy and radiation therapy. Several months after the mastectomy, she presented with metastatic disease and a fungating breast lesion. The major concerns of the Romanian nurses were related to ineffective control of the drainage and foul odor and the patient's perception of her body image. As they changed the patient's dressing at her home, the Romanian nurse described the current approach to Mrs. P's management to the American APN.

The nurse irrigated the area with povidone-iodine (Betadine) and saline and applied wet gauze dressing. Then, petroleum jelly (Vaseline) and crushed metronidazole tablets were applied to reduce odor and prevent infection. Calcium alginate was applied to the edges of the wound to assist with hemostasis.

The APN consultant prepared for the consultation by considering the following questions:

1. How would we manage this type of lesion in the United States?
2. What type of dressings are used in Romania, and why?
3. What solutions are used for irrigating?
4. How can our (U.S.) practice suggestions translate to resources available in Romania, and are there cultural implications?
5. How can nurses communicate with patients with poor body image and compromised sexuality?
6. How do you extend care to family members to inform them about the challenges?

The management issues that were raised for input from the APN consultant included the fact that the wound soaks through the dressing, requiring dressing changes twice daily and resulting in maceration of the wound edges. This then required large amounts of absorbent material and diapers to assist with the drainage. The APN offered the following recommendations considering the materials at hand in Romania:

1. Use gauze made out of a blended material, instead of plain cotton, because it is less likely to stick and may be more absorbent.
2. Consider using K-Y Jelly, because it is water-based, to help prevent the absorbent gauze from sticking to the wound.
3. Replace Vaseline with zinc oxide, if available, around the wound edges, not on the wound.
4. Consider using baking soda between the layers of gauze to assist with odor control.
5. Consider Dakin's solution on the gauze and mix the metronidazole tablets with the zinc oxide to form a paste for protection and to assist with odor control.
6. Use diluted Betadine rinses followed by thorough rinsing of the skin with saline or sterile water.

There was an interactive discussion at the bedside and debriefing following the visit regarding the exploration of which interventions would be useful. The Romanian nurse noted that it is difficult to obtain some of the materials on a consistent basis, such as zinc oxide or alternative dressing materials. Recognizing the limitations in accessing materials for symptom management allowed the consultant to identify areas of creative management, which provided care that was redirected and evidence-based. The eventual outcome was equivalent to using materials that were suggested and available in the United States.

The level of enthusiasm for an integrative consultation program at most institutions is very important. A baseline level of trust and collaborative practice on the part of consultees allows the consultant APN, regardless of specialty, the opportunity to make recommendations with confidence. A setting in which the environment is not open to the consultative use of APN services presents barriers and an unwillingness to use APN expertise. The ground work for implementing an APN consultation program would not be productive prior to laying the foundation of openness and willingness of collaboration.

It is important to consider new settings and potential sources and beneficiaries of advanced practice nursing consultation. APNs from varying specialties can form networks within organizations or geographic locations and identify specific expertise to be shared through consultation among members of the network. APNs in an agency can develop and initiate an explicit process for consultation so that agency staff is clear about how to request an APN consultation and what to expect reasonably from the consultant. When the APN is involved in collaborative relationships, clarification of the possibilities for consultation could be discussed and negotiated to expand APN consultation opportunities. The consultant's services could be made available to interdisciplinary teams in which the APN is a member. Interdisciplinary teams exist in many settings. In addition to working collaboratively on such teams, APNs can offer valuable consultative services. Staff nurses in these settings may be without the benefit of abundant resources to enhance practice and professional development. APNs could offer such opportunities through consultation.

When APNs are the primary providers of care, such as in nursing homes and community health centers, opportunities for consultation may be missed or minimized because the most common interactions are collaborative or comanagerial, or because of time constraints. In these settings, however, the outcome of consultation is often improved patient care. APNs should consider documenting the consultations that they can offer in those settings in somewhat standard and easily retrievable forms, such as computerized databases. If information about these consultations were easier to access, patterns and outcomes of consultation activities would be more apparent and the effectiveness of consultation could be more easily studied.

As APNs move into innovative practices, they should determine which consultative services they will market and which types of APNs and other consultants are available and will be needed. Consultation between APNs offers the additional benefit of collegial networking. APNs are establishing private independent practices that require collaboration and consultation for success. As independent practitioners, they are offering their services in primary care, home health (particularly to assist in the respiratory care of patients who require ventilators), pain clinic, and obstetric care settings. Consultation with other APNs and with other health care professionals in those settings, in addition to the direct care they offer, has the potential to enhance the knowledge and practice of APNs and create comanagement and collaborative possibilities for all the APNs involved.

Issues in Advanced Practice Nurse Consultation

Developing Consultation Skills in Advanced Practice Nurse Students

A variety of advanced skills are central to the development of the APN who begins to consult. Essential core skills of consultation, as identified by Carter and Berlin (2007), are as follows: (1) establishing and maintaining good rapport; (2) structuring the consultation; (3) obtaining and gathering relevant information; (4) prioritizing; (5) using clinical reasoning and judgment; (6) providing information; and (7) developing a management plan. The foundation for the development of these APN consultation skills begins in graduate education.

For APNs to learn the theoretical and practical issues involved in the development of consultative abilities, relevant content must be included in graduate education curricula. Communication and collaboration skills between and within multidisciplinary teams are essential. APNs are expected to influence patients, other providers, and the systems in which they work. Therefore, when APNs graduate, they should be equipped with knowledge, prioritization skills, and confidence in the consultation process. Effective consultation, whether it is sought or provided, enables APNs to establish credibility, build collaborative relationships with other members of the health care team, and influence the processes and outcomes of care. In addition to faculty-initiated experiences with consultation, APN students have much to offer one another as they move through master's and DNP programs. Consulting with peers on challenging clinical issues can offer students experience with the consultation process and help them begin to think of themselves as consultants as their APN role identity is being formed (Goodman, 2012; Morgan, 2007).

Parkin and associates (2006) have examined whether professional-centered consultation training improves outcomes. During the training, each professional was able to identify strengths and areas of their consultation that they thought needed further development. The researchers concluded that when integrated into the curriculum, professional-centered training can be effective in improving the patients' perceptions of the consultation and the students' self-reflection of decision making (Parkin, Barnard, Cradock, et al., 2006).

A similar model of team-based reflection directed at improving consultation was developed by Hirschland (2011). Challenging pediatric cases were brought to staff that helped develop an inclusive and empowering vision of practice and development of new skill to follow through with the consultation (Hirschland, 2011). Reflective practice at all levels improved outcomes for the students and helped nurses form more caring relationships with the children. Reflecting on practice is an important skill and attitude to cultivate in APN students. This reflection on consultation activities can help students begin to understand the depth and breadth of APN consultation over time. Kim (2008) has suggested that research questions could emerge from an analysis of one's own reflections on consultations. In an analysis of her own practice, she believed that clinical judgment skills could be analyzed and reviewed. Encouraging the process of reflection on practice, with a focus on outcomes of care, can help build important practice habits, with benefits beyond the acquisition of consultation skills (Kim, 2008).

Graduate educators and APN students could collaborate on much-needed research to evaluate the effects of consultative activities on patient outcomes. Research related to consultation could serve as an ideal focus for scholarly capstone projects in DNP programs. Learning how to evaluate and consider the implications related to the outcomes of care is of considerable value to students. Documentation of the value and cost-effectiveness of consultation could help inform curricular decisions as the findings of the IOM report are implemented (IOM, 2011). Findings could also be presented by APN educators and students to insurers and policymakers who determine policy and payment for health care services.

Using Technology to Provide Consultation

The use of new technologies to enhance care delivery has affected every aspect of the health care delivery system. APNs should review how consultation activities delivered through these new modalities can enhance the capacity to effect care. Equally important is thoughtful consideration of the potential concerns that might arise in embracing these mechanisms to enhance patient care through consultation. Clarity about the definition of telehealth activities and understanding current legal and ethical issues related to access, privacy, confidentiality, security, jurisdiction, and licensure standards are essential for APNs.

There have been several programs implemented using APN consultation and telehealth. Miller and coworkers (2008) assessed consults completed in the emergency room (ER) by ANPs over a 1-year period. The ANPs tended to minor injuries with the assistance of a telemedicine network, if necessary. Of these consults, 60% were found to be appropriate for APNs (Miller, Alam, Fraser, et al., 2008). This figure increased to 84% if children younger than 14 years and those with shoulder injuries were excluded.

A team of clinical nurse specialists has been gathering clinical data from the electronic health record (EHR) about falls, delirium, and the use of restraints prior to consultation with geriatric patients (Purvis & Brenny-Fitzpatrick, 2010). They are using these computer-generated, high-risk indicators to facilitate nursing practice guidelines, nursing plans of care, and real-time indicators prior to consultation (Purvis & Brenny-Fitzpatrick, 2010).

Consultation is not limited to the physical setting. Some of the care provided by APNs in retail clinics, minor emergency areas, and rural health clinics can be carried out within the digital arena (Lee, 2011). APNs have branched out beyond triaging patients in call centers. In a California study, nurses used two-way audio and visual systems to collect and transmit vital signs and provided "palliative care, rehabilitation, and chronic disease management" to patients suffering from HIV/AIDS (Lee, 2011). During a 4-month period, telehealth monitors were placed in patients' homes and, at the end of the trial, patients reported being satisfied with their care.

Privacy, security, and access to telehealth are additional ongoing concerns. Documentation parameters for security and privacy go beyond the patient, caregivers, and third-party payers; the need for security related to the online sharing of private medical information deserves special attention. Ohler & Daine (2001) have considered risks related to the security of health-related e-mail communication following consultation. Providing information through e-mail and telecommunication across state lines raised concerns about liability and differences in state nurse practice acts regarding scope of practice. They suggested that documentation guidelines and protocols be established for the application of any telecommunication and recommended further research on confidentiality and security issues in telehealth practice.

Reimbursement for telehealth and telehealth consultation remains unclear (Koeniger-Donohue, 2012). The Patient Protection and Affordable Care Act (PPACA; Public Law 111–148), signed into law on March 23, 2010, addresses the use of telehealth as a means of delivering efficient and effective health care in the United States (Lee & Harada, 2012). This national health care reform presents a unique opportunity for clinicians and therapists to become identified as eligible to provide telehealth consultation services. However, several barriers need to be overcome if telehealth will become mainstream as a means of health care delivery. More detailed information regarding the American Telemedicine Association may be obtained online (http://www.telmedinsurance.com/news.html). Solomons (2006) discussed the need for the teleconsultation to be part of the physician's prescribed plan of care in order for Medicare to reimburse for services. Medicaid reimbursement, although funded through federal grants, allows for more discretion at the state level in relation to payment for services, occurring mostly in rural areas with dire need for services. Solomons (2006) noted that 26 states have initiatives related to payment for telehealth services. However, covered services and rates of payment continue to vary greatly from state to state.

APNs are currently leaders in telenursing practice and should be aware of important policy issues to advance the use of telehealth further (Schlachta-Fairchild, Varghese, Deickman, et al., 2010), including consultation. Issues such as technology selection and implementation principles, interstate licensure, malpractice, and telehealth reimbursement are important to advancing telenursing further. In addition, evidence-based strategies for demonstrating caring using technology in patient interactions are key for advancing telenursing in APN practice. Finally, APNs should be aware of how telenursing can affect the nursing shortage in the United States, providing access to care irrespective of geographic location of provider and patients (Schlachta-Fairchild et al., 2010).

Teleconferencing has been used successfully in consultation, medical education, supervision, and simulation. It has been used in transcultural consultation on palliative care between APNs in an established collaborative relationship in Brasov, Romania, the University of Rhode Island, and Simmons College (Gerzevitz, Ferszt, Vosit-Steller, et al., 2009). Once collegial and trusting relationships were established, teleconferencing was used among the three sites to consult on difficult cases from the hospice in Romania. Electronic communication presented the opportunity to advance practice methods and provide validation for nursing actions (Gerzevitz et al., 2009).

In a similar manner, midwestern Veterans Affairs Medical Centers (VAMCs) have created a link by teleconference and an electronic medical record. The collective Bariatric Surgery Department's conducted the initial consultations for patients who resided distances more than 300 miles away by this system (Sudan, Salter, Lynch, et al., 2011). The satisfaction rate for patients who used the system was 82%; the rate of surgical outcomes and satisfaction was 96.6% (Sudan et al., 2011).

The application of technology in delivering health-related information continues to be studied in terms of process and outcomes. APNs should consider the potential opportunities that exist to enhance consultation activities with these modalities, but should exercise caution regarding their implementation until legislative and policy initiatives related to access, security and mutual recognition of APN practice across state lines are more fully developed, and future research elucidates specific processes, outcomes, and concerns related to telehealth strategies and practices.

Documentation and Legal Considerations

Although it has been stressed that the consultee remains clinically responsible for the patient who is the focus of the consultation, it is critical to appreciate that APN consultants are accountable for their practices relative to the consultation problem. Nurse attorney Kim Larkin (2003, 2007, 2012) has emphasized to APNs that once a consultant-consultee relationship has been established, scope of practice is implied and responsibility is assumed. This is initiated once the patient has been seen, recommendations have been rendered, and documentation has been entered into the patient chart (Larkin, 2003, 2007, 2012). The duty of care and the legal responsibility to

follow up on the consultation is of principal importance. The initial consultation should end with a summary communication to the consultee. This communication should ideally echo the documented recommendations, but should be presented in person to the consultee or by telecommunication. Whether the consultee adopts the recommendations is entirely optional, according to professional skill and standard in the specialty.

APN consultation is influenced by factors such as professional standards of practice within the specialty, state and certification regulations, nurse practice acts, and institutional and group policies (Christensen, 2009). If malpractice were to be questioned involving consultation, it would be these specific documents and regulations that would be used to determine duty of care, standard of care, and/or damages, and with which type of provider the consultation is most appropriate.

Inherent in the consultation process is the ability to communicate effectively, but little emphasis is placed on written communication through consultation notes. The art of writing a consultation note is learned primarily through trial and error or through mentorship with a senior practitioner (Stichler, 2002). Documentation is the best defense for the APN consultant, whether the patient is seen or not. If the consultation is on the telephone, sidebar questions have been answered, or medical information interpreted about a patient, an event note should be entered into the chart. Larkin (2003, 2007, 2012) has stressed the importance of establishing a formal consultation relationship. The EHR has shifted legal trends to a more formal level. Legal action has been taken against APNs and APN consultants for informal consultation and the establishment of a relationship between the consultant and patient has been carefully examined (Larkin, 2012). The current trend for APN consultation is more formal than informal. This is likely because of the electronic medical record and increasingly complex billing for specialty consultative services (Burroughs, Dmytrow, & Lewis, 2007).

As the role of APN consultant has expanded, it brings with it greater risk of professional liability in a litigious society. It is advisable that APNs be aware of their malpractice coverage and, if employed in a high-risk area, be aware of the elements that constitute malpractice and plan for the management of risks involved. Nurse practitioners often work with other health care professionals in collaborative settings. The laws governing the degree of supervision and protocol vary by state. These agreements address the level of physician oversight and consultation allowed independently by the APN. In the most constructive settings, collaborative practice results in optimal patient care. Collaborative practice may create a lack of cooperation among physicians, nurse practitioners, health care entities, and pharmacies in the course of defending themselves against allegations of malpractice. These consultative situations raise complex issues in the event of a professional liability claim. For example, the ability to release and review patient health information records on a timely basis may be jeopardized (Burroughs et al., 2007). In addition, evidence to substantiate claims regarding prescribing practices may be difficult to obtain. Because the APN has the ability to examine, diagnose, and establish treatment plans for patients, friction may develop among the various health care professionals. Should these professionals become codefendants in professional liability litigation, an adversarial situation may result. In some jurisdictions, physicians may carry lower limits of professional liability coverage than a nurse practitioner. In such cases, the nurse practitioner may become the focus of the defendant's claim in an effort to collect from the nurse practitioner's additional liability insurance coverage (Burroughs et al., 2007).

Some APNs prefer to purchase additional liability insurance. When obtaining insurance, the APN consultant must consider the following: the practice setting; types of policies; components of the policy; costs; and the means to obtain adequate coverage (Scott & Beare, 1993). The best protection during a consultation includes good client communication and individualized client contracts. A well-written contract serves as a legal document to delineate responsibilities and outcomes, provide a professional image, and protect against possible negative developments.

Discontinuing the Consultation Process

There are circumstances in which an APN has initiated the consultative process and recognition of safety or necessity warrants the closure of a consult. If the APN has become aware that she or he or the patient is in a dangerous situation, and the consultee is not willing to intervene, the consultant would need to assume responsibility for ensuring safety needs and step out of the consultation role (Barron, 1983, 1989). Such a situation is described in Exemplar 9-6.

Developing the Practice of Other Nurses

Consultation can clearly enhance the clinical knowledge and practice of nurses requesting consultation. An outcome of APN consultation, especially over time, is to enhance the professional development and practice of nurse consultees (Barron & White, 2009). One of the most rewarding aspects of the consultative process is to observe the growth in consultees and the mastering of new skills (Stichler, 2002). The increasing number of DNPs in practice has significantly supported the confidence of engaging and effective consultation as a critical part of practice (Christensen, 2009).

 EXEMPLAR 9-6   **Transition from Consultation to Ongoing Collaboration**

Vosit-Steller, an oncology NP, was consulted by the hospitalist team for a palliative care consult regarding pain control for a 58-year-old man with a past medical history of rheumatoid arthritis (RA), anemia, vertebral compression fractures and recent biopsies of his right great toe being positive for methicillin-resistant *Staphylococcus aureus* (MRSA). He was having pain control issues, had developed hallucinations during the night shift, and staff were not sure that his pain medication was dosed appropriately. The patient was taking Oxycontin, 40 mg three times daily, and oxycodone, 20 mg every 6 hours, as needed. He regularly took the break-through medication. Prior to the admission for the biopsy, he was to begin Rituximab every 6 months for treatment for his RA.

On meeting the patient and his wife, he was not oriented to time or place. His wife described a pattern of increased delusions and hallucinations as the long-term and short-term opioids peaked at home. She also mentioned that last night, he struck one of the nursing assistants who was watching him. On examination, his midback was tender bilaterally and his right great toe, although bandaged, was very tender to touch. After assessment, the NP recommended to taper the Oxycontin by 10 mg in 3-day intervals to decrease delirium, evaluating the patient's pain response. After one cycle, the patient's pain was well controlled, yet he continued to display combative and delusional behavior—pulling his Foley catheter out and striking the staff. At this point, the palliative consultant remained involved to evaluate effectiveness of the taper of the pain medication to a reasonable dose for the patient's condition. A psychiatry consult was requested to evaluate the delusions and combative behavior. The APN consultation documentation was finalized, but she would remain available to the patient and family if future symptom management issues became problematic.

Christensen (2009) has emphasized the importance of self-evaluation following consultation. The approach and process of APN consultation largely follows a medical model, focused on symptoms, at times excluding the fact that nurses possess the best traits of empathy, compassion, and holism. As consultants, APNs are in a position to use the reflection skills they develop as graduate students and contribute to the consultation as a whole, being mindful of identifying the awareness of a therapeutic interpersonal relationship with patients. This process can enhance the learning of the consultee and the consultant, contributing in a meaningful way to the process (Barron & White, 2009). It is through critical reflection of the consultative process that nursing practice is advanced. The reflective nature of this element of advanced practice work promotes the development of future APNs (Christensen, 2009).

Consultation Practice Over Time

APNs whose practices involve substantial consultation can make observations over time about the evolution and extent of their consultations. Initially, the demonstration of expertise and marketing skills (see Chapter 20) are necessary to earn the interest and trust of potential consultees. As the number of consults increases and relationships develop across disciplines, communication systems should be developed to prioritize and triage consults. This is a wonderful entrepreneurial opportunity for APNs across systems and subspecialties. A sustainable relationship based on clinical and personal trust is the catalyst for an ongoing consultant-consultee relationship (Memmott, Coverston, Heise, et al., 2010).

There are several examples of how an experienced consultant can develop relationships with other APNs and expand his or her practice. For example, partnerships for consultation could include areas such as oncology, palliative and hospice care, acute care, emergency room care, midwifery, holistic health, incontinence care, and adolescent health. Development of an in-hospital or continuing education unit (CEU) educational program promoting progressive practice techniques that can be translated into primary care, as well as specialty practice, are common requests for APN consultation; examples include review of the care of patients with renal disease, diabetes, or multiple comorbidities and cancer care. In addition, written materials, such as practice guidelines, protocols, personal digital assistant (PDA) applications for the bedside or office, and smartphone applications are being advocated in areas such as cardiology, oncology, palliative care, obstetrics, dermatology, and psychiatry.

Over time, staff and colleagues will recognize the APN's skill and the APN may need to develop strategies to deal with large numbers of requests. Setting priorities and identifying alternative resources when the consultant's caseload is full are important activities as the consultation practice becomes more recognized and valued. Identifying other APNs who can consult on similar issues may be a useful strategy for balancing requests with availability.

Clarifying the availability and timing of responses to requests is essential if consultees are to continue to consider consultation as a helpful and timely option for assistance with complex clinical situations. Negotiating directly with the consultee at the time of the request (or shortly thereafter) allows the consultant to express to the consultee the importance and worth of the request, even if the consultant cannot meet the need directly. It also provides the opportunity to consider appropriate alternative resources to assist the consultee in addressing the clinical problem. The consultant must have established back-up resources who are available to handle emergencies when the consultant is not available. Establishing such resources at the beginning of the consultant's practice is essential. Consultees should always know whom to contact in the event of a clinical emergency.

Over time, the number of consultee-centered requests may increase. After the consultee establishes trust with the consultant, the consultee may feel more comfortable and able to focus on specific problems in the clinical situation. After a while, the consultee may be willing to examine lack of understanding, skill, or objectivity. Ensured professional development can result from that level of self-examination, but trust usually needs to be developed firmly before such self-examination can take place with the consultant.

The consultant may find that the consultees' requests become more sophisticated over time. The consultee who initially requested basic assistance with care may develop skill, understanding, and confidence with basic issues so that future requests for consultation reflect more expert levels of concern and understanding. These requests may involve more complex or unusual situations and can be catalysts for the consultant's ongoing professional growth. Experiencing the development of the consultee's professional practice is exciting and satisfying.

Conversely, boredom with requests may be an issue for the established consultant. Especially in settings in which turnover of staff is high, the consultant may focus repeatedly on the same clinical concerns. Seeking support from a trusted colleague may help the consultant cope with frustration and avoid communicating frustration to consultees inappropriately. Communicating a lack of interest with concerns presented by consultees is a sure way to derail the specific consultation and the use of consultation as a means to address clinical problems. The consultant may also consider developing an educational program to address, in a different way, the needs commonly being expressed in consultation requests. If the problem is common, the consultant may also want to develop written guidelines, protocols, or care plans to share with consultees.

Recently, there has been a strong emphasis on interdisciplinary consultation. This refers to several intraprofessionals consulting on a case simultaneously. It could involve an 82-year-old patient who is having acute or chronic abdominal pain, with a 10-pound weight loss over the past month. The multidisciplinary consulting team may consist of a geriatrician, palliative care consultant, nutritionist, gastroenterologist, speech pathologist (speech and swallow testing), and oncologist. For a child with asthma, it could also involve communication among the parents, primary care NP, pulmonologist, respiratory therapist, and school nurse to provide care together for the child. The coordination of all the consultations would be monitored and coordinated by the consultee.

Billing for Consultation

Payment for consultation services is improving in some APN roles, but APNs need a clear understanding of the requirements for payment. The types of APNs who are consulting in hospital settings are increasing. Traditionally, the CNS, CNM, and CRNA were not only consulted, but were considered collaborative essential team members in the specialty units in which they were employed. However, these APNs did not bill or were not reimbursed for their services (Buppert, 2012). In 2005, the Centers for Medicare and Medicaid Services decided that the shared visit rules for billing do not apply to consultation (Buppert, 2012). Specifically, consultations cannot be billed "incident to." There are, however, specific CMS criteria that must be met for APNs to bill individually for consultation (Box 9-1).

The reason for requesting a consultation may be to obtain a physician's or qualified APN's advice, opinion, recommendation, suggestion, direction, or counsel in evaluating or treating a patient because the individual has expertise in a specific medical area beyond that of the requesting professional's. Consultations may be billed based on time if the counseling and coordination of care constitute more than 50% of the face-to-face encounter between the physician or qualified APN and the patient. The preceding requirements (request, evaluation or counseling and coordination, and written report) shall also be met when the consultation is based on time for counseling and coordination (Buppert, 2012).

When billing a consultation, one must select the current procedural terminology (CPT) code that

---

BOX 9-1 CMS Criteria to Bill for Consultation

1. Specifically, a consultation service is distinguished from other evaluation and management (E/M) visits because it is provided by a physician or qualified nonphysician practitioner (NPP) whose opinion or advice regarding evaluation and/or management of a specific problem is requested by another physician or other appropriate source.

2. The qualified APN may perform consultation services within the scope of practice and licensure requirements for APNs in the state in which he or she practices. Applicable collaboration and general supervision rules (by state) apply as well as billing rules.

3. A request for a consultation from an appropriate source and the need for consultation (i.e., the reason for a consultation service) shall be documented by the consultant in the patient's medical record and included in the requesting physician or qualified APN's plan of care in the patient's medical record.

4. After the consultation is provided, the consultant shall prepare a written report of her or his findings and recommendations, which shall be provided to the referring physician. There are five levels of CPT code for consultations.

Adapted from Buppert, C. (2012). Update on consultation billing: Legal limits. *Journal for Nurse Practitioners, 5,* 730–732. doi: 10.1016/j.nurpra.2009.09.007; and Burroughs, R., Dmytrow, B., & Lewis, H. (2007). Trends in nurse practitioner professional liability: An analysis of claims with risk management recommendations. *Journal of Nursing Law, 11,* 53–60.

---

is supported by documentation under Medicare's documentation guidelines. The following are two resources for the documentation requirements:

- Medicare's Documentation Guidelines for Evaluation and Management (E/M) http://www.cms.gov/Outreach-and-Education/Medicare-Learning-Network-MLN/MLNProducts/downloads/eval_mgmt_serv_guide-ICN006764.pdf
- Medicare administrative contractors have published their audit score sheets for E/M on their websites.

It is best to check the website of your local contractor or agency billing representative.

Evaluation of the Consultation Competency

Evaluation of the APNs competency to complete a consultation successfully is determined by the overall effectiveness of the consultation. Feedback from supervisors, collaborators, peers, administrators, self-evaluation, review of documentation of the consults, and annual evaluation all reflect APN competency for consultation. Individual self-evaluation is the final step in the consultation process. It allows the practitioner review of performance and realistic development of goals for future consultative role performance. APNs should consider strategies that will help them determine their overall effectiveness and their specific effectiveness in relation to consultation.

Guidelines in areas of specialty will dictate the practices of individual APNs and will vary considerably about which questions and criteria are considered relevant to the evaluation of consultation skills. (See Chapter 24 for a comprehensive discussion of evaluation of advanced practice nursing.) The following questions will need to be addressed:

- Are the consultant recommendations appropriate for the patient situation and result in improved patient outcomes?
- Is the consultant recontacted after the initial consultation?
- Are consultation requests becoming more sophisticated over time?
- Was the APN able to respond to all requests for consultation?
- Do glaring issues or needs seem to be going unaddressed?
- Do there seem to be patterns in terms of the theme, number, or location of consultations?
- Are there delays in doing consultation triage?

Productivity is now being measured as a benchmark in any performance review. APN roles differ in consultation, so the consultation evaluation or competency will have various levels of success, depending on the setting, level of collaboration and/or autonomy.

Clinical competency, competency in applying the consultation process, interpersonal skills, improved patient outcomes, and professionalism are all areas to be considered in the evaluation process. Identifying the appropriate people to be involved in the evaluation and developing a systematic approach to data collection regarding the consultation aspects of an APN's practice are important. Evaluation can guide the APN's individual professional growth and ultimately validate the need for the APN's service and skills in the specific work setting, and beyond.

Conclusion

APNs have had a long tradition of being involved in various aspects of direct and indirect patient care activities, including consultation. Consultation has the potential to improve care processes and patient outcomes. It can be exciting, invigorating, and challenging and can bring satisfaction to APNs as they experience personal growth and development through consultative practice. The power of consultative activities to inform and advance practice compels all APNs to consider consultation as an integral aspect of role performance. Consultation offers APNs the opportunity to share and acquire the clinical expertise necessary to meet the increasingly challenging and diverse demands of patient care.

This chapter has defined consultation, identified various types of consultation, and distinguished consultation from comanagement and referral. An ecologic model of the APN consultation competency was presented and issues related to implementation of the consultative process have been highlighted. It remains imperative that the term *consultation* be used appropriately and that APNs participate in defining this competency further and understanding its impact on care processes and patient outcomes. The concept of consultation has been clarified because conceptual clarity will enhance its appropriate use in practice and in the literature.

APN consultation contributes to positive patient outcomes and may promote more appropriate use of scarce health care resources in today's global health market. These assumptions must be tested through quality improvement studies, cost-benefit studies, and research that examines the processes and outcomes of care. Outcomes of consultation activities can then be effectively measured. Ongoing discussion regarding this important topic will assist in the much-needed clarification of the other terms used to characterize relationships with other professionals. APNs can contribute to this discussion, and to research, by sharing their experiences as recipients and providers of consultation. Consultation can facilitate comprehensive and specialty-related knowledge available to all patients in a more efficient manner, and therefore should be an expected and integral aspect of APN role performance. The opportunities to develop and the ability to consult successfully continue to grow as the health care industry evolves and requires highly experienced professionals to assist colleagues and advance patients in quality of life.

Acknowledgment

We wish to acknowledge Anne-Marie Barron and Patricia A. White for their exceptional authorship of this chapter in all previous editions.

References

American Association of Colleges of Nursing (AACN). (2006). Essentials of doctoral education for advanced nursing practice (www.aacn.nche.edu/publications/position/DNPEssentials.pdf).

American Association of Colleges of Nursing (AACN). (2011). Essentials of Master's Education in Nursing (www.aacn.nche.edu/education-resources/MastersEssentials11.pdf).

American Association of Nurse Anesthetists. (2005). Guidelines for core clinical privileges: Certified registered nurse anesthetist (http://www.canainc.org/compendium/pdfs/H%203%20core_clinical_privileges.pdf).

American College of Nurse Midwives. (2011). Position statement. Standards for the practice of midwifery (www.midwife.org/ACNM/files/ACNMLibraryData/UPLOADFILENAME/0000000000/Standards_for_Practice_of_Midwifery_Sept_2011.pdf).

American College of Nurse Midwives. (2012). Core competencies for basic midwifery practice (www.midwife.org/ACNM/files/ACNMLibraryData/UPLOADFILENAME/000000000050/Core%20Competencies%20June%202012.pdf).

Barron, A. M. (1983). The clinical nurse specialist as consultant. In A. B. Hamric & J. A. Spross (Eds.), The clinical nurse specialist in theory and practice (pp. 91–113). New York: Grune & Stratton.

Barron, A. M. (1989). The clinical nurse specialist as consultant. In A. B. Hamric & J. A. Spross (Eds.), The clinical nurse specialist in theory and practice (2nd ed., pp. 125–146). Philadelphia: WB Saunders.

Barron, A. M., & White, P. (1996). Consultation. In A. B. Hamric, J. A. Spross, & C. M. Hanson (Eds.), Advanced nursing practice: An integrative approach (pp. 165–183). Philadelphia: WB Saunders.

Barron, A. M., & White, P. (2009). Consultation. In A. B. Hamric, J. A. Spross, & C. M. Hanson (Eds.), Advanced practice nursing: An integrative approach (3rd ed., pp. 191–216). Philadelphia: WB Saunders.

Benson, L., Mitchell, C., Linke, M., Carlson, G., & Fisher, J. (2008). Using an advanced practice nursing model for a rapid response team. Joint Commission Journal on Quality and Patient Safety, 34, 743–747.

Buppert, C. (2012). Update on consultation billing: Legal limits. Journal for Nurse Practitioners, 5, 730–732. doi: 10.1016/j.nurpra.2009.09.007

Burroughs, R., Dmytrow, B., & Lewis, H. (2007). Trends in nurse practitioner professional liability: An analysis of claims with risk management recommendations. Journal of Nursing Law, 11, 53–60.

Caplan, G. (1970). The theory and practice of mental health consultation. New York: Basic Books.

Caplan, G., & Caplan, R. (1993). Mental health consultation and collaboration. San Francisco: Jossey-Bass.

Carter, F., & Berlin, A. (2007). Using the clinical consultation as a learning opportunity (www.faculty.londondeanery.ac.uk/e-learning/feedback/files/Using_the_clinical_consultation_as_a_learning_opportunity.pdf).

Christensen, M. (2009). The consultative process used in outreach: A narrative account. Nursing in Critical Care, 14, 17–25. doi: 10.1111/j.1478-5153.2008.00310.x

Dias, M. H., Chambers-Evans, J. & Reidy, M. (2010). The consultation component of the clinical nurse specialist role. Canadian Journal of Nursing Research, 42, 92–104.

Dryer, L. A. (2006). Interventional radiology: New roles for nurse practitioners. Nephrology Nursing Journal, 33, 565–570, 592.

Gerzevitz, D., Ferszt, G. G., Vosit-Steller, J., & Mitrea, N. (2009). Cross-cultural consultation on palliative care: The use of teleconferencing. Journal of Hospice & Palliative Nursing, 11, 239–244.

Goodman, J. H., Reidy, P., & Cartier, J. (2012). Role preparation for advanced practice nursing: Practicing consultation and collaboration. Journal of Nursing Education, 51, 59–60.

Hamric, A. B., Spross, J. A., & Hanson, C. M. (2009). Advanced nursing practice: An integrative approach (4th ed.). St. Louis: Saunders.

Hanson, C. M., & Spross, J. A. (1996). Collaboration. In A. B. Hamric, J. A. Spross, & C. M. Hanson (Eds.), Advanced practice nursing: An integrative approach (pp. 229–248). Philadelphia: WB Saunders.

Hirschland, D. (2011). Training, consultation, and mentoring: Supporting effective responses to challenging behavior in early care and education settings. Zero to Three, 32, 18–24.

Institute of Medicine. (IOM). (2011). The future of nursing: Leading change, advancing health. Washington DC: National Academies Press.

Kim, D. D. (2008). Critical reflective inquiry as a tool to improve critical care nursing practice. CONNECT: The World of Critical Care Nursing, 6, 6.

Koeniger-Donohue, R. (2012). Personal communication.

Larkin, K. (2003, 2007, 2012). Personal communications.

LeBuhn, R., & Swankia, D. A. (2010). Reforming scopes of practice—a white paper (www.ncsbn.org/ReformingScopesofPractice-WhitePaper.pdf).

Lee, A. C. W., & Harada, N. (2012). Telehealth as a means of health care delivery for physical therapist practice. Physical Therapy, 92, 463–468. doi: 10.2522/ptj.20110100

Lee, S. (2011). In support of the abolishment of supervisory and collaboration clauses. Journal for Nurse Practitioners, 7, 764–769. doi: 10.1016/j.nurpra.2011.07.011

Lewandowski, W., & Adamle, K. (2009). Substantive areas of clinical nurse specialist practice: A comprehensive review of the literature. Clinical Nurse Specialist, 23, 73–90.

Lipowski, Z. J. (1974). Consultation-liaison psychiatry: An overview. American Journal of Psychiatry, 131, 623–630.

Lipowski, Z. J. (1981). Liaison psychiatry, liaison nursing and behavioral medicine. Comprehensive Psychiatry, 22, 554–561.

Lipowski, Z. J. (1983). Current trends in consultation-liaison psychiatry. Canadian Journal of Psychiatry, 28, 329–338.

Memmott, R. J., Coverston, C. R., Heise, B. A., Williams, M., Maughan, E. D., Kohl, J., et al. (2010). Practical considerations in establishing sustainable international nursing experiences. Nursing Education Perspectives, 31, 298–302.

Miller, D. R., Alam, K., Fraser, S., & Ferguson, J. (2008). The delivery of a minor injuries telemedicine service by emergency nurse practitioners. *Journal of Telemedicine and Telecare, 14,* 143–144.

Minarik, P., & Price, L. (1999). Collaboration? Supervision? Direction? Independence? What is the relationship between the advanced practice nurse and the physician? States legislative and regulatory reform III. *Clinical Nurse Specialist, 13,* 34–37.

Morgan, P., Fogel, J., Hicks, P., Wright, L., & Tyler, I. (2007). Strategic enhancement of nursing students information literacy skills: Interdisciplinary perspectives. *ABNF Journal, 18*(2), 40–45.

National CNS Task Force. (2010). Clinical nurse specialist core competencies 2006-2008. Executive summary (www.aacn.org/WD/Certifications/Docs/corecnscompetencies-exec-summ.pdf).

National Association of Clinical Nurse Specialists. (2004). *Statement on clinical nurse specialist education and practice* (2nd ed.). Harrisburg, PA: Author.

National Organization of Nurse Practitioner Faculty. (2011). Nurse practitioner core competencies (www.nonpf.com/associations/10789/files/IntegratedNPCoreComps FINALApril2011.pdf).

Ohler, L., & Daine, V. (2001). Potential telecommunication risks: Cautions and suggestions for the team. *Progress in Cardiovascular Nursing, 16,* 172–176.

Parkin, T., Barnard, K., Cradock, S., Pettman, P., & Skinner, T. C. (2006). Does professional-centred training improve consultation outcomes? *Practical Diabetes International, 23,* 253–256.

Perry, G. (2011). Conducting a nurse consultation. *British Journal of Cardiovascular Nursing, 6,* 433–438.

Purvis, S., & Brenny-Fitzpatrick, M. (2010). Innovative use of electronic health record reports by clinical nurse specialists. *Clinical Nurse Specialist: The Journal for Advanced Nursing Practice, 24,* 289–294. doi: 10.1097/NUR.0b013e3181f8724c

Scott, L., & Beare, P. (1993). Nurse consultant and professional liability. *Clinical Nurse Specialist, 7,* 331–334.

Schlachta-Fairchild, L., Varghese, S. B., Deickman, A., & Castelli, D. (2010). Telehealth and telenursing are live: APN policy and practice implications. *Journal for Nurse Practitioners, 6,* 98–106. doi: 10.1016/j.nurpa.2009.12.019

Solomons, N. (2006). *Are home health agencies using telehealth and states with telehealth initiatives the little engine that could save Medicare?* Unpublished manuscript, Portland, ME: University of Southern Maine.

Skinner, J. P., & Foureur, M. (2010). Consultation, referral, and collaboration between midwives and obstetricians: Lessons from New Zealand. *Journal of Midwifery & Women's Health, 55,* 28–37. doi: 10.1016/j.jmwh.2009.03.015

Stichler, J. (2002). The nurse as consultant. *Nursing Administration Quarterly, 26,* 52–68.

Sudan, R., Salter, M., Lynch, T., & Jacobs, D. O. (2011). Bariatric surgery using a network and teleconferencing to serve remote patients in the Veterans Administration Health Care System: Feasibility and results. *American Journal of Surgery, 202,* 71–76.

Vosit-Steller, J., Morse, A. B., & Mitrea, N. (2011). Evolution of an international collaboration: A unique experience across borders. *Clinical Journal of Oncology Nursing, 15,* 564–566. doi: 10.1188/11.CJON.564-566

Vosit-Steller, J. (2012). Personal communication.

Wand, T., & Fisher, J. (2006). The mental health nurse practitioner in the emergency department: An Australian experience. *International Journal of Mental Health Nursing, 15,* 201–208.

Van Der Watt, G. (2010). Consultation-liaison nursing: A personal reflection. *Contemporary Nursing, 34,* 167–176.

Xu, X., Lori, J. R., Siefert, K. A., Jacobson, P. D., Ransom, S. B. (2008). Malpractice liability burden in midwifery: A survey of Michigan certified Nurse-Midwives. *Journal of Midwifery & Women's Health, 53,* 19–27.

Evidence-Based Practice

Mikel Gray

CHAPTER CONTENTS

Evidence-based practice (EBP) is defined as the conscientious, explicit, and judicious use of current best research-based evidence when making decisions about the care of individual patients (Sackett et al., 1996). It has evolved into a dominant approach for clinical decision making and a core competency for advanced practice nursing (see Chapter 3). Although components tend to overlap, three levels of this core competency can be identified: (1) interpretation and use of EBP principles in individual clinical decision making; (2) interpretation and use of EBP principles to determine policies for patient care; and (3) use of EBP to evaluate clinical practice.

Evidence-based practice is based on a four-step process: (1) formulation of a clinical question; (2) identification and retrieval of pertinent research findings based on literature review; (3) extraction and critical appraisal of data from pertinent studies; and (4) clinical decision making based on results of this process. Principles of EBP are used for clinical decision making for individual patients, constructing and applying clinical practice guidelines, and determining policies for delivering care to large groups (Gerrish et al., 2011; Stiffler & Cullen, 2010). Despite widespread acceptance of the concept of EBP, clinician understanding of this process and its application to direct patient care remains limited. For example, a cross-sectional analysis of 37 primary care practices revealed that when caring for patients with heart failure, 87% and 62% appropriately prescribed an angiotensin-converting enzyme inhibitor or beta blocker, respectively, but only 16% and 8% reached the target dose recommended by the clinical practice guideline for managing this condition (Peters-Klimm et al., 2008). Similarly, a cross-sectional survey of 720 primary care physicians revealed that only 26.9% and 4.3% adhered fully to evidence-based guidelines for managing acute lower back pain with and without sciatica (Webster et al., 2005). A number of factors are thought to influence clinician acceptance and application of this problem-solving approach to direct patient care, including a lack of knowledge of the principles of EBP. This chapter will define EBP, differentiate it from concepts of research and quality improvement, and define three levels of advanced practice nurse competency related to EBP: (1) use of evidence in individual APN practice; (2) use of evidence to change practice; and (3) use of evidence to evaluate practice (Table 10-1). Exemplars 10-1, 10-2, and 10-3 provide examples of each of these EBP-related competencies.

The term *evidence-based practice* represents a blending of several related concepts, including evidence-based nursing and evidence-based medicine. The original term, *evidence-based medicine,* traces its historical roots to a strategy for educating medical students developed by the faculty at McMaster Medical School in Hamilton, Ontario (Rosenberg & Donald, 1995). Evidence-based nursing is defined as the process that nurses use to make clinical decisions using the best available research evidence, their clinical expertise, and patient preferences (Dicenso, Cullum, & Ciliska, 2002). The explicit inclusion of patient

TABLE 10-1   Overview of Evidence-Based Practice Competencies and Levels

Competency	Fundamental Level	Expanded Level
I: Interpretation and use of research and other evidence in clinical decision making	Incorporate evidence-based practice (EBP) principles and processes into individual practice.	Incorporate EBP practices and principles on a unit, clinic, department, facility, health care system, national, or international level; function as member of an expert panel on a facility, health care system, national, or global level to create clinical practice guidelines of best practice statements.
II: Changing practice	Incorporate best practice changes according to EBP principles into own practice.	Design and implement a process for changing practice beyond the scope of individual practice on a unit, clinic, facility, health care system, or national basis.
III: Evaluation of practice	Identify benchmarks for evaluating own practice.	Design and implement a process to evaluate pertinent outcomes of practice beyond the scope of individual practice (e.g., generic nursing practice, group APN practice, interdisciplinary team practice, facility-wide or health care system–wide practice).

EXEMPLAR 10-1   Level I: Interpretation and Use of Evidence-Based Practice in Individual Clinical Decision Making

The most basic level of EBP competency is the application of the four steps for clinical decision making in an individual patient. This proficiency requires more than formulation of a clinical question and identification of pertinent studies needed to determine best available evidence. The advanced practice nurse (APN) must combine knowledge of best evidence with an assessment of individual patient factors likely to affect treatment effects, such as the presence of comorbid conditions, psychosocial and cultural factors such as locus of control, preference and impact on quality of life, and cost considerations.

Example: As an APN in a urology department, I am often asked by patients and physician colleagues whether cranberry juice or supplements (including cranberry capsules) should be prescribed to prevent urinary tract infection. This persistent query led me to formulate a clinical question, "Are cranberry juice or cranberry products effective in the prevention or management of urinary tract infection?" A systematic literature review based on current best evidence available in 2002 suggested that regular consumption of cranberry juice reduces the incidence of urinary tract infections in community-dwelling women and residents of long-term facilities but does not reduce the risk in patients who undergo intermittent or indwelling catheterization (Gray, 2002). However, more recent evidence has emerged that influences the conclusions I reached at that time. Specifically, two randomized controlled

trials (RCTs) published in 2011 and 2012 found that cranberry juice was no more effective than antimicrobial therapy or cranberry flavored placebo drink for preventing urinary tract infection (UTI; Barbosa-Cesnik et al., 2011; Stapleton et al., 2012). On initial consideration, this evidence appeared to support discontinuing recommendations of consumption of cranberry for women seeking to prevent recurrent UTIs. However, additional evaluation of findings from one of the studies, a study using a placebo group (Barbosa-Cesnik et al., 2011), revealed that both groups experienced a considerably lower incidence of UTIs than anticipated. In a subsequent interview with one of the investigators, the researchers acknowledged a possibility that the placebo-flavored drink might have contained some of the ingredients hypothesized to exert an antimicrobial effect in the urine (Larson, 2010). In addition, I considered the fact that consumption of cranberry juice twice daily is not associated with any known harmful side effects. I also considered the fact that cranberry juice is relatively inexpensive compared with dietary supplement cranberry capsules. As a consequence of all these factors, cranberry juice is preferred as a natural means for preventing UTIs among many women in my practice.

This example of basing individual clinical decisions on an EBP process illustrates several important points. It points out the importance of remaining abreast of emerging evidence and the real possibility that newer

EXEMPLAR 10-1 Level I: Interpretation and Use of Evidence-Based Practice in Individual Clinical Decision Making—*cont'd*

evidence may significantly alter our understanding of the benefits or harmful effects associated with a specific intervention. In addition, this case illustrates the role of patient preference in clinical decision making. Clinical experience strongly suggests that a significant proportion of women prefer nonpharmacologic interventions for preventing UTIs, and regular consumption of cranberry juice tends to increase overall fluid intake and provide possibly beneficial effects without associated adverse side effects. Therefore, given the absence of harm, low direct cost, and mixed evidence of a possible preventive effect, I discuss consumption of cranberry juice with women as a possibly effective intervention, free from harmful side effects. However, I also counsel women to consider engaging in behavioral interventions for the prevention of UTIs, including adequate daily fluid intake based on recent recommendations from the Institute of Medicine, daily consumption of a dietary source of the probiotic lactobacillus, and consideration of avoiding use of a diaphragm and vaginal spermicide as birth control strategies (Salvatore et al., 2011).

This case also illustrates the time-consuming and rigorous demands of basing individual clinical decisions on the EBP process. Fortunately, APNs have access to various evidence-based resources. For example,

the *Cochrane Database of Systematic Reviews* is the world's largest single source of systematic reviews and meta-analyses addressing multiple aspects of APN practice (Cochrane Library, 2012). The U.S. Preventive Services Task Force has also produced a large number of systematic reviews linked to various clinical topics of special interest to APN practice, with its focus on primary and secondary intervention to promote optimal health (Trinite, Cherry, & Marion, 2009).

In addition to these resources, a growing number of professional societies have generated evidence-based clinical practice guidelines that address measurable clinical questions with thorough and extensive systematic reviews of existing evidence to formulate clinical recommendations covering comparatively broad topics such as heart failure, diabetes mellitus, chronic obstructive pulmonary disease, breast cancer, end-stage renal disease, osteoporosis, and other topics of special interest to APN practice. In addition to searching the resources of the appropriate professional association's web page, the National Clearinghouse of Practice Guidelines, operated by the Agency for Healthcare Research and Quality (AHRQ), houses a large collection of evidence-based clinical practice guidelines that can be accessed at http://www.guideline.gov.

 EXEMPLAR 10-2 Level II: Interpretation and Use of Evidence-Based Practice to Create Policies for Patient Care

For many APNs, the growing demand to formulate evidence-based policies and protocols needed to prevent the growing list of "never events" provides an opportunity to master the second level, interpretation and use of EBP to create policies for patient care.

Example: Fineout-Overholt and colleagues (2010a, b, c) have described the EBP process needed to answer a clinical question about whether a rapid response team affects the number of cardiac arrests and unplanned intensive care unit admissions in hospitalized adults. Based on this question, the authors described the process used to search the evidence for pertinent studies, code and extract data from these studies using a standardized protocol, and synthesize data to implement policies needed to launch a rapid response team at their facility. Based on this process, the team

concluded that there is sufficient evidence to justify developing policies and committing the resources needed to form a rapid response team at their facility. In addition to providing an example of the EBP described in this chapter, this series of articles describes the processes required to implement such a program. Although a detailed discussion of this translation from research-based evidence to clinical practice is beyond the scope of this chapter, the authors identify and briefly review essential components of this step in the implementation process, including engaging stakeholders in their facility, securing administrative support, preparing a campaign to launch the rapid response team, including staff education and changes in care protocols, and measuring outcomes following implementation of the practice change.

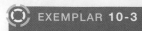

EXEMPLAR 10-3   **Level III: Evaluation of Evidence-Based Practice to Determine Standards of Care**

Participation in an interdisciplinary team to evaluate and determine standards of care using EBP is the third and most advanced level of the EBP competency for APN practice. Generation of an evidence-based clinical practice guideline requires identification of a number of clinically measurable questions required for establishing and evaluating clinical practice in a broad area of patient care, along with an extensive systematic review of pertinent studies. This often encompasses major assessment strategies related to the management of a particular disorder and first-line and alternative interventions for management.

Example: An interdisciplinary group, including two APNs, urologists, urogynecologists, and a medical librarian with extensive experience in systematic literature reviews, was charged with producing an evidence-based clinical practice guideline for treating interstitial cystitis–painful bladder syndrome (IC-PBS) for the American Urological Association (AUA, 2011). This broad topic was broken into clinical questions focusing on assessment strategies and the interventions used to relieve the pain and associated lower urinary tract symptoms associated with this poorly understood syndrome. After the IC-PBS working group reached consensus on pertinent clinical questions, a systematic literature review was completed that covered studies and related articles published between January 1, 1983, and July 22, 2009. The initial electronic database searches retrieved approximately 1130 articles, from which 86 articles were identified for further review. Members of the IC-PBS working group were assigned to review articles for coding and data extraction and the APNs were charged with studies evaluating behavioral interventions, including fluid and dietary strategies for managing bladder pain and related lower urinary tract symptoms (e.g., use of dietary supplements such as calcium glycerophosphate), and pelvic floor muscle training. Because of the generally low levels of supporting evidence, the IC-PBS work group determined that meta-analysis was not feasible. Nevertheless, the group found sufficient evidence to identify and create recommendations for clinical practice for first- through sixth-line treatments (AUA, 2011). Conservative interventions were advocated as first-line treatments because of their combination of moderate benefit combined with few to no harmful side effects. Although the strength of recommendations for clinical practice generated by this interdisciplinary group varied from moderate to low, the production of this clinical practice guideline illustrates the process used to evaluate and create standards of care using the EBP process in an interdisciplinary setting.

preference and clinical expertise are significant for APNs because they reflect the holistic approach central to nursing practice while maintaining the focus on current, research-based evidence.

EBP offers several advantages for clinical decision making when compared with previous models. For example, tradition-based practice is based on clinical and anecdotal experience, combined with received tradition from experienced clinicians, and expert opinion. Tradition-based clinical decision making is based on received wisdom, often provided by instructors or clinical preceptors and expert opinion from those perceived as experts in a given area of care. By substituting a standard of current best evidence for received wisdom or expert opinion, EBP encourages the advanced practice nurse to update and refine clinical practice continually as newer evidence is generated and published. EBP also offers distinctive advantages when compared with rationale-based clinical decision making. Rationale-based clinical decision making relies on identifying a rational explanation for an intervention (Gray et al., 2002). This form of clinical decision making relies on findings from a wide variety of studies, including the following: pathophysiologic research designed to identify the principal action of an intervention or the main reason it exerts a particular effect; and in vitro or in vivo research models that measure outcomes in animals, tissues, or individual cell lines. Although these types of studies are enormously valuable to our overall understanding of health, disease, and the reasons that interventions exert a particular effect, EBP limits its search for evidence to studies that directly measure the efficacy or effectiveness of a particular intervention, predictive power of diagnostic studies, and presence and severity of adverse side effects.

EBP differs from research and quality improvement (QI) projects. Research can be defined as a systematic investigation designed to generate or contribute generalizable knowledge to health care or advanced practice nursing in particular (Arndt & Netsch, 2012). EBP combines findings from multiple research studies that focus on the efficacy of a particular intervention or accuracy of a specific assessment technique to aid APNs and other clinicians when making decisions about the care of an individual patient or group of patients. EBP has been described as the study of studies; its goal is the synthesis of existing knowledge generated from multiple research studies, whereas the goal of an individual research study is to generate new knowledge about an intervention or assessment technique (Gray et al., 2002).

QI is a systematic activity guided by outcome data to achieve rapid improvements in health care delivery in a specific setting (Arndt & Netsch, 2012; Glasziou, Ogrinc, & Goodman, 2010). Both QI projects and research studies are driven by outcome data but QI is an intensely localized activity. The data generated during a QI project is designed to improve specific outcomes within a local facility, clinic, or community. Unlike the data generated by a research study, the results of a QI project can only be generalized to the specific patient population that comprised the project setting.

Despite these differences, the APN should remember that research, EPB, and QI projects share a common goal—improvement of patient care. Further, research, EBP and QI should be viewed as complementary and combined in a manner that improves individual clinical decision making and care processes affecting an entire facility, health care system, or larger community. For example, an acute care APN may observe that the ventilator-associated pneumonia (VAP) incidence in her facility's critical care unit is higher than published benchmarks. As a result, the APN elects to complete a QI project designed at reducing the incidence of VAP. Initially, the APN should review the unit's current prevention protocol to determine whether it is based on current best evidence, such as routine oral hygiene, regular evaluation for readiness to extubate, elevation of the head of the bed, and prophylaxis for peptic ulcer disease and deep vein thrombosis (Tablan et al., 2004). This review may incorporate principles of EBP and findings from individual research studies to answer two questions:

- Are the preventive interventions used by local staff based on current best evidence?
- Does existing research suggest that combining these interventions into a prevention bundle actually reduce the incidence of ventilator-associated pneumonia?

In reference to the first question, a review of current best evidence suggests that bundled interventions are effective for reducing the incidence of VAP (Ramirez, Bassi, & Torres, 2012; Wip & Napolitano, 2009). When examining individual interventions, the acute care APN may note that current best evidence supports regular oral hygiene that incorporates chlorhexidine as effective for preventing VAP (Wip & Napolitano, 2009). In contrast, limited evidence suggests that ongoing elevation of the head of the bed may not affect VAP incidence, even though it is associated with an increased likelihood of sacral pressure ulcer formation. Finally, the APN also may identify findings from an individual study, the NASCENT randomized clinical trial. This study demonstrated that a silver-coated endotracheal tube reduced the incidence of VAP (Kollef et al., 2008) in 9417 critically ill adults from 54 facilities in North America.

Thus, the APN has synthesized essential research-based knowledge using principles of EBP to provide a platform for a QI project. Depending on existing policies in the local critical care unit, the APN may collaborate with others to create a modified or novel prevention bundle and measure VAP incidence before and following implementation of this bundle. Findings of this process comprise a QI project, although these results cannot be generalized to every critical care unit, they can be used to evaluate care processes in the local critical care unit.

Evidence and Current Best Evidence: Historical Perspective

Although the concept of "best evidence" may appear transparent on initial consideration, a more careful analysis of the historical roots of evidence generation in health care is needed. The Oxford English Dictionary Online (2012) defines evidence as an object or document that serves as proof. Within the context of EBP, the objects that clinicians seek to establish evidence for the efficacy and safety of an intervention, or the predictive power of an assessment, are studies. Although the search for evidence can be traced back more than 2000 years, definitions for what constitutes sufficient evidence to reach these conclusions have evolved significantly over time.

The gold standard research design for generating evidence in the twenty-first century remains the RCT (Yoshika, 1998). This research design is based on three critical elements: (1) manipulation of an experimental intervention; (2) comparison of the experimental intervention to a control or comparison group that receives a placebo, sham device, or standard intervention, depending on ethical considerations; and (3) random assignment of subjects to the intervention or control group. Random allocation, advocated since the early 1930s, is an essential element of an RCT because it is the most effective technique for spreading potentially confounding factors evenly among treatment and control groups (Hill, 1937). A well-known RCT that compared streptomycin with standard care at the time (bed rest) is usually cited as the world's first, large-scale, controlled trial (Streptomycin treatment, 1948). Randomization was achieved using a closed envelope system and subjects were blinded to treatment group. However, at least one trial was completed and published before this landmark study. Amberson and associates (1931) compared the antibiotic sanocrysin for the treatment of pulmonary tuberculosis with a placebo. In addition to random allocation of subjects by flipping a coin, they also blinded physician data collectors to group assignment to minimize bias, another important design feature of the modern RCT.

Based on this historical legacy and guided by the pioneering efforts of Archibald Cochrane, current best evidence is now defined as the best available studies evaluating the efficacy and safety of an active or preventive intervention or the predictive accuracy of an assessment (Gray et al., 2004; van Rijswijk & Gray, 2012). These studies must directly evaluate the effect of an intervention, compare the intervention with a placebo, standard care, or sham device, and document adverse side effects associated with the intervention. Studies used to establish current best evidence must be executed in human (rather than animal) subjects and must measure the most direct outcome of treatment, rather than relying on interim outcomes based on convenience. For example, a study of the efficacy of a topical wound therapy should measure wound closure rather than concluding efficacy based on the percentage of wound closure completed at an arbitrary point after the initiation of treatment (van Rijswijk & Gray, 2012).

This definition of current best evidence raises a corollary question: What criteria must be fulfilled to define an intervention as "evidence-based?" At least two major regulatory groups, the U.S. Food and Drug Administration (FDA) and European Medicines Agency (EMEA), have established specific criteria for labeling an intervention as evidence-based (Cormier, 2011). For a drug to receive an indication for clinical use, the FDA requires results from two well-designed RCTs with consistent results, both of which must compare the agent with a placebo- or sham-based control group. The EMEA criteria are similar (EMEA, 2000).

Although these groups provide well-defined criteria for defining an intervention (administration of a drug) as evidence-based, achieving this level of evidence is complex and enormously costly. For example, the total costs of achieving a new drug indication are estimated to vary from $55 million to more than $800 million (U.S. dollars; Adams and Brantner, 2006; DiMasi et al., 2003). Based on these rigid criteria, only a minority of interventions that APNs use to manage their patients would qualify as evidence-based, and limited research in this area has suggested that 40% of clinical decisions used in daily practice are unsupported by evidence (Gray, 2002; Greenhalgh, 2001). As a result, APNs often must search the literature and identify relevant evidence to support clinical decision making in a particular case, or retrieve this information from EBP resources, such as clinical practice guidelines or best practice documents. This chapter will describe the four steps of the evidence-based process and identify resources that the APN can identify and use when making clinical decisions.

Steps of the Evidence-Based Process

Step 1: Formulate a Measurable Clinical Question

Clinical decision making using the EBP process begins with the formulation of a measurable clinical question. Questions arise from various sources. For example, many APNs will formulate their first clinical questions as part of an EBP process when planning a capstone project as part of their Doctor of Nursing Practice degree. Individual clinical practice provides another rich source for clinical questions.

The APN also may be tasked with formulating, and answering clinical questions in response to the need to formulate evidence-based policies for prevention of never events. For example, in 2008, the Centers for Medicare and Medicaid Services (CMS) began a list of "never events" to reduce potentially preventable facility-acquired conditions that included VAP; this list continues to be updated (Chicano & Drolshagen, 2009). For example, in 2007, Gastmeier and Geffers reported on the work of a group of clinicians, including APNs, who were asked which interventions were effective for the prevention of ventilator-associated pneumonia. Their original search for current best evidence identified clinical practice guidelines first released in 2003 and published in 2004 (Tablan et al., 2004). However, they also queried whether newer evidence warranted changes or additions to the preventive interventions recommended in these guidelines. They specifically questioned whether two interventions—oral decontamination via topical chlorhexidine and drainage of subglottic secretions—delay the onset of or prevent VAP. A subsequent literature search revealed recent evidence supporting these interventions that was not included in the 2003 clinical practice guidelines.

Clinical questions may arise from a need to identify evidence supporting the role of the APN in response to a specific disease or disorder. For example, Evans (2010) asked about the effect of adding a follow-up telephone intervention by an APN on blood glucose control when compared with standard treatment. This question was used to identify and retrieve evidence from five RCTs and one systematic literature review to design and implement a protocol that resulted in clinically relevant and statistically significant reductions in fasting blood glucose levels in patients receiving the APN-directed intervention.

After identifying the general topic to be scrutinized, the APN must formulate a measurable question that can be meaningfully addressed using evidence-based clinical decision strategies. Results of several studies have suggested that application of the PICO model aids nurses in formulating clinically relevant and measurable questions

⊚ TABLE 10-2	PICO Model for Generating EBP Clinical Questions
Component	**Definition**
P	**P**atient population—identify the population of interest. **P**roblem—identify the primary problem.
I	**I**ntervention—identify the intervention(s) to be considered.
C	**C**omparison—identify to what the intervention will be compared.
O	**O**utcome—identify the goal of the intervention(s).
T*	**T**ime—time frame for measuring outcomes.

*, Optional.

Adapted from Smith-Strom, H., & Nortvedt, M. W. (2008). Evaluation of evidence-based methods used to teach nursing students to critically appraise evidence. *Journal of Nursing Education, 47,* 372–375; and Sackett, D. L., Strauss, S. E., Richardson, W. S., Rosenberg, W., & Haynes, R. B. (2000). *Evidence-based medicine: How to practice and teach EBM.* (2nd ed.). London: Churchill-Livingstone.

(Balakas & Sparks, 2010; LaRue, Draus & Klem, 2009; Smith-Strom & Nortvedt, 2008; Table 10-2). PICO stands for:

P: Who is the *p*atient *p*opulation?

I: What is the potential *i*ntervention or area of *i*nterest?

C: Is there a *c*omparison intervention or *c*ontrol group?

O: What is the desired *o*utcome?

Thus, as shown, the P in PICO indicates patient or population (Sackett, et al., 2000), although the P is sometimes expanded to include primary problem (Balakas & Sparks, 2010). This element of the formula alerts the APN to define the population to be studied and the nature of the problem to be scrutinized carefully. The population may comprise a subgroup of patients in a facility, such as critically ill patients receiving artificial ventilation or all patients with an indwelling urinary catheter, but it often incorporates much larger populations, such as any individual with a wound or any patient recently diagnosed with diabetes mellitus. As these examples illustrate, identification of the primary problem is closely tied to the population under scrutiny. Examples of primary problems may be a disease such as sinusitis, a disorder such as chronic osteoarthritis, or a predisposition to a potentially preventable condition such as a pressure ulcer.

The I in the PICO model represents the main intervention to be considered. In many cases, the APN will examine a single intervention such as the follow-up telephone intervention for reduction of the fasting blood

glucose level in patients with diabetes mellitus described earlier (Evans, 2010). In contrast, the combined effect of more than one intervention used to prevent or treat a specific disorder will be evaluated. In this case, the APN will identify a protocol or bundle of interventions and analyze their effect on a given outcome. Searching for evidence that evaluates the combined effect of multiple interventions is clinically useful, but presents unique challenges. For example, Hagiwara and coworkers (2011) studied whether decision support tools decrease the time to receive definitive care in acutely ill or trauma patients prior to hospital admission. They operationally defined decision support tools as active knowledge systems that use two or more items to generate case-specific advice. They further classified these tools as electronic or nonelectronic. However, their literature search retrieved only 2 of 33 studies that specifically addressed this clinically relevant question. Despite the use of a well-accepted definition for decision support tools, the authors observed that a number of studies were excluded because it was not possible to classify the study intervention as a decision support tool.

Nayan and coworkers (2011) faced a similar challenge when studying whether smoking cessation rates were higher in oncology patients who receive smoking cessation interventions as compared with usual care. Their initial search identified a meta-analysis of data from eight RCTs that detected no differences in self-reported cessation rates when these interventions were compared with usual care. However, subclassifying smoking interventions into pharmacologic, behavioral, and combined interventions suggested that cessation protocols that combine pharmacologic and behavioral interventions appeared to increase cessation rates when compared with usual care or single-intervention protocols.

The C in the PICO model represents the approach used as a basis for comparison to the intervention undergoing scrutiny. This approach, sometimes called a bundled intervention, is frequently described in research reports as standard care or usual care. Although these terms are descriptive, it is essential that the APN specifically define the intervention(s) that comprise standard care and ensure that the studies retrieved enable adequate differentiation of this standard care from the intervention under scrutiny, especially when evaluating the effect of a bundled intervention or protocol.

The O in PICO represents the outcome, or intended goal of the intervention. When determining the outcome, it is important to identify and evaluate the most direct result indicating clinical efficacy and avoid reliance on indirect outcomes that are more easily measured. Careful consideration of the most direct and clinically relevant outcome is essential when constructing a clinically

TABLE 10-3   Electronic Databases for Identifying and Retrieving Pertinent Research

Name	Description	URL
MEDLINE	Largest online database for nursing, medical, and allied health journals	http://medline.cos.com/
PubMed	Freely accessible online version of MEDLINE database; lacks the robust Boolean features of MEDLINE	http://www.ncbi.nlm.nih.gov/sites/entrez?db=PubMed
Cumulative Index for Nursing and Allied Health Literature (CINAHL)	Largest database for nursing and allied health literature; includes multiple nursing journals not indexed in the MEDLINE database	http://www.ebscohost.com/biomedical-libraries/the-cinahl-database
Education Resource Information Center (ERIC)	Linked to more than 320,000 articles from 1966 to the present; focuses on educational literature, including undergraduate and graduate nursing	http://www.eric.ed.gov/
PsycINFO	Contains more than 3 million resources dating back to 1888; excellent resource for the APN who specializes in providing mental health care	http://www.apa.org/pubs/databases/psycinfo/index.aspx
MD Consult	Incorporates approximately 80 health care journals; includes access to patient education handouts and clinical practice guidelines; accessible via smartphone; administered by Elsevier	http://www.mdconsult.com/php/327720868-2/home.html
Web of Science	Includes journals in the basic and clinical sciences drawn from approximately 9300 journals with impact factors; administered by Thomson-Reuter	http://thomsonreuters.com/products_services/science/training/wos/

relevant question. For prevention studies, the most direct outcome is generally a reduction in the incidence of the disease or disorder under scrutiny. For example, an APN evaluating the effect of a prevention protocol on surgical site infection rates should base conclusions of efficacy on incidence rates, rather than on interim outcomes, such as differences in a nurse's knowledge after education on prevention or self-reported changes in practice following in-service training.

A final element, T, indicating time, may be added to the PICO conceptual framework. The time frame is meant to indicate the relevant observation period for outcomes; it may be short, such as the first 24 to 48 hours following surgery, or long, such as years to decades following the onset of a chronic condition such as dementia or diabetes mellitus (Balakas & Sparks, 2010; LaRue, Draus, & Klem, 2009; Smith-Strom & Nortvedt, 2008).

Step 2: Search the Literature for Relevant Studies

Evidence-based clinical decision making relies on identifying research-based evidence. Therefore, it is essential for the APN to develop expertise in searching the literature to identify and retrieve appropriate studies. Fortunately, the development of modern electronic databases has revolutionized our ability to search the published literature rapidly and access pertinent research reports. A number of electronic databases are now available to the APN (Table 10-3). Although full access to these databases usually requires a paid subscription, APNs may access these electronic databases via a facility-based subscription. Specifically, the vast majority of health system, university, or college libraries maintain institutional subscriptions to OVID, ensuring access to multiple electronic databases such as MEDLINE or CINAHL. In addition, access to PubMed, a service of the MEDLINE database, is available without charge on the Internet.

MEDLINE and PubMed

Administered by the U.S. National Library of Medicine, MEDLINE is the world's largest electronic database of health-related research and literature (U.S. National Library of Medicine, 2012). There are articles from a number of professions, including medicine, nursing, dentistry, veterinary medicine, and associated disciplines such as physiology, pharmacology, and molecular biology. Approximately 5600 journals are indexed. MEDLINE can be accessed via various strategies, including keywords. However, the MEDLINE database is primarily organized around MESH terms (*me*dical *s*ubject *h*eadings). Entering a MESH term, such as "coronary artery disease" or "osteoporosis," will trigger a number of subheads that are potentially useful to identify evidence for answering a clinical question, such as "diagnosis," "drug therapy," "diet therapy," and "nursing." The MEDLINE database may also be searched using various keywords that are not official MESH terms; these searches retrieve articles that include the keyword in its title, abstract, or list of identifying keywords, but they will not provide the subheads available when a MESH term is accessed. The MEDLINE database includes articles published in 39 languages; 91% are printed in English and 83% of those published in other languages have English language abstracts, greatly increasing access for English-speaking searchers.

MEDLINE has particularly robust Boolean functions, allowing the APN to focus or narrow a search based on combining two or more MESH terms or keywords using the functions "AND," "OR," and "NOT" (U.S. National Library of Medicine, 2012). For example, an APN might pose a question about the effectiveness of administering an angiotensin-converting enzyme (ACE) inhibitor for the prevention of mortality and disease progression in patients with heart failure. In this case, the APN might initially select the MESH term "heart failure" along with the MESH term "angiotensin-converting enzyme inhibitors." By using the "AND" Boolean function, the database will retrieve articles that merge the intervention (ACE inhibitor agents) with the primary patient problem under scrutiny (heart failure).

A second Boolean function, "OR" allows the searcher to retrieve articles that contain either of two keywords or MESH terms. This function is useful when terms that are recently coined or historically relevant differ from the corresponding MESH term. For example, an APN may be seeking information about patients who experience chronic lower urinary tract pain not associated with bacterial infection. The MESH term for this condition is "interstitial cystitis." However, a more recent term (painful bladder syndrome) has been increasingly used to describe this condition; combining the MESH term "interstitial cystitis" with the keyword "painful bladder syndrome" retrieves more citations that entering either term alone.

A third Boolean function, "NOT," allows the APN to limit a search by eliminating articles that do not address the intervention, assessment, or patient population under scrutiny. For example, an APN interested in prevention of central line infections might enter the MESH term "indwelling catheters," which will retrieve studies focusing on infections associated with multiple types of catheters, including urinary and peritoneal dialysis catheters. Use of the "NOT" Boolean function will enable the APN to eliminate articles about various types of catheters not pertinent

to a clinical question focusing on hospital-acquired central line infections.

The MEDLINE database allows searches via multiple alternative fields, including author, journal, publication type (e.g., review article), language, experimental approach (human, in vivo, or in vitro), gender, age range, and publication year. These options are useful for focusing searches based on the parameters specified in the clinical question.

The PubMed web page provides free access to the MEDLINE database; it can be accessed at http://www.ncbi.nlm.nih.gov/pubmed. The basic search engine will retrieve articles based on keywords. Clinicians searching PubMed can click on an advanced search icon and access a site that allows combination of keywords or keyword and author or journal using the Boolean function "AND." However, the PubMed database does not have the robust search functions characterized by MEDLINE. In addition, although a limited number of articles can be downloaded directly from the PubMED site, access to most articles is restricted to the complete citation and abstract.

Cumulative Index for Nursing and Allied Health Literature

The Cumulative Index for Nursing and Allied Health Literature (CINAHL) is an electronic database containing more than 2.6 million elements from approximately 3000 nursing and allied health journals and books. CINAHL was originally published as a bound set of reference books entitled *Cumulative Index to Nursing Literature* in the early 1960s and was expanded to include other health professions in 1977. Similar to MEDLINE, the CINAHL database is available online as a subscription service typically accessed as part of an OVID subscription maintained by larger health care facilities and universities. Articles can be searched using keywords; the CINAHL database also contains the Boolean features "AND," "OR," "NOT" and multiple search fields similar to those described earlier. CINAHL also indexes doctoral dissertations, an important source for grey literature (unpublished documents) in the field of nursing. Additional electronic databases useful for advanced practice nursing are listed in Table 10-3.

Online Evidence-Based Resources

In addition to retrieving individual research reports from electronic databases such as MEDLINE and CINAHL, the APN should also search online evidence-based documents such as the *Cochrane Library for Systematic Reviews*, Essential Evidence Plus, and PubMed Health. The *Cochrane Library* is part of the Cochrane Collaboration; it is administered by a nonprofit organization and reviews are generated by more than 28,000 volunteers from across the globe (Cochrane Collaboration, 2012). The *Cochrane Library* contains multiple resources for identifying current best evidence including the *Cochrane Database of Systematic Reviews* and Cochrane Central Register of Controlled Trials. The *Database of Systematic Reviews* contains more than 5000 systematic literature reviews based on clinical questions covering almost every specialty practice area in contemporary health care. Whenever possible, these reviews include a meta-analysis of data pooled from comparable studies. The systematic reviews can be accessed by multiple search fields, including keywords found in the title or abstract and author. Systematic reviews can be retrieved as a summary, standard report, or full report. A plain language summary provides a brief synopsis of the review's main findings. A standard report provides more detailed information, including a structured abstract of the review, plain language summary (see earlier), background, objectives, methods, results, and discussion, along with reference lists for included and excluded studies. Systematic reviews are also available as a full report that incorporates all the elements of the standard report plus a detailed summary of all analyses generated for the review.

The plain language summary is useful as a quick reference when the APN is only interested in a succinct summary of the main findings of a systematic review; this document may also be shared with a patient or family with a college-level education who may wish to know more about evidence supporting a particular intervention or assessment strategy. The full summary provides the more detailed information necessary when the APN is evaluating current best evidence for individual decision making or generation of recommendations for practice. The detailed report also may be used for this purpose; study of this longer version is especially recommended for the novice APN who is learning to synthesize evidence for clinical decision making or generating evidence-based documents such as a plan for a capstone project.

Other online resources include the Joanna Briggs Institute, Essential Evidence Plus, and PubMed Health. The Joanna Briggs Institute is an international collaboration of nurses and other allied health care professionals, including the Cochrane Nursing Care Field and Cochrane Qualitative Research Methods Group, which provides evidence-based resources for nursing (Joanna Briggs Institute, 2012). Essential Evidence Plus is a subscription service administered by Wiley-Blackwell Publishers (Essential Evidence Plus, 2012) that enables users to access multiple electronic databases, including the Cochrane Library, to obtain evidence-based resources and information. An individual or institutional subscription to Essential Evidence Plus also provides access to *p*atient-*o*riented *e*vidence that *m*atters (POEMS). POEMS are regularly updated synopses of evidence from individual studies and an archive of more than 3000 previously posted summaries. They may be downloaded online, to a smart phone, or viewed via podcast.

PubMed Health is an electronic database for evidence-based resources administered by the National Center for Biotechnology Information, U.S. National Library of Medicine (2012). This electronic database includes reviews of clinical effectiveness research; reviews are available in brief reports designed for use by consumers, along with full reports designed for use by clinicians such as APNs. In addition to its link to the extensive MEDLINE–PubMED database, PubMed Health is linked to evidence-based resources from the *Cochrane Library*, AHRQ, National Cancer Institute, National Institute for Health and Clinical Excellence (NICE) guidelines program, and National Institute for Health Research Health Technology Assessment Program. Table 10-4 summarizes additional online resources for EBP.

Clinical Practice Guidelines

This search of electronic databases should also incorporate the identification and retrieval of existing clinical practice guidelines or best practice documents. Clinical practice guidelines may be enormously helpful to the APN because they represent a systematic review of existing evidence based on measurable clinical questions and recommendations for management of the disease, disorder, or condition (Fletcher, 2008). The National Guideline Clearinghouse is the largest online resource for clinical practice guidelines (http://guideline.gov/faq.aspx). Administered by the AHRQ, this database houses more than 3000 clinical practice guidelines formulated within the past 5 years. The APN should also search the web page of the appropriate nursing and medical society for relevant clinical practice guidelines. The number of professional societies producing clinical practice guidelines has grown from a few pioneers, including the American Academy of Pediatrics and Oncology Nursing Society, to the vast majority of societies and organizations, including many smaller subspecialty groups.

The APN should also search for best practice documents pertaining to the clinical question under scrutiny. Best practice guidelines are a synthesis of expert and clinical opinions when higher levels of evidence are not available to guide clinical decision making (Triano, 2008). Although these documents often do not provide the systematic review and evidence-based recommendations of care incorporated into the clinical practice guideline, they can provide an excellent source of current knowledge of a specific intervention or assessment technique. In addition to housing clinical practice guidelines, the National Guideline Clearinghouse also indexes best

TABLE 10-4 Additional Online Resources for Evidence-Based Practice

Name	Description	URL
Clinical Practice Guidelines		
Agency for Healthcare Research and Quality (AHRQ)	Evidence report topics, technical reviews, and clinical guidelines	www.ahcpr.gov
National Guideline Clearinghouse (NGC)	Evidence-based clinical practice guidelines and measurement tools	www.guideline.gov
Institute for Healthcare Improvement	List of published articles about developing and using evidence-based protocols	www.ihi.org
General Sites with Links to Other EBP Sites		
Academic Center for Evidence-Based Nursing (ACE)	Comprehensive list of EBP resources	www.acestar.uthscsa.edu
Centre for Health Evidence	Users' guides for EBP series from the *Journal of the American Medical Association*	www.cche.net/che/home.asp
Centre for Evidence-Based Nursing	Lists of reviews and evidence research reports	www.york.ac.uk/healthsciences/centres
Centre for Evidence-Based Medicine (CEBM)	Links to evidence-based resources, tools, continuing education, and discussion groups	www.cebm.net
Economic and Social Research Council Evidence Network	Lists evidence-based resources in social policy fields	http://evidencenetwork.org/index.html
Joanna Briggs Institute	Privately owned EBP site with some free resources and subscription pages	www.joannabriggs.edu.au/about/home.php
Advanced Practice Nursing	Subscription site for evidence-based resources	www.enursescribe.com

practice documents produced within the past 5 years. The Registered Nurses' Association of Ontario (RNAO) is another excellent resource for best practice guidelines that affect multiple areas of nursing care, including many areas pertinent to advanced practice nursing.

Strategies for Searching Electronic Databases

Because of their robust size and ability to identify potential resources in a matter of seconds to minutes, any hunt for best current evidence begins with a search of several electronic databases. However, the search must not end with this essential initial strategy. Studies have suggested that a competent search using appropriate databases will identify approximately 25% to 50% of all studies pertaining to a clinical question (Hersh & Hickham, 1998; McManus et al., 1998). A more recent randomized controlled trial found that the efficiency of identification and retrieval of studies is significantly improved when a medical librarian is consulted (Gardois et al., 2011). Several factors probably contribute to the incomplete retrieval of pertinent studies when relying solely on searches of electronic databases. Challenges related to keywords are postulated to be a primary cause of incomplete retrieval. Many conditions and interventions are referred to by multiple names and these terms evolve over

time. For example, the chronic wound referred to as a pressure ulcer was historically labeled a bed sore, and this term was later changed to decubitus ulcer or pressure sore before the current term was popularized and added to the MESH term taxonomy. In addition to this limitation, electronic databases typically identify keywords for search purposes from the title, abstract, and a short list of key terms provided by the author and/or publisher. Although authors and publishers share the goal of maximizing the number of times an article is read and cited in subsequent peer-reviewed publications, even subtle changes in narrative or selection of less widely used terms limit the likelihood that a particular study report will be identified in subsequent searches.

Although the lag time between publication and indexing in the major databases has decreased dramatically over the past 5 years, the significant growth in production of clinical studies by scholars from a number of health care fields means that newer research pertinent to a clinical question typically appear within a matter of months to 1 year of a focused search. In addition, electronic databases are heavily weighted toward published documents. Publication bias is defined as the tendency for studies with positive results to achieve favorable peer review and acceptance for publication as compared with research reporting negative results (Smith, 1956). The magnitude of this effect is hypothesized to be substantial (Guyatt et al., 2011). For example, Sutton and colleagues (2000) carried out meta-analyses of 48 systematic reviews and reported that 20% were found to have omitted or missed studies reporting negative results. Electronic databases are also limited by the relative paucity of grey literature, which is especially significant in nursing research. The term *grey literature* is defined as unpublished results of studies available as abstracts or short reports in conference proceedings or journal supplements. Sparse research has suggested that the magnitude of nursing studies that remain unpublished despite completion is substantial. For example, Hicks (1995) reported that 16 of a group of 161 British nurses who completed a study and presented results at a professional conference submitted their findings for publication in a peer-reviewed journal and only 14 (9%) were ultimately published.

Several strategies can be used to increase the proportion of pertinent studies identified during a literature search for current best evidence. They include doing ancestry searches, searching grey literature sources, consulting experts in the field, and using Internet-based search engines. Ancestry searches are completed by reviewing the reference list of individual research reports, review articles, or systematic reviews identified during a literature search (Melnyk & Fineout-Overholt, 2010). In my experience, ancestry searches typically reveal multiple studies that are missed during electronic database searches. Identifying pertinent grey literature sources remains a challenge. Hand searches of one or more peer-reviewed journals that publish research abstracts in a supplement to or regular issue of the society's official journal, or abstracts made available to conference attendees as a proceedings booklet or in an electronic format, may serve as a rich source of pertinent studies. Although these sources may identify many potentially pertinent studies, they typically contain limited details of the study design and analyses of findings, significantly limiting their value as evidence-based resources. In contrast, the CINAHL, PsycINFO, and ERIC databases index doctoral theses and dissertations that provide intensely reviewed and detailed reports of graduate students' supervised research.

Internet-based search engines, such as Google Scholar, act as an increasingly robust source of published and unpublished studies. They are particularly useful when attempting to retrieve full reprints of older articles not yet incorporated into the major electronic databases. Nevertheless, considerable caution must be used when relying on unpublished information from the Internet, especially if the source material has not undergone peer review.

Consulting with an experienced researcher or clinical experts in a particular field can also lead to identification of pertinent studies. For example, McManus and colleagues (1998) reported results of a systematic review that compared laboratory results obtained using a point of care testing technique—defined as obtaining and analyzing a sample at the location the patient received care—with laboratory results obtained by forwarding the sample to a certified laboratory. The final search identified 1057 references; 102 high-quality research reports were ultimately identified that formed the final systematic reviews. Searching via electronic databases alone revealed only 49% of the 102 reports included in the final systematic review. Formal queries of experts in the field via mailed surveys identified an additional 29% of the pertinent studies and the remaining 22% were identified by ancestry search. In addition to serving as a reliable resource for identifying pertinent studies, collaborating with clinical experts also provides the novice APN with an opportunity to contact and network with more experienced colleagues who share an interest in the topic undergoing an evidence-based review.

Step 3: Critically Appraise and Extract Evidence

Although a careful search of the literature using the strategies described will recover pertinent studies, it will also retrieve much information that does not comprise evidence of effectiveness, predictive accuracy, or safety. Therefore, the APN must critically appraise the various documents for their contribution to current best evidence, extract pertinent data, and set aside findings that do not address the clinical question under scrutiny. This process begins with separation of individual research reports and systematic reviews summarizing research findings from secondary sources, such as integrative review articles, or editorials. An integrative review is a comprehensive discussion of research, expert opinion, and theoretical knowledge about a topic (Gray & Bliss, 2005). Although the integrative review typically includes studies that may provide valuable sources of evidence when subjected to an ancestry search, it is ultimately a synthesis of knowledge about a given topic, rather than an evidence-based review of studies intended to establish efficacy or predictive accuracy. Similarly, opinion-based articles such as editorials are eliminated because they report expert opinion rather than original research data.

Evidence Pyramid

After eliminating articles that do not report or systematically review original data, the remaining studies are evaluated based on a pyramid of evidence (Bracke et al., 2008; Fig. 10-1). The pyramid provides a taxonomy for ranking a study's potential contribution to evidence based on its design. The base of this pyramid is typically identified as

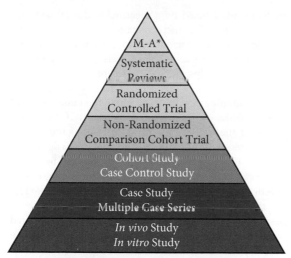

FIG 10-1 Pyramid illustrating levels of evidence used to evaluate efficacy of an intervention. *MA,* Meta-analysis.

containing laboratory-based studies using animals (in vivo model), tissue samples, cell lines, or chemical media (in vitro models). Although these studies are typically well designed and apply much more rigid controls than those used in clinical research, they are nevertheless eliminated because their findings do not yield evidence about efficacy, safety, or predictive value when an intervention is applied to human subjects in a clinical setting.

The second rung up from the base of the evidence pyramid is typically occupied by individual or multiple case series. A case study is a detailed description of results when an individual patient, family, inpatient care unit, long-term care facility, health care system, or community is subjected to an intervention or intervention bundle (protocol; Casey & Houghton, 2010; Crowe et al., 2011). Case studies may look forward prospectively to describe events and observe the outcome, or a retrospective format may be used to look backward and speculate on the influence of various interventions on the outcome. Multiple case series summarize results from more than one patient with a similar condition when exposed to a common intervention or intervention bundle. The results of case studies or multiple case series can be used as evidence that an intervention is feasible, offers an attractive alternative to usual care, can be applied safely in a selected patient or patients, and merits further investigation to determine clinical effectiveness. However, individual case studies or multiple case series do not compare the intervention of interest with standard care and their results cannot be used to reach conclusions about efficacy, effectiveness, or predictive power. The APN must remain aware that findings from these designs tend to favor positive effects of the

intervention and often imply evidence of efficacy or effectiveness. In addition, results of individual case studies (sometimes labeled testimonials) are frequently used in marketing campaigns to imply a positive effect when a particular product is used. Nevertheless, case studies and multiple case series do not compare the intervention under scrutiny to a placebo or to standard (usual) care, and their results cannot be used to establish efficacy or predictive power.

The higher rungs of the evidence pyramid are occupied by the RCT, nonrandomized comparison cohort trials, and cohort or case-control studies. Depending on the nature of the clinical question and availability of research-based evidence, results of one or more of these designs will be used to define current best evidence. The nonrandomized comparison cohort trial shares certain similarities with the RCT; it compares outcomes from at least two groups, including one cohort that is exposed to an experimental intervention, and a second group exposed to usual care, sham device, or placebo (Charpentier, Bogardus, & Inouye, 2001). However, this study design uses non-randomly selected groups because of ethical, financial, or other considerations. Because the nonrandomized comparison cohort trial lacks random assignment, the potential for bias in group membership is high and the likelihood that these differences will influence study findings is significant.

A cohort study, sometimes called a longitudinal or follow-up study, is an observational design in which a large sample is identified and followed over time to determine which participants will develop the disease or disorder under scrutiny (Dunn, Lyman, & Marx, 2003). During this prolonged observation period, the incidence of the disease or disorder is measured prospectively. A cohort study allows researchers to identify new (incident) cases and temporal relationships between preventive interventions or constitutional factors and incidence can be analyzed. Although the cohort study provides valuable results, data collection requires an extended observation period, resulting in a comparatively high likelihood of subject dropout and significant cost. The case-control study, sometimes called the nested case-control design, provides a more restrained alternative to the cohort study. It is characterized by comparison of two groups, one with the condition under study and the other free from the condition at a single point in time. This cross-sectional technique allows the researcher to identify and analyze potential factors associated with presence or absence of the disease or disorder being studied (Dunn, Lyman, & Marx, 2003; Essebag et al., 2003). The nested case-control study uses retrospective analysis of data from a sample population participating in a parallel group or factorial RCT (Essebag et al., 2003). These study designs differ from that of the RCT because they are observational rather than interventional in nature. Study findings can be used to identify relationships between the presence of a given factor and the likelihood of the condition being studied, but they cannot be used to establish a cause and effect relationship between the associated factor and disease or disorder needed to determine efficacy.

The most powerful research design is the RCT, which is considered the gold standard for measuring the efficacy of an intervention or the predictive power of an assessment strategy (Sackett et al., 1996). Efficacy is defined as the likelihood that an intervention will achieve the desired outcome in a group of subjects based on evaluation in a research setting that controls for random effects produced by extrinsic factors. The concept of efficacy must be clearly differentiated from effectiveness, which is defined as the effect of a specific intervention when administered to a particular patient at a given point during the course of an illness or condition.

Several types of RCTs are commonly reported in the health care literature (Stolberg, Norman, & Trop, 2004). The parallel design RCT assigns subjects randomly to an experimental group exposed to the intervention under scrutiny or to a control group exposed to a placebo, sham device, or standard intervention based on ethical considerations. A crossover RCT is characterized by random assignment of subjects to an experimental or control group, followed by crossing the subject over to the alternative group after a washout period designed to remove (wash away) initial exposure effect. Although the crossover RCT potentially needs to enroll fewer total subjects and may incur less cost than the parallel group design, it is performed less often because of the potential for contamination of findings caused by residual effects when subjects are crossed over. The factorial RCT compares two or more experimental interventions with a control group treated with a placebo or sham versus a group receiving usual care or some alternative intervention. Because the RCT is the most powerful study design, it should be routinely included when reviewing the literature for current best evidence; it is generally considered to be of higher quality than designs that do not involve randomization of subjects, such as the cohort or case control study.

Systematic Reviews and Meta-Analyses

Even though the RCT is considered the most powerful individual research design, the highest rungs of the evidence pyramid are occupied by systematic reviews and meta-analyses. These designs form the apex of the evidence pyramid because they combine the results of multiple studies to determine the effect created by a specific intervention. A systematic review uses a structured methodology to comprehensively seek out, select, appraise and analyze studies based on a measurable clinical question (Engberg, 2008). The methods used for generating a systematic review are comparable to those used to identify current best evidence for clinical decision making and the rise of EBP closely parallels the recent explosion of systematic review articles published in the professional literature. Combining results from multiple studies is more powerful than consideration of a single RCT because it allows for the qualitative analysis of results produced by multiple researchers in various study settings to determine whether the effects of the intervention are beneficial (greater than placebo or standard care), mixed (no more effective than placebo in some studies versus more effective than control group findings in others), or ineffective (less effective than placebo or standard care, or associated with adverse side effects that exceed its beneficial effects).

The meta-analysis the highest rung of the level of evidence pyramid because it provides a quantitative technique for pooling and analyzing results from more than one study to determine the direction and magnitude of an intervention's effect (Engberg, 2008). Although the benefits of meta-analysis are apparent, studies must be carefully analyzed before completing this type of statistical analysis. This evaluation is based on data extraction and consideration of the sample populations of the various studies, experimental intervention, study methods, and outcome variables used to determine treatment effect. The outcomes of a meta-analysis based on a dichotomous (nominal) outcome measure are usually expressed as an odds ratio, relative risk, or absolute risk reduction, depending on the nature of the clinical question. The results of a meta-analysis based on a continuous outcome variable will be based on the weighted mean difference and standardized mean difference, sometimes referred to as effect size. The precision of the magnitude of the effect size is expressed by the accompanying confidence interval (CI).

The level of the evidence pyramid is useful for the APN engaging in EBP because it provides a taxonomy for categorizing studies based on underlying design for their potential contribution to current best evidence needed to answer a clinical question. Nevertheless, research design alone cannot be used to judge the quality of individual studies or their contribution to current best evidence (Petticrew & Roberts, 2003). Although RCTs provide excellent designs for minimizing bias in the evaluation of some forms of interventions, such as a medication designed to improve hemodynamic instability, physical manipulation, such as insertion of a catheter for parenteral fluid replacement, or positioning to prevent ventilator-associated pneumonia, it may not be feasible or desirable to limit a systematic review seeking current best evidence to RCT alone. In many cases, the APN will find that there are insufficient RCTs to define current best evidence. As a result, nonrandomized trials or observation epidemiologic studies examining the association between preventive or interventional measures and the outcome of interest may be included because they provide the best available evidence. In other cases, the quality of one or more RCTs may be compromised, limiting the APN's ability to extract data and reach meaningful conclusions about efficacy from these studies. Ogilvie and colleagues (2005) evaluated systematic reviews of evidence related to the efficacy of psychosocial interventions and observed that the inclusion of RCTs alone might miss most pertinent evidence because these interventions tend to be embedded or applied along with physical interventions in many RCTs. In this case, measuring only direct outcomes produced in RCT may paradoxically miss results from alternative studies that examine the effect of the psychosocial interventions that comprise an essential component of APN practice.

Critical Appraisal
Individual Studies

After eliminating studies that do not contribute to determining current best evidence, the APN must evaluate the quality of individual studies and determine their potential to provide evidence for clinical decision making. In selected circumstances, this evaluation may be used to eliminate studies that do not meet criteria for meta-analysis or contain sufficient flaws that severely compromise the generalizability of findings. However, studies must not be eliminated because they report negative findings or the study is not an RCT. Although no standardized form for evaluating study quality exists, several models

have been developed that provide a useful framework for evaluating the quality of individual studies. Melnyk and Fineout-Overholt (2010) have advocated a Critical Appraisal Guide for Quantitative Studies (Table 10-5). Alternatively, the CONSORT (Consolidated Standards of Reporting Trials) criteria for improving reporting the results of RCTs, and the STROBE (Strengthening Reporting of Observational Studies in Epidemiology) criteria for reporting the results of observational studies in epidemiology, can be adapted to enable systematic assessment of the quality of individual studies and their contribution to evidence-based clinical decision making (Moher, Schulz, & Altman, 2001; von Elm et al., 2007). Figure 10-2 is the individual study form used by the Cochrane Collaboration for evaluating individual studies as part of their production of a systematic review of current best evidence. It is based on a three-level ranking—0 to 2—in which a score of 2 indicates that the criterion was clearly met, a score of 1 indicates that it was partially met, and a score of 0 indicates that it was not met. Tables 10-6 and 10-7 summarize criteria for an initial evaluation of study quality adapted from the CONSORT and STROBE statements, respectively (Moher, Schulz, & Altman 2001; von Elm et al, 2007). These statements are designed to serve as a guide when publishing individual study results in a peer-reviewed scholarly journal; they can be easily adapted as a guide for evaluating individual study quality as part of an EBP process.

Systematic Reviews and Meta-Analyses

Because systematic review and meta-analytic techniques are much newer than the design techniques used to generate RCTs, nonrandomized comparison cohort trials, or

---

TABLE 10-5 Critical Appraisal Guide for Quantitative Studies

Question	Evaluation Criteria
Why was the study done?	Does the study include clearly stated research questions, aims, hypotheses, or purpose statements?
What is the sample size?	Did the study enroll enough subjects to allow statistical analysis so that results did not occur by chance?
Are the instruments used to measure major variables valid and reliable?	Were the outcome measures of the study clearly defined? Were instruments used to measure these outcomes valid and reliable?
How were data analyzed?	What statistical tests were used to determine whether the study purpose was achieved?
Were there any untoward events during the study?	Did subjects withdraw before completing the study; if so, why did they withdraw?
How do results fit with previous research in this area?	Did the researchers base their work on a thorough literature review?
What does this research mean for clinical practice?	Is the study purpose an important clinical issue?

Adapted from Melnyk, B. M., Fineout-Overholt, E. (2010). *Evidence-based practice in nursing and healthcare: A guide to best practice.* Philadelphia: Wolters-Kluwer.

Review:
Quality Assessment Tool
Study ID #___   Raters initials: ___   Date___

	Scoring	Score	Query	A/B/C
A: Was the assigned treatment adequately concealed prior to allocation?	2 = Method did not allow disclosure of assignment 1 = Small but possible chance of disclosure of assignment or unclear 0 = quasirandomized or open list/tables Clearly yes = A Not sure = B Clearly no = C			
B: Were the outcomes of patients who withdrew described and included in the analysis (intention to treat)?	2 = withdrawals well described and accounted for in analysis 1 = withdrawals described and analysis not possible 0 = no mention, inadequate mention or obvious differences and no adjustment			
C: Were the outcome assessors blinded to treatment status?	2 = effective action taken to blind assessors 1 = small or moderate chance of unblinding of assessors 0 = not mentioned or not possible			
D: Were the treatment and control group comparable at entry?	2 = good comparability of groups, or confounding adjusted for in analysis 1 = confounding small; mentioned but not adjusted for 0 = large potential for confounding, or not discussed			
E. Were the subjects blind to the assignment status after allocation?	2 = effective action taken to blind subjects 1 = Small or moderate chance of unblinding of subjects 0 = not possible, or not mentioned (unless double-blind) or possible but not done			
F. Were the treatment providers blind to assignment status?	2 = effective action taken to blind treatment providers 1 = Small or moderate chance of unblinding of treatment providers			

FIG 10-2 Individual study quality assessment tool. *(From the Cochrane Collaboration, 2012.)*

	0 = not possible, or not mentioned (unless double-blind) or possible but not done		
G: Were care programmes, other than the trial options, identical?	2 = Care programmes clearly identical 1 = Clear but trivial differences 0 = Not mentioned, or clear and important differences in care programmes		
H. Were the inclusion and exclusion criteria clearly defined?	2 = clearly defined 1 = inadequately defined 0 = not defined		
I. Were the interventions clearly defined?	2 = clearly defined 1 = inadequately defined 0 = not defined		
J. Were the outcome measures used clearly defined?	2 = clearly defined 1 = inadequately defined 0 = not defined		
	Outcome 1:		
	Outcome 2:		
	Outcome 3:		
	Outcome 4:		
	Outcome 5:		
K. Were diagnostic tests used in outcome assessment clinically useful?	2 = optimal 1 = adequate 0 = not defined, not adequate		
	Outcome 1:		
	Outcome 2:		
	Outcome 3:		
	Outcome 4:		
	Outcome 5:		
L. Was the surveillance active, and of clinically appropriate duration?	2 = optimal 1 = adequate 0 = not defined, not adequate		
	Outcome 1:		
	Outcome 2:		
	Outcome 3:		
	Outcome 4:		
	Outcome 5:		

FIG 10-2, cont'd

observational epidemiologic studies, models for evaluating their quality have not yet been well standardized. A technical report prepared for the AHRQ identified more than 20 guidelines for evaluating the quality of systematic reviews, but only two were considered high quality (West et al., 2002). Nevertheless, this report identified common factors that should be incorporated into any evaluation of the quality of these documents including a clinical question, methods for searching the literature and extracting data, and recommendations for practice or policy based on evidence identified (Table 10-8).

The APN should evaluate the systematic review for sources of potential bias associated with study retrieval. Several common sources of bias have been identified, including time-, language- and geography-related bias, as well as publication bias (discussed earlier; Schlosser, 2007).

Time-related bias is created when systematic reviews limit the time frame for study inclusion. Although systematic reviewers are understandably concerned with limiting their reviews to the best current evidence, searches must use original research reports rather than summaries of

TABLE 10-6 Evaluating Quality of the Randomized Controlled Trial and Nonrandomized Comparison Cohort Trial

Criterion Section of the Research Report	Evidence that Criterion Was Met
Study purpose (introduction and background)	The purpose of the study is clearly stated. A rationale for the study is clearly stated and supported by appropriate literature.
Study participants (methods)	Inclusion and exclusion criteria for study participants are described, along with the study setting.
Study aims (methods)	Measurable research aims, questions, or hypotheses are stated. These statements include measurable study outcomes consistent with the stated purpose of the study.
Sample size (methods)	The authors describe how the sample size was determined. Ideally, sample size is based on a power analysis to determine the number of subjects needed to determine group differences. The sample size recruited may be slightly larger than the minimum group size suggested by the power analysis to account for subjects who withdraw prior to completion of data collection.
Random allocation (methods)	Methods used to achieve random allocation are described, the success of randomization may be illustrated in a table comparing demographic and key clinical characteristics between experimental and control groups, and inferential analysis should identify no significant differences between groups. Procedures for group selection in the nonrandomized comparison cohort trial are described. Absence of randomization in group assignment is clearly acknowledged and a table comparing demographic and key clinical characteristics of intervention and comparison group is provided.
Blinding (methods)	Study participants and data collectors are blinded to group assignment whenever feasible; blinding is not feasible for multiple nursing interventions, such as education or counseling.
Statistical methods (methods)	Appropriate statistical methods are used to compare primary and secondary outcomes. Descriptive statistics and inferential statistical analyses are based on considerations of level of measurement (nominal, ordinal or continuous) and distribution of data. Multivariate analyses are used when multiple outcome measures are analyzed. Intention to treat analysis is used, when indicated.
Participant flow (methods and results)	Study procedures are thoroughly described in the methods section; a diagram of participant flow may be placed in the results section. The number of subjects who do not complete data collection is stated, and reasons for early study withdrawal are clearly stated. Ideally, the proportion of patients who do not complete the study is ≤15%.
Outcomes (results)	Outcomes based on research questions or aims are stated for each group and the precision of the outcomes are measured using a 95% CI.
Adverse events	Adverse events are reported, along with their impact on study completion.
Generalizability	Results are interpreted in the context of current evidence along with limitations of study, including potential sources of bias. Limitations associated with multiple analyses are discussed.

Adapted from Moher, D., Schulz, K. F., & Altman, D. (2001). The CONSORT statement: Revised recommendations for improving the quality of reports of parallel-group randomized trials. *Journal of the American Medical Association, 285,* 1987–1991.

TABLE 10-7 Evaluating Quality of Observational Studies: Adapted from the STROBE Statement

Criterion Section of the Research Report	Evidence that Criterion Was Met
Study purpose (introduction and background)	The purpose of the study is clearly stated. A rationale for the study is clearly stated and supported by appropriate literature.
Study participants (methods)	Eligibility criteria for study participation and follow-up criteria are clearly described for the cohort study. Criteria for cases and controls are described for the case-control study; criteria used to match cases and controls are clearly described.
Study outcomes (methods)	Outcome variables are clearly defined, along with confounding factors and potential associated (predictive) factors. Diagnostic criteria for differentiating cases and controls are clearly described for cohort and case control studies.
Bias (methods)	Potential sources of bias are acknowledged.
Statistical methods (methods)	Appropriate statistical methods are used to analyze primary and secondary outcome measures. Descriptive statistics and inferential statistical analyses are based on considerations of level of measurement (nominal, ordinal or continuous) and distribution of data. Multivariate analyses are used when multiple outcome measures are analyzed. An explanation of methods used to control for confounding factors and how missing data were managed is provided.
Participants (results)	Demographic and pertinent clinical characteristics of cases and controls are described.
Outcome data (results)	For the cohort study, a report of incidence or summary measures over time should be reported. For the case-control study, outcomes of variables potentially associated with likelihood of status as a case or control subject are reported. Association between outcome as a case or control should be based on multivariate analysis when multiple factors are analyzed.
Generalizability (discussion)	Key findings are presented based on study questions or aims. Limitations of the study are clearly acknowledged, including sources of bias and inability to determine cause and effect based on the presence of statistically significant associations. Limitations associated with multiple inferential analyses are acknowledged.

Adapted from von Elm, E., Eggar, M., Altman, D. G., Egger, M., Pocock, S. J., Gotzsche, P. C., et al. (2007). Strengthening the Reporting of Observational Studies in Epidemiology (STROBE) statement: Guidelines for reporting observational studies. Strengthening the reporting of observational studies in epidemiology (STROBE) statement: guideline for reporting observational studies. *British Medical Journal, 335,* 806–808.

studies contained in integrative or systematic reviews. Therefore, decisions about time frames in systematic reviews should include the latest publications at the time the review was conducted and extend backward to a meaningful point in time. This time frame may be based on a landmark event, such as passage of legislation, development of an intervention or diagnostic technology, or publication of a phase 3 RCT and approval of a drug for clinical use. Gaps in the timeline for searches should not be present.

Language-related bias is common in systematic reviews. Although English is the predominant language of

science (Meneghini & Packer, 2007), and most articles in MEDLINE and CINAHL are published in English, many studies are only published in other languages and the potential for language-related bias associated with the use of English language–only sources should be acknowledged in the methods section or discussion of a systematic review.

Limiting studies based on geography is rarely justified, but may be appropriate if a certain treatment is used only in a small number of regions worldwide. The systematic review should contain explicit acknowledgment that data were extracted based on a standardized protocol, along

TABLE 10-8   Criteria for Evaluation of a Systematic Review, With or Without a Meta-Analysis

Criterion	Evidence that Criterion Was Met
Study question	A clearly defined clinical question is provided; the question should define the patient population and problem, intervention or assessment strategy under scrutiny, comparison treatment, and outcomes indicating intervention effect or predictive power of the assessment strategy.
Inclusion or exclusion criteria	Search methods are clearly described. Techniques used to identify studies include electronic database searches along with techniques to increase the efficiency of the search, such as ancestry search, consultation with experts in the field of inquiry, web engine searches, trial registries, and conference proceedings. Inclusion and exclusion criteria for studies are clearly stated. Potential sources of bias in selection criteria (time-, language-, and geography-related) are acknowledged and minimized.
Data extraction	The process for data extraction from individual studies is clearly described. A standardized protocol for data extraction is included in the methods section of the systematic review. This protocol specifies persons involved in data extraction and procedures for coding data, ranking study quality, building consensus about data extraction, and resolving conflicts in individual study coding. Incorporation of an independent coder is used to measure reliability (interrater agreement rates) similar to that used for reporting original data when multiple data collectors participate in a research protocol. Interrater agreement rates should vary from 75%-100%. A persuasive rationale for excluding studies based on methodologic quality is provided and excluded studies are clearly identified. The process used to weight evidence (e.g., results of meta-analysis, ranking of evidence) is clearly defined. The process for determining study quality, including weighting of the study for purposes of evidence ranking or meta-analysis, is clearly explained. Evidence ranking is based on consensus among authors and a process for resolving disagreements concerning quality rankings via consensus is clearly described.
Recommendations for clinical practice.	Recommendations for clinical practice are supported by evidence extracted from the systematic review. The strength of recommendations should be specified and the process for determining strength of recommendation clearly explained. Ideally, evidence ranking and determination of strength of recommendations for clinical practice are based on validated and published ranking systems.

Adapted from Schlosser, R. W. (2007). Appraising the quality of systematic reviews (http://www.ncddr.org/kt/products/focus/focus17/index.html); and West, S., King V., Carey, T. S., Lohr, K. N., McKoy, N., Sutton, S. F., et al. (2002). *Systems to rate the strength of scientific evidence*. Evidence Report–Technology Assessment No. 47. AHRQ Publication 02-E016. Rockville, MD: Agency for Healthcare Research and Quality.

with a brief explanation of who was involved in data extraction and coding. Minimally, this procedure should include an explanation of how persons coding the various studies reached consensus on study quality and how disagreements were resolved. Inclusion of an independent coder is optimal because it enables a measurement of reliability (interrater agreement rates) among persons extracting data from the various studies.

Data Extraction

The decision making process associated with EBP relies on more than simply retrieving studies and basing a clinical decision on a generalized assumption of reported findings. Instead, the APN should use a consistent process to extract only pertinent outcomes based on criteria determined in the clinical question posed in step 1. To ensure consistency, study review and data extraction should follow a predetermined protocol, just as original research adheres to established study procedures, regardless of whether results will be used for writing a formal systematic review, evaluating existing evidence for the purposes of a QI project, or formulating new policies in a local facility. The process used to extract data varies based on the nature of the clinical question. For example, the protocol used to extract data from a group of RCTs—possibly combined with results of one or more nonrandomized trials—to determine the efficacy of a given intervention will differ from data coded and extracted for a review of the predictive accuracy of a diagnostic examination. The Cochrane Collaboration (http://bjmtg.cochrane.org/resources-developing-review) provides excellent resources for coding forms enabling a standardized protocol for data extraction. Figure 10-3 is a data extraction form used for coding data from an individual study evaluating the efficacy of a single experimental intervention. This form can be used when measuring outcomes of trials comparing two groups, one of which was exposed to the intervention of interest and the other exposed to a placebo, sham device, or standard care. The web page also provides a standardized form designed to aid the clinician when extracting data from RCTs comparing the effects of multiple interventions.

Step 4: Implement Useful Findings in Clinical Decision Making

Implementing useful findings is a deceptively complex process that goes beyond simply combining study results to create a protocol for implementation of a given intervention or assessment strategy. This process occurs on multiple levels, including clinical decision making when caring for an individual patient, creation and implementation of policies on a facility- or community-wide level, and creation of evidence-based clinical practice guidelines designed to set standards of care on a national or global level. Implementing EBP when caring for individual patients, establishing local policies for clinical practice, or establishing guidelines for practice on a national or global basis requires a synthesis of knowledge of the intervention's predictive power or efficacy, consideration of individualized physical and psychosocial factors likely to have an impact on effectiveness when applied to an individual patient, and knowledge of its direct cost or economic impact (van Rijswijk & Gray, 2012). For example, whereas a new drug may be shown to be effective in an RCT when compared with patients receiving a placebo, its adaptation into an evidence-based clinical practice guideline must also address its comparative effectiveness to existing agents with similar pharmacologic actions, the frequency and nature of the adverse side effects associated with the drug, and its cost. The increased cost associated with a new drug may be justified if it proves more effective than existing agents in the same class or is associated with a lower risk of adverse side effects. In contrast, the novelty of a drug does not provide justification for inclusion in evidence-based clinical practice guidelines or protocols if it does not offer clinically relevant advantages in terms of the efficacy or safety needed to justify the increased patient cost likely to be associated with a newer agent.

The process of implementing findings from an EBP process begins with the generation of recommendations for clinical practice, which are derived from the data extracted from pertinent studies. However, just as the strength of individual evidence underlying assessment strategies or interventions varies, so must the strength or associated recommendations for clinical practice. Similar to the various systems used to grade evidence, a review of the literature reveals that more than 60 different taxonomies for grading the strength of practice recommendations have been incorporated into various clinical practice guidelines and best practice documents (Garcia, Alvarado, & Gaxiola, 2010). Predominant systems include the Strength of Recommendation Taxonomy (SORT) scale, Grading of Recommendations Assessment, Development and Evaluation (GRADE) scales, NICE scale, Center for Preventive Medicine scale (developed in Oxford), and Scottish Intercollegiate Guideline Network (SIGN) taxonomy. Garcia and colleagues (2010) have compared the effect of evidence-based clinical decision making in a child with diarrhea using four scales (NICE, GRADE, Centre for Evidence-Based Medicine [CEBM], and SIGN scales) in a group of 216 novice physicians (pediatric residents). A significant number of physicians changed their recommendation for management of the index case based on review of the various clinical recommendations. Of the four scales recommended, the GRADE scale was found to exert the greatest influence on clinical decision making.

The GRADE scale was developed by a group of clinicians to rank the strength of clinical recommendations based on current best evidence (Brozek et al., 2009; GRADE Working Group, 2004). The GRADE Work Group has recommended evaluating the quality of evidence based on a four-point ordinal scale:

1. High evidence indicates a small likelihood that additional research is unlikely to change confidence of the direction or magnitude of the effect size associated with a specific intervention.
2. Moderate evidence indicates that additional research may significantly influence the magnitude of treatment effect.
3. Low evidence indicates that new research may affect the direction and magnitude of treatment effect.
4. Very low evidence indicates insufficient evidence to determine treatment effect.

Using this underlying scale for grading evidence, the GRADE Working Group advocates a scale for recommendations for clinical practice in which the highest grade indicates benefits that clearly outweigh potential for harm, the second level indicates that benefits of treatment must be carefully weighed against potential adverse sides effects,

{Review name}- Basic information for study ID: ....

Method

Randomisation	Blinding	Intention to treat - Loss to Follow-up

Participants

N	Age	Sex	Type of injury:
Country	Hospital	Period of Study	Other participants (not review?)

Inclusion criteria	Exclusion Criteria

Interventions

Intervention (including description, when started, frequency, duration & when stopped etc)

Overall length of follow-up:

Outcomes

Outcomes	Tick if available	How measured	When done

Notes - see over   **Reviewer:**

FIG 10-3 Data extraction form of individual studies comparing two groups. *(From the Cochrane Collaboration, 2012.)*

TABLE 10-9 **U.S. Preventive Services Task Force Scale for Strength of Recommendations for Clinical Practice**

Rank	Description	Recommendation for Practice
A	The service* is recommended and supported by evidence of substantial benefit.	The APN should offer or provide this service when indicated.
B	The action is recommended and supported by strong evidence of moderate benefit associated with the service, or moderate-level evidence suggesting moderate to substantial benefit from the service.	The APN should offer or provide this service when indicated.
C	Evidence suggests that the service provides only a small benefit.	The APN should offer or provide this service only when other considerations support offering or providing this service.
D	Evidence demonstrates no benefit from the service or potential harm outweighs the service.	The APN should discourage use of the service.
I	Current evidence is insufficient to assess the balance between harm and benefit of the service.	The APN should counsel patients about the uncertainty of the balance between benefit and harm before offering or providing this service.

*Service is defined as an intervention, intervention bundle, or assessment strategy. From Trinite, T., Cherry, C. L., & Marion, L. (2009). The U.S. Preventive Services Task Force: An evidence-based prevention resource for nurse practitioners. *Journal of the American Academy of Nurse Practitioners, 21,* 301–306.

the third level indicates that balance between benefit and harm cannot be clearly distinguished based on best available evidence, and the lowest grade level indicates that the best available evidence suggests the intervention is likely to produce more harm than benefit.

A second ranking system likely to be familiar to many APNs practicing in North America has been promulgated by the U.S. Preventive Services Task Force. This scale uses grades A to D, with a fifth category labeled I (Trinite, Cherry, & Marion, 2009). Similar to the rankings advocated by the GRADE working group, recommendations for practice are linked to the direction, magnitude, and balance between benefit and harm. Table 10-9 summarizes the Task Force scale for recommendations for clinical practice.

From Policy to Practice: Tips for Achieving Meaningful Changes in Practice Based on Current Best Evidence

Although the EBP process is effective for identifying current best evidence, completion of the process does not guarantee meaningful changes in practice needed to achieve desired clinical outcomes. Instead, evidence strongly suggests that introducing a new policy or directing clinicians to alter their current practice is unlikely to lead to meaningful or sustained changes in practice (West, 2001). Instead, many evidence-based practice innovations introduced through the efforts of one or

more clinician advocates tend to result in short-term adoption by a limited number of clinicians that is not likely to be sustained over time (Stetler, 2003). To overcome this problem, the APN must be aware of successful strategies to design and implement a structured program for translating practice innovations into meaningful and sustained changes.

Rogers' Diffusion of Innovation Theory provides a useful framework for the APN seeking to implement successful and sustained changes in practice based on EBP processes (Rogers, 2003). This theoretical framework describes four stages that an individual clinician or group will experience when evaluating and deciding to adopt or reject a practice innovation. The first phase, described as the knowledge stage, occurs when clinicians are made aware of the innovation and its potential impact on practice and patient outcomes. For many clinicians, knowledge may be introduced through continuing education activities, announcement of a practice innovation, or informal communication from colleagues or informal clinical leaders. Historically, many clinicians have believed that simply introducing a practice innovation is sufficient to ensure a sustained practice change, but research utilization studies have repeatedly proven this assumption false (Rogers, 2003; Stetler, 2003).

The second stage is characterized by a process of persuasion. During this stage, clinicians will form a favorable or unfavorable attitude toward a practice innovation. Although the decision making process is highly individualized, formation of a positive attitude toward a practice innovation is primarily determined by two major factors—the perceived benefit of the practice change on patient outcomes and the perceived investment associated with the practice change as compared with current practice. Outcomes of research studies tend to focus on benefits to patients, but the APN must also carefully consider the impact of a proposed practice innovation on existing practice. Such considerations are particularly relevant when an evidence-based practice innovation comprises a bundle of interventions. For example, current best evidence reveals that prevention of facility-acquired pressure ulcers is based on a number of preventive interventions, including regular skin assessment, pressure ulcer risk assessment, selective use of support surfaces, and regular patient turning and repositioning (WOCN Pressure Ulcer Panel, 2003). Research has also demonstrated that pressure ulcer risk assessment is more effective when based on a validated instrument as compared with an individual clinician's judgment. Various pressure ulcer risk instruments have been validated, but the Braden Scale for Pressure Sore Risk has emerged as being predominant in North America (Bolton, 2007). This is not based on its predictive power alone; a number of scales have been shown to exert robust predictive power in evaluating pressure ulcer risk. Rather, clinical experience overwhelmingly suggests that the parsimony of the Braden scale profoundly influences it predominance in clinical practice, especially when compared with other scales that require far longer to complete.

The third phase (decision stage) occurs when individual clinicians reach a decision about the proposed practice innovation (Rogers, 2003). At this point, the clinician will elect to support (accept) the practice innovation as valuable and worthy of implementation or reject the innovation as offering insufficient benefit for the patient or being too costly when compared with outcomes achieved using current practice patterns. Historically, the decision to accept or oppose a practice innovation when reached by a key decision maker, such as a physician or nurse administrator, was thought to be the same as adopting or rejecting it, but the rise of EBP and interdisciplinary care teams has led to a more transparent separation of individual decision making from adoption of a practice innovation.

The final stage of innovation diffusion is adoption into daily clinical practice. Similar to the other stages of innovation diffusion, successful adoption requires more than assent to integrate the innovation into practice. It also requires varying levels of adapting or restructuring the practice environment in a manner that enables clinicians to engage in the behavioral changes needed to adopt an innovation. When planning to introduce an evidence-based practice innovation, the APN should consider the following factors: (1) its relative advantage; (2) its compatibility with current practice patterns; (3) the degree to which the innovation can be adapted on a trial basis; and (4) the degree to which results of the innovation can be observed (Rogers, 2003). Judging the relative advantage of a practice innovation requires comparing the time required to execute its various assessments and innovations as compared with the time and effort committed to existing practice patterns. Demonstrating the relative advantage of an evidence-based practice innovation is particularly challenging when it requires a greater time investment than current practice patterns. In this case, the APN should clearly communicate and emphasize advantages to patient outcomes. Additional factors that favor adoption of an evidence-based practice innovation include support from organizational administration, clinical leadership at the inpatient unit or clinic level, and manipulation of the practice environment to enhance adoption of new practices.

The degree to which a practice innovation can be adopted on a trial basis can also enhance the likelihood of its successful and sustained adoption (Rogers, 2003). For example, implementation of a facility-acquired pressure ulcer prevention program might include risk assessment using the Braden Scale for Pressure Sore Risk. In this case, integration of the Braden scale into the hospital's electronic medical record, combined with an online training program, allows nurses to familiarize themselves with use of the instrument prior to officially adopting this assessment into routine practice (Magnan & Maklebust, 2008, 2009).

Adoption of an evidence practice innovation is also enhanced by the degree to which results are observable. Meaningful feedback has traditionally been reserved for administrators or selected clinical leaders. However, front-line clinicians must be included in this feedback loop if they are to adopt practice changes on a sustained basis.

The process of implementing evidence-based practice in the APN's local facility must be individualized based on existing practice patterns, staffing and resources of the facility, and organizational culture of the facility (Carlson, Rapp, & Eichler, 2012; Ferlie & Shortell, 2001; Kimball, 2005; Stetler et al., 2003). Nevertheless, experience and existing research provide insights into key elements needed for achieving a successful and sustained change in practice patterns: (1) identification of an interdisciplinary team of stakeholders needed to plan and implement the practice innovation; (2) support from the organization's administration; (3) clinical leadership structure that supports EBP principles; and (4) feedback data for monitoring improvement and rewarding clinician stakeholders.

Stakeholder Engagement

Formation of an interdisciplinary team of key stakeholders is essential to the implementation of a successful and sustained evidence-based practice innovation (Gallagher-Ford, Fineout-Overholt, Melnyk, & Stillwell, 2011; Powell et al., 2012). This group should include key clinical leaders who will be affected by the proposed practice innovation, such as clinical nursing leaders, physicians, and other clinicians (e.g., physical or occupational therapists, case managers). This group will be most directly responsible for completing the initial EBP process to identify current best evidence or using available resources, such as clinical practice guidelines, to aid with this determination. This group should also take primary responsibility for determining how the practice innovation should be incorporated into existing practice patterns. The key stakeholder group must consider a number of factors when designing an implementation strategy, including potential facilitators and barriers to implementation. Although evidence is limited, Weiner and associates (2008) have provided a detailed description of strategies that have proven effective for assessing organizational culture and barriers or facilitators likely to influence introduction of an evidence-based practice innovation. This core group should also design strategies to gain administrative support and support from key clinical leaders essential to the implementation of an evidence-based practice innovation. An APN is often the coordinator or leader of this interdisciplinary team.

Organizational Support

In some cases, administrative personnel may approach the APN concerning the need for a practice innovation based on regulatory changes, such as the introduction of "never events" by the Centers for Medicare and Medicaid Services in 2008 (Drake-Land, 2008). However, clinical experience strongly suggests that most evidence-based practice innovations are initiated by a clinician seeking to improve patient care outcomes. Ensuring administrative support involves more than merely informing them of an intention to change organizational practice based on EBP principles (Bradley et al., 2001). Instead, the APN must work with other key stakeholders to formulate a proposal that provides key administrative personnel with knowledge of the rationale for the recommended practice innovation, its anticipated impact on patient outcomes, and associated costs, a number of resources will vary, depending on the practice innovation proposed. Essential resources usually include a commitment to clinical leaders and staff education about the proposed practice innovation, alterations to the electronic medical record system needed to facilitate the innovation, disposable supplies or durable medical equipment needed to implement the practice change, and a system for measuring outcomes and providing staff and stakeholders with meaningful feedback about outcomes.

Clinical Leadership Support

The presence of a corporate culture and clinical leadership structure that supports EBP principles may be the single most important factor influencing the adoption of EBP innovations (Fixsen et al., 2005; Rapp et al., 2010). Rapp and coworkers (2010) have evaluated barriers to the implementation of EBP initiatives and observed that the behavior of clinical supervisors forms a substantial barrier to statewide EBP innovation projects. Specifically, they found that although clinical leaders did not oppose the use of EBP principles for clinical decision making, they did not set expectations among front-line clinicians, relying instead on informal methods of practice adoption. Although this approach may not act as a barrier to select clinicians who share an inherent interest in EBP and practice innovation, it ultimately favors maintenance of the status quo rather than organizational adoption of EBP principles and associated practice innovations.

Fortunately, several strategies have been identified to avoid this potential barrier to the adoption of EBP innovations. Obtaining magnet status is another strategy for promoting an organizational environment that promotes EBP in nursing practice. Magnet status from the American Nurses Credential Center requires the integration of EBP principles into nursing care (Reigle et al., 2008). Although obtaining magnet status is a major undertaking that goes well beyond the implementation of a single EBP innovation, it has been shown to aid facilities when transforming an organizational culture to one that promotes the principles of EBP among clinical nursing leaders and front-line clinicians.

In addition, the involvement of unit- or clinic-based champions has been shown to facilitate adoption of EBP innovations in multiple health care settings (Slaunwhite et al., 2009; Taggart et al., 2012). The unit- or clinic-based champion is a clinician who practices on the unit in question and agrees to act as a mentor for the implementation of the EBP innovation. Selection of the proper individual is critical; Rogers (2003) noted that group adoption of innovation occurs in a step-wise manner, with some individuals acting as early adopters, followed by most group members who adopted the innovation based on positive results and feedback from early adopters, followed by a second minority of individuals (late adopters) who change practice only after it becomes apparent that the innovation is inevitable. Clinicians who are early adopters, and who are recognized on their units as influential practitioners, are preferred to the appointment of clinicians who are not persuaded that the innovation is advantageous when compared with current practice patterns.

Evidence-Based Practice Innovation Feedback

Providing meaningful feedback to all stakeholders involved in an EBP innovation is critical to an evaluation of the impact of the strategy on clinical outcomes and cost, including organizational administration, clinical leaders, and front-line clinicians. This feedback should be easily interpretable to all stakeholders and should be provided on a regular basis to promote sustained changes in practice based on a track record of improved clinical and other outcomes. For example, feedback may include regular reporting of facility-wide pertinent clinical outcomes, such as reduction in surgical site infections or indwelling catheter days, or it may include individual provider or unit outcomes. Some studies have revealed that clinical leaders are reluctant to criticize individual providers based on clinical outcomes (Rapp et al., 2010). Reporting negative outcomes is also essential to continue to strive for optimal patient care.

Future Perspectives

The identification and evaluation of studies to identify current best evidence is currently based on a hierarchy that identifies the RCT as the most powerful study design for generating evidence, along with systematic reviews and meta-analytic techniques that combine data from multiple RCTs to reach conclusions about the strength of evidence. Although the RCT clearly provides the best research design for evaluating the efficacy of an intervention, it does not necessarily follow that determination of efficacy indicates that the intervention will prove effective when applied in daily clinical practice as opposed to the rigidly controlled clinical trial setting (van Risjwijk & Gray, 2012). In addition, evaluations of current best evidence do not incorporate other real-world factors that influence treatment effectiveness when applied to the management of individual patients, including patient preference and the impact of cost. To account for the influence of these factors on clinical decision making and health care policy more fully, Congress passed the Patient Protection and Affordable Care Act (PPACA; U.S. Department of Health and Human Services, 2011), which has focused economic resources and attention on the

development and generation of comparative effectiveness research (CER), defined as the comparison of existing health care interventions to determine which treatment works best, for whom, and under what circumstances. This approach differs from traditional EBP processes because it seeks to measure clinical effectiveness based on considerations of treatment efficacy, patient preference, and resource allocation. Whereas the EBP process focuses on data generated from RCTs, CER seeks to generate data from real-world trials (Wilkins & Mullins, 2011). Optimal techniques for generating a well-designed, real-world trial have not yet been developed, but basic principles include comparison of existing options for treatment, enrolling participants with few inclusion and exclusion criteria, minimal or no manipulation of treatment interventions outside individual clinical judgment, and consideration of treatment effect, cost, and patient preference. The growth of large electronic databases are hypothesized to provide a basis for generation of data for this type of real-world trial, although the nature of widespread clinician and patient participation in such a trial has not been well developed in the private sector. Principles of CER remain poorly developed, as do techniques for generating high-quality data from a well-designed, real-world trial; nevertheless, this form of inquiry should be especially attractive to the APN who regularly engages in clinical decision making that incorporates these considerations. Although the future of this emerging trend in using EBP for clinical decision making remains unclear, it seems likely that APNs will play a pivotal role in its evolution and benefit from the knowledge gained from this attempt to study and evaluate more systematically the impact of multiple factors on the effectiveness of our interventions.

Conclusion

Evidence-based practice involves the generation of a clinically measurable question, identification of pertinent research findings, coding and extraction of essential data, and implementation of findings. Intimate knowledge of this process is critical for the APN to master three core levels of the EBP competency, application to individual clinical decision making, formulating policies for patient care in a local facility, or evaluating evidence in order to establish standards of care via clinical practice guidelines. These competencies are increasingly essential as the APN functions as a team member, leader and decision maker within an interdisciplinary health care team.

References

Adams, C. P., & Brantner, V. V. (2006). Estimating the cost of new drug development: Is it really $802 million? *Health Affairs (Millwood)*, *25*, 420–428.

Amberson, J., McMahon, B., & Pinner, M. (1931). A clinical trial of sanocrysin in pulmonary tuberculosis. *American Review of Tuberculosis*, *21*, 401–435.

American Urological Association (AUA) Guideline. (2011). Diagnosis and treatment of interstitial cystitis/painful bladder syndrome (http://www.auanet.org/content/guidelines-and-quality-care/clinical-guidelines/main-reports/ic-bps/diagnosis_and_treatment_ic-bps.pdf).

Arndt, J. V., & Netsch, D. S. (2012). Research study or quality improvement project? *Journal of Wound, Ostomy, and Continence Nursing*, *39*, 371–375.

Atkins, D., Best, D., Briss, P. A., Eccles, M., Falck-Ytter, Y., Flottorp, S., et al; GRADE Working Group. (2004). Grading quality of evidence and strength of recommendations. *British Medical Journal*, *328*, 1490.

Balakas, K., & Sparks, L. (2010). Teaching research and evidence-based practice using a service-learning approach. *Journal of Nursing Education*, *49*, 691–695.

Barbosa-Cesnik, C., Brown, M. B., Buxton, M., Zhang, L., DeBusscher, J., & Foxman, B. (2011). Cranberry juice fails to prevent recurrent urinary tract infection: results from a randomized placebo-controlled trial. *Clinical Infectious Disease*, *52*, 23–30.

Bolton, L. (2007). Evidence-based report card. Operational definition of moist wound healing. *Journal of Wound Ostomy Continence Nursing*, *34*, 23–29.

Bracke, P. J., Howse, D. K., & Keim, S. M. (2008). Evidence-based Medicine Search: A customizable federated search engine. *Journal of the Medical Library Association*, *96*, 108–113.

Bradley, E. H., Holmboe, E. S., Mattera, J. A., Roumanis, S. A., Radford, M. J., & Kromholz, H. M. (2001). A quantitative study of increasing β-blocker use after myocardial infarction: why do some hospitals succeed? *Journal of the American Medical Association*, *285*, 2604–2611.

Brozek, J. L., Akl, E. E., Alonso-Coello, P., Lang, D., Jaeschke, R., Williams, J. W., et al. (2009). Grading quality of evidence and strength of recommendations in clinical practice guidelines. *Allergy*, *64*, 669–677.

Carlson, L., Rapp, C. A., & Eichler, M. S. (2012). The experts rate: Supervisory behaviors that impact the implementation of evidence-based practices. *Community Mental Health Journal*, *48*, 179–186.

Casey, D., & Houghton, C. (2010). Clarifying case study research: Examples from practice. *Nurse Researcher*, *17*, 41–51.

Charpentier, P. A., Bogardus, S. T., & Inouye, S. K. (2001). An algorithm for individual matching in a non-randomized clinical trial. *Journal of Clinical Epidemiology*, *54*, 1166–1173.

Chicano, S. G., & Drolshagen, C. (2009). Reducing hospital-acquired pressure ulcers. *Journal of Wound, Ostomy, and Continence Nursing*, *36*, 45–50.

Cochrane Collaboration. (2012). About the Cochrane Library (http://www.thecochranelibrary.com/view/0/AboutTheCochraneLibrary.html).

Cormier, J. W. (2011). Advancing FDA's regulatory science through weight of evidence evaluations. *Journal of Contemporary Health Law and Policy*, *28*, 1–22.

Crowe, S., Cresswell, K., Robertson, A., Huby, G., Avery, A., & Sheik, A. (2011). The case study approach (http://www.biomedcetnral.com/1471-2288/11/100).

Dicenso, A., Cullum, N., & Ciliska, D. (2002). Implementing evidence-based nursing: Misconceptions. *Evidence-Based Nursing*, *5*, 4–5.

DiMasi, J. A., Hansen, R. W., & Grabowski, H. G. (2003). The price of innovation: New estimates of drug development costs. *Journal of Health Economics*, *22*, 141–185.

Drake-Land, B. (2008). CMS never events (www.aha-solutions.org/…/rlsolutions-cmsneverevent-021611.pdf).

Dunn, W. R., Lyman, S., & Marx, R. (2003). Research methodology. *Arthroscopy*, *19*, 870–873.

Education Resources Information Center. (2012). About the ERIC program (http://eric.ed.gov/ERICWebPortal/resources/html/about/about_eric.html).

Engberg, S. (2008). Systematic reviews and meta analysis: Studies of studies. *Journal of Wound, Ostomy and Continence Nursing*, *35*, 258–265.

Essebag, V., Genest, J., Suissa, S., & Pilote, L. (2003). The nested case control study in cardiology. *American Heart Journal*, *146*, 581–590.

Essential Evidence Plus. (2012). At a glance (http://www.essentialevidenceplus.com/product).

European Medicines Agency. (2000). Points to consider on switching between superiority and non-inferiority (http://www.emea.europa.eu/docs/en_GB/document_library/Scientific_guideline/2009/09/WC500003658.pdf).

Evans, M. M. (2010). Evidence-based practice protocol to improve glucose control in individuals with type-2 diabetes mellitus. *Medical-Surgical Nursing*, *19*, 317–322.

Ferlie, E. B., & Shortell, S. M. (2001). Improving the quality of healthcare in the United Kingdom and United States. A framework for change. *Milbank Quarterly*, *79*, 281–315.

Fineout-Overholt, E., Melnyk, B. M., Stillwell, S. B., & Williamson, K. M. (2010a). Evidence-based practice: Step by step. Critical appraisal of the evidence: Part I. *American Journal of Nursing*, *110*, 47–52.

Fineout-Overholt, E., Melnyk, B. M., Stillwell, S. B., & Williamson, K. M. (2010b). Evidence-based practice: Step by step. Critical appraisal of the evidence: Part II. *American Journal of Nursing*, *110*, 41–48.

Fineout-Overholt, E., Melnyk, B. M., Stillwell, S. B., & Williamson, K. M. (2010c). Evidence-based practice: Step by step. Critical appraisal of the evidence: Part III. *American Journal of Nursing*, *110*, 43–51.

Fixsen, D. L., Naoom, S. F., Blase, K. A., Friedman, R. M., & Wallace, F. (2005). *Implementation research: A synthesis of the literature*. Tampa, FL: University of South Florida, Louis de la Parte Florida Mental Health Institute, National Implementation Research Network.

Fletcher, R. H. (2008). Clinical practice guidelines (http://www.themgo.com/content/CIguidelines.PDF).

Gallagher-Ford, L., Fineout-Overholt, E., Melnyk, B. M., & Stillwell, S. B. (2011). Evidence-based practice, step by step:

Implementing an evidence-based practice change. *American Journal of Nursing, 111,* 54–60.

Garcia, C. A. C., Alvarado, K. P. P., & Gaxiola, G. P. (2010). Grading recommendations in clinical practice guidelines: randomized experimental evaluation of four different systems. *Archives of Disease in Childhood, 96,* 723–728.

Gardois, P., Calabrese, P., Colomib, N., Deplano, A., Lingua, C., Longo, F., et al. (2011). Effectiveness of bibliographic searches preformed by pediatric residents and interns assisted by librarians. A randomized controlled trial. *Health Information and Libraries Journal, 28,* 273–284.

Gastmeier, P., & Geffers, C. (2007). Prevention of ventilator-associated pneumonia: Analysis of studies published since 2004. *Journal of Hospital Infection, 67,* 1–8.

Gerrish, K., Nolan, M., McDonnell, A., Tod, A., Kirshbaum, M., & Guillame, L. (2011). Factors influencing advanced practice nurses' ability to promote evidence-based practice among frontline nurses. *Worldviews on Evidence-Based Nursing, 9,* 30–39.

Glasziou, P., Ogrinc, G., & Goodman, S. (2010). Can evidence-based medicine and clinical quality improvement learn from each other? *BMJ Quality & Safety, 20*(Suppl 1), i13–i17.

Gray, G. E. (2002). Evidence-based medicine: An introduction for psychiatrists. *Journal of Psychiatric Practice, 8,* 5–13.

Gray, M. (2002). Are cranberry juice or cranberry products effective for prevention or management of urinary tract infections? *Journal of Wound, Ostomy and Continence Nursing, 29,* 122–126.

Gray, M., Beitz, J., Colwell, J., Bliss, D. Z., Engberg, S., Evans, E., et al. (2004). Evidence-based nursing practice II. Advanced concepts for WOC nursing practice. *Journal of Wound, Ostomy and Continence Nursing, 31,* 53–61.

Gray, M., & Bliss, D. Z. (2005). Preparing a grant proposal—part 2: Reviewing the literature. *Journal of Wound, Ostomy and Continence Nursing, 32,* 83–86.

Gray, M., Bliss, D. Z., Bookout, K., Colwell, J., Dutcher, J. A., Engberg, S., et al. (2002). Evidence-based practice: A primer for the WOC nurse. *Journal of Wound, Ostomy and Continence Nursing, 29,* 283–286.

Greenhalgh, T. (2001). *How to read a paper: The basics of evidence-based medicine.* (2nd ed.). London: BMJ Books.

Guyatt, G. H. Oxman, A. D., Montori, V., Vist, G., Kunz, R., Brozek, J., et al. (2011). GRADE Guidelines 5. Rating the quality of evidence—publication bias. *Journal of Clinical Epidemiology, 64,* 1277–1282.

Hagiwara, M., Henricson, M., Jonsson, A., & Suserud, B. O. (2011). Decision support tool in prehospital care: A systematic review of randomized trials. *Prehospital and Disaster Medicine, 26,* 319–329.

Hersh, W. R., & Hickham, D. H. (1998). How well do physicians use electronic information retrieval systems? *Journal of the American Medical Association, 280,* 1347–1352.

Hicks, C. (1995). The shortfall of published research: A study of nurses' research and publication activities. *Advanced Nursing, 21,* 594–604.

Hill, A. B. (1937). Principles of medical statistics. I. The aim of the statistical method. *Lancet, 1,* 41–43.

Joanna Briggs Institute. (2012). Welcome to the Joanna Briggs Institute (http://www.joannabriggs.edu.au).

Kimball, B. (2005). Cultural transformation in health care (http://www.rwjf.org/files/publications/NursingCulturalTrans.pdf).

Kollef, M. H., Afessa, B., Anzueto, A., Veremakis, C., Kerr, K. M., Margolis, B. D., et al. (2008). Silver-coated endotracheal tubes and incidence of ventilator-associated pneumonia: The NASCENT randomized trial. *Journal of the American Medical Association, 300,* 805–813.

Larson, N. F. (2010). Cranberry juice may not prevent urinary tract infection (http://www.medscape.com/viewarticle/734360).

Larue, E. M., Draus, P., & Klem, M. L. (2009). A description of a web-based educational tool for understanding PICO framework in evidence-based practice with a citation ranking system. *Computers, Informatics, Nursing: CIN, 27,* 44–49.

Magnan, M. A., & Maklebust, J. (2008). The effect of Web-based Braden Scale training on the reliability and precision of Braden Scale pressure ulcer risk assessments. *Journal of Wound, Ostomy and Continence, 35,* 199–208.

Magnan, M. A., & Maklebust, J. (2009). The effect of web-based Braden Scale training on the reliability of Braden Subscale ratings. *Journal of Wound, Ostomy & Continence Nursing, 36,* 51–59.

McManus, R. J., Wilson, S., Delaney, B. C., Fitzmaurice, D. A., Hyde, C. J., Tobias, R. S., et al. (1998). Review of the usefulness of contacting other experts when conducting a literature search for systematic reviews. *British Medical Journal, 317,* 1562–1563.

Melnyk, B. M., & Fineout-Overholt, E. (2010). *Evidence-based practice in nursing and healthcare: A guide to best practice.* Philadelphia: Wolters-Kluwer.

Meneghini, R., Packer, A. L. (2007). Is there science beyond English? Initiatives to increase the quality and visibility of non-English publications might help to break down language barriers in scientific communication. *EMBO Reports, 8,* 112–116.

Moher, D., Schulz, K. F., & Altman, D. (2001). The CONSORT statement: Revised recommendations for improving the quality of reports of parallel-group randomized trials. *Journal of the American Medical Association, 285,* 1987–1991.

Nayan, S., Gupta, M. K., & Sommer, D. D. (2011). Evaluating smoking cessation interventions and cessation rates in cancer patients: A systematic review and meta-analysis. *ISRN Oncology,* 849023.

Ogilve, D., Egan, M., Hamilton, V., & Petticrew, M. (2005). Systematic review of health effects of social interventions: 2. Best available evidence: How low should you go? *Journal of Epidemiology and Community Health, 59,* 886–892.

Oxford English Dictionary (OED) Online. (2012). Evidence (http://www.oed.com/view/Entry/65368?rskey=AJuEt8&result=1&isAdvanced=false#eid).

U.S. Department of Health and Human Services. (2011). Patient Protection and Affordable Care Act (PPACA) (http://www.healthcare.gov/law/index.html).

Peters-Klimm, F., Muller-Tasch, T., Schellberg, D., Remppis, A., Barth A., Holzapfel, N., et al. (2008). Guideline adherence for pharmacotherapy of chronic systolic heart failure in general practice: A closer look on evidence-based therapy. *Clinical Research in Cardiology, 97,* 244–252.

Petticrew, M., & Roberts, H. (2003). Evidence hierarchies and typologies: Horses for courses. *Journal of Epidemiology and Community Health, 57,* 527–529.

Powell, H. P., Doig, E., Hackley, B., Leslie, M. S., & Tillman, S. (2012). The midwifery two-step: A study on evidence-based midwifery practice. *Journal of Midwifery and Women's Health, 57,* 454–460.

National Center for Biotechnology Information, U.S. National Library of Medicine. (2012). PubMED health (http://www.ncbi.nlm.nih.gov/pubmedhealth).

Ramirez, P., Bassi, G. L., & Torres, A. (2012). Measures to prevent nosocomial infections during mechanical ventilation. *Current Opinion in Critical Care*, 18, 86–92.

Rapp, C. A., Etzel-Wise, D., Marty, D., Coffman, M., Corlson, L., Asher, D., et al. (2010). Barriers to Evidence-based practice in a implementation: results of a qualitative study. *Community Mental Health Journal*, 46, 112–118.

Reigle, B. S., Stevens, K. R., Belcher, J. V., Hugh, M. M., McGuire, E., & Mals, D. (2008). Evidence-based practice and the road to magnet status. *Journal of Nursing Administration*, 38, 97–102.

Rogers, E. M. (2003). *Diffusion of innovation*. (5th ed.). New York: Simon & Schuster.

Rosenberg, W., & Donald, A. (1995). Evidence-based medicine: An approach to clinical problem-solving. *British Medical Journal*, 310, 1122–1126.

Sackett, D. L., Rosenberg, W. M., Gray, J. A., Haynes, R. B., & Richardson, W. S. (1996). Evidence-based medicine: What it is and what it isn't. *British Medical Journal*, 312, 71–72.

Sackett, D. L., Strauss, S. E., Richardson, W. S., Rosenberg, W., & Haynes, R. B. (2000). *Evidence-based medicine: How to practice and teach EBM* (2nd ed.). London: Churchill-Livingstone.

Salvatore, S., Salvatore, S., Cattoni, E., Siesto, G., Serati, M., Sorice, P., et al. (2011). Urinary tract infections in women. *European Journal of Obstetrics, Gynecology and Reproductive Biology*, 156, 131–136.

Schlosser, R. W. (2007). Appraising the quality of systematic reviews (http://www.ncddr.org/kt/products/focus/focus17/index.html).

Slaunwhite, J. M., Smith, S. M., Fleming, M. T., Strang, R., & Lockhart, C. (2009). Increasing vaccination rates among health care workers using unit champions as a motivator. *Canadian Journal of Infection Control*, 24, 159–164.

Smith, M. B. (1956). Editorial. *Journal of Abnormal and Social Psychology*, 52, 4.

Smith-Strom, H., & Nortvedt, M. W. (2008). Evaluation of evidence-based methods used to teach nursing students to critically appraise evidence. *Journal of Nursing Education*, 47, 372–375.

Stapleton, A. E., Dziura, J., Hooton, T. M., Cox, M. E., Yarova-Yarovaya, Y., Chen, S., et al. (2012). Recurrent urinary tract infection and urinary Escherichia coli in women ingesting cranberry juice daily: A randomized controlled trial. *Mayo Clinic Proceedings*, 87, 143–150.

Stetler, C. B. (2003). Role of the organization in translating research into evidence-based practice. *Outcomes Management*, 7, 97–103.

Stiffler, D., & Cullen, D. (2010). Evidence-based practice for nurse practitioner students: a competency-based teaching framework. *Journal of Professional Nursing*, 26, 272–277.

Stolberg, H. O., Norman, G., & Trop, I. (2004). Randomized controlled trials. *American Journal of Roentgenology*, 183, 1539–1544.

Streptomycin treatment of pulmonary tuberculosis. (1948). *British Medical Journal*, 2, 769–782.

Sutton, A. J., Duvall, S. J., Tweedie, R. L., Abrams, K. R., & Jones, D. R. (2000). Empirical assessment of effects of publication bias in meta-analysis. *British Medical Journal*, 320, 1574–1577.

Tablan, O., Anderson, L., Besser, R., Bridges, C., & Hajjeh, R.; CDC; Healthcare Infection Control Practices Advisory Committee. (2004). Guidelines for preventing health-care-associated pneumonia, 2003. *MMWR Recommendations and Reports*, 53(RR-3), 1–36.

Taggart, E., McKenna, J., Stoelting, J., Kirkbride, G., & Mottar, M. (2012). More than skin deep: Developing a hospital-wide wound ostomy continence unit champions. *Journal of Wound, Ostomy and Continence Nursing*, 39, 385–390.

Triano, J. J. (2008). What constitutes evidence for best practice? *Journal of Manipulative and Physiological Therapeutics*, 31, 637–643.

Trinite, T., Cherry, C. L., & Marion, L. (2009). The U.S. Preventive Services Task Force: An evidence-based prevention resource for nurse practitioners. *Journal of the American Academy of Nurse Practitioners*, 21, 301–306.

U.S. National Library of Medicine. (2012). MEDLINE (http://www.ncbi.nlm.nih.gov/pubmed).

von Elm, E., Eggar, M., Altman, D. G., Egger, M., Pocock, S. J., Gotzsche, P. C., et al. (2007). Strengthening the Reporting of Observational Studies in Epidemiology (STROBE) statement: Guidelines for reporting observational studies. Strengthening the reporting of observational studies in epidemiology (STROBE) statement: guideline for reporting observational studies. *British Medical Journal*, 335, 806–808.

van Rijswijk, L., & Gray, M. (2012). Evidence, research and clinical practice: A patient-centered framework for progress in wound care. *Journal of Wound, Ostomy and Continence Nursing*, 39, 35–44.

Webster, B. S., Courtney, T. K., Huang, Y. H., Matz, S., & Christiani, D. C. (2005). Physicians' initial management of acute low back pain versus evidence-based guidelines. Influence of sciatica. *Journal of General Internal Medicine*, 20, 1132–1135.

Weiner, B. J., Amick, H., & Lee, S. Y. (2008). Conceptualization and measurement of corporate readiness for change. A review of the literature in health services research and other fields. *Medical Care Research and Review*, 65, 379–436.

West, S., King, V., Carey, T. S., Lohr, K. N., McKoy, N., Sutton, S. F., et al. (2002). *Systems to rate the strength of scientific evidence*. Evidence Report–Technology Assessment No. 47. AHRQ Publication 02-E016. Rockville, MD: Agency for Healthcare Research and Quality.

West, E. (2001). Management matters: The link between hospital organization and quality of patent care. *Quality Health Care*, 10, 40–48.

Wilkins, R. J., & Mullins, D. (2011). "Ten commandments" for conducting comparative effectiveness research using "real-world data." *Journal of Managed Care Pharmacy*, 17, S10–S15.

Wip, C., & Napolitano, L. (2009). Bundles to prevent ventilator-associated pneumonia: How valuable are they? *Current Opinion in Infectious Disease*, 22, 159–168.

Wound, Ostomy, and Continence Nurses Society. (2003). *Guideline: Prevention and management of pressure ulcers*. Cherry Hill, NJ: Wound, Ostomy, and Continence Nurses Society.

Yoshika, A. (1998). Use of randomization in the Medical Research Council's clinical trial of streptomycin in pulmonary tuberculosis in the 1940s. *British Medical Journal*, 317, 1220–1223.

Mary Fran Tracy • Charlene M. Hanson

CHAPTER CONTENTS

Mmore than ever before, the flattening of the world through global interactions (Friedman, 2006), the rate with which change occurs, and the unsettled status of health care make leadership skills a necessity for successful advanced practice nurses (APNs). Leadership is a core competency of advanced practice nursing, but the concept has some unique characteristics in the APN context. Our conceptualization of APN leadership involves three distinct defining characteristics—mentoring, innovation, and activism. Calls for systems redesign and transformation (Institute of Medicine [IOM], 2011, 2001, 2000; Institute for Healthcare Improvement [IHI], 2011; Leape, Berwick, Clancy, et al., 2009), changes in health professional education (American Association of Colleges of

Nursing [AACN], 2006), and core interdisciplinary competencies for health professionals (Canadian Interprofessional Health Collaborative [CIHC], 2010; Greiner & Knebel, 2003; Health Sciences Institute, 2005; Interprofessional Collaborative Initiative [IPEC], 2011) have important implications for the leadership competency in APN education and practice. To provide leadership in individual patient care situations, APNs must be able to assess the clinical microsystems in which they provide care, understand the macrosystems that influence the smaller systems, determine the need for redesign to improve safety, quality, and reliability, and evaluate the results. In short, systems leaders must be able to identify the need for innovation and change and implement strategies to achieve it. In partnership with others, APNs craft approaches to evaluate, reassess, and implement systems redesign and innovation.

APNs exercise leadership in four key domains—in clinical practice environments, in the nursing profession at the systems level, and in the health policy arena. APNs may exercise leadership activities at local, regional, and/ or national levels; their activities may range from taking a stand on behalf of an individual patient to advocating for a change in national health policy. The leadership competency depends on and interacts with other APN competencies. Specific leadership skills should be discussed, nurtured, and developed during graduate education through refinement of communication skills, supported risk taking, reflective learning, and interactions with nurse leaders, mentors, and role models. The recommended movement of APN education to the Doctorate of Nursing Practice (DNP) has implications for the APN's leadership competency (AACN, 2004). For example, the DNP essential requiring expertise in systems leadership means that the organizational and professional leadership components of advanced practice nursing curricula will need to expand (AACN, 2006).

The purposes of this chapter are to describe the defining characteristics and domains of the leadership competency, provide useful literature and resources on leadership and change, describe characteristics of effective leaders, identify obstacles to effective leadership, and discuss strategies for developing leadership skills. This chapter will help APNs define their need for leadership skills and develop a plan for acquiring the necessary skills appropriate to their particular positions and professional goals.

Context in Which Advanced Practice Nurses Exercise Leadership Competency

Leading in today's health care environment is a task of unprecedented complexity for APNs, administrators, and policymakers. To understand the need for APN leadership across the four domains, it is important to understand the factors that are shaping this competency in the twenty-first century. The IOM has issued a number of reports, all of which call for a radical redesign and transformation of the health care system. The groundbreaking report by the IOM, *The Future of Nursing: Leading Change, Advancing Health* (2011) states that is essential for nurses to be full partners and leaders in the transformation of health care. In addition, the education of those in the health professions is being transformed. Such changes have not occurred quickly, in part because they require a significant rethinking of how care is delivered, the roles of patients and education of

providers, effective channels for diffusing innovation, how health care is financed, and which provider activities count and should be reimbursed (Greiner & Knebel, 2003; see Chapters 19 and 22).

Health Care System Transformation

The IOM's call to transform the health care system is predicated on six national quality aims—safety, effectiveness, patient-centeredness, timeliness, efficiency, and equity (IOM, 2001). This far-reaching report has led to numerous assessments and initiatives. For example, the IOM noted that nursing homes are at high risk for the occurrence of adverse events, yet numerous institutional barriers to reporting these events still exist, such as long-standing cultures around naming and blaming individuals rather than exploring gaps in systems of care and organizational culture (Wagner, Capezuti, & Ouslander, 2006). Leaders have come to realize that errors occur because of a continuum of reasons. David Marx, a systems safety engineer, has developed a model to encourage leaders to use open communication and accountability at all levels to optimize organizational safety (Just Culture Community, 2012). Leaders can use these principles to facilitate the evaluation of errors, near misses, and questionable behavior to determine root causes of situations in which employee behavior does not match organizational values. Causes for these situations can range from organizational culture to defective systems and processes to bad choices on the part of employees. The Agency for Healthcare Research and Quality (AHRQ) has highlighted a number of innovative examples of health care organizations using Just Culture principles to improve response to errors (AHRQ, 2010).

The IHI launched a campaign to save 100,000 lives from medical error (Berwick, Caulkins, McCannon, et al., 2006; Patient Safety and Quality Health Care, 2005). This campaign was so successful, with an estimated 122,000 lives saved, that a new goal was promoted to save 5 million lives, which has had a significant impact on patient outcomes through the reduction of morbidity and mortality (IHI, 2007, updated 2012). Many health care systems are participating in these efforts to improve safety and quality, such as Magnet recognition or participating in the IHI campaign. A recent survey has found that opinion leaders would like nurses to have more influence in the transformation of health care in areas such as reducing medical errors, improving the quality of care, and promoting wellness (Blizzard, Khoury, & McMurray, 2010). These leaders suggest that nurses should take on more leadership roles to have their voices heard. APNs not only have a stake in these efforts, but also have the clinical expertise and leadership that can ensure success.

Redesign of Health Professional Education

Greiner and Knebel (2003), the Health Sciences Institute (2005), and the AACN (2006) have identified competencies that health professionals must have, including APNs, and many of these relate to the leadership competency. The Josiah Macy Jr. Foundation, in a 2010 national conference, promulgated recommendations concerning how health care providers need to be trained to meet the needs of primary health care (Cronenwett & Dzau, 2010; Pohl, Hanson, Newland, et al., 2010). A review of research shows that there is no clear data yet regarding the impact that interprofessional education has had on provider practice and outcomes for patients; however, there is enough indication of potential that further rigorous research is warranted (Reeves, Zwarenstein, Goldman, et al., 2009). Although the recommendations for leadership competencies affect primarily educators and the curricula that they design, they have significant implications for APNs already practicing and for the environments in which APN students learn.

Interdisciplinary Competencies

The IOM has identified five competencies that all health professionals must possess if the redesign and transformation of the U.S. health care system is to be realized: provide patient-centered care, work in interdisciplinary teams, use evidence-based practices, apply quality improvement principles, and use informatics (Greiner & Knebel, 2003). The Health Sciences Institute (2005) has published a model of Continuous Chronic Care and identified five levels of change. At the provider level of change, they identified three major competencies: promote health and prevent disease; manage diseases and disease impacts; and promote consumer independence and life quality. More recently, there has been a resurgence of interest in major competencies to encourage interprofessional collaboration for health care providers (CIHC, 2010; IPEC, 2011). This movement, led by our Canadian colleagues, has an important impact for health care in the United States, and specifically for APNs. APN leaders will participate in creating environments in which these interdisciplinary competencies are not merely supported but can flourish. When APNs and others can implement these competencies fully, the transformation will be underway.

Advanced Practice Nurse Competencies

In the AACN's *The Essentials of Doctoral Education for Advanced Nursing Practice* (2006), several specific competencies relate to leadership for all DNP graduates, including APNs. Of the eight essentials, four inform the leadership competency—organizational and system leadership for quality improvement and systems thinking, clinical scholarship and analytic methods, information systems and technology and patient care technology for the improvement and transformation of health care, and clinical prevention and population health for improving the nation's health. Recent core competencies by the National Association of Clinical Nurse Specialists (NACNS, 2010) and National Organization of Nurse Practitioner Faculties (NONPF, 2012) also address leadership requirements of clinical nurse specialists (CNSs) and nurse practitioners (NPs). The reader will note that several of these essentials and competencies are consistent with the competencies being expected of all health professionals just described.

In summary, numerous contextual and educational factors that require APN leadership have been identified in calls for the redesign and transformation of the health care system. Certain themes are apparent—in particular, patient-centeredness (see Chapter 7), teamwork (see Chapter 12), quality improvement (Cronenwett, Sherwood, Pohl, et al., 2009; Sherwood, 2010), the use of information technology (IT), and complexity. These factors must be considered in APN graduate and continuing education so that APNs acquire the knowledge and skills they need to lead effectively.

Leadership Domains of Advanced Practice Nurses

Although the need for leadership in health care settings is well recognized (Aduddell & Dorman, 2010; Carlson, Klakovich, Broscious, et al., 2011; NACNS, 2011, 2004; NONPF, 2012), the topic has not been well studied, and research on effective leadership is needed (Falk-Rafael, 2005). Not all APNs are comfortable with the idea of being leaders, but leadership is not an optional activity. As noted, the APN leadership competency can be conceptualized as occurring in four primary domains or areas: in clinical practice with patients and staff, within professional organizations, within health care systems, and in health policymaking arenas. The extent to which individual APNs choose to lead in each of these areas depends on patients' needs, APNs' personal characteristics, interests, and commitments, institutional or organizational priorities and opportunities, and priority health policy issues in nursing as a whole and within one's specialty (Carroll, 2005; Leavitt, Chaffee, & Vance, 2007). There is considerable overlap in the knowledge and skills needed across the four domains; for example, developing skills in the clinical leadership domain will enable the APN to be more effective at the policy level.

Clinical Leadership

Clinical leadership focuses first on the patient and his or her needs, ensuring that quality patient care is achieved. Clinical leadership is a foundational component to attaining and maintaining a productive environment in which safe and excellent care is provided and professionals assume self-accountability (Murphy, Quillinan, & Carolan, 2009). It occurs when APNs learn with and from others about how to build appropriate working relationships with health care team members, how to instill confidence in patients and colleagues, and how to problem-solve as part of a team (Bally, 2007). APN leaders are role models and mentors who empower patients and colleagues. They propose and implement change strategies that improve patient care and enhance others' perceptions of the value of advanced practice nursing. Some clinical leadership skills are part of the competencies of consultation (see Chapter 9) and collaboration (see Chapter 12) and are portrayed in the exemplars in the role chapters (see Part III) as well. The most common clinical leadership roles APNs can expect to play are those of advocate (for patient, family, staff, or colleagues), group leader, and systems leader. APNs may advocate for a particular patient or family, as when an acute care nurse practitioner (ACNP) advocates with the attending physician about the need for a better explanation of the side effects of an elective surgery. Writing articles and presenting talks on clinical topics are other ways of expressing clinical leadership and influencing others.

Group leadership may be informal, as when an APN agrees to coordinate multiple referrals for a patient with complex care needs or has expertise in a particular clinical problem such as pain management and assumes a team leadership role because of this expertise. APNs may also have more formal leadership responsibilities; for example, an APN may lead a weekly team meeting or agree to convene a group and lead the development of a new practice protocol to bring care into line with new standards. One function of the APN leader is to motivate colleagues and facilitate their use of new knowledge and/or the adoption of new practices.

APNs often exercise leadership to ensure that clinical problems are addressed by administrative leaders at a systems level. Brown (1989) called this role the "shuttle diplomat" because APNs move between clinical and administrative arenas, interpreting the needs of one to the other. Advancing clinical excellence requires financial, creative, and political skills to promote innovative care and collaborate with others (Murphy, Quillinan, & Carolan, 2009). Having these additional skills improves the success of shuttle diplomacy and the compelling translation of ideas between distinct perspectives. APNs recognize the clinical problems related to their specialty that require attention or intervention from the larger (macro) system of which they are a part. For example, when a CNS called a patient to learn why he had not kept his appointment at the heart failure clinic, she learned that he could not find parking nearby because of hospital construction, did not know that a shuttle would take him from the satellite lot to the clinic, and did not have the energy to walk from the satellite lot. The CNS knew that this could be a problem for other clinic patients and worked with administrators to make sure patients had knowledge of and access to the resources that were needed and available. She understood the clinical implications (patients might experience more complications requiring readmission) and systems implications (e.g., lower quality, increased risks for patients, higher costs, missed appointments) of construction-related, missed appointments for her patient population.

APNs who lead patient care teams well and who perform effectively as shuttle diplomats find that their interdisciplinary leadership skills are in demand. Covey (1989) has indicated that he considers interdisciplinary leadership a high-level skill. For example, an APN who was successful in leading a quality improvement (QI) initiative to improve care of asthmatics admitted to the hospital was invited to chair a national task force of health care professionals developing practice guidelines for the treatment of asthma. The ability to provide clinical interdisciplinary leadership requires a firm grasp of clinical and professional issues and differences within nursing while responding to the challenges of other disciplines and the larger society. As APNs gain skill in clinical leadership, they develop the attributes needed to lead in other domains.

Professional Leadership

Mentorship, empowerment, and active participation in organizations are particularly important within the professional domain. First, to be an effective leader, the APN must be able to collaborate with colleagues (see Chapter 12). Second, they must be able to recognize situations in which they themselves need mentoring and in which colleagues can benefit from being mentored and empowered. In the professional domain, APN leaders facilitate the growth of other nurses.

Mentoring needs of the APN change over time and more than one mentor may be needed as different aspects of the role are developed. APNs agree that mentorship in professional development is helpful (Doerksen, 2010). Novice or experienced APNs seeking new challenges look for mentors who will foster their professional development. A prospective protégé may recognize and seek an APN's guidance on clinical or professional development issues. Sometimes, it is the APN who recognizes a potential protégé and offers her or him opportunities to learn and grow. APNs have a responsibility to mentor and prepare the next generation of advanced practice clinicians.

Professional leadership is also exercised by participation in professional organizations. Novice APNs may begin by seeking membership on a committee of a local or national nursing or interdisciplinary organization. As APNs become more experienced, they may seek opportunities to apply the leadership skills that they have learned in their work organizations to their professional organizations. Most APNs are members of one or more nursing and interdisciplinary organizations. These memberships provide myriad leadership opportunities including organizing continuing education offerings, presenting at national conferences, chairing a committee, and running for the board of directors. In these situations, APNs exercise more choice as to whether and when they will participate in leadership activities than in their employee roles.

Professional leadership begins at the grassroots level and proceeds upward to state, national, and international levels. To acquire leadership skills and experience, it is helpful for novice APNs to become involved in the leadership and committee work of local advanced practice nursing coalitions and organizations and move into state and regional leadership roles as they develop their style and strengths as APN leaders. The ability to place APN leaders in key local, state, and national positions is critical to the visibility and credibility of APNs and to the establishment of their roles within nursing and the larger health care community. In addition to informal leadership development opportunities, there are also formal programs in which APNs can develop the skills to lead in positions such as board membership (Carlson, Klakovich, Broscious, et al., 2011).

Systems Leadership

Systems leadership means leading at the organizational or delivery system level—a skill that requires a multidimensional understanding of systems. Within health care organizations, APNs may lead clinical teams, chair committees, chair or serve as members of boards, manage projects, and direct other initiatives aimed at improving patient care and/or the clinical practice of nurses and other professionals. Systems leadership overlaps the professional domain in situations in which leaders are formally or informally elected or appointed to positions of authority or power within defined organizations and groups. For example, APNs may identify an increase in the rate of patient falls

and create a task force to evaluate the problem and design corrective interventions. A critical care CNS or ACNP may initiate interdisciplinary rounds to monitor patients on mechanical ventilation and gather data on clinical variables such as complication rate and time to weaning. APNs may be asked to participate in or lead standing or ad hoc interdisciplinary committees (e.g., medical credentialing, ethics, institutional review board, pharmacy and therapeutics) to ensure that a nursing perspective will be articulated. APNs may be asked by administrators to participate in organizational reengineering or other activities aimed at improving the environment in which nurses practice. APNs, whether in a line or supervisory position, should have the authority to provide systems leadership related to the delivery of clinical care by virtue of their clinical credibility and specific APN job responsibilities. Education strategies for systems leadership are a core responsibility for APN education (Thompson & Nelson-Martin, 2011).

Although most APNs will not be entrepreneurs, they need to be aware that the characteristics of successful entrepreneurs are desirable and valued in systems leaders. The term *entrepreneurial leadership* refers to those leaders who go outside of traditional employment systems to create new opportunities to exercise their special abilities (Shirey, 2004). When these leaders use the entrepreneurial skills of innovation and risk taking, and assume responsibility for achieving specific targets in an organization, they are termed *intrapreneurs*. Because this leadership style is consistent with the call for health care system redesign, it is worth reviewing characteristics associated with entrepreneurial leadership. Shirey (2007b) has stated that nurse entrepreneurs have a desire to make a difference and see opportunities in situations in which others see barriers or challenges. Blanchard and colleagues (2007) have developed tools for leaders to assess their entrepreneurial strengths and have identified 20 attributes of entrepreneurs (e.g., resourceful, purposeful, risk taker, problem solver, visionary, innovative, communicative, determined). Universities that prepare APNs are offering coursework on innovation, entrepreneurship, and out of the box thinking to prepare entrepreneurial and intrapreneurial APN leaders (Shirey, 2007a). APNs frequently underestimate their transferable skills, which can be used in entrepreneurial or intrapreneurial opportunities (Shirey, 2009). Recognition of those skills will assist the intrapreneurial APN to build a case for how their services can assist the organization in achieving innovative clinical excellence (Shirey, 2007b). Entrepreneurial leadership skills are illustrated in Exemplar 11-1, which also illustrates the evolving nature of the advanced practice nursing leadership competency and how it expands in breadth over time.

◉ EXEMPLAR 11-1 **Entrepreneurial Leadership in Advanced Practice Nursing**

Ellie's dream and goal on entering a graduate family NP program was to open a practice in the rural community where she and her family lived. She used her health policy course requirements to conduct a needs assessment and to set up interviews with the regional hospital to propose an outreach clinic that would be sponsored by the hospital (entrepreneurial leadership [EL]; health policy leadership [HPL]). She planned to see patients independently and would contract with her physician preceptor to visit once a week for collaboration and to see patients who were beyond her scope of practice. Ellie's entrepreneurial leadership skills allowed her to negotiate with the managed care owner of the hospital and with the medical staff, and the outreach clinic was established. Over time, her community-based practice was viewed as a model of excellence for other NPs, and she served as a mentor and role model for many (clinical leadership [CL]; professional leadership [PL]). As her clinic gained prominence, Ellie was nominated by the governor to represent APNs and rural interests on the state board of nursing (HPL, PL). She also wrote a column for the local weekly newspaper about prevention and wellness.

After 3 years in practice, Ellie wanted to use extra space in her clinic to broaden the services she offered, so she set up a meeting with members of a midwifery group in an adjoining town to invite them to use her office as a satellite clinic once a week. She also invited two CNSs who were seeing mental health and oncology patients in the area to do the same (EL; systems leadership [SL]). Her vision and excellent communication skills offered new alliances with other APNs and brought new services for rural patients. The visibility of her successful clinic led to her nomination to become a member of the National Rural Health Advisory Committee, which advises the Secretary of Health and Human Services on matters of rural health care. This nationally based committee work allowed Ellie to use her well-developed leadership skills to influence the health care system (HPL, PL).

For more on entrepreneurs and intrapreneurs, see Chapter 19.

Willingness to Name Difficult Organizational Problems

A common human characteristic in organizations is to operate around the periphery of problems and not in the heart of them. It is a rare leader who directly acknowledges and names dysfunctional activities that are deeply embedded in organizations. A key role of APNs is to name, in a nonblaming way, what everybody is thinking but not saying. Collaborative leadership brings problems into the light without the burden of having to solve it. In this way, the APN is inviting others into the conversation for a better understanding of blocks to true collaborative practice and state of the art patient-centered care. For example, if office staff thinks that they are not empowered to make scheduling and patient flow work better, the APN can name this problem and invite members of the organization to explore it further to see whether it resonates with others as being true and to explore how it may be affecting the practice. The willingness for APNs to enter into these courageous conversations is a key skill set to effective collaboration. When there are high-stakes issues with high emotions, it is tempting to focus instead on peripheral issues.

Here is another example. For years, a primary care practice has had a significant number of complaints about waiting times to see a physician who was excellent, but older. She was always behind in her appointment times and could not keep pace with the demands of primary care. This created conflict in the waiting room and with support staff as patients frequently waited more than 2 hours to be seen for a scheduled appointment. The newly hired APN was able to name the problem and the impact on the entire system, including paying overtime for medical assistants to work late. This naming of a problem that had been going on for years greatly relieved the organization and everybody effected by it who had not felt empowered to speak up. Once the problem and its dimensions were defined, the physician became aware of the impact that these long waits had on the entire office, as well as her patients. The team came up with an approach that allowed this particular physician to have longer appointments and, soon after, she retired from practice. Although initially she felt defensive, the manner in which the APN raised the quality concerns made it safe because it was always in the context of patient care.

APNs can apprentice themselves to entering these conversations by naming troubling dynamics or environmental threats. This is truly advanced practice nursing as we apply the skills of assessment in the organizational realm. One can not solve a patient's problem without having its dimensions clearly defined. The same holds true for organizational leadership and the need to foster more collaboration and unity at the systems level. This type of acknowledgment of issues and willingness to name problems (real or potential) without having to solve them is a powerful way for APNs to model true leadership.

Health Policy Leadership

Although some APNs may not see themselves as being particularly interested in or talented at political advocacy, all APNs have a vested interest in policymaking that affects nursing generally and advanced practice nursing specifically. This domain is becoming increasingly important as more laws and regulations are enacted with implications for APN practice (see Chapters 21 and 22). APNs should be aware of and must often respond to local, state, and national policymaking efforts likely to affect these laws and regulations (Donelan, Buerhaus, DesRoches, et al., 2010; Gilliss, 2011; NACNS, 2011). To be a leader at the level of health policy requires an ability to analyze health care systems, an understanding of the personal qualities associated with effective leadership, and the skill to use these understandings to act strategically.

Across these four domains of leadership, APNs use their clinical expertise, team building, and collaborative skills to build community around shared values such as patient-centeredness and commitment to quality. They also build the capability of individuals and systems to respond promptly and efficiently to meet patient needs and improve outcomes (Spross, 2001). The defining characteristics of APN leadership—mentoring and empowerment, innovation and change agency, and activism—may be apparent in all four domains, but the emphasis accorded to each one depends on the particular leadership demands. By outlining these various leadership domains early in the chapter, we want to encourage readers to reflect on the leadership opportunities that they encounter, consider those that align with their clinical interests and personal characteristics, and begin to develop a leadership portfolio. We hope to challenge readers to rethink their ideas about leadership and to integrate a personally meaningful concept of leadership into their identity as an APN.

Leadership: Definitions, Models, and Concepts

The nursing, sociology, and business literatures are rich sources of leadership definitions, models, and concepts that can help APNs develop as effective and dynamic leaders.

Definitions of Leadership

Contemporary definitions of leadership generally fit into one of two categories, transformational (Vance & Larson,

2002) or situational (Grohar-Murray & DiCroce, 1992). Barker (1994) has defined the term *transformational leadership* as a process whereby "the purposes of the leader and follower become fused, creating unity, wholeness and a collective purpose" (p. 83). Transformational leadership can lead to changes in values, attitudes, perceptions, and/or behaviors on the part of the leader and the follower and lays the groundwork for further positive change. Thus, transformational leadership occurs when people interact in ways that inspire higher levels of motivation and morality among participants. How do leaders do this? Transformational leaders analyze a situation to understand the particular leadership needs and goals; they use this information, together with their interpersonal skills, to motivate, stimulate, share with, conciliate, and satisfy their followers in an interdependent interactional exchange. DePree (1989) has described leadership as an art form that frees (empowers) people "to do what is required of them in the most effective and humane way possible" (p. 1) and contended that contemporary leadership may be viewed simply as a process of moving the self and others toward a shared vision that becomes a shared reality. Successful transformational leadership is relational, driven by a common goal or purpose, and satisfies the needs of leader and follower. It is the leadership style often associated with effective change agents. Schwartz and colleagues (2011) have studied the effects of transformational leadership on the Magnet designation for hospitals. Other authors who have described a transformational approach to leadership include Wang and associates (2012), who studied transformational leadership with Chinese nurses, Heifetz (1994), Secretan (1999, 2003), Senge (2006), and Covey (1989).

The term *situational leadership* is defined as the interaction between an individual's leadership style and the features of the environment or situation in which he or she is operating. Leadership styles are not fixed and may vary based on the environment. Situational leadership depends on particular circumstances, with leaders and followers assuming interchangeable roles according to environmental demands (Fiedler, Chermers, & Mahar, 1976; Lynch, McCormack, & McCance, 2011; Solman, 2010; Stogdill, 1948). The role of follower is important to any discussion about APN leadership because APNs will find themselves in both roles at a given time. Grohar-Murray and DiCroce (1992) and DePree (1989) enlarged on this idea and used the term *roving leadership* to describe a participatory process that legitimizes the situational leadership of empowered followers through the support and approval of the hierarchical leader. This notion of leadership is relevant because APNs' work in collaborative health care teams requires that the roles of leader and follower be interchangeable to meet the complex needs of the patient.

Inherent in this discussion of transformational and situational leadership is the importance of vision. The APN as a leader, with a vision of collaboration among health care team members, may facilitate an atmosphere that supports individuals (followers) to assume leadership roles in various situations. The APN does not cease being the leader by empowering colleagues to appropriately assume a leadership role. In fact, across the domains of leadership, APNs must be capable of both sharing a vision and sharing power, issues discussed later in this chapter.

Leadership Models That Lead to Transformation

APNs can draw on numerous models of leadership and change processes to inform their leadership development. Leadership models or frameworks that include the following concepts seem most applicable in these unsettled times:

- Empowerment of colleagues and followers
- Engagement of stakeholders within and outside nursing or one's agency in the change process
- Provision of individual and system support during change initiatives

Leadership models that informed this chapter are summarized in Table 11-1. Models are organized by their focus on transformational leadership or change. The many national initiatives calling for system redesign means that change, transformation, and uncertainty are constants. We believe that the models in Table 11-1 have the most promise for helping APNs survive and thrive under these circumstances because individuals and the organizations in which they work are considered. Table 11-1 highlights elements of each model that relate to APN leadership. Readers are encouraged to consult original sources for full descriptions of each model.

The Fifth Discipline

The Fifth Discipline (Senge, 1990, 2006) includes concepts that will be useful to APNs as they strive to master the APN leadership competency. Whereas certain people may have innate gifts for leadership, others can develop these proficiencies through practice and commitment to the task. To become an effective leader, Senge's definition implies that one must practice and commit to lifelong learning. In this case, APN leaders are constantly striving to become effective team members who empower others and facilitate change to create effective learning organizations.

Senge outlines five disciplines or practices associated with leadership; the framework provides a structure APNs can use to understand leadership and change within complex structures and environments. The five disciplines (Senge, 1990, 2006) are as follows:

- **Personal mastery.** This is the act of continually redefining and clarifying one's personal vision, refocusing energies, maintaining objectivity, and committing to personal goals and objectives. The importance of personal growth and development is vital to attaining the leadership competency.
- **Mental models.** These are the images that influence how one views the world and attains new insights. Leaders must be aware of their mental models and be willing to examine them and hold them up for inquiry and scrutiny by others. This discipline speaks to the need for clear vision about advanced practice nursing and the ability to defend this viewpoint.
- **Shared vision.** This refers to the leader's ability to help a team develop and sustain a common image of what the team seeks to create in the future; it is the ability to share a vision with others rather than dictate that vision. The ability to empower others to share the dream and implement change is critical to this discipline.
- **Team learning.** This is the ability to suspend one's own assumptions, listen to other viewpoints, and genuinely think together.
- **Systems thinking.** This is the fifth discipline, a framework for leadership based on the ability to see the whole picture rather than the isolated parts. It helps us see how our own actions influence what is happening in the larger system (health care). This discipline is an important concept for APNs, who must be able to view advanced practice within the overall context of health care as one member of a team of professionals and patients.

Senge and colleagues (1999) have noted that challenges are inherent in the change process, challenges such as delays, competition, and fragmented management that thwarts new productive relationships. By nature, change is dynamic, nonlinear, and characterized by complexity. Senge and colleagues (1999) have defined the term *systems citizens* as persons who have a perspective and an awareness of the entire world rather than just the local areas in which they live. Catastrophes such as Hurricane Katrina and bridge collapses may not touch us directly, but they do influence our thinking about how to make changes in health care and safety. Unexpected and unplanned events, large and small, can make it difficult to predict the trajectory that a change initiative will take and highlight the importance of a flexible, responsive leadership style. Such a style fosters cohesion, collaboration, and communication among team members, enabling

TABLE 11-1   Useful Models of Transformational Leadership and Change

Author (Year)	Title or Model	Relevant Concepts	APN Use
Senge (1990, 2006)	*The Fifth Discipline*	Describes five actions or processes that characterize effective teams and organizations that manage change well: • Personal mastery • Awareness of mental models • Shared vision • Team learning • Systems thinking	APNs can use these concepts to identify: • Personal leadership goals • Strengths and needs of the teams and organizations with whom they work • Strategies to enhance team development and collaboration
Covey (2006)	*The Seven Habits of Highly Effective People*	Development of a personal mission statement to live by as one develops independence and interdependence. The seven characteristics that foster acquisition of leadership skills are: • Be proactive. Take the initiative, choose your response. • Begin with the end in mind. Define success. • Put first things first; personally manage yourself. • Think win-win, with a willingness to cooperate. • Seek first to understand and then to be understood. • Synergize; the whole is greater than the sum of its parts. • Sharpen the saw; renew your physical, mental, spiritual, and social dimensions.	APNs can use these characteristics to: • Acquire leadership skills • Attain interdependence by fully incorporating one's personal mission statement into practice • Use influence and inspiration as a creative catalyst for change
Nelson et al. (2002)	Microsystems in health care: High-performing clinical units	Studied 20 varied microsystems; identified nine common success characteristics associated with delivery of high-quality, cost-efficient care: • Leadership • Culture • Organizational support • Patient focus • Staff focus • Interdependence of care team • Information and information technology • Process improvement • Performance patterns	APNs can use these characteristics to assess one's system and identify gaps in and opportunities for leadership.
Massoud et al. (2006)	A Framework for Spread	Model evolved by the IHI to understand phases of successful system change. Key elements: • Prepare for spread. • Establish aim for spread. • Develop an initial spread plan. • Execute and refine plan.	APNs can use ideas for each phase of spread. Also useful for: • Understanding the importance of leadership in planning for spread. • Detailing elements of the aim and initial plan for spread (addresses the who, what, when, where).
Cooperrider et al. (2008)	*Appreciative Inquiry Handbook*	Uses a 4D cycle to seek positive attributes to build on through conversations and relationships building rather than focusing on problem areas: • Discovery • Dream • Design • Destiny	APNs can use these concepts to: • Motivate and inspire colleagues to excellence in practice. • Develop partnerships to capitalize on positive attributes of individual team members to solve complex problems in health care.

them to approach problem identification and solutions with candor, commitment, and creativity.

The Seven Habits of Highly Effective People

Stephen Covey's 1989 best-seller presented personal and interdependent characteristics that foster acquisition of leadership skills. In creating a personal view of leadership, Covey suggested that the most effective way to "keep the end in mind" is to create a personal mission statement that becomes a standard to live by as one progresses to new levels of independence and subsequent interdependence. In Covey's model, interdependence is achieved only after one has defined and integrated this personal mission or standard into one's practice. He described attributes of those who lead from a philosophy of interdependence: listening twice as much as you speak, remaining trustworthy by never compromising honesty, maintaining a positive attitude, and keeping a sense of humor. Interdependence allows one to hear and understand the other person's viewpoint, leading to a synergistic or win-win level of communication. In 2004, Covey expanded on this leadership model by proposing an eighth habit—leaders need to find their voice and help others to find theirs. He noted that leaders at any level can use their inspiration and influence to overcome negativity and use creativity to move the organization to greatness; this type of leader can be a catalyst for change. Covey (2006) developed leadership ideas in light of managing people in the information age. A key concept in this update is that leaders must be aware that the ways in which they lead will influence workers' choices. He described five choices, ranging from rebel or quit to creative excitement. This can be considered an empowerment model; leadership of knowledge workers "will be characterized by those who find their own voice and who, regardless of their formal position, inspire others to find theirs" (p. 15).

Leadership Models That Address Systems Change and Innovation

Change is a constant in today's clinical environments. Efforts to transform the health care system are generally focused in three areas, diffusion of innovation, clinician behavior change, and patient behavior change. The reality is that change is messy and not always welcome, even when it seems straightforward. Leaders must be able to stay focused, listen, and manage multiple and changing contingencies. Since the call for redesign and transformation of the health care system, efforts to understand the messiness of systems redesign and transformation have redoubled. For example, an integrative review of diffusion and dissemination of innovations reveals why redesign and transformation are messy—they are exceedingly complex (Greenhalgh, Robert, MacFarlane, et al., 2004)!

Microsystems in Health Care: High-Performing Clinical Units

Nelson and colleagues (2002) have stated that clinical microsystems, defined as the front-line units in which patients and providers interface, are the foundation for providing safe and high-quality care within large organizations. Transforming care at the front-line unit is essential to optimizing care throughout the continuum. They studied the processes and methods of 20 high performing sites and identified nine characteristics that were related to high performance: leadership, organizational culture, macro-organizational support of microsystems, patient focus, staff focus, interdependence of the care team, information and IT, performance improvement, and performance patterns.

APNs practice at the patient-provider interface and their leadership can contribute greatly to the optimization of other successful characteristics. APNs are skilled at creating cohesive teams, identifying and advocating patient and staff needs, leading performance improvement efforts at the front-line interface, and contributing to a positive organizational culture.

Spread of Innovation

Massoud and colleagues (2006) have developed a model for IHI to address the difficulty in spreading effective innovation beyond the immediate environment. With today's imperative to implement best practices throughout health care, diffusion within and among health care organizations is key. Founded on Everett Rogers' definition of diffusion, this framework for spread is based on four main components—preparing for spread, establishing an aim for spread, developing an initial spread plan, and executing or refining the spread plan. Leadership is essential in preparing a plan to spread innovation. As a leader, the APN must take an active role, beginning with the preparation phase and continuing throughout implementation and maintenance of the plan. Identifying the target population, improvements to be made, and target time frame is the focus of establishing the aim. During the development of the spread plan, the leader oversees the project and may take an active role in developing the plan. Finally, the APN leader needs to ensure collection and use of feedback and data about the effectiveness of the plan, supporting course correction as needed. IHI has provided an example of improved waiting times in 1800 Veterans Affairs outpatient clinics by using the spread of innovation model (Massoud, Nielsen, Nolan, et al., 2006). Leaders in this project were enthusiastic about improving access for patients, ensuring adequate resources, providing incentives, and closely tracking the outcomes of the spread (Massoud et al., 2006). APNs are particularly well prepared as leaders to promote the spread of innovative best practices in health care.

When considering these models of leadership and change, several common themes emerge that are discussed in the remainder of this chapter. Effective leadership requires sound knowledge of oneself and one's organization with regard to values, strengths, and weaknesses, as well as expert communication and relationship-building skills and the ability to think and act strategically.

Appreciative Inquiry

Appreciative inquiry (AI) is a leadership model that is predicated on the focus of seeking positives through appreciative conversations and relationship building (Cooperrider, Whitney, & Stavros, 2008). Rather than focusing on a problem, the model encourages a focus on what is working well and what the organization does well, and builds on this. When we expand what we do best, problems seem to fall away or are outgrown. Leading through positive interactions results in people working together toward a shared vision and preferred future, without the burden of being weighed down by problems. Leaders using this leadership model are open to inquiry without having a preconceived outcome in mind; rather, they facilitate a search for shared meaning and build and expand on what is working well. For example, faculty at a graduate program for APNs wanted to create a DNP program, but there were quality concerns about some of their existing MSN programs. Through an AI process, the faculty decided to build a DNP program based solely on the certified registered nurse anesthetist (CRNA) role, because that was their strongest program. Moreover, through this process, they decided to phase out two of their Master of Science in Nursing (MSN) programs because they were not up to the same level of quality. Over time, the CRNA program was recognized as one of the nation's top programs. So, rather than investing solely on fixing what's broken, the appreciative inquiry model directs resources and visioning to an organization's greatest strengths. This leadership model uses a 4D cycle:

- *D*iscovery—an exploration of what is; finding organizational strengths and processes that work well
- *D*ream—imagining what could be; envisioning innovations that would work even better for the organization's future
- *D*esign—determining what should be; planning and prioritizing those processes
- *D*estiny—creating what should be; implementing the design

AI uses a positive perspective that can be motivational and inspirational for employees with the goal of increasing

exceptional performance. This model can work well for the APN who is skilled in developing partnerships, which can be symbiotic in this model building in regard to the ideas and innovations of each partner to solve problems in the complex health care environment (Sherwood, 2006). Although evidence for the effectiveness of this leadership model is low level and primarily anecdotal, there is enough evidence to support further rigorous research (Jones, 2010). The consequences of leading with an emphasis on defects are that it lacks vision, places attention to yesterday's causes, and can lead to narrow and fragmented solutions. The AI model shifts from asking "What is the biggest problem?" to "What possibilities exist that we have not yet considered?" This approach quickly leads individuals to a shared purpose and vision. Recent studies are all informative in our use of the AI model, including one by Rapede (2011), who used a model of participatory dreaming and journaling to understand the life struggles of women abused as children, one by Richer and associates (2009), who used case study research to look at the reorganization of health care services, and one by Smythe and coworkers (2009), who researched optimal service in a rural primary birthing center.

Concepts Related to Change

In this section, change is used to refer to any of the various types of initiatives aimed at improving the quality and safety of practice, whether by revising policies or helping clinicians master new knowledge and change behavior. In other words, change is seen as any clinical or systems effort to encourage the adoption and diffusion of innovation, including but not limited to quality improvement, product rollouts, clinician education, and skill development. Change does not have a discrete beginning and end but, instead, appears to be a series of continuous transitions that overlap one another. Because of this, change agency must be woven into the fabric of an APN's everyday life and work. As with patient assessment to effect individual behavior change, APNs must be skilled at assessing and reassessing their organizations and the complex forces that drive the health care system to be effective change agents. Systems innovation requires leadership that is continuous and flexible and demands ongoing attention to and redefinition of appropriate strategies (Greenhalgh et al., 2004; Klein, Gabelnick, & Herr, 1998; Massoud et al., 2006; Thompson & Nelson-Martin, 2011).

Opinion Leadership

One specific change strategy associated with leading a change initiative is opinion leadership (Greenhalgh et al., 2004; Locock, Dopson, Chambers, et al., 2001;

Oxman, Thomson, Davis, et al., 1995; Soumerai et al., 1998; Thomson et al., 1999). Opinion leaders are clinicians who are identified by their colleagues as likeable, trustworthy, and influential (Doumit, Gattellari, Grimshaw, et al., 2007; Oxman et al., 1995) A clinician is likely to listen to the opinion leader and might make a change in practice based on what he or she has learned from the opinion leader. The role of an opinion leader parallels that of the maven described by Gladwell (2000). One study of opinion leaders in several different clinical settings has indicated that contextual factors influenced the ability of an opinion leader to promote guideline adoption by colleagues (Locock et al., 2001). Shirey (2008) has stated that "opinion leaders must not only be knowledgeable, respected, trusted, and well-connected within the organization, they must also be generous with their time and giving of their expertise." As APNs become recognized for their accurate clinical decision making, they become opinion leaders. They are sought out by others and, when the APN speaks, others listen. Thus, a staff nurse may ask a CNS to look at a wound and advise, or an NP returns to her practice from a conference and, when she shares what she has learned, colleagues are eager to try the new information. This finding suggests the importance of attending to environmental cues when change is planned. Although studies of opinion leaders have been done, findings about their effectiveness are mixed, in part because the activities of opinion leaders have not been well described (Oxman et al., 1995).

Driving and Restraining Forces

Driving and restraining forces are useful concepts for APNs as they plan for change and evaluate both planned and unplanned changes. For example, as APNs extend their practices across state lines, the movement toward multistate licensure is gaining momentum (Young et al., 2012; see Chapter 12, Fig. 12-1, for an illustration of driving and restraining forces). Depending on existing policies and procedures for reimbursement and prescriptive authority within states, these forces can serve as driving or restraining influences for APNs. As multistate licensure for APNs evolves, telehealth may be considered a driving force and states' rights may be a restraining force. Driving and restraining forces are also useful for analyzing the organizational settings in which APNs work. For example, an organizational assessment of these various forces is useful in determining an institution's level of commitment to diversity.

At times, physicians have been perceived as restraining forces for change. Experienced APNs know that one of the challenges in system redesign and transformation has been engaging physicians in the work of improving quality as a team member rather than in a silo (Shortell & Singer, 2008). Physicians themselves have begun to recognize this and have made specific recommendations that administrators and APNs can use for engaging physicians in this important work (Reinertsen, Gosfield, Rupp, et al., 2007). For example, physicians and APNs together can request support through workshops and on-site experts in making a major institutional change, such as implementation of electronic medical records.

Pace of Change

A major concern for health care stakeholders at all levels is the rapidity with which change is occurring in the health care field. Even when one develops detailed plans for a change, events may occur that reshape process and progress so that what gets implemented may not be exactly the same as the original proposal. As the rapidity of change increases, the time frame to accomplish change strategies shortens. This phenomenon makes change more difficult for individuals and organizations to manage. As a consequence, many of the traditional models still being used to implement change will not work. Planned versus unplanned change is based predominantly on issues of time (Senge, 2006)—time to plan for and think through the desired change, time to orient and allow stakeholders to become comfortable with change, and time to educate and allow the change process to occur. In most health care systems, people perceive a poverty of time; this barrier requires creativity to transcend.

O'Connell (1999) has questioned whether health care organizations can sustain fast-paced change unless a "culture of change" is in place that assists and supports adaptation to new systems and ways of knowing and doing. A culture of change requires several components, including learning about change and change strategies, encouraging dialogue, valuing collaboration, and being committed to enacting change. O'Connell proposed the following strategies for promoting a culture of change within an organization:

- Maintain momentum toward change.
- Emphasize managerial support in the process of changing work flow and practice patterns.
- Encourage the question "why" and exercise tolerance for the results.
- Emphasize the importance of personal concerns and address them.
- Find new and different ways to demonstrate administrative support.

APNs can use one or more of the models of leadership described here to assess their systems. Knowing where one's system is in terms of readiness for change and identifying the forces that will support or restrain adoption of an innovation can help the APN design strategies that will work. It is also helpful to consider the techniques

BOX 11-1   Leadership Strategies for Moving Through Change

- Spark a passion; believe in what you are doing; shine a light on activities that inspire and excite.
- Understand the organizational culture.
- Create a vision.
- Get the right people involved.
- Hand the work over to the champions of change.
- Let values serve as the compass for where you are headed.
- Change people first; organizations evolve.
- Seek and provide opportunities for professional renewal and regeneration.
- Maintain a healthy balance.

Adapted from Kerfoot, K., & Chaffee, M. W. (2007). Ten keys to unlock policy change in the workplace. In D. J. Mason, J. K. Leavitt, & M. W. Chaffee (Eds.), *Policy and politics in nursing and health care* (pp. 482–484). Philadelphia: Saunders; and Kerfoot, K. (2005). On leadership: Building confident organizations by filling buckets, building infrastructures, and shining the flashlight. *Dermatology Nursing, 17,* 154–156.

TABLE 11-2   Characteristics and Core Elements of the Leadership Competency

Defining Characteristic	Core Elements (Knowledge and Skills)
Mentoring	• Shared vision • Seeks mentors and serves as a mentor • Willing to share power • Empowering self and others • Self-reflection
Innovation	• Knowledge of models of leadership and change • Systems thinking • Systems assessment skills • Flexibility • Risk taking • Expert communication • Credibility • Change agent
Activism	• Knowledge and understanding of factors driving change in the health care system • Involvement in policy arenas, whether local, regional, national, or global • Advocacy for patients, advanced practice nurses, and the nursing profession

used for implementing change, such as building alliances, creating a shared vision, being assertive, negotiating conflict (Norton & Grady, 1996), and managing transitions (see Chapter 8) as they relate to providing a positive culture for change. As leaders, APNs can use their so-called shuttle diplomacy skills to translate the need for and perspectives on change between clinicians and executives. In addition, APN leaders need to be prepared to use their voice in identifying when it is not in an organization's best interest to pursue a change based on context, environment, inadequate problem solving, or unresolved barriers. Repetitive rapid change can take a toll on engagement and productivity and potentially on patient safety, particularly if implications and consequences are not thoroughly considered. Most importantly, leaders need to understand the personal implications of change if a culture of change is to be realized. Box 11-1 provides a useful set of strategies for APN leaders who are helping their organizations and colleagues work through change transitions.

Defining Characteristics of the Advanced Practice Nurse Leadership Competency

The three defining characteristics of APN leadership—mentoring , innovation, and activism—are listed, along with their core elements, in Table 11-2. These are discussed separately to help readers understand the differences among them. However, there is considerable overlap in the knowledge and skills needed for each characteristic. Experienced APNs can demonstrate these characteristics

in all four leadership domains. Although they have beginning competence in leading within each domain, novice APNs tend to exercise leadership in the clinical domain. Over time, they expand their leadership activities into other areas.

Mentoring

The responsibility to mentor is central to all the definitions of leadership and change outlined earlier and is a key element of the APN leadership competency. The ability to help others grow and encourage them toward self-actualization requires competent caring leaders who are interested in the success and well-being of their followers. Mentoring is required to ensure the development of future nursing leaders (McCloughen, O'Brien, & Jackson, 2010). Mentoring bridges the gap between education and real-world experience (Barker, 2006). Coaching and guiding, leading by example, and role modeling with awareness and attentiveness to the needs and concerns of followers are basic characteristics of successful leaders. The ideas behind the colloquial statements of "taking someone under your wing" or "giving a colleague a leg up" are grounded in the mentoring process. Mentors have been defined as being competent and self-confident, having qualities that epitomize success in their own careers, and having the ability and desire to help others succeed. A number of characteristics have been identified in successful mentors—inspiring, confident, committed to the development of others, and being willing to share. Mentors take on responsibility for the development of mentee skills, such as flexibility, adaptability, judgment, and creativity (McCloughen et al., 2010). Protégés (or mentees) are viewed as individuals who exhibit a desire to learn, are committed to the long course of events, and are open to the process of trial and error. Successful protégés have high self-esteem, can self-monitor, and are resilient risk takers (Tourigny & Pulich, 2005). The reward for the mentor is to step back and enjoy the success and achievements of the protégé. APNs who have had the benefit of mentoring have stated that it affected the progression of their career and hastened their leadership development (McCloughen et al., 2009).

Two types of mentoring are described in the literature. The first, termed *formal mentoring,* has the approval and support of the organization with objectives, selection process, and mentoring contract. Mentors are chosen from the ranks of experienced clinicians and provide exposure to clinical situations that offer opportunities to demonstrate competence, coaching, and role modeling and afford protection in controversial situations (Tourigny & Pulich, 2005). Many professional organizations, such as Sigma Theta Tau, offer formal mentoring programs. Readers can consult their professional and specialty organizations' websites for information on formal mentoring programs. The term *informal mentoring* has been defined as a mutual attraction that is unstructured and mutually beneficial; the experiences usually last longer and are self-selected (Tourigny & Pulich, 2005). Good mentors foster growth rather than dependency and instill the internal strengths to enable protégés to traverse rough spots in their career development. Mentors lead mentees on a journey of self-discovery and help them find the value they bring to the role and to nursing leadership (Vos, 2009). As mentoring relationships progress, the protégé is given more freedom to try new behaviors and develops confidence in trying new skills, always with the knowledge that someone is behind them.

Mentoring relationships can be developed based on specific needs of the APN mentee (e.g., writing for publication, developing professional presentation skills) or on the general development of career and leadership skills. Harrington (2011) has reported that mentoring new NPs will accelerate their development as primary care providers. Finding a mentor in your geographic location may not be feasible, depending on the skill to be developed. In today's technologic world, it behooves APN leaders to remember that long-distance mentoring can be a rewarding experience as well. Use of conference calls, video conferencing, and networking at professional conferences can all be feasible means to support a long-distance mentoring relationship.

It is important to note that there are two parts to the APN mentorship equation, APNs who are seeking to be mentored by those they aspire to emulate, and APNs who can serve as mentors. Unfortunately, some APN leaders are reluctant to mentor, perhaps thinking that the protégé will compete with them, overshadow their expertise, or not work as hard as they did to be successful. However, Vance (2002) has asserted that the current, chaotic, health care environment makes mentoring support more important than ever. She suggested that mentors and protégés adopt a mentoring philosophy that encourages collaboration with others, not competition. Novice APNs are fortunate if they can find a mentoring relationship that lasts over time. The APN mentor creates a safety net in which the protégé can expose vulnerabilities and be coached to develop confidence in new skills (Davis, Little, & Thornton, 1997). Mentoring is a gift that allows new APN leaders to emerge.

An interrelationship exists among the concepts of mentoring, organizational culture, and leadership. Bally (2007) has described organizational culture as the values, norms, and rituals that make up an organization and set the rules for its members. A positive organizational culture offers social support and a sense of well-being and empowerment that fosters the mentoring process (Bally, 2007; Harrington, 2011; Shirey, 2004). Thus, APNs should seek opportunities to mentor or be mentored and articulate the benefits of mentoring activities to their organization.

Empowering Others

As the word implies, the term *empowerment* is defined as giving power to another, encouraging, or giving authority. APNs operationalize empowerment by sharing power with other nurses, colleagues, and patients or enabling them to access or assert their own power. Empowerment as a leadership strategy is guided by the shared vision of the leader and follower and a willingness of the leader to delegate authority to others. Visionary leaders who empower their followers greatly increase the influence of APNs within nursing and beyond nursing's boundaries.

Empowerment requires more than just giving others permission to act on their own. It is a developmental process that a good leader fosters over time; it encourages constituents to feel competent, responsible, independent, and authorized to act. Rajotte (1996) has offered a useful six-step method for advanced practice nursing leaders to use to empower others, whether patients, nurses, or members of other disciplines:

1. Educate to empower through increasing the individual's knowledge base.
2. Use inspiration, motivation, and encouragement.
3. Provide structure that offers protection and security as one moves into new territory.
4. Provide resources to support others' growth and development.
5. Mentor to give the support and direction necessary for change toward empowerment.
6. Foster actualization, empowering others to evoke change.

For example, a certified nurse-midwife (CNM) empowers pregnant women by putting them in control of the birthing process through education, mentoring, and providing resources for parenting that nurture self-esteem and enhance family structure.

Innovation

As the prior discussion suggests, initiating change and diffusing and sustaining innovation are critical elements of the APN leadership competency. Covey's work (1989) with interdisciplinary groups is instructive to APNs who are learning change agent skills. Change occurs at the system and personal levels, and one must deal with core values to change or serve as an agent for change successfully. Covey contended that people have a changeless core inside them that they need if they themselves are to be able to change. Thus, one key to the ability of people to change is a changeless sense of who they are, what they are about, and what they value. Real change comes from the inside out. This observation is relevant to APNs. First, APNs need to identify their own core values to become effective in leading change. Second, Covey's insight can help APNs who encounter resistance to change initiatives, especially when it persists. The resistance may come from the sense that a core value is being threatened.

There is an affective dimension to change (Greenhalgh et al., 2004). Although many people are excited by the prospect of change, some changes are difficult and painful, and any change contains an element of loss. Senge (2006) described this feeling as an emotional tension associated with holding a vision that differs from the current reality. Mastering emotional tension during change requires perseverance, patience, and compassion. At best, change can be described as challenging and invigorating (Norton & Grady, 1996). Lazarus and Fell (2011) have suggested that it is important to cross the gap in creativity and use innovation as a process to induce change in health care. To understand change in today's health care environment, APNs must explore the dynamics of change and the culture in which it occurs.

Taken together, this discussion suggests that APNs must consider several factors when they are experiencing or trying to introduce change—the relevance of power and influence, stakeholders' concerns and interests, contextual factors, individuals' values, and the affective dimensions of change. Understanding these important factors is integral to the APN leadership competency.

Political Activism

As doctorally prepared APNs hone their skills for systems leadership and change, political activism and advocacy will become even more important. Many of the skills needed to navigate successfully in political waters are closely associated with good leadership. The core elements that define contemporary leadership, such as shared vision, systems thinking, and the ability to engage in high-level communication within the context of a changing environment, are all basic to political effectiveness. Again, change is the common denominator that drives APNs to advocate for advanced practice and patient issues. There is little room for discussion about whether APNs need to take on the mantles of policymaker and patient advocate as part of their leadership role (see Chapter 22). For many, this falls within the context of a moral imperative: "Nurses practice at the intersection of public policy and the personal lives (of their patients); they are, therefore, ideally situated and morally obligated to include sociopolitical advocacy in their practice" (Falk-Rafael, 2005, p. 222). Working for social justice is seen as part of the ethical decision making competency of APNs (see Chapter 13). APNs must position themselves strategically at the policy table to advocate for access to care and appropriate interventions for everyone. There is also little question about whether APNs are up to the task. Great strides have been made in developing nurses' skill and acuity as policymakers (see Chapter 22, Exemplar 22-2). Rapidly evolving policy situations mean that APNs are often faced with trial by fire learning when it comes to activism and advocacy. Identifying trusted mentors with whom to debrief and developing a plan of action can help APNs develop the poise and skills needed to respond effectively in unexpected, chaotic, and tense political situations.

Although activism is frequently associated with advocacy in the political realm, activism can also occur in the clinical and system environments as well. The same leadership skills apply in those settings when advocating for issues such as access to care, ethical decision making, and resolving injustice.

Attributes of Effective Advanced Practice Nurse Leaders

Several personal attributes are deemed necessary for successful leadership (Box 11-2). These qualities are very broad; all leaders should demonstrate these qualities because they are needed in the interdisciplinary context of today's health care. No longer do nurse leaders have the luxury of leading only in nursing circles. The history of advanced practice nursing (see Chapter 1) demonstrates that nurse leaders have led outside the realm of organized nursing education and practice.

Vision

Vision, the ability to anticipate the future and communicate that image to others, is often perceived as the most important component of leadership and the talent that is most coveted (Carroll, 2005). Vision encompasses a long-range view of personal and collective goals that can be shared and that empower others to move forward. Innovation is associated with and closely linked to vision. It is the ability to think big or think outside the box, the capability to see alternatives to current thinking on a given issue. In some graduate schools, teaching APNs innovation and thinking outside the box is a program goal (Shirey, 2004). Vision is also grounded in a deep knowledge of the subject and brings with it the responsibility to stay abreast of trends and issues in the field. However, having vision is not enough. A leader must be able to articulate and develop a shared vision, one that others can embrace as their own (Christopher, Miller, Beck, et al., 2002; Senge, 2006). To do this well, a visionary leader must not get too far out in front of his or her followers because teamwork is critical to shared vision. Tornabeni (1996), a nurse leader, has noted that she would not have been able to "hold onto the vision" (p. 65) had she not broadened her scope of influence to include others outside of the discipline of nursing. Another important element of vision is the ability to set priorities so that there is a clear path to the ultimate goal. Rychnovsky (2011) has described Dr. Ruth Lubic's contributions as a visionary leader in maternal-child health. Among her many accomplishments, Dr. Lubic was particularly recognized for her influential work in helping found the first free-standing maternity care center, the first of more than 150 subsequent free-standing birth centers to be established.

Leaders are involved with change at many points in the change process. Anticipating and preparing for change can help ensure success. Visionary change makers intervene early in the change process, before change occurs, and set the stage for the events that follow. They provide the guiding principles and assumptions for the proposed

BOX 11-2   Attributes of Nurse Leaders

Expert Communication Skills
- Articulate in speech and in writing
- Able to get one's point across
- Uses excellent listening skills
- Desires to hear and understand another's point of view
- Stays connected to other people

Commitment
- Gives of self personally and professionally
- Listens to one's inner voice
- Balances professional and private life
- Plans ahead; makes change happen
- Engages in self-reflection

Developing One's Own Style
- Gets and stays involved
- Sets priorities
- Manages boundaries
- Uses technology
- Engages in lifelong learning
- Maintains a good sense of humor

Risk Taking
- Gets involved at any level
- Demonstrates self-confidence and assertiveness
- Uses creative and big picture thinking
- Willing to fail and begin again
- Has an astute sense of timing
- Copes with change

Willingness to Collaborate
- Respects cultural diversity
- Desires to build teams and alliances
- Shares power
- Willing to mentor

Adapted from Hanson, C., Boyle, J., Hatmaker, D., & Murray, J. (1999). *Finding your voice as a leader.* Washington DC: American Academy of Nursing.

change and begin to introduce themes that position the organization and its members in a positive direction toward the new events. Change implementers, as defined by Kantor and colleagues (1992), have the difficult task of making it happen.

Timing

A good sense of timing may be an inherent gift, but for most people it requires painstaking development and practice. APN leaders know when to act and when to hold back. They recognize the need for urgency at times as, for example, during an unexpected legislative vote in Congress; they also know to take the time to develop a carefully thought-out plan with deliberate strategy when a change in scope of practice is being considered. The notion of timing is apparent when APNs use mandated change as an opportunity to introduce other changes. For example, institutions applying for accreditation by The Joint Commission (TJC) are expected to demonstrate compliance with TJC's current evidence-based standards for specific health care problems (TJC, 2012). Many institutions use these mandated changes to launch a variety of initiatives aimed at improving care management.

Self-Confidence and Risk Taking

Taking risks is inherent in the leadership process and is tied inextricably to self-confidence and vision. The willingness to take a chance, try, and occasionally fail is the mark of a true leader. The mantra, "take a risk, make a decision, pay the price," coined by Helen Mannock in 1959, is worth keeping in mind (Norton & Grady, 1996). Risk-taking behaviors differentiate APNs who will be recognized as leaders and change drivers from other capable nurses. By learning to take risks, APNs enhance their leadership repertoire, allowing for more spontaneity and flexibility in response to conflict, resistance, anger, and other reactions to change and high-risk situations (Norton & Grady, 1996). Motivation, which can be described as the desire to move forward, can also be viewed as a component of risk. Wheatley (2005) has affirmed that another component of risk taking is the willingness to be disturbed. Certainty is more comfortable. Staying put is rarely as risky as taking the chance to move ahead. Risk taking should be differentiated from risky leadership behaviors. Taking risk involves evaluating all types of evidence available at the time and making educated decisions based on that information. It also involves trying to anticipate consequences of actions, having a plan in place to evaluate the implementation, be willing to accept that the risk was not successful, and learning from the experience. Risky behavior, on the other hand, is making decisions impetuously without fully exploring available information or having a strategy to address unintended consequences.

It is not accidental that several of the key attributes in Box 11-2 incorporate some form of the word *willingness*. The abilities to be open, willing to take what comes, and work through differences are key to all levels of leadership. Leadership is about negotiation and interactions with others to reach common goals. To do this may mean failing and trying again and again to reach the desired outcome. This quality of personal hardiness—the ability to pick oneself up and start again—is seen repeatedly in biographies of successful leaders who have made change happen in difficult times.

Expert Communication and Relationship Building

The relevance of expert communication skills and collegial relationships to quality health care has received significant attention in the past few years (Castledine, 2008; Houghton, 2003; Rider, 2002). APNs must be able to communicate effectively to collaborate with other professionals (see Chapter 12) and participate in the identification and resolution of clinical and ethical conflicts among team members (see Chapter 13). The successful leader must have superb communication skills to build the trust and cooperation necessary to negotiate difficult intraprofessional and interprofessional issues. The ability to understand another's viewpoint and respect opposing views is key to effective communication and ultimately to reaching a mutually satisfactory outcome. Covey (1989) has suggested that one should "seek first to understand and then to be understood" (p. 235). Good leaders listen and really try to hear the other person's viewpoint before they speak. The charisma that is associated with many natural-born leaders is often simply outstanding listening and communication skills. The ability to influence, a key power strategy used to gain the cooperation of others, is an outcome of excellent communication. A second part of expert communication is relationship building. The art of building strong alliances and coalitions with others and staying connected with colleagues and groups is basic to the sense of community needed to lead effectively. Building relationships within the work environment can minimize the impact of organizational structures that hinder one's ability to collaborate and solve problems (Wheatley, 2005). These alliances are important, whether at the highest levels of international policymaking or at the local level when building a coalition to address a recurring patient issue. Building relationships is central to the effectiveness of a team who cares for patients. Not only must APNs establish effective relationships with their coworkers, but they are often in a position to strengthen relationships among other members of the team through role modeling and mediation.

Thought leaders use conversational leadership as a way to bring key stakeholders together to raise critical questions and issues and gain collective intelligence leading to innovation and wise actions. Open conversations are one way in which leaders share what they know with colleagues and create new ways of knowing and doing (Hurley & Brown, 2009). This type of open conversation may lead to having the courageous conversations that are sometimes needed to name a problem so that the communication can move forward. Building relationships is also central to another advanced practice nursing communication skill, conflict negotiation (see Chapter 12). Advanced practice nursing students may come to their graduate programs having been socialized to be silent or suppress their opinion in situations of conflict. Specific approaches to identifying conflicts and resolving them successfully have been identified and used successfully in business (Fisher, Ury, & Patton, 2002) and in health care (Longo & Sherman, 2007). Readers are referred to the following websites for resources and information on conflict negotiation: the Conflict Resolution Network (www.crnhq.org); and the Program on Negotiation at Harvard Law School (www.pon.org).

Boundary Management

Managing boundaries refers to how APNs limit or extend various aspects of advanced practice nursing, such as scope of practice, workload, and interpersonal boundaries. Sometimes, APNs are in the position of guarding the boundary, such as when they are approached to undertake a task that is not within their scope of practice. Productivity requirements mean that APNs must be clear about the numbers and types of patients that they care for on a given day. Often, managing boundaries means extending them—building a bridge that enables the APN to partner with other groups or expanding a boundary as other patient or health care needs are identified, an idea increasingly recognized in calls for core health professional competencies (Greiner & Knebel, 2003; Health Sciences Institute, 2005). For example, although CRNAs may not need prescriptive authority in a given state, they assist their colleague NPs in their quest for state prescriptive authority. Extending a boundary may also mean expanding one's scope of practice at an agency level so that patient needs can be better met. Knowing the current boundaries of nursing practice and making strategic decisions about going beyond them are other ways to define risk taking.

As boundary managers, APNs recognize communications and behaviors that breach or enhance interpersonal relationships (see later, "Horizontal Violence" and "Dysfunctional Leadership Styles"). APN leaders also teach others how to collaborate with colleagues in other disciplines, build coalitions, and set limits while maintaining their own boundaries—a fine distinction, but strategically important. For example, a CNM may delicately negotiate the boundaries or responsibilities among the neonatologist, obstetrician, and nurse-midwifery staff. Clinical leadership and professional leadership require the negotiation of boundaries, regardless of whether the borders are drawn around professional roles, patient populations, or organizations.

Respect for Cultural Diversity

Cultural competence and valuing diversity are significant attributes of APN leaders. These attributes require awareness of one's own biases and of damaging attitudes and behaviors that surface at all levels of interaction and in all settings. An APN leader needs to serve as a role model by demonstrating respect for the cultural, racial, and ethnic differences of individuals and constituencies in any given situation. When a systems framework is used for understanding a complex concept such as culturally competent leadership, four levels can be identified—societal, professional, organizational, and individual. For the APN, the responsibility for culturally competent care includes all four of these levels. A useful aid for developing a sound respect for cultural diversity can be found in the Interprofessional Education Collaborative (IPEC) competencies developed in 2011 (see Chapter 12, Box 12-1, for this resource). Culturally competent care is delivered with knowledge, sensitivity, and respect for the patient's and family's cultural, racial, and ethnic background and practices. Cultural competence is an ongoing process that involves accepting and respecting differences and not letting personal beliefs get in the way (Giger et al., 2007). This definition is built on the assumption that care providers are fully aware of and sensitized to their own cultural, racial, and ethnic backgrounds and that they are able to integrate this sensitivity into their delivery of care. The interactive nature of caregiving requires the authentic engagement of the provider with the patient to appreciate and respond to differences that may affect giving or receiving care. A good example of the challenge that culturally competent care presents has been provided by Wheatley (2005). In this example, a group practice offered free car seats and training in their use to parents but no one took advantage of the gift. On debriefing, the providers learned that for Asian parents, using a car seat was an invitation to God to cause a car accident. Differences are issues for every member of the human race and they become even more important when one becomes a leader and role model. Working with colleagues who are different provides APNs with opportunities for soliciting information about others' experiences. Box 11-3 presents strategies for enhancing cultural awareness.

Global Awareness

The world is becoming more interconnected and interdependent every day; this affects the APN leader because issues such as patient safety and quality care are global issues that are not confined to any particular geographic region. There is a global workforce crisis, natural and human catastrophes occur with regularity, and there are

BOX 11-3   Strategies to Achieve Cultural Competence

- Explore and learn about your own racial and ethnic culture and background.
- Explore and learn about the different racial and ethnic cultures most frequently encountered in your practice.
- Read ethnic newspapers, magazines, and books.
- Listen to the music from a different culture.
- Learn the language of a different culture. Become bilingual with the verbal and nonverbal behavior of the culture.
- Take advantage of training opportunities to increase your cultural awareness and sensitivity.
- Be able to identify personal biases and develop strategies to manage, eliminate, or sublimate those potentially damaging attitudes and behaviors.
- When faced with a difficult patient, consider whether unconscious biases may be operating for you or your colleagues.

Adapted from Hanson, C. M., & Malone, B. (2000). Leadership: Empowerment, change agency, and activism. In A. B. Hamric, J. A. Spross, & C. M. Hanson (Eds.), *Advanced nursing practice: An integrative approach* (pp. 279–313; 2nd ed.). Philadelphia: Saunders.

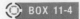 **BOX 11-4   Global Competencies for Nursing Leaders**

Develop global mindset and worldview:
- Global environmental awareness
- Cultural adaptation
- Awareness of social, political, and economic trends

Understand needs of technology:
- Enhanced ability of communication and technology
- Create global networks
- Individuals can now drive change just as businesses used to drive change

Respect diversity and cultivate cross-cultural competencies:
- Institutional mergers and growth
- Multicultural work force
- Multicultural patient populations

Adapted from Nichols, B., Shaffer, F., & Porter, C. (2011). Global nursing leadership: A practical guide. *Nursing Administration Quarterly, 35,* 354–359.

- International Council of Nurses
- World Health Organization
- Sigma Theta Tau International
- Pan American Health Organization

fewer barriers to interactions between countries (Abbott & Coenen, 2008). Minimally, APN leaders interface with a multicultural workforce in their immediate setting or through professional organizations, and they are asked to lead multicultural teams (Nichols, Shaffer, & Porter, 2011). APNs may look to other countries for problem-solving ideas or may be asked for consultation in person or via technology (e.g., teleconferencing, Skype) from health care providers across the globe.

The sharing of new techniques, therapies, and knowledge resources is imperative as we work together to address global issues such as the global chronic illness epidemic, infectious diseases, and common health crises (Abbott & Coenen, 2008). Nichols and coworkers (2011) have identified global competencies for nursing leaders, outlined in Box 11-4. In addition, they have outlined areas for nurse leaders to consider in development of a world view that includes sense of self and space, cultural dress, family relationships and decision making, values and beliefs, nutrition habits, and religious preferences (Nichols et al., 2011). Friedman (2006) has termed this view *global citizenship* and suggested that individuals and groups in leadership positions have a responsibility to think and act as global citizens. There are several organizations that have a global perspective in their mission, which can be accessed for resources:

Balance in Personal and Professional Life

Most people know when they have overextended themselves; their bodies give clues such as fatigue, stress signals, feelings of frustration, and even physical illness. One of the negative aspects of being a good leader is the provocative realization that one is being asked to play many important cutting edge roles at the same time. These invitations are exciting and seductive because they open new opportunities and speak to the high regard that others have for the leader. For these reasons, it is easy for good leaders to overextend their activities well beyond manageable, realistic boundaries. The skills of being able to delegate tasks, say no and mentor others to take on some of the load, and enlarge the circle of leaders, strategists, and followers are integral to effective leadership. Unfortunately, the inability to set realistic personal boundaries paves the way for stress, frustration, and burnout. It is not easy to be a leader and competent APN provider, but it can be done. This skill requires the APN to say "no" when a request is made that the APN is not willing to do or cannot do because of competing responsibilities. Skillful practice with saying "no" uses the sandwich technique. It begins with articulating the larger "yes"—what the APN is currently reaching for in the practice or trying to accomplish, followed by a firm "no"—and ends with a hopeful statement such as "Perhaps I can help you find somebody else" or "Maybe I can help in the future." The goal is to leave the requester with a sense of respect and a better understanding of the APN. For example, "I am really trying to build the prenatal care outreach service to underserved women. So, I cannot serve on the hospital CEO search committee. Perhaps I can help you find another qualified CNM to serve".

The process of self-reflection is useful for APNs to figure out which personal and work characteristics seem to set off imbalances. We offer three strategies, which are simple in concept but can be complicated in execution. First, expecting perfection is often a setup for imbalance. Keeping in mind the axiom, "Perfect is the enemy of good," may help APNs establish realistic expectations. Another strategy is for APNs to examine what makes them say "yes" or "no." It is easy to think, "If I just do this one more thing, everything will be fine." One APN kept a Post-it note on her phone that read, "The answer is no." This reminded her to decline something that would tip the scales to overcommitment or to buy time by asking, "Can I think about it and call you tomorrow?" One colleague avoids commitments that are perceived as distant elephants; these are invitations for activities months or even years in the future. Such activities may not appear to threaten one's usual commitments and deadlines but, as the time to fulfill the commitment approaches, distant elephants can become as threatening as an impending stampede. The challenge for the APN is to ensure that adequate time to plan for, develop, and organize the work is budgeted well in advance of the due date. The third strategy is to make appointments with oneself for important personal and professional activities. By putting these appointments on a calendar, APNs can lessen the risk of giving away time that they need to maintain balance. Using "the three things rule" may be helpful; identify the three most important things that must be done before any new commitments are made or started.

Developing Skills as Advanced Practice Nurse Leaders

When considering a leadership development plan, there are formal and informal strategies. Students must have formal and informal opportunities to develop leadership skills in each domain. These can occur in the classroom, clinical practice, student leadership, and health-related service projects. In general, lessons learned in one domain will apply to leadership situations in other domains. Health policy leadership is discussed separately because it has specific features that are somewhat different from the APN's everyday leadership activities.

Factors Influencing Leadership Development

Power Resources

A common myth is that leaders are born and not made. Trent (2003) has asserted that this is not true and that individuals can learn to lead by understanding and using "power resources," as described by Rost (1993). Power resources include many of the attributes described in this chapter, such as education, experience, expert communication, networking, assertiveness, and collaboration and are clearly demonstrated in the studies of leadership discussed in the following sections. Zaccaro (2007) has argued that with increases in conceptual and methodologic resources, combinations of inborn traits and learned attributes are more likely to predict leadership than once was believed. Leadership represents complex patterns of behavior explained in part by multiple leader attributes (Zaccaro, 2007). In this section, we explore leadership traits and attributes that are innate and those that can be learned as APNs develop their leadership competence.

Personal Characteristics and Experiences

Allen (1998) explored perceptions of 12 nurse leaders regarding the primary factors and individual characteristics that influenced their leadership development. Self-confidence, traced to childhood and subsequent risk-taking behaviors, was perceived as a critical factor. Feedback from significant others led to enhanced self-confidence over time. The nurse leaders also spoke about having innate qualities and tendencies of leaders, such as being extroverted or bossy and wanting to take charge, and about having roles as team captains and officers in organizations. They were seen as people who rise to the occasion. A third important factor was a progression of experiences and successes that were pivotal in moving them forward. Being at the right place at the right time and taking advantage of opportunities presented in those situations allowed them to grow as leaders. Closely aligned with this factor was the influence of significant people, such as mentors, role models, faculty, and parents, who had the ability to encourage and provide opportunities for advancement. A final set of factors identified in this study were personal life factors, defined as situations in which time, family, health, and work schedules influenced their development to a greater or lesser degree. For example, study participants who had supportive spouses and relatives who assisted with family and home responsibilities and employers who were flexible found these factors to be important to the leadership development process.

Zaccaro and colleagues (2004) have developed a model that described distal attributes (personality, cognitive abilities, motives, values) and proximal attributes (social appraisal skills, problem-solving skills, expertise, tacit knowledge) as they relate to a leader's emergence, effectiveness, and advancement. In this model, the leader's operating environment influences the trajectory toward success, which supports the importance of organizational culture described by Bally (2007) in the mentoring section. Carroll (2005) identified six factors that were present in women leaders and nurse executives: personal integrity, strategic vision and action orientation, team-building and communication skills, management and technical competencies, people skills (collaboration, empowering others, valuing diversity), and personal survival skills. Note the similarity with the attributes in Box 11-2.

Strategies for Acquiring Competency as a Leader

Formal educational opportunities such as those experienced during graduate school fit well into the process of leadership development. Opportunities to work with role models and mentors help students acquire leadership skills and further reinforce their self-confidence. Running

for graduate student office or local leadership positions in professional organizations and serving on local and national coalitions are other good strategies for developing this competency (Grossman, 2006; Sandrick, 2006). Also, leadership conferences that foster effective communication and interaction are beneficial. Exemplar 11-2 shows how students can practice their leadership development during graduate education.

Leadership skills are developed and perfected over time and in myriad ways. Communication is one of the strengths often attributed to nurses; it is a skill that can be augmented through practice. Many other skills and attributes listed in Box 11-2 are familiar to APNs and just need to be framed within the context of leadership. For example, the notion of staying connected is important for busy APNs and can be operationalized in a variety of ways, from e-mail lists and shared projects to attending conferences that allow for time to interact and problem-solve with colleagues about similar professional issues (Hanson, Boyle, Hatmaker, et al., 1999). A sense of timing was described by one leader in the study by Hanson and colleagues as negotiating child care duties with her spouse for time to lobby for

---

 EXEMPLAR 11-2   **Mentoring an Advanced Practice Nurse Student to Develop Health Policy Skills**

Joan was beginning her second year as a student APN. She had completed her core courses, which gave her a good foundation in the theoretical concepts related to role development, health policy, and research. Now she was ready to move on to the clinical component of her program and complete her scholarly project. Joan had thought carefully about this and wanted to focus her project on developing her leadership skills in the policy arena. She knew that one member of her faculty, Dr. Wesson, who had taught her health policy course, was a respected state and national leader who was actively engaged in the process of gaining primary care provider (PCP) status for APNs. Joan made an appointment to talk with Dr. Wesson about how she could help with the PCP issue and at the same time complete her scholarly project. Dr. Wesson had three suggestions: (1) Joan should use the Internet to become familiar with and articulate about the proposed legislation; (2) she could accompany Dr. Wesson to the next statewide meeting of APNs and offer to carry out the phone survey of APNs that was needed by this group; and (3) she could develop the research proposal, implement the survey methodology, and present the findings as part of testimony at the

hearing at the state capitol in the spring. These activities would allow Joan to interact with leader role models, try out her new leadership skills, and complete her research assignment. Dr. Wesson also suggested that Joan apply for the student scholarship offered by a national advanced practice nursing organization to attend the Washington DC–based APN Summit.

Throughout the fall and winter, Joan implemented the phone survey with the advanced practice nursing community. She interacted with many practicing APNs and learned a great deal about advanced practice nursing. The APN leaders at the state meeting were excellent role models and Dr. Wesson served as an excellent mentor throughout the year. Joan was extremely proud of her contribution to advanced practice nursing when she presented her findings at the hearing. Throughout the process, she had used many of the skills that she had read about in her leadership class, such as communication, networking, vision, and timing. Because Joan had a husband and 4-year-old child, she also learned about balance and boundary management. Her most lasting recollection was how important it was to have a mentor to guide her through the process.

prescriptive authority, with the understanding that she would increase her family responsibilities at the end of the legislative session. For faculty and students in graduate programs to become involved with raising the visibility of advanced practice nursing roles in their institutions and communities, it is extremely important to build a community of advanced practice nursing leaders. For APNs who already have some leadership experience, the Robert Johnson Executive Nurse Fellows Program is a highly motivating experience (Robert Wood Johnson Foundation, 2012).

To acquire leadership skills and experience, novice APNs need to become involved in the leadership and committee work of local advanced practice nursing coalitions and organizations and move into state and regional leadership roles as they develop their style and strengths as APN leaders. The ability to place nurse leaders in key positions is critical to the visibility and credibility of APNs and to the establishment of roles for APNs in nursing and the larger health care community.

Developing Leadership in the Health Policy Arena

Health policy issues affecting APNs and their patients, including strategies for political advocacy, are explored in Chapter 22. The following section describes how APNs can develop skills to influence health policy through creative leadership and political advocacy, whether by means of local grassroots endeavors or directly through congressional involvement. The term *advocacy* can be defined as the act of pleading another person's cause; it is multifaceted, with diverse activities (Halpern, 2002; Kendig, 2006); "the endpoint of advocacy is the health and welfare of the public" (Leavitt, Chaffee, & Vance, 2007, p. 37). APNs are being called on, collectively and individually, to make their voices heard as the nation and individual states struggle with budget constraints and difficult decisions about health policies and the funding of health care programs.

Becoming an Astute Political Activist: The Growth Process

In the political arena, developing power and influence is an imperative that tests one's leadership skills. Leadership strategies used by APNs in the political arena include developing influence with policymakers, influencing contacts, motivating colleagues to stay abreast of current issues, and providing bridges to other leaders who have access to important resources. Mentoring APNs to understand their power and influence in the health

policy arena is a key role for the APN leader. The developmental process for becoming a political activist can begin as early as primary school when children are first introduced to government and the political system. However, serious involvement often begins in graduate school, when health policy is offered as one of the core courses in the curriculum (see Exemplar 9-2). During graduate education, APN students are coached to understand the power inherent in policymaking, the power of politics to influence practice, and the ways that they can influence the system, individually and collectively, to better their own practice and be high-level patient advocates. Faculty members need to serve as resource persons to keep students informed about key legislative issues and introduce them, through role modeling, to the role of political advocacy. Inviting APNs to accompany faculty who are giving testimony at a legislative hearing is an appropriate way to model the advocacy role. Many professional organizations also offer tools about how to engage in the political process, such as the American Association of Nurse Anesthetists (AANA), 2012; NACNS, 2011; Zenti, 1998).

Depth of Involvement

There is no question that influencing policy is costly in terms of commitment, time, and energy. Timing is an important consideration. It is important for APNs to ask themselves several personal and professional questions to determine the degree of involvement and level of sophistication at which advocacy is to be undertaken, including the following:

- What are my personal responsibilities related to wage earning, small children, dependent parents, single parenthood, health issues, school, and gaining initial competence as an APN?
- How can I best serve the APN community at this time?
- What learning opportunities will help me be an effective APN advocate?
- How can I develop short-term and long-term plans for becoming a more politically astute advocate for myself, my patients, and nursing?
- What am I able to commit to, based on the response to these questions?

Once APNs have made a decision about the depth of involvement to which they can commit, they need to find an appropriate mentor. Advanced practice nursing has a wealth of effective nursing leaders and advocates who are willing and able to move new advocates into positions to make positive changes in health policy. Opportunities for input and influence exist at various levels of the legislative process (Larson, 2004; Park & Jex, 2011; Winterfeldt, 2001; see Chapter 22).

Using Professional Organizations to the Best Advantage

For APNs, close contact with their professional organizations is an important link for staying abreast of national and state policy agendas, finding a support network of like-minded colleagues, and accessing information about changes in credentialing and practice issues. In today's complex world, this may mean being an active member of more than one affiliate organization to stay on the cutting edge of pertinent issues. Most APNs are aligned with at least one nursing organization; those who aspire to an active role in influencing policy will need to have membership in several. As new graduates move from the educational milieu into diverse practice settings, they must align with the advanced practice nursing organizations that best meet their needs and offer the strongest support, choosing to engage actively in some and remaining on the periphery in others.

Choosing the "right" organizations to belong to is a very personal decision based on particular needs, comfort level, specialty, and experience. Many APNs belong to one organization that meets their particular clinical needs (e.g., the Oncology Nursing Society [ONS] or AANA) and to another that offers cutting edge access to pressing professional issues (e.g., NONPF or American Nurses Association [ANA]). Others use the local, regional, or state affiliate of a professional organization as a support group that offers nurturing and professional sustenance, a group that understands local advanced practice nursing concerns.

The critical factor in interfacing with organizations is getting and staying involved in a definitive way. At a minimum, APNs will need to stay current on the issues by reading the organization's publications, frequently accessing their website and supporting the organization financially. Reading newsletters and journals, being part of an e-mail list or chat room, attending meetings and conferences, participating on committees or expert panels, and working up the ladder to leadership positions represent different levels of involvement. Professional organizations offer an important source of leadership and collective wisdom necessary to stay the course in today's political and policy arena. The notions of strength in numbers and speaking with one strong voice are not new concepts but are essential to the success of advanced practice nursing.

Political Action Committees

A political action committee (PAC) is the arm of an organization that finances political campaigns. Federal guidelines dictate how donations and funds are raised and administered (Clark, 2011; Malone & Chafee, 2007). PACs are required to be structured as a separate entity. PAC contributions do not buy votes but they do buy access to candidates and visibility in a campaign, which is critical to the advocacy process (Malone & Chafee, 2007). Decisions about endorsements are complex and are made at the national professional organization level based on careful research and candidates' past support for nursing and health care interests that align with the organization's professional priorities and values. Fundraising to support candidates is a major function of PACs and requires nursing support at every level. PACs are important to APN leaders at the national and state levels because the decisions about Medicare and Medicaid that undergird APN reimbursement are at stake.

Internships and Fellowships

One excellent way to develop the skills necessary to move into the role of advanced practice nursing policy advocate is to apply for a national or state policy internship or fellowship. These appointments, which last from several days to 1 or 2 years, offer a wide range of health policy and political experiences that are targeted to novice and expert APNs. For example, the Nurse in Washington Internship (NIWI), sponsored by the Nursing Organizations Alliance, is a 4-day internship that introduces nurses to policymaking in Washington DC (www.nursing-alliance.org). This internship serves as an excellent beginning step in learning the APN policy role. The National Rural Health Association also offers fellowships from time to time. Federal fellowships and internships that link nurses to legislators or to the various branches of federal and state government are invaluable in assisting APNs to understand how leaders are developed and how the system for setting health policy operates. Recently, two NPs, sponsored by supporters of the Nurse Practitioner Healthcare Foundation (NPHF), completed internships in the U.S. Surgeon General's Office.

Raising Awareness Through Communication

The ability of APNs to influence public policy rests with the individual nurse and with collective groups of APNs. The ability to communicate with others accurately, efficiently, and in a timely manner is a driving force in the world of policy and politics. Never before have people had such an opportunity to share information in its original form and to engage with others at a distance (Wakefield, 2003). Face to face, one on one interaction and on-site networking are always the best ways to ensure successful communication that satisfies all parties. Time and distance are no longer serious obstacles to communication. The multiple modes of Internet access make virtual communication a reality.

Today's communication networks are wonderful resources for gaining awareness and keeping current on policy initiatives and concerns from a wide variety of perspectives. Probably the most useful tool available to APNs is the Internet, which makes it possible for APN leaders to influence policy change from their own homes. It is possible to follow committee sessions in Congress via television or computer as they happen or later the same day via cable networks such as CNN and C-SPAN. Conference calls save countless hours on the road or in the air. Often, APNs at the grassroots level must push for this type of interaction with major policy activists and organizations. It is important for APNs in busy practices to press for distance access to engage directly in policy activities without disruptions in delivering patient care.

General Political Strategies

APNs have come a long way in demonstrating their political acumen at the state and national levels and have considerable power to achieve positive change if they capitalize on their newfound status. An important cohesiveness within nursing has emerged in response to health care system changes. The nursing profession as a whole has begun to recognize its strength at the policy table (see Chapter 22). Politics and ethics are inherent in relationships at all systems levels and, most obviously, in policy development. Therefore, nursing's ethical stance on social mandates that support poor and underserved populations needs to be clearly articulated (Falk-Rafael, 2005; Javitt, Berkowitz, & Goslin, 2008; Sarikonda-Woitas, 2002). Advanced practice nursing leaders have a responsibility to bring their views and perspectives to decision making and policy forums. They need to turn competitors into partners to make changes that will result in a less fragmented and more interdisciplinary system.

Dialogue about health care reform initiatives may cause some physicians and other important health care stakeholders to retrench, leading to a heightened perception of APNs as a threat. This has made the current political arena extremely sensitive. The political agenda that is carried out at the professional level (ANA–American Medical Association [ANA-AMA]) and among APN specialty organizations differs greatly from the agenda at the grassroots level. There is evidence that locally practicing physicians and nurses have strong collaborative relationships and are frustrated by the lack of cohesion among professional organizations when it comes to policymaking. APNs must closely monitor policy issues through all avenues open to them. New initiatives and recommendations (see earlier) provide an important strategy for the removal of barriers to APN practice. Also, the resurgence of a team approach to care is positive for the nursing agenda. Creating local networks of APNs and close interaction with collaborating physicians and leaders of local health care entities are crucial to removing barriers and developing workable practice guidelines. The Consensus Model for the Regulation of APRNs (see Chapter 21) will help states that continue to seriously constrain advanced practice nurses.

Nurses have a formidable voting power base of more than 3.5 million. This is an incredible strength for nurses but requires cohesiveness within the ranks to make positive change for advanced practice nursing. The notion that someone else will carry the flag is not realistic. Developing political acumen and competence is a required skill for all practicing APNs, and most certainly for APN leaders, that is nurtured through time and experience. Peters (2002) has asserted that nursing is facing an important policy window triggered by the nursing shortage, decreased access to care, and skyrocketing health care costs that provides an opportunity for nurses to gain leverage in the policy arena. Today, this same policy window exists (IOM, 2011; IPEC, 2011; U.S. Department of Health & Human Services, 2011). It will be important for APNs to take advantage of this opportunity.

Obstacles to Leadership Development and Effective Leadership

Professional and System Obstacles

There are several obstacles to achieving competence as an APN leader. Most of the obstacles result from conflict or competition among individuals, groups, or organizations. Professional turf issues have plagued APNs since the early days of their clinical practice. A lack of legal empowerment to practice to the fullest extent of knowledge and skills has been a dominant barrier to the optimal practice of APNs for decades. CNMs and CRNAs have the longest track record in dealing with these issues and have many successes to their credit. Competition can be intraprofessional, as between APN groups, and interprofessional, as between physicians and nurses. Grensing-Pophal (1997) has identified several barriers to good leadership and offered this advice. Being respected rather than being liked is one desired criterion for leadership; for most people, this is a difficult reality because being accepted and popular with others is important. Trying to do it all rather than delegating to others is a common trap that plagues busy leaders. As noted, a good leader can encourage a shared workload that recognizes the talents and abilities of followers.

Dysfunctional Leadership Styles

Leadership is often a lonely place and successful leadership requires careful nurturing. Although good leaders are sought after and desired, we have all experienced the other side of the coin—a dysfunctional leader. There are a multitude of traits and styles that can be attributed to a dysfunctional leader, such as micromanager, passive-aggressive, narcissistic personality, a quest for personal power, a game player. It is easy to recognize the dictatorial leader or the leader who is most interested in building his or her empire. Dysfunctional leaders often have poor self-control, have no time for others, and/or fail to accept responsibility for their own actions. At its worst, dysfunctional leadership moves into the realm of horizontal violence.

Horizontal Violence

Horizontal violence in nursing is described as an aggressive act carried out by one nursing colleague toward another (Longo & Sherman, 2007). This type of behavior is often seen among oppressed groups as a way for individuals to achieve a sense of power. Although there are many barriers to leading effectively and creating community, several constellations of behaviors that are particularly destructive have been identified. Nurses may be vulnerable to these destructive behaviors because of the profession's historical marginalization as being female and a relatively powerless group in health care. The culture of an organization, as described earlier, is also a factor in the development of these dysfunctional styles. These behaviors undermine successful APN leadership. APNs must avoid engaging in such behaviors and intervene assertively when they do occur. Three manifestations of horizontal violence in workplace culture limit the ability of APNs to lead, termed *star complex, queen bee syndrome,* and *failure to mentor* ("eating one's young"). These behaviors are of particular concern when the profession needs to recruit and mentor younger nurses to help them have satisfying careers and pass on the legacy of a satisfying career to future generations of nurses. Faculty and advanced practice nursing preceptors need to be alert to the appearance of such behaviors in students and coach them to understand their destructive impact on patients and colleagues. Readers are referred to the articles by Anderson (2011), Longo & Smith (2011), King (2002), Rider (2002), Longo and Sherman (2007), and Bally (2007) for specific suggestions on strategies for communicating with students and colleagues who demonstrate these negative interpersonal styles.

Abandoning One's Nursing Identity: Star Complex

An effective APN leader is proud of his or her identity as a nurse. Those with a star complex deny their nursing identity or minimize their affiliation with nursing when being identified as a nurse might diminish their influence (e.g., some nurse authors use only their academic credentials in publications within and outside of nursing). The star complex is a condition that is seen in some experienced APNs or in APNs who have not been well socialized into nursing as a profession. Although the psychology of this phenomenon is beyond the scope of this chapter, individuals with a star complex are those whose sense of self and identity depend a great deal on the opinions of powerful others. Acknowledging or promoting their identity as nurses is seen to diminish their power or the opinions that powerful others hold about them. As an example, consider Janice, an expert APN who provides superior patient-focused care. Physician colleagues consider her to be a partner in the delivery of care, but staff and other APNs gave up consulting with her because her self-promotion often interfered with patient and colleague interactions. In a recent conversation, a well-respected physician colleague told her how impressed he was with her practice. "In fact," he stated, "you're really not a nurse. You're different from all the other nurses I know." Janice graciously accepted this compliment, knowing that stardom, although overdue, had finally arrived. She had ascended to the heights of provider status and crashed through the nursing ceiling into a zone beyond nursing. Clearly, Janice's understanding of herself as an APN was dormant.

APNs are particularly vulnerable to being seduced into believing that they are something other (more) than a nurse. Advanced practice nursing specialties that have expanded roles may seek the status of medicine. This vulnerability stems from the historical lack of recognition of nursing by physicians, other disciplines, and even other nurses, the need for approval, and a lack of personal mastery.

A primary strategy for the management of this obstacle is effective mentoring by a powerful APN with an intact nursing identity. An APN with a star complex may have been mentored exclusively by individuals outside of nursing. The affirmation of the APN's expert clinical skills and even personal mastery are thus validated by a reference group outside of nursing. An additional essential strategy is to use clear and concise communication skills to provide an appropriate response to a colleague who believes that it is a compliment to be identified as other than a nurse. An appropriate response for Janice to have made would have been, "Thank you, but I'm proud to be an APN. It is good that we can work together to help our patients." The existence of a star complex may represent a more fundamental problem for the APN than good communication skills can address. The issue is whether the APN truly desires to be identified as a nurse, performing at the boundaries of nursing practice and accepted by other nurses as a valued member of the nursing profession. As APNs are increasingly recognized as valued members of the health care team and as mentoring and empowerment become understood as core elements of leadership, star complex behavior will become unnecessary and less frequent.

Hoarding or Misusing Power: Queen Bee Syndrome

An effective leader is generous, looking for opportunities to lift colleagues up by sharing opportunities, knowledge, and expertise and acknowledging the contributions of others. Queen bees hoard all the visible leadership tasks for themselves. Like those with a star complex, the effort to garner power is a theme. In this case, power derives not from powerful others but from the queen bee's own knowledge and expertise. Such APNs are threatened by strong individuals and tend to denigrate them instead of sharing power. This type of leader prefers to be surrounded by servile individuals who will not challenge her or his authority. For example, Jackie, an experienced wound and ostomy APN, makes sure that she sees every patient and that patients know she is the authority on wounds and ostomies. Staff nurses who are competent in these skills report that Jackie undermines them with patients by saying that the care should have been done a certain way. Jackie was not happy when the staff on a surgical unit, who had tried unsuccessfully to involve her in a unit project, conducted a quality improvement project during which both physicians and patients identified some service delivery issues relative to ostomy care. These staff members had the support of an assertive new CNS and nurse manager and, over time, slowly changed the way wound and ostomy services were managed.

The antidote to a queen bee syndrome is to use knowledge and expertise to move away from hoarding power toward collaborative, empowered leadership. Queen bee behavior is the antithesis of good leadership and, unfortunately, is not uncommon among women and nurses. As advanced practice nursing leaders become more confident in their leadership abilities and as more APNs join the circle of leaders, queen bees will have more difficulty remaining as leaders and keeping positions of power. All effective leaders empower others.

Failure to Mentor

The most distressing form of horizontal violence is, unfortunately, the most common. "Nurses eat their young" is an epithet that characterizes the experience of many novice nurses and APNs, as well as of some older, more experienced nurses (Baltimore, 2006). Nurses who advance in their profession may forget their roots and leave novice nurses behind or, worse, actively undermine their advancement. For example, nurses are often criticized by other nurses for continuing their education and moving into APN roles. This denigration of important values and

goals by colleagues is dispiriting and discouraging; it can hamper nurses from moving forward in their careers. In another example, the orientation process for a new position may become a survival test to see whether the new APN can survive without mentoring or a supportive network. Because perceived powerlessness is at the root of this behavior, an important antidote is empowerment. The common practice of mentoring, apprenticing, and "giving a leg up" to the least experienced is not as common in nursing as it is in many other professions.

Failure to mentor may be evident in the following behaviors (Baltimore, 2006; Longo & Sherman, 2007; Longo & Smith, 2011):

- Gossiping or bad mouthing
- Criticizing
- Failure to give assistance when needed
- Setting up road blocks by withholding information
- Bullying
- Scapegoating
- Undermining performance

Bullying is a severe form of horizontal violence attributed to oppressed group behavior. Hutchinson and colleagues (2005), Longo and Sherman (2007), and Keefe (2007) have suggested that horizontal violence is a more complex phenomenon and includes those external to nursing who make up the organization's culture and add to stress in the work setting. Curran (2006) has reported that with the baby boomer generation, there will be more career nurses vying for leadership positions and that forms of horizontal violence such as bullying will worsen. Bullying is not a one-time event but, instead, is a subtle, deliberate, ongoing behavior that accumulates over time and leaves the victim feeling hurt, vulnerable, and powerless (Anderson, 2011; Hutchinson et al., 2005; Longo & Sherman, 2007).

Personal and organizational symptoms of horizontal violence are job dissatisfaction, increased stress levels, and physical and psychological illness. If the broader cause is a negative organizational culture, then the most effective leadership strategy to prevent its occurrence is to adopt a zero tolerance policy and a shared set of values with the staff (Longo & Sherman, 2007; Longo and Smith, 2011) that support positive behaviors. For example, fostering mentoring opportunities and enhancing the transition of colleagues into new positions of leadership can create a positive culture that does not tolerate horizontal violence. See Box 11-5 for suggested leadership strategies to eliminate horizontal violence.

Negative behaviors that are expressed as failure to mentor, bullying, and disenfranchising others may continue to be present in an increasingly stressful health care environment (McAvoy & Murtagh, 2003; Thomas, 2003). It is not an overstatement to claim that the future health

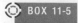 **BOX 11-5** | **Leadership Strategies to Stop the Cycle of Horizontal Violence**

- Examine the organizational culture for symptoms of horizontal violence.
- Name the problem as horizontal violence when you see it.
- Educate staff to break the silence.
- Allow victims of horizontal violence to tell their stories.
- Enact a process for dealing with issues that occur.
- Provide training for conflict and anger management skills.
- Empower victims to defend themselves.
- Engage in self-reflection to ensure that your leadership style does not support horizontal violence.
- Encourage a culture of zero tolerance for horizontal violence.

Adapted from Longo, J., & Sherman, R. O. (2007). Leveling horizontal violence. *Nursing Management, 38,* 34–37, 50–51.

of the profession depends on overcoming this barrier and relegating it to history. It is the role of APN leaders as role models to create a more empowering and humane work environment for their colleagues and those who follow them.

Strategies for Implementing the Leadership Competency

Developing a Leadership Portfolio

Throughout this chapter, definitions, attributes, and components of leadership and key strategies for developing competency in APN leadership have been presented. These approaches will help new APNs acquire leadership skills. Developing a leadership component as part of a marketing portfolio is helpful to novice APNs who desire to individualize continuing development of the leadership competency consistent with their personal vision, goals, timeline, and APN role in the practice setting. An Australian study in 2010 reported increased knowledge, skill sets, and outcomes in clinicians and leaders who used portfolios to enhance their effectiveness (Dadich, 2010). Falter (2003) has suggested the use of a strategy map that includes vision, goals, and objectives that outline steps to achieve a particular strategy. Portfolios are designed to meet the needs of individual APNs and should be consistent with clinical and personal interests and professional goals and provide a timeline that allows for personal and professional balance and boundary setting. Chapter 20 provides the elements of a marketing portfolio.

Promoting Collaboration Among Advanced Practice Nursing Groups

At different times, each subgroup of APNs has emerged as a leader for the nursing profession. Psychiatric CNSs were among the first entrepreneurial APNs to hang out their shingle, despite the litigious climate in which they could be threatened with lawsuits for "practicing medicine." CNMs and CRNAs have led the way in using data effectively to justify their practice and attain appropriate scopes of practice. Early in their history, both groups began to record the results of their practices, showing the quality and suitability of their care (see Chapter 1). In the 1990s, NPs, with their flexible, community-based primary care practices, stood at the forefront of the changing health care delivery system. Although these subgroups of APNs have made impressive strides for advanced practice nursing, an obstacle to effective leadership is the tendency for APN specialty groups to separate and establish rigid boundaries that distinguish them from one another, thereby fragmenting APN groups and blocking opportunities for the increased power that unity would bring.

The tension and fragmentation created by rigid boundaries require leaders who can transcend APN roles and specialties. APNs must manage and bridge boundaries among other nursing groups and within the ranks of the various APN constituencies. Although the uniqueness of each type of APN must be protected, a professional structure that provides a forum for discussing issues pertinent to all types of APNs also needs to be created. This structure may simply be an annual meeting for APNs or a permanent entity residing within an existing or new professional organization. Consensus groups at the national level have been meeting to discuss policy issues in which the power of the collective numbers of all APN groups speaking with one voice cannot be overemphasized (see Chapters 2, 12, and 21). An excellent example of professional collaboration among nursing leaders is the Consensus Model work (Chapter 21). APN organizations have joined to speak out collaboratively about state regulations regarding reimbursement, prescriptive authority, and managed care empanelment.

It is critical that each APN, regardless of specialty, takes on the responsibility of moving toward an integrative and unified understanding of advanced practice nursing. Creating community in the current health care environment is particularly challenging because of the realignment of clinical decision making, scopes of practice for APNs and physicians, and new roles that blur boundaries between nursing and medicine.

An understanding of change, effective communication, coalition building, shared vision, and collaborative practice leads to the development of structures on which unity is built. These five building blocks form the foundation of interdisciplinary leadership and practice.

Motivating and Empowering Others

Motivation and empowerment are core elements of the APN leadership competency. Empowerment was defined earlier as the ability of the leader to give followers the freedom and authority to act. However, truly empowering others requires more than just giving them permission to act on their own. Empowerment is a developmental process; over time, a good leader encourages their constituents' sense of responsibility and competence, thus reinforcing their autonomy and authority to act. Wheatley (2005) has affirmed the importance of motivation and empowerment in developing innovators and has noted that older notions of power and control are things of the past, as has Senge (2006). Today's APN leaders need to use the tools of empowerment and motivation to mentor future leaders who can lead with creativity, innovation, and caring.

Networking

Networking is an essential technique used by leaders to stay informed and connected regarding APN issues. Networking, formal and informal, is not a new strategy for APN leaders. Formal networks take the form of committees, coalitions, and consortia of people who come together to share information, collaborate, and plan strategy regarding mutual issues. Formal networks open doors to new opportunities and provide shared resources that ensure a competitive edge in the organization (Carroll, 2005; Montgomery, 2011). Informal networking is a behind the scenes strategy that allows for contact with APNs and others who speak the same language, have the same viewpoints, and can offer support and feedback at critical times. The ability of APNs to stay connected to important practice and education issues through networking is key to the leadership competency. The most effective strategy for becoming an insider is networking with colleagues within the circle of APN peers and with other health care providers who have a stake in the outcomes of a particular issue. Montgomery (2011) has suggested that it is important to make your "net" work!

Engaging Others in Planning and Implementing Change

The skills outlined earlier, "Attributes of Effective Advanced Practice Nurse Leaders," on personal attributes of successful leaders (p. 281) are integral to leading innovation and change. However, other strategies also assist in the process. It is important to analyze the situation and explore the need for change. If change is warranted, one must craft an implementation plan that involves everyone. Box 11-1 lists leadership strategies that are useful for moving through these transitions. Bonalumi and Fisher (1999) have suggested that an important component of leadership during times of change is the ability to foster and encourage resilience in change recipients. O'Connell (1999) and, more recently, Grafton and associates (2010) have defined resilient people as being positive and self-assured in the face of life's complexities, having a focused, clear vision of what they want to achieve, and having the ability to be organized but flexible and proactive rather than reactive. Helping colleagues and followers develop resilience should be a major focus for advanced practice nursing leaders who seek to facilitate the growth of their followers.

The second DNP essential for advanced nursing practice education addresses the provision of sophisticated leadership that "emphasizes practice, ongoing improvement of health outcomes and ensuring patient safety"; to accomplish these goals, APNs will need "expertise in assessing organizations, identifying systems issues and facilitating organization-wide changes in practice delivery" (AACN, 2006, p. 10).

Institutional Assessment Regarding Readiness for Change

With the emphasis on evidence-based practice and the knowledge that evidence-based guidelines and therapies are underused (IOM, 2001; McGlynn et al., 2003), overused, or misused (IOM, 2001), APNs have an important systems leadership role in improving care. This can be accomplished by leading and collaborating with nurses and interdisciplinary colleagues to ensure the adoption of best practices (Duffy, 2002; Spencer & Jordan, 2001; Spross & Heaney, 2000; Weaver, Salas, & King, 2011). An institutional assessment of specific factors will help the APN identify facilitators of and barriers to change. These data can then be used to design a plan for change in collaboration with others. Box 11-6 lists key assessment questions to consider.

Followship

As APNs focus on developing their leadership skills, they cannot ignore the importance of being a good follower. It takes skill to recognize when one should be a follower rather than a leader—when another is more skilled or more appropriate to lead a particular situation, or when it is appropriate to let another who is developing his or her leadership skills take the lead on a project. Successful

BOX 11-6   Assessment Questions to Evaluate Readiness for Change

- What is the nature of the change (e.g., policy, procedure, new skill, behavior)?
- Is the issue significant? For all stakeholders or just one group?
- Is a national policy, guideline, or standard the focus of the change? Is it a mandate with which the agency must be in compliance?
- Is the change simple or complex? Will different stakeholders perceive its simplicity or complexity differently?
- Do you foresee major problems associated with change, such as an increase in errors or resistance on the part of a group?
- Will it be possible to address these major problems?
- Are there vested interests—who is likely to gain from the change, who will view the change as a loss (e.g., of power)?
- Are there opinion leaders who will promote the change? Do you anticipate strong opposition?
- Have you observed a gap between public statements and private actions (e.g., a colleague agrees to serve on a committee but never shows up or participates in the committee's work)?
- Are there resource implications? What are the costs (e.g., staffing, materials, lost revenue)?

Adapted from the University of York National Health Centre for Reviews and Dissemination. (1999). Getting evidence into practice. *Effective Health Care Bulletin, 5,* 1–16.

collaboration and teamwork require not just leadership, but skilled followers as well. Expert followers know how to accept direction, be forthcoming with pertinent information that is valuable to the team, seek clarification, and provide appropriate constructive feedback.

Conclusion

The health care system is constantly changing. Despite the challenges of change, the future is bright for APNs as clinical, professional, health policy, and systems leaders. APNs can define the scope of their leadership influence in far-reaching ways, from the bedside to the White House. The evolution of APNs in all the various roles has had significant influence on this country's health care system, as well as on nursing itself, at every level. APNs exercise leadership when they present ideas or dilemmas and offer solutions to colleagues, whether on an e-mail list or at a national meeting. Many small changes contribute to a big change, so APNs should not underestimate the impact of leadership exercised at the bedside or in the clinic and with patients, colleagues, and administrators. It is important for all APNs to consider how they can lead, make a difference, and commit to doing so, knowing that they can redefine the scope of their leadership influence in response to opportunities or changing life circumstances. The dynamic, ever-changing environment of health care sets the stage for ceaseless opportunities for APNs to innovate and lead.

Nursing care is based on an interactive style that empowers patients and colleagues. This foundation holds APN leaders in good stead as they move into the interdisciplinary paradigm to come. As APNs contemplate the demands and opportunities for leadership that the future holds, they must work toward identifying, clarifying, and demystifying the health care system of today, for within today's reality lies the basis of tomorrow's change. APNs are change specialists who operate at the boundary between today's health care system and that of tomorrow. The attributes, goals, and vision of APN leaders put them at the forefront of the health care frontier.

References

Abbott, P. A., & Coenen, A. (2008). Globalization and advances in information and communication technologies: The impact on nursing and health. *Nursing Outlook, 56,* 38–246.

Aduddell, K. A., & Dorman, G. E. (2010). The development of the next generation of nurse leaders. *Journal of Nursing Education, 49,* 168–171.

Agency for Healthcare Research and Quality (AHRQ). (2010). Comprehensive program to promote "fair and just principles" improves employee perceptions of how a health system responds to errors (www.innovations.ahrq.gov/content.aspx?id=2588).

Allen, D. W. (1998). How nurses become leaders: Perceptions and beliefs about leadership development. *Journal of Nursing Administration, 28,* 15–20.

American Association of Colleges of Nursing (AACN). (2004). *Position statement on the practice doctorate in nursing.* Washington, DC: Author.

American Association of Colleges of Nursing (AACN). (2006). *The essentials of doctoral education for advanced nursing practice.* Washington, DC: Author.

American Association of Nurse Anesthetists (AANA). (2012). Federal government affairs. (www.aana.com/Advocacy/federalgovernment affairs/Pages/default.aspx

Anderson, K. (2011). Work place aggression and violence: Midwives and nurses say no. *Australian Nursing Journal, 26,* 1320–1385.

Bally, J. M. G. (2007). The role of nursing leadership in creating a mentoring culture in acute care environments. *Nursing Economic$, 25,* 143–148.

Baltimore, J. (2006). Nurse collegiality: Fact or fiction. *Nursing management, 37,* 28–36.

Barker, A. (1994). An energy leadership paradigm: Transformational leadership. In E. I. Hein & M. J. Nicholson (Eds.), *Contemporary leadership* (pp. 81–86, 4th ed.). Philadelphia: JB Lippincott.

Barker, E. R. (2006). Mentoring: A complex relationship. *Journal of the American Academy of Nurse Practitioners, 18,* 56–61.

Berwick, D. M., Caulkins, D. R., McCannon, C. J., & Hackbarth, A. D. (2006). The 100000 lives campaign: Setting a goal and a deadline for improving health care quality. *Journal of the American Medical Association, 295,* 324–327.

Blanchard, K., Hutson, D., & Willis, E. (2007). *The one minute entrepreneur: Discover your entrepreneurial strengths.* Mechanicsburg, PA: Executive Books.

Blizzard, R., Khoury, C., & McMurray, C. (2010). Nursing leadership from bedside to boardroom: Opinion leaders' perceptions (http://www.thefutureofnursing.org/sites/default/files/Research%20Brief-%20Nursing%20Leadership%20from%20Bedside%20to%20Boardroom.pdf).

Bonalumi, N., & Fisher, K. (1999). Health care change: Challenge for nurse administrators. *Nursing Administration Quarterly, 23,* 69–73.

Brown, S. J. (1989). Supportive supervision of the CNS. In A.B. Hamric & J.A. Spross (Eds.), *The clinical nurse specialist in theory and practice* (pp. 285–298, 2nd ed.). Philadelphia: WB Saunders.

Canadian Interprofessional Health Collaborative (CIHC). (2010). A national interprofessional competencies framework (www.cihc.ca/files/CIHC_IPCompetencies_Feb1210.pdf).

Carlson, E. A., Klakovich, M., Broscious, S. K., Delock, S., Roche-Dean, M., Hittle, K., et al. (2011). Board leadership development: The key to effective nursing leadership. *Journal of Continuing Education in Nursing, 42,* 107–113.

Carroll, T. L. (2005). Leadership skills and attributes of women and nurse executives: Challenges for the 21st century. *Nursing Administration Quarterly, 29,* 146–153.

Castledine, S.G. (2008). Dealing with difficult doctors. *British Journal of Nursing, 17,* 1305.

Christopher, M. A., Miller, J., Beck, T., & Toughill, E. (2002). Working with the community for change. In D. Mason, J. Leavitt, & M. Chaffee (Eds.), *Policy and politics in nursing and health care* (pp. 933–946, 4th ed.). Philadelphia: WB Saunders.

Clark, S. (2011). The importance of nursing political action committees. *Illinois Nurse, 7,* 10.

Cooperrider, D. L., Whitney, D., & Stavros, J. M. (2008). *Appreciative inquiry handbook* (2nd ed.). Brunswick, OH: Berrett-Koehler.

Covey, S. (1989). *The seven habits of highly effective people: Powerful lessons in personal change.* New York: Simon & Schuster.

Covey, S. (2004). *The 8th habit. From effectiveness to greatness.* New York: Free Press.

Covey, S. (2006). Leading in the knowledge worker age. *Leader to Leader Journal, 41,* 11–15

Cronenwett, L., & Dzau, V. (2010). In B. Culliton & S. Russell (Eds). *Who will provide primary care and how will they be trained? Proceedings of a conference sponsored by the Josiah Macy Jr. Foundation.* Durham, NC: Josiah Macy Jr. Foundation.

Cronenwett, L., Sherwood, G., Pohl, J., Barnsteiner, J., Moore, S., Sullivan, D. T., et al. (2009). Quality and safety education for advanced practice nurses. *Nursing Outlook, 57,* 338–348.

Curran, C. (2006). Boomers: Bottlenecked, bored, and burned out. *Nursing Economic$, 24,* 57, 93.

Dadich, A. (2010). From bench to bedside: Methods that help clinicians use evidence-based practice. *Australian Psychologist, 45,* 197–211.

Davis, L. L., Little, M. S., & Thornton, W. L. (1997). The art and angst of the mentoring relationship. *Academic Psychiatry, 21,* 61–71.

DePree, M. (1989). *Leadership is an art.* New York: Doubleday.

Doerksen, K. (2010). What are the professional development and mentorship needs of advanced practice nurses? *Journal of Professional Nursing, 26,* 141–151.

Donelan, K., Buerhaus, P., DesRoches, C., & Burke, S. (2010). Health policy thought leaders' views of the health workforce in an era of health reform. *Nursing Outlook, 58,* 175–180.

Doumit, G., Gattellari, M., Grimshaw, J., & O'Brien, M. (2007). Local opinion leaders: Effects on professional practice and health care outcomes. *Cochrane Database of Systematic Reviews,* (1), CD000125.

Duffy, J. R. (2002). The clinical leadership role of the CNS in the identification of nursing-sensitive and multidisciplinary quality indicator sets. *Clinical Nurse Specialist, 16,* 70–76.

Falk-Rafael, A. (2005). Speaking truth to power: Nursing's legacy and moral imperative. *Advances in Nursing Science, 28,* 212–223.

Falter, E. (2003). Successful leaders map and measure. *Nurse Leader, 1,* 40–42, 45.

Fiedler, F. E., Chermers, M. M., & Mahar, L. C. (1976). *Improving leadership effectiveness: The leader match concept.* New York: John Wiley.

Fisher, R., Ury, W., & Patton, B. (2002). *Getting to yes: How to negotiate an agreement without giving in* (2nd ed.). New York: Penguin Putnam.

Friedman, T. L. (2006). *The world is flat.* New York: Farrar, Straus, & Giroux.

Giger, J., Davidhizar, R., Purnell, L., Taylor-Harden, J., Phillips, J., & Strickland, O. (2007). Understanding cultural language to enhance cultural competence. *Nursing Outlook, 55,* 212–213.

Gilliss, C. (2011). Developing policy leadership in nursing: Three wishes. *Nursing Outlook, 59,* 179–181.

Gladwell, M. (2000). *The tipping point: How little things can make a big difference.* Boston: Little Brown.

Greenhalgh, T., Robert, G., Macfarlane, F., Bate, P., & Kyriakidou, O. (2004). Diffusion of innovation in service organizations: Systematic review and recommendations. *The Millbank Quarterly, 82,* 581–629.

Grafton, E., Gillespie, B., & Henderson, S. (2010). Resiliance: The power within. *Nursing Oncology Forum, 37,* 698–705.

Greiner, A., & Knebel, E. (Eds.). (2003). Health professions education: A bridge to quality. Washington, DC: Institute of Medicine.

Grensing-Pophal, L. (1997). Improving your leadership skills: Seven common pitfalls to avoid. *Nursing, 27,* 41–42.

Grohar-Murray, M. E., & DiCroce, H. R. (1992). *Leadership and management in nursing.* Norwalk, CT: Appleton & Lange.

Grossman, D. (2006). Fostering leadership through collaboration: Move over physicians. Nurses belong on health care boards too. *Reflections on Nursing Leadership* (www.reflectionsonnursingleadership.org).

Halpern, I. M. (2002). Reflections of a health policy advocate: The natural extension of nursing activities. *Oncology Nursing Forum, 29,* 1261–1263.

Hanson, C. M., Boyle, J., Hatmaker, D., & Murray, J. (1999). *Finding your voice as a leader.* Washington, DC: American Academy of Nursing.

Harrington, S. (2011). Mentoring new nurse practitioners to accelerate their development as primary care providers. *Journal of the American Academy of Nurse Practitioners, 23,* 168–174.

Health Sciences Institute. (2005). Chronic care competency model (www.chroniccare.org/documents/FullCCPCompetency Model.pdf).

Heifetz, R. (1994). *Leadership without easy answers.* Cambridge, MA: Belknap Press.

Houghton, A. (2003). Bullying in medicine. *British Medical Journal, 326,* S125.

Hurley, T. J., & Brown, J. (2009). Conversational leadership: Thinking together for change (http://www.theworldcafe.com/articles/Conversational-Leadership.pdf).

Hutchinson, M., Vickers, M., Jackson, D., & Wilkes, L. (2005). Workplace bullying in nursing: Toward a more critical organizational perspective. *Nursing Inquiry, 13,* 118–126.

Institute for Healthcare Improvement (IHI). (2007, updated 2012). Protecting 5 million lives (http://www.ihi.org/offerings/Initiatives/PastStrategicInitiatives/5MillionLivesCampaign/Pages/default.aspx).

Institute for Healthcare Improvement (IHI). (2011). Transforming care at the bedside (http://www.ihi.org/offerings/Initiatives/PastStrategicInitiatives/TCAB/Pages/default.aspx).

Institute of Medicine (IOM). (2000). *To err is human: Building a safer health system.* Washington, DC: National Academy Press.

Institute of Medicine (IOM). (2001). *Crossing the quality chasm: A new health system for the 21st century.* Washington, DC: National Academy Press.

Institute of Medicine. (IOM). (2011). *The future of nursing: Leading change, advancing health.* Washington, DC: National Academy Press.

Interprofessional Collaborative Initiative (IPEC). (2011). Core competencies of interprofessional collaborative practice (www.aacn.nche.edu/education/pdf/IPECreport.pdf).

Javitt, G., Berkowitz, D., & Goslin, L. (2008). Assessing mandatory HPV vaccination. *Journal of Law, Medicine, and Ethics, 36,* 384–395.

Jones, R. S. P. (2010). Appreciative inquiry: More than just a fad? *British Journal of Healthare Management, 16,* 114–119.

Just Culture Community. (2012). About us (http://www.justculture.org/about-us).

Kantor, R. M., Stein, B. A., & Jick, T. D. (1992). *The challenge of organizational change: How companies experience it and leaders guide it.* New York: Free Press.

Keefe, S. (2007). Bullying among nurses. *Advance for Nurses,* July 16, 36–38.

Kendig, S. (2006). Advocacy, action, and the allure of butter: A focus on policy (www.medscape.com/viewarticle/523631).

King, J. (2002). Dealing with difficult doctors. *British Medical Journal, 325,* S43.

Klein, E., Gabelnick, F., & Herr, P. (1998). *The psychodynamics of leadership.* Madison, CT: Psychosocial Press.

Larson, L. (2004). Telling the story: Trustees and grassroots political advocacy. *Trustee, 57,* 6–11.

Lazarus, I. R., & Fell, D. (2011). Innovation or stagnation: Crossing the creativity gap in healthcare. *Journal of Healthcare Management, 56,* 263–267.

Leape, L., Berwick, D., Clancy, C., Conway, J., Gluck, P., Guest, J., et al.; Lucian Leape Institute at the National Patient Safety Foundation. (2009). Transforming healthcare: A safety imperative. *Quality and Safety in Health Care, 18,* 424–428.

Leavitt, J. K., Chaffee, M. W., & Vance, C. (2007). Learning the ropes of policy, politics, and advocacy. In D. J. Mason, J. K. Leavitt, & M. W. Chaffee (Eds.), *Policy and politics in nursing and health care* (5th ed.). Philadelphia: Saunders.

Locock, L., Dopson, S., Chambers, D., & Gabbay, J. (2001). Understanding the role of opinion leaders in improving clinical effectiveness. *Social Science and Medicine, 53,* 745–757.

Longo, J., & Sherman, R. O. (2007). Leveling horizontal violence. *Nursing Management, 38,* 34–37, 50–51.

Longo, J., & Smith, M. (2011). A prescription for disruptions in care: Community building among nurses to address horizontal violence. *Advances in Nursing Science, 34,* 345–356.

Lynch, B., McCormack, B., & McCance, T. (2011). Development of a model of situational leadership in residential care of older people. *Journal of Nursing Management, 19,* 1058–1069.

Malone, P., & Chafee, M. (2007). Interest groups: Powerful political catalysts in health care. In D.J. Mason, J.K. Leavitt, & M. Chaffee (Eds.), *Policy and politics in nursing and health care* (pp. 766–770, 5th ed.). Philadelphia: Saunders.

Massoud, M. R., Nielsen, G. A., Nolan, K., Schall, M. W., & Sevin, C. (2006). A framework for spread: From local improvements to system-wide change. IHI Innovation Series White Paper. Cambridge, MA: Institute for Healthcare Improvement. (available at www.IHI.org).

McAvoy, B., & Murtagh, J. (2003). Workplace bullying: The silent epidemic [letter]. *British Medical Journal, 326,* 776–777.

McCloughen, A., O'Brien, L., & Jackson, D. (2009). Esteemed connection: creating a mentoring relationship for nurse leadership. *Nursing Inquiry, 16,* 326–336.

McCloughen, A., O'Brien, L., & Jackson, D. (2010). More than vision: Imagination as an elemental characteristic of being a nurse leader-mentor. *Advances in Nursing Science, 33,* 285–296.

McGlynn, E. A., Asch, S. M., Adams, J., Keesey, J., Hicks, J., DeCristofaro, A., et al. (2003). The quality of health care delivered to adults in the United States. *New England Journal of Medicine, 348,* 2635–2645.

Montgomery, T. (2011). Going up? Intentional networking works (http://www.reflectionson nursingleadership.org/Pages/Vol37_2_Montgomery.aspx).

Murphy, J., Quillian, B., & Carolan, M. (2009). Role of clinical nurse leadership in improving patient care. *Nursing Management, 16,* 26–28.

National Association of Clinical Nurse Specialists (NACNS). (2004). *Statement on clinical nurse specialist practice and education.* Harrisburg, PA: Author.

National Association of Clinical Nurse Specialists (NACNS). (2010). Organizing framework and CNS core competencies (www.nacns.org/docs/CNSCoreCompetencies.pdf).

National Association of Clinical Nurse Specialists (NACNS). (2011). Starter kit for impacting change at the government level: How to work with your state legislators and regulators (www.nacns.org/html/toolkit.php).

National Organization of Nurse Practitioner Faculties (2012). Nurse practitioner core competencies (www.nonpf.com/associations/10789/files/NPCoreCompetenciesFinal2012.pdf).

Nelson, E. C., Batalden, P. B., Huber, T. P., Mohr, J. J., Godfrey, M. M., Headrick, L. A., et al. (2002). Microsystems in health care: Part 1. Learning from high-performing front-line clinical units. *Joint Commission Journal on Quality Improvement, 28,* 472–493.

Nichols, B., Shaffer, F., & Porter, C. (2011). Global nursing leadership: A practical guide. *Nursing Administration Quarterly, 35,* 354–359.

Norton, S. F., & Grady, E. M. (1996). Change agent skills. In A. B. Hamric, J. A. Spross, & C. M. Hanson (Eds.), *Advanced nursing practice: An integrative approach* (pp. 249–271). Philadelphia: WB Saunders.

O'Connell, C. (1999). A culture of change or a change of culture. *Nursing Administration Quarterly, 23,* 65–68.

Oxman, A. D., Thomson, M. A., Davis, D. A., & Haynes, R. B. (1995). No magic bullets: A systematic review of 102 trials of interventions to improve professional practice. *Canadian Medical Association Journal, 153,* 1423–1431.

Park, Y., & Jex, S. (2011). Work-home boundary management using communication and information technology. *International Journal of Stress Management, 18,* 133–152.

Patient Safety and Quality Health Care. (2005). IHI launches national campaign to save 100,000 lives in U.S. hospitals (http://www.psqh.com/janfeb05/100k.html).

Peters, R. M. (2002). Nurse administrators' role in health care policy: Teaching the elephant to dance. *Nursing Administration Quarterly, 26,* 1–8.

Pohl, J. M., Hanson, C. M., Newland, J. A., & Croenwett, L. (2010). Unleashing nurse practitioners' potential to deliver primary care and lead teams. *Health Affairs, 29,* 900–905.

Rajotte, C. A. (1996). Empowerment as a leadership theory. *Kansas Nurse, 71,* 1.

Rapede, E. (2011). Participatory dreaming: A unitary appreciative inquiry into healing with women abused as children. *Advances in Nursing Science, 34,* 174–197.

Reeves, S., Zwarenstein, M., Goldman, J., Barr, H., Freeth, D., Hammick, M., et al. (2009). Interprofessional education: Effects on professional practice and health care outcomes (https://ipls.dk/pdf-filer/ip_education_cochrane.pdf).

Reinertsen, J., Gosfield, A., Rupp, W., & Whittington, J. (2007). *Engaging physicians in a shared quality agenda.* Cambridge, MA: Institute for Healthcare Improvement.

Richer, M., Ritchie, J., & Marichionni, C. (2009). If we can't do more, let's do it differently: Using appreciative inquiry to promote innovative ideas for better health care work environments. *Journal of Nursing Management, 17,* 947–955.

Rider, F. (2002). Twelve strategies for effective communication and collaboration in medical teams. *British Medical Journal, 325,* S45.

Robert Wood Johnson Foundation. (2012). Robert Wood Johnson executive nurse fellows (http://www.rwjfleaders.org/programs/robert-wood-johnson-foundation-executive-nurse-fellows-program).

Rost, J. C. (1993). *Leadership for the 21st century.* Westport, CT: Praeger.

Rychnovsky, J. (2011). Dr. Ruth Lubic, a timeless and tireless visionary for child-bearing families. *Journal of Obstetric, Gynecologic, and Neonatal Nursing, 40,* 509–511.

Sandrick, K. (2006). The new political advocacy. *Trustee, 59,* 6–10.

Sarikonda-Woitas, C. (2002). Ethical health care policy: Nursing's voice in allocation. *Nursing Administration Quarterly, 26,* 72–80.

Schwartz, D., Spencer, T., Wilson, B., & Wood, K. (2011). Transformational leadership: Implications for nursing leaders in facilities seeking magnet designation. *AORN Journal, 93,* 737–748.

Secretan, L. (1999). *Inspirational leadership: Destiny, cause and calling.* Ontario, Canada: Secretan Center.

Secretan, L. (2003). *Reclaiming higher ground: Creating organizations that inspire the soul.* Ontario, Canada: Secretan Center.

Senge, P. (1990). *The fifth discipline: The art and practice of the learning organization.* New York: Doubleday.

Senge, P. (2006). *The fifth discipline: The art and practice of the learning organization (revised edition).* New York: Doubleday.

Senge, P., Kleiner, A., Roberts, C., Ross, R., Roth, G., & Smith, B. (1999). *The dance of change: The challenges of sustaining momentum in learning organizations.* New York: Doubleday.

Sherwood, G. (2006). Appreciative leadership. Building customer-driven partnerships. *Journal of Nursing Administration, 36,* 551–557.

Sherwood, G. (2010). New views of quality and safety offer new roles for nurses and midwives. *Nursing and Health Sciences, 12,* 281–283.

Shirey, M. R. (2004). Social support in the workplace: Nurse leader implications. *Nursing Economic$, 22,* 313–319.

Shirey, M. R. (2007a). AONE leadership perspectives. Competencies and tips for effective leadership: From novice to expert. *Journal of Nursing Administration, 37,* 167–170.

Shirey, M. R. (2007b). An evidence-based understanding of entrepreneurship in nursing. *Clinical Nurse Specialist, 21,* 234–240.

Shirey, M. R. (2008). Influencers among us: A practical approach for leading change. *Clinical Nurse Specialist, 22,* 63–66.

Shirey M. R. (2009). Transferable skills and entrepreneurial strategy. *Clinical Nurse Specialist, 23,* 128–130.

Shortell, S. M., & Singer, S. J. (2008). Improving patient safety by taking systems seriously. *Journal of the American Medical Association, 299,* 445–447.

Smythe, L., Payne, D., & Wynyard, S. (2009). Warkworth Birthing Centre: Exemplifying the future. *New Zealand College of Midwives Journal, 41,* 7–11.

Solman, A. (2010). Director of nursing and midwifery leadership: Informed through the lens of critical social science. *Journal of Nursing Management, 18,* 472–476.

Soumerai, S. B., McLaughlin, T. J., Gurwitz, J. H., Guadagnoli, E., Hauptman, P. J., Borbas, C., et al. (1998). Effect of local medical opinion leaders on quality of care for acute myocardial infarction: A randomized controlled trial. *Journal of the American Medical Association, 279,* 1358–1363.

Spencer, J., & Jordan, R. (2001). Educational outcomes and leadership to meet the needs of modern health care. *Quality and Safety in Health Care, 10*(Suppl 2), 38–45.

Spross, J. A. (2001). Harnessing power and passion: Lessons from pain management leaders and literature (www.edc.org/lastacts).

Spross, J. A., & Heaney, C. A. (2000). Shaping advanced nursing practice in the new millennium. *Seminars in Oncology Nursing, 16,* 12–24.

Stogdill, R. M. (1948). Personal factors associated with leadership in a survey of the literature. *Journal of Psychology, 25,* 35–71.

The Joint Commission (TJC). (2012). Joint Commission vision statement (www.jointcommission.org/about_us/about_the_joint_commission_main.aspx).

Thomas, S. P. (2003). Anger: The mismanaged emotion. *Dermatology Nurse, 15,* 351–357.

Thomson, M. A., Oxman, A. D., Haynes, R. B., Davis, D. A., Freemantle, N., & Harvey, E. L. (1999). *Local opinion leaders to improve health professional practice and health care outcomes.* Oxford: Cochrane Library.

Tornabeni, J. (1996). Changes in the advanced practice of administration: A personal perspective of the changes affecting the role. *Advanced Practice Nursing Quarterly, 2,* 62–66.

Tourigny, L., & Pulich, M. (2005). A critical examination of formal and informal mentoring among nurses. *The Health Care Manager (Frederick), 24,* 68–76.

Trent, B. A. (2003). Leadership myths. *Reflections on Nursing Leadership, 29,* 8.

Thompson, C., & Nelson-Martin, P. (2011). CNS Education: Actualizing the systems leadership competency. *Journal of Advanced Nursing Practice, 25,* 133–139.

U.S. Department of Health & Human Services. (2011). Patient Protection and Affordable Care Act. (http://www.healthcare.gov/law/full/index.html).

Vance, C. (2002). Mentoring at the edge of chaos. *Creative Nursing, 8,* 7, 14.

Vance, C., & Larson, E. (2002). Leadership research in business and health care. *Journal of Nursing Scholarship, 34,* 165–171.

Vos, T. C. (2009). Leadership begins with you. *Gerontology Nursing, 32,* 374–375.

Wagner, L. M., Capezuti, E., & Ouslander, J. G. (2006). Reporting near-miss events in nursing homes. *Nursing Outlook, 54,* 85–93.

Wakefield, M. K. (2003). Change drivers for nursing and health care. *Nursing Economic$, 21,* 150–151.

Wang, X., Chontawan, R., & Nantsupawat, R. (2012). Transformational leadership: Effect on the job satisfaction of registered nurses in a hospital in China. *Journal of Advanced Nursing, 68,* 444–451.

Weaver, S., Salas, E., & King, H. (2011). Twelve best practices for team training evaluation in healthcare. *Joint Commission Journal on Quality and Patient Safety, 37,* 341–349.

Wheatley, M. J. (2005). *Finding our way: Leadership for uncertain times.* San Francisco: Berrett-Koehler.

Winterfeldt, E. (2001). Influencing public policy. *Topics in Clinical Nutrition, 16,* 8–16.

Young, H., Siegel, E. O., McCormick, W. C., Fulmer, T., Harootyan, L. K., & Dorr, D. A. (2012). Interdisciplinary collaboration in geriatrics: Advancing health for older adults. *Nursing Outlook, 59,* 243–251.

Zaccaro, S. J. (2007). Trait-based perspectives of leadership. *American Psychologist, 62,* 6–16.

Zaccaro, S. J., Kemp, C., & Bader, P. (2004). In J. Antonakis, A. T. Cianciolo, & R. J. Sternberg (Eds.), *The nature of leadership* (p. 122). Thousand Oaks, CA: Sage.

Zenti, D. (1998). Getting politically involved. *Journal of the American Association of Nurse Anesthetists, 66,* 19–22. (www.aana.com/newsandjournal/Documents/washington_scene_0298_p019.pdf)

Collaboration

Charlene M. Hanson • Michael Carter

CHAPTER CONTENTS

The collaboration competency is important in that it is fundamental to successful APN practice. The presence or absence of collaborative relationships affects patient care, including the cost and quality of care. Patients assume that their health care providers communicate and collaborate effectively; thus, patient dissatisfaction with care, unsatisfactory clinical outcomes, and clinician frustration can often be traced to a failure to collaborate with other members of the health care team. Collaboration depends on clinical and interpersonal expertise and an understanding of factors that can promote or impede efforts to establish collegial relationships. The primary focus of this chapter is on collaboration between and among individuals and work groups within organizations and across larger health care delivery systems. Our goal in this chapter is to define collaboration and make more explicit the values, behaviors, structures, and processes that facilitate effective collaboration. Furthermore, the current trends in health care promulgated by the IOM Futures of Nursing report (2011) and the Patient Protection and Affordable Care Act (PPACA; U.S. Department of Health and Human Services [HHS], 2011) and recent education initiatives toward a rebirth of interprofessional collaboration will be described.

Definition of Collaboration

Some background on our definition of collaboration is warranted. When we began writing about collaboration, extant definitions of collaboration were inadequate to describe the process we experienced as clinicians (Hanson & Spross, 1996, 2000; Spross, 1989). The term *collaboration* is often associated with teamwork and partnership. The description of collaboration in the American Nurses Association's (ANA's) *Social Policy Statement* (ANA, 2003) and the American College of Nurse-Midwives' (ACNMs') collaboration statement (ACNM, 2011; see Chapters 7 and 17) have informed our conceptualization and definition of collaboration. The ANA recognized that the boundaries of each health care professional's practice change and that high-quality care depends on a common focus, recognition of each other's expertise, appreciation for the skills and knowledge shared across disciplines, and the collegial exchange of ideas and knowledge. However, none of these definitions in these resources adequately represents the concept of collaboration as it exists or should exist in the provision of health and illness care.

On the basis of a review of the literature and our experience, this definition of collaboration as a dynamic, interpersonal process was developed for the first edition of this text (Hanson & Spross, 1996): "Collaboration is a dynamic, interpersonal process in which two or more individuals make a commitment to each other to interact authentically and constructively to solve problems and to learn from each other to accomplish identified goals, purposes, or outcomes. The individuals recognize and articulate the shared values that make this commitment possible." (Hanson & Spross, 1996, p. 232).

Characterizing collaboration as an interaction is intended to convey the communicative and behavioral aspects of this competency. Our definition implies partnership, shared values, commitment, and goals and yet allows for differences in opinions and approaches. It also acknowledges that collaboration requires individuals to interact holistically (strengths, weaknesses, emotions) and authentically, to share power, and to remain open to the possibilities for personal and professional transformation that exist within a collaborative relationship. Including the notions of shared values and commitment makes it clear that collaboration is a process that evolves over time. Collaboration engages the head, the heart, and the will (Senge, Scharmer, Jaworski, & Flowers, 2004). These three "thresholds" are the essence of collaboration and are consistent with our definition.

The ability to commit to authentic and constructive interaction suggests that prospective partners must bring certain characteristics and qualities to initial and ongoing encounters. To interact authentically means that partners do not leave some part of themselves behind. For example, partners share the emotional satisfactions and frustrations of clinical work and develop ways of supporting each other. Although not discussed in the literature, we have observed that successful collaboration can lead to an intimacy that arises from working closely together over time. In her sixth year in a collaborative practice, one nurse practitioner (NP) compared the relationship to a marriage in terms of the interpersonal ups and downs that occur and the challenge of dealing with the same person(s) daily over matters of great or negligible, albeit clinical, import. Managing and engaging in conflict and crucial conversations is key to success and requires the skills that we define in our definition of collaboration.

By definition, collaboration describes relationships that are positive and work well for professionals, patients, and communities. There is room for disagreement in collaborative relationships; partners and teams develop strategies for dealing with disagreement that are mutually satisfactory and enhance collaboration. The other types of interactions described in the following sections do not always require collaboration as it is described here, although a collaborative relationship is likely to enhance many of these interactions. It is important to note that collaboration is an interpersonal and developmental process that demands a fairly sophisticated level of communication; collaboration cannot be mandated, legislated, or regulated.

Collaboration: What It Is Not

Collaboration can be thought of as one of several modes of interaction that occur between and among clinicians during the delivery of care—it is probably the most sophisticated and complicated interaction that occurs in practice. In addition to collaboration, we have observed other interactions between clinicians in practice. Parallel communication may be the simplest form of communication but is likely to be the least effective for facilitating optimal outcomes, and collaboration is the most complex and most effective.

Parallel Communication. Providers interact with a patient separately; they do not talk together before seeing a patient nor do they see the patient together. There is no expectation of joint interactions. For example, the staff registered nurse, medical student, and attending physician all ask the patient about his or her medications. In this example, the three different interactions are burdensome, if not frustrating, to the patient. At best, the patient is inconvenienced; at worst, an error may occur because each clinician elicits different information and subsequent clinical decisions are made on information that may be incomplete or inaccurate. Moreover, this is an inefficient use of the health care workforce.

One-Sided Compromise. The APN is overly agreeable, consistently yields to the other health care providers, and senses a lack of integrity in the care she or he is providing as a result. This yielding results in compromised care and falls below the standard of care of that with which the APN is comfortable. This occurs when the APN lacks the will or skill to engage in a collaborative negotiation.

Faux Collaboration. The person in a position of authority believes that they are being collaborative when those around them are agreeing with or not engaging in meaningful dialogue.

Parallel Functioning. Providers care for patients, addressing the same clinical problem, but do not engage in any joint or collaborative planning. For example, nurses, physical therapists, and physicians document their interventions for pain in separate parts of the patient record. The effect of such interactions is the same as for parallel communication.

Information Exchange. Informing may be one-sided or two-sided and may or may not require action or decision making. If action is needed, the decision is unilateral, not a result of joint planning. Information exchange may be sufficient and exert a neutral or beneficial effect on care processes and outcomes. If the situation actually requires joint planning and decision making, there is a risk of miscommunication.

Coordination. This lends structure to communication and actions to minimize duplication of effort but not interaction. The charge nurse role is an example.

Consultation. The clinician who is caring for a patient seeks advice regarding a patient's concern but retains primary responsibility for care delivery (see Chapter 9)

Comanagement. Two or more clinicians provide care and each professional retains accountability and responsibility for defined aspects of care. This process usually arises from consultation in which a problem requires management that is outside the scope of practice of the referring clinician (see Chapters 9 and 17). Providers must be explicit with each other about their responsibilities. Comanagement may also be a process used by interdisciplinary teams, such as palliative care.

Referral. The advanced practice nurse (APN) directs the patient to a physician or other practitioner for management of a particular problem or aspect of the patient's care when the problem is beyond the APN's expertise (see Chapters 9 and 17).

With the exceptions of parallel communication and parallel functioning, the processes just described require some level of interaction and communication among providers but may not involve collaboration. For particular situations, information exchange, coordination, consultation, comanagement, and referral may be sufficient for the purposes of achieving clinical goals. For these processes to work to benefit patients, minimize errors, and enhance quality, clinicians must engage in effective and timely communication. By comparing these types of communication with our definition of collaboration, readers should be able to appreciate the complexity of collaboration and the exquisite interpersonal skills needed to be a collaborator.

Domains of Collaboration in Advanced Practice Nursing

APNs execute the collaboration competency in several domains—between or among individuals, work groups, and organizations. The collaboration competency is often executed at the same time as other competencies, as the description of the domains illustrates. It is a dynamic competency, shifting as the particulars of a situation change.

Collaboration with Individuals

Collaboration with patients, families, and colleagues in the delivery of direct care is the primary domain in which collaboration is practiced. For example, in forming partnerships with patients (see Chapter 7), APNs aim to understand how the patient wants to work with the APN and other providers. APNs collaborate with patients and families when they set and revise goals and determine barriers to adherence; these activities are aimed at uncovering a common purpose, a hallmark of collaboration. APNs also collaborate with individual clinicians. For example, the diabetes clinical nurse specialist (CNS) may collaborate with the cardiac CNS and a staff nurse to determine who will carry out which aspects of patient education for a patient. The collaborative process may include determining the order and timing of content to be taught. In this case, the APN is also executing the direct care (interacting with the patient to assess learning needs) and coaching (coaching patients in lifestyle changes) competencies.

Collaboration with Teams and Groups

Another common domain in which APNs implement collaboration is in their work with clinical teams and on departmental and institutional committees. These groups may be comprised of individuals from one or more disciplines. A key function of the collaborative competency is the facilitation of teamwork to ensure the delivery of effective, safe, high-quality care leading to positive outcomes. The literature and our experience suggest that APNs play key roles in facilitating and leading interdisciplinary teams. As APNs become more experienced, their skill in facilitating collaboration in groups grows. Thus, APNs often lead interdisciplinary performance improvement teams, an activity that requires integration of the collaboration and leadership competencies (see Chapter 11).

Collaboration in the Organizational and Policy Arenas

In this domain, the focus of collaboration extends beyond the delivery of care to individuals and groups. The organizational and policy forces shaping advanced practice nursing and clinical care require that even novice APNs attend to collaboration in this area. Initiatives aimed at clarifying credentialing requirements, making it easier to practice across state lines, and improving reimbursement for APNs require APNs to use their status as clinicians, citizens, and members of professional organizations to collaborate with organizational leaders and policymakers. See national APN websites and that of the Nursing Alliance for Quality Care (www.gwumc.edu/healthsci/departments/nursing/naqc).

Collaboration in Global Arenas

Global or international collaboration is becoming an essential collaborative domain within the APN collaboration competency (American Association of Colleges of Nursing [AACN], 2006; Institute of Medicine [IOM],

2011; National Organization of Nurse Practitioner Faculties [NONPF], 2011). See Chapter 6.

Friedman (2005) has argued that global communication and collaboration will be the keys to successful living, working, and economic success over the next century, and we believe that this is true for health care. There is evidence that globalization is already affecting practice; the APN covering the emergency room at night may be communicating with a radiologist in Australia about a diagnostic image that was sent electronically to be interpreted in real time. In addition, APNs' experiences with volunteerism in other countries (e.g., Doctors without Borders, mission trips to Haiti and Africa) are shaping APN goals and opportunities. Nursing leaders across the globe are meeting to further nursing's contributions to education and practice (see www.icn.ch).

Types of Collaboration

The terms *multidisciplinary, interdisciplinary,* and *transdisciplinary* and, most currently, *interprofessional collaboration* are often used interchangeably. There are subtle but important differences among these terms; the prefix actually indicates the level and depth of interactions to which the term refers. The differences were best expressed in work by Alberto and Hearth (2009), D'Amour, Ferrada-Videla, Rodriguez, et al. (2005), and Garland, McConigel, Frank, et al. (1989). A key difference among the terms is reflected in the philosophy of team interaction. In a multidisciplinary team, the philosophy of team interaction is a simple recognition of the importance of the contributions of other disciplines. In an interdisciplinary team, members willingly share responsibility for providing care or services to patients. In a transdisciplinary team, members are committed to teaching each other, learning from each other, and working across boundaries to plan and provide integrated services to clients (Garland et al., 1989). Interprofessional collaboration takes these types of collaboration a bit further to eliminate traditional prescribed boundaries through negotiation and interaction (Alberto & Hearth, 2009; Bainbridge, Nasmith, Orchard, et al., 2010; Interprofessional Education Collaborative [IPEC], 2011).

Interprofessional collaboration has been described as the "interactions of two or more disciplines involving professionals who work together with intention, mutual respect and commitment for the sake of a more adequate response to a human problem." (Harbaugh, 1994, p. 20). More recently, Petri (2010) has suggested that it is an interpersonal process characterized by health care professionals with shared objectives, decision making responsibility, and power working together to solve patient care problems. IPEC (2011; Schmitt, 2011), a partnership made up of the AACN, American Association of Colleges of Osteopathic Medicine, American Association of Colleges of Pharmacy, American Dental Education Association, Association of American Medical Colleges, and Association of Schools of Public Health furthers this definition with their goal to prepare all health professions students to work together deliberatively to build a safer and better patient- and community-centered health care system in the United States. To this end, IPEC has developed core domains and competencies for interprofessional collaborative practice based on four domains, described in Box 12-1. Each IPEC domain has several behaviors that further define the competency (IPEC, 2011).

The move to reintroduce team approaches to care is evident across the spectrum of health care today (Clausen, Strohschein, Farems, et al., 2012; HHS, 2011; IOM, 2011; Young, Siegel, McCormick, et al., 2011). APNs should aspire and help teams achieve interprofessional collaboration. Interprofessional and transdisciplinary work foster the development of new understanding and new fields of inquiry in clinical care. We propose that this level of interaction leads to new insights in the interpretation of assessments and creative and effective clinical problem solving, leading to successful outcomes.

Interprofessional Collaboration

There is a heightened urgency to ensure that collaboration occurs. The need for collaboration among health care professionals is not a new concept, but has been a serious concern over many years (Bainbridge et al., 2010; Dumez, 2011; Petri, 2010; World Health Organization, 1978). Efforts to transform the health care system to improve reliability of care, safety, quality, efficiency, and cost-effectiveness will fail if clinicians, teams, and administrators do not undertake the important collaborative work necessary to effect this transformation.

Several phenomena have coalesced to bring the struggles to attain interprofessional collaboration to a critical point. The IOM report on quality and safety in the late 1990s (IOM, 2001), identified shortages, especially in primary care, and the need for team approaches through community-based care, ACOs (accountable care organizations), and nurse-managed clinics proposed in the PPACA. In addition, the latest IOM report (2011), *The Future of Nursing,* has urged teamwork among health care providers. These have all led to a resurgence of the need to foster interpersonal and interprofessional competency for all health care providers. The pressing need for collaboration among health care professionals led to the development of specific interprofessional competencies in 2011 (Canadian Interprofessional Health Collaborative [CIHC], 2010; HHS, 2011; IPEC, 2011).

BOX 12-1   Interprofessional Collaborative Initiative Domains and Competencies

Competency Domain 1: Values and Ethics for Interprofessional Collaboration

- Place patients and populations at center of care.
- Respect dignity and privacy of patients and confidentiality of team members.
- Embrace cultural diversity.
- Respect unique cultures, values, and roles.
- Work in cooperation with patients and providers and those who support care.
- Develop trusting relationships with patients, families, and team members.
- Demonstrate ethical conduct and quality care as a member of the team.
- Manage ethical dilemmas in interprofessional care situations.
- Act with honesty and integrity.
- Maintain personal and professional competence.

Competency 2: Roles and Responsibilities for Collaboration

- Communicate role and responsibilities clearly to patients and professionals.
- Recognize skill, knowledge, and ability limitations.
- Engage with professionals who complement one's practice.
- Explain roles and responsibilities of other team members.
- Use the full scope of the knowledge, skills, abilities of all team members.
- Communicate with the team to clarify roles and responsibilities.
- Forge interdependent relationships.
- Engage in continuous interprofessional development.
- Use unique and complementary abilities of all members to optimize care.

Competency 3: Interprofessional Communication

- Choose effective communication tools to enhance team function.
- Communicate information to patients and team members, avoiding discipline-specific terminology.

- Express knowledge and opinions to team with confidence, respect, and clarity to ensure common understanding.
- Listen actively and encourage ideas and opinions of other team members.
- Give timely, sensitive, and instructive feedback to team members about their performance and respond respectively to feedback from others.
- Use respectful language in difficult situations or interprofessional conflict.
- Recognize one's own uniqueness and contributions to effective communication, conflict resolution, and positive working relationships.
- Consistently communicate the importance of patient-centered care.

Competency 4: Interprofessional Teamwork and Team-Based Care

- Describe the process of team and role development and the role and practice of effective teams.
- Develop consensus on ethical principles to guide all aspects of patient care and teamwork.
- Engage other health professionals in shared, patient-centered problem solving.
- Integrate knowledge and experience of other professions to inform care decisions while respecting the patient's and community's values and priorities.
- Apply leadership practices that support collaborate practice.
- Engage self and others to manage disagreements constructively about values, roles, and goals of care.
- Share accountability with other professions, patients, and communities for relevant health care outcomes.
- Reflect on individual and team performance to improve individual and team performance.
- Use process improvement strategies to improve the effectiveness of interprofessional teamwork and practice.
- Use available evidence to inform effective teamwork and team-based practice.
- Perform effectively on teams and in different team roles in a variety of settings.

Adapted from Interprofessional Collaborative Initiative (IPEC). (2011). Core competencies of interprofessional collaborative practice (www.aacn.nche.edu/education/pdf/IPECreport.pdf).

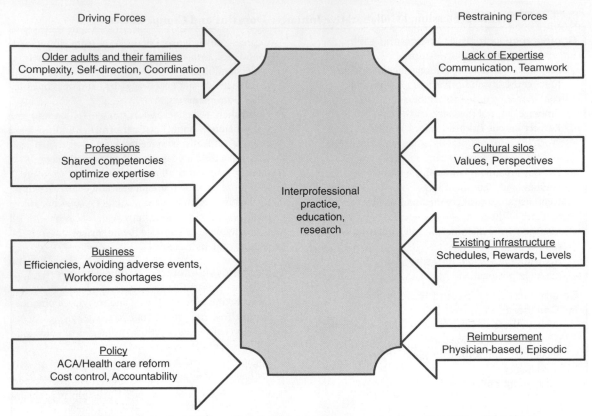

FIG 12-1 Driving and restraining forces for interprofessional practice, research, and education. *(From Young, H. M., Siegel, E. O., McCormick, W. C., Fulmer, T., Harootyan, L. K., & Dorr, D. A. [2012]. Interdisciplinary collaboration in geriatrics: Advancing health for older adults.* Nursing Outlook, 59, *243–250.)*

A paradox of the contemporary health care system is that there are incentives and disincentives for members of different disciplines, work groups, and organizations to collaborate. Incentives and disincentives may be equally powerful, so that motivation to collaborate can be diminished or eliminated by a compelling counterforce (Fig. 12-1; Young et al., 2012). An understanding of this paradox can help APNs and their colleagues approach opportunities for collaboration strategically and build and sustain clinical environments that support collaboration. Numerous clinical initiatives aimed at improving quality and safety, the need to eliminate health care disparities, and an increasing proportion of nonphysician health care professionals underscore that interprofessional collaboration at the educational, clinical, and institutional levels is essential in the current health care marketplace (American College of Graduate Medical Education, 2002; Cronenwett & Dzay, 2010; Disch, 2002; IOM, 2011; Schmitt, 2011; Pohl, Hanson, Newland, et al., 2010; Lindeke, 2005). The ability to collaborate is essential if future APNs are to implement interdisciplinary practice

models and analyze complex health problems in an interactive environment (AACN, 2006; Cronenwett & Dzay, 2010; IOM, 2011; Pohl et al., 2010).

Characteristics of Effective Collaboration

The definitions of collaboration and interprofessional collaboration proposed in this chapter invite exploration of the characteristics that make up a successful collaborative relationship. Personal- and setting-specific attributes are pivotal to successful professional collaborations. Some characteristics of collaboration have long been recognized and promulgated, but too often clinicians and organizations have resisted adopting the philosophy, commitment, and behaviors necessary to develop collaborative practices. Steele's analysis (1986) of collaboration among NPs and physicians has revealed several characteristics—mutual trust and respect, an understanding and acceptance of each other's disciplines, positive self-image, equivalent professional maturity arising from education and experience, recognition that the partners are not substitutes for each other, and a willingness to negotiate. In their program of research, Baggs and Schmitt (1988, 1997), noted the following characteristics of collaboration between registered nurses and physicians: assertiveness, shared decision making, communication, planning together, and coordination. Petri (2010) and Hughes and Mackenzie (1990) have outlined four characteristics of NP-physician collaboration: collegiality, communication, goal sharing, and task interdependence. Spross (1989) has described three essential elements of collaboration: a common purpose, diverse and complementary professional knowledge and skills, and effective communication processes. Although this is not an exhaustive summary of the literature on collaboration, it is clear that certain core elements characterize collaboration, these are listed in Box 12-2. The domains and competencies described by IPEC and the CIHC further explicate the attributes and competencies of interprofessional collaboration.

The discussion of characteristics of collaboration that follows elaborates on each of these elements. However, the reader will notice their overlapping and interlinked nature because many are mutually dependent on others for full collaboration to be realized. Collaboration requires clinical competence, common purpose, and effective interpersonal and communication skills (or a willingness to learn them). Trust, mutual respect, and valuing each other's knowledge and skills are equally important but develop fully only over time. For these characteristics to develop, prospective partners must approach encounters with a willingness to trust, commitment to respect each other, and assumption that the other's knowledge and skills are valuable. In one sense, these characteristics are therefore prerequisites; however, they are fully realized only after many constructive and productive interactions. Finally, a sense of humor among team members serves many functions in helping team members stay committed to each other's collaborative practice (Balzer, 1993; Hanson, 1993).

◉ BOX 12-2   Essential Characteristics of Collaboration

- Clinical competence and accountability
- Common purpose
- Interpersonal competence and effective communication
- Trust
- Mutual respect
- Recognition and valuing of diverse, complementary knowledge, and skills
- Humor

Clinical Competence and Accountability

Clinical competence is perhaps the most important characteristic underlying a successful collaborative experience among clinicians; without it, the trust and desire needed to work together are not possible. Trust and respect are built on the assurance that each member is able to carry out his or her role, function in a competent manner, and be accountable for his or her practice. Clinical competence is a critical element of collaboration and has been validated in research (Bosque, 2011; Hanson, Hodnicki, & Boyle, 1994; Prescott & Bowen, 1985), yet stereotyped views of nursing and medical practice may interfere with collaborative efforts. Physicians are sometimes perceived as all-knowing and as having ultimate responsibility for patient care, whereas nurses may be viewed as nonintellectual, second-best substitutes for excellent health care (Fagin, 1992; Sands, Stafford, & McClelland, 1990) who have little authority or responsibility for patient care outcomes (Larson, 1999). The status of advanced practice nursing is still such that nurses must prove their competence to the profession and to society (Fagin, 1992; Hanson, Hodnicki, & Boyle, 1994; Prescott & Bowen, 1985; Safriet, 2002, 2010).

When collaborating clinicians can rely on each other to be clinically competent, mutual trust and respect develop. Partners recognize that leadership is problem-based, not team- or role-based, and are open to sharing power. Instead of one person always being the team leader, leadership can shift among partners in a departure from the traditional captain of the team approach. Thus, the person with the most expertise, interest, or talent can respond to the particular demands of the situation or problem. The recent ACO and Medical Home concepts (American Academy of Family Physicians [AAFP], American Academy of Pediatrics, American College of Physicians, American Osteopathic Association, 2007; HHS, 2011) are excellent examples of how this approach could work (see Chapter 22). The trust and respect among collaborators is such that they can count on satisfactory resolution of the problem, even when they know as individuals that they might have approached the issue differently. This openness to shared leadership and alternative solutions allows partners to learn from each other. For example, APNs usually have expertise in educating patients about their illnesses and lifestyle choices, and physicians are often expert diagnosticians. Therefore, collaboration offers APNs and physicians opportunities to model their varied assessment and intervention strategies, which fosters mutual learning and appreciation for the contributions of each to the care of patients and families.

Being accountable for practice enhances collaboration. APNs who share in planning, decision making, problem solving, goal setting, and assuming responsibility are modeling full partnership on caregiving teams (Baggs & Schmitt, 1988; Clausen, Strohschein, Farems, et al., 2012; IPEC, 2011).

Common Purpose

The notion that a common purpose must be the basis for collaboration has been well supported in the literature (Alberto & Herth, 2009; Murray-Davis, Marshall, Gordon, et al., 2011; Nolan, Resar, Haraden, et al., 2004; Petri, 2010; Spross, 1989). Even if partners have not discussed the purposes and goals of their interactions, the organizations in which they work usually have an explicit mission and goals. Goals can be the starting point for identifying the purposes of clinical collaboration. Common purposes may range from ensuring that an underserved patient gains access to preventive services, such as mammography, to a more ambitious quality improvement agenda to improve the management of heart failure patients across settings.

One of the paradoxes of collaboration is that the partners are autonomous (self-governing, accountable) but interdependent, reflecting a reciprocal reliance on each other for support in carrying out their responsibilities. Recognizing their interdependence, team members can combine their individual perceptions and skills to synthesize care plans that are more complex and comprehensive than what they could have created working alone. Like other characteristics, the common purpose that initially brought partners together may change over time. The situation that brought two clinicians together may become secondary to the deep personal commitment to work together in ways that improve patient care and are interpersonally and professionally satisfying. In addition to a common purpose, partners who are guided by a shared vision of the possibilities inherent in collaboration, believe in the value of collaboration, and committed to achieving the relationship's potential (Lindeke, 2005; Young et al., 2012) will be most able to move toward transdisciplinary and interprofessional collaboration. Developing a shared vision does not negate the differences among partners' ideas, opinions, and actions. On the contrary, it permits— and may even value—such differences.

Interpersonal Competence and Effective Communication

Interpersonal competence is the ability to communicate effectively with colleagues in a variety of situations, including uncomplicated, routine interactions. disagreements. unique cultural value conflicts. and stressful situations. It is imperative that nurses understand and articulate to team members the skills and knowledge that they bring.

The key to demonstrating interpersonal competence is the APN's ability to communicate openly, clearly, and convincingly, orally and in writing.

In light of corporate, governmental, and research scandals, the concept of transparency of communication and behavior has emerged in health care today. The IOM's Crossing the Quality Chasm lists transparency as one of the rules for the twenty-first century health care system (IOM, 2001). The term *transparency* can be defined as the honest and open sharing of information and ideas. It includes open communication among parties, keeping everyone in the loop. It also means that one does not dissemble or pretend that everything is fine when it is not. Transparent communications are closely linked to accountability; transparency engenders trust and thus is an underlying requisite for collaboration. After clinical competence, interpersonal competence and effective communication may be the most important characteristics needed for APNs to establish collaborative relationships.

Assertiveness is a key element of interpersonal competence and APN students need to learn and practice assertiveness skills. A range of qualities may be required for APNs to be able to do the following: take risks; discuss honest disagreements in clinical judgment and agree to criteria for resolving such conflicts; be able to avoid a near miss, such as an error in prescribing or interpretation of clinical data; and admit that a mistake, miscommunication, or oversight has happened. Assertiveness is not sufficient in certain situations and environments and, in these cases, courage will be required to confront the problem. Over time, experience and confidence increase an APN's interpersonal competence.

Trust and Mutual Respect

Implicit in discussions of collaboration is the presence of mutual trust, mutual respect, and personal integrity— qualities evinced in the nature of interactions between partners. The development of trust and respect depends on clinical competence; it is difficult to trust and respect a colleague whose clinical competence is questionable. This does not mean that novice APNs cannot establish collaborative relationships. However, the environments in which advanced practice nursing students and new graduates work must support their "novicehood" so that they can learn and mature clinically. Trust and assertiveness seem to act reciprocally in collaboration; as individuals trust each other more, their ability to engage in difficult communication successfully increases. Responding assertively in situations of risk and keeping the focus on the patient's welfare can enhance trust.

Respect for others' practice and knowledge is key to successful collaboration because it enhances shared decision making. Respect extends to acknowledgment and appreciation for each other's time and competing commitments.

Recognizing and Valuing Diverse, Complementary Culture, Knowledge, and Skills

There must be a belief, at a personal level, that the complementary knowledge other team members have will enhance one's own personal plan for patient care. Appreciation for the diverse and complementary knowledge each party brings to the work, commitment to quality and patient-centeredness, and willingness to invest in the partnership or team are all necessary for collaboration to become the normative process in team interactions.

A lack of knowledge about another's discipline is thought to be a barrier to developing effective teamwork (Dumez, 2011; Gilbert, Camp, Cole, et al., 2000). Partners must recognize and value the overlapping and diverse skills and knowledge that each discipline brings to the team (CIHC, 2010; IPEC, 2011; Spross, 1989) so that mutual trust and respect can develop and deepen over time. Partners observe that patients benefit from their combined talents and efforts. They come to depend on each other to use good clinical judgment and to take appropriate actions.

Initially, collaborators have limited knowledge of each other as individuals and as professionals; collaboration is a "conscious, learned behavior" that improves as team members learn to value and respect one another's practice and expertise (IPEC, 2011; Moeller, Vezeau, & Carr, 2007). The first step is to recognize these differing contributions. Medicine and nursing, although overlapping disciplines, are culturally distinct and have diverse goals for patient care. In many cases, they complement each other in their quest to restore patients to health. These complementarities also extend to other disciplines. Collaboration is built on the respect and valuing of the contributions of each profession to the common goal of optimal health care delivery.

Humor

A final important aspect of the collaborative process is humor. Humor in which the intent is positive and non-threatening is a creative way to set the stage for effective communication and problem solving among members of different disciplines (Balzer, 1993; Hanson, 1993). In collaborative practice, humor serves to decrease defensiveness, invite openness, relieve tension, and deflect anger. It helps individuals keep perspective and acknowledge the lack of perfection, and it sets the tone for trust and acceptance among colleagues so that difficult situations can be reframed (Balzer, 1993). Ciesielka, Conway, Penrose, & Risco (2005) suggested that humor is essential to successful collaboration because it is a bridge to different backgrounds. The use of humor helps defuse the need for persons to argue their own point of view and allows them to refocus on how they can work together to meet common goals (Hill & Hewlett, 2002). Graduate students can be encouraged to observe how humor is used by preceptors and colleagues and identify those uses that seem effective for improving communication and defusing conflict situations.

Although this list of characteristics of effective collaboration may seem daunting to the novice, a consistent commitment to and practice of collaboration can develop this competency over time in an APN's practice. Exemplar 12-1 showcases the elements of collaboration in an individual APN's practice. APNs and their professional colleagues need to recognize that an important component of clinical practice is investing the time and energy to build these relationships. The high levels of interchange of ideas and expertise that become possible when all of these characteristics come together is one of the great satisfactions of collaborative practice.

Impact of Collaboration on Patients and Clinicians

Experience and evidence suggest that collaboration works, but effective collaboration eludes many clinicians. Why? Some authors link barriers to the history of the health care professions, traditional gender roles, disciplinary heritage, ineffective communication, and hierarchical relationships (Christman, 1998; Larson, 1999; Reuben, Levy-Storms, Yee, et al., 2004; Rosenstein & O'Daniel, 2005; Zwarenstein & Reeves, 2002). Over the years, there have been many reports of successful collaborative relationships involving APNs (Brooten, Youngblut, Blais, et al., 2005; Cowan, Shapiro, Hays, et al., 2006; Lindeke, 2005; Naylor, Brooten, Campbell, et al., 2004.). The importance of collaboration in various aspects of advanced practice nursing continues to be recognized (Bosque, 2011; Ingersoll, McIntosh, & Williams, 2000; Kleinpell, Faut-Callahan, Lauer, et al., 2002; Sheer, 2007; Young, et al., 2011).

Although few studies of collaboration have measured patient outcomes systematically (Litaker, Mion, Planavsky, et al., 2003; McCaffrey, Hayes, Stuart et al., 2010; Wooton, Lee, Jared, et al., 2011; see Chapter 24), patient and provider benefits have been documented. Patients are sensitive to the relationships among caregivers and are quick to pick up on the lack of respect or trust among their providers. Some research has suggested that collaborative relationships among interdisciplinary health

EXEMPLAR 12-1   **Elements of Collaboration in One Advanced Practice Nurse's Practice**

Mary Q and two physicians are part of a group primary care practice in a small community. The caregivers in this clinic are committed to high-quality health care for their patients. Mary is a competent nurse practitioner and an able diagnostician. The physicians trust and respect Mary's ability to care for patients. She and her physician colleagues have many of the same values and ideas about good patient care. Although Mary carries her own panel of patients very successfully, she consults with the physicians if she is concerned about a complex patient and they, in turn, ask for her expertise concerning some of the older patients that she has been following closely and knows well. Mary and her physician colleagues function as a team and have all learned from each other's knowledge and skill. They communicate effectively to solve problems in their practice. Mary's nursing expertise brings an added dimension to this primary care team. Most importantly, Mary is a team player; all the members of the group practice enjoy her quick wit and willingness to share her expertise. The physicians have many years of experience and gladly share their pearls of health care wisdom. At first, one of the partners did not want a nurse practitioner to join the group, but Mary won him over with her professional and interpersonal competence.

In this example of interprofessional practice, the patients and their families are cared for by a professional team that combines all of their talents in order to achieve the best outcome.

care providers can ameliorate some of these negative effects (Remonder, Koch, Link, et al., 2010; Weinstein, McCormack, Brown, et al., 1998). Successful collaborative practices are those in which patients easily move back and forth between providers as their care and situations dictate. Collaboration requires an ability to transform competitive situations into opportunities for working together that are mutually beneficial, and in which all parties can imagine the possibility of creating a win-win situation.

Studies of the impact of APNs on disease management and care transition interventions indicate that there are positive outcomes for patients. Collaboration is implied based on the fact that the APNs in these studies typically communicated with other providers, but collaboration is rarely identified or measured (these studies are discussed in Chapter 24). Table 12-1 illustrates the types of patient and provider benefits that have been ascribed to clinical collaboration. Collaboration competencies have been in place for APNs for several years (AACN, 2006; NONPF 2011). New competencies required by the American College of Graduate Medical Education (ACGME) for participants in medical residency programs include behaviors related to interdisciplinary teamwork, group problem solving, and communication across settings. These collaborative expectations were adopted in 2002 by the ACGME.

Evidence That Collaboration Works

Over time, these essential characteristics of collaboration may lead to improved physician collaboration with other clinicians, as seen in Exemplar 12-2.

 TABLE 12-1   **Benefits of Collaboration**

Who Benefits?	Benefits
Patients	Improved quality of care Increased patient satisfaction Lower mortality rate Improved patient outcomes Patients feel more secure, cared for, closer to health care providers Empowers patients and family to become team members
Providers	Improved trust and respect for care givers Improved communication and clarity of message Increased sharing of responsibility Increased sharing of expertise Mutually satisfying problem solving Improved communications Increased personal satisfaction Increased quality of professional life Enhanced mutual trust and respect Bridges care-cure dichotomy Expands horizons of providers Avoids redundant care and ensures coverage Empowers providers to influence health policy

Adapted from Sullivan, T.J. (1998). *Collaboration: A health care imperative* (pp. 26–27). New York: McGraw-Hill Health Professionals Division.

Research Supporting Interprofessional Collaboration

Research studies, although far from definitive, have supported the premise that collaboration results in better patient outcomes, including patient satisfaction,

◎ EXEMPLAR 12-2   Collaboration Works for Patients and Clinicians

While a CNS at a tertiary hospital, JS noted that patients who were admitted directly from the oncology clinic for a short admission were receiving their chemotherapy late at night because members of the house staff were not taking the patients' histories and performing physical examinations until last. Lengths of stay were longer, treatments that could have been prepared and given during the better staffed day shift were burdening the evening and night staff, and patients were dissatisfied. House staff left these admissions until last because the patients tended to be clinically stable and, to the interns, this was an appropriate way of triaging their workload. The CNS and nurse manager met with the physician director of hematology-oncology to propose that short-stay chemotherapy admissions be handled differently from other admissions, an idea for which there was no precedent. The physician director had also recognized the problem and willingly collaborated with the

nursing leaders to craft a solution. Previously, all admissions and examinations had been done by the interns and residents. Under the new arrangement, patients came to the unit directly from the clinic, with their admission orders written by the attending physician. IV lines were initiated immediately, examinations were completed by the APN, prescriptions were filled by the pharmacy as the orders came down, and nurses were able to initiate teaching and other interventions in a timely fashion.

The outcomes of this new plan included increased patient, nurse, and house staff satisfaction and decreased time from admission to beginning chemotherapy. Patient length of stay also decreased. Perhaps most importantly, the success of the joint problem solving in this case provided a precedent for increased interdisciplinary collaboration on the hematology-oncology service.

---

and provides personal and professional satisfaction for clinicians (Bosque, 2011; Brooten, et al., 2005; Cowan, Shapiro, Hays et al., 2006; Makowsky, Schindel, Rosenthal et al., 2009). Adoption of interprofessional models for care has been slow to develop over the years, despite interest (Alberto & Hearth, 2009; Young, et al., 2011) APNs must have or acquire interpersonal communication skills and behaviors that make collaboration possible among a broad range of professionals and patients.

Historically, discussions about collaboration in the health field have focused on the relationship between physicians and nurses because that is where the most serious tensions have occurred (Cowan, et al., 2006; Lindeke, 2005; Safriet, 2002; Schmitt, 2001). However, it is increasingly important that any discussion of collaborative relationships address interprofessional collaboration among nurses, collaboration between nurses and members of other disciplines, collaboration among work groups, agencies, and communities, and collaboration with patients. Although collaboration is recognized by many as central to improving the quality and effectiveness of health care, publications about implementing collaborative processes have, until recently, not kept pace with the number of national initiatives that require effective collaboration. Global literature, especially from Canada, provides incentives for us to move forward (CHIC, 2010; Dumont, Briere, Morin, et al., 2010; Rice, Zwarenstein, Conn, et al., 2010). Of note, publications that address interdisciplinary collaboration (particularly with physicians) and APNs specifically have increased significantly with the recent

health care reform work and IPEC development of interprofessional competencies. Important ideas about collaboration from leaders in other disciplines have informed this discussion of collaboration (Bainbridge, et al., 2010; Dumez, 2011; Palinkas, Ell, Hansen, et al., 2011). In addition to updating the literature, our aim is to help readers understand what collaboration looks like in practice, strengthen this competency in their practice, enhance their leadership of collaborative teams and initiatives, and increase the motivation of clinicians and institutions to adopt structures and processes that support the collaboration competency.

Primary Care: Impact on Chronic Disease Management

Efforts to improve the management of chronic diseases, such as diabetes, heart failure, and hypertension, will increasingly involve an APN, usually an NP or a CNS. For example, Litaker, et al, (2003) conducted an experiment to compare the care provided to diabetics and hypertensive patients by a physician-NP team, with usual care provided by primary care physicians. Despite higher costs, the investigators found statistically and clinically significant improvements in hemoglobin A1c (HbA1c) and high-density lipoprotein (HDL) levels, as well as increased satisfaction (e.g., general satisfaction, communication with provider, and interpersonal care). There were no observed significant differences in total cholesterol and quality of life. The authors observed that the increased costs of care (usual care was about one-third less than that of the physician-NP team) may be justified because the improved clinical indicators are associated with better longer term outcomes, such as reduction in disease complications, rehospitalizations, and mortality.

Outcomes of Intensive Care Unit Stays

One of the first studies to identify the impact of nurse-physician communication on patient outcomes indicated that the most significant factor associated with decreased mortality rates in intensive care units (ICUs) was effective nurse-physician communication patterns (Knaus, Draper, Wagner, et al., 1986). The investigators reported that another factor associated with lower mortality rates was the presence of a comprehensive nursing education support system in which CNSs had responsibility for staff development. Hospitals with lower mortality rates had systems that ensured excellent nurse-physician communication.

In an extension of this research, a study of 17,440 patients in 42 ICUs provided additional evidence that interactions among caregivers affect patient care (Shortell, Zimmerman, Rousseau, et al., 1994). Effective caregiver interactions were associated with lower risk-adjusted length of stay, lower nurse turnover, better quality of care, and greater ability to meet family member needs. In the analytic model that the investigators used, caregiver interaction included the culture, leadership, coordination, communication, and conflict management abilities of the unit's staff. Greater availability of technology, a measure of state of the art treatment, was also associated with lower risk-adjusted mortality rates.

Effects of Physician and Advanced Practice Nurse Collaboration on Costs

One study has compared 627 control patients who received usual care with 1207 hospitalized medical patients who received care from physician-NP teams. The researchers compared multidisciplinary team-based planning, expedited discharge, and assessment after discharge with usual patient management. They found that multidisciplinary care management reduced the length of hospital stay, lowered hospital stay costs, and improved hospital care without altering readmissions or mortality (Cowan, et al., 2006). More recently, Burke and O'Grady (2012) have reported that group visits carried out by transdisciplinary health care teams are efficacious and hold promise for improved outcomes and better cost containment. Similarly, an integrative review of the impact of transdisciplinary teams on the care of the underserved demonstrated other benefits, such as better primary care access and quality for underserved populations (Ruddy & Rhee, 2005).

Brooton, Youngblut, Blais, et al. (2005) have reported the positive effects of APN and physician collaboration on caring for women with high-risk pregnancies. The frequency of urgent care visits to a geriatric primary care clinic was decreased through collaborative care provided by NPs and physicians (Sears, Maxwell, & Townsend, 2003). Jackson and coworkers (2003) have reported that fewer fiscal resources were required when obstetricians and certified nurse-midwives (CNMs) worked within a collaborative care birth center model.

Some commentators have noted that collaboration may actually cost more in the short run (Litaker, et al., 2003). Kinnaman and Bleich (2004), from an administrative perspective, observed that collaboration is a more complex and labor- and resource-intensive problem-solving strategy. One of the challenges of evaluating cost-effectiveness when it comes to clinical collaboration is to measure change over an appropriate time-horizon. As the Litaker study suggested, a 1-year collaborative intervention is enough to change patient behaviors in ways that reduced important clinical markers but was not sufficient to assess and measure the impact of complications and disease-related comorbidities on the disease trajectory over time. The fact that the 1-year intervention was insufficient to sustain the behavior changes that led to the reduced clinical markers supports our conceptualization of collaboration as a process that evolves and matures over time and has suggested that our understanding of long-term changes in patient behavior and clinical outcomes may depend on a more complete empirical understanding of collaborative processes.

Bourbonniere and Evans (2002), in an integrative review of the impact of APN outcomes on care, have affirmed that interdisciplinary collaboration is an important function of APNs. In 2012, the Robert Wood Johnson Foundation (RWJF) reported examples of increased quality of life and safety in patients who were cared for by health care professionals who had overcome professional boundaries to work together. Readers are encouraged to review current literature on chronic disease management because this is an area in which APNs are practicing and participating in research. Results from such studies will continue to shape our understanding of collaboration and coaching competencies of APNs (see Chapters 7 and 8).

Other Evidence

Earlier work on the importance of collaboration to effective, accessible health care has been recognized by several philanthropies that support health care initiatives. The report of the Pew Health Professions Commission (1995) has identified collaborative care core competencies (improved communication and relationships among patients, practitioners, and the community) needed for future health professionals (Gelman, O'Neil, & Kimmey, 1999).

RWJF has supported projects that provide further evidence that collaboration works. RWJF's Partnerships for Quality Education (PQE) project, conducted from 1998 to 2003, included a program that helped NPs and medical residents learn how to work together (Johnson-Pawlson, Posey, Dalal, et al., 2003).

The Institute for Health Care Improvement (IHI) has published a series of white papers, a number of which relate to collaboration, including "Transforming Care at the Bedside" (TCAB; RWJF partnered with IHI on this project; Rutherford, Lee, & Greiner, 2004) and "Engaging Physicians in a Shared Quality Agenda" (Reinertsen, Gosfield, Rupp, et al., 2007). Although specific recommendations from these documents are presented throughout this chapter, a few points are worth making here. The TCAB recommendations are built on a framework of four main themes: safety and reliability, patient-centeredness, care team vitality, and increased value. Care team vitality has been described by Rutherford and associates (2004) as being within an environment that nurtures joyfulness, support, and career development. There is also evidence that institutions can create structures to facilitate collaboration. Although much has been made of the application of crew resource management (CRM) principles to facilitate collaboration and cooperation among health care team members, Zwarenstein and Reeves (2002) have noted that health care organizations are bigger, more complex, and more widely dispersed geographically than many of the industries, such as aviation, in which they have been tested. Even so, there is evidence that organizationally supported teams, such as rapid response teams, can improve patient outcomes (Morse, Warshawsky, Moore, et al., 2006; Nolan, Resar, Haraden, et al., 2004; Sheer, Wilson, Wagner, et al., 2012).

In recent years, there have been many fine examples of collaboration initiatives leading to positive changes in health care and collaborative interactions among the health care disciplines. In 2007, boards of nursing, pharmacy, medicine, occupational therapy, physical therapy and social work joined in a collaborative effort to assist regulatory bodies and legislators to make joint decisions about scope of practice for the health care professions (National Council of State Boards of Nursing [NCSBN], 2006). New competencies for education and practice that include collaboration and team work have been developed (AACN, 2006; ACGME, 2002; IPEC, 2011). Both the IOM Future of Nursing Committee (2011) and the Josiah Macy Foundation recommendations for training primary care providers include strong recommendations for collaboration among health care professionals (Cronenwett &

Dzau, 2010). Language in the Patient Protection and Affordable Care Act (PPACA) is clear about the need for heightened interprofessional collaboration in health care education and in practice. These efforts are encouraging; new positive strides in preparing health professions students for collaborative practice will be fulfilled.

Effects of Failure to Collaborate

Effects on Organizations

Failure to collaborate has implications for organizations and individuals. The anthrax scare after the events of 9/11 provided health care professionals with a compelling example of the failure of organizations and agencies to collaborate. The Centers for Disease Control and Prevention (CDC) and other parts of the U.S. Public Health Service failed to share data and resources with other agencies that would have ensured timely, broad-based solutions to the anthrax problem. Conversely, in February 2003, effective collaboration and coordination between the World Health Organization and several nations in dealing with the severe acute respiratory syndrome (SARS) outbreak received worldwide acclaim (Hotez, 2003). A current example is the exemplary collaboration among federal, state, and local law enforcement agencies in the Boston Marathon bombings (www.cnn.com/2013/04/20/us/Boston-area-violence/index.html). studies and initiatives are aimed at understanding the impact of organizational processes such as teamwork, handoffs, continuity of care, and disruptive behaviors. Rosenstein and O'Daniel (2005) have noted that more is known about the impact of disruptive behaviors on job satisfaction but that the impact of work relationships on patient outcomes has not been well studied until rather recently. Although a review of this body of work is beyond our scope here, we see this as evidence that accrediting organizations, health care executives, administrators, and researchers are paying attention to the collaborative and communication processes that undermine institutional bottom lines—positive patient and financial outcomes. The most important result of failure to collaborate is its negative effect on patient care.

Effects on Individuals

The failure to communicate and collaborate affects individual patients, families, communities, and clinicians. Failure to collaborate contributes to inefficiencies in the delivery of patient care (Cooper, Henderson, & Dietrich, 1998; Cronenwett & Dzay, 2010; Gordon, 2011; IOM, 2011). Alpert, Goldman, Kilroy, and associates (1992) have found that job satisfaction and attitude are negatively affected when collaboration fails and that territoriality and competitiveness increase. The absence of collaboration has been identified as a source of distress to nurses (Aiken, Smith, & Lake, 1994; Fagin, 1992). Lack of collaboration and the diminished autonomy that often accompanies it may contribute to job dissatisfaction and staff turnover and, more recently, was believed to contribute to the nursing shortage (Rosenstein & O'Daniel, 2005). Job dissatisfaction and turnover among staff nurses are serious concerns, especially during a nursing shortage, and are particularly relevant to the CNS. Although APNs may experience these effects of failure to collaborate, APNs usually have more autonomy and advanced communication skills than staff nurses and can work within the work setting to improve collaboration.

Imperatives for Collaboration

We believe that organizations and individual clinicians have a moral obligation to collaborate, but collaboration cannot be mandated. The following sections present a set of imperatives that we believe clinicians must consider as they make decisions about collaboration and collaborative relationships. The effects of collaboration or failure to collaborate can be seen in the way that ethical and institutional dilemmas are resolved and how research is conducted. Providers must be willing to negotiate and transcend disciplinary boundaries in all activities aimed at improving the quality, safety, and reliability of care for individuals and populations.

Ethical Imperative to Collaborate

Some have suggested that the failure to collaborate is an ethical issue. The clinical imperative of the APN role to collaborate is embedded within the ethical imperative. IPEC (2011) has recommended that all future health professionals assert the values and ethics of interprofessional practice by placing the needs and dignity of patients at the center of health care delivery and include a specific ethics domain and competencies (Box 12-1). Compassionate and ethical patient care that provides a healing environment requires collaborative working relationships between physicians and nurses (Larson, 1999; Petri, 2010; Schmitt, 2011). As noted in Chapters 1 and 13, communication and collaboration problems are often components of ethical dilemmas. Thus, environments that foster collaboration may also create a more supportive context for addressing ethical issues.

Larson (1999) has identified key beliefs about collaboration on which nurses and physicians differ—the importance of relationships, what constitutes effective and desirable communication, the degree to which communication and shared decision making occur, the authority that nurses have to make decisions, and which strategies

would improve communication. The failure of physicians and nurses to understand each other's perspectives, a prerequisite for collaboration, results in a difficult work environment and contributes to uncoordinated unsafe care (Larson, 1999).

Collaboration is a moral imperative; good patient care requires it, collaboration reinforces commitment to a common goal and reaffirms the message that patient welfare is the goal, and collaboration enhances shared knowledge as physicians and nurses repeatedly educate each other about the patient.

Institutional Imperative to Collaborate

The evidence that collaboration works has suggested that there are structural and interpersonal dimensions to collaboration. That is, although institutional policies or standards do not guarantee collaboration, they can establish expectations for communication and collaboration. These institutional expectations can provide a structure that facilitates interpersonal communication and relationship building (D'Amour, et al., 2005; IOM, 2011; PPACA, 2011). The mutual goal of good patient care and the ethical imperative to collaborate should be at the center of any interprofessional efforts that provide care or resolve conflicts in approaches to care for patients. For example, institutions that apply for Magnet status are expected to have a structure in place for effective communication among nurses, physicians, and administrators as one of five key characteristics (McClure & Hinshaw, 2002; North Shore Long Island Jewish Health System, 2010). The incentive for hospitals to move to Magnet status has never been higher, with the current emphases on nurse retention, quality, and safety. Institutions that have applied for the American Nurses' Credentialing Center (ANCC, 2012) Magnet credential must demonstrate that they meet 14 characteristics (McClure & Hinshaw, 2002). These criteria have been associated with the ability to attract and retain nurses. Of the 14 criteria, several relate to collaboration, such as interdisciplinary relationships and professional models of care. APNs are usually intimately involved in efforts to seek Magnet status: they have led quality improvement initiatives, facilitated professional development of staff, and contributed to the establishment of policies and procedures that support nurses' autonomy, efforts that shape an environment in which effective collaboration can occur.

Finally, incentives and mandates to reduce error and increase the reliability of care by adopting evidence-based practices constitute another significant institutional imperative to foster collaboration. Improvements that result from such initiatives are often tied to reimbursement (e.g., pay for performance, merit pay).

An example of the institutional imperative to collaborate is the rapid progression of the Doctorate in Nursing Practice (DNP). The national concerns about the quality and safety of health care (IOM, 2001) have informed the development of the DNP and helped form consensus among schools, faculty, and other stakeholders (AACN, 2004). The DNP *Essentials* (AACN, 2006) have affirmed the importance of collaboration as a core competency. The document includes numerous mentions of the terms *collaboration* and *collaborative* in the competencies that will need to be met by all who seek a DNP, including APNs. Examples of situations from the DNP *Essentials* that require collaborative competencies include the ability to create change in health care delivery systems, need to collaborate across settings to enhance population-based health care, and need for interprofessional collaboration to implement practice guidelines and peer review processes (AACN, 2006). Current competencies for all APN groups include competencies based on high-level communication and interprofessional practice skills (see APN websites and competencies).

Research Imperative to Study Collaboration

In 2011, Schmitt suggested that collaboration be examined as an intermediate outcome when health care is evaluated. In a review of the literature, Schmitt cited a number of challenges faced by health services researchers in trying to understand collaboration and its impact on outcomes. Methodological challenges include the need for more robust, well-designed studies, including clinical trials to provide more conclusive evidence about the impact of collaboration on patient outcomes. In addition, sample selection, measurement of collaboration, and outcome measurement pose dilemmas for those interested in studying the phenomenon. A major limitation of existing knowledge is that much of it comes from hospital-based practice and, according to Schmitt, studies of collaboration and its outcomes are underdeveloped. Schmitt (2011, p. 63) noted that "If there is an important place for interprofessional collaboration in health care delivery, then it is a high-priority task to get on with the research, difficult as it is, that demonstrates what mix of collaborators, for what purposes, for whom, with what outcomes and at what costs matters." These words have been noted and collaborative outcomes research has been finding its way into the literature, although more is needed (see Chapter 24).

Institutional imperatives to collaborate and the research imperative to study collaboration are becoming more closely aligned. For example, the Agency for Healthcare Research and Quality (AHRQ) has become an important resource for funding and disseminating the results of research on quality improvement, patient safety, adoption of evidence-based practices, and other issues associated with the delivery of safe and reliable health care (see www.ahrq.gov/QUAL/advances). In addition, the National Institutes of Health's (NIH's) Common Fund (https://commonfund.nih.gov) continues to expect collaboration among clinical investigators. Drenning (2006) has urged collaboration among nurses, APNs, and nurse researchers to understand and implement evidence-based practice (EBP) changes likely to improve patient care.

Collaboration among providers with different perspectives results in a creative and multidimensional intelligence that is emotionally rewarding because patients do better and clinicians derive personal and professional gratification from this work. This has implications for APNs, administrators, physicians, researchers, and others. APNs and their administrative and clinical colleagues need to assess the collaborative climate, determine facilitators and barriers, and work together to strengthen relationships while building an organizational culture that values collaboration. Researchers must help APNs and administrators understand the structures and processes associated with collaboration and the extent to which collaboration affects patient and utilization outcomes.

Context of Collaboration in Contemporary Health Care

The pressures on APNs, physicians, and others to improve quality, work more efficiently, and allow others (e.g., insurers) to be involved in decisions about patient care could be expected to foster collaboration among clinicians. Paradoxically, these same factors may undermine collaboration. As APNs have become more educated and better prepared to practice autonomously and collaboratively, physicians have experienced multiple pressures, including the increasing supply of APN providers (Cooper, Henderson, & Dietrich, 1998; Phillips, Harper, Wakefield, et al., 2002), which apparently or actually encroach on a physician's autonomy and willingness to collaborate. The mounting pressures on physicians may lead them to fear undifferentiation, that no one will be able to tell them from physician assistants, APNs, or other providers, which might underlie turf battles. These same pressures generate concern about relinquishing authority and power, fears that may cause individuals to withdraw from or sabotage efforts to collaborate. Thus, the transition to a presumably more effective, accessible, and efficient health care system may actually undermine collaboration, a process many leaders believe is central to achieving the goal of a health care system that is accessible, effective, and affordable.

In addition, confusion about scope of practice can be damaging to collaboration for all involved. Physicians may ask themselves the following (LaVizzo-Mourey, 2012; Safriet, 2002):

- What's in it for me to collaborate?
- What areas of my work do I get to expand because other providers can do things that I have traditionally done?

APNs may be uncertain about their scope of practice when a physician or institution asks them to assume responsibility for a new skill, such as performing an invasive procedure. The reality is that payment structures and regulatory initiatives are rearranging practice boundaries almost daily. These changes are often at the heart of the tension associated with collaboration among players as the roles and boundaries of disciplines have blurred and expanded.

Incentives and Opportunities for Collaboration

Efforts to reduce costs and improve quality of health care actually provide APNs, physicians, and administrators with common goals toward which to work and with opportunities for learning from each other. Medicare guidelines that are used to document care for coding and billing purposes are structured to encourage physicians and APNs to work together to provide the appropriate level of care necessary to meet the standards for reimbursement. National interdisciplinary guidelines and standards of care are intended to reduce unwarranted, often expensive, variations in health care. Many guidelines specify interdisciplinary collaboration as a critical component of effective care. Standards and guidelines developed and agreed on by interdisciplinary groups, whether at the local (office or institution) or national level, offer a sound starting point for jointly determining patient care goals, processes, and outcomes. Accreditation activities offer another opportunity to build collaborative relationships. The Joint Commission (TJC; http://www.jointcommission.org/standards_information/joint_commission_requirements.aspx) requires documentation that demonstrates collaborative, interdisciplinary practice to help providers develop stronger interdisciplinary approaches to care. The need for a highly coordinated system of chronic care management led the Health Sciences Institute to promulgate interdisciplinary competencies. The goals for chronic illness care, which include promoting health and preventing disease, managing disease and disease impacts, and promoting consumer independence and life quality, are centered around a model of interdisciplinarity in which all players are valued for their contributions and collaborative effort (Health Sciences Institute, 2005, 2007).

The move toward a more community-based, health promotion and disease prevention model of care has also been creating new opportunities for collaborative practice in primary care (Bodenheimer & Grumbach, 2012). Also, the use of telehealth and electronic medical records offers creative opportunities for interaction. For these systems to work, APNs, physicians, and other clinicians need to be involved in selecting, piloting, modifying, and implementing new technologies. From the selection of vendors to full deployment of the technology, the adoption of new technologies offers opportunities for clinicians to develop collaborative learning communities. In the current global market, innovative new alliances among advanced practice nursing groups and between advanced practice nursing groups and physician groups need to be developed and nurtured (McCaffrey, Hayes, Stuart, et al., 2010; Young et al., 2012).

Barriers to Collaboration

Implementing effective collaborative professional relationships in the workplace can be challenging. Barriers to collaboration exist and can be characterized as professional, sociocultural, organizational, and regulatory. Several authors have suggested that team members see themselves primarily as representatives of their own discipline rather than as members of a collaborative team (D'Amour, et al., 2005; Reuben, Levy-Storms, Yee, et al., 2004).

Disciplinary Barriers

Silos in health science education have long been barriers to successful collaboration. Each profession is a culture with its own values, knowledge, rules, and norms (Lindeke, 2005; Reuben, Levy-Storms, Yee, et al., 2004). Often, clinicians differ in their basic philosophy of care based on how they have been socialized into the system. For example, allopathic medicine is oriented toward biomedical research, technical solutions, hierarchical relationships, and a strong sense of personal responsibility for patient outcomes. This sense of responsibility is apparent even among physicians who support APNs but imply or explicitly indicates that physician oversight of APNs' practice is necessary (American Medical Association [AMA], 2012). Fagin (1992) has asserted that the stance preferred by physicians is not to collaborate with anyone, a strong statement that might seem inflammatory. However, the Pew-Fetzer Task Force (1994), most of whose members were physicians, has also acknowledged that collaboration is a particular challenge for physicians. Current efforts to place certified registered nurse anesthetists (CRNAs) under physician supervision (see Chapter 18) also suggest that collaboration is difficult for physicians. In an evaluation of the Hartford Foundation initiative to strengthen interdisciplinary team training in geriatrics (Reuben, Levy-Storms, Yee, et al., 2004), faculty and students in advanced practice nursing, medicine, and social work were found to be influenced by disciplinary attitudes and cultural factors that were obstacles to teamwork, a phenomenon the authors termed *disciplinary split*. They observed that disciplinary heritage and a differential willingness to participate in teamwork characterized disciplinary split and constituted a significant obstacle to implementing effective interdisciplinary teamwork in geriatrics training.

There are few opportunities for interdisciplinary education as health care providers learn their professions. The RWJF Partnerships for Training initiative (Rice, Zwarenstein, Conn, et al., 2010; RWJF, 2003; Young, et al., 2012) identified many of the stresses inherent in building and sustaining interdisciplinary academic-community partnerships. Stresses encountered by participants as they developed partnerships centered on money, differing agendas, systems that were not integrated, varying philosophies, and long-held beliefs about how things should be done.

Collaboration at the community grassroots level is easier to implement and maintain than at the professional organizational level. Although collaboration happens daily among practicing clinicians, at national levels, where it is really needed, collaboration may be nonexistent, impeding efforts to move toward a coordinated health care system. The positions espoused by so-called old guard policymakers from all disciplines may be based on stereotyped beliefs about disciplinary roles and responsibilities, rather than reflecting consideration of the issues or what is best for consumers. These factors make it increasingly important for APNs and physicians practicing at local levels who have learned the art of collaboration to take an active role in bringing their perspectives and experiences to policymaking at institutional, community, state, and national levels to foster collaboration (Hanson, Spross, & Carr, 2000). A broader statutory definition of professional autonomy for APNs than what is found in many states is necessary if the more complex autonomy of interdependent collaborators is to be exercised effectively (Lugo, O'Grady, Hodnicki, et al., 2007; Pearson, 2012; Safriet, 2002).

Despite these existing challenges to collaboration, there is evidence of progress. The U.S. Preventive Services Task Force, which is part of the federal AHRQ, is made up of an interdisciplinary group of providers and researchers who develop, disperse, and revise evidence-based recommendations on screening and prevention for a variety of health care concerns (U.S. Preventive Services Task Force, 2012).

Ineffective Communication and Team Dysfunction

Communication styles may also be a barrier to collaboration. Dysfunctional styles of interactions among health care professionals that particularly undermine collaboration have been identified. These styles have been characterized as being difficult, bullying, or abusive (Anderson, 2011; Houghton, 2003; McAvoy & Murtagh, 2003; Rider, 2002). More recently, the term *disruptive behavior* has been used to include these and other intimidating behaviors. Clinicians whose behavior is disruptive display the attitudinal and behavioral problems (e.g., arrogance, rudeness, and poor communication) of those who are unable to work as part of a team (Longo & Smith, 2011; Rosenstein & O'Daniel, 2005; Saxton, Hines & Enriquez, 2009). Although these individuals may be clinically competent, if their behavior is harassing, coercive, or abusive, they put patients at risk, in part because other clinicians may be unwilling to deal with them in regard to nonclinical behaviors or actions (Longo & Smith, 2011; Rosenstein & O'Daniel, 2005). APNs have a responsibility to recognize disruptive behavior as risks to collaboration and safe patient care and to develop a repertoire of interpersonal and system strategies with which to address these behaviors directly and promptly.

Lencioni, a business consultant on team effectiveness, has proposed a model of team dysfunction (2005). The field guide (Lencioni, 2005) will be of practical use to APNs. In this model, the first four of the five dysfunctions reflect the absence of key components of our conceptualization of collaboration: (1) absence of trust; (2) fear of conflict; (3) lack of commitment; (4) avoidance of accountability; and (5) inattention to results. The fifth dysfunction, inattention to results, is consistent with the observation that efforts within health care to improve safety, reliability, and quality represent an opportunity to foster teamwork and collaboration by examining the processes and outcomes of care, attending to results.

Sociocultural Issues

Tradition, role, and gender stereotypes are obstacles to collaboration (Rafferty, Ball, & Aiken, 2001). Safriet (1992) has suggested that the field of medicine staked out broad turf early on and considers any movement into this turf by other clinicians, at any level, to be unacceptable. Thus, turf issues have been a major stumbling block to successful interactions between nurses and physicians. Nurses are highly valued for the physical care, nurturing, and psychosocial support that they provide for patients whereas physicians are valued as the decision makers about treatment.

Nursing remains a predominantly female profession and, despite the influx of women into medicine, pharmacy, and dentistry, gender role stereotypes still exist and affect collaboration. Gender stereotypes dominate images of staff nurses in the media and APNs are rarely portrayed on television. Media bias and the nursing profession's inability to market itself adequately make nursing and advanced practice nursing invisible (Fagin, 1992). The so-called doctor-nurse game, a phenomenon influenced by roles and gender, first described in the 1970s, continues to operate in many institutions. However, it is apparent that the rules are changing and nurses do not want to play anymore (Rafferty, Ball, & Aiken, 2001; Rosenstein & O'Daniel, 2005). Stereotypical images and the invisibility of APNs influence how nursing is viewed by health care professionals and consumers: at best, nurses are viewed as kind and nice; at worst, as unintelligent and incompetent. Thus, APNs often find that they must actively counter low expectations with interactions and practices that convey their intelligence, competence, confidence, and trustworthiness.

Organizational Barriers

Competitive situations arise that can interfere with collaboration among and between APNs and those in other disciplines at the level of systems and organizations. In her extensive work in the field of health policy, one of the authors (CH) has observed one group of APNs who became aligned around a common viewpoint early in a debate, whereas members of other advanced practice nursing groups used precious time debating fine points, delaying or eliminating the possibility of unity on a policy issue that would affect all advanced practice nursing groups. Competitive stances and polarizing statements, whether they occur within or between disciplines, are barriers to collaboration.

Federal APN policies and organizational fragmentation make collaboration difficult and may contribute to unproductive competition. For example, the intent of Medicare billing requirements is to foster cooperation among clinicians, but they also discourage collaborative relations between health care providers and may actually serve as disincentives. Incident-to billing (see Chapter 19) requires that patient care services provided by APNs be directly supervised by physicians and offer reimbursement inequities, severely hampering a collaborative environment (Centers for Medicare and Medicaid Services [CMS], 2012).

Regulatory Barriers

Legislation and regulations have been barriers to the implementation of collaborative roles (Lugo, et al., 2007; Pearson, 2012). In the early days of advanced practice nursing, the overlap in APNs' and physicians' scopes of practice was often addressed by requiring physician supervision of aspects of an APN's practice. An outcome of this historical accident is that supervision of APNs by physicians is often mentioned explicitly or implicitly in some advanced practice nursing literature on collaboration and in state practice acts and regulations. In the past 20 years, there has been a slow but steady movement away from language requiring physician supervision and reference to protocols and toward emphasizing consultation, collaboration, peer review, and use of referral (Lugo, et al., 2007; Pearson, 2012).

In addition, some state statutes and regulations support a hierarchical structure that impedes collaboration between nurses and physicians (Hodnicki, Dietz, McNeil et al., 2004; Lugo, et al., 2007; Pearson, 2012). A scope of APN practice based on joint purposes and the public interest is more likely to foster collaboration between the professions (HHS, 2011; IOM, 2011; Safriet, 2002). The view advanced here is that a supervision requirement precludes the development of a collaborative relationship and that physicians cannot truly supervise advanced practice nursing.

Addressing regulatory barriers to collaboration will become more important for several reasons. As telehealth technologies expand, consumers and clinicians will be interacting across state lines, whether via e-mail, smartphones, telephone, or some other type of remote monitoring. In addition, consumers are becoming increasingly likely to consult quality score cards, licensing boards, websites, blogs, and other Internet resources to identify agencies and individual clinicians who provide the best health care. Adopting a multistate licensure compact for APNs will become important to ensure that collaboration and continuity of care can occur (Philipsen & Haynes, 2007).

Opportunities to create collaborative relationships can be lost in the morass of money, political power, and control issues that arise when too rapid changes in health care delivery systems occur (Remonder, Koch, Link, et al., 2010; Young et al., 2012). Furthermore, nurses and other stakeholders who are confronting their own professional concerns may not fully appreciate the stresses that physicians experience in today's volatile market. This factor is a serious deterrent to collaborative relationships.

Although conflicts with the medical community regarding regulation can make collaborative practice difficult for APNs, collaboration within the APN nursing community is also problematic at times. Overall, there are four dimensions of APN regulation—education, certification, accreditation, and licensure. Often, language and policy barriers make it difficult for the groups responsible for each of these to collaborate. These groups are making a concerted effort to enter into a truly collaborative network that allows them to match their individual organizational priorities to the priorities for APNs overall.

A Shared Vision for the Future Education and Regulation of Advanced Practice Nurses

For several years, two groups of advanced practice nursing leaders—the Advanced Practice Registered Nurse (APRN) Consensus Group, made up of representatives of educators, certifiers, accreditors, and professional groups, and the National Council of State Boards of Nursing APRN Advisory Committee—have been working to create a new vision for APRN regulation. Early on, both these groups had disparate beliefs about how the process and vision for APRN regulation should unfold. Two markedly diverse studies were under development.

Two years later, after failure to reach common ground, the two groups decided to meet as a joint dialogue group, with representation from both groups. Ground rules of conduct, including a group charter, were developed, including several tenets of collaboration—respect, transparency, trust, coming to common ground, a common purpose. The goal was to establish a vision of the future that was complementary, not divisive, and promote effective communication among the four regulatory bodies (licensure, accreditation, certification, education; LACE).

The group met several times over the next 2 years. Members were faithful to the process and few, if any, missed a meeting. The work began by establishing areas of agreement and consensus about APN regulation. This was the easy part. After each joint dialogue meeting, the decisions were brought back to the constituent groups for validation. As time progressed, areas of disagreement surfaced and were negotiated until agreement was reached. Over time, members of the group began to hear the concerns voiced by committee members from other organizations. They began to view the issue from a stance that was above what was right for themselves and see how a collaborative decision was needed to embrace all four APN roles (NP, CNM, CRNA, CNS) and LACE. At times, this was difficult work, but the commitment to collaborate to achieve a successful outcome carried the group along.

Since the last edition of this text, significant progress has been made. An electronic network with the ability to dialogue virtually has been implemented and 28 organizations have paid memberships to be part of the LACE community to ensure ongoing communication and dialogue around APRN regulatory issues. A public website has been developed for public access (http://aprnlace.org). At the same time, the NCSBN has established a Campaign for Consensus to assist the states in the implementation of the consensus model for regulation.

The process is still unfolding, but great strides have been made in developing a new vision for regulation of APNs. The most important is that the group has decided that one collaborative vision for APN regulation is needed, rather than the two visions that were originally planned.

Exemplar 12-3 describes this current effort and illustrates how an initial failure to collaborate can turn into a win-win situation for all involved.

Processes Associated with Effective Collaboration

Recurring Interactions

In addition to the characteristics discussed, several processes enable effective collaboration. A theme implicit in those writing about their positive experiences with collaboration is that establishing a trusting and collaborative relationship is a developmental process that depends on recurring, meaningful interactions (Alberto and Herth, 2009; Alpert, et al., 1992; D'Amour, et al., 2005). Although this concept of development over time is relevant to all aspects of collaboration, it is particularly important to establishing trust. The fact that effective collaboration is developmental and time-dependent explains why collaborative relationships are difficult to develop in organizations in which there is a high staff turnover or frequent rotation of clinicians, such as with house physicians. A physician wrote that the process seemed to be related to how well the nurse and physician know each other (Alpert, et al., 1992). Thus it seems likely that a series of less-complicated interactions (such as information exchange and coordination) that have been meaningful and clinically or personally satisfactory will contribute to the development of collaborative relationships. Team members need recurring interactions to acquire an understanding of each other's backgrounds, roles, and functions and develop patterns of interaction that are constructive, productive, and supportive. Projects focused on quality and outcomes of care that involve joint collection and analysis of data build collegiality and foster collaboration. In our experience, membership on such interdisciplinary committees as pharmacy and therapeutics, performance improvement, institutional review boards, ethics, and others with a patient care focus also foster communication and collegiality.

Effective Conflict Negotiation and Resolution Skills

As individuals, teams, and organizations work more closely together on their shared goals, inevitably, conflict will arise. APNs need to have some general approaches to conflict negotiation and resolution. As they work with particular partners with whom they will have relationships over time, it is wise to anticipate and discuss the criteria that the partners, team, or organization will use to address conflicts and disagreements. Box 12-3 lists some key conflict resolution skills (Conflict Resolution Network, 2012). Extensive detail on these skills and how to apply them is available on the internet (http://www.crnhq.org).

Bridging and Appreciative Inquiry

The work of Krumm (1992) has identified bridging as a component of collaboration. She did not define bridging

but implied that it is the ability to develop connections that support positive outcomes for individuals and populations of patients. She described one bridging skill as the "ability to recognize and rearrange boundaries within the practice setting" (p. 24). Appreciative inquiry (AI) is another strategy for building bridges and may keep conflict from escalating. Partners and teams work together to identify what is working in the situation and what needs to improve (note: the focus is not on what is wrong) This technique helps improvise new ways to achieve success and reframe toward the positive. AI focuses on examples of excellence and ways to emulate them. (See www.appreciativeinquiry.org.)

An example of bridging is the regulatory document, *Changes in Health Care Professions Scope of Practice: Legislative Considerations* (NCSBN et al., 2006). This study is the outcome of a collaborative effort of the disciplines of social work, physical therapy, nursing, medicine, pharmacy, and occupational therapy to remove turf battles from scope statements and focus on patient safety. These six disciplines have collaborated to develop guidelines to assist legislators and regulatory bodies to make decisions about scope of practice that focus on the provision of safe health care to patients, rather than perpetuate clinicians' boundaries. Their ability to do this work is a fine example of the progression of collaboration across disciplines and portrays our collaboration conceptualizations of shared goals and partnering to reach mutual outcomes.

Consensus building goes beyond bridging. Leaders identify anyone who has a stake in the outcome (as many as possible) to participate in the process. Stakeholders work together to identify common ground in issues that cross disciplinary boundaries and may or may not have been divisive.

Partnering and Team Building

It is only recently that health care leaders have begun to examine ways to improve the functioning of teams (Bosque, 2011; IPEC, 2011; Moeller, Vezeau, & Carr, 2007; Sennour, Counsell, Jones, et al., 2009). Effective models of teamwork have been used in subspecialties in psychology and health care (e.g., child development, rehabilitation). As health care leaders engage in the redesign and transformation of health care delivery, APNs can draw on the lessons learned in these fields. Some of the processes that have been associated with effective team building and conflict negotiation listed in Box 12-3 are further illustrated in Exemplar 12-3.

Implementing Collaboration

APNs may believe that they are the only ones with an active commitment to collaboration (Spross, 1989). Of all

---

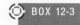 **BOX 12-3   Conflict Resolution Network's 12 Skills Summary***

- Win-win approach (identify attitude shifts to respect all parties' needs).
- Creative response (transform problems into creative opportunities).
- Empathy (develop communication tools to build rapport; use listening to clarify understanding).
- Appropriate assertiveness (apply strategies to attack the problem, not the person).
- Cooperative power (eliminate "power over" to build "power with" others).
- Managing emotions (express fear, anger, hurt, and frustration wisely to effect change).
- Willingness to resolve (name personal issues that cloud the picture).
- Mapping the conflict (define the issues needed to chart common needs and concerns).
- Development of options (design creative solutions together).
- Introduction to negotiation (plan and apply effective strategies to reach agreement).
- Introduction to mediation (help conflicting parties to move toward solutions).
- Broadening perspectives (evaluate the problem in the broader context).

*Adapted from Conflict Resolution Network. (2012). 12 skills summary: Conflict resolution skills (http://www.crnhq.org/pages.php?pID=10).

the competencies required for advanced practice, collaboration may be the most difficult to accomplish because it is mediated by social processes such as attitudinal and cultural factors that are ingrained in their professions or society in general. Efforts to change the environment to one that is more collaborative involve proving oneself over and over and challenging colleagues' behaviors that restrain attempts to work together. These intrapersonal demands, along with the clinical demands of one's job, can be exhausting. Therefore, APNs need to evaluate the potential for collaboration when seeking career opportunities. Questions about how clinicians work together, the interpersonal climate and organizational structures that support collaboration, should be a high priority. A realistic appraisal of the existence of or potential for collaboration is needed to determine whether APNs can provide the standard and quality of care characteristic of advanced practice nursing and whether they can expect a reasonable level of job satisfaction.

Assessment of Personal, Environmental, and Global Factors

APNs bring many personal attributes to a professional partnership. Assessment of their current attributes against the characteristics of collaboration listed in Box 12-4 can help beginning APNs to determine the areas in most need of development.

Covey (1989) has offered a perspective on moving toward a higher level of interdependence with colleagues. He portrayed interdependence as a higher level of performance than independence. Only individuals who have gained competence and confidence in their own expertise are able to move beyond autonomy and independence

BOX 12-4 Personal Strengths and Weaknesses Questionnaire

- Am I clear about my role in the partnership?
- What values do I bring to the relationship?
- What do I expect to gain or lose by collaborating?
- What do others expect of me?
- Do I feel good about my contribution to the team?
- Do I feel self-confident and competent in the collaborative relationship?
- Are there anxieties causing repeated friction that have not been addressed?
- Has serious thought been given to the boundaries of the collaborative relationship?

Adapted from Rider, E. (2002). Twelve strategies for effective communication and collaboration in medical teams. *British Medical Journal, 325*, S45.

toward the higher synergistic level of collaboration. Collaboration appears to have the same meaning as interdependence in Covey's work. This view is provocative when one considers the hierarchical context that often frames clinical collaboration. The notion that interdependence is the higher level of performance is supported in the evolution of advanced practice nursing. A number of clinical specialties are evolving to such a stage as disciplines mature and identify a shared interdisciplinary component to their work. For example, in the specialty of diabetes, advanced diabetes management involves interprofessional collaboration and is recognized by a certification examination open to a number of disciplines (see Chapter 5).

It must not be forgotten that teams collaborate with patients and their families; this collaborative relationship can be problematic for clinicians or for patients. When patients are abrasive or ill-equipped to deal with conflict, Saxton and colleagues (2009) suggested that clinicians remember to treat patients with dignity and respect, even when disagreeing with them, and to remember that a patient is more than his or her illness. In addition, illness can interfere with or diminish a patient's normal or effective communication skills. When patients have difficulty because their clinicians lack compassion, are abrasive, or otherwise fail to communicate with and care for them, Crocker and Johnson (2006) found that patients assert themselves by honoring their body's' wisdom and firing noncompassionate caregivers. Self-assessment is one important component to consider when embarking on a new professional relationship or evaluating the success or failure of current or potential collaborative relationships. The self-directed questions in Box 12-4 may help individuals identify their personal strengths and weaknesses in regard to collegiality. In addition to understanding personal characteristics that affect collaboration, APNs should consider contextual factors in the systems in which they practice.

Administrative leadership plays a key role in the development of collaborative relationships between organizational members. Administrators who support team and interdisciplinary administrative models, and who are themselves good communicators, can do a great deal to increase the momentum of new collaborations. Differing philosophies and standards of care within organizational settings can cause conflict between team members and need to be resolved early (Chreim, Williams, Janz, & Dastmalchian, 2010; Spross, 1989). The common vision of quality patient care and provider satisfaction makes collaboration a worthy goal for APNs and nursing administrators.

One environmental factor that needs to be understood is the loci of formal and informal power. Understanding and addressing power differences between groups can equalize the hierarchical differences among members, making collaboration possible if there is sufficient expertise among players (Stichler, 1995).

Global interactions require high levels of individual and organizational collaboration beyond what we can envision. "Systems citizenship refers to seeing the systems we have shaped and in turn, how they shape us and our decisions" (Senge, 2006, p. 343). APNs that recognize the need for global participation and collaboration at the personal, organizational, and systems levels are more likely to become the systems citizens of which Senge speaks.

Strategies for Successful Collaboration

Individual Strategies

Box 12-5 lists strategies that are thought to promote collaboration (Rider, 2002). Students and practicing APNs can examine their interactions for opportunities to implement these ideas and strengthen their interpersonal competence.

One strategy is for APNs to promote their exemplary nursing practices to help other health professionals and

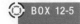 **BOX 12-5   Strategies to Promote Effective Communication and Collaboration**

- Be respectful and professional.
- Listen intently.
- Understand the other person's viewpoint before expressing your opinion.
- Model an attitude of collaboration, and expect it.
- Identify the bottom line.
- Decide what is negotiable and non-negotiable.
- Acknowledge the other person's thoughts and feelings.
- Pay attention to your own ideas and what you have to offer to the group.
- Be cooperative without losing integrity .
- Be direct.
- Identify common, shared goals, and concerns.
- State your feelings using "I" statements.
- Do not take things personally.
- Learn to say "I was wrong" or "You could be right."
- Do not feel pressure to agree instantly.
- Think about possible solutions before meeting and be willing to adapt if a more creative alternative is presented.
- Think of conflict negotiation and resolution as a helical process, not a linear one; recognize that negotiation may occur over several interactions.

consumers better understand the strengths of APNs as health care providers (Fagin, 1992; Pohl, et al., 2010). Participating in interdisciplinary quality improvement initiatives and development and evaluating EBP guidelines (see Chapter 10) are other ways to engage with colleagues within and across disciplines. It is useful for APNs to model their practice strategies for other nurses to facilitate intranursing collaboration and consultation. One way to share excellence in practice in grand rounds or a team conference is to include the opportunity for each care team member to describe her or his own decision making about patients and suggest new strategies for care to the team.

Working together on joint projects is an excellent way to facilitate good collaboration. Collaborative research and scholarly writing projects, as well as community service projects that tap into the strengths of various members, open people's eyes to the benefits of collaboration. Federal and private agencies are currently supporting interdisciplinary collaborative studies. Reporting the results in the literature will illustrate the considerable advantages of collaborative interactions. In addition, social opportunities at conferences and receptions allow camaraderie to develop and help reinforce the bond between members of the partnership (Hanson, 1993; Hanson, Spross, & Carr, 2000). These strategies move across lines from personal life to organizational settings and from education to practice arenas. New models that foster joint medical and nursing care are needed in primary care and within specialty practice in all settings. More importantly, collaboratively developed practice guidelines improve communication and clarify clinicians' roles in patient treatment (Cooper, 2007; U.S. Preventive Services Task Force, 2012; www.NAP.org).

Team Strategies

A primary focus for groups is to develop effective teams; the development of effective teams was one of the IOM's recommendations (2001) for improving health care quality (HHS, 2011). The health care environment is at an optimal point for those in the health professions to work together. Lencioni's field guide (2005) provides activities aimed at helping team members overcome the team dysfunctions described earlier, noting that there are two important questions team members must ask themselves:
- Are we really a team?
- Are we ready to do the heavy lifting that will be required to become a team?

If a group of collaborators can respond affirmatively to both questions, they will be able to use the field guide to advantage. The activities are aimed at helping teams address each of the five dysfunctions by helping them build trust, master conflict, achieve commitment, embrace accountability, and focus on results.

One serious challenge to collaboration is team members who are uninterested in developing collaborative teams. In this type of situation, APNs must step up and operate from a stance and expectation of collaboration; that is, APNs should model collaboration in all interactions and expect the same from all other members of the team. Building a group of like-minded colleagues can also increase the momentum toward collaboration as the expected style of interaction within a team. APNs should understand that collaboration as defined here is not routinely taught in health profession schools. Consequently, they must be prepared to teach this process to others.

A recent concept is the idea of a group visit by a collaborative group of providers. The group visit can be understood as an extended office visit during which not just physical and medical needs are met, but educational, psychological, and social concerns are also addressed by a collaborative group of caregivers invested in caring for the patient (Burke & O'Grady, 2012; Young et al., 2012). A suggested starter group kit might include ways to plan ahead before starting collaborative group visits, how to let patients know about the new change, who needs to be part of the collaborative provider group, who does what, and an agenda for the visit (Bodenheimer & Grumbach, 2012). An example of a group visit practice that includes an NP, CNS and CNM is "Centering Pregnancy: A New Program for Adolescent Prenatal Care" (Moeller, Vezeau, & Carr, 2007). The great significance of the group visit is the inclusion of the patient as part of the group and the cost-effective use of resources to address multiple aspects of the patient's care.

Organizational Strategies

The numerous initiatives to improve safety and quality that have evolved from the IOM reports in the past 10 years can help health administrators and leaders create organizational structures that will facilitate collaboration while attending to important quality and safety goals. The IHI's white papers, TJC and Magnet requirements for evidence of interdisciplinary collaboration in patient care, toolkits for interdisciplinary education, and clinical and organizational toolkits to facilitate the adoption of EBP guidelines (e.g., from the Registered Nurses Association of Ontario [rnao.org]) are available. These toolkits often include assessments that can be done to identify the location of the barriers and the opportunities for improvement. APNs, physicians, and other clinical colleagues and leaders can use these assessments to develop strategic plans for improving the collaborative environment.

Depending on the results of the assessment, clinicians may need professional development to enable them to collaborate.

Organizational leaders must take seriously reports of disruptive behavior and take action to eliminate this behavior (Rosenstein & O'Daniel, 2005). It is incumbent on APNs to report these and other organizational factors that impede collaboration and expect action. Kinnaman and Bleich (2004) have observed that collaboration is "the highest developmentally, and most complex and resource-intensive interdisciplinary behavior" (p. 316). The authors posited that collaboration requires more resources and suggested that the type of problem-solving behavior should be matched to the degree of complexity and uncertainty inherent in the problem. As APNs practice and collaborate with administrators and physicians, it will be useful to pay attention to the costs (e.g., time, money, resources, patient outcomes) of collaborating and not collaborating, or of coordinating (or delegating coordinating functions). Documenting positive and negative patient and institutional outcomes of collaboration or its absence can contribute to identifying which clinical resources are needed to achieve clinical and institutional goals.

Fagin (1992) and Hanson (1993) have identified several strategies that foster successful collaboration at all levels. As noted, there needs to be a move toward interdisciplinary educational programs that allow for face to face interaction and problem solving among health science students (Alberto & Herth, 2009; Bainbridge, et al., 2010; Petri, 2010). Definitive changes in the structure of clinical education and sequencing of content will be required. Given the entrenched bureaucracies involved, this will be a difficult task, requiring stronger interactions among educational programs. Health care providers need to be learning about health policy issues from a perspective that offers broad stroke solutions. Faculty across programs need to be evaluating and treating patients and supervising students together. It is important to introduce joint appointments of nursing, medicine, pharmacy, dental, and other faculty to provide faculty with opportunities to model advanced practice nursing care and build rapport.

National and state health professional organizations must endorse the shift toward a collaborative model (Fagin, 1992; Hanson, 1993; NCSBN et al., 2006). Strategies that facilitate this shift, such as retreats, social interactions, communication workshops, joint practice committees, and sensitivity training sessions aimed at consensus building, are imperative. As noted, there are some successful models of consensus building in some sectors of health care. These models, across diverse stakeholders, must be replicated more widely in health care if barriers to successful interprofessional collaboration are to be reduced.

Exemplar 12-4 is an example of how APNs from different specialties can work together to alter a hospital policy. They pooled the expertise in their particular specialty and their knowledge of the political issues that often surround hospital-based work. They knew that if they wanted to make this change, the key players in the decision making process would have to buy into the idea. The usual pattern is not to change because past policy and procedures have been in place and there is substantial pressure not to change something that is viewed as working. The pull of the familiar was in place, yet it was not working for the mothers who wanted different options available to them.

These APNs all knew that in their facility, policy approval was the purview of the medical staff. They would have to be included to make this change. Also, the hospital was governed by the strong department chairs in medicine and they would also have to agree. These APNs well understood that science, although critically important, was not sufficient to bring about this change. All the stakeholders had to be included. The APNs knew which parts of the policy were open for negotiation and which were not, and crafted their proposal cleverly. This change did not happen quickly; several months were required to gain the support of all the key players. However, in the end, the women who used the birthing center were

 EXEMPLAR 12-4   **Collaboration in Quality Improvement: Improved Analgesia and Anesthesia Options During Labor**

Ms. Smith is a CNM who provides full-scope midwifery services to women who choose this approach for pregnancy and delivery. The birthing center at which Ms. Smith attends the delivery of her patients has a policy that women must choose no analgesia during labor and delivery or they must have an epidural. Many of the women were not happy with having only two choices. Some women believed that they might need some help with the discomfort of delivery but did not want to be confined to labor in a bed by use of the traditional epidural anesthesia. Ms. Smith has investigated this issue and the policy seems to have been developed in the past by a committee that consisted of OB-GYN physicians and anesthesiologists. The policy was approved by the medical staff. No mothers, CNMs, or CRNAs were part of the policy making. There have been a number of advances in care since this policy was developed and Ms. Smith wishes to bring about a change to improve care to the mothers and their families.

In this particular facility, only anesthesia providers (physician or CRNA) were credentialed to administer any analgesic or anesthetic agents, a practice touted as necessary for the quality of care for recipients of these agents. Ms. Smith did not believe that she would be able to alter this policy, nor did she really wish to do so. However, she wanted to provide an expanded set of options for her mothers. Although many of the mothers did not choose to receive any analgesia for labor or delivery, they wanted to have the option available prior to needing it.

Ms. Smith consulted with a CRNA colleague who specialized in obstetric anesthesia. They met and discussed a number of options and decided that there were types of epidural approaches that could allow the mother

to continue to walk while in labor and thereby improve the likelihood of a normal vaginal birth. Also, additional approaches were added to the list of available agents. One was a hand-held device that delivered inhaled nitrous oxide when the mother thought she needed it. The services of the pediatric nurse practitioner (PNP) were requested because the APN believed that the substantial literature on the topic indicated that newborns have better outcomes if the mother does not receive a standard epidural and that normal vaginal birth could be encouraged.

This trio of APNs crafted the new policy proposal, engaged support from the Chair of OB-GYN, Chair of Pediatrics, Chair of Anesthesiology and nursing supervisor, and advanced the change in policy to the medical staff committee. After a great deal of argument, discussion, and negotiation, the policy was changed and approved by the hospital board. Now, women could choose from a variety of approaches that best met their wishes and particular situation. This group of APNs knew that there were some parts of the policy that would not change, including the administration by anesthesia providers only. Also, all the anesthesiologists and CRNAs who provided obstetric anesthesia were not equally adept at all the new approaches, so the CRNA provided in-service education for them. The nursing staff of the birthing center needed additional training and the CNM provided this education, along with the CRNA. Although the change in policy was created to accommodate the wishes of the midwifery practice, the outcome was that all women who delivered in the facility now had options that improved their satisfaction and quality of care. In addition, all the APN caregivers believed that they had enhanced the labor experience of their maternity patients.

greatly advantaged by the collaborative efforts of all involved.

Conclusion

Many of the barriers to successful collaboration occur because of values, beliefs, and behaviors that have until recently gone unchallenged in society and in the organizations in which nurses practice. Radical change is needed if the conditions conducive to collaboration are to become the norm. Collaborative relationships not only are professionally satisfying, but also improve access to care and patient outcomes. Although APNs collaborate with many individuals within and outside of nursing, and do so successfully, they may find that one of their most important collaborative relationships—with physicians—may also be the most challenging. Despite the fact that there are many successful individual APN-physician collaborative practices, including many with evidence demonstrating their beneficial effects on health care, tradition and stereotypes are often powerful negative influences on policymaking and in health care and professional organizations.

To meet the demands for cost-effectiveness and quality, clinicians from all disciplines have been meeting together to discuss the care they provide and to define ways to deliver it to maximize quality and minimize duplication of effort. These interactions foster the trust and respect required for mature collaboration. They enable collaborators to recognize their interdependence and value the input of others, thus creating a synergy that improves the quality of clinical decision making (Health Sciences Institute, 2005). Systems citizenship starts with seeing the systems we have shaped and that in turn shape us (Friedman, 2005). Collaboration becomes a priority as global interconnectedness enters our everyday interactions in the complex health care arena in which APNs practice. In today's health care environment, collaboration may flourish, regardless of the barriers identified in this chapter. However, there is an urgent need for a better understanding of the organizational structures, communication processes, and interactive styles that enable clinicians to collaborate in ways that benefit clinical processes and outcomes. APNs can contribute to this understanding in several ways: (1) by documenting and analyzing their experiences with collaboration in published case studies; (2) by precepting students and helping them develop the skills essential for collaboration; and (3) by working with researchers who are studying the characteristics and clinical implications of collaboration. Effective collaboration must be at the heart of any redesign of the health care delivery system, whether that redesign occurs in a unit, in a clinic, within and between organizations, or globally.

References

Aiken, L. H., Smith, H. L., & Lake, E. T. (1994). Lower Medicare mortality among a set of hospitals known for good nursing care. *Medical Care, 32,* 771–787.

Alberto, J., & Herth, K., (2009). Interprofessional collaboration within faculty roles: Teaching, service, and research. *OJIN,* 2009, May; *14,* 1–14.

Alpert, H., Goldman, L., Kilroy, C., & Pike, A. (1992). 7 Gryzmish: Toward an understanding of collaboration. *Nursing Clinics of North America, 27,* 47–59.

American Academy of Family Physicians, American Academy of Pediatrics, American College of Physicians, American Osteopathic Association. (2007). *Joint principles of the patient-centered medical home.* Washington DC: Author.

American Association of Colleges of Nursing (AACN). (2004). *AACN position statement on the practice doctorate in nursing.* Washington, DC: Author.

American Association of Colleges of Nursing (AACN). (2006). *The essentials of doctoral education for advanced nursing practice.* Washington, DC: Author.

American College of Graduate Medical Education. (2002). ACGME outcome competencies (http://www.acgme.org/acgmeweb/Portals/0/PDFs/commonguide/IVA5_EducationalProgram_ACGMECompetencies_Introduction_Explanation.pdf).

American College of Nurse Midwives. (2011). Ob-Gyns and midwives seek to improve health care for women and their newborns: Groups issue collaborative practice statement (www.midwife.org/Ob-Gyns-Midwives-Seek-to-Improve-health-care-for-women-and-their-newborns).

American Medical Association (AMA). (2012). House of Delegates resolution 317. (www.ama-assn.org/resources/doc/council-on-med.../res317a08.pdf).

American Nurses Association (ANA). (2003). *Nursing's social policy statement* (2nd ed.). Washington, DC: Author.

American Nurses Credentialing Center (2012). Magnet recognition program (www.nursecredentialing.org/Magnet.aspx).

Anderson, K. (2011). Work place aggression and violence: Midwives and nurses say no. *Australian Nursing Journal, 26,* 1320–1385.

Baggs, J. G., & Schmitt, M. H. (1988). Collaboration between nurses and physicians. *Image: The Journal of Nursing Scholarship, 20,* 145–149.

Baggs, J. G., & Schmitt, M. H. (1997). Nurses' and resident physicians' perceptions of the process of collaboration in an MICU. *Research in Nursing & Health, 20,* 71–80.

Bainbridge, L., Nasmith, L., Orchard, C., & Wood, V. (2010). Competencies for interprofessional collaboration. *Journal of Physical Therapy Education, 24,* 6–11.

Balzer, J. (1993). Humor: A missing ingredient in collaborative practice. *Holistic Nursing Practice, 7,* 28–35.

Bodenheimer, T., & Grumbach, K. (2012). *Improving primary care.* New York: McGraw-Hill Lange.

Bosque, E. (2011). A model of collaboration and efficiency between neonatal nurse practitioner and neonatologist: Application of collaboration theory. *Advances in Neonatal Care, 11,* 108–113.

Bourbonniere, M., & Evans, L. (2002). Advanced practice nursing in the care of frail older adults. *Journal of the American Geriatrics Society, 50,* 2062–2076.

Brooten, D., Youngblut, J., Blais, K., Donahue, D., Cruz, I., & Lightbourne, M. (2005). APN-physician collaboration in caring for women with high-risk pregnancies. *Journal of Nursing Scholarship, 37,* 178–184.

Burke, R. E., & O'Grady, E. T. (2012). Group visits hold great promise for improving diabetic care and outcomes, but best practices must be developed. *Health Affairs, 31,* 1, 103–109.

Canadian Interprofessional Health Collaborative (CHIC). (2010). A national interprofessional competencies framework (www.cihc.ca/files/CIHC_IPCompetencies_Feb1210.pdf).

Centers for Medicare and Medicaid Services (CMS). (2012). Medicare claims processing manual. Physician/nonphysician practitioners (http://www.cms.gov/Regulations-and-Guidance/Guidance/Manuals/Downloads/clm104c12.pdf).

Chreim, S., Williams, B. E., Janz, L., & Dastmalchian, A. (2010). Change agency in a primary health care context: The case of distributed leadership. *Health Care Management Review, 35,* 187–199.

Christman, L. (1998). Advanced practice nursing: Is the physician's assistant an accident of history or a failure to act? *Nursing Outlook, 46,* 56–59.

Ciesielka, D., Conway, A., Penrose, J., & Risco, K. (2005). Maximizing resources: The share model of collaboration. *Nursing Education Perspectives, 26,* 224–226.

Clausen. C., Strohschein, F. J., Farems, S., Bateman, D., Posel, N., & Fleiszer, D. M. (2012). Developing an interprofessional care plan for an older adult women with breast cancer: From multiple voices to a shared vision. *Oncology Nursing, 16,* E18–E25.

Conflict Resolution Network. (2012). 12 skills summary: Conflict resolution skills (http://www.crnhq.org/pages.php?pID=10).

Cooper, R. A. (2007). New directions for nurse practitioners and physician assistants in an era of physician shortages. *Academic Medicine, 82,* 827–828.

Cooper, R. A., Henderson, T., & Dietrich, C. L. (1998). Roles of nonphysician clinicians as autonomous providers in patient care. *Journal of the American Medical Association, 280,* 795–800.

Covey, S. R. (1989). *The seven habits of highly effective people.* New York: Simon & Schuster.

Cowan M. J., Shapiro M., Hays R. D., Afifi A., Vazirani S., Ward C. R., et al. (2006). The effect of multidisciplinary hospitalist/physician/advanced practice nurse collaboration on hospital costs. *Journal of Nursing Administration, 36,* 79–85.

Crocker, L., & Johnson, B. (2006). *Privileged presence: Personal stories of connections in health care.* Boulder, CO: Bull Publishing.

Cronenwett L., & Dzay, V. (2010). Who will provide primary care and how will they be trained? Proceedings of a conference sponsored by the Josiah Macy Jr. Foundation (http://www.macyfoundation.org/docs/macy_pubs/JMF_PrimaryCare_Monograph.pdf).

D'Amour, D. D., Ferrada-Videla, M., Rodriguez, L. S., & Beaulieu, M. (2005). The conceptual basis for interprofessional collaboration: Core concepts and theoretical frameworks. *Journal of Interprofessional Care, 19*(Suppl 1), 116–131.

Disch, J. (2002). Collaboration is in the eye of the beholder. *The Joint Commission Journal on Quality Improvement, 28,* 233–234.

Drenning, C. (2006). Collaboration among nurses, advanced practice nurses, and nurse researchers to achieve evidence based practice. *Journal of Nursing Care Quality, 21,* 298–301.

Dumez, A. G. (2011). There is need for broader and more effective cooperation among the health service professions. *American Journal of Pharmaceutical Education, 75,* 99.

Dumont, S., Briere, N., Morin, D., Houle, N., & Hoko-Fundi, M. (2010). Implementing an interfaculty series of courses on interprofessional collaboration in prelicensure health science curriculums. *Education for Health, 23,* 1–12.

Fagin, C. (1992). Collaboration between nurses and physicians: No longer a choice. *Nursing and Health Care, 13,* 354–363.

Friedman, T. L. (2005). *The world Is flat: A brief history of the 21st century.* New York: Farrar, Straus and Giroux.

Garland, C. G., McGonigel, J. J., Frank, A., & Buck, D. (1989). *The transdisciplinary model of service delivery.* Lightfoot, VA: Child Development Resources.

Gelman, S., O'Neill, E., & Kimmey, J.; The Task Force on Accreditation for Health Professions Education. (1999). *Strategies for change and improvement: The report of the Task Force on Accreditation of Health Professions Education.* San Francisco: Center for the Health Professions, University of California at San Francisco.

Gilbert, J. H. V., Camp, R. D., Cole, C. D., Bruce, C., Fielding, D. W., & Stanton, S. J. (2000). Preparing students for interprofessional teamwork in health care. *Journal of Interprofessional Care, 14,* 223–235.

Gordon, S. (2011). Team intelligence—language is a good place to start (http://suzannecgordon.com/team-intelligence-a-much-needed-concept).

Hanson, C. M. (1993). Our role in health care reform: Collegiality counts. *American Journal of Nursing, 93,* 16A–116E.

Hanson, C. M., Hodnicki, D. R., & Boyle, J. S. (1994). Nominations for excellence: Collegial advocacy for nurse practitioners. *Journal of the American Academy of Nurse Practitioners, 6,* 471–476.

Hanson, C. M., & Spross, J. A. (1996). Collaboration. In A. B. Hamric, J. A. Spross, & C. M. Hanson (Eds.), *Advanced nursing practice: An integrative approach* (pp. 229–248). Philadelphia: WB Saunders.

Hanson, C. M., Spross, J. A., & Carr, D. B. (2000). Collaboration. In A. B. Hamric, J. A. Spross, & C. M. Hanson, (Eds.), *Advanced nursing practice: An integrative approach* (pp. 315–347; 2nd ed.). Philadelphia: WB Saunders.

Harbaugh, G. (1994). Assumptions of interprofessional collaboration: Interrelatedness and wholeness, In R. M. Casto & M. C. Julia (Eds.), *Interprofessional care and collaborative practice* (pp. 13–23). Pacific Grove, VA: Brooks/Cole.

Health Sciences Institute. (2005). Chronic care competency model (www.chroniccare.org/documents/FullCCPCompetency Model.pdf).

Health Sciences Institute. (2007). Chronic care professional certification program (www.chroniccare.org/profdev_CCcert.htm).

Hill, M. N., & Hewlett, P. O. (2002). Getting to the top: Martha Hill, President American Heart Association. In D. J. Mason, J. K. Leavitt, & M. W. Chaffee. (Eds.), *Policy and politics in nursing and health care* (pp. 621–625). Philadelphia: WB Saunders.

Hodnicki, D.R., Dietz, A., McNeil, F., & Miles, K. (2004). Prescriptive authority: Medication-ordering patterns of advanced practice registered nurses in Georgia. *American Journal for Nurse Practitioners, 8*, 9–24.

Hotez, P. (April 13, 2003). For the latest disease, a faster response. *Washington Post*, pp. B1, B4.

Houghton, A. (2003). Bullying in medicine. *British Medical Journal, 326*, S125.

Hughes, A., & Mackenzie, C. (1990). Components necessary in a successful nurse practitioner–physician collaborative practice. *Journal of the American Academy of Nurse Practitioners, 2*, 54–57.

Ingersoll, G. L., McIntosh, E., & Williams, M. (2000). Nurse-sensitive outcomes of advanced practice. *Journal of Advanced Nursing Practice, 32*, 1272–1281.

Institute of Medicine (2011). *The future of nursing: Leading change, advancing health*. Washington DC: National Academy Press.

Institute of Medicine (IOM), Committee on Quality Health Care in America. (2001). *Crossing the quality chasm: A new health system for the 21st century*. Washington, DC: National Academy Press.

Interprofessional Collaborative Initiative (IPEC). (2011). Core competencies of interprofessional collaborative practice (www.aacn.nche.edu/education/pdf/IPECreport.pdf).

Jackson, D. J., Lang, J. M., Swartz, W. H., Ganiats, T. G., Fullerton, J., Ecker, J., et al. (2003). Outcomes, safety, and resource utilization in a collaborative care birth center program compared with traditional physician-based perinatal care. *American Journal of Public Health, 93*, 999–1006.

Johnson-Pawlson, J., Posey, L., Dalal, A., & Page, J. (2003). *Educating primary care practitioners in their home communities: Partnerships for training*. Washington, DC: Partnerships for Training, Association for Academic Health Centers.

Kinnaman, M. L. R., & Bleich, M. R. P. (2004). Collaboration: Aligning resources to create and sustain partnerships. *Journal of Professional Nursing, 20*, 310–322.

Kleinpell, R. M., Faut-Callahan, M., Lauer, K., Kremer, M., Murphy, M., & Sperhac, A. (2002). Collaborative practice in advanced nursing in acute care. *Critical Care Nursing Clinics of North America, 14*, 307–313.

Knaus, W. A., Draper, E. A., Wagner, D. P., & Zimmerman, J. E. (1986). An evaluation of outcome from intensive care in major medical centers. *Annals of Internal Medicine, 104*, 410–418.

Krumm, S. (1992). Collaboration between oncology clinical nurse specialists and nursing administrators. *Oncology Nursing Forum, 19*(Suppl. 1), 21–24.

Larson, E. (1999). The impact of physician-nurse interaction on patient care. *Holistic Nursing Practice, 13*, 38–46.

Lavizzo-Mourey, R. (2012). The nurse education imperative (www.medscape.com/viewarticle/757397).

Lencioni, P. (2005). *Overcoming the five dysfunctions of a team: A field guide for leaders, managers, and facilitators*. San Francisco: Jossey-Bass.

Lindeke, L. (2005). Nurse-physician workplace collaboration. *Online Journal of Issues in Nursing, 10*, 1–7.

Litaker, D., Mion, L. C., Planavsky, L., Kippes, C., Mehta, N., & Frolkis, J. (2003). Physician–nurse practitioner teams in chronic disease management: The impact on costs, clinical effectiveness, and patients' perception of care. *Journal of Interprofessional Care, 17*, 223–237.

Longo, J., & Smith, M. (2011). A prescription for disruptions in care: Community building among nurses to address horizontal violence. *Advances in Nursing Science, 34*, 345–356.

Lugo, N. R., O'Grady, E. T., Hodnicki, D. R., & Hanson, C. M. (2007). Ranking state NP regulation: Practice environment and consumer health care choice. *American Journal for Nurse Practitioners, 11*, 8–23.

Makowsky, M. J., Schindel, T., Rosenthal, M., Campbell, K., Tsuyuki, R. T., & Madill, H. M. (2009). Collaboration between pharmacists, physicians, and nurse practitioners: A qualitative investigation of working relationships in the inpatient medical setting. *Journal of Interprofessional Care, 23*, 169–184.

McAvoy, B., & Murtagh, J. (2003). Workplace bullying: The silent epidemic [letter]. *British Medical Journal, 326*, 776–777.

McCaffrey, R. G., Hayes, R., Stuart, W., Cassell, A., Farrell, C., Miller-Reyes, C., et al. (2010). A program to improve communication between nurses and medical residents. *Journal of Continuing Education in Nursing, 41*, 172–178.

McClure, M., & Hinshaw A. (Eds.). (2002). *Magnet hospitals revisited: Attraction and retention of professional nurses*. Washington, DC: American Nurses Association.

Moeller, A. H., Vezeau, T. M., & Carr, K. C. (2007). Centering pregnancy: A new program for adolescent prenatal care. *American Journal for Nurse Practitioners, 11*, 48–56.

Morse, K. J., Warshawsky, D., Moore, J. M., Pecora, D. C. (2006). A new role for the ACNP: The rapid response team leader. *Critical Care Nursing Quarterly, 29*, 137–146.

Murray-Davis, B., Marshall, M., & Gordon, F. (2011). What do midwives think about interprofessional working and learning? *Midwifery, 27*, 376–381.

National Council of State Boards of Nursing (NCSBN), Association of Social Work Boards, Federation of State Boards of Physical Therapy, Federation of State Medical Boards, National Association of Boards of Pharmacy, National Board for Certification in Occupational Therapy. (2006). *Changes in healthcare professions' scope of practice: Legislative considerations (brochure)*. Chicago: Author.

National Organization of Nurse Practitioner Faculties. (2011). Nurse practitioner core competencies (www.goshen.edu/nursing/files/2011-core-competencies.pdf).

Naylor, M. D., Brooten, D. A., Campbell, R. L., Maislin G., McCauley K. M., & Schwartz J. S. (2004). Transitional care of older adults hospitalized with heart failure: A randomized, controlled trial. *Journal American Geriatric Society, 52*, 675–684.

Nolan, T., Resar, R., Haraden, C., & Griffin, F. A. (2004). *Improving the reliability of health care.* Cambridge, MA: Institute for Healthcare Improvement.

North Shore Long Island Jewish Health System. (2010). Magnet award (www.northshorelij.com/NSLIJ/Quality+Awards+and+Recognition).

Palinkas, L. A., Ell, K., Hansen, M., Cabassa, L., & Wells, A. (2011). Sustainability of collaborative care interventions in primary care settings. *Journal of Social Work, 11,* 99–117.

Pearson, L. (2012). The Pearson report (http://www.pearsonreport.com).

Petri, L. (2010). Concept analysis of interdisciplinary collaboration. *Nursing Forum, 45,* 73–82.

Pew Health Professions Commission. (1995). *Critical challenges: Revitalizing the health professions for the twenty-first century (3rd report).* San Francisco: University of California—San Francisco Center for the Health Professions.

Pew-Fetzer Task Force on Advancing Psychosocial Health Education. (1994). *Health professions education and relationship-centered care.* San Francisco: Pew Health Professions Commission.

Philipsen, N. C., & Haynes, D. R. (2007). The multi-state nursing licensure compact: Making nurses mobile. *Journal for Nurse Practitioners, 3,* 36–40.

Phillips, R. L., Harper, D. C., Wakefield, M., Green, L. A., & Fryer, G. E. (2002). Can nurse practitioners and physicians beat parochialism into plowshares? *Health Affairs, 21,* 133–142.

Pohl, J. M., Hanson, C. M., Newland, J. A., & Croenwett, L. (2010). Unleashing nurse practitioners' potential to deliver primary care and lead teams. *Health Affairs, 29,* 900–905.

Prescott, P., & Bowen, S. (1985). Physician-nurse relationships. *Annals of Internal Medicine, 103,* 127–133.

Rafferty, A. M., Ball, J., & Aiken, L. H. (2001). Are teamwork and professional autonomy compatible and do they result in improved hospital care? *Quality in Health Care, 10*(Suppl 2), ii32–ii37.

Reinertsen, J., Gosfield, A., Rupp, W., & Whittington, J. (2007). Engaging physicians in a share quality agenda (www.ihi.org/IHI/Results/WhitePapers/EngagingPhysiciansWhitePaper.htm).

Remonder, J., Koch, S., Link, J., & Graham, C. (2010). Lessons learned—4 years outcomes: The need for collaboration, utilization and projection. *Child Welfare, 89,* 251–267.

Reuben, D. B., Levy-Storms, L., Yee, M. N., Lee, M., Cole, K., Waite, M., et al. (2004). Disciplinary split: A threat to geriatrics interdisciplinary team training. *Journal of the American Geriatrics Society, 52,* 1000–1006.

Rice, K., Zwarenstein, M., Conn, L. G., Kenaszchuk, C., Russell, A., & Reeves, S. (2010). An intervention to improve interprofessional collaboration and communications: A comparative qualitative study. *Journal of Interprofessional Care, 24,* 350–361.

Rider, E. (2002). Twelve strategies for effective communication and collaboration in medical teams. *British Medical Journal Career Focus, 325,* S45.

Robert Wood Johnson Foundation (RWJF). (2003). Partnerships for training: Educating primary care practitioners in their home communities (www.pftweb.org/pft_brochure_web.pdf).

Robert Wood Johnson Foundation (RWJF). (2012). Interdisciplinary collaboration improves safety, quality of care, experts say (www.rwjf.org/pr/product.jsp?id=71488).

Rosenstein, A. H., & O'Daniel, M. (2005). Disruptive behaviors and clinical outcomes: Perceptions of nurses and physicians, and administrators say that clinicians' disruptive behavior has negative effects on clinical outcomes. *Nursing Management, 36,* 18–28.

Ruddy, G., & Rhee K. (2005). Transdisciplinary teams in primary care for the underserved: A literature review. *Journal of Health Care for the Poor and Underserved, 16,* 248–256.

Rutherford, P., Lee B., & Greiner A. (2004). Transforming care at the bedside (www.ihi.org/IHI/Results/WhitePapers/TransformingCareattheBedsideWhitePaper.htm).

Safriet, B. J. (1992). Health care dollars and regulatory sense: The role of advanced practice nursing. *Yale Journal on Regulation, 9,* 417–487.

Safriet, B. J. (2002). Closing the gap between "can" and "may" in health care providers' scopes of practice: A primer for policymakers. *Yale Journal on Regulation, 19,* 301.

Safriet, B. J. (2010). Federal options for maximizing the value of advanced practice nurses (http://www.webnponline.com/articles/article).

Sands, R., Stafford, J., & McClelland, M. (1990). "I beg to differ": Conflict in the interdisciplinary team. *Social Work in Health Care, 14,* 55–72.

Saxton, R., Hines, T., & Enriquez, M. (2009). The negative impact of nurse/physician disruptive behavior on patient safety. *Journal of Patient Safety, 5,* 180–183.

Schmitt, M. H. (2001). Collaboration improves the quality of care: Methodological challenges and evidence from U.S. health care research. *Journal of Interprofessional Care, 15,* 47–66.

Schmitt, M. H. (2011). Fostering the development of interprofessional competency. *Nurse Practitioner World News, 16,* 18–19.

Sears, L., Maxwell, W., & Townsend, C. (2003). Urgent-care visits to a geriatric primary care clinic. *American Journal for Nurse Practitioners, 7,* 15–18.

Senge, P. M. (2006). *The Fifth Discipline: The art and practice of the learning organization (revised and updated).* New York: Currency/Doubleday.

Senge, P. M., Scharmer, C. O., Jaworski, J., & Flowers, B. S. (2004). *Presence: An exploration of profound change in people, organizations, and society.* New York: Currency/Doubleday.

Sennour, Y., Counsell, S. R., Jones, J., & Weiner, M. (2009). Development and implementation of a proactive geriatrics consultation model in collaboration with hospitalists. *Journal of the American Geriatrics Society, 57,* 2139–2145.

Sheer, B. (2007). ICN advanced practice nurses network meets in Japan. *Nurse Practitioner World News, 12,* 1, 10–11.

Scheer, K., Wilson, D. M., Wagner, J., & Haughian, M. (2012). Evaluating a new rapid response team: NP-led versus intensivist-led comparisons. *AACN Advanced Critical Care, 23,* 32–43.

Shortell, S. M., Zimmerman, J. E., Rousseau, D. M., Gillies, R. R., Wagner, D. P., Draper, E. A., et al. (1994). The performance of intensive care units: Does good management make a difference? *Medical Care, 32,* 508–525.

Spross, J. A. (1989). The CNS as collaborator. In A. B. Hamric & J. A. Spross (Eds.), *The clinical nurse specialist in theory and practice* (pp. 205–226; 2nd ed.). Philadelphia: WB Saunders.

Steele J. E. (Ed.). (1986). *Issues in collaborative practice*. Orlando, FL: Grune & Stratton.

Stichler, J. F. (1995). Professional interdependence: The art of collaboration. *Advanced Practice Nursing Quarterly, 1*, 53–61.

U.S. Department of Health and Human Services (HHS). (2011). Patient Protection and Affordable Care Act (http://www. healthcare.gov/law/full/index.html).

U.S. Preventive Services Task Force. (2012). About the USPSTF (http://www.uspreventive servicestaskforce.org).

World Health Organization (1978). *Alma-Ata 1978: Primary health care. Report of the International Conference on Primary Health Care. 6-12 September 1978, Alma-Ata, USSR.* Geneva: Author.

Young, H., Siegel, E. O., McCormick, W. C., Fulmer, T., Harootyan, L. K., & Dorr, D. A. (2012). Interdisciplinary collaboration in geriatrics: Advancing health for older adults. *Nursing Outlook, 59*, 243–251.

Weinstein, M. E., McCormack, B., Brown, M. E., & Rosenthal, D. S. (1998). Build consensus and develop collaborative practice guidelines. *Nursing Management, 29*, 48–52.

Wooton, K. T., Lee, J., Jared, H., Boggess, K., & Wilder, R. (2011). Nurse practitioners and CNMs: Knowledge, opinions and practice behaviors regarding periodontal disease and adverse pregnancy outcomes. *Journal of Dental Hygiene, 85*, 122–131.

Zwarenstein, M., & Reeves, S. (2002). Working together but apart: Barriers and routes to nurse-physician collaboration. *The Joint Commission Journal on Quality and Patient Safety, 28*, 1–7.

Ethical Decision Making

Ann B. Hamric • *Sarah A. Delgado*

CHAPTER CONTENTS

Changes in interprofessional roles, advances in medical technology, privacy issues, revisions in patient care delivery systems, and heightened economic constraints have increased the complexity of ethical issues in the health care setting. Nurses in all areas of health care routinely encounter disturbing moral issues, yet the success with which these dilemmas are resolved varies significantly. Because nurses have a unique relationship with the patient and family, the moral position of nursing in the health care arena is distinct. As the complexity of issues intensifies, the role of the advanced practice nurse (APN) becomes particularly important in the identification, deliberation, and resolution of complicated and difficult moral problems. Although all nurses are moral agents, APNs are expected to be leaders in recognizing and resolving moral problems, creating ethical practice environments, and promoting social justice in the larger health care system. It is a basic tenet of the central definition of advanced practice nursing (see Chapter 3) that skill in ethical decision making is one of the core competencies of all APNs. In addition, the Doctor of Nursing Practice (DNP) essential competencies emphasize leadership in developing and evaluating strategies to manage ethical dilemmas in patient care and organizational arenas (American Association of Colleges of Nursing [AACN], 2006). This chapter explores the distinctive ethical decision-making competency of advanced practice nursing, the process of developing and evaluating this competency, and barriers to ethical practice that APNs can expect to confront.

Characteristics of Ethical Dilemmas in Nursing

In this chapter, the terms *ethics* and *morality* or *morals* are used interchangeably (see Beauchamp & Childress, 2009, for a discussion of the distinctions between these terms). A problem becomes an ethical or moral problem when issues of core values or fundamental obligations are present. An *ethical* or *moral dilemma* occurs when obligations require or appear to require that a person adopt two (or more) alternative actions, but the person cannot carry out all the required alternatives. The agent experiences tension because the moral obligations resulting from the dilemma create differing and opposing demands (Beauchamp & Childress, 2009; Purtilo & Doherty, 2011). In some moral dilemmas, the agent must choose between equally unacceptable alternatives; that is, both may have elements that are morally unsatisfactory. For example, based on her evaluation, a family nurse practitioner (FNP) may suspect that a patient is a victim of domestic violence, although the patient denies it. The FNP is faced with two options that are both ethically troubling—connect the patient with existing social services, possibly straining the family and jeopardizing the FNP-patient relationship, or avoid intervention and potentially allow the violence to continue. As described by Silva and Ludwick (2002), honoring the FNP's desire to prevent harm (the principle of beneficence) justifies reporting the suspicion, whereas respect for the patient's autonomy justifies the opposite course of action.

Jameton (1984, 1993) has distinguished two additional types of moral problems from the classic moral dilemma, which he termed *moral uncertainty* and *moral distress*. In situations of moral uncertainty, the nurse experiences unease and questions the right course of action. In *moral distress*, nurses believe that they know the ethically appropriate action but feel constrained from carrying out that action because of institutional obstacles (e.g., lack of time or supervisory support, physician power, institutional policies, legal constraints). Noting that nurses and others often take varied actions in response to moral distress, Varcoe and colleagues (2012) have proposed a revision to Jameton's definition: "moral distress is the experience of being seriously compromised as a moral agent in practicing in accordance with accepted professional values and standards. It is a relational experience shaped by multiple contexts, including the socio-political and cultural context of the workplace environment" (p. 60). The phenomenon of moral distress has received increasing national and international attention in nursing and medical literature. Studies have reported that moral distress is significantly related to unit-level ethical climate and to health care professionals' decisions to leave clinical practice (Corley, Minick, Elswick, et al., 2005; Epstein & Hamric, 2009; Hamric, Borchers, & Epstein, 2012; Hamric, Davis, & Childress, 2006; Pauly, Varcoe, Storch, et al., 2009; Schluter, Winch, Hozhauser, et al., 2008; Varcoe, Pauly, Webster, & Storch, 2012). APNs work to decrease the incidence of moral uncertainty and moral distress for themselves and their colleagues through education, empowerment, and problem solving.

Although the scope and nature of moral problems experienced by nurses and, more specifically APNs, reflect the varied clinical settings in which they practice, three general themes emerge when ethical issues in nursing practice are examined. These are problems with communication, the presence of interdisciplinary conflict, and nurses' difficulties with managing multiple commitments and obligations.

Communication Problems

The first theme encountered in many ethical dilemmas is the erosion of open and honest communication. Clear communication is an essential prerequisite for informed and responsible decision making. Some ethical disputes reflect inadequate communication rather than a difference in values (Hamric & Blackhall, 2007; Ulrich, 2012). The APN's communication skills are applied in several arenas. Within the health care team, discussions are most effective when members are accountable for presenting information in a precise and succinct manner. In patient encounters, disagreements between the patient and a family member or within the family can be rooted in faulty communication, which then leads to ethical conflict. The skill of listening is just as crucial in effective communication as having proficient verbal skills. Listening involves recognizing and appreciating various perspectives and showing respect to individuals with differing ideas. To listen well is to allow others the necessary time to form and present their thoughts and ideas.

Understanding the language used in ethical deliberations (e.g., terms such as beneficence, autonomy, and utilitarian justice) helps the APN frame the concern. This can help those involved to see the components of the ethical problem rather than be mired in their own emotional responses. When ethical dilemmas arise, effective communication is the first key to negotiating and facilitating a resolution. Jameson (2003) has noted that the long history of conflict between certified registered nurse anesthetists (CRNAs) and anesthesiologists influences how these providers communicate in practice settings. In interviews with members of both groups, she found that some transcended role-based conflict whereas others became mired in it, particularly in the emotions around perceived threats to role fulfillment. She recommended enhancing communication through focus on the common goal of patient care, rather than on the conflicting opinions about supervision and autonomous practice. In other words, focusing on shared values rather than the values in conflict can promote effective communication.

Interdisciplinary Conflict

The second theme encountered is that most ethical dilemmas that occur in the health care setting are multidisciplinary in nature. Issues such as refusal of treatment, end-of-life decision making, cost containment, and confidentiality all have interprofessional elements interwoven in the dilemmas, so an interprofessional approach is necessary for successful resolution of the issue. Health care professionals bring varied viewpoints and perspectives into discussions of ethical issues (Hamric & Blackhall, 2007; Piers, Azoulay, Ricou, et al., 2011; Shannon, Mitchell, & Cain, 2002). These differing positions can lead to creative and collaborative decision making or to a breakdown in communication and lack of problem solving. Thus, an interdisciplinary theme is prevalent in the presentation and resolution of ethical problems.

For example, a clinical nurse specialist (CNS) is writing discharge orders for an older woman who is terminally ill with heart failure. The plan of care, agreed on by the interprofessional team, patient, and family, is to continue oral medications but discontinue IV inotropic support and all other aggressive measures. Just prior to discharge, the social worker informs the CNS that medical coverage for the patient's care in the skilled nursing facility will only be covered by the insurer if the patient has an IV in place. The attending cardiologist determines that the patient can be discharged to her daughter's home because she no longer requires skilled care and the social worker agrees to proceed with this plan. However, the CNS is concerned that the patient's need for physical assistance will overwhelm her daughter and believes that the patient is better off returning to the skilled nursing facility. Although each team member shares responsibility to ensure that the plan of care is consistent with the patient's wishes and minimizes the cost burden to the patient, they differ in how to achieve these goals. Such legitimate but differing perspectives from various team members can lead to ethical conflict.

Multiple Commitments

The third theme that frequently arises when ethical issues in nursing practice are examined is the issue of balancing commitments to multiple parties. Nurses have numerous and, at times, competing fidelity obligations to various stakeholders in the health care and legal systems (Chambliss, 1996; Hamric, 2001). Fidelity is an ethical concept that requires persons to be faithful to their commitments and promises. For the APN, these obligations start with the patient and family but also include physicians and other colleagues, the institution or employer, the larger profession, and oneself. Ethical deliberation involves analyzing and dealing with the differing and opposing demands that occur as a result of these commitments. An APN may face a dilemma if encouraged by a specialist consultant to pursue a costly intervention on behalf of a patient, whereas the APN's hiring organization has established cost containment as a key objective and does not support use of this intervention (Donagrandi & Eddy, 2000). In this and other situations, APNs are faced with an ethical dilemma created by multiple commitments and the need to balance obligations to all parties.

The general themes of communication, interdisciplinary conflict, and balancing multiple commitments are prevalent in most ethical dilemmas. Specific ethical issues may be unique to the specialty area and clinical setting in which the APN practices.

Ethical Issues Affecting Advanced Practice Nurses

Primary Care Issues

Situations in which personal values contradict professional responsibilities often confront NPs in a primary care setting. Issues such as abortion, teen pregnancy, patient nonadherence to treatment, childhood immunizations, regulations and laws, and financial constraints that interfere with care were cited in one older study as frequently encountered ethical issues (Turner, Marquis, & Burman, 1996). Ethical problems related to insurance reimbursement, such as when implementation of a desired plan of care is delayed by the insurance authorization process or restrictive prescription plans, are an issue for APNs. The problem of inadequate reimbursement can also arise when there is a lack of transparency regarding the specifics of services covered by an insurance plan. For example, a patient who has undergone diagnostic testing during an inpatient stay may later be informed that the test is not covered by insurance because it was done on the day of discharge. Had the patient and nurse practitioner (NP) known of this policy, the testing could have been scheduled on an outpatient basis with prior authorization from the insurance company and thus be a covered expense.

Viens (1994) found that primary care NPs interpret their moral responsibilities as balancing obligations to the patient, family, colleagues, employer, and society. More recently, Laabs (2005) has found that the issues most often noted by NP respondents as causing moral dilemmas are those of being required to follow policies and procedures that infringe on personal values, needing to bend the rules to ensure appropriate patient care, and dealing with patients who have refused appropriate care. Issues leading to moral distress included pressure to see an excessive number of patients, clinical decisions being made by others, and a lack of power to effect change (Laabs, 2005). Increasing expectations to care for more patients in less time are routine in all types of health care settings as pressures to contain costs escalate. APNs in rural settings may have fewer resources than their colleagues working in or near academic centers in which ethics committees, ethics consultants, and educational opportunities are more accessible.

Issues of quality of life and symptom management traverse primary and acute health care settings. Pain relief and symptom management can be problematic for nurses and physicians (Oberle & Hughes, 2001). APNs must confront the various and sometimes conflicting goals of the patient, family, and other health care providers regarding the plans for treatment, symptom management, and quality of life. The APN is often the individual who coordinates the plan of care and thus is faced with clinical and ethical concerns when participants' goals are not consistent or appropriate.

Acute and Chronic Care

In the acute care setting, APNs struggle with dilemmas involving pain management, end-of-life decision making, advance directives, assisted suicide, and medical errors (Shannon, Foglia, Hardy, & Gallagher, 2009). Rajput and Bekes (2002) identified ethical issues faced by hospital-based physicians, including obtaining informed consent, establishing a patient's competence to make decisions, maintaining confidentiality and transmitting health information electronically. APNs in acute care settings may experience similar ethical dilemmas. Recent studies of moral distress have revealed that feeling pressured to continue aggressive treatments that respondents thought were not in the patients' best interest or in situations in which the patient was dying, working with physicians or nurses who were not fully competent, giving false hope to patients and families, poor team communication, and lack of provider continuity were all issues that engendered moral distress (Hamric & Blackhall, 2007; Hamric, Borchers, & Epstein, 2012).

APNs bring a distinct perspective to collaborative decision making and often find themselves bridging communication between the medical team and patient or family. For example, the neonatal nurse practitioner (NNP) is responsible for the day-to-day medical management of the critically ill neonate and may be the first provider to respond in emergency situations (Juretschke, 2001). The NNP establishes a trusting relationship with the family and becomes aware of the values, beliefs, and attitudes that shape the family's decisions. Thus, the NNP has insight into the perspectives of the health care team and family. This "in-the-middle" position, however, can be accompanied by moral distress (Hamric, 2001), particularly when the team's treatment decision carried out by the NNP is not congruent with the NNP's professional judgment or values. Botwinski (2010) conducted a needs assessment of NNPs and found that most had not received formal ethics content in their education and desired more education on the management of end-of-life situations, such as delivery room resuscitation of a child on the edge of viability. Knowing the best interests of the infant and balancing those obligations to the infant with the emotional, cognitive, financial, and moral concerns that face the family struggling with a critically ill neonate is a complex undertaking. Care must be guided by an NNP and health care team who understand the ethical principles and decision making related to issues confronted in neonatal intensive care unit (NICU) practice.

Societal Issues

Ongoing cost containment pressures in the health care sector have significantly changed the traditional practice of delivering health care. Goals of reduced expenditures and services and increased efficiency, although important, may compete with enhanced quality of life for patients and improved treatment and care, creating tension between providers and administrators, particularly in managed care systems in which providers find that their clinical decisions are subject to outside review before they can be reimbursed. Ulrich and associates (2006) surveyed NPs and physician assistants to identify their ethical concerns in relation to cost containment efforts, including managed care. They found that 72% of respondents reported ethical concerns related to limited access to appropriate care and more than 50% reported concerns related to the quality of care. An earlier study of 254 NPs revealed that 80% of the sample perceived that to help patients, it was sometimes necessary to bend managed care guidelines to provide appropriate care (Ulrich, Soeken, & Miller, 2003). Most respondents in this study reported being moderately to extremely ethically concerned with managed care; more than 50% said that they were concerned that business decisions took priority over patient welfare and more than 75% stated that their primary obligation was shifting from the patient to the insurance plan. Although the passage of the Patient Protection and Affordable Care Act (PPACA; U.S. Department of Health & Human Services [HHS], 2011) may help with these concerns to some extent, the ethical tensions that underlie cost containment pressures and the business model orientation of health care delivery may continue.

An example of how cost containment goals can create conflict is a situation in which a NP wishes to order a computed tomography (CT) scan to evaluate a patient complaining of abdominal pain. The NP knows that the patient has a history of diverticulosis resulting in abscess formation and the current presentation with fever and abdominal tenderness justifies this testing; however, the insurance approval process takes a minimum of 24 hours. By sending the patient to the emergency room, the test can be done more quickly, but the patient will also face a long wait and a high copay if she does not require subsequent hospital admission. Limiting access to CT scans is based on containing costs and avoiding unnecessary testing, which are two laudable goals. However, in this situation, the lengthy approval process means that the NP does not have needed information to direct the treatment plan and alleviate the patient's suffering in a timely manner. The use of the emergency room to obtain essential clinical information is a greater burden on the patient and may ultimately prove more expensive to the system.

Technologic advances, such as the rapidly expanding field of genetics, are also challenging APNs (Caulfield, 2012; Harris, Winship, & Spriggs, 2005; Horner, 2004; Pullman & Hodgkinson, 2006). As Hopkinson and Mackay (2002) have noted, although the potential impact of mapping the human genome is immense, the challenge of how to translate genetic data rapidly into improvements in the prevention, diagnosis, and treatment of disease remains. To counsel patients effectively on the risks and benefits of genetic testing, APNs need to stay current in this rapidly changing field (a helpful resource for this and other issues is the text by Steinbock, Arras, and London, 2012). As one example, genetic testing poses a unique challenge to the informed consent process. Patients may feel pressured by family members to undergo or refuse testing, and may require intensive counseling to understand the complex implications of such testing; APNs are also involved in post-test counseling, which raises ethical concerns regarding the disclosure of test results to other family members (Erlen, 2006). Because genetic information is crucially linked to the concepts of privacy and confidentiality, and the availability of this information is increasing, it is inevitable that APNs will encounter legal issues and ethical dilemmas related to the use of genetic data.

APNs may engage in research as principal investigators, co-investigators, or data collectors for clinical studies and trials. In addition, leading quality improvement (QI) initiatives is a key expectation of the DNP-prepared APN (AACN, 2006). Ethical issues abound in clinical research, including recruiting and retaining patients in studies, protecting vulnerable populations from undue risk, and ensuring informed consent, fair access to research, and study subjects' privacy. As APNs move into QI and research initiatives, they may experience the conflict between the clinician role, in which the focus is on the best interests of an individual patient, and that of the researcher, in which the focus is on ensuring the integrity of the study (Edwards & Chalmers, 2002).

Access to Resources and Issues of Justice

Issues of access to and distribution of resources create powerful dilemmas for APNs, many of whom care for underserved populations. Issues of social justice and equitable access to resources present formidable challenges in clinical practice. Trotochard (2006) noted that a growing number of uninsured individuals lack access to routine health care; they experience worse outcomes from acute and chronic diseases and face higher mortality rates than those with insurance. McWilliams and colleagues (2007) found that previously uninsured Medicare beneficiaries require significantly more hospitalizations and office visits when compared with those with similar health problems who, prior to Medicare eligibility, had private insurance. The PPACA, when fully enacted, will help improve access to quality care and decrease the incidence of these dilemmas. However, as noted, the escalating costs of health care represent ethical challenges to providers and systems alike, regardless of the population's insurance status.

The allocation of scarce health care resources also creates ethical conflicts for providers; regardless of payment mechanisms, there are insufficient resources to meet all societal needs (Bodenheimer & Grumbach, 2012; Trotochard, 2006). Scarcity of resources is more severe in developing areas of the world and justice issues of fair and equitable distribution of health care services present serious ethical dilemmas for nurses in these regions (Harrowing & Mill, 2010). A further international issue is the "brain drain" of nurses and other health professionals who leave underdeveloped countries to take jobs in developed countries (Chaguturu & Vallabhaneni, 2007; Dwyer, 2007).

Allocation issues have been described in the area of organ transplantation but dilemmas related to scarce resources also arise in regard to daily decision making, for example, with a CNS guiding the assignment of patients in a staffing shortage, or an FNP finding that a specialty consultation for a patient is not available for several months. Whether in community or acute care settings, APNs must, on a daily basis, balance their obligation to provide holistic, evidence-based care with the necessity to contain costs and the reality that some patients will not receive needed health care. As Bodenheimer and Grumbach (2012) have noted, "Perhaps no tension within the U.S. health care system is as far from reaching a satisfactory equilibrium as the achievement of a basic level of fairness in the distribution of health care services and the burden of paying for those services" (p. 215).

One of the value-added components that APNs bring to any practice setting is creativity and a wide range of patient management strategies, which are crucial in caring for large numbers of uninsured and underinsured persons. It is not uncommon for an APN to encounter a patient who has been forced to stop taking certain medications for financial reasons. Although many practitioners prescribe generic forms of medications, if available, some patients still have to pay an exorbitant price for their medications. For example, an acute care nurse practitioner (ACNP) managing an underinsured patient with chronic lung disease and heart failure discovers that the patient is unable to pay for all the medications prescribed and has elected to forego the diuretic and an angiotensin-converting enzyme inhibitor (ACE-I). Because the ACNP knows that ACE-Is are associated with reduced morbidity and mortality rates, and that diuretics control symptoms and prevent rehospitalization, these changes are discouraged. Instead, the ACNP helps the patient make more suitable choices when altering medications, such as dosing some medications on an every-other-day basis. The ACNP has helped the patient cope with the situation but must face the morally unsettling fact that this plan of care is medically inferior.

Finally, as APNs broaden their perspectives to encompass population health and increased policy activities, both essential competencies of the DNP-prepared APN (AACN, 2006), they will experience the tension between caring for the individual patient and the larger population (Emanuel, 2002). Caregivers are increasingly being asked to incorporate population-based cost considerations into individualized clinical decision making (Bodenheimer & Grumbach, 2012). Population-based considerations present a challenge to the moral agency of APNs, who have been educated to privilege the individual clinical decision.

Legal Issues

Over the last 30 years, the complexity of ethical issues in the health care environment and the inability to reach agreement among parties has resulted in participants turning to the legal system for resolution. A body of legal precedent has emerged, reflecting changes in society's moral consensus. Ideally, moral rights are upheld or protected by the law. For example, the Culturally and Linguistically Appropriate Services (CLAS) Standards established by the HHS mandate that health care institutions receiving federal funds provide services that are accessible to patients regardless of their cultural background (HHS, Office of Minority Health, 2001). These standards provide a legislative voice for the ethical obligation to respect all persons, regardless of their cultural background and primary language. In a different voice, the PPACA (HHS, 2011) has mandated that persons who can afford health insurance purchase it or pay a penalty, starting in 2014. According to this law, societal beneficence, in the form of limiting high expenditures on the care of uninsured persons, is preferred over individual autonomy (Trautman, 2011).

APNs must use caution and not conflate legal perspectives with ethical decision making. In many cases, there is no relevant law and thoughtful deliberation of the ethical issues offers the best hope of resolution. In addition, looking to the judicial system for guidance in ethical decision making is troubling because the judicial aim is to interpret the law, not to satisfy the ethical concerns of all parties involved. In addition, clinical understanding may be absent from the judicial perspective. Involvement of the media may further confuse the situation, as was evident in the Schiavo case (Gostin, 2005). The legal guidelines in that case were clear; the Florida court system repeatedly upheld the right of Ms. Schiavo's spouse to refuse nutrition and hydration on her behalf. However, advocacy groups, politicians, and Ms. Schiavo's parents used the media to offer a variety of interpretations of the case and wielded political power to prevent removal of the feeding tube and to have it replaced twice after it was removed. Clearly, the legal perspective did not satisfy the moral concerns of all involved. Unfortunately, much of the publicity focused on the emotional experience of the parents fearing the loss of their daughter and not on careful consideration of the ethical elements.

Sometimes, the law not only falls short of resolving ethical concerns, but contributes to the creation of new dilemmas. Changes in the Medicare hospice benefit under the PPACA (HHS, 2011) offer a clear example. Designed to prevent hospice agencies from enrolling and re-enrolling patients who do not meet criteria, the new regulations require a face-to-face assessment by a health care provider to recertify hospice eligibility at set intervals after the initial enrollment (Kennedy, 2012). Often, patients with dementia or another slowly progressive disease state who enroll in hospice experience an initial period of stability, likely because they have improved symptom management and access to comprehensive services. If this stability extends to the next certification period, the patient may face disenrollment. For the practitioner conducting the assessment, this creates the ethical dilemma of wanting to be truthful regarding the patient's status and at the same time avoid removing a service that is benefiting the patient and family.

Ethical Decision Making Competency of Advanced Practice Nurses

There are a number of reasons why ethical decision making is a core competency of advanced practice nursing. As noted, clinical practice gives rise to numerous ethical concerns and APNs must be able to address these concerns. Also, ethical involvement follows and evolves from clinical expertise (Benner, Tanner, & Chesla, 2009). Another reason why ethical decision making is a core competency can be seen in the expanded collaborative skills that APNs develop (see Chapter 12). APNs practice in a variety of settings and positions but, in most cases, the APN is part of an interprofessional team of caregivers. The team may be loosely defined and structured, as in a rural setting, or more definitive, as in the acute care setting. The recent re-emergence of an interprofessional care model is changing practice for all providers (Interprofessional Collaborative Initiative [IPEC], 2011). Regardless of the structure, APNs need the knowledge and skills to avoid power struggles, broker and lead interdisciplinary communication, and facilitate consensus among team members in ethically difficult situations.

Phases of Core Competency Development

The core competency of ethical decision making for APNs can be organized into four phases. Each phase depends on

TABLE 13-1	Phases of Development of Core Competency for Ethical Decision Making	
Phase and Title	**Knowledge**	**Skill or Behavior**
1. Knowledge Development—Moral Sensitivity	Ethical theories	Sensitivity to ethical dimensions of clinical practice
	Ethical issues in specialty	Values clarification
	Professional code	
	Professional standards	Sensitivity to fidelity conflicts
	Legal precedent	Gather relevant literature related to problems identified
	Moral distress	Evaluate practice setting for congruence with literature
		Identify ethical issues in the practice setting and bring to the attention of other team members
2. Knowledge Application—Moral Action	Ethical decision-making frameworks	Apply ethical decision making models to clinical problems
	Mediation and facilitation strategies	Use skilled communication regarding ethical issues
		Facilitate decision making by using select strategies
		Recognize and manage moral distress in self and others
3. Creating an Ethical Environment	Preventive ethics	Role model collaborative problem solving
	Awareness of environmental barriers to ethical practice	Mentor others to develop ethical practice
		Address barriers to ethical practice through system changes
		Use preventive ethics to decrease unit-level moral distress
4. Promoting Social Justice Within the Health Care System	Concepts of justice	Ability to analyze the policy process
	Health policies affecting a specialty population	Advocacy, communication, and leadership skills
		Involvement in health policy initiatives supporting social justice

the acquisition of the knowledge and skills embedded in the previous level. Thus, the competency of ethical decision making is understood as an evolutionary process in an APN's development. Phase 1 and beginning exposure to Phase 2 should be explicitly taught in the APN's graduate education. Phases 3 and 4 evolve as APNs mature in their roles and become comfortable in the practice setting; these phases represent leadership behavior and the full enactment of the ethical decision making competency. Phase 4 relies on competencies required of DNP-prepared APNs; the knowledge and skills needed for Phases 3 and 4 should be incorporated into DNP programs. Although an expectation of the practice doctorate, all APNs should develop their ethical knowledge and skills to include elements of all four phases of this competency. The essential elements of each phase are described in Table 13-1.

Phase 1: Knowledge Development

The first phase in the ethical decision making competency is developing core knowledge in ethical theories and principles and the ethical issues common to specific patient populations or clinical settings. This dual knowledge enables the APN student to integrate philosophical concepts with contemporary clinical issues. The emphasis in this initial stage is on learning the language of ethical discourse and achieving cognitive mastery. The APN learns the theories, principles, codes, paradigm cases, and relevant laws that influence ethical decision making. With this knowledge, the APN begins to compare current practices in the clinical setting with the ethical standards described in the literature.

Phase 1 is the beginning of the APN's personal journey toward developing a distinct and individualized ethical framework. The work of this phase includes developing sensitivity to the moral dimensions of clinical practice (Weaver, 2007). A helpful initial step in building moral sensitivity is understanding one's values, in which students clarify the personal and professional values that inform their care (Fry & Johnstone, 2008). Engaging in this work uncovers personal values that may have been internalized and not openly acknowledged, and is particularly important in our multicultural world.

Another key aspect of this phase is developing the ability to distinguish a true ethical dilemma from a situation of moral distress or other clinically problematic situation. This requires a general understanding of ethical theories, principles, and standards that help the APN define and discern the essential elements of an ethical dilemma. Novice APNs should be able to recognize a moral problem and seek clarification and illumination of the concern. The APN identifies ethical issues and formulates the concerns about which others are uneasy. This step earns credibility and enables the APN to gain self-confidence by bringing the issue to the awareness and attention of others. If the issue remains a moral concern after clarification, the APN should pursue resolution, seeking additional help if needed.

Formal education in ethical theories and concepts should be included in graduate education programs for APNs. Although some beginning graduate students will have had significant exposure to ethical issues in their undergraduate programs, most have not. A 2008 U.S. survey of nurses and social workers found that only 51% of the nurse respondents had formal ethics education in their undergraduate or graduate education; 23% had no ethics training at all (Grady, Danis, Soeken, et al., 2008). APN students with no ethics education will be at a disadvantage in developing this competency because graduate education builds on the ethical foundation of professional practice. The current master's essentials (AACN, 2011) do not address ethics education directly but include competencies in the use of ethical theories and principles. *The Essentials of Doctoral Education for Advanced Nursing Practice* (AACN, 2006) contains explicit ethical content in five of the eight major categories (Box 13-1). Even categories that do not explicitly list necessary ethical content imply it in referring to issues such as improving access to health care, addressing gaps in care, and using conceptual and analytic skills to address links between practice and organizational and policy issues.

Exposure to ethical theories, principles, and concepts allows the APN to develop the language necessary to articulate ethical concerns in an interprofessional environment. It is important, however, that knowledge development extend beyond classroom discussions. Clinical practicum experiences also need to build in discussions of ethical dimensions of practice explicitly rather than assume that these discussions will naturally occur. In one study of the clinical experiences of graduate students from four graduate programs, only 4 of 20 students were identified as having experience with an ethical dilemma and only 2 of 22 preceptors noted any exposure to ethical dilemmas for students (Howard & Steinberg, 2002). The authors concluded that this apparent void in clinical education may have been a function of limited recognition of

 BOX 13-1 Ethical Competencies in the DNP Essentials*

- Integrate nursing science with knowledge from ethics and biophysical, psychosocial, analytic, and organizational sciences as the basis for the highest level of nursing practice. (I)
- Develop and/or evaluate effective strategies for managing the ethical dilemmas inherent in patient care, the health care organization, and research. (II)
- Design, direct, and evaluate quality improvement methodologies to promote safe, timely, effective, efficient, *equitable* (emphasis added), and patient-centered care. (III)
- Provide leadership in the evaluation and resolution of ethical and legal issues within health care systems relating to the use of information, information technology, communication networks, and patient care technology. (IV)
- Advocate for social justice, equity, and ethical policies within all health care arenas. (V)

*Essential number in parentheses.
From American Association of Colleges of Nursing. (2006). *The essentials of doctoral education for advanced nursing practice.* Washington, DC: Author.

ethical decision making processes by APN students and preceptors. In another study, Laabs (2005) noted that 67% of NP respondents claimed that they never or rarely encountered ethical issues. Some respondents showed confusion regarding the language of ethics and related principles. In a later study, Laabs (2012) found that APN graduates, most of whom had had an ethics course in their graduate curriculum, indicated a fairly high level of confidence in their ability to manage ethical problems, but their overall ethics knowledge was low. These three studies provide compelling commentary on the need for Phase 1 activity in graduate curricula.

The core knowledge of ethical theories should be supplemented with an understanding of issues central to the patient populations with whom the APN works. As APNs assume positions in specific clinical areas or with particular patient populations, it is incumbent upon them to gain an understanding of the applicable laws, standards, and regulations in their specialty, as well as relevant paradigm cases. This information may be garnered from current literature in the field, continuing education programs, or discussions with colleagues. Information on legal and policy guidelines should be offered during graduate practicum experiences in the area of clinical concentration.

Although Phase 1 is the building block for the other phases of this competency, it is also an ongoing process. APNs will gain core knowledge in graduate education but, as societal issues change and new technologies emerge, new dilemmas and ethical problems arise. The ability to be a leader in creating ethical environments involves a commitment to lifelong learning about ethical issues, of which professional education is just the beginning.

Developing an Educational Foundation

As noted, education in ethical theories, principles, rules, and moral concepts provides the foundation for developing skills in ethical reasoning. Because the APN will apply these theoretical principles in actual encounters with patients, it is imperative that consideration of the context in specific situations be strengthened. A portion of graduate ethics education should involve discussion of typical issues encountered by APNs, rather than issues that receive extensive media attention but occur infrequently. Howard and Steinberg (2002) maintained that graduate curricula need to go beyond traditional ethical issues to encompass building trust in the APN-patient relationship, professionalism and patient advocacy, resource allocation decisions, individual versus population-based responsibilities, and managing tensions between business ethics and professional ethics. The latter three areas are crucial for developing the Phase 4 level of the ethical decision making competency.

Continuing education programs are also effective and necessary forums in which current information can be provided in a rapidly changing health care environment. As technology changes and new dilemmas confront practitioners, the APN must be prepared to anticipate conditions that erode an ethical environment. Knowledge and skills in all phases of this competency depend on the application of current ethical knowledge in the clinical setting; ethical reasoning and clinical judgment share a common process and each serves to teach and inform the other (Dreyfus, Dreyfus, & Benner, 2009). Therefore, the importance of clinical practice cannot be overemphasized.

Overview of Ethical Theories

Principle-Based Model. Although ethical decision making in health care is extensively discussed in the bioethics literature, two dominant models are most often applied in the clinical setting. The first model of decision making is a principle-based model (Box 13-2), in which ethical decision making is guided by principles and rules (Beauchamp & Childress, 2009). In cases of conflict, the principles or rules in contention are balanced and interpreted with the contextual elements of the situation. However, the final decision and moral justification for actions are based on an appeal to principles. In this way,

> **BOX 13-2**   **Principles and Rules Important to Professional Nursing Practice**
>
> - Principle of respect for autonomy: The duty to respect others' personal liberty and individual values, beliefs, and choices
> - Principle of nonmaleficence: The duty not to inflict harm or evil
> - Principle of beneficence: The duty to do good and prevent or remove harm
> - Principle of formal justice: The duty to treat equals equally and treat those who are unequal according to their needs
> - Rule of veracity: The duty to tell the truth and not to deceive others
> - Rule of fidelity: The duty to honor commitments
> - Rule of confidentiality: The duty not to disclose information shared in an intimate and trusted manner
> - Rule of privacy: The duty to respect limited access to a person
>
> Adapted from Beauchamp, T. L., & Childress, J. F. (2009). *Principles of biomedical ethics* (6th ed.). New York: Oxford University Press.

the principles are binding and tolerant of the particularities of specific cases (Beauchamp & Childress). The principles of respect for persons, autonomy, beneficence, nonmaleficence, and justice are commonly applied in the analysis of ethical issues in nursing. The American Nurses Association (ANA) *Code of Ethics for Nurses* (2001) has endorsed the principle of respect for persons and underscores the profession's commitment to serving individuals, families, and groups or communities. The emphasis on respect for persons throughout the code implies that it is not only a philosophical value of nursing, but also a binding principle within the profession.

Although ethical principles and rules are the cornerstone of most ethical decisions, the principle-based approach has been criticized as being too formalistic for many clinicians and lacking in moral substance (Gert, Culver, & Clouser, 2006). Other critics have argued that a principle-based approach conceals the particular person and relationships and reduces the resolution of a clinical case simply to balancing principles (Rushton & Penticuff, 2007). Because all the principles are considered of equal moral weight, this approach has been seen as inadequate to provide guidance for moral action (Gert et al., 2006; Strong, 2007). In spite of these critiques, bioethical principles remain the most common ethical language used in clinical practice settings.

Casuistry. The second common approach to ethical decision making is the casuistic model (Box 13-3), in

BOX 13-3 Alternative Ethical Approaches

Casuistry
- Direct analysis of particular cases
- Uses previous paradigm cases to infer ethical action in a current case
- Analogues in common law and case law
- Values practical knowledge rather than theory (pretheoretical)
- Privileges experience

Narrative Ethics
- Supplements principles by emphasizing importance of full context
- Gathers views of all parties to provide more complete basis for moral justification
- Story and narrator substitute for ethical justification, which emerges naturally
- Privileges stories

Virtue-Based Ethics
- Emphasizes the moral agent, not the situation or the action
- Right motives and character reveal more about moral worth than right actions
- Character more important than conformity to rules
- Right motives make for right actions
- Privileges actor's values and motives

Feminist Ethics
- Views women as embodied, fully rational, and having experiences relevant to moral reasoning
- Emphasizes view of the disadvantaged—women and other underrepresented groups
- Emphasizes importance and value of openness to different perspectives
- Concerned with power differentials that create oppression
- Emphasizes importance of attention to the vulnerable and to resulting inequalities
- Privileges power imbalances

Care-Based Ethics
- Emphasizes creating and sustaining responsive connection with others
- Emphasizes importance of context and subjectivity in discerning ethical action
- Sees individuals as interdependent rather than independent; focuses on parties in a relationship
- Privileges relationships

---

which current cases are compared with paradigm cases (Beauchamp & Childress, 2009; Jonsen & Toulmin, 1988; Toulmin, 1994). The strength of this approach is that a dilemma is examined in a context-specific manner and then compared with an analogous earlier case. The fundamental philosophical assumption of this model is that ethics emerges from human moral experiences. Casuists approach dilemmas from an inductive position and work from the specific case to generalizations, rather than from generalizations to specific cases (Beauchamp & Childress, 2009).

Concerns have also been raised regarding the use of a casuistic model for ethical decision making. As a moral dilemma arises, the selection of the paradigm case may differ among the decision makers and thus the interpretation of the appropriate course of action will vary. In nursing, there are few paradigm cases of ethical issues on which to construct a decision making process. Furthermore, other than the reliance on previous cases, casuists have no mechanisms to justify their actions. The possibility that previous cases were reasoned in a faulty or inaccurate manner may not be fully considered or evaluated (Beauchamp & Childress, 2009). In spite of these concerns, the case-based moral reasoning used in casuistry appeals to clinicians because it mimics clinical reasoning, in which providers often appeal to earlier similar cases to

make clinical judgments. Artnak and Dimmitt (1996) applied the casuistic model to an analysis of a complex case, concluding that the use of this approach allows fuller consideration of the contextual particulars of the case and provides a systematic approach for organizing and analyzing the facts of the case. An adaptation of this approach has been developed by Jonsen and colleagues (2010), sometimes referred to as the "four box" approach. These authors have advocated clustering patient information according to four key topics—medical indications, patient preferences, quality of life, and contextual features—and then using that information to resolve a dilemma.

Narrative Ethics. Because neither of these theoretical approaches have been seen as fully satisfactory, alternatives have emerged (see Box 13-3). Narrative approaches to ethical deliberation have evoked considerable interest (Charon & Montello, 2002; Nelson, 2004; Rorty, Werhane, & Mills, 2004). Narrative ethics emphasizes the particulars of a case or story as a vehicle for discerning the meaning and values embedded in ethical decision making. The argument is that all knowing is bound up in a narrative tradition and that all participants in ethical deliberations need the coherence and singular meaning given to a particular situation that only narrative knowledge can provide. Narrative ethics begins with a patient's story and has some similarities with casuistry in its inductive particularistic approach. Critics of this approach have argued that although narrative is a necessary element in ethical analysis, it cannot supplant principle- or theory-based ethics (Arras, 1997; Childress, 1997). There is, however, recognition that careful consideration of patient's stories can enlarge and enrich ethical deliberations. In commenting on narrative versus principle-based approaches, Childress (1997) noted that "We need both in any adequate ethics" (p. 268). As with casuistry, narrative-based approaches appeal to nurses, who find much of the meaning in their work through entering into the stories of their patient's lives.

Care-Based Ethics. Other approaches, such as virtue-based ethics, feminist ethics, and care-based ethics, provide alternative processes for moral reflection and argument (Beauchamp & Childress, 2009; Wolf, 1996). Historically, nursing ethics was virtue-based, with an emphasis on qualities necessary to be a virtuous nurse. Although this is no longer a dominant theme in nursing literature, it can still be seen. For example, Gallagher and Tschudin (2010) based their understanding of ethical leadership in professional values and virtues.

The ethics of care has emerged as relevant to nursing (Cooper, 1991; Edwards, 2009; Lachman, 2012). The care perspective constructs the central moral problem as sustaining responsive connections and relationships with important others, and consequently focuses on issues surrounding the intrinsic needs and corresponding responsibilities that occur in relationships (Gilligan, 1982; Little, 1998). In this approach, moral reasoning requires empathy and emphasizes responsibilities rather than rights. The response of an individual to a moral dilemma emerges from important relationship considerations and the norms of friendship, care, and love. Viens (1995) reported that NPs she interviewed used a moral reasoning process that mirrored Gilligan's model in the major themes of caring and responsibility.

Although every ethical theory has some limitations and problems, an understanding of contemporary approaches to bioethics enables the APN to appeal to a variety of perspectives in achieving a moral resolution. In the clinical setting, ethical decision making most often reflects a blend of the various approaches rather than the application of a single approach. Although there is some danger in oversimplifying these rich and complex approaches, Exemplar 13-1 shows how they can be reflected in ethical decision making. A more thorough discussion of ethical theory is beyond the scope of this chapter, but the reader is referred to the references cited for more detail.

 EXEMPLAR 13-1   **Clinical Situation Demonstrating Differing Ethical Approaches**

To illustrate the different ethical approaches, consider the case of a 64-year-old man, GB, who is unable to speak for himself because of an aggressive brain tumor. He had seen a neurosurgeon 1 month prior to the current hospital admission and was told that the tumor was inoperable. He has been undergoing outpatient radiation treatment and is now taken to his local hospital because of altered mental status. In the emergency room, his condition worsens; he is unable to communicate or breathe so he is started on mechanical ventilation and transferred to the ICU. Imaging shows that the tumor has continued to progress, despite radiation. The patient's daughter requests that the patient be transferred to another facility for a second opinion from a different neurosurgeon. The social worker has a copy of the patient's advance directive, completed prior to starting radiation, which states that he does not desire aggressive medical treatment if there is little hope of recovery. The team caring for the patient, including a staff nurse, resident, attending physician, social worker, and CNS apply different ethical theories when they approach this case.

The nurse adopts a principle-based approach, favoring patient autonomy and respect for persons, as emphasized in the *Code of Ethics for Nurses* (ANA, 2001). He recognizes the daughter's distress but believes that her desire to seek a second opinion comes from her own fear of losing her father and is not based on her knowledge of the patient's wishes. Because the patient should be respected as a person, keeping him on life support or transferring him to another institution as a means to alleviate his daughter's fears is unethical. The nurse believes that the daughter's inability to support her father's advanced directive renders her an inappropriate decision maker. The advance directive, as an indication of the patient's autonomous wishes, should guide care. Because it clearly states the patient that does not wish to be kept alive with little hope of recovery, he favors withdrawal of ventilator support and institution of comfort measures only.

The resident had a case a year ago, when she was still a medical student, in which a patient's cancer was thought to be inoperable but a second opinion was sought and the patient went on to survive surgical intervention. This case, occurring early in her career in health care, profoundly influences her to support second opinions on complicated surgical cases. Applying a casuistry-based approach, the resident supports the daughter's request and agrees to help her explore avenues for transferring the patient for consultation with a different neurosurgeon on the slim chance that he may be eligible for additional treatment to prolong his life. She consults the social worker to assist in investigating the feasibility of transferring the patient.

The attending physician adopts a care-based approach, privileging the relationships within the patient's family. He himself has a long-standing relationship with the neurosurgeon who was previously consulted, and he trusts that a second opinion at an outside facility will not yield a different prognosis. He favors keeping the patient in his current setting, because transferring him to a distant facility will take him far from his family, and their time with him is essential. He does not see any reason to withdraw mechanical ventilation but he also believes that initiating cardiopulmonary resuscitation (CPR) would be futile and would disrupt the peaceful atmosphere his family deserves as they struggle with the loss of their father and grandfather. He therefore convinces the patient's daughter to agree to a do not resuscitate (DNR) order, and closes the discussion by encouraging her and the rest of the family to stay with the patient and to "be together at this crucial time." He also asks the ICU staff to relax the regulations regarding family visitation so that the daughter and her children can spend more time at GB's bedside.

The social worker completes a lengthy assessment of the patient and family in response to the consult requested by the resident. In the process, she learns that the family has limited financial resources and that the patient's daughter has a 10th-grade education. Prior to GB's diagnosis, her only interactions with the health care system were the births of her three children. Her mother died when she was teenager and, for the past few years, her father has assisted her in the care of her children. The social worker views the attending physician as condescending, and she hears one of the ICU nurses describe the daughter as "totally clueless." Interpreting the case from a feminist viewpoint, she worries that the family's socioeconomic status and the daughter's educational background are creating a bias against honoring the request for transfer. She is determined to advocate for the patient's daughter to correct this power imbalance.

The CNS's involvement in the case begins when the nurse consults her because his appeals to the resident and attending physician have failed to result in what he believes is the right course of action—namely withdrawal of the ventilator. The CNS listens to the nurse's story and attends carefully to the details he gives. She then seeks out the resident, attending physician, and social worker to hear their perspectives. She adopts a narrative-based approach and wants to hear all the contextual features of the case before coming to a conclusion about the best course of action. When she speaks to GB's daughter, she learns about the conversation that she had with her father shortly before he became unresponsive, in which he expressed a desire to attend her oldest child's high school graduation. It is this conversation that led the patient's daughter to request a transfer for a second opinion: "I know he wants to live," she explains, "no matter what it says on that paper."

Resolution of the Case

The CNS calls a team meeting. She asks the members to work toward a consistent message that can be given to GB's family because the contrasting views are clearly creating confusion. This request results in careful review of the clinical aspects of the case, including the most recent magnetic resonance imaging (MRI) scan, and brings the team to an agreement that the patient's prognosis is poor and a second opinion from an outside neurosurgeon is not necessary to confirm this. The social worker has an opportunity to ask questions and is thus assured that the team was unaware of the daughter's educational background and economic status and are not basing their care on these factors. The CNS then moves forward to establish a mutually acceptable plan of care.

In a subsequent family meeting, the team explains the patient's prognosis to the patient's daughter using layman's terms and simple pictures to clarify the growth of the tumor and its position. After addressing the family's questions, the CNS presents two options—withdrawing intensive care interventions or continuing to provide this care with the DNR order in place. She explains that the team has met separately to consider carefully the daughter's request for transfer GB and determined that the risks of such a plan outweigh potential benefits. The CNS ends the meeting with the family by offering them additional time to discuss their options and ask any further questions. After several days, the family elects to withdraw the ventilator and initiate comfort measures.

Professional Codes and Guidelines

The ANA's *Code of Ethics for Nurses* (2001) describes the profession's philosophy and general ethical obligations of the professional nurse. It describes broad guidelines that more reflect the profession's conscience than provide specific directions for particular clinical situations. It provides a framework that delineates the nurse's overriding moral obligations to the patient, family, community, and profession.

Professional organizations delineate standards of performance that reflect the responsibilities, obligations, duties, and rights of the members. These standards also can serve as guidelines for professional behavior and define desired conduct. Although the general principles are relatively stable, professional organizations often reflect on specific or contemporary issues and take a proactive position on pivotal concerns. For example, the American Association of Critical-Care Nurses (2008) has issued a position paper on moral distress, acknowledging that it negatively affects quality of care and influences nurses who are considering leaving the profession. The paper then lists the responsibilities of nurses to address moral distress, some resources that can be helpful to them, and the obligations of nurses' employers to offer support, such as employee assistance programs and ethics committees, to assist with managing moral distress. An additional example is the International Association of Forensic Nurses' position paper (2009) supporting the use of emergency contraception for victims of sexual assault. This document provides ethical and clinical rationales for policies that permit dispensing of these medications.

Personal and Professional Values

Individuals' interpretations and positions on issues are a reflection of their underlying value system. Value systems are enduring beliefs that guide life choices and decisions in conflict resolution (Ludwick & Silva, 2000). Viens (1995) found that values were an essential feature of the everyday practice of the 10 primary care NPs she interviewed. Values of caring, responsibility, trust, justice, honesty, sanctity and quality of life, empathy, and religious beliefs were articulated by the study participants, often as ideals that motivated their actions. An awareness of personal values generates more consistent choices and behaviors; it can also assist APNs to be aware of the boundaries of their personal and professional values so that they can recognize when their own positions may be unduly influencing patient and family decision making.

Values awareness should include an understanding of the complex interplay between cultural values and ethical decision making (Buryska, 2001; Ludwig & Silva, 2000). When patient and family decisions contradict traditional Western medical practice, health care providers may resort to coercive or paternalistic measures to influence patient's choices to be more consistent with the provider's values. APNs and other health care providers must understand that the assumptions they make may be based on their own cultural values and biases and understand how these assumptions may influence their recommendations of particular treatments. As health care professionals gain an understanding of factors that guide a person's decisions, treatment plans that reflect the patient's value preferences are more easily developed. For example, a patient from a Southeast Asian culture may show respect to authority figures by obeying the APN's treatment suggestions, even if he or she disagrees with the plan. In this situation, the APN could assure the patient that questions about the plan of care are welcomed and are not disrespectful.

By the same token, claims made in the name of religious and cultural beliefs are not absolute. Buryska (2001) offered helpful guidelines for clinicians to assess the defensibility of patient and family claims made in the name of cultural or religious considerations. For example, he maintained that spiritual or cultural claims grounded in an identifiable and established community are more defensible than those that are idiosyncratic to the person making the claim. Although it is critical for caregivers to respond with respectful dialogue, support, and compassionate care, patient and family demands for treatment must be considered in relation to other claims that also have ethical weight—the professional integrity of providers, legal considerations, economic realities, and issues of distributive justice.

Professional Boundaries

In their professional capacity, APNs have access to personal and private patient information and may develop long-term therapeutic relationships with many of their patients. The atmosphere of intimacy in the nurse-patient relationship, coupled with the need to touch the patient during a physical examination, sets up a power differential that accentuates the patient's vulnerability (Holder & Schenthal, 2007). Boundaries must be established that acknowledge the appropriate and necessary use of this patient information and intimacy to meet the patient's needs and provide care. The obligation to maintain professional boundaries within a therapeutic relationship is shared with all nurses (ANA, 2001), but APNs are also in a position to observe for boundary violations by others and to intervene when they occur.

Boundary violations, in which the APN or another health care professional inadvertently or purposely breaches the limits and expectations of the relationship, may profoundly alter the foundation of a therapeutic relationship. Such transgressions may be subtle, such as the APN sharing excessive personal information, or blatant, as in sexually seductive behavior. Regardless of the magnitude of the violation, the behavior must be confronted immediately and the culpable individual must be removed from interaction with the patient. Other members of the health care team should strive to restore the patient's integrity and trust, involving the help of others as necessary (National Council of State Boards of Nursing, 2009).

Phase 2: Knowledge Application

The second phase of the core competency is applying the knowledge developed in the first level to the clinical practice arena. Phase 2 continues the APN's journey in assessing ethical problems and being actively involved in the process of resolving ethical dilemmas. As APNs acquire core ethical decision making knowledge, the responsibility to take moral action becomes more compelling. Rather than retrospectively analyzing ethical dilemmas, the APN takes moral action, which implies that the APN recognizes, pursues, and responds to ethical issues. Often, the inequities toward or infringements on other persons are enough to motivate moral action and a timely response can change the course in present and future situations. Therefore, moral action should not be underestimated as a core APN skill and should be recognized, fostered, and valued by others. *Once an advanced nursing role is assumed, the APN accepts the responsibility to be a full participant in the resolution of moral dilemmas rather than simply an interested observer or one of many parties in conflict.*

Although the core knowledge of ethical concepts provides the foundation for moral reasoning, the application of these concepts enables the APN to develop the practical wisdom of moral reasoning. It is the experience in the practice setting and the courage of the APN to discuss sensitive issues openly that enable the APN to assume an active role in dispute resolution. The success and speed with which the APN gains these behavioral skills is related to the presence of mentors in the clinical setting and the willingness of the APN to become immersed in ethical discussions.

Institutional resources, such as ethics committees and institutional review boards, provide valuable opportunities for APNs to participate in the discussion of ethical issues. Typically, hospital ethics committees serve three functions—policy formation, case review, and education. As a member of the ethics committee, the APN exchanges ideas with colleagues and gains an understanding of ethical dilemmas from a variety of perspectives. In addition, the APN is informed of current legislation, regulations, and hospital policies that have ethical implications.

This is an extremely valuable experience that can accelerate the development of ethical decision making skills.

Unfortunately, most APNs do not have the opportunity to serve on interdisciplinary ethics committees and, in some cases, may have few professional colleagues available to mentor and develop the skills of ethical decision making. Thus, the APN must advance this phase by actively seeking opportunities to engage in ethical dialogue with professional colleagues. Professional organizations offer materials such as *The 4 A's to Rise Above Moral Distress* (American Association of Critical Care Nurses, 2004) and workshops in which case studies are discussed and analyzed. This format is helpful to the inexperienced APN who needs guidance in applying knowledge to clinical cases.

Ethical Decision Making Frameworks

Several authors have proposed a stepwise approach to ethical decision making (McCormick-Gendzel & Jurchek, 2006; Purtilo & Doherty, 2011; Rushton & Penticuff, 2007; Spencer, 2005; Weuste, 2005). In Box 13-4, the steps suggested by Purtilo and Doherty (2011) are listed as an example. The reader will note that this framework uses many elements of the various ethical approaches discussed earlier in considering contextual factors, seeking full information on a case, and specifying a step that explicitly appeals to ethical theory. This framework for ethical decision making is intended for all health professionals and therefore is applicable to a wide variety of situations.

Most frameworks for ethical decision making include information gathering as a key step. Generally, information about the clinical situation, the parties involved, their obligations and values, and legal, cultural, and religious factors are needed. However, this factual information is not sufficient unless tempered with the contextual features of each case. Identifying the cause of the problem and determining why, where, and when it occurred, and who or what was affected, will help clarify the nature of the problem.

Problem identification is also a common step in most frameworks. Strong emotional responses to a situation can be the first signal that ethical conflict exists. However, many conflicts that arise in the clinical setting generate powerful emotional responses but may not be ethical issues. Ethical issues are those that involve some form of controversy about conflicting moral values and/or fundamental duties or obligations. The APN must distinguish and separate moral dilemmas from other issues, such as administrative concerns, communication problems, and lack of clinical knowledge. For example, a communication problem between a staff nurse and physician may be resolved if an APN acts as a facilitator, ensuring that each

BOX 13-4   Sample Ethical Decision Making Framework

1. **Gather information:**
   - Clarify the additional information needed.
   - Categories of information to consider include clinical indications, patient preferences, quality of life, and contextual factors.
   - Caution is advised not to make this step an end in itself.
2. **Determine that the problem is an ethical one and identify the type:**
   - Locus of authority—conflict involves determining who should make a decision.
   - Ethical dilemma—conflict in which two opposing courses of action are both ethically justifiable but cannot both be satisfied.
   - Moral distress—conflict in which the ethical course of action seems clear but the agent feels unable to carry it out.
3. **Use ethical theories or approaches to analyze the problem:**
   - A utilitarian approach would focus on the consequences of potential actions.
   - A deontological approach would focus the duties of involved parties.
   - Various ethical theories provide additional perspectives (see "Overview of Ethical Theories" and the references cited)
4. **Explore the practical alternatives:**
   - Imagination is required to ensure that a wide range of alternatives are identified.
   - Diligence in assessing the feasibility of identified actions is also essential.
5. **Complete the action:**
   - Once determined, motivation to carry out the ethical action is essential.
   - Not to act at this point is a conscious choice, with consequences.
6. **Evaluate the process and outcome:**
   - What went well, and why?
   - To what other situations might this experience apply?
   - What do the patient, family, and other providers say about the course of action taken?

Adapted from Purtilo, R. B. & Doherty, R. (2011). *Ethical dimensions in the health professions* (5th ed.). Philadelphia: Saunders.

understands the perspective of the other. In this case, ethical decision making may not be needed; the conflict does not result from a difference in values but rather a failure to communicate. As noted, effective and compassionate communication skills undergird this competency.

Although a framework provides structure and suggests a method of examining and studying the ethical issues, the essential component of resolution of ethical dilemmas is moral action. Simply knowing the right course of action does not guarantee that a person has the motivation or courage to act (LaSala & Bjarnason, 2010; Rest, 1986; Rushton & Penticuff, 2007).

Strategies for Resolution of Ethical Conflict

The challenge in most cases of ethical disputes is to have all involved parties listen to each other's perspective to understand the basis of the disagreement and work together to create a collaborative solution. In cases in which conflict is intense and resolution seems difficult, it may be helpful to solicit help from a member of the institution's ethics committee or another professional colleague not involved in the case. However, in many cases, the APN must serve as a facilitator for the parties in dispute. The objective of successful facilitation in ethical disputes is to achieve an integrity-preserving solution that is satisfactory to all parties. In reality, however, that is

not always possible. The issues of time, cost, available resources, level of moral certainty, and perceived value of the relationship play important roles in the strategy used and likelihood of reaching a desired outcome (Spielman, 1993).

Two decades ago, Spielman (1993) identified five strategies for resolving ethical conflicts, of which collaboration is the preferred approach. Her typology is useful for evaluating ethical conflict resolution. As described in Chapter 12, collaboration is a core competency of advanced practice nursing. Recent attention to interprofessional competencies has also emphasized the importance of collaboration (Canadian Interprofessional Health Collaborative, 2010; Interprofessional Education Collaborative Expert Panel, 2011). In ethical conflicts, a collaborative approach is the most likely to result in a solution that preserves the integrity of all involved parties.

Collaboration, however, is not always possible in resolving ethical disputes. Other approaches include the following:

- Compromise is an appropriate approach to ethical decision making when the parties involved are committed to preserving their relationship and each possesses a high moral certainty about their position.
- Alternatively, accommodation occurs when one party is more committed than the other to

preserving the relationship; the committed party defers to the other, with the result that only one perspective directs the outcome. Accommodation is unlikely to promote the integrity of all involved parties and should be used only when time is limited or the issue is trivial.

- Coercion is also a strategy unlikely to result in an integrity-preserving outcome. In this approach, the more powerful party, who has a strong commitment to a particular position, determines the outcome of the conflict through an aggressive stance.

- Avoidance is the most dangerous of the strategies considered by Spielman (1993), because the less powerful party does not articulate their ethical concerns.

Exemplar 13-2 provides examples of each of these strategies in a situation that evoked considerable ethical conflict.

 EXEMPLAR 13-2   **Strategies Used in Resolving Ethical Conflict**

An ACNP in a hospital-based clinic provides comprehensive care to patients with HIV/AIDS. TD, a 44-year-old female patient, also has a history of diabetes mellitus, hypertension, cigarette smoking, and depression. She arrives at the clinic after missing multiple appointments. In the interval since her last visit, she has been placed on house arrest because of pleading guilty to fraud. TD accepted government aid without reporting a change in income that rendered her ineligible for this support.

At this visit, the patient reports that she has not taken medications for diabetes or hypertension because she ran out of pills and had no mechanism for refilling them. She is depressed, hyperglycemic, and dehydrated, and is given 2 liters of IV fluids in the clinic because she refuses hospital admission. She is fearful of violating the conditions of her house arrest; she is only permitted to leave her home for prescheduled medical appointments. She is scheduled to return in 1 week's time and given prescriptions for an antidepressant, oral hypoglycemic, and glucose monitoring supplies.

The following day, a pharmacist calls the clinic to report that the prescriptions given to him by TD have been altered. The frequency of the antidepressant has been changed from once to twice a day, and the number of refills for the hypoglycemic agent has been changed from three to 18. Furthermore, the pharmacist is annoyed with the patient because her behavior in the pharmacy was disruptive. He states that he plans to refuse to dispense medications for her if this continues. On hearing about this incident, the clinic nurse, who has worked with the patient over a long period of time, becomes angry and states her view that this is consistent with the patient's past behavior in clinic. She suggests that the ACNP tell the patient that her alteration of the prescriptions can be reported to the Department of Corrections and that further incidents like this will result in termination from care at this clinic. The social worker, whose ongoing contact with the patient was instrumental in getting her to return to clinic after a long absence, advises the ACNP that no report to the correction officer is required. She states her belief that even to mention this to the patient would result in the patient ceasing to come to clinic.

The ACNP notes the emotional responses of the interprofessional team members, which signal an ethical conflict. Her initial thought is to wait until TD's scheduled return visit to identify a course of action. This strategy is an example of avoidance. Another avoidance option would be to send the patient to another provider for her medications. For example, an endocrinologist could be consulted for the diabetes medication. The ACNP considers, but does not select, these courses of action.

In communications with the pharmacist, the ACNP uses accommodation as a strategy for managing ethical conflict. She validates his concern about the negative impact of the patient's behavior on the other costumers and agrees that he can refer her to another pharmacy if her behavior continues to be inappropriate. The pharmacist agrees to accept corrected prescriptions faxed directly from the ACNP, and to dispense these to the patient, if she is not disruptive when she returns the next day. He also agrees to notify the ACNP if she is disruptive and therefore does not get her medications.

The strategy favored by the social worker is also an example of accommodation. She believes that the obligation of the clinic staff is the delivery of patient care, not upholding the legal regulations around the handling of prescriptions. She suggests not providing prescriptions to TD again, but adopting a policy of calling or faxing all prescriptions for her directly to a pharmacy. In this way, TD's unethical behavior is accommodated by a change in clinic practice.

The clinic nurse's strategy is an example of coercion. In coercive strategies, the ethical decision maker resolves the conflict by exerting a controlling influence on another party whose actions or values are fueling the conflict. Suggesting to the patient that her actions will

EXEMPLAR 13-2   **Strategies Used in Resolving Ethical Conflict—*cont'd***

be reported and that these actions may affect her access to the care she needs can be expected to influence her behavior. The disadvantage of this type of strategy is the powerlessness it imposes.

When the patient arrives for her follow-up appointment the next week, the ACNP uses collaboration to manage the ethical conflict. She informs the patient that the pharmacist called about the prescriptions and that this created concern among the providers at the clinic. She tells the patient, "I do not want you to be in trouble, and changed prescriptions can get you in trouble. I want to work with you to help you stay well." She asks the patient for her story. The patient then explains her fear of again running out of the hypoglycemic agent she knows she needs, and of being unable to afford medication refills. TD mistakenly thought that by altering the prescriptions, she would get a larger supply of the medicines. The ACNP agrees to help TD identify strategies to obtain her medications through prescription assistance programs and

the patient agrees not to alter prescriptions she is given.

Another conflict evident in this case is between the nurse and social worker. Compromise is needed to maintain an effective working relationship because the two provide care to the same patient population. Compromise can be achieved if the two parties focus on a common goal and relinquish control of some elements of the final decision. In this case, the ACNP meets with both parties and they identify that their common goal is efficient delivery of quality health care. Through compromise, the nurse recognized the value that the social worker placed on keeping the patient in care and relinquished her desire to report the patient to the Department of Corrections. Similarly, the social worker recognized that the nurse wanted to avoid disruptive behavior that upsets other clinic patients. She agreed to relinquish her accommodating approach to the patient's behavior if it negatively affected the clinic's operation in the future.

There is an additional dynamic that may be operating in environments in which avoidance is the norm in dealing with ethical conflict. In a series of observational qualitative studies of hospital-based nurses, Chambliss (1996) documented a phenomenon he called "routinization" of the moral world (p. 38). In routinization, nurses became enmeshed in the tasks and routines of care delivery and, over time, became accustomed and desensitized to the ethical conflicts around them. The routine blunted the nurses' moral sensitivity and moral agency so that moral difficulties were not recognized; nurses commented, "You just get used to it." Chambliss (1996) also noted that nurses were aware of problems but often did not see them as "ethics problems", and neither did those in authority. The great ethical danger in such environments is not that nurses would make the wrong choice when faced with an important decision, but that they would never realize that they are facing a decision at all. APNs must be alert for signs of routinization of the moral dimension of practice in the environments in which they practice. Identifying and addressing features of the system that blunt or dismiss the moral sensitivity of any care provider is a critical part of APN leadership and moves the APN into Phase 3 of the ethical decision making competency.

Phase 3: Creating an Ethical Environment
As the APN becomes more skilled in the application of ethical knowledge, the third phase of competence begins

to develop. The quality of the ethical environment is a critical factor in whether ethical problems are productively addressed. In one study of NPs, the participants' perception of the ethical environment was the strongest predictor of ethical conflict in practice; the more ethical the environment, the lower was the ethical conflict (Ulrich, Soeken, & Miller, 2003). The APN's level of influence needs to extend beyond the individual patient encounter to create a climate in which ethical concerns are routinely addressed.

Role modeling, mentoring others regarding ethical decision making, and creating an ethical environment are leadership behaviors seen in the practice of the mature APN. Once the APN transforms ethical knowledge into moral action, the role of mentoring others emerges. Too often, other nurses and members of the health care team remain silent about ethical issues (Gordon & Hamric, 2006). In a mentoring capacity, the APN helps colleagues deal with moral uncertainty and develop the ability to voice ethical concerns. In this way, the APN supports and empowers other team members to develop confidence and fosters an environment in which diverse views are expressed and problems are moved toward resolution. The experienced APN also initiates informal learning opportunities for nurses and other professional colleagues. Ethics rounds and case review are two ways to engage colleagues in the discussion of moral issues.

In a classic article, Shannon noted that the roots of interdisciplinary conflict in the clinical setting are often based on preconceived stereotypes of the moral viewpoints of other disciplines and perceptions of the moral superiority of one's own discipline (Shannon, 1997). The APN can help professionals from other disciplines understand the perspectives and socialization of nurses. In addition, the APN models successful negotiation with other disciplines. Teaching and mentoring activities of the mature APN often focus on other professional colleagues to prepare them proactively to communicate openly with patients about ethical concerns. One way for APNs to maintain the trust and respect of professional colleagues is to acquire ethical knowledge and expertise in their specialty area.

This phase also encompasses aspects of coaching and teaching patients and families in ethical decision making. It is not sufficient for the APN simply to provide information to patients and families facing difficult moral choices and expect them to arrive at a comfortable decision. The ethical competency is linked closely with the ability to mobilize patients and the APN's colleagues so that those who need help move through the necessary steps to reach resolution.

APNs should strive to develop environments that encourage patients and caregivers to express diverse views and raise questions. Thoughtful ethical decision making arises from an environment that supports and values the critical exchange of ideas and promotes collaboration among members of the health care team, patients, and families. A collaborative practice environment, in turn, supports shared decision making, shared accountability, and group participation, fostering relationships based on equality and mutuality. The APN is integral to the development and preservation of a collaborative culture that inspires and empowers individuals to respond to moral dilemmas.

The current nature of health care delivery in inpatient and outpatient settings creates a climate in which many workers feel overwhelmed, stressed, and discouraged by the lack of time to care for patients and their increased acuity levels. Combined with a sense of powerlessness and routinization (Chambliss, 1996), these factors can result in nurses retreating from a stance of moral agency. An ethically sensitive environment is one in which providers are encouraged to acknowledge when they feel overwhelmed and seek help when they need it (Hamric, Epstein & White, in press). The *Code of Ethics for Nurses* (ANA, 2001) has affirmed the importance of nurses contributing to an ethically sensitive health care environment, as well as preserving personal integrity. One provision states that "The nurse owes the same duties to self as to others, including the responsibility to preserve integrity

and safety" (p. 4). Only when care providers recognize and attend to their personal needs will they be better able to detect and nurture the needs of others.

As APNs become more competent and capable in ethical reasoning, they are able to anticipate situations in which moral conflicts will occur and recognize the more subtle presentations of moral dilemmas. The ability to look beyond the immediate situation and foresee potential issues directs the APN down a path of preventive ethics.

Preventive Ethics

Phase 2 concentrates on the resolution of current and ongoing issues rather than on preventing the recurrence of moral dilemmas. An additional important role of the APN in Phase 3 is to extend the concept of ethical decision making beyond problem solving in individual cases and to move toward a paradigm of preventive ethics. The term *preventive ethics* is derived from the model of preventive medicine; the term was coined by Forrow and associates (1993). It emphasizes developing effective organizational policies and practices that prevent ethical problems from developing (McCullough, 2005). The ability to predict areas of conflict and develop plans in a proactive rather than reactive manner will avert some potentially difficult dilemmas and can lead to more ethically responsive environments (Forrow, Arnold, & Parker, 1993; Fox et al., 2007; McCullough, 2005; Nelson, Gardent, Shulman, et al., 2010).

When value conflicts arise, resolution becomes more difficult because one value must be chosen over another. Preventive ethics emphasizes that all important values should be reviewed and examined prior to the conflict so that situations in which values may differ can be anticipated. In other words, the goals of the health care team should be articulated as clearly as possible to avoid potential misinterpretations. For example, a CRNA should have an understanding of a terminally ill patient's values regarding aggressive treatment in case a cardiopulmonary arrest occurs during surgery. However, the CRNA's moral and legal obligations should be openly discussed so that the patient and professional appreciate and recognize each other's values and moral and legal positions. Modeling this preventive approach in ethical deliberations encourages the early identification of values and beliefs that may influence treatment decisions and allows time to resolve impending issues before problems arise. In much the same way, early anticipation of potential complications in patient trajectories can lead to proactive discussions of ethical issues and restructuring of the care environment to anticipate and avoid ethical conflict.

In addition to the early examination and ongoing dialogue regarding values, a conscientious inspection of other factors that influence the evolution of moral dilemmas is required. A number of environmental factors can become barriers to ethical practice; Chambliss (1996) made the important point that features of the work setting and their role as employees often create moral problems for nurses. The roles and responsibilities of all parties must be clearly defined to expose any existing power imbalance. During this process, issues of powerlessness surface as an area in which the APN can influence change. By providing knowledge, promoting a positive self-image, and preparing others for participation in decision making, the APN empowers individuals. The skill of the APN is used not to resolve moral dilemmas single-handedly, but to mentor others to assume a position of moral accountability and engage in shared decision making. This process of enhancing others' autonomy and providing opportunities for involvement in reaching resolution is a key concept in preventive ethics (Forrow et al., 1993).

Ethically responsive environments are enhanced by a process of ongoing, rather than episodic, ethical inquiry. Throughout this process, the APN incorporates his or her skills, ethical expertise, and clinical background on issues necessary to facilitate dialogue, mediate disputes, analyze options, and design optimal solutions. In this phase, the ethical decision making skills of the APN move the resolution of moral dilemmas beyond individual cases toward the cultivation of an environment in which the moral integrity of individuals is respected. Development and preservation of this ethical environment is the key contribution of the APN. Although ethical issues may develop with little warning, the practice of preventive ethics greatly improves a team's ability to handle these issues in a morally responsible and innovative manner. Exemplar 13-3 provides an example of preventive ethics in addressing staff moral distress.

 EXEMPLAR 13-3   Addressing Staff Moral Distress Through Preventive Ethics*

Dea, a CNS in a neuroscience ICU, seeks to change the management of patients with traumatic brain injury (TBI). She and other members of the staff have noted that the care of this population is inconsistent, and many staff have a fatalistic attitude about these patients' hope of recovery. She is also aware of recent research on the use of a new technology, brain tissue oxygen monitoring, that has shown promise in improving outcomes for these patients. As an initial step, she invites a CNS from another state, an expert in the management of TBI whom she knows to be an inspiring speaker, to give a presentation on brain tissue oxygen monitoring. Dea arranges for staff coverage so that all neuroscience ICU registered nurses (RNs) can attend the presentation, in which the speaker describes how the technology is used to prevent progressive injury in patients with TBI. Members of the respiratory therapy team, staff in the emergency room, and nurses from the trauma ICU are also invited to the presentation, which is highly successful. Dea then collaborates with the nurse manager and administration to implement brain tissue oxygen monitoring in the neuroscience ICU. She obtains key physician support, provides training sessions, supports the staff when the technology is introduced into patient care, and develops algorithms for acting on the information this technology provides. Dea also creates a Wall of Fame, highlighting all unit patients who have recovered, to help staff celebrate successes in caring for this challenging patient population.

As staff develop skills and knowledge related to the management of TBI patients, they notice the improved outcomes in monitored patients as the technology detects changes in cerebral oxygen level; these data promote early aggressive intervention. However, Dea begins to realize that this success itself is creating a new source of moral distress. Although patients with TBI are often managed in the neuroscience ICU, they are also admitted to other ICUs where this technology is not available. In addition, the application of the technology varies depending on the preferences of the attending physician and residents assigned to manage TBI patients. Although some of the medical staff are open to the use of the brain tissue oxygen monitor, others do not agree that it is a valid tool. Because the nurses see the better than expected outcomes of monitored patients as compared with those who do not receive monitoring, they believe that all patients should receive this technology. The staff's moral distress heightens after a particularly troubling case of a young TBI patient who was never monitored with the new technology and subsequently died.

Recognizing an ethical conflict with the potential to recur with increasing frequency, Dea takes action using a preventive ethics approach. She consults a nurse with expertise in ethics to meet with the staff. During that meeting, their moral distress is articulated. The nurses value their growing expertise in brain tissue oxygen monitoring and note that this new technology has served as the impetus for improving the care of TBI patients. However, the nurses are not empowered to maximize its application because decisions about the admission of patients with TBI to an ICU are made without nursing input, and because the medical staff, not the nursing staff, makes the final decision to make use of the brain tissue oxygen monitor.

During the meeting, the staff identify a number of strategies for decreasing their moral distress. One is directing admission of TBI patients to the neuroscience ICU, recognizing at the same time that patients with thoracic and abdominal trauma, as well as TBI, would still be admitted to the trauma ICU; in addition, many TBI patients are first admitted to the trauma ICU while these other problems are ruled out. Better communication between ICU charge nurses was considered as a means to improve nursing input into bed assignment. Another strategy discussed in the meeting was advocacy for patients' needs on the part of the neuroscience nurses with the medical staff. The staff is encouraged to use Dea as a resource when they encounter resistance from their medical colleagues. A final strategy identified at this meeting was to track the outcomes of patients who have received brain tissue oxygen monitoring and thus develop a database to support the value of this tool. Dea agrees to collect the data, review each case, and follow up on quality of care issues.

Dea then works with a colleague in the trauma ICU to improve communication among the neuroscience ICU, trauma ICU, and neurosurgical team. They arrange a meeting with nurses from both ICUs and surgeons from the neurosurgery and trauma teams. At that meeting, the use of aggressive measures in TBI patients, including brain tissue oxygen monitoring, are discussed. In follow-up, Dea and her physician colleagues in neurosurgery and neurocritical care develop algorithms for the management of TBI, identifying patients who may benefit from brain tissue oxygen monitoring and facilitating their admission to the neuroscience ICU. These algorithms are reviewed by the trauma service for incorporation into the trauma manual, a document used by all trauma residents.

Dea also continues to encourage and support her staff to be proactive advocates. She coaches the nurses toward effective advocacy and role-models collaboration and information sharing in her own communications with residents and attending physicians. Over time, Dea begins to see an increased acceptance of the new technology and of an aggressive approach to managing TBI among the neurosurgery teams.

Two members of the nursing staff, with Dea's encouragement and guidance, developed a poster about their moral distress and steps to address it. The poster was accepted and presented at a national conference (Pracher, Moss, & Mahanes, 2006). The nurses attending the conference to present the poster learned that their situation is not unique; other conference attendees noted similar conflicts in their own units and validated the distress experienced as a result.

Although a closer connection between the neuroscience and trauma ICUs is a secondary benefit, concerns about inconsistencies in care continue. Patients with TBI continue to be admitted to the neuroscience and trauma ICUs, and are not always transferred quickly if they need monitoring. Through a collaborative process with the CNS in the trauma ICU, a new approach to standardizing the care of TBI patients is identified and plans are made to incorporate brain tissue oxygen monitoring in the trauma ICU. The database that Dea has maintained demonstrates positive patient outcomes that support this change. Dea lends support to the CNS in that unit as she begins to train the staff in the use of the technology and the algorithms for responding to the information it provides. Two years after the initial educational session on this technology, Dea notes that "there is still work to do to optimize the care of these patients." However, because of her proactive response to the staff's distress, champions for this technology now exist on both units, and an environment for effecting positive change has been created.

*We gratefully acknowledge Dea Mahanes, MSN, RN, Charlottesville, VA, for sharing this exemplar.

This case highlights how the ethical decision making competency of APNs can lessen the reoccurrence of moral problems. In this situation, Dea's actions went beyond resolving a single case of moral distress and focused on the features of the system that were contributing to the distress of the staff. As this exemplar shows, recurring ethical problems, particularly moral distress, are sometimes a result of the structure of care delivery systems in an institution. Dea's case demonstrates that applying a preventive ethics approach to the system requires perseverance and ongoing identification of new strategies to change complex and interrelated system features.

Phase 4: Promoting Social Justice Within the Health Care System

The final phase in the ethical decision making competency is seen in mature APNs who have expanded their focus of concern to incorporate the needs of their larger specialty population. This phase again builds on the previous ones as APNs move their sphere of involvement beyond their institution into the societal sector. Moving into the arena of social justice is an historic legacy and a current imperative. Falk-Raphael (2005) has noted that Nightingale's work bequeathed to professional nursing "a legacy of justice-making as an expression of caring and compassion" (p. 212). Increasing attention to social justice has been seen in nursing literature in the United States and internationally (Bell & Hulbert, 2008; Buettner-Schmidt & Lobo, 2011; Grace & Willis, 2012; Tarlier & Browne, 2011). Although APNs prepared at the master's level may develop Phase 4 practices over time, the AACN's *Essentials of Doctoral Education for Advanced Nursing Practice* (2006) strongly supports APNs moving into a larger arena of ethical decision making, with explicit preparation in DNP programs. The need for nursing to speak to mounting concerns regarding the quality of patient care delivery and outcomes in policy and public forums is one justification for doctoral-level education for APNs. Most of the DNP *Essentials* address the need for systems leadership in these larger forums; one in particular, "Health Care Policy for Advocacy in Health Care," advocates for DNP graduates to "design, implement and advocate for health care policy which addresses issues of social justice and equity in health care. The powerful practice experiences of the DNP graduate can become potent influencers in policy formation" (p. 13).

In a number of hallmark reports, the Institute of Medicine (IOM, 1999, 2001, 2003) has highlighted the fragmentation and systems failures in health care and called for restructuring efforts to achieve safe, effective, and equitable care. Equity is primarily an issue of justice; as noted, concerns about access to and distribution of health care resources are key justice concerns of APNs. In this phase, APNs work as agents of change for justice in the health care system on behalf of their specialty populations.

Nurses in many roles have been increasingly concerned by the current health care system and the gaps in care provision to many of the neediest members of society.

Some have asserted that all nurses should include sociopolitical advocacy in their practice if the profession is to fulfill its social mandate (Falk-Raphael, 2005). This is a tall order; most undergraduate nursing programs do not include the requisite skills needed for this level of advocacy. Even APN curricula may not include such content, so the APN must commit to continued skill development and involvement in national organizations to reach this phase. One distinguishing feature of the APN's activities in this arena as compared with other nurses is the clinical expertise of the APN. The central competency of direct clinical practice and the APN's cutting edge understanding of the clinical needs of her or his patient population provide the platform from which the APN speaks to social justice issues. Nurses in policy, research, or other non-APN roles often call on APNs to provide expert information on the policy and larger system issues that confront their specialty populations.

To enact this level of the ethical decision making competency requires sophisticated use of all of the core competencies of advanced practice nursing. In particular, advocacy, communication, collaboration (see Chapter 12), and leadership (see Chapter 11) are required. APNs active in this phase are often consultants to policy makers or serve on expert panels crafting policies for specialty groups. Essential knowledge needed for this phase includes an understanding of the concepts of justice, particularly distributive justice (the equitable allocation of scarce resources) and restorative justice (the duty owed to those who have been systematically disadvantaged through no fault of their own). In addition, knowledge of the health policy process in general (see Chapter 22) and specific health policies affecting their specialty population are needed by APNs to move into this level of activity.

Exemplar 13-4 describes one APN's development through the phases of the EDM competency, including beginning activity in Phase 4. Chapter 22 also provides examples of Phase 4 actions by nurses who have expanded their concerns about individual patients into working for social justice in the policy arena.

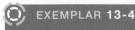 EXEMPLAR 13-4   **Putting It All Together: Development Through the Four Phases of the Ethical Decision Making Competency***

RT is a FNP who is completing a DNP program. Her experience with providing health care to Hispanic migrant farmworkers in rural Virginia has given her many opportunities to use her ethical decision making skills. This exemplar portrays her journey through the phases of ethical decision making as she has developed her APN practice.

One fall evening, RT accompanies a team of outreach workers into a migrant farm camp to screen workers for diabetes and heart disease. Three older men approach her with concerns regarding Antonio, one of the new younger workers. They report that he has been losing weight, sweating all the time, shaking, and appears ill. They are scared for him and a little frightened that he

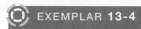 **EXEMPLAR 13-4**   **Putting It All Together: Development Through the Four Phases of the Ethical Decision Making Competency*—*cont'd***

could be contagious. RT encourages the men to have him schedule an appointment with her the following night, because she would be staffing a mobile clinic in the community. The men are concerned that Antonio would be unwilling to give his information to anyone because he lacks legal documentation to be in the United States. The men promise that they will encourage Antonio to make an appointment and reassure him that RT will not report him to the authorities.

The next night, RT waits for someone to come to her with these concerns. When this doesn't happen, she walks outside the mobile clinic and luckily sees Antonio. He is easy to identify because he is sweating profusely and his hands are trembling. RT asks her community health worker to ask him to join her in the mobile clinic and, to her surprise, he agrees. Antonio looks much older than his reported age of 19. He is frail, anxious-appearing, and sweaty. After taking a history and doing an examination, RT suspects that he might have hyperthyroidism. She convinces Antonio to allow her to check some laboratory values.

The laboratory results confirm RT's suspicions. Normally, she could refer a patient with hyperthyroidism to endocrinology for urgent treatment because she is concerned that Antonio could go into a coma or die. Instead, she is faced with many barriers to accessing care for him. He is in this country illegally and uninsured. Although he lives well below the poverty line, he does not qualify for Medicaid. He might qualify for financial assistance but he would be leery of providing any identification or pay stubs. Furthermore, Antonio does not want to see any doctors in the United States, preferring to wait until he returns to Mexico in 6 months to have the issue addressed. He does not want to miss time from work because he thinks he might get fired. In addition, he has transportation and language barriers, which would make it difficult to see a specialist. RT struggles to determine whether the principle of beneficence or the

principle of respect for autonomy should carry the most weight in her decision making.

Stories such as this are common when working with migrant Hispanic farm workers. In Phases 1 and 2 of RT's development in ethical decision making, she would have thought only about the individual situation.

The first two phases solidified knowledge regarding professional obligations and ethical theories that could help her deal with this situation. As she expanded into the third stage, she began to look at the bigger problem, the system. The existing referral system placed most of the burden on patients to obtain appointments with specialists. The referral staff was not allotted the needed time to assist non-English speaking or illiterate patients, such as Antonio, with obtaining financial assistance at the local academic hospital. RT realized that ethical dialogue would need to occur among staff and administration for the health care center's culture to change. Antonio's case helped shape a new system. The outreach coordinator now assists migrant farmworkers with the financial screening process, interpretation, and transportation. Antonio's case was the first success. Although it took three times as long to get him the care he needed, he finally underwent thyroid ablation and is now a healthy 20-year-old.

As RT is developing her practice as a DNP-prepared NP, she is looking for ways to promote social justice within the health care system. She knows that making changes in the ethical practice of one health care center is not enough to make changes across the system. To have a voice in the larger political arena, RT joined the leadership committee of her region's NP organization. She has taken on the role of governmental affairs chairperson. This allows her to be involved in health care legislation that affects APNs and patients. Her hope is that this will become an avenue for addressing the ethical problems associated with caring for undocumented Hispanic migrant farm workers.

*We thank Reagan Thompson Holland, MSN, RN, NP, for her assistance with this exemplar.

Although this phase of the ethical decision making competency may sound daunting to the novice, beginning activities in this arena, such as involvement in institutional or community policymaking groups and sustained efforts to build knowledge in the areas discussed can establish the foundation for larger policy involvement. Many graduate programs and almost all DNP programs have courses dedicated to the development of policy skills. It is often the case that the experience of moral outrage over the

unethical treatment of patients propels the APN into the policy arena as the APN sees the consequences of the gaps in the current health care system.

Evaluation of the Ethical Decision Making Competency

The evaluation of ethical decision making should focus on two areas—the process and the outcome. Process evaluation is important because it provides an overview of the moral disagreement, interpersonal skills used, interactions between both parties in conflict, and problems encountered during the phases of resolution. Whether the APN is the facilitator or a party in conflict, a deliberate and reflective evaluation of the process of resolution should occur. It is useful for the APN to assess the type of issue, interrelational and situational variables, ethical shifts that occurred during the process, and strategies used by all parties during the negotiation phase. Mediation can be a very useful process (Dubler & Liebman, 2011). As the APN reflects on the process, attention should be given to how similar situations could be anticipated and resolved in the future. Debriefing situations with the affected parties is also an important process evaluation strategy. To avoid the debriefing session becoming simply a venting of emotions, the APN must keep the focus on preventive ethics and what needs to change in the environment to avoid or minimize future problems.

Deliberate and consistent review of the process will help the APN assess various approaches to the resolution of ethical dilemmas and identify the onset of moral conflict earlier. This ongoing evaluation of process is particularly important in Phase 4 because it takes years for changes in system-wide health policies that support social justice to be implemented. Evaluating grassroots and legislative efforts as they occur will help identify strategies likely to be successful versus those that ought to be abandoned.

Evaluation of the outcome is also critical because it acknowledges creative solutions and celebrates moral action. Components of the outcome evaluation include the short- and long-term consequences of the action taken and the satisfaction of all parties with the chosen solution. Unfortunately, a successful process does not always result in a satisfactory outcome. Occasionally, the outcome reveals the need for changes in the institution or health care system. The APN may need to become involved in advancing these desired changes or identifying appropriate resources to pursue them. The goal of outcome evaluation is to minimize the risks of a similar event by identifying predictable patterns and thereby averting recurrent and future dilemmas. The questions "What do we want to happen differently if we are confronted with a similar situation?" and "What first steps can we take to achieve this change?" can be helpful in framing the discussion.

Although evaluation of the ethical problem is an important step for preventing future dilemmas and building ethically sensitive environments, tension and uneasiness will remain in some situations. In true ethical dilemmas, even the best process may still result in a course of action that is not seen positively by all participants. It is important for the APN to acknowledge that many

issues leave a "moral residue" that continues to trouble participants involved in the conflict (Epstein & Hamric, 2009). Part of the outcome evaluation must address the reality of these lingering feelings and the related tensions that they create.

Barriers to Ethical Practice and Potential Solutions

A number of factors influence how moral issues are addressed and resolved in the clinical setting. Some barriers are easily corrected, but others may require attention at institutional, state, or even national levels. Regardless of type, the APN must identify and respond to the barriers that inhibit the development of morally responsive practice environments.

Barriers Internal to the Advanced Practice Nurse

Lack of knowledge about ethics, lack of confidence in one's own ability to resolve ethical conflicts, and a sense of powerlessness are potent barriers to the application of the ethical decision making competency. Such moral uncertainty and perceived powerlessness can lead to ethical issues being swept under the rug and unaddressed in clinical settings. To address these barriers, APNs need to seek out opportunities for ethics education through schools of nursing and professional organizations. Values clarification exercises can be helpful for APNs and all members of the health care team who experience conflict. For example, an emergency room NP may be faced with providing care for a criminal injured in a gunfight that killed innocent bystanders. Although it is disturbing and difficult to provide care for an individual who has caused harm to others, the NP's personal views should not interfere with the quality of the care provided. The process of values clarification is helpful when preparing for this situation. Once personal values are realized, the NP can more easily anticipate situations in which these conflicts will arise and develop strategies for managing them.

APNs can empower themselves by role-modeling ethical decision making within their team. For example, in the primary care setting, a clinic nurse mentions to the APN a concern about how a patient situation was handled. In addition to reflective listening and emotional support, the APN questions the nurse, encouraging her to gather all the necessary information, and together they begin to analyze the ethical elements and consider practical solutions. This process demonstrates the process of ethical decision making for the clinic nurse and empowers the APN in the development of this core competency. Including ethical aspects of a patient's case in interdisciplinary rounds, scheduling debriefing sessions after a particularly difficult case, reading and discussing ethics articles specific to the specialty patient group in a journal club, and/or using simulation activities in which caregivers role-play different scenarios are additional strategies that APNs can use to empower themselves and other nurses to examine ethical issues.

Lack of time is often a barrier faced by APNs seeking to enact this competency. In some cases, the APN may need to resolve a presenting dilemma in stages, with the most central issue addressed first. The APN also needs to enlist the aid of administrative and physician colleagues in recognizing the ongoing consequences of lack of time for team deliberations. For example, if a patient is not receiving adequate pain management because the bedside nurse is concerned about hastening death and is unaware of the full treatment plan, the CNS should first focus on relieving the patient's pain. Once the immediate need is addressed, the CNS can help the nurse identify nonpharmacologic interventions to promote comfort and educate the nurse about the dosage and timing of medications to prevent wide fluctuations in pain management. At this point, the administrative leadership may need to be approached about supporting ongoing staff education. An additional strategy, such as arranging for the nurse to rotate to a hospice unit, represents a preventive approach to help avert similar dilemmas in the future.

Interprofessional Barriers

Different approaches among health care team members can pose a barrier to ethical practice. For example, nurses and physicians often define, perceive, analyze, and reason through ethical problems from distinct and sometimes opposing perspectives (Curtis & Shannon, 2006; Hamric & Blackhall, 2007; Shannon, 1997). Although the roles are complementary, these differing approaches may create conflict between a nurse and physician, further separating and isolating their perspectives. A physician may be unaware of the nurse's differing opinion or may not recognize this difference as a conflict (Hamric & Blackhall; Shannon, Mitchell, & Cain, 2002). One study has indicated that physicians and nurses deal with the same ethical problems and use similar moral reasoning but that differences are related to professional roles, the types of responsibilities each group had in the situation, and the resulting different questions each group raised (Oberle & Hughes, 2001). Similar to a ground figure optical illusion, the nurse and physician may look at the same ethically troubling clinical situation but, because of differences in their perspectives, they focus on opposing features and arrive at different conclusions about the appropriate course of action. In such situations, the APN first seeks to understand alternative interpretations of the situation and establish respectful and open communication before seeking resolution of ethical problems.

Open communication, cooperation, demonstrated competence, accountability for both role and actions, and developing trust by the physician and APN will facilitate a successful collaborative relationship. Physicians, nurses, and APNs need to engage in moral discourse to understand and support the ethical burden that each professional carries (Curtis & Shannon, 2006; Hamric & Blackhall, 2007; Oberle & Hughes, 2001). Encouraging examples of interprofessional collaboration include the European MURINET (Multidisciplinary Research Network on Health and Disability) project, which launched a training course for researchers on ethics, human rights, and classification of functionality (Ajovalasit et al., 2012), and the National Consensus Project, comprised of nursing and medical professional organizations that appointed a team of doctors and nurses to revise the *Clinical Practice Guidelines for Quality Palliative Care* (National Consensus Project for Quality Palliative Care, 2009).

A third robust initiative, initiative including multiple professions has been the establishment of the Interprofessional Education Collaborative (IPEC), whose mission is to advance interprofessional education so that students entering the health care professions not only seek collaborative relationships with other providers but view collaboration as the norm and not the exception (IPEC, 2011). An expert panel developed core competencies for interprofessional education; one of the four domains focuses on values and ethics. The emphasis of this domain is developing climates of mutual respect and shared values. Box 13-5 lists the 10 competencies identified.

These statements focus on values shared by all health care disciplines and can serve as a basis for building collaborative interprofessional teams that emphasize preventive ethics. As noted, collaboration is the key strategy for eliminating interprofessional barriers.

Patient-Provider Barriers

Additional barriers to ethical practice arise from issues in the patient-provider relationship. Health care providers, employees of the health care institution, and patients and families all contribute to the settings in which most APNs practice, offering opportunities for both personal enrichment and cultural conflict (Linnard-Palmer & Kools, 2004). For example, parents may inform an NP in a pediatric outpatient setting that for cultural and religious reasons, they do not want their child immunized. In this case, the NP is faced with a belief that places the child and community at risk. The NP wants to preserve the parent's rights and preferences but is concerned about the child's best interests and the potential harm to other children if they are exposed to an illness from a nonimmunized child (Fernbach, 2011). Issues that result from cultural diversity

*Competencies as identified by the Interprofessional Education Collaborative. From Interprofessional Education Collaborative Expert Panel. (2011). *Core competencies for interprofessional collaborative practice: Report of an expert panel.* (p.18). Washington, DC: Interprofessional Education Collaborative.

BOX 13-5   Values and Ethics Competencies*

1. Place the interests of patients and populations at the center of interprofessional health care delivery.
2. Respect the dignity and privacy of patients while maintaining confidentiality in the delivery of team-based care.
3. Embrace the cultural diversity and individual differences that characterize patients, populations, and the health care team.
4. Respect the unique cultures, values, roles and responsibilities, and expertise of other health professions.
5. Work in cooperation with those who receive care, those who provide care, and others who contribute to or support the delivery of prevention and health services.
6. Develop a trusting relationship with patients, families, and other team members.
7. Demonstrate high standards of ethical conduct and quality of care in one's contributions to team-based care.
8. Manage ethical dilemmas specific to interprofessional patient/population-centered care situations.
9. Act with honesty and integrity in relationships with patients, families, and other team members.
10. Maintain competence in one's own profession appropriate to scope of practice.

---

are difficult to resolve without help from others who are more familiar with the specific cultural practices and beliefs. Occasionally, hospital chaplains, local clergy, or individuals from the patient's culture who may teach in the language department in a local university can assist with obtaining an expanded understanding of specific belief systems. Internet-based resources, such as "The Provider's Guide to Quality and Culture" (Management Sciences for Health, 2012), also provide specific information about cultural groups.

Ensuring appropriate care for patients at the end of life is an additional challenge to ethical practice. Although some patients use advance directives to convey their wishes, these forms are not always applicable to specific clinical situations and the appointed decision maker may never have discussed end-of-life care with the patient. APNs in primary care settings should encourage such conversations or guide patients, particularly those with life-limiting conditions, through the process of making their wishes known if they become incapacitated. The "Physician Orders for Life-Sustaining Treatment" (POLST) framework (Center for Ethics in Health Care, 2012) provides an effective approach to discuss and document patient wishes. In acute care settings, particularly ICUs, APNs can broker conversations with families who are facing difficult decisions and ensure that the choices in care are based on what the patient would want and not on anticipatory grief. In a study of families of ICU patients, Ahrens and coworkers (2003) found that 42 of 43 families receiving support and enhanced communication from a CNS–physician team were able to make decisions to withhold or withdraw care at the end of life. The authors noted that "This finding underscores the importance of intentional and well-designed communication and support systems for families making medical and moral decisions" (p. 322). More recently, Curtis and colleagues (2012) reported an evidence-based intervention involving "communication facilitators" to improve interprofessional team and family communications in the ICU (Curtis, Ciechanowski, Downey, et al., 2012).

Another barrier to ethical practice that challenges many APNs is the issue of patient non-adherence. Patients and families may choose not to be actively involved in their care or resist an APN's attempts to improve their well-being, which raises clinical and ethical questions. Managing non-adherent patients is ethically troubling because they consume a disproportionate amount of health care resources, including the APN's time, redirecting these resources from patients who are more amenable to the established plan of care. There are no easy solutions to managing the non-adherent patient (Resnick, 2005); however, full consideration of this issue is beyond the scope of this chapter. In many cases, other factors, such as impaired thinking and concentration, knowledge deficits, financial issues, and emotional disorders, can conflict with the patient's ability to follow the prescribed treatment plan (Bishop & Brodkey, 2006). APNs should seek additional support from resources such as social workers or home health nurses to discover the underlying causes and find solutions.

Organizational and Environmental Barriers

Lack of support for nurses who speak up regarding ethical problems in work settings is a potent barrier to ethical practice. Unfortunately, early research and recent literature have revealed disturbing examples of environments in which nurses' concerns were minimized or ignored by physicians, administrators, and even by other nurses (Ceci, 2004; Gordon & Hamric, 2006; Klaidman, 2007; Ulrich, 2012); such environments can lead to moral distress. Recent studies have revealed significant correlations between the level of moral distress and turnover of nurses and physicians (Hamric, Borchers, & Epstein, 2012; see Schluter et al. [2008] for a review of other studies). These findings lend urgency to the need for APNs to provide leadership in building ethical practice environments. APNs need to assess the level of support that nurses receive from others and work to create environments that are "morally habitable places" (Austin, 2007, p. 86). Consideration should be given to organizational ethics programs, which focus on building structures and processes to deal with conflicts of roles and expectations (Rorty, Werhane, & Mills, 2004; Hamric, White, & Epstein, in press). APNs need to develop skills in collaborative conflict resolution and preventive ethics to build ethical practice environments in which moral distress is minimized and the moral integrity of all caregivers is respected and protected.

APNs should identify resources within and outside the institution to assist with the resolution of ethical problems. Internal resources may include chaplain staff, liaison psychiatrists, patient representatives, social work staff, ethics committees and their members, and ethics consultation services. Resources outside the institution include the ANA's Center on Ethics and Human Rights (www.nursingworld.org/ethics), Veterans Administration's National Center for Ethics in Health Care (www. ethics.va.gov), ethics groups in national specialty organizations, and ethics centers in universities or large health care institutions. The recognition of a moral dilemma does not commit the APN to conducting and managing the process of resolution individually. APNs should engage appropriate resources to address the identified needs and work toward agreement.

As noted, nursing's ethical obligations to patients and their families can also be challenged when organizations implement cost containment practices. Continuity of care and knowing the patient and family are significant issues for APNs in in acute and primary care settings. In outpatient settings, pressures to see more patients in less time can decrease the APN's opportunity for individualized problem solving for patients and families. Thomas and colleagues (2005) noted that NPs' interpersonal skills can enhance the patient's "personhood," an essential part of the caring relationship and the provision of holistic care. Whittemore (2000) has argued that resolving ethical dilemmas requires knowing the patient as a person to be able to recognize the salient aspects of a situation that are important for resolution. However, in time-pressured settings, the emphasis is on efficiency and not on the patient-provider relationship or the provision of holistic care. APNs struggle in these types of environments to balance the needs of individuals with generalized treatment approaches and productivity targets.

However, it is also the case that the costs of the U.S. health care system are unsustainably high and growing (Emanuel et al., 2012). Improving the efficiency and effectiveness of care delivery at a reduced cost can itself be seen as a moral good, one that requires clinicians to work together with administrators to achieve cost-effective goals. Also, there are times when cost-conscious care can enhance accessibility and quality. APNs can bridge clinical and administrative perspectives and collaborate with administrators to help achieve quality patient outcomes at reduced cost to the system. One proposal for decreasing costs involves removing scope of practice barriers to increase the use of APNs in the United States (Emanuel et al., 2012; IOM, 2011). APNs can be instrumental in decreasing the adversarial view between clinicians and administrators that hampers decision making in many settings.

Many institutions are willing to make concessions in the delivery of patient care if there are clear outcome data that support a change in practice. APNs can successfully navigate the cost-conscious health care environment if they effectively demonstrate how their unique contributions to patient care, although more time-intensive, ultimately reduce health care expenditures (see Chapter 23). Because patients have shorter hospital stays, open communication and collaboration with the health care team, patients, and families are essential behaviors for optimal planning. Also, as described in Phase 4, APNs should maintain and affirm patient's rights and articulate strong ethical reasons for the interventions; questioning and challenging features in the health care system that negatively affect the quality of care delivered may be necessary. Finally, there is a need to review patient outcomes consistently and the quality of nursing care provided (see Chapters 23 and 24) because these data can be powerful in building the case for quality changes to promote ethically responsive environments. With its emphasis on cost-effectiveness research and incentives for achieving positive patient outcomes, together with sanctions for underachievement (e.g., charging hospitals for high levels of readmissions), the PPACA is expected to accelerate the reliance on outcome data as a guide to practice.

Box 13-6 lists websites that contain valuable ethics resources for clinicians. Many specialty organizations issue policy statements related to ethical issues or publish guidelines for their members' use in responding to ethical problems. Box 13-6 also contains sites useful

BOX 13-6   Websites for Ethics Resources

Ethics Policy Statements or Guidelines

American Academy of Neurology, Practice Statements: http://www.aan.com/resources.html

American Academy of Pediatrics, Policy Statements: http://www.aap.org/policy

American Association of Nurse-Anesthetists (AANA): http://www.aana.com

American College of Nurse-Midwives: http://www.acnm.org

American College of Medical Genetics, Policy Statements: http://www.faseb.org/genetics/acmg

American College of Physicians, Center for Ethics and Professionalism: http://www.acponline.org/ethics

American College of Surgeons: http://www.facs.org

American Medical Association, Council on Ethical and Judicial Affairs: http://www.ama-assn.org

American Nurses Association, Center for Ethics and Human Rights: http://www.ana.org/ethics

American Society for Law, Medicine and Ethics: http://www.aslme.org

American Society for Reproductive Medicine: http://www.asrm.org

American Society of Anesthesiologists, Policy Statements: http://www.asahq.org/standards

American Society for Transplantation, Policy Statements: http://www.a-s-t.org/index.html

Americans for Better Care of the Dying: http://www.abcd-caring.org

Canadian Resource for Nursing Ethics: http://www.NursingEthics.ca

Institute of Medicine, National Academy of Sciences: http://www4.nas.edu/IOM/IOMHome.nsf

International Centre for Nursing Ethics: http://www.surrey.ac.uk/fhms/research/centres/icne

International Council of Nurses: http://www.icn.ch

Midwest Bioethics Center: http://www.midbio.org

National Bioethics Advisory Commission: http://www.georgetown.edu/research/nrcbl/nbac/

National Catholic Bioethics Center: http://www.ncbcenter.org

National Hospice Organization: http://www.nho.org

National Human Genome Research Institute: http://www.nhgri.nih.gov

National Institutes of Health Resources on Bioethics: http://www.nih.gov/sigs/bioethics/

National Institutes of Health, Office for Protection from Research Risks: http://www.grants.nih.gov/grants/oprr/oprr.htm

Society for Critical Care Medicine: http://www.sccm.org

United Network for Organ Sharing, Policy Statements: http://www.unos.org

University of Pennsylvania Center for Bioethics: http://www.med.upenn.edu/~bioethics

Ethics and Legal Search Sites

Bioethics line database on Internet Grateful Med (literature search): http://www.igm.nlm.nih.gov

Legal Information Institute: http://www.law.cornell.edu

Medical College of Wisconsin Center for the Study of Bioethics, Bioethics Online Service (literature search): http://www.mcw.edu/bioethics

National Reference Center for Bioethics Literature: http://www.georgetown.edu/research/nrcbl

State laws on the Internet: http://www.legalonline.com

U.S. National Library of Medicine, National Institutes of Health: http://www.nlm.nih.gov/medlineplus.bioethics

---

for gathering current literature on legal and ethical issues.

Conclusion

The changing health care environment has placed extraordinary demands on nurses in all care settings. Many forces conflict with nursing's moral imperatives of involvement, connection, and commitment. The ethical decision making competency involves four phases of progressively complex knowledge and skill development necessary to move patient care, caregiving environments, and the larger system toward ethical practices. As a core competency for the APN, ethical decision making reflects the art and science of nursing. The APN is in a key position to assume a more decisive role in managing the resolution of moral issues and helping create ethically responsive health care environments. The identification of patterns in the presentation of moral issues enables the APN to engage in preventive strategies to improve the ethical climate in patient care environments. Ethical decision making skills, together with clinical expertise and leadership, empower the APN to assume leadership roles in public policy processes that promote social justice within the larger health care arena. Preparation for this competency begins in graduate education, but continues throughout the APN's career.

References

Ahrens, T., Yancey, V., & Kollef, M. (2003). Improving family communications at the end of life: Implications for length of stay in the intensive care unit and resource use. *American Journal of Critical Care, 12*, 317–323.

Ajovalasit, D., Cerniauskaite, M., Aluas, M., Alves I., Bosisio Fazzi, L., Griffo, G., et al. (2012). Multidisciplinary research network on health and disability training on the International Classification of Functioning, Disability and Health, Ethics and Human Rights. *American Journal of Physical Medicine and Rehabilitation, 91*(Suppl), S168–S172.

American Association of Colleges of Nursing. (2006). *The essentials of doctoral education for advanced nursing practice*. Washington, DC: Author.

American Association of Colleges of Nursing. (2011). *The essentials of master's education in nursing*. Washington, DC: Author.

American Association of Critical-Care Nurses (2004). *The 4A's to rise above moral distress*. Aliso Viejo, CA: Author.

American Association of Critical-Care Nurses (2008). *Position statement*: Moral distress (http://www.aacn.org/WD/Practice/Docs/Moral_Distress.pdf).

American Nurses Association (ANA). (2001). *Code of ethics for nurses, with interpretive statements*. Washington, DC: Author.

Arras, J. D. (1997). Nice story, but so what? In H. L. Nelson (Ed.), *Stories and their limits: Narrative approaches to bioethics* (pp. 65–88). New York: Routledge.

Artnak, K., & Dimmit, J. H. (1996). Choosing a framework for ethical analysis in advanced practice settings: The case for casuistry. *Archives of Psychiatric Nursing, 10*, 16–23.

Austin, W. (2007). The ethics of everyday practice: Health care environments as moral communities. *Advances in Nursing Science, 30*, 81–88.

Beauchamp, T. L., & Childress, J. F. (2009). *Principles of biomedical ethics* (6th ed.). New York: Oxford University Press.

Bell, S. E., & Hulbert, J. R. (2008). Translating social justice into clinical nurse specialist practice. *Clinical Nurse Specialist, 22*, 293–299.

Benner, P., Tanner, C., & Chesla, C. (2009). *Expertise in nursing practice: Caring, clinical judgment, and ethics* (2nd ed.). New York: Springer.

Bishop, G., & Brodkey, A. C. (2006). Personal responsibility and physician responsibility—West Virginia's Medicaid plan. *New England Journal of Medicine, 355*, 756–758.

Bodenheimer, T. S., & Grumbach, K. (2012). *Understanding health policy: A clinical approach* (6th ed.). New York: Lange Medical/McGraw Hill.

Botwinski, C. (2010). NNP Education in end of life: A needs assessment. *Maternity Child Nursing, 35*, 286–292.

Buettner-Schmidt, K., & Lobo, M.L. (2011). Social justice: A concept analysis. *Journal of Advanced Nursing, 68*, 948–958.

Buryska, J. F. (2001). Assessing the ethical weight of cultural, religious and spiritual claims in the clinical context. *Journal of Medical Ethics, 27*, 118–122.

Canadian Interprofessional Health Collaborative. (2010). *A national interprofessional competency framework*. Available at www.cihc.ca/files/CIHC_IPCompetencies_Feb1210.pdf. Accessed April 23, 2013.

Caulfield, T. (2012). DTC genetic testing: Pendulum swings and policy paradoxes. *Clinical Genetics, 81*, 4–6.

Ceci, C. (2004). Nursing, knowledge and power: A case analysis. *Social Science and Medicine, 59*, 1879–1889.

Center for Ethics in Health Care. (2012). Physician orders for life-sustaining treatment (www.ohsu.edu/polst).

Chaguturu, S., & Vallabhaneni, S. (2007). Aiding and abetting: Nursing crises at home and abroad. *New England Journal of Medicine, 353*, 1761–1763.

Chambliss, D. F. (1996). *Beyond caring: Hospitals, nurses, and the social organization of ethics*. Chicago: University of Chicago Press.

Charon, R., & Montello, M. (2002). *Stories matter: The role of narrative in medical ethics*. New York: Routledge.

Childress, J. F. (1997). Narrative(s) versus norm(s): A misplaced debate in bioethics. In H. L. Nelson (Ed.), *Stories and their limits: Narrative approaches to bioethics* (pp. 252–271). New York: Routledge.

Cooper, M. C. (1991). Principle-oriented ethics and the ethic of care: A creative tension. *Advances in Nursing Science, 14*, 22–31.

Corley, M. C., Minick, P., Elswick, R. K., & Jacobs, M. (2005). Nurse moral distress and ethical work environment. *Nursing Ethics, 12*, 381–390.

Curtis, J. R., Ciechanowski, P. S., Downey, L., Gold, J., Neilsen, E. L., Shannon, S. E., et al. (2012). Development and evaluation of an interprofessional communication intervention to improve family outcomes in the ICU. *Contemporary Clinical Trials, 33*, 1245–1254.

Curtis, J. R., & Shannon, S. E. (2006). Transcending the silos: Toward an interdisciplinary approach to end-of-life care in the intensive care unit. *Intensive Care Medicine, 32*, 15–17.

Donagrandi, M. A., & Eddy, M. (2000). Ethics of case management: Implications for advanced practice nursing. *Clinical Nurse Specialist, 14*, 241–249.

Dreyfus, H. L., Dreyfus, S. E., & Benner, P. (2009). Implications of the phenomenology of expertise for teaching and learning everyday skillful ethical comportment. In P. Benner, C. A. Tanner, & C. A. Chesla (Eds.), *Expertise in nursing practice: Caring, clinical judgment and ethics* (pp. 309–334, 2nd ed.). New York: Springer.

Dubler, N. N., & Liebman, C. B. (2011). *Bioethics mediation: A guide to shaping shared solutions (revised and expanded edition)*. New York: United Hospital Fund of New York.

Dwyer, J. (2007). What's wrong with the global migration of health care professionals? Individual rights and international justice. *Hastings Center Report, 37*, 36–43.

Edwards, M., & Chalmers, K. (2002). Double agency in clinical research. *Canadian Journal of Nursing Research, 34*, 131–142.

Edwards, S. D. (2009). Three versions of the ethics of care. *Nursing Philosophy, 10*, 231–240.

Emanuel, E. J. (2002). Patient v. population: Resolving the ethical dilemmas posed by treating patients as members of populations. In M. Danis, C. Clancy, & L. R. Churchill (Eds.), *Ethical dimensions of health policy* (pp. 227–245). New York: Oxford University Press.

Emanuel, E., Tanden, N., Altman, S., Armstrong, S., Berwick, D., de Brantes, F., et al. (2012). A systemic approach to containing health care spending. *New England Journal of Medicine, 367,* 949–954.

Epstein, E. G., & Hamric, A. B. (2009). Moral distress, moral residue, and the crescendo effect. *Journal of Clinical Ethics, 20*(4), 330–342.

Erlen, J. A. (2006). Genetic testing and counseling: Selected ethical issues. *Orthopaedic Nursing, 25,* 423–426.

Falk-Raphael, A. (2005). Speaking truth to power: Nursing's legacy and moral imperative. *Advances in Nursing Science, 28,* 212–223.

Fernbach, A. (2011). Parental rights and decision making regarding vaccinations: Ethical dilemmas for the primary care provider. *Journal of the American Academy of Nurse Practitioners, 23,* 336–345.

Forrow, L., Arnold, R. M., & Parker, L. S. (1993). Preventive ethics: Expanding the horizons of clinical ethics. *Journal of Clinical Ethics, 4,* 287–294.

Fox, E., Bottrell, M., Foglia, M., & Stoeckle, R. (2007). Preventive ethics: Addressing ethics quality gaps on a systems level (www.ethics.va.gov/integratedethics).

Fry, S. T., & Johnstone, M. J. (2008). *Ethics in nursing practice: a guide to ethical decision making* (3rd ed.). Chichester, England: Wiley-Blackwell.

Gallagher, A., & Tschudin, V. (2010). Educating for ethical leadership. *Nurse Education Today, 30,* 224–227.

Gert, B., Culver, C. M., & Clouser, K. D. (2006). *Bioethics: A systematic approach* (2nd ed.). New York: Oxford University Press.

Gilligan, C. (1982). *In a different voice.* Cambridge, MA: Harvard University Press.

Gostin, L. O. (2005). Ethics, the constitution, and the dying process: The case of Theresa Marie Schiavo. *Journal of the American Medical Association, 293,* 2403–2407.

Gordon, E. J., & Hamric, A. B. (2006). The courage to stand up: The cultural politics of nurses' access to ethics consultation. *Journal of Clinical Ethics, 17,* 231–254.

Grace, P. J., & Willis, D. G. (2012). Nursing responsibilities and social justice: An analysis in support of disciplinary goals. *Nursing Outlook, 60,* 198–207.

Grady, C., Danis, M., Soeken, K. L., O'Donnell, P., Taylor, C., Farrar, A., et al. (2008). Does ethics education influence the moral action of practicing nurses and social workers? *American Journal of Bioethics, 8*(4), 4–11.

Hamric, A. B. (2001). Reflections on being in the middle. *Nursing Outlook, 49,* 254–257.

Hamric, A. B., & Blackhall, L. J. (2007). Nurse-physician perspectives on the care of dying patients in intensive care units: Collaboration, moral distress, and ethical climate. *Critical Care Medicine, 35,* 422–429.

Hamric, A. B., Borchers, C. T., & Epstein, E. G. (2012). Development and testing of an instrument to measure moral distress in healthcare professionals. *AJOB Primary Research, 2,* 1–9.

Hamric, A. B., Davis, W. S., & Childress, M. D. (2006). Moral distress in health care professionals: What is it and what can we do about it? *Pharos of Alpha Omega Alpha Honor Medical Society, 69,* 16–23.

Hamric, A. B., Epstein, E. G., & White, K. R. (In press). Moral distress and the health care organization. In G. Filerman, A. Mills, & P. Schyve (Eds.). *Health care ethics for health care organizations: A moral imperative.* Chicago: Health Administration Press.

Harris, M., Winship, I., & Spriggs, M. (2005). Controversies and ethical issues in cancer-genetics clinics. *Lancet Oncology, 6,* 301–310.

Harrowing, J., & Mill, J. (2010). Moral distress among Ugandan nurses providing HIV care: A critical ethnography. *International Journal of Nursing Studies, 47,* 723–731.

Holder, K. V., & Schenthal, S. J. (2007). Watch your step: Nursing and professional boundaries. *Nursing Management, 38,* 24–29.

Hopkinson, I., & Mackay, J. (2002). The clinical impact of the Human Genome Project: Inherited variants in cancer care. *Annals of Oncology, 13*(Suppl 4), 105–107.

Horner, S. D. (2004). Ethics and genetics: Implications for CNS practice. *Clinical Nurse Specialist, 18,* 228–231.

Howard, E. P., & Steinberg, S. (2002). Evaluations of clinical learning in a managed care environment. *Nursing Forum, 37,* 12–20.

Institute of Medicine. (1999). *To err is human: Building a safer health system.* Washington, DC: National Academies Press.

Institute of Medicine. (2001). *Crossing the quality chasm: A new health system for the 21st century.* Washington, DC: National Academies Press.

Institute of Medicine. (2003). *Health professions education: A bridge to quality.* Washington, DC: National Academies Press.

Institute of Medicine (IOM). (2011). *The future of nursing: Leading change, advancing health.* Washington, DC: National Academies Press.

International Association of Forensic Nurses (2009). The use of emergency contraception post–sexual assult. Position paper (http://www.iafn.org/associations/8556/files/IAFN%20Position%20Statement-Emergency%20Contraception%20Approved.pdf).

Interprofessional Education Collaborative Expert Panel. (2011). *Core competencies for interprofessional collaborative practice: Report of an expert panel.* Washington, DC: Interprofessional Education Collaborative. (Available at www.aacn.nche.edu/education-resources/ipecreport.pdf).

Jameson, J. K. (2003). Transcending intractable conflict in health care: An exploratory study of communication and conflict among anesthesia providers. *Journal of Health Communications, 8,* 563–581.

Jameton, A. (1984). *Nursing practice: The ethical issues.* Englewood Cliff, NJ: Prentice Hall.

Jameton, A. (1993). Dilemmas of moral distress: Moral responsibility and nursing practice. *AWHONN's Clinical Issues in Perinatal and Women's Health Nursing, 4,* 542–551.

Jonsen, A. R., Siegler, M., & Winslade, W. J. (2010). *Clinical ethics: A practical approach to ethical decisions in clinical medicine* (7th ed.). New York: McGraw-Hill.

Jonsen, A. R., & Toulmin, S. (1988). *The abuse of casuistry: A history of moral reasoning.* Berkeley, CA: University of California Press.

Juretschke, L. J. (2001). Ethical dilemmas and the nurse practitioner in the NICU. *Neonatal Network, 20,* 33–38.

Kennedy, J. (2012). Demystifying the role of nurse practitioners in hospice: Nurse practitioners as an integral part of the hospice plan of care. *Home Health Care Nurse, 30,* 48–51.

Klaidman, S. (2007). *Coronary: A true story of medicine gone awry.* New York: Scribner.

Laabs, C. A. (2005). Moral problems and distress among nurse practitioners in primary care. *Journal of the American Academy of Nurse Practitioners, 17,* 76–84.

Laabs, C. A. (2012). Confidence and knowledge regarding ethics among advanced practice nurses. *Nursing Education Perspectives, 33,* 10–14.

Lachman, V. D. (2012). Applying the ethics of care to your nursing practice. *MedSurg Nursing, 21,* 112–115.

LaSala, C. A., & Djarnason, D. (2010). Creating workplace environments that support moral courage (http://www.medscape.com/viewarticle/737896).

Linnard-Palmer, L., & Kools, S. (2004). Parents' refusal of medical treatment based on religious and/or cultural beliefs: The law, ethical principles, and clinical implications. *Journal of Pediatric Nursing, 19,* 351–356.

Little, M. O. (1998). Care: from theory to orientation and back. *Journal of Medicine and Philosophy, 23,* 190–209.

Ludwig, R., & Silva, M. C. (2000). Nursing around the world: Cultural values and ethical conflicts (http://www.nursingworld.org/ojin/ethicol/ethics_4.htm).

Management Sciences for Health. (2012). The provider's guide to quality and culture (http://erc.msh.org/mainpage.cfm?file=1.0.htm&module=provider&language=English).

McCormick-Gendzel, M., & Jurchak, M. (2006). A pathway for moral reasoning in home healthcare. *Home Healthcare Nurse, 24,* 654–661.

McCullough, L. B. (2005). Practicing preventive ethics—the keys to avoiding ethical conflicts in health care. *The Physician Executive, 31,* 18–21.

McWilliams, J. M., Meara, E., Zaslavsky, A. M., & Ayanian, J. Z. (2007). Use of health services by previously uninsured Medicare beneficiaries. *New England Journal of Medicine, 357,* 143–153.

National Council of State Boards of Nursing. (2009). *Professional boundaries: A nurse's guide to the importance of appropriate professional boundaries.* Chicago: Author.

National Consensus Project for Quality Palliative Care (2009). *Clinical practice guidelines for quality palliative care* (2nd ed.). Pittsburgh, PA: Author.

Nelson, H. L. (2004). Four narrative approaches to bioethics. In G. Khushf (Ed.), *Handbook of bioethics: Taking stock of the field form a philosophical perspective* (pp. 163–181). Hingham, MA: Kluwer.

Nelson W.A., Gardent P.B., Shulman E., & Splaine M. E. (2010). Preventing ethics conflicts and improving health care quality through system redesign. *Quality and Safety in Health Care, 19,* 526–530.

Oberle, K. R., & Hughes, D. (2001). Doctors' and nurses' perceptions of ethical problems in end-of-life decisions. *Journal of Advanced Nursing, 33,* 707–715.

Pauly, B., Varcoe, C., Storch, J., & Newton, L. (2009). Registered nurses' perceptions of moral distress and ethical climate. *Nursing Ethics, 16,* 561–573.

Piers, R. D., Azoulay, E., Ricou, R., Ganz, F. D., Decruyenaere, J., Max, A., et al. (2011). Perceptions of appropriateness of care among European and Israeli intensive care unit nurses and physicians. *Journal of the American Medical Association, 306,* 2694–2703.

Pracher, T., Moss, B., & Mahanes, D. (2006). *Moral distress in the care of patients with traumatic brain injury.* Poster presentation, San Diego, CA: American Association of Neuroscience Nurses.

Pullman, D., & Hodgkinson, K. (2006). Genetic knowledge and moral responsibility: Ambiguity at the interface of genetic research and clinical practice. *Clinical Genetics, 69,* 199–203.

Purtilo, R. B., & Doherty, R. (2011). *Ethical dimensions in the health professions* (5th ed.). Philadelphia: Elsevier Saunders.

Rajput, V., & Bekes, C. E. (2002). Ethical issues in hospital medicine. *Medical Clinics of North America, 86,* 869–886.

Resnick, D. B. (2005). The patient's duty to adhere to prescribed treatment: An ethical analysis. *Journal of Medicine and Philosophy, 30,* 167–188.

Rest, J. R. (1986). *Moral development: Advances in research and theory.* New York: Praeger.

Rorty, M. V., Werhane, P. H., & Mills, A. E. (2004). The Rashomon effect: Organization ethics in health care. *HEC Forum, 16,* 75–94.

Rushton, C. H., & Penticuff, J. H. (2007). A framework for analysis of ethical dilemmas in critical care nursing. *AACN Advanced Critical Care, 18,* 323–328.

Schluter, J., Winch, S., Holzhauser, K., & Henderson, A. (2008). Nurses' moral sensitivity and hospital ethical climate: A literature review. *Nursing Ethics, 15,* 304–321.

Shannon, S. E. (1997). The roots of interdisciplinary conflict around ethical issues. *Critical Care Nursing Clinics of North America, 9,* 13–28.

Shannon, S. E., Foglia, M.B., Hardy, M., & Gallagher, T. H. (2009). Disclosing errors to patients: Perspectives of registered nurses. *Joint Commission Journal on Quality and Safety, 35,* 5–12.

Shannon, S. E., Mitchell, P. H., & Cain, K. C. (2002). Patients, nurses, and physicians have differing views of quality of critical care. *Journal of Nursing Scholarship, 34,* 173–179.

Silva, M. C., & Ludwick, R. (2002). Domestic violence, nurses and ethics: What are the links? (http://www.nursingworld.org/ojin/ethicol/ethics_8.htm).

Spencer, E. M. (2005). A case method for consideration of moral problems. In *Fletcher's introduction to clinical ethics* (pp. 339–347, 3rd ed.). Hagerstown, MD: University Publishing Group.

Spielman, B. J. (1993). Conflict in medical ethics cases: Seeking patterns of resolution. *Journal of Clinical Ethics, 4,* 212–218.

Steinbock, B., Arras, J. D., & London, A. J. (2012). *Ethical issues in modern medicine: Contemporary readings in bioethics* (8th ed.). New York: McGraw-Hill.

Strong, C. (2007). Specified principlism: What is it and does it really resolve cases better than casuistry? *Journal of Medicine and Philosophy, 25,* 323–341.

Tarlier, D. S., & Browne, A. J. (2011). Remote nursing certified practice: Viewing nursing and nurse practitioner practice through a social justice lens. *Canadian Journal of Nursing Research, 32,* 38–61.

Thomas, J. D., Finch, L. P., Schoenhofer, S. O., & Green, A. (2005). The caring relationships created by nurse practitioners and the ones nursed: Implications for practice (http://www.medscape.com/viewarticle/496420).

Toulmin, S. (1994). Casuistry and clinical ethics. In E. R. DuBose, R. Hamel, & L. J. O'Connell (Eds.), *A matter of principles?* (pp. 310–318). Valley Forge, PA: Trinity Press International.

Trautman, D. (2011). Health care reform: One year later. *Nursing Management, 42*, 26–31.

Trotochard, K. (2006). Ethical issues and access to health care. *Journal of Infusion Nursing, 29*, 165–170.

Turner, L. N., Marquis, K., & Burman, M. E. (1996). Rural nurse practitioners: Perceptions of ethical dilemmas. *Journal of the American Academy of Nurse Practitioners, 8*, 269–274.

Ulrich, C. (2012). *Nursing ethics in everyday practice*. Indianapolis: Sigma Theta Tau International.

Ulrich, C., Soeken, K., & Miller, N. (2003). Predictors of nurse practitioners' autonomy: Effects of organizational, ethical and market characteristics. *Journal of the American Academy of Nurse Practitioners, 15*, 319–325.

Ulrich, C. M., Danis, M., Ratcliffe, S. J., Garrett-Mayer, E., Koziol, D., Soeken, K., et al. (2006). Ethical conflicts in nurse practitioners and physician assistants in managed care. *Nursing Research, 55*, 391–401.

U.S. Department of Health & Human Services (HHS). (2011). Patient Protection and Affordable Care Act (http://www.healthcare.gov/law/full/index.html).

U.S. Department of Health and Human Services, Office of Minority Health. (2001). National standards for culturally and linguistically appropriate services in health care (http://www.omhrc.gov/assets/pdf/checked/executive.pdf).

Varcoe, C., Pauly, B., Webster, C., & Storch, J. (2012). Moral distress: Tensions and springboards for action. *HEC Forum, 24*, 51–62.

Viens, D. C. (1994). Moral dilemmas experienced by nurse practitioners. *Nurse Practitioner Forum, 5*, 209–214.

Viens, D. C. (1995). The moral reasoning of nurse practitioners. *Journal of the American Academy of Nurse Practitioners, 7*, 277–285.

Weaver, K. (2007). Ethical sensitivity: State of knowledge and needs for further research. *Nursing Ethics, 14*, 141–155.

Whittemore, R. (2000). Consequences of not "knowing the patient." *Clinical Nurse Specialist, 14*, 75–81.

Wolf, S. M. (Ed.). (1996). *Feminism and bioethics: Beyond reproduction*. New York: Oxford University Press.

Wueste, D. E. (2005). A philosophical yet user friendly framework for ethical decision making in critical care nursing. *Dimensions of Critical Care Nursing, 24*(2), 70–79.

CHAPTER

The Clinical Nurse Specialist

14

Garrett K. Chan • Cathy C. Cartwright

CHAPTER CONTENTS

Overview and Definitions of the Clinical Nurse Specialist

The clinical nurse specialist (CNS) role was created for the following reasons: (1) to provide direct care to patients with complex diseases or conditions; (2) to improve patient care by developing the clinical skills and judgment of staff nurses; and (3) to retain nurses who are experts in clinical practice (Cooper, Sparacino, & Minarik, 1990; Hamric & Spross, 1989). Expert clinical practice is the essence, the core value, of the CNS role. Historically, the role has been versatile, evolving, flexing, responsive, and adaptable to patient populations and health care environments, notably the same characteristics that have led to concerns regarding role confusion and ambiguity because of variability in implementation. However, the core strength of the CNS in providing complex specialty care while improving the quality of care delivery has remained central to the understanding of this advanced practice nurse (APN) role. Currently, the CNS is defined as an APN who practices in three substantive areas, as

articulated by Lewandowski and Adamle (2009), to manage the care of complex and vulnerable populations, educate and support nursing and interdisciplinary staff, and facilitate change and innovation in health care systems. Lewandowski and Adamle developed these concepts of the three substantive areas of CNS practice in the context of the evolving health care environment by conducting an extensive literature review, based on the foundational work delineated by the National Association of Clinical Nurse Specialists (NACNS). In their 2004 document, *Statement on Clinical Nurse Specialist Practice and Education,* NACNS described CNSs as practicing in the three interrelated spheres of client direct care, nurses and nursing practice, and organizations and systems. As noted earlier in this text, direct care of patients is the primary distinguishing feature of CNS practice (see Chapter 7) and interventions in the other two spheres are intended ultimately to affect the care of patients. Examples include interventions such as guiding and educating staff nurses in the nurses and nursing practice sphere and leading quality improvement projects and redesigning the delivery of care in the organizations and systems sphere. In the NACNS model, therefore, the client direct care sphere encompasses the interventions of the other two spheres to depict the centrality of the patient care focus. NACNS has been currently revising their statement at the time of this writing. In this chapter, we will use the NACNS spheres of influence and the further refined substantive areas of practice from Lewandowski and Adamle (2009) to illustrate the unique contributions of the role of the CNS and how the CNS role differs from other APN roles.

Exemplar 14-1 describes a typical day in the life of a pediatric clinical nurse specialist.

In spite of a core understanding of the nuances of the CNS role, the activities of CNSs are as varied as their individual specialty practices. The diversity of CNS specialties, differences in their individual practices, and practice differences seen among CNSs in the same institution has created confusion about what CNSs do. Unlike other APNs, whose primary role is to deliver direct patient care, the multifaceted CNS delivers direct patient care specifically to complex and vulnerable populations, educates and supports nurses and interdisciplinary staff, provides leadership to specialty practice program development, and facilitates change and innovation in health care systems (Lewandowski & Adamle, 2009). This variability in CNS practice, even within the same institution, has characterized the role since its creation. The definition of the CNS role has remained deliberately broad so that CNSs can respond to changing clinical environments. For example, a unit- or population-based critical care CNS with an experienced, certified specialty staff may balance his or her time equally among direct patient care activities, educating interdisciplinary staff, and system-wide improvements. Conversely, if a preventive cardiology CNS works in an outpatient clinic in the same institution and sees a panel of patients as a provider of expert specialty care, that CNS practice may focus more on direct patient care and less on education and system-wide improvements. Several clinical, staff, and system variables must be weighed when planning for CNS positions and implementing the role, including the number, type, and background of nurses and other clinical staff, clinical, educational, or institutional resources, and patient population, acuity, and outcomes.

This versatility in CNS practice has continued to challenge the CNS role definition and understanding of the impact of CNSs on clinical outcomes and costs of care. Role confusion and variability, regulatory drivers, and fiscal retrenchment in the last 20 years have resulted in the loss of CNS positions in many parts of the country to save hospitals money without jeopardizing direct care registered nurse (RN) positions. The CNS role is the only APN role to decrease in numbers in the most recent national RN survey (see Chapter 3). CNS clinical practices are shaped by many factors, such as health care agency needs, community needs, payor and other regulatory agency mandates, statutory limitations, supervisor requests, and individual CNS interests. Over the past few decades, CNSs have been able to change their practices in response to these influential forces.

Clarifying the work and core competencies of all CNSs, regardless of specialty, has been complicated historically

---

● EXEMPLAR 14-1   A Day in the Life of a Clinical Nurse Specialist

PM, a pediatric CNS in the department of neurosurgery, started his day by checking the list of patients on the service. After reviewing their charts, he noted that a new brain tumor patient, an 11-year-old boy, was admitted during the night after a seizure. After looking at the head CT scan, checking his vital signs and nurses' notes, he noted that the patient had a Glasgow Coma Scale (GCS) score of 15 and was stable. PM checked to make sure that the patient had been started on appropriate doses of dexamethasone and ranitidine and that he had a brain magnetic resonance imaging (MRI) scan ordered for this morning. PM was mentoring a CNS graduate student and she joined him just before rounds. He reviewed the patients with her, including the 11-year-old boy's head computed tomography (CT) scan, explaining that the seizure was caused by the location of the tumor. He also explained the importance of steroids in treating edema in brain tumor patients.

PM, his CNS student, and the pediatric neurosurgeon made rounds together on the patients, formulating a plan of care for each one for the day. Because the neurosurgeon would be in the operating room most of the day, PM planned to keep him updated on any changes in patient conditions. PM included the staff nurses caring for each patient in rounds so they could contribute to developing the patient's plan for the day.

After documenting daily progress notes on each patient, PM then led a meeting with a group of staff nurses and CNSs from medical-surgical units and the medical-surgical intensive care unit to address issues related to the care of neurosurgical patients throughout the hospital. PM had noticed inconsistencies across units in patient neurologic assessments, documentation of those assessments, and lack of implementation of current guidelines in the care of this population and had formed the group to discuss these concerns. PM had led the group in reviewing the latest evidence in neurosurgical patient care, identifying gaps in the electronic health care record to facilitate accurate documentation and care planning, and performing a learning needs assessment of the staff caring for these patients. The group had identified next steps to take in improving the quality of care and was continuing to meet under PM's leadership to implement identified strategies and assess the effectiveness of these interventions.

After the meeting, PM was called to the preanesthesia testing unit to do a history and physical examination on a 3-year-old boy who was to undergo surgery the next day to release his tethered cord. After examining the child, he answered the mother's many questions about what to expect after surgery, such as activity, pain control, and wound care. PM also arranged for the child life specialist to visit with the child about what to expect because his mother was concerned about his understanding of the hospital stay.

PM received a page from the emergency department (ED) to see a 5-year-old patient with spina bifida who presented with a 1-day history of fever and vomiting. Because he also had a ventriculoperitoneal shunt, the ED physician wanted neurosurgery to evaluate him for shunt malfunction. PM went to the ED, assessed the patient, and ordered a head CT and shunt series x-ray, explaining to his CNS student that although there are many causes of fever and vomiting in a child with spina bifida, he wanted to rule out shunt malfunction. PM also asked the ED physician to order a urinalysis and culture because the patient's mother said that his urine had started to look cloudy. The CT and shunt series were within normal limits for this patient but the urinalysis showed that he had a urinary tract infection, which the ED physician treated with antibiotics.

After grabbing a quick lunch at his desk and writing postoperative orders, PM remembered that he needed to follow up with one of the patient's mothers. He called the nurse caring for the 11-year-old brain tumor patient to see if his mother was available. On hearing that she was, PM and his CNS student went to talk with her in a private conference room about her concerns for surgery to remove his tumor. His mother was insistent that she did not want her son to know about the surgery until the day before because he was such a "worrier." She was upset that so many of the staff kept coming in his room and talking over him like he wasn't there and mentioning all sorts of scary procedures. After letting her verbalize her concerns, PM assured her that because she knew

her son the best and could determine the best time to talk with him about surgery, the team would support her decision to discuss his condition outside of his room. PM communicated this with his primary team, neurosurgery team, and staff nurse caring for him.

PM then left the floor to give a lecture to staff nurses on a medical-surgical unit on how to perform neurologic assessments. He had developed this lecture as one of the interventions identified from the earlier quality improvement group to improve the care and outcomes for the neurologic population.

As PM was returning to the neurologic unit after the lecture, one of the staff nurses stopped him and said she was worried that the 3-year-old with a recurrent brain tumor was less responsive and not drinking as well as yesterday. PM and his CNS student stopped by the patient's room to assess her. After determining that she was responsive but not as alert as yesterday, he ordered a head CT stat to check for hydrocephalus and restarted her IV fluids. He called the neurosurgeon to report his assessment findings and interventions and that the head CT showed an improvement. The neurosurgeon wanted to increase her dexamethasone and obtain an MRI scan of the brain in the morning, so PM placed those orders. He thanked the staff nurse for being alert to the patient's decline and explained the CT scan to her, comparing it with her previous one. He said he would call back in an hour to check on her.

Shortly thereafter, PM received a page from a new staff nurse to come to a patient's room because the patient's ventriculostomy tubing had come apart. The nurse had noted the disconnection right away and clamped the tube so only a minimum amount of cerebrospinal fluid (CSF) drained onto the floor. PM praised the nurse for her quick action and demonstrated how to reattach a new system using sterile technique. Because the nurse was new, PM also took this opportunity to explore and review with her knowledge related to the purpose of a ventriculostomy. He asked about her understanding of the risks and benefits of this treatment, answered other questions for her, and reviewed the plan of care for this patient with this intervention.

Back in his office, PM had time to return phone calls from anxious parents and answer questions his CNS student had about the day. He called the nurse caring for the 3-year-old and was gratified to learn that she had improved. The neurosurgeon was out of surgery at this time, so PM reviewed the patients with him before leaving for the day.

because specialty organizations have established varying educational, competency, and practice standards for CNSs (e.g., critical care, oncology, neuroscience specialties). NACNS was not established until 1995 (see Chapter 1). The NACNS itself has acknowledged that advanced practice organizations for the other three APN roles had a significant head start in defining competencies and influencing health policies related to advanced practice nursing (NACNS, 2004b). The American Nurses Association (ANA), many specialty organizations, and APN leaders have worked hard to define CNS practice, define standards and competencies, and develop CNS curricula (see Chapters 1 and 2). More work, however, is required to educate colleagues, administrators, and the public about the role of the CNS. For reasons outlined later in this chapter, and discussed in Chapter 21, we believe that CNSs and the nursing profession are at a critical juncture for the survival of the role of the CNS. For the purposes of clinical practice and licensure, accreditation, credentialing, and education (LACE), the work and contributions of CNSs as APNs must be made unambiguously clear.

The ANA has defined APNs as nurses who "practice from both expanded and specialized knowledge and skills" (ANA, 2003, p. 9). An expanded knowledge base and skill set refers to the "acquisition of new practice knowledge and skills, including the knowledge and skills that authorize role autonomy within areas of practice that may overlap traditional boundaries of medical practice" (ANA, 2003, p. 9; see Chapter 3). Specialized knowledge and skills are defined as "concentrating or delimiting one's focus to part of the whole field of professional nursing" (ANA, 2003, p. 9). According to the National Council of State Boards of Nursing (NCSBN) Consensus Model for advanced practice registered nurse (APRN) regulation, a defining factor for all APNs is that a significant component of the education and practice be focused on direct care of individuals (NCSBN, 2012b). If CNSs want to be recognized nationally, statewide, or locally as APNs, they must have a significant component of direct care of individuals in their role. If the focus is mainly on educating nursing and/or interdisciplinary staff or process improvement without direct care of individuals, the clinician is not practicing in the role of a CNS (Cronenwett, 2012).

New opportunities for expanded CNS practices have presented themselves with the introduction of the Patient Protection and Affordable Care Act (PPACA; U.S. Department of Health and Human Services [HHS], 2011). Successful CNSs have consistently delivered direct and indirect care that improves patient care quality and outcomes, patient safety, and nursing practice and that ensures efficient use of resources, cost efficiency, cost savings, and revenue generation (NACNS, 1998, 2004b;

Newhouse, Stanik-Hutt, White et al., 2011; see Chapter 23). CNSs' clinical acumen and expertise are not limited to their patients' physiologic and psychological needs. Their clinical expertise permeates the other elements of their multifaceted responsibilities—education, evidence-based practice (EBP), health policy, organizational factors, and political change—and they are highly qualified to lead interdisciplinary teams in health care reform. The purpose of this chapter is to describe the core competencies, current marketplace challenges, and future directions for CNSs.

Clinical Nurse Specialist Practice: Spheres of Influence and Advanced Practice Nursing Competencies

Although other models of CNS practice have been described (see Chapter 2), the NACNS's three spheres of influence and Hamric's seven competencies (see Chapter 3 and Chapters 7 through 13) will primarily be used to organize and explain CNS practice in this chapter. CNS students are encouraged to familiarize themselves with the NACNS *Statement on Clinical Nurse Specialist Practice and Education* (2004b) and with specialty-specific standards (e.g., the Emergency Nurses Association [2011] competencies for clinical nurse specialists) to understand the discussion of spheres and competencies better. In addition, readers should also be aware of the substantive areas of CNS practice reported by Lewandowski and Adamle (2009) to understand a more recent articulation of CNS practice. To be successful, a CNS must understand and apply the seven competencies of advanced practice nursing across the three spheres of influence, regardless of setting or specialty (Sparacino & Cartwright, 2009). The NACNS (2010), along with other nursing organizations, has endorsed a list of comprehensive, entry-level competencies and behaviors expected of graduate programs in the preparation of CNSs (Table 14-1).

Advanced practice competencies are categories of proficient performance and include specific knowledge and skill sets. The direct care of patients and families is the central competency in Hamric's model (see Fig. 2-4) and links every other competency. According to the NACNS model, the impact and influence of CNSs are felt within three spheres of influence—direct care of patients or clients,* nurses and nursing practice, and organizations and systems (NACNS, 2004b; see Fig. 2-2).

Text continued on p. 368

---

*In the NACNS document, this sphere is termed *client direct care*. For clarity in this chapter, this sphere is termed *direct care of patients or clients*.

TABLE 14-1 NACNS Core Competencies

Behavioral Statement	Sphere of Influence	Nurse Characteristics
A. Direct Care Competency Direct interaction with patients, families, and groups of patients to promote health or well-being and improve quality of life, characterized by a holistic perspective in the advanced nursing management of health, illness, and disease state		
A.1 Conducts comprehensive, holistic wellness and illness assessments using known or innovative evidence-based techniques, tools, and direct and indirect methods	Patient	Clinical judgment
A.2 Obtains data about context and causes (including both nondisease– and disease-related factors) necessary to formulate differential diagnoses and plans of care, and identify and evaluate outcomes	Patient	
A.3 Employs evidence-based clinical practice guidelines to guide screening and diagnosis	Patient and system	
A.4 Assesses the effects of interactions among the individual, family, community, and social systems on health and illness	Patient	
A.5 Identifies potential risks to patient safety, autonomy, and quality of care based on assessments across the patient, nurse, and system spheres of influence	Patient, nurse, and system	
A.6 Assesses the impact of environmental and system factors on care	Patient and system	
A.7 Synthesizes assessment data, advanced knowledge, and experience, using critical thinking and clinical judgment to formulate differential diagnoses for clinical problems amenable to CNS intervention	Patient and system	
A.8 Prioritizes differential diagnoses to reflect those conditions most relevant to signs, symptoms, and patterns amenable to CNS interventions	Patient	
A.9 Selects interventions that may include, but are not limited to, the following: A.9.a Application of advanced nursing therapies A.9.b Initiation of interdisciplinary team meetings, consultations, and other communications to benefit patient care A.9.c Management of patient medications, clinical procedures, and other interventions A.9.d Psychosocial support, including patient counseling and spiritual interventions	Patient	
A.10 Designs strategies, including advanced nursing therapies, to meet the multifaceted needs of complex patients and groups of patients	Patient	
A.11 Develops evidence-based clinical interventions and systems to achieve defined patient and system outcomes	Patient, nurse, and system	
A.12 Uses advanced communication skills within therapeutic relationships to improve patient outcomes	Patient	Caring practice
A.13 Prescribes nursing therapeutics, pharmacologic and nonpharmacologic interventions, diagnostic measures, equipment, procedures, and treatments to meet the needs of patients, families and groups in accordance with professional preparation, institutional privileges, state and federal laws, and practice acts	Patient	Clinical judgment
A.14 Provides direct care to selected patients based on the needs of the patient and the CNS's specialty knowledge and skills	Patient	
A.15 Assists staff in the development of innovative, cost effective programs or protocols of care	Patient, nurse, and system	
A 16 Evaluates nursing practice that considers safety, timeliness, effectiveness, efficiency, efficacy and patient-centered care	Patient, nurse, and system	
A.17 Determines when evidence-based guidelines, policies, procedures, and plans of care need to be tailored to the individual	Patient	

Continued

TABLE 14-1   NACNS Core Competencies—*cont'd*

Behavioral Statement	Sphere of Influence	Nurse Characteristics
A.18 Differentiates between outcomes that require care process modification at the individual patient level and those that require modification at the system level	System	Systems thinking
A.19 Leads development of evidence-based plans for meeting individual, family, community, and population needs	Patient and system	Caring practice
A.20 Provides leadership for collaborative, evidence-based revision of diagnoses and plans of care to improve patient outcomes	Patient, nurse, and system	Clinical judgment

B. Consultation Competency
Patient, staff, or system-focused interaction among professionals in which the consultant is recognized as having specialized expertise and assists consultee with problem solving

B.1 Provides consultation to staff nurses, medical staff, and interdisciplinary colleagues	Patient, nurse, and system	Clinical judgment
B.2 Initiates consultation to obtain resources as necessary to facilitate progress toward achieving identified outcomes	Patient	
B.3 Communicates consultation findings to appropriate parties consistent with professional and institutional standards	Patient	Collaboration
B.4 Analyzes data from consultations to implement practice improvements	Nurse and system	Facilitation of learning

C. Systems Leadership Competency
Ability to manage change and empower others to influence clinical practice and political processes within and across systems

C.1 Facilitates the provision of clinically competent care by staff and team through education, role modeling, team building, and quality monitoring	Nurse and system	
C.2 Performs system level assessments to identify variables that influence nursing practice and outcomes, including but not limited to the following:	System	Systems thinking
C.2.a Population variables (age distribution, health status, income distribution, culture)	Patient and system	Response to diversity
C.2.b Environment (schools, community support services, housing availability, employment opportunities)	Patient and system	Systems thinking
C.2.c System of health care delivery	Patient and system	
C.2.d Regulatory requirements	System	
C.2.e Internal and external political influences, stability	System	
C.2.f Health care financing	System	
C.2.g Recurring practices that enhance or compromise patient or system outcomes	Patient, nurse, and system	
C.3 Determines nursing practice and system interventions that will promote patient, family and community safety	Nurse and system	
C.4 Uses effective strategies for changing clinician and team behavior to encourage adoption of evidence-based practices and innovations in care delivery	Nurse and system	
C.5 Provides leadership in maintaining a supportive and healthy work environment	System	
C.6 Provides leadership in promoting interdisciplinary collaboration to implement outcome-focused patient care programs meeting the clinical needs of patients, families, populations, and communities	Patient and system	Collaboration
C.7 Develops age-specific clinical standards, policies and procedures	System	Collaboration and response to diversity

TABLE 14-1 NACNS Core Competencies—*cont'd*

Behavioral Statement	Sphere of Influence	Nurse Characteristics
C.8 Uses leadership, team building, negotiation, and conflict resolution skills to build partnerships within and across systems, including communities	System	Collaboration
C.9 Coordinates the care of patients with use of system and community resources to assure successful health/illness/wellness transitions, enhance delivery of care, and achieve optimal patient outcomes	Patient and system	

C.10 Considers fiscal and budgetary implications in decision making regarding practice and system modifications
    C.10.a Evaluates use of products and services for appropriateness and cost-benefit in meeting care needs
    C.10.b Conducts cost-benefit analysis of new clinical technologies
    C.10.c Evaluates impact of introduction or withdrawal of products, services, and technologies
	System	Systems thinking

C.11 Leads system change to improve health outcomes through evidence-based practice:	Patient, nurse, and system	Systems thinking
C.11.a Specifies expected clinical- and system- level outcomes	Patient, nurse, and system	
C.11.b Designs programs to improve clinical and system level processes and outcomes	Patient, nurse, and system	
C.11.c Facilitates the adoption of practice change	Patient, nurse, and system	
C.12 Evaluates impact of CNS and other nursing practice on systems of care using nurse-sensitive outcomes	Nurse and system	
C.13 Disseminates outcomes of system-level change internally and externally	System	

D. Collaboration Competency

Working jointly with others to optimize clinical outcomes; CNS collaborates at an advanced level by committing to authentic engagement and constructive patient, family, system, and population-focused problem-solving

D.1 Assesses the quality and effectiveness of interdisciplinary, intra-agency, and interagency communication and collaboration	Nurse and system	Clinical inquiry and collaboration
D.2 Establishes collaborative relationships within and across departments that promote patient safety, culturally competent care, and clinical excellence	System	Collaboration and response to diversity
D.3 Provides leadership for establishing, improving, and sustaining collaborative relationships to meet clinical needs	Nurse and system	
D.4 Practices collegially with medical staff and other members of the health care team so that all providers' unique contributions to health outcomes will be enhanced	Nurse and system	
D.5 Facilitates intra-agency and interagency communication	Nurse and system	

E. Coaching Competency

Skillful guidance and teaching to advance the care of patients, families, groups of patients, and the profession of nursing

E.1 Coaches patients and families to help them navigate the health care system	Patient sphere	Advocacy and moral agency

Continued

TABLE 14-1   **NACNS Core Competencies**—*cont'd*

Behavioral Statement	Sphere of Influence	Nurse Characteristics
E.2 Designs health information and patient education appropriate to the patient's developmental level, health literacy level, learning needs, readiness to learn, and cultural values and beliefs	Patient sphere	Facilitation of learning and response to diversity
E.3 Provides education to individuals, families, groups and communities to promote knowledge, understanding, and optimal functioning across the wellness-illness continuum	Patient sphere	
E.4 Participates in pre-professional, graduate and continuing education of nurses and other health care providers: E.4.a. Completes needs assessment as appropriate to guide interventions with staff E.4.b. Promotes professional development of staff nurses and continuing education activities E.4.c. Implements staff development and continuing education activities	Nurse	
E.4.d. Mentors nurses to translate research into practice	Nurse	Facilitator of learning and clinical inquiry
E.5 Contributes to the advancement of the profession as a whole by disseminating outcomes of CNS practice through presentations and publications	Nurse	
E.6 Mentors staff nurses, graduate students, and others to acquire new knowledge and skills and develop their careers	Nurse	Facilitator of learning
E.7 Mentors health professionals in applying the principles of evidence-based care	Nurse and system	
E.8 Uses coaching and advanced communication skills to facilitate the development of effective clinical teams	Nurse and system	Advocacy and moral agency
E.9 Provides leadership in conflict management and negotiation to address problems in the health care system	Patient, nurse, and system	Collaboration

F. Research Competency

The work of thorough and systematic inquiry. Includes the search for, interpretation, and use of evidence in clinical practice and quality improvement, as well as active participation in the conduct of research

F.I Interpretation, Translation, and Use of Evidence

F.I.1 Analyzes research findings and other evidence for their potential application to clinical practice	Patient, nurse, and system	Clinical inquiry
F.I.2 Integrates evidence into the health, illness, and wellness management of patients, families, communities, and groups	Patient	Clinical inquiry
F.I.3 Applies principles of EBP and quality improvement to all patient care	Patient and system	Clinical inquiry
F.I.4 Assesses system barriers and facilitators to adoption of EBPs	System	
F.I.5 Designs programs for effective implementation of research findings and other evidence in clinical practice	Patient, nurse, and system	
F.I.6 Cultivates a climate of clinical inquiry across spheres of influence:	Patient, nurse, and system	Clinical inquiry, systems thinking
F.1.6.a Evaluates the need for improvement or redesign of care delivery processes to improve safety, efficiency, reliability, and quality	Patient, nurse, and system	
F.1.6.b Disseminates expert knowledge	Patient, nurse, and system	Facilitation of learning

F.II. Evaluation of Clinical Practice

F.II.1 Fosters an interdisciplinary approach to quality improvement, EBP, research, and translation of research into practice	Nurse/Team	Collaboration

⊙ TABLE 14-1 NACNS Core Competencies—*cont'd*

Behavioral Statement	Sphere of Influence	Nurse Characteristics
F.II.2 Participates in establishing quality improvement agenda for unit, department, program, system, or population	System	Clinical inquiry
F.II.3 Provides leadership in planning data collection and quality monitoring	System	
F.II.4 Uses quality monitoring data to assess the quality and effectiveness of clinical programs in meeting outcomes	Patient, nurse, and system	
F.II.5 Develops quality improvement initiatives based on assessments	System	
F.II.6 Provides leadership in the design, implementation, and evaluation of process improvement initiatives	System	
F.II.7 Provides leadership in the system-wide implementation of quality improvements and innovations	System	

F.III. Conduct of Research
F.III.1 Participates in conduct of or implementation of research, which may include one or more of the following:
  F.III.1.a Identification of questions for clinical inquiry
  F.III.1.b Conduct of literature reviews
  F.III.1.c Study design and implementation
  F.III.1.d Data collection
  F.III.1.e Data analysis
  F.III.1.f Dissemination of findings
	Patient, nurse, and system	Clinical inquiry

G. Ethical Decision Making, Moral Agency, and Advocacy Competency

Identifying, articulating, and taking action on ethical concerns at the patient, family, health care provider, system, community, and public policy levels

Behavioral Statement	Sphere of Influence	Nurse Characteristics
G.1 Engages in a formal self-evaluation process, seeking feedback regarding own practice, from patients, peers, professional colleagues, and others	Nurse	Clinical inquiry
G.2 Fosters professional accountability in self or others	Nurse and system	Advocacy and moral agency

G.3 Facilitates resolution of ethical conflicts:
  G.3.a Identifies ethical implications of complex care situations
  G.3.b Considers the impact of scientific advances, cost, clinical effectiveness, patient and family values and preferences, and other external influences
  G.3.c Applies ethical principles to resolving concerns across the three spheres of influence
	Patient, nurse, and system	Response to diversity

G.4 Promotes a practice climate conducive to providing ethical care	Nurse and system	Moral agency
G.5 Facilitates interdisciplinary teams to address ethical concerns, risks or considerations, benefits, and outcomes of patient care	Nurse and system	Advocacy and collaboration
G.6 Facilitates patient and family understanding of the risks, benefits, and outcomes of proposed health care regimen to promote informed decision making	Patient	Facilitator of learning

G.7 Advocates for equitable patient care by the following:
  G.7.a Participating in organizational, local, state, national, or international level of policymaking activities for issues related to their expertise
  G.7.b Evaluating the impact of legislative and regulatory policies as they apply to nursing practice and patient or population outcomes
	Patient and system	Advocacy and moral agency

Continued

TABLE 14-1   NACNS Core Competencies—*cont'd*

Behavioral Statement	Sphere of Influence	Nurse Characteristics
G.8 Promotes the role and scope of practice of the CNS to legislators, regulators, other health care providers, and the public:	Nurse and system	Advocacy and facilitator of learning
G.8.a. Communicates information that promotes nursing, the role of the CNS and outcomes of nursing and CNS practice through the use of the media, advanced technology, and community networks	Nurse and system	
G.8.b. Advocates for the CNS-APRN role and for positive legislative response to issues affecting nursing practice	Nurse and system	

From the National Association of Clinical Nurse Specialists. (2010). Clinical nurse specialist core competencies (www.nacns.org/docs/CNSCoreCompetenciesBroch.pdf).

Both the Hamric and NACNS models emphasize the importance of direct care; clinical expertise and direct care are basic to CNS practice. For this reason, the direct care of patients or clients sphere is the largest sphere in the NACNS model and encompasses the other two spheres. For examples of activities in this sphere, as expanded on by Lewandowski and Adamle (2009), see Box 14-1.

CNSs demonstrate all seven competencies across the three spheres of influence and often execute some competencies simultaneously. They exert influence in the nurses and nursing practice sphere by caring for patients directly and by serving as coaches, guides, and role models for nursing staff and other caregivers. They provide consultation. They demonstrate EBP competencies by working with staff to develop, implement, and evaluate EBPs. They may collaborate in clinical research, an activity likely to affect all three spheres of influence. Similarly, they collaborate and facilitate team development, assess and intervene to alleviate the moral distress inherent in clinical care, and create environments that support clinicians' ethical decision making. See Box 14-2 for examples, as described by Lewandowski and Adamle (2009). CNSs exert influence in the organizations and systems sphere by providing clinical and systems leadership in many ways, whether articulating nursing issues to team members, advocating for a patient, taking a stand on behalf of nurses, or evaluating the quality and cost-effectiveness of technologies and care processes. Box 14-3 lists activities in this sphere (Lewandowski & Adamle, 2009).

Throughout all three spheres, CNSs apply the nursing process; assessment, planning, implementation, and evaluation activities are designed to improve the care of patients, develop nurses, and improve the systems in which nurses work and care is delivered. Experienced CNSs understand that activities in each sphere of influence and their advanced practice competencies exert reciprocal influences on each other. Implementing competencies across the three spheres can result in improvements in clinical outcomes, patient safety, patient-family

BOX 14-1   Manage the Care of Complex and/or Vulnerable Populations

Expert Direct Care
1. Provide expert, in-depth, specialized assessment.
   a. Develop and implement assessment tools.
2. Provide evidence-based and/or theory-driven treatment and care of illness, symptoms, and responses to illness using advanced concepts related to the nursing process.
3. Provide patient and family education.
4. Develop methods of risk identification.
5. Use strategies that promote health and wellness.
6. Monitor and prescribe medication.
7. Order and interpret laboratory and diagnostic tests.
8. Perform advanced procedures.

Care Coordination and Collaboration
1. Facilitate movement of patients and families through and across health care settings.
2. Facilitate health care system access.
   a. Identify proactively high-risk patients and families.
   b. Provide case management.
   c. Provide outcomes management.
   d. Provide discharge planning.
   e. Provide community follow-up.
3. Advocate for patient and family.
   a. Serve as liaison between the patient and family and nurse and interdisciplinary team.
4. Facilitate communication among interdisciplinary team members.

Adapted from Lewandowski, W., and Adamle, K. (2009). Substantive areas of clinical nurse specialist practice: A comprehensive review of the literature. *Clinical Nurse Specialist, 23,* 73–90.

BOX 14-2 **Educate and Support Interdisciplinary Staff**

Education

1. Educate interdisciplinary staff.
   a. Provide formal classes.
   b. Provide informal, bedside teaching.
   c. Provide and/or facilitate patient care conferences.
   d. Provide and/or facilitate teaching rounds.
   e. Provide orientation for new staff.
   f. Conduct unit-based research forums.
2. Provide role modeling, preceptorship, and mentoring.
3. Disseminate knowledge through publication and conference presentations.

Consultation

1. Provide case consultation.
2. Provide administrative consultation.
   a. Develop forums for staff communication.
   b. Assist in conflict resolution among staff.
   c. Inform staff of organizational changes.
3. Evaluate and introduce new technology.

Collaboration

1. Serve as communication link between researcher and practitioner.
   a. Assist in developing evidence-based plans of care.
   b. Assist with research utilization.
2. Collaborate with nurse manager.
   a. Assist with financial planning for units.
   b. Assist in recruiting and retaining staff.
   c. Contribute to formal and informal evaluation of nursing staff.
   d. Coordinate work activities on unit.
   e. Serve as unit spokesperson.
3. Collaborate on clinical research projects.
4. Collaborate with academic institutions to educate undergraduate and graduate nurses.

Adapted from Lewandowski, W., and Adamle, K. (2009). Substantive areas of clinical nurse specialist practice: A comprehensive review of the literature. *Clinical Nurse Specialist, 23*, 73–90.

 BOX 14-3 **Facilitate Change and Innovation Within Health Care Systems**

Change Agency

1. Assess needs of patients, families, communities, nurses, and organizations.
2. Develop research-based protocols, policies/procedures, clinical pathways, and standards of care.
3. Cultivate unit culture that values research utilization and EBP.
4. Promote quality improvement.
   a. Identify and prioritize quality improvement issues.
   b. Develop indicators and methods to measure patient outcomes.
   c. Perform unit-based quality improvement studies.
   d. Perform audits.
5. Introduce innovative models of care.
6. Develop, implement, and evaluate programs.
7. Participate on advisory and policymaking boards and committees.

Adapted from Lewandowski, W., and Adamle, K. (2009). Substantive areas of clinical nurse specialist practice: A comprehensive review of the literature. *Clinical Nurse Specialist, 23*, 73–90.

changes in health care, reimbursement, and credentialing that have affected advanced practice nursing, CNSs have remained focused on championing excellence in nursing practice and on improving clinical care and the systems in which the care is delivered.

Without sustained engagement in direct care (direct care of patients or clients sphere), it would be difficult, if not impossible, to continue to be effective in the other two spheres, because the effectiveness depends on the CNS's clinical credibility. However, because CNSs provide more than just direct care, maintaining their commitment to patient care is often challenged as organizational priorities change. In the following sections, the ways in which CNSs implement the seven competencies across three spheres of influence are described.

Direct Clinical Practice

Specialization was the genesis of the CNS role, but expert clinical practice—and direct patient care—is its heart. The central competency of direct clinical practice is explicitly linked to the patient-client sphere of influence; the insights and outcomes of providing direct care influence the CNS's work in the other two spheres of nursing practice and systems.

satisfaction, resource allocation, professional nursing staff knowledge and skills, health care team collaboration, and organizational efficiency (Murray & Goodyear-Bruch, 2007; Ryan, 2009; Vollman, 2006).

The variety of activities, the challenge of in-the-moment problem solving that characterizes clinical work, and intermediate- and long-range planning efforts to improve the care of patients attract CNSs to this work. Throughout the history of CNS practice, and despite the

CNS practice includes advanced assessment skills and the integration of "biophysical, psychosocial, behavioral, sociopolitical, cultural, economic, and nursing science" (American Association of Colleges of Nursing [AACN], 2006b, p. 16) into specialized, expert nursing practice. Skills (clinical, advanced communication, and relational) and knowledge (theoretical, practical, and particular) are essential, but practical wisdom is a hallmark of advanced practice nursing (Oberle & Allen, 2001). Many authors have described strategies for successfully implementing the expert clinician dimension, building on the conceptual foundations of previous authors (Duffy, Dresser, & Fulton, 2009; Fulton, Lyon, & Goudreau, 2010; Zuzelo, 2010). Each strategy is highly dependent on the individual CNS and his or her practice setting and can fluctuate from year to year in relation to the prevailing health care environment. It is easy for the direct care component of the role to be overemphasized or underemphasized because of institutional priorities and competition for CNS expertise. The unique skill set of CNSs may result in them being continually pulled away from direct care to lead projects that are of high priority for the institution. Conversely, if an institution recognizes value only in the revenue generation component of direct care, the CNS may be required to focus exclusively on that component of the role. The CNS role is optimally enacted when CNSs have the opportunity to use what they have learned from direct clinical practice to improve care for individual patients, families, and patient populations, whether that occurs at the patient-CNS interface, through nursing personnel, or through organizational improvements.

Although clinical expertise is the cornerstone of CNS practice, a CNS's success will not be measured by clinical knowledge or technical expertise alone. Providing regular and consistent direct patient care is essential for the CNS to do the following:

- Evaluate the quality, effectiveness, efficiency, and safety of patient care and determine whether inadequacies are the result of a lack or ineffective use of nursing resources, insufficient equipment and supplies, or systems' inefficiencies; this assessment by CNSs has been characterized as surveillance (Brooten, Youngblut, Deatrick, et al., 2003; see Chapter 7).
- Demonstrate one's clinical competency and maintain clinical expertise, thereby role modeling clinical behaviors, establishing credibility, and maintaining team relationships and collegial trust.
- Identify nursing staff learning needs, including knowledge and skill development.
- Refine one's clinical expertise and reflective abilities.
- Maintain CNS credentials and certification.

Direct care, or direct clinical practice, refers to CNS activities and responsibilities that occur within the patient-nurse interface (see Chapter 7). For many years, a CNS's direct clinical practice was not clearly linked to measureable goals, such as patient outcomes or resource use. Thus, few data were available to justify the role and correlate its expense with the cost avoidance and quality improvement aspects of the role when health care institutions were restructuring their operating systems. However, most patients requiring the expertise of a CNS are sicker, more frail, and in need of specialized expert care. Clinical studies with high-risk patients, such as very-low-birth-weight (VLBW) infants, women with a high-risk pregnancy, and older adults with cardiac diagnoses, have consistently shown improved patient outcomes and reduced health care costs when CNSs and other APNs were directly involved with patient care, including assessing, teaching, counseling, and negotiating systems (Dejong & Veltman, 2004; Murray & Goodyear-Bruch, 2007; Ryan, 2009; Vollman, 2006).

A CNS is most likely to care directly for a patient whose diagnosis or care is complex, unique, or problematic. Examples of complex or problematic patients include a VLBW infant, frail older person with multiple hospital readmissions, child with complex congenital heart disease, young pregnant woman with a transplanted organ, or man diagnosed with bipolar disorder who has survived a suicide attempt but who requires prolonged physical rehabilitation. Examples of unique situations include the care of a child with a rigid external distraction device for midface advancement, evaluation and implementation of a new intervention, such as teletechnology to assess the efficacy of preventive interventions for pressure ulcers, and introduction of an experimental chemotherapeutic agent. CNSs have the advanced skills to care for these challenging patients by incorporating a holistic perspective, forming therapeutic partnerships, and using expert clinical thinking and skillful performance to optimize outcomes. The CNS has the access and ability to evaluate the latest evidence and apply it in diverse ways to manage complex cases.

Direct care also affords a CNS the opportunity to assess the quality of care for a specific patient population. This qualitative assessment enhances the interpretation of quantitative data and directs changes in care processes. For example, a CNS might notice a pattern of frequently missed clinic appointments for a heart failure patient. Through the therapeutic partnership, the CNS may determine that a lack of clinic parking results in a barrier for this patient to keep appointments. The outcome is not one of a noncompliant patient but a logistical failure that requires immediate resolution for the benefit of all clients with heart failure. When a home care nurse notes that older patients are not taking medications consistently, a CNS's engagement with those patients can provide a more detailed and complex assessment. The result of such an assessment may be that older patients are cognitively impaired and forget to take their medications, the medication regimen may be too complex, causing a patient to miss doses, or the medication may be too expensive and not covered by supplemental insurance or Medicaid, causing a patient to halve or skip doses and let prescriptions go unfilled. The CNS's evaluation might integrate advanced assessment skills, such as cognitive screening, into the admission assessment of all older patients, might identify therapeutic alternatives, such as a simpler or more economical medication regimen, to improve compliance, or might introduce other creative interventions to promote health and quality of life.

A CNS's clinical practice interventions may be continuous, in which the CNS carries a consistent caseload, or time-limited, regular, or episodic, in which the CNS cares for complex cases as they arise (Koetters, 1989). Examples of regular ongoing care include the following: providing care for high-risk newborns in a pediatric special care clinic; providing psychotherapy, medication management, and other specialized nursing care for patients requiring mental health care; delivering total patient care to the first patients in an innovative surgery program; or providing yearly comprehensive neurologic care for children with spina bifida in a hospital-based clinic. Episodic care helps a CNS assess and intervene in a particular problem. Examples of episodic care include planning and coordinating a patient's complex hospital discharge, facilitating a support group for families of children with hydrocephalus, and providing total patient care (similar to a staff nurse but with a different lens) to determine the feasibility of proposed changes in patient care or other system changes. Involvement in regular or episodic care enables CNSs to identify systems problems that interfere with care and require CNS intervention. Examples include lack of staff knowledge, the need for clinical policies or procedures, and the need for conflict mediation among team members. For each clinical situation, a CNS takes a comprehensive approach, using discriminative judgment, advanced knowledge, and expert skills, including expertise in the technical, humanistic, and organizational aspects of care. In these situations, CNSs are particularly skilled at the use of surveillance, quickly identifying patient and system issues and intervening to avoid further complications. A CNS intervention may be as simple as assisting a patient and family navigate a hospital's bureaucracy. A CNS knows how and when to break the rules and when to bypass organizational or philosophical roadblocks, thus ensuring the focus on the patient and family and a successful outcome.

If clinical skills (e.g., particularly psychomotor ones, such as administering chemotherapy and troubleshooting external ventricular drains) are not used periodically, CNSs become less proficient. Regular clinical practice helps a CNS maintain the expertise and clinical competence needed to practice and develop the skills of other nurses. In addition to maintaining and refining clinical skills, direct clinical practice is imperative at two pivotal points—during a CNS's orientation to establish credibility and before and occasionally throughout the implementation of organizational change to assess the impact of the change on patient care. CNSs must weigh the benefits and costs of different ways to implement direct care. Advantages, such as developing credibility with staff or maintaining one's skills, are evaluated against potential disadvantages, such as competing demands or time pressures. For example, the pediatric oncology CNS may need to prioritize responsibilities, such as talking with parents of a child newly diagnosed with neuroblastoma, performing a lumbar puncture on a 3-year-old with leukemia, teaching the pediatric chemotherapy class, and visiting the school of a child who has been treated with radiation and chemotherapy for a brain tumor and now has learning disabilities. In addition to episodic involvement with particular patients, a critical care CNS could schedule 8 hours of staff nursing per month to maintain clinical skills, assess staff needs and the quality of teamwork and communication, and identify obstacles to the delivery of care. This hands-on involvement helps a CNS understand the conditions under which nurses are expected to implement standards of care and ensure quality.

Clinical practice can also occur indirectly. For example, a CNS may delegate direct care to a staff nurse but still guide the care. A CNS's goal is always to improve the direct care skills and knowledge of staff nurses. A CNS may select a patient population in which there are recurrent problems, poor outcomes, or recidivism and then collaborate with members of the health care team to develop and implement standards of care, clinical pathways, clinical procedures, and/or quality or performance improvement plans. Implementation of and adherence to recommended practice changes should be evaluated to assess the impact of the change on outcomes, refine algorithms or guidelines, improve clinical management, and promote consistent adherence. Algorithms and guidelines are rarely self-sustaining and require a champion who continuously facilitates their implementation, constantly evaluating new evidence that may result in the need for revisions. This role is imperative if the algorithm or guideline is to be successful and achieve its intended outcome. A CNS is often the person to fulfill the champion role.

System responsibilities for evaluating technology and its impact on patients and resources is another facet of the CNS's indirect clinical practice. Technologic advances have accelerated changes in health care delivery. These advances, however, coupled with the pressure of cost containment, increased competition, heightened consumer expectations, and capped budgets, create conflicting demands and priorities. Technologic advances have provided the objective data necessary to make clinical judgments (e.g., medication titration based on hemodynamic indices), devices to remotely assess a patient (e.g., telemonitoring of vital signs and weights), and interventional alternatives to treat disease (e.g., fiberoptic, robotic, and virtual reality surgery). However, technology warrants close scrutiny, because with it comes responsibility to evaluate its impact on budgets, quality of care, the environment, risk-benefit ratios, staff, and patients.

Patient safety is integral to all aspects of direct and indirect clinical practice, including CNS availability to and support of novice nurses (Altmiller, 2010; Ebright, Urden, Patterson, et al., 2004). The CNS's familiarity with National Patient Safety Goals, the Agency for Health Research and Quality (AHRQ) patient safety network, teaching strategies from Quality and Safety Education in Nursing (QSEN), and Open School at the Institute for Healthcare Improvement (IHI) are resources that can help the CNS keep abreast of patient safety issues (AHRQ, 2012; IHI, 2012; QSEN, 2012; The Joint Commission [TJC], 2012). It is this direct clinical practice that empowers a CNS to assume a leadership role in evaluating patient safety, exploring root cause analyses, and preventing adverse events. A CNS facilitates change, influences others, and builds an atmosphere of trust in situations in which adverse events are investigated.

Although providing direct care to patients is a core competency, how CNSs provide direct care varies across CNS specialties and practice settings; it is determined by population needs, influenced by the expertise of other nursing personnel, and affected by regulatory designations of CNSs as APNs and their scopes of practice. When, how, for whom, and with whom direct care is given are fluid and are negotiated and renegotiated with professional nursing staff and organizational leadership, based on patients' needs and the knowledge and clinical skill of nursing personnel.

Exemplar 14-2 illustrates how one of the authors (CC), a pediatric CNS, uses her professional competencies to provide expert care to a specific patient population and demonstrates the importance of direct care to execution of the other CNS competencies. CC coordinates health care services for a large pediatric craniofacial population, specifically infants with craniosynostosis. The pediatric neurosurgeon with whom CC works uses a new, less invasive technique to correct craniosynostosis in young infants. To inform families and referring health care providers about craniosynostosis treatment in her hospital, CC has developed and maintains a craniosynostosis link on the institution's website. This minimally invasive surgical treatment—and its follow-up—has drawn patients from a large geographic area.

Guidance and Coaching

One of the essential components of the CNS role is that of expert coach. This role of coach, guide, or educator is one that facilitates transition from one situation to another and depends on the interaction of technical, clinical, and interpersonal competencies and self-reflection (see Chapter 8). Its development is also influenced by scholarly inquiry and the use, interpretation, and application of

---

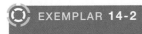 **EXEMPLAR 14-2**   **Direct Clinical Practice and Core Competencies of the Clinical Nurse Specialist**

I (CC) perform the preoperative history and physical examination in the clinic, order appropriate radiographs, laboratory tests, and consultations, and obtain cephalometric measurements and photographs for patients undergoing surgery for craniosynostosis. On the day of surgery, I notify the staff nurses who will be caring for the patient about pertinent findings and specific needs. Postoperatively, I assess the patient for adequate pain control, dietary needs, vital sign changes, incision status, swelling, and neurologic function. I facilitate discussions about these findings, staff nurses' concerns, parents' concerns and plan of care among care team members. I adapt standing orders for each patient in collaboration with the neurosurgeon.

Consultation
I am frequently consulted by staff nurses, referring physicians, or other APNs to assess misshapen heads by physical assessment or reviewing radiographs. These consultations provide opportunities to teach health care professionals how to recognize the differences between positional plagiocephaly and craniosynostosis, leading to earlier referrals for improved outcomes.

Guidance and Coaching
The Internet can be an excellent resource for families seeking health care information about medical conditions and treatment options. To help families learn more about craniosynostosis, I created a website that describes

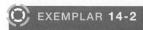 **EXEMPLAR 14-2**   **Direct Clinical Practice and Core Competencies of the Clinical Nurse Specialist—*cont'd***

the various types of craniosynostosis and treatment options, including a new, less invasive technique. As a result, I receive many inquiries from families seeking information about this new technique for their babies. Providing accurate information on the website is critical so that families can make informed decisions about surgery. Much of the preoperative teaching is done by telephone or in the clinic because parents and other family members have many questions.

I have educated nurses about the early recognition of craniosynostosis, surgical options, and positional plagiocephaly through professional journal articles, a book chapter, presentations at national nursing conferences, teaching at the school of nursing, and in-service education programs for the staff nurses. Mentoring graduate students has provided additional opportunities for role modeling.

Evidence-Based Practice

Collaboration on research with the pediatric neurosurgeon has yielded data demonstrating that the new surgical technique decreases patients' hospital stays, lowers costs, and improves patient outcomes. When parents noticed a sharp decrease in fussiness in their baby immediately after surgery, I developed a questionnaire to survey parents' perceptions of fussiness and irritability in their baby before and after surgery. Statistically significant decreases in fussiness and irritability were found postoperatively, suggesting that babies with craniosynostosis experience increases in intracranial pressure.

Leadership

In this unique role, I can provide care throughout the continuum, using clinical pathways to help families navigate the hospital system in an efficient manner. Bringing a baby to an unfamiliar city for surgery by surgeons that they have never met is a daunting experience for most parents. My leadership skills are put to the test coordinating preoperative donor-directed blood, arranging lodging at the Ronald McDonald House,

scheduling preoperative workups and follow-up appointments with the neurosurgeon, plastic surgeon, ophthalmologist, and anesthesiologist, and coordinating the postoperative molding helmet.

Collaboration

Collaboration occurs at many levels. First, I have a collaborative practice agreement with the pediatric neurosurgeon, as required by hospital policy and the state board of nursing. I collaborate with the staff nurses who care for the babies with craniosynostosis, providing in-service educational programs about the disorder and conducting rounds with them on the postoperative patients. Collaboration also occurs with other members of the craniofacial team, such as ophthalmologists, genetic counselors, plastic surgeons, and orthotic designers. I confer with referring health care providers to provide continuity after the patient leaves the hospital and between follow-up visits.

Ethical Decision Making

Although this new surgical treatment for craniosynostosis results in minimal blood loss, an infant will occasionally present with a low hemoglobin level or experience excessive intraoperative blood loss. Some families refuse blood transfusions for religious reasons, requiring more intensive preoperative preparation to minimize the need for a blood transfusion. Being present for the conversations that the neurosurgeon has with the family who refuses blood transfusion assists in understanding the reasons for refusing a blood transfusion and allows the CNS to reinforce the plan of care should the child need blood during or after surgery. A protocol for preoperative erythropoietin injections can be sent to the patient's pediatrician in an attempt to increase the hemoglobin level.

A great deal of preparation is required for a family to bring their baby to the hospital for this type of surgery. The CNS is instrumental in facilitating this process, using the core competencies and spheres of influence.

---

relevant research. CNSs use formal and informal coaching and teaching strategies with patients and families, nurses and nursing personnel, graduate nursing students, other clinical nurse specialists, health professionals, consumer groups, and organizations or systems (see Chapter 8).

Patients and Families

A CNS's expert coaching and guidance are pivotal in providing or influencing patient and family education. CNS

coaching and teaching complement the care given to a patient and family by other nurses and health professionals. CNSs continually seek better ways to coach patients and families using combinations of cognitive, educational, and behavioral strategies to improve patient education and adherence to interventions. However, a CNS cannot teach every patient and family and so must assess whom to teach. For example, a CNS could mentor a case manager or presurgical program educator to provide routine preoperative teaching for cardiac surgical patients. A CNS could then allocate more time to coach high-risk, complex, unusual, or challenging patients, such as a teenage girl with a recurrent brain tumor who is scared that she will die if she undergoes surgery again, or a young pregnant mother whose fetal MRI scan shows that her baby has spina bifida and must prepare to give birth to a child with special needs. A CNS may demonstrate to staff nurses how to facilitate difficult conversations with patients and their families by supporting the parents of a newborn who has died, working with a patient and family on end-of-life decisions, or "translating" a physician's technical explanation into lay terms.

As health care systems are restructured, there is increasing emphasis on patients' accountability for their own health. This means that in addition to coaching individuals, CNSs are even more likely to be involved in educational program planning and implementation aimed at helping groups of patients manage chronic illnesses and associated symptoms. Many patients know that they need to be better informed and educated about the health risk determinants, preventive self-care, treatment options, and risks and benefits of treatments, but their health care behaviors are influenced by many personal, psychological, and sociocultural factors. Because a patient is not always able or willing to change his or her lifestyle or to adhere to health care recommendations, a CNS must determine which patient or patient population is most appropriate for the advanced coaching requiring a CNS, such as a prenatal patient with poor social support living in an economically depressed community, an African American woman at risk of contracting human immunodeficiency virus (HIV), or a teenager who engages in risky behaviors. With many consumers seeking health care from nontraditional providers (Tindle, Davis, Phillips, et al., 2005), CNSs often help patients and providers integrate conventional and integrative therapies into care plans.

Nurses and Nursing Personnel

A CNS is a role model for nurses, demonstrating the practical integration of theory and EBP. Whereas nurse practitioners (NPs) and certified nurse-midwives (CNMs) primarily coach patients and families, a CNS strives continuously to improve clinical practice and integrate new knowledge into practice, thereby influencing the further development of the proficient and expert nurse and enhancing the staff nurse's accountability and self-sufficiency (Cronenwett, 2012). A CNS cannot be effective when she or he is or is perceived to be territorial, omnipotent, or omniscient (see Chapter 11). A CNS's time is often better spent by teaching others the why, what, and how of common patient care interventions rather than repeatedly

personally providing those same interventions. For example, a well-developed, standardized nursing care plan that details the assessment of different wound types and stages, with stage-specific interventions, will enable the nursing staff to provide consistent and evidence-based care to patients with the simpler types of wounds. The CNS is then appropriately consulted for complex wounds. Developing standards for patient education and providing resources to ensure consistency across populations are equally important CNS educational activities. As a staff nurse applies the new knowledge and skills taught by a CNS, the CNS can attend to new or more complex responsibilities. A staff nurse can become the role model for the skill mastered or the knowledge gained, and so a CNS's influence will continue to improve patient care. This notion of extending the reach of the CNS's expertise can be considered a defining characteristic of the coaching competency of CNS practice. The cycle of enrichment and growth is never complete. Whenever major staff turnover occurs or a CNS enters a new practice setting, the cycle must begin anew.

Students

A CNS has a professional responsibility to educate graduate nursing students and, when the opportunity arises, to be their mentor. In working with graduate nursing students in the classroom or clinical setting, a CNS shares knowledge, models the integration of practical and scientific knowledge into expert clinical practice, and demonstrates the level of advanced practice nursing to which a student can aspire. A CNS can provide opportunities for a graduate nursing student to do a clinical practicum or residency; the reward of working with an excellent student is being able to do more, extend one's influence more broadly, and make advanced practice expertise more widely available. In addition to providing patient care, a student completes projects (e.g., writing patient education materials or clinical procedures) or tasks (e.g., a literature review to support proposed changes in clinical practice) that also benefit the practice setting. A CNS may also be involved in the education of undergraduate nurses and other health professionals.

Other Health Care Providers and the Public

A CNS has many opportunities to educate other health care providers and consumer groups, usually more than one can reasonably fulfill. When considering such an opportunity, a CNS must determine whether the topic is within his or her specialty, the size of the audience or the number who can be reached, visibility (internal or external to the institution), and the potential for cost savings or revenue. For example, the CNS might volunteer to provide on-site care to campers attending specialty summer camps, such as a camp for those with spina bifida, diabetes, or cancer. Sometimes, such requests are opportunities to expand one's area of expertise. When the content is outside a CNS's specialty, however, the CNS has to prepare extensively to compensate for inexperience and risks overcommitment. In any case, a CNS must carefully balance teaching obligations within her or his practice setting with teaching requests outside the practice setting or immediate community. The more a CNS is pulled away from the practice setting, the higher the risk of becoming an invisible and, therefore an unnecessary, health care provider.

Consultation

The nursing literature offers classic descriptions of the essential components of consultation and strategies for ensuring the success of a CNS as a consultant (Barron, 1983, 1989; Gurka, 1991; Hamric, 1983b; Noll, 1987; Sneed, 1991; Sparacino & Cooper, 1990). Skill as a consultant cannot be assumed, although it is an expected CNS competency, and each CNS's consultative proficiency and the need to use this competency varies. The CNS can be in consultation to the patient; however, consultation also occurs when the CNS requests advice from another member of the health care team yet retains primary responsibility for that patient's care (see Chapter 9).

The consultation competency affects all three spheres of CNS influence. As a content expert, a CNS can suggest a wide range of alternative approaches or solutions to clinical or systems problems, whether internal or external to the practice setting. As a consultant, the CNS often directs staff to other resources (e.g., other colleagues, community resources, practice guidelines) that enable nurses and others to make decisions based on relevant and appropriate alternatives. A CNS is a process consultant and facilitates change so that decisions can be made for immediate and future situations (Sparacino & Cooper, 1990). Process activities and outcome achievement are two critical and measurable elements of the CNS consultation competency. Documenting consultations and linking them to outcomes are important. An example of this connection has been described by Gurka (1991), who used four consultative process activities (the fact finder, educator, informational expert, and advocate modes) from Lippitt and Lippitt's consultation model and measured three major outcomes (prevention of complications, maintenance or development of standards of care, and improvement in staff nurses' clinical judgment skills).

A CNS is both an internal and external consultant. Because consultation is becoming an increasingly important role for the CNS, care must be taken to optimize opportunities to mentor other staff in following through

with recommendations; otherwise, the CNS may be pulled in too many directions.

Internal Consultation

Internal consultation includes assisting staff and facilitating organizational development in one's own practice setting, especially through the creative use of resources and alternative strategies to overcome or eliminate perceived system obstacles. A CNS may determine that a request for internal consultation requires the collaboration of a number of consultants, including other CNSs and members of other disciplines. A CNS often initiates the plan, mobilizes the resources, convenes team meetings, defuses the politics, and facilitates the resolution. Examples of CNS consultation from the literature and our own experiences include the following:

- A liaison psychiatric CNS consults with an obstetric-gynecologic department to screen and provide treatment for mental health problems in women (D'Afflitti, 2004).
- A pediatric CNS (neurosurgery) consults with a pediatric CNS (endocrine) about hormone replacement for a 13-year-old girl who recently underwent resection of a pituitary tumor and now has panhypopituitarism.
- A behavioral health CNS and critical care CNS collaborate and lead a multidisciplinary team to implement a standardized assessment tool and treatment protocol for alcohol withdrawal (Phillips, Haycock, & Boyle, 2006).
- An oncology CNS who rarely cares for patients with brain tumors consults a neurology or neurosurgery CNS when brain tumor patients are admitted for assistance in developing a care plan that addresses neurologic deficits and ensures the effective monitoring of potential complications.
- A neurologist consults with a cardiovascular surgery CNS for assistance in preparing a patient admitted with a brain abscess and a previously undiagnosed congenital cardiac anomaly for urgent cardiac surgery.
- A maternal child CNS consults with a pediatric CNS (neurosurgery) before assisting the parents of a 24-week premature baby with grade IV intraventricular hemorrhage and hydrocephalus with treatment decisions.

External Consultation

External consultation occurs apart from the CNS's practice or employment setting. External consultation offers approaches or solutions to specific problems to assist the nursing profession, a specialty organization, other health care providers, and health systems. External consultation may require ongoing intensive interaction to effect significant change (Rantz, Popejoy, Petroshki, et al., 2001). Examples of external consultation include the following

- A geriatric care CNS consults with nursing homes about the clinical decision making processes involved in preventing falls and reducing restraint use (Wagner, Capezuti, Brush, et al., 2007).
- A pediatric CNS (neurosurgery) in a children's hospital provides consultation for the medical-surgical CNS in an adult clinic about transitioning care of the 18-year-old spina bifida patient with shunted hydrocephalus.
- The local chapter of Pilot International asks the pediatric CNS (neurosurgery) to speak at local skate parks to skateboarders and their parents about the dangers of skateboarding head injuries and the importance of wearing a helmet.

Unless internal or external consultation is a CNS's primary responsibility (e.g., the internal consultation provided by a psychiatric liaison CNS), problems may arise if a CNS's time is used more for consultations than for direct care. The impact on patient care is less visible unless the content and process of consultations are well documented and the outcomes are measured. See Chapter 9 for further discussion of documenting and evaluating the consultation competency.

Evidence-Based Practice

In implementing the EBP competency, CNSs involvement in the evaluation and improvement of nursing practice and activities may range from scholarly inquiry to formal scientific investigation. The Doctor of Nursing Practice (DNP) degree adds to the knowledge base of traditional master's programs for CNSs by expanding depth in EBP and quality improvement (AACN, 2012). DNP-prepared CNSs can implement the science developed by nurse researchers, such as those with a PhD or Doctor of Nursing Science (DNS) degree (AACN, 2012). There has been increasing collaboration between PhD-prepared nurses and CNSs in the clinical setting, in which the CNS lends clinical expertise to the research component (Fulton, 2011). The three specific EBP competencies, each of which has basic and advanced levels of activity, are interpretation and use of research findings (evidence- or research-based practice), participation in collaborative research, and evaluation of practice (see Chapter 10).

CNSs have the knowledge, skills, and clinical expertise to use EBP to transform the work environment and support clinical practice. Nurse-sensitive indicators have been defined that capture nursing's unique contributions to patient outcomes. Assuming responsibility for

identifying nursing-sensitive and multidisciplinary quality indicators (Duffy, 2002; Kleinpell & Gawlinski, 2005), and using outcome data to improve patient care delivery are prime opportunities for a CNS to assess patient care strategies and community systems, analyze interdisciplinary communication and collaboration, coordinate care, and monitor patient and system progress. Much work has yet to be done, however, to develop the science linking nursing, health care processes, available measures, and quality outcomes (Naylor, 2007). There has been an increase in collaboration between CNSs in clinical practice and school of nursing faculty, which serves to support EBP in practice settings (Fulton, 2011). All CNSs must demonstrate the EBP competency and have ongoing accountability for monitoring and improving their practice and the practice of other nurses (NACNS, 1998, 2004b). CNSs implement this competency in a variety of ways, depending on experience, expertise, circumstances, setting, and resources. The following discussion illustrates how CNSs implement the EBP competency.

Interpretation and Use of Research and Evidence in Practice

Evidence-based practice has become an umbrella term for research utilization, research-based practice, or outcomes research (Jennings, 2000; see Chapter 10). Integration of new scientific findings and science-based knowledge influences the development and evaluation of new approaches to clinical practice (AACN, 2006b).

For CNSs, the interpretation and use of research and evidence often begins with a clinical question identified by the CNS or staff with whom he or she works. Knowledge is the basis for practice but, too frequently, routine practice may not be based on sound evidence. The foundation of improved quality of care and patient outcomes is the analysis of research-based evidence and consensus-dependent practice changes to ensure best practice and achieve quality patient care. Inherent in the CNS role is the evaluation of the appropriateness of evidence and the application of its findings to clinical practice. A CNS is the ideal clinician to assess factors that are barriers and facilitators to change and to develop, implement, and evaluate EBP. EBP is integrated into clinical procedures, administrative policies, educational materials for patients and staff, and clinical pathways. A CNS's involvement in developing policies and procedures means that evidence informs clinical processes and standards.

A CNS who develops an evidence-based guideline of care for a patient population promotes improved patient outcomes throughout the three spheres of influence. The patient's physical or mental function improves, treatment is safer and with fewer complications, there is continuity of care across the health care continuum, and nursing practice improves (McCabe, 2005). Multiple examples of CNS-led evidence-based practice can be found in the literature. CNS contributions to improving patient outcomes by providing evidence-based care include the following: implementation of scheduled oral care for ventilator patients that decreased the incidence of ventilator-associated pneumonia in the neurointensive care unit to zero (Fields, 2008); reduction of CNS prescribing errors (O'Malley, 2007); the design of a weight management program for African Americans (Walker-Sterling, 2005); and an innovative quality initiative to facilitate transition between the intensive care unit (ICU) and the medical wards (St-Louis & Brault, 2011). One Western academic hospital system used a CNS-led council to mentor staff nurses in promoting evidence-based nursing care (Becker, Dee, Gawlinski, et al., 2012). CNSs had a leadership role in transforming a policy and procedure committee into a clinical practice council in which nursing practice was evidence-based.

Evaluation of Practice

At the most basic level, this competency requires that a CNS evaluate her or his practice across spheres of influence. Several authors have discussed CNS evaluation from a variety of perspectives, including self-evaluation, staff evaluation, and peer review (Cooper & Sparacino, 1990; Girouard, 1996; Girouard & Spross, 1983; Hamric, 1983a, 1989). Peer review is not institutional performance evaluation. In a peer review, the key participants are other practicing CNSs; essential elements are clinical practice, leadership, and professional behaviors (Briggs, Heath, and Kelley, 2005). Although many CNS specialties develop practice setting–specific evaluation tools, a standardized tool should be developed for expected competencies and the assurance of outcome quality. Lunney and colleagues (2007) have designed a tool for graduate students to use for self-evaluation of CNS competency development, which could be adapted for practicing CNSs. Portfolios can be used as a tool to evaluate CNS practice, as exemplified by the model developed in Ohio that merges the APRN standards, relationship-based care, and Magnet forces to recognize professional development (Hespenheide, Cottingham, & Mueller, 2011).

CNSs may document the components of their clinical practice, including the following: numbers of patients seen, types and frequencies of interventions, and outcomes achieved; educational activities for staff, including one-on-one coaching, in-service programs, orientation, and continuing education; and system initiatives, such as quality improvement activities and interdisciplinary rounds (AACN, 2006b). To evaluate one's ability and effectiveness in exercising influence, a CNS may ask nursing and interdisciplinary colleagues to comment on his or her communication and collaboration skills. CNSs may use this information for self-assessment to determine whether the allocation of activities is consistent with personal, professional, and institutional goals, to prepare quarterly reports, or to assemble a portfolio for one's annual evaluation. Tracking these data enables CNSs to identify recurring events that may require an intervention at the staff or system level and midcourse corrections if schedule demands require a shift in goals or a realignment of expectations.

In the early days of CNS practice, few studies documented the impact of CNSs on patient and family outcomes. The evidence is mounting, however, and the positive impact on patient outcome is irrefutable (see Chapter 24). Some hospitals hire CNSs specifically for their positive impact on patient outcomes (Scherff & Siclovan, 2009). One should expect optimal patient outcomes when CNS competencies complement patient needs or characteristics (Becker, Kaplow, Muenzen, et al., 2006). Outcome studies can help CNSs document their activities and their effects on patient and family outcomes. Classic studies include evaluation of the impact of CNS interventions on LBW infants and older patients in the hospital (Brooten, Kumer, Brown, et al., 1986; Neidlinger, Kennedy, & Scroggins, 1987). CNSs are positioned by their direct patient care to evaluate protocols and use National Patient Safety Goals to prevent errors. More recent studies have shown the impact of CNS interventions on causes of medication errors (Flanders & Clark, 2010) and, specifically, in regard to revising a policy on labeling medications and solutions on the sterile field in the operating room (Brown-Brumfield & DeLeon, 2010). As these topics suggest, CNSs can identify relevant structure, process, and outcome variables that can be used to assess the CNSs' contributions to quality patient care. How CNSs use clinical practice guidelines and their effect on clinical outcomes should also be evaluated. The relationship between implementation and outcomes may depend on the recency of the scientific evidence (Cunningham, 2006) and sensitivity of outcomes to nursing practice, such as symptom experience, functional status, prevention of adverse events, and psychological distress (Gobel, Beck, & O'Leary, 2006).

Evaluation of CNS practice often includes outcomes management (AACN, 2006b). One component of outcomes management is the analysis of data regarding care efficiency and cost-effectiveness, the results of which guide systematic and continuous process and performance improvement. Examples include evidenced-based ventilator-acquired pneumonia prevention programs (Fields, 2008; Murray & Goodyear-Bruch, 2007) and a CNS-directed program to reduce pressure ulcers in vulnerable intensive care patients (Vollman, 2006). CNSs have also been instrumental in developing a hospital-wide process that promoted EBP guidelines through research, patient safety workshops, nursing staff orientation, professionalism, quality of work life, and prevention of falls (Ford, Rolfe, & Kirkpatrick, 2011).

Practice evaluation must be integrated into one's daily work. Although researchers have begun to identify the interventions used most often by APNs, most of this work has been done in the evaluation of primary care or as part of programs evaluating the interventions of CNSs and NPs providing transitional care to discharged patients (Brooten, Kumer, Brown, et al., 1986; Brooten, Naylor, York, et al., 2002; see Chapter 23 for additional research evidence of APN impact).

Participation in Collaborative Research

Although the number of PhD-prepared CNSs with the training to conduct research is increasing, most CNSs are prepared at the master's and DNP level and can be partners in collaborating on research relevant to practice. Collaborative research between a CNS and researcher facilitates the application of research findings to clinical practice. Researchers provide CNSs with new evidence for patient care practices and the assessment of their impact. The PhD-prepared CNS collaborates with peer CNSs by using advanced research skills to appraise journal articles critically and set up research designs, as well as facilitate contacts with other faculty. They are the bridge between bench and bedside. In turn, CNSs stimulate researchers to investigate the science that explains their observations of patients and populations. A CNS-led initiative to foster collaboration between hospital staff nurses and university faculty resulted in increased partnerships between faculty and nursing staff and the initiation of research projects focusing on quality improvement (Zinn, Reinert, Bigelow, et al., 2011).

Typically, novice CNSs are not involved in collaborative research because the competencies that are directly related to patient care should be mastered first. For experienced CNSs, collaborative research is often a realistic CNS goal. Whether novice or experienced CNSs become involved in research depends on the setting, pregraduate and graduate school experience, resources within the setting, and access to research expertise. Many CNSs find satisfaction with involvement in research as a consultant or co-investigator. A CNS is the clinical expert, understands clinical issues, has access to patients, and can anticipate clinical and system challenges that may occur throughout the research process. A nurse researcher is a research expert, knows research methodology, and has access to the resources that support the research. The CNS is optimally positioned to stimulate a researcher's interest

because of her or his direct clinical association with patients or participant populations (Nelson, Holland, Derscheid, et al., 2007). Before participating in a research project, a CNS must determine whether there is readiness and receptiveness in the practice setting and administrative support, and whether research activities are a realistic performance goal.

Interdisciplinary collaborative research offers opportunities and benefits, including an enriched practice environment, examination of clinically relevant issues, and policy and practice improvements (Disch, Chlan, Mueller, et al., 2006). CNSs know the organizational and social facilitators and barriers to clinical research, can bridge the academic-clinical gap, and can assist in recruiting and retaining research participants (Fitzgerald, Tomlinson, Peden-McAlpine, et al., 2003; Nelson et al., 2007). Whatever the model, a CNS is a key player in developing and implementing relevant nursing-sensitive and multidisciplinary quality indicators for measuring patient and system outcomes.

In addition to applying research findings to clinical practice, CNSs can use research to influence public policy. Although conducting prospective research to address statutory or regulatory initiatives has rarely been carried out, research results can provide substantive and objective facts that are more powerful and meaningful than impassioned pleas. There is extensive data in professional, state, and national data banks but these data must be translated into language that is understandable and easily communicated.

CNSs have an important role in helping a hospital achieve and maintain Magnet status (Walker, Urden, & Moody, 2009). Hospital-based CNSs are in a unique position to contribute to Magnet status of the hospital because of their education in the three spheres of influence (Newhouse, 2009). Although sometimes known as an invisible champion, the CNS is often able to identify quality and systems issues and, using EBP, lead interdisciplinary teams to improve patient outcomes and decrease costs (Kleinpell, 2007; LaSala, Connors, Pedro, et al., 2007).

Leadership

CNSs serve as leaders of multidisciplinary quality improvement teams because of their unique preparation at the graduate level with master's degrees, practice doctorate degrees, or research doctorates (Purvis, Brown, Chan, et al., 2012). The CNS uses advanced communication and leadership skills to evaluate practice and effect change in complex health care delivery systems (AACN, 2006b). It is because of these very leadership skills that CNSs are often pulled away by administration to lead other initiatives. There are different domains, types, and attributes of leadership (see Chapter 11). Leadership is integral to the role because a CNS has responsibility for clinical innovation and change within the patient care system. A CNS has significant formal and informal impact and must be visionary yet practical. Through a CNS's clinical and systems leadership, change strategies are implemented and nursing practice and patient care improve. A CNS is the link between many disciplines and resources and asserts clinical and professional leadership in the practice setting or health care system, in health care policy and delivery decisions, and in the administration of direct care programs. A CNS identifies the need for practice changes and leads the development and implementation of clinical procedures, practice guidelines, and clinical pathways, designs and directs performance improvement initiatives, chairs interdisciplinary committees or manages clinical projects, and influences or guides institutional health care policy decisions. Clinical and professional leadership competencies are integrated with the other CNS competencies to support an organization's purpose and goals.

Most health care organizations are a bureaucratic maze. A CNS works with and advocates for staff, patients, and families to help them understand the complexities and wend their way through the system. Because of the CNS's communication skills and knowledge of diplomacy, a CNS can be a facilitator among staff, administration, and patients during organizational change, problem solving, or conflict resolution. A CNS can facilitate the design, implementation, and evaluation of a clinical information system, leading the collaboration between computer designers and users, integrating the needs of clinicians and patients, and facilitating innovative practice changes (Roggow, Solie, & Tracy, 2005). As leaders, CNSs also help the members of one discipline understand the priorities of another discipline and often negotiate agreements that bring diverse perspectives into alignment. This mediation benefits patients, promotes communication, and creates an environment that fosters collaboration, as discussed in the next section.

Collaboration

CNSs must be skilled at collaboration because so many people regularly work and interact with a CNS (see Chapter 12). A CNS collaborates with nurses, physicians, other health care providers, and patients and their families, providing an interface among them (AACN, 2006b). The Institute of Medicine (IOM) report, *The Future of Nursing: Leading Change, Advancing Health,* has recommended that opportunities be expanded for nurses to "lead and diffuse collaborative improvement efforts"

(IOM, 2011, p. 11). Many patients have such complex health care needs that no one health care professional can manage them all. CNSs understand the knowledge and skills of other team members and actively participate in or lead interdisciplinary teams and rounds. A CNS can assist a patient and family members determine their needs; help them ask questions and assess treatment options; and facilitate timely referrals to other disciplines to ensure a positive outcome. Throughout his or her interactions with patients and colleagues, a CNS models the communication and collaboration skills that help teams mature.

A CNS can be thought of as an attending nurse, teacher, and role model for nursing staff. CNSs often identify potential or actual conflicts, and CNS advocacy often prevents adversarial situations and their negative sequelae. A CNS must be skilled in helping team members address and negotiate conflicts to optimize patient care. The outcome of CNS-coordinated collaboration is the empowerment of nurses and recognition of the nurse as a critical member of the health care team. This results in team building, synergy, and integrative solutions. CNSs and physicians also collaborate, although some practice settings and working relationships are more conducive to partnership than others. The IOM report on the *Future of Nursing* has recommended that nurses be educated with physicians and other health care professionals as students and that interdisciplinary experiences occur throughout their careers (IOM, 2010). Collaboration between a CNS and organizations outside the health care realm, such as academia and industry, can be mutually beneficial and improve patient care (Benedict, Robinson, & Holder, 2006; Kerfoot, Rapala, Ebright, et al., 2006). Patient health problems have become increasing complex and require more interdependence to manage (Brooten, Youngblut, Hannan, et al., 2012). Ongoing research has shown that quality care and patient outcomes improve when CNSs collaborate as equals with other health care providers (Naylor, 2011).

Collaboration between a CNS and other health care professionals leads to effective and efficient health care, especially for complex patient populations. CNSs can integrate the insights of many individuals with different perspectives, with each providing theoretical and applied knowledge. Collaboration is an essential competency— the well-earned result of clinical competence, effective communication, mutual trust, the valuing of complementary knowledge and skills, collegiality, and a favorable organizational structure (Benedict et al., 2006; D'Afflitti, 2004; Phillips et al., 2006; see Chapter 12). For example, a pediatric CNS for neurosurgery collaborated with the pediatric hospitalist in the care of a 16-year-old adolescent with a recently resected pituitary tumor and a history of anorexia; their goal was to maintain her independence and still provide optimum nutrition. Further collaboration with the pediatric CNS for endocrinology was essential to coordinate hormone replacement therapy with other therapies. A transitional care model (TCM) is a nurse-led, evidenced-based approach to transitioning chronically ill, high-risk adults from the hospital to home, which requires interdisciplinary collaboration and coordination, an ideal role for the CNS (Naylor, 2011).

Blurring of boundaries can occur as the CNS role develops. These boundaries can overlap between the CNS and staff nurse or even between the CNS and another APN. As a pediatric CNS teaches the mother of a child with traumatic brain injury how to comfort him without raising his intracranial pressure, she is delivering direct patient care and role modeling for the orientee caring for that child. Blurred boundaries are also evident when a pediatric neurosurgery CNS and pediatric oncology CNS collaborate to plan the comprehensive discharge care for a 10-year-old child with a recently resected brain tumor who required radiation therapy, chemotherapy, and a plan for reintegration into his school. Such collaboration with others in the health care system enables a CNS to influence their colleagues to improve patient care across specialties, not just for the particular patient but in future situations in which patients' needs are similar. CNSs must avoid being territorial; this limits their effectiveness and they are unlikely to develop positive relationships that could help patients and families navigate the health care system efficiently.

Ethical Decision Making

CNSs often identify or consult on ethical issues and facilitate their resolution. In some cases, a CNS is consulted on what staff perceive is a clinical issue but really turns out to be an ethical concern. Being able to recognize, name, and address the moral distress and ethical concerns that are inherent in clinical care is a crucial part of CNS practice. A CNS can significantly influence the negotiation of moral dilemmas, direction of patient care, access

to care, and allocation of resources. CNSs consider numerous factors when making ethical decisions, including professional and religious codes, cultural values, bioethical principles, and ethical theories (see Chapter 13). The CNS also has ethical responsibilities when conducting, facilitating, or collaborating in research activities, such as adhering to ethical standards for research and obtaining informed consent (Steinke, 2004).

CNSs have similar responsibilities when applying ethical decision making skills to patient and organizational issues. They recognize clinicians' experiences of moral distress and articulate moral dilemmas, often serving as advocates for patients, families, and staff. They interpret and mediate patient, family, and team members' views to ensure as complete a discussion of the dilemma as possible. They recognize the need to consult an ethics committee and often initiate that consult. When necessary, CNSs validate staff nurses' concerns and help nurses present their concerns to other team members, ensuring that the nursing perspective is considered when ethical issues are discussed. When CNSs are excluded from interdisciplinary ethical decisions, opportunities for effective nursing care are minimized and outcomes, such as timely and appropriate end-of-life care, are compromised (Oddi & Cassidy, 1998). Because CNSs facilitate optimal care for frailer and sicker patients, the ethical challenge is to balance the expectations for quality care with the limitations of appropriate care and articulate the moral dilemmas for patients, nursing personnel, and organizations.

Exemplar 14-3, a composite case, illustrates the multidimensional and complex nature of CNS practice, implementing the substantive clinical areas of CNS practice and including the seven competencies across three spheres of influence. Exemplar 14-3 discusses a critically ill woman with complex medical problems, her distraught and divided family, a concerned but overwhelmed physician, and many caring but inexperienced nursing staff members. Key elements, including pragmatic implementation of CNS competencies and the impact of the CNS in a

---

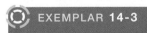 **EXEMPLAR 14-3**   **Advanced Practice Competencies and Spheres of Influence: Clinical Nurse Specialist Practice with a Complex Patient***

HH, an 82-year-old woman, was brought by paramedics to the emergency department with acute abdominal pain and severe pulmonary congestion. For the past few weeks, HH had been experiencing dyspnea on exertion and was unable to walk more than a few steps. These symptoms progressively worsened. She was having severe respiratory distress at rest and slept elevated on three pillows.

HH's medical history included insulin-dependent diabetes mellitus, hypertension, atrial fibrillation, coronary artery disease, critical aortic stenosis, severe heart failure, mild chronic obstructive pulmonary disease (COPD), chronic renal insufficiency, chronic urinary tract infections, and obesity. On admission, HH was alert and oriented but somnolent, and she had labored breathing. Pertinent diagnostic results from the chest

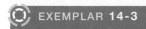

EXEMPLAR 14-3   **Advanced Practice Competencies and Spheres of Influence: Clinical Nurse Specialist Practice with a Complex Patient*—cont'd**

x-ray examination showed mild cardiac enlargement, pulmonary edema, left pleural effusion, and calcification of the aortic valve. A cardiac catheterization showed severe calcification of the aortic valve not amenable to valvuloplasty.

In discussing the results of the examinations with HH, it became clear that she wanted the valve replaced surgically, despite the extensive risks of the surgery at her age and in her condition. The surgeon and staff nurses expressed discomfort with the patient's request; therefore, the CNS (PSAS) was consulted.

PSAS met the patient and her family to assess the situation. HH seemed withdrawn and had poor eye contact and limited interaction. PSAS also recognized that English was the patient's second language. The son was very vocal about preferences for his mother's care, but the older daughter had multiple personal crises and tended to defer to her two sons (HH's grandsons). The younger daughter was hesitant to voice opinions about medical decisions. HH stated that she did not want to continue living as a "cardiac cripple" and continued to demand the surgery.

PSAS believed that several interventions needed to occur to ensure that HH was making an informed decision and that appropriate consideration of risks had been taken by everyone involved. PSAS facilitated a health team care conference with all disciplines to review the case and clarify the risks of proceeding with the surgery. Because there was concern about the language barrier, PSAS also facilitated a care conference with the health care team, HH, her family, and an interpreter. This satisfied the health care team that HH clearly understood her options.

PSAS performed a literature search and spoke with the surgeon to clarify the risks versus benefits of this surgery in an octogenarian. She initiated an ethics committee consult with the staff to discuss concerns related to moral distress about performing surgery in an older patient with such a high risk for a poor outcome. She held multiple in-services to discuss the literature search results and ethical principles involved in proceeding with the surgery. She used the expertise of her psychiatric CNS colleague to help staff identify communication techniques for maintaining optimal relationships with the patient and family.

PSAS also recognized that HH had not completed an advance directive. She initiated a consult with the palliative care team, who discussed with HH how she envisioned her postoperative care. As a result, HH completed an advance directive and made her wishes

known not to be indefinitely dependent on external life support.

HH had the surgery to replace her aortic valve with a tissue valve. Her postoperative course was complicated by another surgery to control bleeding, hypotension requiring pharmacologic support, complete heart block requiring a pacemaker, and low urine output. Because of her COPD, HH was difficult to wean from the ventilator and required a percutaneous tracheostomy placement. Because of her diabetes, her sternal wound failed to heal. An episode of sepsis resulted in renal failure, requiring continuous renal replacement therapy (CRRT). PSAS was active in assisting the novice and experienced nurses to provide direct care to this challenging patient and teaching them new procedures, such as assisting with placement of a tracheostomy at the bedside, managing fluid balance in a cardiac patient with CRRT, and managing skin care needs for a sacral pressure wound.

HH's family continued to have difficulty reaching a consensus and showed frustration with the situation. They had unrealistic expectations related to the likelihood of HH's recovery and believed that staff should "cure her," despite the extensive discussions before surgery regarding the high surgical risks and poor prognosis. PSAS facilitated multiple care conferences with the health care team and family to keep communication lines open.

Approximately 6 weeks after surgery, it became clear that HH would likely never be weaned from the ventilator and would need to be placed in a long-term care facility. PSAS facilitated one final care conference with the health care team and family to discuss HH's poor likelihood of improvement and review her advance directive. With assistance from the health care team, the family decided that in accordance with HH's wishes, she should be transitioned to comfort care and have the ventilator removed and dialysis discontinued. PSAS reassured the family that the patient's pain would be well managed, and she spoke with them about the rituals important to them in facilitating end-of-life care. PSAS ensured that HH's wishes were honored, such as having spiritual music played in the room and a bedside prayer service led by her pastor. With her extended family present, HH died several days after the transition to comfort care.

Commentary
Direct Care
PSAS demonstrated skill in performing direct care for HH, including tracheostomy care, complex sternal

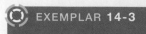

EXEMPLAR 14-3   **Advanced Practice Competencies and Spheres of Influence: Clinical Nurse Specialist Practice with a Complex Patient*—cont'd**

wound care, and CRRT, in expert communication skills in the original assessment of patient and family needs, and in ongoing discussions of difficult issues with the family, staff, and interdisciplinary team (direct care of patients or clients sphere). Because of her advanced illness, English as a second language, and complex family dynamics, this patient was deemed as a complex and vulnerable patient who could benefit from CNS intervention (direct care sphere).

Guidance and Coaching

PSAS was active in role modeling and coaching staff nurses in the complex care required by HH and her family. She tailored her coaching interventions to the experience level of the nurse. She also coached the family as they worked to make decisions about HH's care (direct care of patients or clients sphere, nurses and nursing practice sphere).

Consultation

PSAS maintained good communication with the staff nurses and interdisciplinary team, creating an environment in which they felt comfortable consulting in a difficult situation. PSAS sought consultation from colleagues to ensure optimal care (all three spheres).

Evidence-Based Practice

PSAS used her skills in searching and evaluating the literature to clarify the risks of this type of surgery in an octogenarian. She used evidence to support implementation of new treatments (direct care of patients or clients sphere, nurses and nursing practice sphere).

Leadership

PSAS demonstrated leadership across several competencies and spheres of influence. She knew when and how to bring consultants into the case. She made certain that the nurses' concerns were represented in discussions with the physician and she facilitated team meetings so that staff felt empowered to participate and communicate with colleagues. She ensured continuity of care and communication during HH's prolonged hospital stay, demonstrating both clinical and systems leadership (organization and systems sphere).

Collaboration

PSAS facilitated interactions with multiple individuals—patient, family members, staff, physicians, and consultants. The case demonstrates aligning multiple, conflicting perspectives to maintain appropriate care as everyone's central purpose (nurses and nursing practice sphere, organization and systems sphere).

Ethical Decision Making

PSAS's expertise in ethical decision making enabled her to remain objective and to elicit and discuss staff nurses' moral distress, interpret their concerns to team members, and explain the ethical principles underlying all decisions. This enabled the staff to provide good care and respect HH's autonomy (all three spheres).

*We wish to thank Patricia S. A. Sparacino, PhD, RN, FAAN, for this exemplar.

complex and uncertain situation, are emphasized. The commentary explains how the author applied the competencies across the spheres of influence.

Current Marketplace Forces and Concerns

The CNS has been viewed as an expert nurse; role contributions have focused on improving outcomes primarily for populations of patients through process improvements and education of staff. CNS contributions in the areas of nursing education and systems improvements have improved patient care, specifically in the areas of decreasing lengths of stay in the hospital, decreasing costs, reducing complications, and increasing patient satisfaction (Newhouse et al., 2011). These outcomes are vitally important in the new era of health care reform and should continue to be a part of the CNS role. Also, at the same time, these activities are not solely in the

domain of advanced practice nursing. There are many very qualified and exceptional nurses (e.g., quality and performance improvement nurses, nurse administrators, and nurse educators) and non-nurses who contribute to the improvements within the health care system, similar to the CNS. So, this leads to the question, what are the unique contributions of a CNS at the APN level? Until now, the CNS community has debated the issue with mixed results and has had difficulty articulating the difference clearly as a unified voice. In 2012, current challenges lie predominantly in the domain of regulatory and statutory debates. Events over the past decade have exemplified these challenges. However, before the issues related to CNS licensure and regulation of practice can be understood, it is important to understand the concepts of scope of practice and delegated authority (see Chapter 21 for a detailed discussion of these concepts).

Scope of Practice and Delegated Authority

A scope of practice is a state-based legal framework (i.e., statutes, codes, and regulations) that defines who is authorized to provide clearly delineated services, to whom and under what circumstances those services can be provided, and who can be reimbursed for those services. All health professions have an autonomous domain of practice and a delegated authority within the medical domain (Lyon, 2004). The autonomous domain of nursing practice "encompasses the diagnosis of health conditions (e.g., nursing diagnoses) that are amenable to nursing interventions [and] therapeutics, the implementation of interventions, and evaluation of the effectiveness of nursing interventions [and] therapeutics" (Lyon, 2004, p. 9).

Historically, the medical profession developed a broad, overarching scope of practice that encompassed almost all health care activities (see Chapter 1; Safriet, 2010). As a consequence, other health professionals (e.g., nurses, physical therapists, pharmacists) have had to carve out their scopes of practice out of the medical scope of practice. The ANA's restrictive 1955 definition of nursing reinforced the practice of nursing as having independent functions and being dependent on and delegated to by the profession of medicine. It also prohibited nurses from diagnosing and prescribing.

This history has contributed to a false dichotomy of what constitutes nursing practice and medical practice. As Chapter 1 has demonstrated, the practice of nursing has evolved over time to take on more responsibility and skills once considered to be the sole domain of medicine. As discoveries about health and illness continue to progress, the knowledge and skills of professional nurses and other health professionals will continue to evolve in their own right and the professional practice will advance into traditional boundaries of medicine

(Standards for supervision of nursing practice, 1983). Physicians will need to become specialists and treat the most complicated or complex patients. Therefore, nursing scopes of practice, educational curricula, and competency validation need to stay flexible to evolve over time (Hartigan, 2011).

For CNSs specifically, delegated authority continues to pose an issue as APNs establish their independent scopes of practice. In order for CNSs to provide specialty care in an expanded role to meet the needs of more patients who will need care under the PPACA, CNSs will need an independent scope of practice. Inefficiencies in the health care system will be created and patients will not be able to obtain timely care if physician supervision is required.

Institute of Medicine *Future of Nursing* Report

The 2010 Institute of Medicine report, *The Future of Nursing: Leading Change, Advancing Health* (IOM, 2011), clearly articulated four key messages and eight recommendations as a blueprint for change in nursing and advanced practice nursing in the United States to meet the health needs of Americans in the era of health care reform (see Chapter 22 for a detailed discussion). NACNS (2012c) has formulated a response to address the eight recommendations from the perspective of CNSs (Table 14-2). This section will address the key messages and recommendations as they pertain to CNSs.

Key Message 1

Nurses should practice to the fullest extent of their education and training.

The two recommendations that fall under this key message are to remove scope of practice barriers and implement nurse residency programs. APN residency

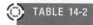

TABLE 14-2 **NACNS Strategies for Enacting Institute of Medicine's *Future of Nursing* Recommendations Related to the Clinical Nurse Specialist Role**

IOM Key Message	NACNS Recommendations for Enactment
1. Nurses should practice to the fullest extent of their education and training.	• Amend Nurse Practice Acts to allow CNSs to diagnose and treat health conditions. • Eliminate requirements for physician "collaborative practice agreements." • Remove prescribing restrictions or limitations imposed by required physician oversight, collaboration, or signature. • Amend requirements for hospital participation in the Medicare program to ensure that CNSs are eligible for clinical privileges, admitting privileges, and membership on medical staffs. • Advocate for all insurers, including but not limited to Medicare, Medicaid, and third-party insurers, to include coverage of CNS services that are within their scope of practice under state law. • Amend the Medicare and Medicaid programs to authorize CNSs to perform admission assessments, certify patients for home health care services, and admit patients to hospitals, hospice, and skilled nursing facilities.

Continued

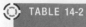 **TABLE 14-2** **NACNS Strategies for Enacting Institute of Medicine's *Future of Nursing* Recommendations Related to the Clinical Nurse Specialist Role—*cont'd***

IOM Key Message	NACNS Recommendations for Enactment
2. Nurses should achieve higher levels of education and training through an improved education system that promotes seamless academic progression.	• Advocate for academic institutions to offer research and practice doctorates that support CNS specialty-focused advanced practice nursing. • Advocate for CNS-focused courses in doctoral programs. • Develop Bachelor of Science in Nursing (BSN)–to–PhD and BSN-to-DNP programs for CNSs to streamline the process for preparing research and clinical scholars. • Recommend options for seamless progression to DNP preparation for CNSs.
3. Nurses should be full partners, with physicians and other health care professionals, in redesigning health care in the United States.	• Promote interdisciplinary education at the graduate level to optimize collaboration skills. • Support entrepreneurial opportunities for CNSs in the design, implementation, and evaluation of innovative care models. • Optimize education related to technology and technology evaluation. • Revise or amend regulatory language to recognize CNSs as primary care providers for patients with chronic health problems related to medical diagnoses such as diabetes, heart failure, and mental health or chronic conditions such as chronic wounds, chronic pain, or impaired mobility. • Actively engage CNSs in health care policy decisions. • Advocate for organizational support to increase CNSs' responsibility in implementing system improvements. • Encourage accountable care organizations (ACO) to include CNS services among all the services provided. • Facilitate the delivery of CNS specialty services in novel health care delivery systems. • Foster the use of CNS leadership skills in the redesign of health care delivery across settings. • Encourage CNSs to design, implement, and evaluate new systems of providing care to specialty populations. • Advocate for CNS opportunities for continued development of leadership skills (life-long learning). • Encourage and mentor CNSs to participate in policy and regulatory bodies.
4. Effective workforce planning and policymaking require better data collection and an improved information infrastructure.	• Ensure that the criteria for all future survey designs include CNSs. For example, the Workforce Commission and the Health Resources Services Administration may want to develop an APRN survey focusing on the underserved and vulnerable populations. It is critical that CNSs provide the necessary consultation to ensure that CNS-sensitive outcomes are captured within such a survey. • Include CNSs in the design of all workforce standardized minimum data sets (MDS), including work by state licensing boards. • Increase the sample size and fielding the survey to every other year, facilitating expanding the data collected on APRNs, and release survey results more quickly. • Include recommendations by CNSs when establishing a monitoring system that uses data from the MDS to measure systematically and project nursing workforce requirements by role, skill mix, region, and demographics. • Integrate CNSs when coordinating workforce research efforts with the Department of Labor, state and regional educators, employers, and state nursing workforce centers to identify regional health care workforce needs and when establishing regional targets and plans for appropriately increasing the supply of health professionals.

Adapted from National Association of Clinical Nurse Specialists. (2012c). Response to the Institute of Medicine's Future of Nursing report (http://www.nacns.org/html/papers.php).

programs are vital to helping new graduate CNSs understand and develop a practice to the fullest extent of their education, training, and licensure under the guidance of more experienced CNSs. Mentors must be careful to have the new graduate CNS fully embrace the NCSBN and ANA definitions of advanced practice and have a significant component of their practice in the direct care of complex and vulnerable individuals at the specialist level.

Key Message 2

Nurses should achieve higher levels of education and training through an improved education system that promotes seamless academic progression.

Two recommendations related to CNSs fall under this key message—double the number of nurses with a doctorate by 2020 and ensure that nurses engage in lifelong learning. CNSs, by definition, are prepared at the graduate level, primarily master's preparation at this point in time. With the rapid evolution of health care in technology and scientific evidence, options for doctoral level training, at the DNP or PhD level, are increasing and should continue to be facilitated (NACNS, 2012c). This includes encouragement of new CNSs to obtain doctoral degrees for initial preparation as well as encouraging master's-prepared CNSs to return to school for a doctoral degree (NACNS, 2012). This will require a significant investment on the part of educational institutions to develop these seamless opportunities.

The professional development of nurses in clinical practice settings is a key distinguishing feature of the CNS. CNSs' abilities to guide and mentor nurses toward stronger specialty practice can reduce turnover, improve patient safety, and support enhanced patient outcomes (Muller, Hujcs, Dubendorf, et al., 2010). CNSs have an important role in helping a hospital achieve and maintain Magnet recognition by the American Nurses Credentialing Center (Muller et al., 2010). This so-called nurse influence dimension of the CNS is already recognized by many hospitals seeking to obtain or maintain Magnet status and should make this role even more valuable in the future. Hospital-based CNSs skilled in the three spheres of influence and the activities as delineated by Lewandowski and Adamle (2009) contribute positively to projects that meet the Magnet standards. Particular strengths lie in the areas of nursing education, EBP, and process improvement, which are key concerns for attaining Magnet status (Muller et al., 2010).

Key Message 3

Nurses should be full partners, with physicians and other health care professionals, in redesigning health care in the United States.

Recommendations subsumed in this key message include expanding opportunities for nurses to lead and diffuse collaborative improvement efforts and preparing and enabling nurses to lead change to advance health care. CNSs are in a unique position to promote these recommendations by the IOM. CNSs are educated and trained to lead process improvement and collaborative improvement projects. In addition, they are able to mentor and coach staff in a variety of disciplines to lead changes to improve health care systems. CNS skills in leadership, collaboration, integration of current evidence, and development and evaluation of innovative interventions make them particularly well suited to lead these efforts actively.

Key Message 4

Effective workforce planning and policymaking require better data collection and an improved information infrastructure.

Building an infrastructure for the collection and analysis of interprofessional health care workforce data is the only recommendation in this key message. This is an important IOM recommendation for CNSs because they have been excluded from federal governmental data collection. Every 10 years, the Office of Management and Budget in the federal government revises their standard occupational classification (SOC). The SOC is a uniform classification system designed to help federal agencies organize the data that they collect, analyze, and disseminate to inform public policy. Data collected for the SOC includes items such as the number of persons by occupation and salary. In 2008, a request for public comment was made related to the revised list of standard occupations. In the revised list, under the broad group of registered nurses, the detailed occupations of nurse anesthetists, nurse midwives, and NPs were added; however, CNSs were excluded. This lack of recognition at the federal level initiated a letter-writing campaign to include CNS as its own detailed occupation. Despite the information given to the SOC, the Standard Occupational Classification Revision Policy Committee did not create a separate detailed occupation and stated, "even though education for Clinical Nurse Specialists is different from that of Registered Nurses, the task of Clinical Nurse Specialists are not sufficiently unique from those of Registered Nurses who 'assess patient health problems and needs, develop and implement nursing care plans, and maintain medical records' " (Cosca & Emmel, 2010, p. 36).

Without understanding the numbers of CNSs in geographic regions, their practice settings, and salaries, it is difficult to know the steps required to increase the number of specialist APNs to meet the need for safe and high-quality care. A minimum data set for CNSs could be created and required when licensees seek renewal of their licensure by the boards of nursing as a way to start tracking CNSs in the field (IOM, 2011).

NCSBN Consensus Model for Advanced Practice Registered Nurse Regulation and Implications for the Clinical Nurse Specialist

In early discussions surrounding the development of the NCSBN Consensus Model for APRN regulation, some CNS leaders had strongly asserted that CNSs prefer to practice within the RN scope of practice (Hartigan, 2011), and that contributions of CNSs focus more on the nursing aspect of care (Lyon, 2005; Nelson, 2006) rather than a practice that is expanded to include aspects of medical practice. This opinion, combined with CNSs not clearly articulating their expanded practice at the advanced nursing practice level, resulted in the NCSBN not recommending, from a regulatory perspective, that CNSs be included as APNs in their vision paper of 2006 (Chan & Hackenschmidt, 2006). Through an intensive campaign from professional organizations and within the CNS community, comments and evidence were provided to the NCSBN regarding the need to include CNSs among the four APN roles to be included in standardized regulatory language for expanded practice. Although the NCSBN does not have regulatory authority over the states, it has been a leader in working to standardize regulations and legal scope of practice for APRNs across the United States.

The NCSBN Consensus Model for APRN regulation (hereafter referred to as the consensus model; NCSBN, 2012b) is described in greater detail in Chapters 2 and 21. The main purposes of the Consensus Model are to delineate the scope of practice for APRNs and define the regulation of APRNs in the areas of licensure, accreditation of educational programs, certification, and educational program requirements. This section will focus on the implications of the Consensus Model as it relates to the CNS role. It is important to note that this important regulatory understanding of APRNs does not encompass a full conceptual understanding of advanced practice nursing (see Chapter 3). Some of the debates regarding the CNS role in relation to other APRN roles may trace their points of contention to the differences between a regulatory and conceptual approach to the CNS. Scopes of practice for CNSs are highly variable from state to state. The Consensus Model clarifies that all APRNs have a patient-focused practice and should include the legal authority to perform acts of advanced assessment, diagnosing, prescribing, and ordering. If CNSs move away from direct patient care and focus more on nursing education and systems improvements, they are at risk for not being recognized as APRNs

in state regulations (Cronenwett, 2012; NCSBN, 2012b). CNS practices must incorporate direct care of individuals, especially in specialty patients and families that are complex or vulnerable, to reclaim the public and professional recognition that CNSs are APNs.

Currently, not all state boards of nursing (BON) authorize the full role of the CNS. Psychiatric–mental health CNSs (PMHCNS), however, are recognized by at least 30 BONs, and many of these states allow prescriptive authority for PMHCNSs (Oleck, Retano, Tebaldi, et al., 2011). The Consensus Model requires title protection for CNSs, which would be a step forward for states not having this basic regulatory requirement. A grandfather clause (i.e., recognizing and granting authority to APRNs who graduated from accredited programs and were in practice before the implementation date of the Consensus Model) is included in the model regulatory language. This grandfather clause is important for CNSs because certification examinations are not available for all population foci (see later, "National Certification for Clinical Nurse Specialists"). Certification of APRNs at the role and population focus levels will be required for all APNs who seek licensure for practice at the advanced practice level. New certification examinations starting in 2013 will match the CNS role and three of the six population foci: adult-gerontology, pediatrics, psychiatric–mental health (adult and pediatrics). Specialty certification will be voluntary and outside the licensure of APRNs once an individual state adopts the Consensus Model. This certification plan poses a challenge for CNSs because most CNS programs educate at the specialty level rather than at the generalist level (see Chapter 3). CNS programs will need to ensure that some level of "generalist education" regarding the continuum of health and illness is incorporated into curricula.

Regional and Local Variations in Clinical Nurse Specialist Regulation

As noted, variability continues among the states with regard to CNS scope of practice. In 2012, 11 states and the District of Columbia allowed independent prescriptive authority and 23 other states allow prescriptive authority with supervision for CNSs (NCSBN, 2012a). Medicaid and other state health insurance companies and exchanges have traditionally not recognized CNSs as providers of care to be reimbursed and have denied them the ability to be listed as care providers or have a panel of patients.

At the local or organizational level, there is an overwhelming lack of uniform credentialing of CNSs in organizations (especially hospitals). In May 2012, the Centers of Medicare and Medicaid Services (CMS) changed the Conditions of Participation to allow APNs to be eligible candidates for membership of the medical staff organization of hospitals. If CNSs have a large part of their practice in direct care of individuals and are involved in assessing, diagnosing, prescribing, and/or ordering for patients at the advanced level, they should consider recognition and membership in their institution's medical staff organization.

Availability and Standardization of Educational Curricula for Clinical Nurse Specialists

The Consensus Model delineates educational requirements of programs such as ensuring that the three Ps (advanced physical and health assessment, advanced pharmacology, and advanced physiology and pathophysiology) be included in the educational program. Faculty credentials, preceptor credentials, and other course content are also delineated. CNS programs need academic faculty and clinical preceptors who have detailed knowledge of the role or who are practicing CNSs. This poses a challenge for CNS students because the number of CNSs practicing may be limited in their area.

The goal of graduate-level education is to prepare a nurse to think critically and abstractly, assess patient and clinical situations at an advanced level, and use and integrate research into clinical practice. The knowledge, skills, and clinical experience acquired in a graduate program should prepare a CNS to practice at an advanced level, regardless of setting or patient population. Experience in direct patient care is desirable before entering a CNS program because it provides a foundation on which to develop advanced clinical expertise. Identifying and reaching consensus on a core body of knowledge for practice has been the challenge in defining appropriate CNS education. The intent of developing a core curriculum is to ensure standardization. Without common standards for the educational preparation of a CNS, it is difficult to define uniform standards of practice, provide uniform certification at the advanced level, and define standards for credentialing. Early efforts to standardize CNS education arose within specialties; the focus in this chapter is on the profession's efforts to address this issue of standardization.

The ANA's Council of Clinical Nurse Specialists, and subsequently its Council for Advanced Practice Nursing, NACNS, and AACN have worked toward the standardization of APN curricula. For many years, the AACN's *The Essentials of Master's Education for Advanced Practice Nursing* (AACN, 1996) was the blueprint for APN education. The NACNS (1998, 2004b) also recommended the inclusion of 13 core content areas necessary for developing CNS competencies and 18 guidelines for evaluating CNS programs (NACNS, 2004c; see Table 14-1).

CNS graduate students must complete a minimum of 500 clinical hours (NACNS, 2004b). This recommendation coincides with the requirements for other APN master's programs and for CNS certification. Clinical practice that offers sufficient opportunities to master and apply knowledge and skills and begin the maturation from competency to expertise in a selected area of clinical practice is a critical and integral part of CNS educational preparation. The NACNS has further specified that a student's experience should be "consistent with the conceptual framework of the three spheres of influence" (NACNS, 2004b, p. 53).

Despite these efforts to standardize CNS graduate preparation, programs vary substantially (NACNS, 2004b). To ensure that the CNS continues to be a recognized advanced practice nursing role, the need is urgent to clarify competencies, standardize CNS curricula, and reach a rational consensus on how to credential CNSs from multiple specialties. Many initiatives are underway that will directly or indirectly affect future CNS preparation, credentialing, and practice. The Society of Clinical Nurse Specialist Education (SCNSE) was formed in 2010 specifically to support education in academic and practice settings. Recommendations from the Consensus Model were included to guide new and existing programs as they modify or compose their curricula with the purpose of preparing CNSs to provide expert care to patients and improve patient outcomes through education and system changes. According to NACNS, there are 217 CNS programs throughout the United States (NACNS, 2012a). NACNS published the *Statement on Clinical Nurse Specialist Practice and Education* (NACNS, 2004), and NACNS also created core competencies for CNSs, regardless of specialty, to help standardize education and practice for the new graduate CNS (NACNS, 2010; see Table 14-1).

Recent initiatives are challenging traditional CNS education. The AACN's DNP initiative and the goal of requiring new APNs to have a practice doctorate (AACN, 2006) have engendered considerable debate and discussion within the CNS community. Although the DNP initiative is considered by many to have already been done, there is debate about its consequences, some of which may be unintended (Chase & Pruitt, 2006; NACNS, 2005a). Concerns that it may result in fewer students preparing to be CNSs to meet at least geographic pockets of shortages have been discussed in the literature. The length of the DNP curriculum and inability of some universities to offer doctorates poses a challenge for academic institutions (Chase & Pruitt, 2006). There is also concern that there is a focus on disease management at the expense of philosophy of science or metatheoretical issues (Fulton & Lyon, 2005). The separation of the profession's practice and research missions, differences in master's- and doctorate-prepared CNS competencies, the acronym's suggestion that a DNP is an NP, and regulatory considerations are additional concerns about the DNP (Chase &Pruitt, 2006; Fulton & Lyon, 2005; Meleis & Dracup, 2005). Another concern about the DNP degree is that the focus on disease management displaces the significance of wellness management and the CNS-sensitive impact on human responses to health and illness (Fulton & Lyon, 2005). Despite the increase in DNP programs, the range of concerns expressed by some nursing leaders and APN organizations suggests that the question of the appropriateness of DNP preparation for APNs, including CNSs, is still undecided.

The most controversial issue in the DNP *Essentials* is the plan to have the ultimate degree for APNs be the practice doctorate (AACN, 2006). In 2006, the NACNS convened meetings with national specialty organizations to discuss the implications of DNP preparation for CNS practice (NACNS, 2006). In their *Position Paper on the Nursing Practice Doctorate* (NACNS, 2009), NACNS supported education of CNSs at the master's or practice doctorate level but did not support the elimination of master's degree programs in favor of DNP programs. Some colleges and universities may not allow the granting of doctoral degrees, which could limit the accessibility to CNS programs.

National Certification for Clinical Nurse Specialists

Certification for CNSs by examination is available through the American Nurses Credentialing Center (ANCC) or the certification boards of specialty organizations (e.g., Oncology Nursing Society, American Association of Critical-Care Nurses). However, certification examinations are not available for many CNS specialties, such as cardiovascular, neuroscience, and perinatal nursing, and currently these specialty certification examinations do not meet the role and population focus as articulated in the NCSBN Consensus Model Regulatory Language. The lack of certification is a major regulatory barrier for many CNS specialties, especially in the era of the Consensus Model. Although ANCC created and offered a CNS certification examination in the population focus of the family and individual across the life span, it was only offered twice before it was suspended indefinitely. Such a generic certification is ill matched to the reality of CNS practice, which is by definition specialty-specific. If states are going to adopt the Consensus Model, it is imperative that nationally recognized CNS certification examinations be developed for the role to survive. Unfortunately, in 2002, the NCSBN decided to remove alternative mechanisms for

granting APRN licensure, such as a portfolio or clinical practice evaluation (Hartigan, 2011). Today, NACNS encourages states to analyze how the lack of a certification examination for all population foci for CNSs will have an impact on practice within each state before fully implementing the Consensus Model (NACNS, 2012b).

Variability in Individual Clinical Nurse Specialist Practices and Prescriptive Authority

The evolution of the CNS role has been dynamic. CNSs who pioneered the role were specialists in psychiatry and mental health. The CNS was initially conceptualized as an expert clinician, consultant, educator, and researcher (Hamric & Spross, 1989). Direct care, although central, was not the only focus. Integrating these role manifestations was difficult but essential to sustain the role's effectiveness, yet differentiating these elements has not been sufficient to describe what CNSs do.

Historically, CNSs have debated the individuality of CNS practices. Various and seemingly different positions have been published in the literature. Articles and position statements that have been written clearly outline the debate; some have taken a neutral position, trying to support both sides of the argument, whereas others indicate a negative stance against colleagues (Lyon, 2003). A classic example of this is the prescriptive authority debate (NACNS, 2005). Some CNSs want prescriptive authority, others do not, and both sides have been adamant about their positions rather than saying that it is a privilege that an individual CNS can exercise based on her or his preference and practice. This latter approach is how NPs handled this issue—they want prescriptive authority; whether they will use it or not is up to the individual. Physicians are also the same; most use it, some do not, but all have the authority. The key to moving forward is to publicly support prescriptive authority for CNSs and discuss the positive contributions to patient outcomes based on that authority. This consistent messaging will help regulators and other professionals outside the CNS community understand the possibilities for the role.

Understanding the Similarities and Differences Between Clinical Nurse Specialists and Nurse Practitioners

The origins of the CNS and NP roles arose from very different needs in health care when the roles were created. In response to a need for nurses with specialized knowledge and training in psychiatric nursing, Peplau (1952) created the first CNS educational program (see Chapter 1). In the 1960s, clinical nurse specialization, specifically in psychiatry and mental health as well as in critical care units, took its modern form as a result of three forces in health care: (1) an increase in specialty-related information; (2) new technologic advances; and (3) a response to public need and interest. In coronary care units, nurses expanded their knowledge and skills by learning how to identify cardiac arrhythmias, administer intravenous medications, and defibrillate patients. These nurses were, in fact, diagnosing and treating patients (Keeling, 2004). Therefore, the origin of the CNS role was born out of a need for specialty practices.

Concurrently, in the 1960s, the role of the pediatric nurse practitioner was formed to help relieve the shortage of physicians in poor rural and urban areas. Physicians were increasingly drawn to medical specialties and leaving primary care. Diagnosing, treating, and providing primary care to patients in outpatient settings were beginning to come under the purview of nurse practitioners and were some of the defining characteristics, later termed *competencies,* of the role (see Chapter 1). Today, more NPs are entering specialty practice as the need for specialists has grown (Kleinpell, Ely, & Grabenkort, 2008; McCorkle, Engleking, Lazenby, et al., 2012).

In the 1990s, forces in health care, such as a downturn in the fiscal health of hospitals, layoffs or repurposing of CNSs into quality managers, case managers, or nurse educator roles, increased emphasis on primary care, rapid growth of NP programs, and introduction of acute care nurse practitioners led to a sharp decrease in the number of nurses entering CNS programs (see Chapter 1). The image of the CNS as quality manager, case manager, or nurse educator, combined with CNS leaders insisting that CNSs practice in the domain of nursing and not in medicine (Hartigan, 2011) persists today despite NACNS's efforts to publicize core competencies and activities (NACNS, 2004, 2010).

CNSs and NPs in the specialties of psychiatric and mental health (Oleck, Retano, Tebaldi, et al., 2011; Rice, Moller, DePascale, et al., 2007), critical care (Becker, Kaplow, Muenzen, et al., 2006), and emergency advanced practice nursing (Chan & Garbez, 2006), as well as generically (Elder & Bullough, 1990; Fenton & Brykczynski, 1993; Lincoln, 2000; Stark, 2006; Williams & Valdivieso, 1994), have found that their role activities, competencies, and educational preparation have much overlap and many similarities. For example, in direct care, CNSs and NPs in the state of Minnesota spent an average amount of their daily work activity in planning treatment (80.8% versus 97.4%), initiating treatment (63.8% versus 95.2%), managing treatment (72.3% versus 94.7%), evaluating treatment (87.7% versus 97.9%), prescribing medications (23.8% versus 95.8%), and teaching staff (85.4% versus 68.8%) (Lincoln, 2000). As noted, Commission on Collegiate Nursing Education (CCNE) accreditation mandates that

all APN students receive the three Ps (AACN, 1995, 2006). Knowledge of the pathophysiology of sepsis, assessment, and treatment is no different if a clinician is a CNS, NP, or physician.

There are differences, however, between the two roles. Significantly, the amount of time spent performing a particular competency or activity is different for each. CNSs spend time among the three substantive areas of practice, as outlined by the NACNS (2004; Lewandowski & Adamle, 2009) whereas NPs spend most of their time in direct care management of patients (Becker, Kaplow, Muenzen, et al., 2006; Rice, Moller, DePascale, et al., 2007). With the introduction of the DNP degree, core competencies for APNs who graduate from these programs will have a balance of direct care management education and didactic instruction in education and systems changes to produce a more well-rounded clinician. Perhaps we will see CNSs receive more instruction about direct care management and NPs receive more instruction about education and influencing system-level changes. A helpful way to differentiate the role of a CNS from that of an NP is to recall the three substantive areas of practice of CNSs—managing the care of complex and vulnerable populations, educating and supporting interdisciplinary staff, and facilitating change and innovation in health care systems (Lewandowski & Adamle, 2009).

In 2007, the American Psychiatric Nurses Association (APNA) and the International Society of Psychiatric Mental Health Nurses (ISPN) published a job analysis between psychiatric mental health CNSs (PMH-CNS) and psychiatric mental health NPs (PMH-NP) that found there was 90% commonality in the two roles (Rice, Moller, DePascale, et al., 2007). However, a subsequent analysis of the items in the job analysis revealed that there was a heavy emphasis on direct care activities and fewer items related to health care system changes, organizational consultation, consultation with nursing personnel, and research, which falls heavily in the CNS domain (Jones & Minarik, 2012). For psychiatric–mental health APNs, competency must be attained in the APN, medical, and psychotherapy domains. PMH-CNSs have a strong history of in-depth psychotherapy training, whereas PMH-NPs have more training in psychopharmacology. Based on the job analysis findings, APNA and ISPN have endorsed the recommendation that educational programs prepare psychiatric mental health APNs as NPs educated across the life span (APNA, 2011). The National Organization of Nurse Practitioner Faculties (NONPF), which created the standards for NP education, has recognized that there is a transition phase and has acknowledged the expertise and contributions of PMH-CNS faculty and clinicians (NONPF, 2012). Criterion I.B of the *Criteria for Evaluation of Nurse Practitioner Programs* (NONPF,

2012) states that "The faculty member who provides direct oversight for the nurse practitioner educational component or track is nationally certified in the same population-focused area of practice" (p. 4). Specifically, a nationally certified PMH-CNS can oversee a PMH-NP track. Criterion III.F states that "Post-graduate students must successfully complete graduate didactic and clinical requirements of an academic graduate NP program" (p. 9). However, a qualifier for PMH-CNSs has been given (NONPF, 2012, p. 9):

> PMH CNSs returning for a postgraduate certificate or an academic degree as a PMH NP: To address a period of transition and consistency with the Consensus Model on APRN Regulation, consideration for challenging selected courses and experiences may be given to those Psychiatric-Mental Health CNSs who are seeking national certification as a Psychiatric-Mental Health NP. However, didactic and clinical experiences shall be sufficient for the student to master the NP competencies and meet the criteria for certification as a PMH NP. These students should complete a sufficient number of direct patient care clinical hours to establish/demonstrate competency in the role and population-focused area of practice. Programs must document credit granted for prior didactic and clinical experiences for individual students through a gap analysis.

The NONPF criteria are likely to stay in effect until transitions of programs and certification mechanisms from PMHCNS to PMHNP have been complete. As APNA and ISPN continue to consider implications for CNSs and NPs in psychiatric and mental health, it will be important to continue to incorporate core competencies of the two roles, which include medical, psychiatric, and psychotherapy treatment modalities, educating and supporting interdisciplinary staff, and facilitating change and innovation in health care systems to provide improved access to high quality mental health care.

Future Directions

Three powerful forces have been converging to influence the practice and regulation of APRNs: the IOM report on the *Future of Nursing* (IOM, 2011), the NCSBN Consensus Model for APRN regulation (NCSBN, 2012b), and health care reform. There are many exciting opportunities for CNSs to reinvigorate their roles and ensure a unique place in the health care system. At the same time, the CNS role is threatened by wide variability in philosophy, education, and operationalization that continues role confusion or ambiguity among those in the CNS community, regulators, educators, employers, and the public. To combat the

forces that threaten the survival of the role, CNSs must engage in five action areas:

1. CNSs need to unify around the NCSBN regulatory affirmation of CNSs as being APRNs, with a significant component of practice in the direct care of individuals and an expanded scope of practice that includes advanced assessment, diagnosing, prescribing, and ordering (NCSBN, 2012b). A cohesive voice from the CNS community must advocate for all activities to be legally permissible in state scopes of practice and in individual practices, regardless of individual practices or preferences. Use of common language shared by all APN groups is essential for identifying shared knowledge, skills, and practices. This reduces the perception of infighting and advances the CNS as an APN role in collaboration with other APNs. There is strength in numbers and internal unity.

2. CNSs must clearly articulate their contributions to patients, families, and the health care system in the three spheres of influence (NACNS, 2004) and the substantive areas of practice as described by Lewandowski and Adamle (2009). By claiming the definition of CNS practice defined at the beginning of the chapter, CNSs can differentiate themselves from other APNs and still provide direct and indirect care to patients to improve health outcomes in specialty populations (Goudreau, Baldwin, Clark, et al., 2007).

3. CNSs must ensure that educational curricula and continuing education programs prepare current and future CNSs with the knowledge and skills to have an expanded practice at the advanced level with specialty populations, educating interdisciplinary staff and facilitating change and innovation in health care systems. Adherence to the AACN essentials for DNP and master's APRN education (AACN, 1995, 2006) is mandatory for the accreditation of APN programs and serve as the basis for educational standards, according to the NCSBN Consensus Model for APRN regulation (NCSBN, 2012b). The standard competencies developed by NACNS should serve as a guide to didactic courses and clinical practica, with an additional focus area on disease management. Preceptors must have CNS students engage in activities in these three substantive areas of CNS practice to prepare them for a future successful practice (Lewandowski &Adamle, 2009). CNSs have a strong history of continuing educational conferences focused on nursing education and systems or process improvement. Continuing education programs for CNSs should increase the course offerings to include care

management of specialty populations, including disease and medication management.

4. CNSs need to be involved in conducting and publishing comparative effectiveness studies that test the efficacy of CNS interventions in complex and vulnerable specialty populations and patient outcomes. Comparative effectiveness research (CER) "is designed to inform health-care decisions by providing evidence on the effectiveness, benefits, and harms of different treatment options. The evidence is generated from research studies that compare drugs, medical devices, tests, surgeries, or ways to deliver health care" (AHRQ, 2012). CNSs continue to need to establish that patient outcomes are improved, safe, and high quality as a result of their interventions compared with other practice models. In a recent systematic review of the literature, NPs and CNMs compared their patient care outcomes with physician patient care outcomes in the years 1990 to 2008 (Newhouse, Stanik-Hutt, White, et al., 2011). It was found that NPs and CNMs provide effective, safe, and high-quality patient care. When the authors reviewed the CNS literature, they found that CNSs compared their interventions with usual or standard care; one study investigated CNS care compared with physician assistants (Newhouse, Stanik-Hutt, White, et al., 2011). More studies need to be carried out to compare CNS effectiveness in achieving patient outcomes and system-wide improvements, with CNSs managing care as the intervention.

5. CNSs need to seek recognition as APNs locally, statewide, nationally, and internationally through involvement in policymaking and health care reform efforts. Local recognition can be obtained by seeking institutional credentialing and privileging and ensuring that institutional job descriptions incorporate the three spheres of influence, with particular attention to the direct care of individuals.

CNSs must become involved in passing regulations and legislation using Consensus Model language and including CNSs as APRNs in state regulations or statutes. CNSs must lobby and advocate for national certification mechanisms that accurately reflect CNS practice. In addition, CNSs need to monitor national changes to regulation in agencies such as the CMS to ensure that CNSs continue to be recognized as APNs for purposes of reimbursement.

The International Council of Nurses (ICN) has established the International Nurse Practitioner–Advanced Practice Nursing Network (INP-APNN; see Chapter 6). The goal, aims, and objectives of this group are to become an international resource for nurses practicing in NP or APN roles, and interested others (e.g., policymakers, educators, regulators, health planners) by doing the following: (1) making relevant and timely information about practice, education, role development, research, policy and regulatory developments, and appropriate events widely available; (2) providing a forum for sharing and exchanging knowledge expertise and experience; (3) supporting nurses and countries who are in the process of introducing or developing NP or APN roles and practice; and (4) accessing international resources that are pertinent to this field (ICN, 2012; Pulcini, Jelic, Gul, et al., 2010).

CNS titling, education, and regulatory issues continue to be a challenge to establishing the role internationally; however, there are many driving forces that support role creation (Schober & Affara, 2006). More support for nursing colleagues in the form of educational exchange programs and teaching and practicing internationally should be given by CNSs to improve patient outcomes globally.

Conclusion

CNSs have a strong and tumultuous history. Over the past 20 years, the departure from direct patient care as being a main focus to working predominantly in the nursing education and systems improvement domains has created confusion within nursing and the public because non-CNSs (e.g., nurse educators, quality improvement managers) function in the same capacity. However, CNSs are uniquely educated to provide advanced practice and specialist expertise when working directly with complex and vulnerable patients, educating and supporting interdisciplinary staff, and facilitating change and innovation in health care systems that those in other roles in health care cannot.

As health care reform continues to gain momentum to improve the health care system, there will be many new opportunities for CNSs. As masters of flexibility and creativity, CNSs can develop new roles to meet the needs of patients and health care systems. For example, in nurse-managed clinics, perhaps NPs could deliver the primary care to patients in the management of hypertension. Once first- or second-line therapies or interventions are found to be ineffective, a referral could be placed to the cardiovascular CNS for specialized pharmacologic and nonpharmacologic treatment. Also, the cardiovascular CNS could integrate the latest evidence to create educational materials for patients and other health care professionals. Perhaps a CNM who is caring for a pregnant woman who develops gestational diabetes, preeclampsia, and is in breech position could ask the perinatal CNS to comanage the patient by following the patient and fetus or neonate in the prenatal setting through hospital discharge into the postpartum phase. The perinatal CNS could establish interagency processes to facilitate care delivery across practice settings to provide seamless transitions of care. The possibilities are endless if CNSs understand their role, improve understanding of the importance of this role in advanced practice nursing, and maximize the driving forces and minimize the restraining forces in the health care system.

*The authors wish to acknowledge Patricia S. A. Sparacino for her authorship of this chapter in previous editions.

References

Agency for Healthcare Research and Quality. (2012). Patient safety network (http://psnet.ahrq.gov).

Agency for Healthcare Research and Quality. (2012). What is comparative effectiveness research? (http://effectivehealthcare.ahrq.gov/index.cfm/what-is-comparative-effectiveness-research1).

Altmiller, G. (2010). Quality and safety education for nurses competencies and the clinical nurse specialist role: Implications for preceptors. *Clinical Nurse Specialist, 25*, 28–32.

American Association of Colleges of Nursing. (1996). *The essentials of master's education for advanced practice nursing.* Washington, DC: Author.

American Association of Colleges of Nursing. (2006). The essentials of doctoral education for advanced nursing practice (http://www.aacn.nche.edu/DNP/pdf/Essentials.pdf).

American Association of Colleges of Nursing. (2012). DNP fact sheet (http://www.aacn.nche.edu/media-relations/fact-sheets/dnp).

American Nurses Association. (2003). *Nursing's social policy statement* (2nd ed.). Washington, DC: Author.

American Psychiatric Nurses Association. (2011). APNA / ISPN Joint Task Force Recommendations on the implementation of the "Consensus model for APRN regulation: Licensure, accreditation, certification and education" (http://www.apna.org/i4a/pages/index.cfm?pageid=4495).

Barron, A. M. (1983). The clinical nurse specialist as consultant. In A. B. Hamric & J. A. Spross (Eds.), *The clinical nurse specialist in theory and practice* (pp. 91–113). New York: Grune & Stratton.

Barron, A. M. (1989). The clinical nurse specialist as consultant. In A. B. Hamric & J. A. Spross (Eds.), *The clinical nurse specialist in theory and practice* (2nd ed., pp. 125–146). Philadelphia: WB Saunders.

Becker, E., Dee, V., Gawlinski, A., Kirkpatrick, T., Lawanson-Nichols, M., Lee, B., et al. (2012). Clinical nurse specialists shaping policies and procedures via an evidence-based clinical practice council. *Clinical Nurse Specialist, 26*, 74–86.

Becker, D., Kaplow, R., Muenzen, P. M., & Hartigan, C. (2006). Activities performed by acute and critical care advanced practice nurses: American Association of Critical-Care Nurses study of practice. *American Journal of Critical Care, 15*, 130–148.

Benedict, L., Robinson, K., & Holder, C. (2006). Clinical nurse specialist practice within the Acute Care for Elders interdisciplinary team model. *Clinical Nurse Specialist, 20*, 248–252.

Briggs, L. A., Heath, J., & Kelley, J. (2005). Peer review for advanced practice nurses: What does it really mean? *AACN Clinical Issues, 16*, 3–15.

Brooten, D., Kumer, S., Brown, L. P., Butts, P., Finkler, S. A., Bakewell-Sachs, S., et al. (1986). A randomized clinical trial of early hospital discharge and home follow-up of very-low-birth-weight infants. *New England Journal of Medicine, 315*, 934–939.

Brooten, D., Naylor, M. D., York, R., Brown, L. P., Munro, B. H., Hollingsworth, A. O., et al. (2002). Lessons learned from testing the Quality Cost Model of Advanced Practice Nursing (APN) Transitional Care. *Journal of Nursing Scholarship, 34*, 369–375.

Brooten, D., Youngblut, J. M., Deatrick, J., Naylor, M., & York, R. (2003). Patient problems, advanced practice nurse (APN) interventions, time and contacts among five patient groups. *Journal of Nursing Scholarship, 35*, 73–79.

Brooten, D., Youngblut, J. M., Hannan, J., & Guido-Sanz, F. (2012). The impact of interprofessional collaboration of the effectiveness, significance, and future of advanced practice nurses. *Nursing Clinics of North America, 47*, 283–294.

Brown-Brumfield, D., & DeLeon, A. (2010). adherence to a medication safety protocol: Current practice for labeling medications and solutions on the sterile field. *Association of Operating Room Nurses Journal, 91*, 610–617.

Centers for Medicare and Medicaid Services. (2012). 42 CFR parts 482 and 485. Medicare and Medicaid programs; reform of hospital and critical access hospital conditions of participation; final rule (http://www.gpo.gov/fdsys/pkg/FR-2012-05-16/html/2012-11548.htm).

Chan, G. K., & Garbez, R. O. (2006). Education of advanced practice nurses for emergency care settings: Emphasizing shared competencies and domains. *Advanced Emergency Nursing Journal, 28*, 216–225.

Chan, G. K., & Hackenschmidt, A. (2006). Understanding the influences that determine nursing practice and the opportunities for involvement: A study of the NCSBN vision paper. *Journal of Emergency Nursing, 32*, 350–353.

Chase, S. K., & Pruitt, R. H. (2006). The practice doctorate: Innovation or disruption? *Journal of Nursing Education, 45*, 155–161.

Cooper, D. M., & Sparacino, P. S. A. (1990). Acquiring, implementing, and evaluating the clinical nurse specialist role. In P. S. A. Sparacino, D. M. Cooper, & P. A. Minarik (Eds.), *The clinical nurse specialist: Implementation and impact* (pp. 41–75). Norwalk, CT: Appleton and Lange.

Cosca, T., & Emmel, A. (2010). Revising the standard occupational classification system for 2010 (www.bls.gov/opub/mlr/2010/08/art3full.pdf).

Cronenwett, L. R. (2012). Molding the future of advanced practice nursing. *Nursing Outlook*, *60*, 241–248. doi: S0029-6554(12)00146-7 [pii] 10.1016/j.outlook.2012.06.010.

Cunningham, R. S. (2006). Clinical practice guideline use by oncology advanced practice nurses. *Applied Nursing Research*, *19*, 126–133.

D'Afflitti, J. G. (2004). A psychiatric clinical nurse specialist as liaison to OB/GYN practice. *Journal of Obstetric, Gynecologic, and Neonatal Nursing*, *34*, 280–285.

DeJong, S., & Veltman, R. H. (2004). The effectiveness of CNS-led community-based COPD screening and intervention program. *Clinical Nurse Specialist*, *18*, 72–79.

Disch, J., Chlan, L., Mueller, C., Akinduoto, T., Sabo, J., Feldt, K., et al. (2006). The Densford Clinical Scholars Program: Improving patient care through research partnerships. *Journal of Nursing Administration*, *36*, 567–574.

Duffy, J. R. (2002). The clinical leadership role of the CNS in the identification of nursing-sensitive and multidisciplinary quality indicator sets. *Clinical Nurse Specialist*, *16*, 70–76.

Duffy, M., Dresser, S., & Fulton, J. S. (2009). *Clinical nurse specialist toolkit: A guide for the new clinical nurse specialist*. New York: Springer.

Ebright, P. R., Urden, L., Patterson, E., & Chalko, B. (2004). Themes surrounding novice nurse near-miss and adverse-event situations. *Journal of Nursing Administration*, *34*, 531–538.

Elder, R. G., & Bullough, B. (1990). Nurse practitioners and clinical nurse specialists: Are the roles merging? *Clinical Nurse Specialist*, *4*, 78–84.

Emergency Nurses Association. (2011). *Competencies for clinical nurse specialists in emergency care*. Des Plaines, IL: Author.

Fenton, M. V., & Brykczynski, K. A. (1993). Qualitative distinctions and similarities in the practice of clinical nurse specialists and nurse practitioners. *Journal of Professional Nursing*, *9*, 313–326.

Fields, L. B. (2008). Oral care intervention to reduce incidence of ventilator-associated pneumonia in the neurologic intensive care unit. *Journal of Neuroscience Nursing*, *40*, 291–298.

Fitzgerald, M., Tomlinson, P. S., Peden-McAlpine, C., & Sherman, S. (2003). Clinical nurse specialist participation on a collaborative research project: Barriers and benefits. *Clinical Nurse Specialist*, *17*, 44–49.

Flanders, S., & Clark, A. P. (2010). Interruptions and medication errors. *Clinical Nurse Specialist*, *24*, 281–285.

Ford, P. E. A., Rolfe, S., & Kirkpatrick, H. (2011). A journey to patient-centered care in Ontario, Canada. *Clinical Nurse Specialist*, *25*, 198–206.

Fulton, J. S. (2011). Across the years. *Clinical Nurse Specialist*, *25*, 273–274.

Fulton, J. S., & Lyon, B. L. (2005). The need for some sense making: doctor of nursing practice. *Online Journal of Issues in Nursing*, *10*, 4. doi: topic28/tpc28_3.htm [pii].

Fulton, J. S., Lyon, B. L., & Goudreau, K. A. (2010). *Foundations of clinical nurse specialist practice*. New York: Springer.

Girouard, S. A. (1996). Evaluating advanced nursing practice. In A. B. Hamric, J. A. Spross, & C. M. Hanson (Eds.), *Advanced nursing practice: An integrative approach* (pp. 569–600). Philadelphia: Saunders.

Girouard, S. A., & Spross, J. (1983). Evaluation of the clinical nurse specialist: Using an evaluation tool. In A. B. Hamric & J. A. Spross (Eds.), *The clinical nurse specialist in theory and practice* (pp. 207–218). New York: Grune and Stratton.

Gobel, B. H., Beck, S. L., & O'Leary, C. (2006). Nursing-sensitive patient outcomes: The development of the putting evidence into practice resources for nursing practice. *Clinical Journal of Oncology Nursing*, *10*, 621–624.

Goudreau, K. A., Baldwin, K., Clark, A., Fulton, J., Lyon, B., Murray, T., et al., National Association of Clinical Nurse Specialists. (2007). A vision of the future for clinical nurse specialists: Prepared by the National Association of Clinical Nurse Specialists, July 2007. *Clinical Nurse Specialist*, *21*, 310–320.

Gurka, A. M. (1991). Process and outcome components of clinical nurse specialist consultation. *Dimensions of Critical Care Nursing*, *10*, 169–175.

Hamric, A. B. (1983a). A model for developing evaluation strategies. In A. B. Hamric & J. A. Spross (Eds.), *The clinical nurse specialist in theory and practice* (pp. 187–206). New York: Grune and Stratton.

Hamric, A. B. (1983b). Role development and functions. In A. B. Hamric & J. A. Spross (Eds.), *The clinical nurse specialist in theory and practice* (pp. 39–56). New York: Grune and Stratton.

Hamric, A. B. (1989). A model for CNS evaluation. In A. B. Hamric & J. A. Spross (Eds.), *The clinical nurse specialist in theory and practice* (pp. 83–104, 2nd ed.,). Philadelphia: WB Saunders.

Hamric, A. B., & Spross, J. A. (Eds.), (1989). *The clinical nurse specialist in theory and practice* (2nd ed.). Philadelphia: WB Saunders.

Hartigan, C. (2011). APRN regulation: The licensure-certification interface. *AACN Advanced Critical Care*, *22*, 50–65.

Hespenheide, M., Cottingham, T., & Mueller, G. (2011). Portfolio use as a tool to demonstrate professional development in advanced nursing practice. *Clinical Nurse Specialist*, *25*, 312–320.

Institute for Healthcare Improvement. (2012). Open school (http://www.ihi.org/IHI/Programs/IHIOpenSchool).

Institute of Medicine (IOM). (2011). *The future of nursing: Leading change, advancing health*. Washington, DC: The National Academies Press.

International Council of Nurses. (2012). Aims and objectives (http://www.icn-apnetwork.org).

Jennings, B. M. (2000). Evidence-based practice: The road best traveled? *Research in Nursing & Health*, *23*, 343–345.

Jones, J. S., & Minarik, P. A. (2012). The plight of the psychiatric clinical nurse specialist: The dismantling of the advanced practice nursing archetype. *Clinical Nurse Specialist*, *26*, 121–125. doi: 10.1097/NUR.0b013e318256855a00002800-201205000-00002 [pii]

Keeling, A. W. (2004). Blurring the boundaries between medicine and nursing: Coronary care nursing, circa the 1960s. *Nursing History Review*, *12*, 139–164.

Kerfoot, K. M., Rapala, K., Ebright, P., & Rogers, S. M. (2006). The power of collaboration with patient safety programs. *Journal of Nursing Administration*, *36*, 582–588.

Kleinpell, R. M. (2007). APNs invisible champions? *Nursing Management, 38*, 18–22.

Kleinpell, R. M., Ely, E. W., & Grabenkort, R. (2008). Nurse practitioners and physician assistants in the intensive care unit: An evidence-based review. *Critical Care Medicine, 36*, 2888–2897. doi: 10.1097/CCM.0b013e318186ba8c.

Kleinpell, R., & Gawlinski, A. (2005). Assessing outcomes in advanced practice nursing: The use of quality indicators and evidence-based practice. *AACN Clinical Issues, 16*, 43–57.

Koetters, T. L. (1989). Clinical practice and direct patient care. In A. B. Hamric & J. A. Spross (Eds.), *The clinical nurse specialist in theory and practice* (pp. 107–124, 2nd ed.). Philadelphia: WB Saunders.

LaSala, C. A., Connors, P. M., Pedro, J. T., & Phipps, M. (2007). The role of the clinical nurse specialist in promoting evidence-based practice and effecting positive patient outcomes. *Journal of Continuing Education in Nursing, 38*, 262–270.

Lewandowski, W., & Adamle, K. (2009). Substantive areas of clinical nurse specialist practice: A comprehensive review of the literature. *Clinical Nurse Specialist, 23*, 73–90. doi: 10.1097/NUR.0b013e31819971d000002800-200903000-00008 [pii].

Lincoln, P. E. (2000). Comparing CNS and NP role activities: A replication. *Clinical Nurse Specialist, 14*, 269–277.

Lyon, B. L. (2003). Advanced practice registered nurse compact: A call to action with a primer on the regulation of CNS practice. *Clinical Nurse Specialist, 17*, 185–187. doi: 00002800-200307000-00013 [pii].

Lyon, B. L. (2004). The CNS regulatory quagmire—we need clarity about advanced nursing practice. *Clinical Nurse Specialist, 18*, 9–13.

Lyon, B. L. (2005). Reflecting on getting back on track: Nursing's autonomous scope of practice. *Clinical Nurse Specialist, 19*, 25–27. doi: 00002800-200501000-00009 [pii].

Lunney, M., Gigliotti, E., & McMorrow, M. E. (2007). Tool development for evaluation of clinical nurse specialist competencies in graduate students. *Clinical Nurse Specialist, 21*, 145–151.

McCabe, P. J. (2005). Spheres of clinical nurse specialist practice influence evidence-based care for patients with atrial fibrillation. *Clinical Nurse Specialist, 19*, 308–317.

McCorkle, R., Engelking, C., Lazenby, M., Davies, M. J., Ercolano, E., & Lyons, C. A. (2012). Perceptions of roles, practice patterns, and professional growth opportunities. *Clin Journal of Oncology Nursing, 16*, 382–387. doi: H4583313J0524187 [pii]10.1188/12.CJON.382-387.

Meleis, A. I., & Dracup, K. (2005). The case against the DNP: History, timing, substance, and marginalization. *Online Journal of Issues in Nursing, 10*, 3. doi: topic28/tpc28_2.htm [pii].

Muller, A. C., Hujcs, M., Dubendorf, P., & Harrington, P. T. (2010). Sustaining excellence: clinical nurse specialist practice and magnet designation. *Clinical Nurse Specialist, 24*, 252–259. doi: 10.1097/NUR.0b013e3181effe0f00002800-201009000-00007 [pii].

Murray, T., & Goodyear-Bruch, C. (2007). Ventilator-associated pneumonia improvement program. *AACN Advanced Critical Care, 18*, 190–192.

National Association of Clinical Nurse Specialists (NACNS). (1998). *Statement on clinical nurse specialist practice and education.* Glenview, IL: Author.

National Association of Clinical Nurse Specialists. (2004). *NACNS statement on clinical nurse specialist practice and education* (2nd ed.). Harrisburg, PA: Author.

National Association of Clinical Nurse Specialists. (2005). NACNS position statement on advanced pharmacology: Practice, curricular and regulatory recommendations (http://www.nacns.org/html/papers.php).

National Association of Clinical Nurse Specialists (NACNS). (2006). Executive summary: 2006 CNS summit, July 21–22, Indianapolis, IN. *Clinical Nurse Specialist, 21*, 50–51.

National Association of Clinical Nurse Specialists. (2009). Position statement on the nursing practice doctorate (http://www.nacns.org/html/papers.php).

National Association of Clinical Nurse Specialists. (2010). Clinical nurse specialist core competencies (www.nacns.org/docs/CNSCoreCompetenciesBroch.pdf).

National Association of Clinical Nurse Specialists. (2012a). CNS program directory (http://www.nacns.org/html/student.php).

National Association of Clinical Nurse Specialists. (2012b). NACNS statement on APRN consensus model implementation (http://www.nacns.org/html/papers.php).

National Association of Clinical Nurse Specialists. (2012c). Response to the Institute of Medicine's Future of Nursing report (http://www.nacns.org/html/papers.php).

National Council of State Boards of Nursing. (2012a). Independent prescribing—CNS (https://www.ncsbn.org/2579.htm).

National Council of State Boards of Nursing. (2012b). NCSBN consensus model for APRN regulation (https://www.ncsbn.org/aprn.htm).

National Organization of Nurse Practitioner Faculties. (2012). Criteria for evaluation of nurse practitioner programs (http://www.nonpf.org/displaycommon.cfm?an=1&subarticle nbr=15).

Naylor, M. D. (2007). Advancing the science in the measurement of health care quality influenced by nurses. *Medical Care Research and Review, 64*, 144S–169S.

Naylor, M. D. (2011). Viewpoint: Interprofessional collaboration and the future of health care. *American Nurse Today, 6*. accessed January 27, 2013, from http://www.americannursetoday.com/Article.aspx?id=7908&fid=7870.

Neidlinger, S., Kennedy, L., & Scroggins, K. (1987). Effective and cost efficient discharge planning for hospitalized elders. *Nursing Economic$, 5*, 225–230.

Nelson, R. (2006). NCSBN 'Vision Paper' ignites controversy. Second licensure exam proposed; clinical nurse specialists excluded from advanced practice model. *American Journal of Nursing, 106*, 25–26. doi: 00000446-200607000-00019 [pii].

Nelson, P. J., Holland, D. E., Derscheid, D., & Tucker, S. J. (2007). Clinical nurse specialist influence in the conduct of research in a clinical agency. *Clinical Nurse Specialist, 21*, 95–100.

Newhouse, R. P. (2009). Nursing's role in engineering a learning healthcare system. *Journal of Nursing Administration, 39*, 260–262.

Newhouse, R. P., Stanik-Hutt, J., White, K. M., Johantgen, M., Bass, E. B., & Zangaro, G. (2011). Advanced practice nurse outcomes 1990-2008: A systematic review. *Nursing Economic$, 29*, 230–250.

Noll, M. (1987). Internal consultation as a framework for clinical nurse specialist practice. *Clinical Nurse Specialist, 1*, 46–50.

Oberle, K., & Allen, M. (2001). The nature of advanced practice nursing. *Nursing Outlook, 49*, 148–153.

Oddi, L. F., Cassidy, V. R. (1998). The message of SUPPORT: Study to Understand Prognosis and Preferences for Outcomes and Risks of Treatment. Change is long overdue. *Journal of Professional Nursing, 14*, 165–174.

Oleck, L. G., Retano, A., Tebaldi, C., McGuinness, T. M., Weiss, S., & Carbray, J. (2011). Advanced practice psychiatric nurses legislative update. State of the States, 2010 *Journal of the American Psychiatric Nurses Association, 17*, 171–188. doi: 17/2/171 [pii]10.1177/1078390311402331.

O'Malley, P. (2007). Order no harm: Evidence-based methods to reduce prescribing errors for the clinical nurse specialist. *Clinical Nurse Specialist, 21*, 68–70.

Peplau, H. E. (1952). *Interpersonal relations in nursing: A conceptual frame of reference for psychodynamic nursing.* New York: Putnam.

Phillips, S. J. (2006). Legislative update: A comprehensive look at the legislative issues affecting advanced nursing practice. *Nurse Practitioner, 31*, 6–38.

Pulcini, J., Jelic, M., Gul, R., & Loke, A. Y. (2010). An international survey on advanced practice nursing education, practice, and regulation. *Journal of Nursing Scholarship, 42*, 31–39. doi: JNU1322 [pii]10.1111/j.1547-5069.2009.01322.x.

Purvis, S., Brown, E., Chan, G. K., Dresser, S., Fulton, J. S., Koyama, K., et al.; National Association of Clinical Nurse Specialists task force members (2012). The National Association of Clinical Nurse Specialists response to the Institute of Medicine's The Future of Nursing report. *Clinical Nurse Specialist, 26*, 222–224.

Quality and Safety Education for Nurses. (2012). Teaching strategies (http://www.qsen.org/view_strategies.php).

Rantz, M. J., Popejoy, L., Petroshki, P. F., Madsen, R. W., Mehr, D. R., Zwygart-Stauffacher, M., et al. (2001). Randomized clinical trial of a quality improvement intervention in nursing homes. *Gerontologist, 41*, 525–538.

Rice, M. J., Moller, M. D., DePascale, C., & Skinner, L. (2007). APNA and ANCC collaboration: Achieving consensus on future credentialing for advanced practice psychiatric and mental health nursing. *Journal of the American Psychiatric Nurses Association, 13*, 153–159.

Roggow, D. J., Solie, C. J., & Tracy, M. F. (2005). Clinical nurse specialist leadership in computerized provider order entry design. *Clinical Nurse Specialist, 19*, 209–214.

Ryan, M. (2009). Improving self-management and reducing readmissions in heart failure patients. *Clinical Nurse Specialist, 23*, 216–221.

Safriet, B. J. (2010). Federal options for maximizing the value of advanced practice nurses in providing quality, cost-effective health care (http://thefutureofnursing.org/IOM-Report).

Scherff, P., & Siclovan, D. (2009). Organizational strategies to recruit clinical nurse specialists. *Journal of Nursing Administration, 39*, 14–18.

Schober, M., & Affara, F. (2006). *International Council of Nurses: Advanced nursing practice.* Oxford, UK: Blackwell.

Sneed, N. V. (1991). Power: Its use and potential for misuse by nurse consultants. *Clinical Nurse Specialist, 5*, 58–62.

Sparacino, P. S. A., & Cartwright, C. C. (2009). The clinical nurse specialist. In A. B. Hamric, J. A. Spross, & C. M. Hanson (Eds.), *Advanced practice nursing. An integrative approach* (4th ed). St Louis: Elsevier.

Standards for supervision of nursing practice—Sermchief v. Gonzales, 660 S.W.2d 683 (Mo. 1983) (1983). (http://biotech.law.lsu.edu/cases/medmal/Sermchief_v_Gonzales.htm).

Stark, S. W. (2006). The effects of master's degree education and the role choices, role flexibility, and practice settings of clinical nurse specialists and nurse practitioners. *Journal of Nursing Education, 45*, 7–15.

Steinke, E. E. (2004). Research ethics, informed consent, and participant recruitment. *Clinical Nurse Specialist, 18*, 88–95.

St-Louis, L., & Brault, D. (2011). A clinical nurse specialist intervention to facilitate safe transfer from the ICU. *Clinical Nurse Specialist, 25*, 321–326.

The Joint Commission. (2012). Home page (http:/www.jointcommission.org).

Tindle, H. A., Davis, R. B., Phillips, R. S., & Eisenberg, D. M. (2005). Trends in use of complementary and alternative medicine by U.S. adults. *Alternative Therapies in Health and Medicine, 11*, 42–49.

U.S. Department of Health and Human Services (HHS). (2011). Patient Protection and Affordable Care Act (http://www.healthcare.gov/law/full/index.html).

Vollman, K. (2006). Ventilator-associated pneumonia and pressure ulcer prevention as targets for quality improvement in the ICU. *Critical Care Nursing Clinics of North America, 18*, 453–467.

Wagner, L. M., Capezuti, E., Brush, B., Boltz, M., Renz, S., & Talerico, K. A. (2007). Description of an advanced practice nursing consultative model to reduce restrictive siderail use in nursing homes. *Research in Nursing and Health, 30*, 131–140.

Walker, J. A., Urden, L. D., & Moody, R. (2009). The role of the CNS in achieving and maintaining magnet status. *Journal of Nursing Administration, 39*, 515–523.

Walker-Sterling, A. (2005). African-Americans and obesity: Implications for clinical nurse specialist practice. *Clinical Nurse Specialist, 19*, 193–198.

Williams, C. A., & Valdivieso, G. C. (1994). Advanced practice models: a comparison of clinical nurse specialist and nurse practitioner activities. *Clin Nurse Spec, 8*(6), 311–318.

Zinn, J., Reinert, J., Bigelow, A., Ellis, W., French, A. F., Milner, F., et al. (2011). Innovation in engaging hospital staff and university faculty in research. *Clinical Nurse Specialist, 25*(4), 193–197.

Zuzelo, P. R. (2010). *The clinical nurse specialist handbook* (2nd ed.). Sudbury, MA: Jones and Bartlett.

Joanne M. Pohl • Tsui-Sui Annie Kao

CHAPTER CONTENTS

This chapter provides an overview of the primary care nurse practitioner (NP) role. The primary care NP provides care for patients in diverse settings, including community-based settings such as private and public practices, acute, and long-term care settings across the life span. This chapter explores the historical context and evolution of primary care NP roles and settings and relates the NP role to the Institute of Medicine (IOM) definition of primary care (1996). Nurse practitioner competencies (National Organization of Nurse Practitioner Faculties [NONPF], 2012) are used to operationalize NP practice in our ever-changing U.S. health care system, including the patient-centered medical home (PCMH) and accountable care organizations (ACOs). Exemplars of primary care practice are provided to demonstrate the integration of NP competencies into diverse primary care settings. Finally, information about role implementation and key issues confronting current primary care NPs is presented.

Historical Roots of Primary Care in the United States

Primary care had its origins in Britain about 100 years ago and is the foundation of most international health care systems, yet the vision for and outcomes of primary care in the United States actually lags far behind those of other developed countries (Macinko, Starfield, & Shi, 2003; Starfield, 1992) (See Figure 1). Historians remind us that at one time, all health care was once really primary care, and that in reality the United States, unlike other countries, developed a fixation on specialty care in the last century (Howell, 2010). Before World War II, most Americans' health care was provided by a generalist physician and specialists would be seen only if referred. Throughout the 1930s and 1940s, primary care expanded to include pediatricians, internists, and public health nurses (IOM, 1996). The use of the term *primary care* began in the late 1960s; at the same time, there was a growth in specialist physician care. It wasn't until 1969 that family medicine was approved as a specialty, just after the first NP program started.

The triad of circumstances in the 1960s—President Kennedy's assassination, President Johnson's "War on Poverty," and the women's movement—sparked a widespread commitment to public service and instigated a revaluing of nursing that encompassed women's work, caring, ethics, and knowledge. These social forces, coupled with a physician workforce misdistribution, provided a powerful social context to lay the groundwork for a demonstration project at the University of Colorado to build on and reclaim the role of the public health nurse. Thus, the role of NPs began and was historically rooted in primary care. This emerging NP model was extraordinarily patient-centered. It was distinct from the medical model of that time in that it focused on prevention, health and wellness, patient education, and including the patient as a partner in making clinical decisions and cost-benefit alternatives so that patients were empowered to weigh treatment options.

The 1970s brought a rapid influx of capitated group practice models, or health maintenance organizations (HMOs), which emphasized primary care and lower hospitalization rates. The expansion of the HMO grew out of the Health Maintenance Organization Act of 1973, which intended to control expenditures for employers who offered health insurance benefits. Despite these efforts, primary care did not flourish for a number of reasons, one of which was that the role of primary care as gatekeeper was perceived as a barrier for patients' access to specialty care by physicians. Today, patients who enroll in HMOs are often assigned to a primary care physician. Each full-time physician is assigned, or empanelled, with approximately 1500 patients to care for (Murray, Davies, & Boushon, 2007). Some HMOs and other third-party insurers do not empanel NPs or list them as primary care providers, rendering NPs' contribution to primary care invisible. NP empanelment would provide a basis for measuring the effectiveness of NPs more accurately, whose services are often now significantly underestimated because they are recorded as being provided by their collaborating physicians (Naylor & Kurtzman, 2010; Pohl, Hanson, & Newland, 2010).

More recently, the PCMH concept has been highly acclaimed as improving outcomes and management of complex chronic diseases (Nutting, Crabtree, Jaen, et al., 2009). It is a model of health care that embodies the full spectrum of primary care based on patient-centered care, clearly defined provider-patient relationships, and primary care standards of accessibility, continuity, comprehensiveness, integrated care, and interdisciplinary care (Keckley & Underwood, 2008). Most of primary care practice has been considered a cottage industry, with many small businesses (physician practices that employ NPs) that are not integrated vertically with other sectors of the health care system. Historically, NPs worked as employees in group physician practices who operated in a predominantly fee-for-service delivery system. With the move toward ACOs, this trend is likely to change. The relationship of NPs as employees of private, physician-owned businesses has led to the lack of data on NP primary care practice. Some

primary care NPs are associated with academic or medical center primary care services, although a few are also connected with nurse-managed health centers (NMHCs) and other nurse-led primary care practices.

Since the first primary care NP role, which focused on the care of children, a variety of primary care NP foci have emerged over 4 decades, emphasizing care to specific populations such as families, adults, older adults, and women. All these roles were conceived to increase access to primary care and address the needs of underserved populations. NPs have been acknowledged as high-quality, cost-effective providers of primary care (Brown & Grimes, 1993; Cook & Nolan, 1996; Laurant et al., 2005; Mundinger et al., 2000; Newhouse et al., 2011).

Federal Government and Primary Care

The Patient Protection and Affordable Care Act (PPACA), passed in 2010, has far-reaching goals to address access to care and emphasize primary care, including health promotion (U.S. Department of Health and Human Services [HHS], 2011). It will be phased in over time, with comprehensive implementation by 2014, and will give an estimated 32 million more people in the United States access to health care. Because of its emphasis on primary care and the significant shortage of primary care physicians, NPs and other advanced practice nurses (APNs) will play a major role in providing access to quality care under the PPACA. It is expected that the PPACA will expand opportunities for the PCMH, community health centers (CHCs), NMHCs, and ACOs. These will be discussed later in the chapter.

Health Resources and Services Administration

The Health Resources and Services Administration (HRSA), an agency of the HHS, is the primary federal agency for improving access to health care services for people who are uninsured, isolated, or medically vulnerable. HRSA's Bureau of Primary Care funds grants that build a safety net infrastructure in high-poverty counties, such as CHCs that provide primary health care, regardless of the person's ability to pay. The Bureau of Health Professions funds grants to schools of nursing through its nursing education, practice, quality, and retention grants; their purpose is to provide support for academic, service, and continuing education projects, in part to increase nurse retention and strengthen the nursing workforce (HRSA, 2012a). Although this funding is not directed solely to primary care, it has helped fund NMHCs that provide primary care; often, these centers serve the underserved.

Health Professional Shortage Areas Designation

About 20% of the U.S. population (60 million people) reside in health professional shortage areas (HPSAs). One criterion for this shortage designation is a community that has a population of 3500 but only one full-time primary care physician in one of the four primary care specialties—general or family practice, general internal medicine, pediatrics, and obstetrics and gynecology (Council of State Governments, 2008; HRSA, 2012b). Of those 60 million people living in HPSAs, about 34 million are considered to be medically underserved. Currently, NPs, certified nurse-midwives (CNMs), and physician assistants (PAs) are not included in the counts of primary care providers for the HPSA designation, for several reasons, but they are critically important for the APN community. First, there is concern that counting NPs and CNMs would render communities ineligible for a shortage designation because they would raise the eligibility ratio higher for communities that had APN(s) to more than the population-to-provider ratio of 3500:1, thus creating a catch-22. Second, the outdated state practice acts governing NP and CNM practice vary widely; some state laws permit independent APN practice, whereas others are highly restrictive. This variability across states introduces systematic bias in counting them as full-time equivalent primary care providers, because an APN in a restrictive state is not able to practice to full capacity because of restrictive laws. Finally, and perhaps most importantly, there is a substantial lack of data on the location and practice patterns of NPs. The IOM report, *The Future of Nursing* (2011), has identified this lack of data as critical for sound decision making. Individual NP organizations have tried to track data on their members, but there is no comprehensive national data set on NPs or APNs.

Centers for Medicare & Medicaid Innovation

The Centers for Medicare & Medicaid Innovation was established by the PPACA, is intended to revitalize and sustain Medicare, Medicaid, and the Children's Health Insurance Program (CHIP), and ultimately improve the health care system for all Americans. The Innovation Center has the resources and flexibility to test innovative care and payment models rapidly and encourage the widespread adoption of practices that deliver better health care at lower cost. This Center will be significant for establishing new models of care and has potential for testing nurse-led models, as well as innovations in which nursing is a significant part of the team. Some of these models will be addressed later in this chapter.

Primary Care Workforce Composition

The National Sample Survey of Registered Nurses in 2010 (based on data from 2008; Table 15-1) estimated that there were 250,527 registered nurses (RNs) prepared as APNs in one or more areas. Of these, 220,494 were employed in nursing (HRSA, 2010). NPs represented the largest group of APNs, approximately 154,000; this includes NPs who identify themselves as both a clinical nurse specialist (CNS) and NP. However, this figure is only an estimate of the NP primary care workforce because no national data have analyzed practicing NPs by specialty or focus (e.g., acute care, gerontology, family). The 2012 graduation data (American Association of Colleges of Nursing [AACN] & NONPF, 2013), shown in Table 15-2, suggest that most NP graduates (82%) select primary care specialties. Although these graduation data do not fully inform the current workforce composition, they do suggest that most NPs choose primary care as their focus and are potential primary care workforce providers. The enrollment and graduation rate of NPs over the past 3 years continues to rise, with an annual graduation rate increasing overall by more than 1000 annually, and with most of the graduates prepared in primary care. This is a different picture from physician

TABLE 15-1   Composition of the Primary Care Workforce

Primary Care Workforce	Estimated Number
Nurse practitioners (2010)*	155,000
Physician assistants (2010)[†]	83,540
Family medicine physicians (2010)[‡]	87,650
General internal medicine physicians (2010)[‡]	93,655
General pediatric physicians (2010)[‡]	49,642
Geriatric physicians (2010)[‡]	3,260
Total	482,510

*From U.S. Department of Health and Human Services, Health Resources and Service Administration (HRSA). (2010). The registered nurse population: Findings from the March 2008 national sample survey of registered nurses (http://bhpr.hrsa.gov/healthworkforce/rnsurvey2008.html).

This survey is a sample of the registered nurse population, not the subpopulation of NPs, making the accuracy of the NP estimate less reliable. Moreover, this estimate reflects all NPs in all specialties and settings, making it an overestimate for the primary care workforce. There are no national workforce data on NPs by specialty certification.

[†]Bureau of Labor Statistics. (2011). Occupational employment and wages, May 2011: 29-1071 Physician assistants (http://www.bls.gov/oes/current/oes291071.htm).

[‡]Agency for Healthcare Research and Quality Primary Care. (2011). Workforce facts and stats no. 1. The number of practicing primary care physicians in the United States (http://www.ahrq.gov/research/ pcwork1.htm).

TABLE 15-2 2012 Graduates of Masters, Post-Masters, and Post-Baccalaureate DNP-Level Nurse Practitioner Programs*

Clinical Track/Certificate Examination	Graduates N (total % for each category)
Family NP	7,400 (57.0% of all Masters NPs—Primary Care and Non Primary Care)
Post-Masters	583 (47.9% of all Post Masters NPs—Primary Care and Non Primary Care)
DNP Post-Baccalaureate	121 (54.5% of all DNP Post Baccalaureate NPs—Primary Care and Non Primary Care)
Adult NP	1,677 (13.1%)
Post-Masters	176 (14.4%)
DNP Post-Baccalaureate	14 (6.3%)
Pediatric NP	826 (6.5%)
Post-Masters	34 (2.8%)
DNP Post-Baccalaureate	28 (12.6%)
Gerontological NP	66 (0.5%)
Post-Masters	15 (1.2%)
DNP Post-Baccalaureate	0
Adult Gerontology Primary Care NP	372 (2.9%)
Post-Masters	22 (1.8%)
DNP Post-Baccalaureate	4 (1.8%)
Women's Health NP	397 (3.1%)
Post-Masters	21 (1.7%)
DNP Post-Baccalaureate	5 (2.3%)
PRIMARY CARE TOTAL MASTERS NPs	**10,741**
PRIMARY CARE TOTAL POST-MASTERS	**851**
PRIMARY CARE TOTAL DNP POST-BACCALAUREATE	**172**
TOTAL PRIMARY CARE NP GRADUATES	**11,764**

The above primary care specialties account for 84 % of all specialties selected by masters graduates, 70% of all specialties selected by post-masters graduates, and 78% of all specialties selected by post-baccalaureate DNP graduates in 2012.

Adult Acute Care NPs	803 (6.3 %)
Post-Masters	79 (6.5%)
DNP Post-Baccalaureate	21 (9.5%)
Neonatal NPs	233 (1.8%)
Post Masters	20 (1.6)
DNP Post-Baccalaureate	2 (0.9%)
Pediatric Acute Care NPs	130 (1.0%)
Post-Masters	44 (3.6%)
DNP Post-Baccalaureate	2 (0.9%)
Adult Gerontology Acute Care NPs	94 (0.7%)
Post-Masters	7 (0.6%)
DNP Post-Baccalaureate	8 (3.6%)
Adult Psychiatric & Mental Health NP	267 (2.1%)
Post-Masters	68 (5.6%)
DNP Post-Baccalaureate	3 (1.4%)
Family Psychiatric and Mental Health NP	334 (2.6%)
Post-Masters	139 (11.4%)
DNP Post-Baccalaureate	5 (2.3%)
NP Dual Track/Other NP	187 (1.5%)
Post-Masters	10 (0.8%)
DNP Post-Baccalaureate	9 (4.1%)

Continued

TABLE 15-2   **2012 Graduates of Masters, Post-Masters, and Post-Baccalaureate DNP-Level Nurse Practitioner Programs*—*cont'd***

Clinical Track/Certificate Examination	Graduates N (total % for each category)
TOTAL NON PRIMARY CARE MASTERS	2,048
TOTAL NON PRIMARY CARE POST-MASTERS	367
TOTAL NON PRIMARY CARE DNP POST-BACCALAUREATE	50
TOTAL NON PRIMARY CARE NPs	2,465
TOTAL ALL NP GRADUATES 2012	14,401

From American Association of Colleges of Nursing and National Organization of Nurse Practitioner Faculties. (2013). *Annual survey*. Washington, DC: Authors.
NP = Nurse Practitioner.
*Percentages may not total 100 due to rounding.

data. Family practice, for example, is the largest primary care specialty in medicine. Over the last 2 years, only 1184 and 1317 U.S. medical students each year chose residencies in family medicine (American Academy of Family Physicians [AAFP], 2011), compared with closer to about 12,000 primary care NPs graduating in 2012 (AACN & NONPF, 2013). These estimates, and the dearth of data on the NP workforce, make a compelling case for more robust workforce data on NP practice patterns, distribution, and impact on outcomes. However, the data we do have are compelling in terms of the key role that NPs will need to play in addressing the primary care needs of the nation with the implementation of the PPACA.

The Doctor of Nursing Practice

In response to the need to support the advanced educational needs of the APN, the Doctor of Nursing Practice (DNP) is the expected requirement for APN preparation in the future. Endorsed by AACN, the DNP is a practice-focused doctorate designed to "prepare experts in specialized advanced nursing practice" (AACN, 2004). Foundational competencies and competencies in areas of specialization and role are included in DNP preparation. The DNP *Essentials* (AACN, 2006) outline specific foundational competencies and learning experiences in a variety of settings so that the broad consequences of decision making can be identified. These competencies are central to current APN practice and are particularly salient to primary care advanced practice. Many DNP programs started out as post-masters programs, but there are increasing numbers of post-baccalaureate programs that include NP preparation in their course of study. Although the numbers are still very small, they were included in the data presented in Table 15-2.

Nurse Practitioner Role and Competencies in Primary Care

Nurse Practitioners in Primary Care: A Role in Advanced Practice Nursing

Foundational to NP graduates overall, and specifically NPs in primary care, is that they have knowledge, skills, and abilities essential to independent and direct clinical practice (see Chapter 7, NONPF, 2012). The NP core competencies are acquired throughout an NP's educational program through mentored patient care experiences, with emphasis on independent and interprofessional practice; analytic skills for evaluating and providing evidence-based, patient-centered care across settings, and advanced knowledge of the health care delivery system. Doctorally prepared NPs apply knowledge of scientific foundations in practice for quality care. They are able to apply skills in technology and information literacy and engage in practice inquiry to improve health outcomes, policy, and health care delivery. Areas of increased knowledge, skills, and expertise include advanced communication skills, collaboration, complex decision making, leadership, and the business of health care. The NONPF core competencies build on the APN competencies described in Chapter 3 and throughout this text. They also build on previous work that identified knowledge and skills essential to Doctor of Nursing Practice (DNP) competencies (AACN, 2006; NONPF & National Panel, 2006) and are consistent with the recommendations of the IOM report on *The Future of Nursing* (2011). Box 15-1 cross-maps the seven APN competencies from Chapter 3 and the nine NP core competencies (NONPF, 2012). The competencies described in the following section reflect some of the selected core competencies for all APNs, as presented in Chapter 3, as well as the nine NONPF core competencies for all NPs relevant to the NP in primary care

BOX 15-1 Cross Mapping of Advanced Practice Nurse Competencies and National Organization of Nurse Practitioner Faculties Nurse Practitioner Competencies

APN Competencies (see Chapter 3)	NONPF NP Core Competencies
Direct clinical practice (see Chapter 7) • Use of holistic perspective • Formation of therapeutic partnerships with patients • Expert clinical thinking and skillful performance • Use of reflective practice • Use of evidence as a guide to practice • Use of diverse approaches to health and illness management	**Independent practice competencies** • Functions as a licensed independent practitioner • Demonstrates the highest level of accountability for professional practice • Practices independently managing previously diagnosed and undiagnosed patients 　• Provides the full spectrum of health care services to include health promotion, disease prevention, health protection, anticipatory guidance, counseling, disease management, palliative, and end-of-life care 　• Uses advanced health assessment skills to differentiate among normal, variations of normal, and abnormal findings 　• Uses screening and diagnostic strategies in the development of diagnoses 　• Prescribes medications within scope of practice 　• Manages the health and illness status of patients and families over time • Provides patient-centered care, recognizing cultural diversity and the patient or designee as a full partner in decision making 　• Works to establish a relationship with the patient; characterized by mutual respect, empathy, and collaboration 　• Creates a climate of patient-centered care that includes confidentiality, privacy, comfort, emotional support, mutual trust, and respect 　• Incorporates the patient's cultural and spiritual preferences, values, and beliefs into health care 　• Preserves the patient's control over decision making by negotiating a mutually acceptable plan of care **Scientific foundation competencies** • Critically analyzes data and evidence for improving advanced nursing practice • Integrates knowledge from the humanities and sciences within the context of nursing science • Translates research and other forms of knowledge to improve practice processes and outcomes • Develops new practice approaches based on the integration of research, theory, and practice knowledge
Coaching and guidance (see Chapter 8)	Independent practice competencies (see above) Technology and information literacy competencies (see below)
Consultation (see Chapter 9)	Independent practice competencies (see above) Scientific foundation competencies (see above) Ethics competencies (see below)
Collaboration (see Chapter 12)	Independent practice competencies (see above) Scientific foundation competencies (see above) Ethics competencies (see below) Leadership competencies (see below)

Continued

BOX 15-1   Cross Mapping of Advanced Practice Nurse Competencies and National Organization of Nurse Practitioner Faculties Nurse Practitioner Competencies—*cont'd*

APN Competencies (see Chapter 3)	NONPF NP Core Competencies
Evidence-based practice (see Chapter 10)	**Quality competencies** • Uses best available evidence to improve quality of clinical practice continuously • Evaluates the relationships among access, cost, quality, and safety and their influence on health care • Evaluates how organizational structure, care processes, financing, marketing, and policy decisions affect the quality of health care • Applies skills in peer review to promote a culture of excellence • Anticipates variations in practice and is proactive in implementing interventions to ensure quality **Practice inquiry competencies** • Provides leadership in the translation of new knowledge into practice • Generates knowledge from clinical practice to improve practice and patient outcomes • Applies clinical investigative skills to improve health outcomes • Leads practice inquiry, individually or in partnership with others • Disseminates evidence from inquiry to diverse audiences using multiple modalities • Analyzes clinical guidelines for individualized application into practice **Scientific foundation competencies (see above)**
Leadership (see Chapter 11)	**Leadership competencies** • Assumes complex and advanced leadership roles to initiate and guide change • Provides leadership to foster collaboration with multiple stakeholders (e.g., patients, community, integrated health care teams, policy makers) to improve health care • Demonstrates leadership that uses critical and reflective thinking • Advocates for improved access, quality, and cost-effective health care • Advances practice through the development and implementation of innovations incorporating principles of change • Communicates practice knowledge effectively orally and in writing • Participates in professional organizations and activities that influence advanced practice nursing and/or health outcomes of a population focus **Health delivery system competencies** • Applies knowledge of organizational practices and complex systems to improve health care delivery • Effects health care change using broad-based skills, including negotiating, consensus building, and partnering • Minimizes risk to patients and providers at the individual and systems levels • Facilitates the development of health care systems that address the needs of culturally diverse populations, providers, and other stakeholders • Evaluates the impact of health care delivery on patients, providers, other stakeholders, and the environment • Analyzes organizational structure, functions, and resources to improve the delivery of care • Collaborates in planning for transitions across the continuum of care **Policy competencies** • Demonstrates an understanding of the interdependence of policy and practice • Advocates for ethical policies that promote access, equity, quality, and cost • Analyzes ethical, legal, and social factors influencing policy development • Contributes in the development of health policy • Analyzes the implications of health policy across disciplines • Evaluates the impact of globalization on health care policy development

BOX 15-1 **Cross Mapping of Advanced Practice Nurse Competencies and National Organization of Nurse Practitioner Faculties Nurse Practitioner Competencies**—*cont'd*

APN Competencies (see Chapter 3)	NONPF NP Core Competencies

Ethical decision making (see Chapter 13)	**Ethics competencies**
	• Integrates ethical principles in decision making
	• Evaluates the ethical consequences of decisions
	• Applies ethically sound solutions to complex issues related to individuals, populations and systems of care
	
	Technology and information literacy competencies
	• Integrates appropriate technologies for knowledge management to improve health care
	• Translates technical and scientific health information appropriate for various users' needs
	  • Assesses the patient's and caregiver's educational needs to provide effective, personalized health care
	  • Coaches the patient and caregiver for positive behavioral change
	• Demonstrates information literacy skills in complex decision making
	• Contributes to the design of clinical information systems that promote safe, quality, and cost-effective care
	• Uses technology systems that capture data on variables for the evaluation of nursing care

Adapted from National Organization of Nurse Practitioner Faculties (NONPF). (2012). Nurse practitioner core competencies (http://nonpf.org/associations/10789/files/NPCoreCompetenciesFinal2012.pdf).

(NONPF, 2012). The NONPF core competencies were developed by integrating existing Master's and Doctor of Nursing Practice (DNP) core competencies. They are guidelines for educational programs preparing NPs to implement the full scope of practice as licensed independent practitioners. The competencies are essential proficiencies for all NPs and should be demonstrated on graduation. The competencies are specific to the NP role and prepare NPs, regardless of the population focus, to meet the complex challenge of translating rapidly expanding knowledge into practice and enable NPs to function in a changing health care environment. We will apply the APN and NP core competencies to the NP in primary care.

Advanced Practice Nurse Core Competencies

Direct Clinical Practice

As with other advanced practice roles, direct clinical practice is the foundation of the work of the primary care NP, which unfolds around the premise that individuals seek care for a broad range of health care concerns over time and across the life span. Relationships evolve over time, which facilitates a sense of mutual respect and trust. In that relationship, a deep understanding of the patient's life and the meaning of the illness or health issue at hand develops. Knowing patients and their family members,

their jobs and careers, and their challenges in raising children and caring for aging parents is part of accompanying patients through the transitions of life. Every exemplar included in this chapter illustrates the central competency of direct clinical practice. Readers will also see the extensive use of the APN competencies of expert coaching and guidance, consultation, and collaboration, as well as the overlap of the APN competencies with the NONPF core NP competencies.

For primary care NPs, one day is as varied as the next. Some days are filled with episodic visits and some days are spent predominantly on health care maintenance and education. The complexity of care and the NP's familiarity with patients are cultivated over longitudinal encounters. Although the hallmark of the primary care NP's practice is the breadth of health issues encountered, the privilege of patient-NP relationships occurs over time. This enables the NP to be patient-centered, tailor evidence-based interventions to the individual, and sustain a holistic practice. Characteristics of direct clinical practice, including the use of a holistic perspective, formation of therapeutic partnerships, expert clinical thinking, use of reflective practice, use of evidence as a guide to practice, and use of diverse approaches to guide practice are evidenced in the six exemplars in this chapter. Box 15-1 cross-maps direct clinical practice with the NONPF NP core competencies of independent practice and scientific foundations.

Reflective Practice: A Component of Direct Patient Care

Expert clinical thinking and skillful performance are cultivated through repeated evaluation of similar sets of health and illness scenarios and formulating plans of care based on patient expectations, standards of care, experience, clinical judgment, and current research. Experienced APNs incorporate this practical wisdom into their decision making, taking actions that they might have been unlikely to take as novice practitioners. Practical wisdom involves knowing what to do and when to do it.

- When is a patient ready to begin home glucose monitoring?
- When is it time to suggest respite or home health care?
- What is the right time to address sexuality issues with a preteen or teenager?
- What is the right time to address an issue directly, and when is it time to back off from confronting difficult issues?

Often, an assessment of the chief complaint unearths many issues; the patient may not be aware of some of these. The skilled practitioner helps the patient sift and sort through issues, establish priorities, and understand the interconnectedness of these priorities. Practical wisdom guides the practitioner to use expert clinical thinking and skillful interviewing to develop a plan of care that is likely to improve health and quality of life and be carried out by the patient. NPs are expert clinical thinkers who listen carefully to the story that the patient tells them.

Partnerships with patients and families develop over time. Relationships with patients should be therapeutic, regardless of whether or not it is the first or hundredth encounter. As partnerships deepen, the relationship becomes an even more important clinical tool. Patients are more likely to comply with medical recommendations if they are given a part in the decisions made about their care.

Another important strategy for reflective practice is peer review if done in a supportive collaborative way and is included in the NONPF NP competency (see Box 15-1). Open transparent sharing and review of difficult and complex patient situations can lead to important self-reflection.

Holistic Perspective

The development of a holistic perspective is another feature of direct clinical practice. With increasing evidence of the importance of patient-centered care, and the broad definitions of primary care, a holistic, patient-centered approach is key for NPs in primary care. The exemplars in this chapter address this perspective extensively. In practice, APN core competencies (see Chapter 3) are often executed simultaneously to achieve the best outcome. However, for purposes of didactic discussion, specific competencies are discussed in the individual exemplars for clarity. The exemplars reflect the extent to which the core competencies enhance direct clinical practice, the core of primary care.

Coaching and Guidance

The relationship between the primary care NP and the patient creates a strong foundation for the coaching and guidance competency (see Chapter 8). The coaching and guidance competency overlaps with the independent practice competencies and technology and information literacy NONPF NP competencies.

A challenge for the primary care provider is to identify serious illness and involve other disciplines in the care of the complex patient. Exemplar 15-2, with LM, illustrates the coaching competency. It also shows how the NP collaborates with other health care professionals to provide comprehensive care to complex patients. In this case, LM's NP may be the first provider to see the young adult with an eating disorder.

Coaching and guidance is exemplified in Exemplar 15-1, in which CL (the NP) addresses the broad array of developmental and age-related concerns of a young adult who she has followed since her late teens. High-risk behaviors had been addressed in earlier years and prevention is consistently emphasized. A strong relationship has developed, with an emphasis on coaching and guidance. CL also uses NP competencies, such as scientific foundations and health delivery system competencies. Over the years, CL continues to develop the partnership with the patient. NPs have a deep knowledge of the change process and a menu of tools to use, depending on where the patient is in the cycle of change. Time is another tool for the primary care NP. As in the case of KI, the primary care NP is available to her longitudinally as she moves through developmental stages and health issues.

Consultation

Consultative relationships are critical to primary care NP practice. Relationships with other APNs, physicians, nurses, social workers, and other health care providers ensure that patients have access to comprehensive care. The exemplars illustrate different consultative relationships. In Exemplar 15-3, in which care is delivered in a nurse-managed health center, consultation is clearly evident through the use of technology and an electronic health record (EHR), making care seamless. Consultation can be formal, as reflected in Exemplar 15-3, or informal, with colleagues in one's practice. This informal style is a frequent part of the daily rhythm of a nurse-managed center, as well as many primary care practices, and includes elements of the collaboration competency and independent practice. NPs in a smaller or solo practice may have to develop methods of consultation, as described in Exemplar 15-3. The increased use of technology in practice makes this more possible today.

NPs in primary care use other APNs as a consultant in their specialty areas. For example, the primary care NP might initiate a consultation with a psychiatric NP or CNS to evaluate depression in a hospitalized patient. In Exemplar 15-2, psychiatric consultation was sought to address an eating disorder. A referral for consultation with a CNM for preconception counseling provides valuable information to the woman ready to start a family. Newly diagnosed patients with type 2 diabetes benefit from consultation with a CNS whose specialty is diabetes management, and the expertise of home health nurses is critical in discharge planning. Community health nurses have a wealth of knowledge regarding other community resources and insurance coverage for home care services. NPs often initiate consultations with other health care professionals, including physicians, pharmacists, physical therapists, occupational therapists, speech therapists, nutritionists, and social workers.

Collaboration

The IOM definition of primary care (1996) implies the use of professional collaboration to deliver "integrated" and "accessible" care for all health care providers. The fiscal realities of practicing solo, in addition to the restrictions on NP practice imposed by state regulations, make a team approach the preferred choice for physicians and many nurses in primary care. Effective collaboration results in more comprehensive, patient-focused care (Bodenheimer & Grumbach, 2007) and it promotes high-quality, cost-effective outcomes (Cowan, Shapiro, & Hays et al., 2006). Most NPs practice in settings with physicians who are in a private practice or publicly funded practice, such as community health centers, the Veterans Administration (VA), or other government practices, including local health departments. Collaboration is seen as a professional ethic, central to primary care, and not easily regulated. All health professions collaborate on a regular basis to address the complex needs presented in primary care. It is an expected norm of primary care and not unique to NP practice. With the growth of the PCMH, collaborative and team practice will no doubt have an increasing prominence in primary care.

Most of the exemplars in this chapter include some form of collaboration, but Exemplar 15-6 describes a gerontology practice based on collaboration among physicians, NPs, other nurses, pharmacists and social workers. The practice is intentionally interdisciplinary, exceptionally collaborative, and team-based. Patients benefit from a team approach although an NP or physician may be the leader of a group of patients. This exemplar demonstrates independent practice (NP NONPF competency) of an NP within a strong team–collaborative model of care. Patients clearly benefit from this approach to care and, in primary care, it is increasingly becoming more common in a PCMH.

Nurse Practitioner Core Competencies

Independent Practice Competencies

The work of the primary care NP is based on the premise that individuals seek care for a broad range of health care concerns over time across the life span. Relationships evolve over time (e.g., Exemplars 15-1 and 15-6), which facilitates a sense of mutual respect and trust (NONPF, 2012). Within that relationship, a deep understanding of the patient's life and the meaning of the illness or health issue at hand develops. It is essential for NPs to know their patients' lives, including their family members, their jobs and careers, and their challenges in raising children, as well as caring for aging parents.

As clinicians, leaders, and role models, primary care NPs bring a holistic approach to care, an approach that directly affects the lives of individuals, families, and even whole communities. There are many social forces that emerge to shape the future health and professional practice environment for primary care NPs. Most importantly, the primary care NP needs to be prepared to function as a licensed independent practitioner and demonstrate the highest level of accountability for professional practice. In their practice, primary care NPs independently manage previously diagnosed and undifferentiated or undiagnosed patients and provide a full spectrum of health care services, including health promotion, disease prevention, health protection, anticipatory guidance, counseling, disease management, palliative care, and end-of-life care. The primary care NP is capable of using advanced health assessment skills to differentiate between normal, variations of normal, and abnormal findings and uses screening and diagnostic strategies in the development of diagnoses. Furthermore, she or he prescribes medications within the scope of practice and manages the health and illness status of patients and families over time.

Primary care NPs also need to be able to provide patient-centered care, recognizing cultural diversity and the patient or designee as a full partner in decision making. They should work to establish patient relationships characterized by mutual respect, empathy, and collaboration. They need to create a climate of patient-centered care that includes confidentiality, privacy, comfort, emotional support, mutual trust, and respect. They should incorporate patients' cultural and spiritual preferences, values, and beliefs into their care. Finally, they should preserve a patient's control over decision making by negotiating a mutually acceptable plan of care. The competency of independent practice is very similar to that of the APN's direct clinical practice. It implies that every NP is responsible for the care that he or she delivers, including the quality of that care and the practice of collaboration and consultation.

Scientific Foundation Competencies

Complexity of care and an NP's familiarity with patients is cultivated over a series of encounters. Although the hallmark of the primary care NP's practice is the breadth of health issues encountered, the privilege of developing a patient-NP relationship occurs over time. This enables the NP to tailor evidence-based interventions to the patient and to sustain a holistic practice. As with other advanced practice roles, primary care NPs needs to have the ability to analyze data and evidence critically for improving advanced nursing practice. The scientific underpinnings of practice provide a basis of knowledge for advance nursing practice. Primary care NPs need to be able to integrate knowledge from the humanities and sciences within the context of nursing science. In particular, the primary NP should have a scientific foundation derived from the natural and social sciences and that might include human biology, physiology, and psychology.

Nursing science foundations have contributed to the discipline of nursing, which is characterized by a "unique perspective, a distinct way of viewing all phenomena, which ultimately defines the limits and nature of its inquiry" (Donaldson & Crowley, 1978, p. 113). According to the AACN *DNP Essentials* (2006), specific middle-range theories should be used to guide the practice of NPs. Primary care NPs may use middle-range theory to guide their assessment, decision making, and interventions, particularly when situations call for them (Lenz, 1998). Historically, nursing professionals have struggled to close the theory-practice gap because of lack of knowledge, understanding, and applicability of nursing theory to guide nursing practice (Kenny, 2006). Doctorally prepared NPs, in particular, should be capable of understanding middle-range theory and translating research and other forms of information to improve practice processes and outcomes. Ultimately, primary care NPs must be able to develop new practice approaches based on the integration of research, theory, and practice knowledge.

Leadership Competencies

Primary care NPs, particularly doctorally prepared NPs, are expected to assume complex and advanced leadership roles to initiate and guide change. This competency is similar to the APN competency of clinical, professional and systems leadership (see Chapter 11). Their leadership should foster collaboration with multiple stakeholders (e.g. patients, families, community, integrated health care teams, policymakers) and demonstrate critical and reflective thinking. Collaboration and leadership are closely linked in the effort to improve health care. In primary care, for example, the NP's direct clinical practice with expert coaching and guidance exemplifies a collaborative relationship between patient and NP. The 1996 IOM definition of primary care implies the use of professional collaboration to deliver integrated and accessible care. Effective collaboration results in more comprehensive, patient-focused care (Bodenheimer & Grumbach, 2007) and promotes high-quality, cost-effective outcomes (Cowan et al., 2006). The NP's expert coaching and guidance also require the establishment of a collaborative relationship between patient and provider (Dick & Frazier, 2006).

Moreover, primary care NPs should be capable of advocating for improved access, better quality, and cost-effective health care for all populations. They are able to use the development and implementation of innovations that incorporate principles of change to advance practice. They should also be able to communicate practice knowledge effectively, orally and in writing. At the local practice level, for example, NPs enact leadership roles when they guide and support staff, triage patients, and oversee the appropriate use of resources. NPs must ensure that primary care practices have an evidence base and that they use meaningful, systematic, quality improvement initiatives. On a broader level, primary care NPs engaged in clinical and professional leadership must also use effective collaborative skills to assist groups and organizations to envision preferred futures, achieve consensus, and implement change.

The essence of primary care is the sustained continuity of health care for patients and their families. As the long-term member of the entire team that provides continuity and stability in the care and management of patients over long periods, primary care NPs often emerge as leaders in health care settings. Additionally, the primary care NP's role as a leader in the community via membership on boards of health and education, and as an influential policymaker, cannot be underestimated.

Quality Competencies

Rapidly rising health care costs are leading to a variety of changes in the U.S. health care system and are placing patients and providers in jeopardy. Patients risk losing out on effective, albeit costly, care. Increasing consumer desire for care oriented toward prevention, primary care NPs are presented with unique opportunities to contribute significantly in improving the quality and measurement of health care delivery and the patient's health outcome. Ongoing monitoring and continuous improvement of practice outcomes is essential for all NPs, including those in primary care.

Primary care NPs are expected to use the best available evidence to improve the quality of clinical practice continuously. Ongoing evaluation of the relationships among access, cost, quality, and safety and their influence on health care is essential to the role that NPs play in health care. Primary care NPs need to be competent in evaluating how organizational structures, care processes, financing, marketing, and policy decisions affect the quality of health care. To ensure quality, primary care NPs need to apply skills in peer review to promote a culture of excellence and anticipate variations in practice. Also, they need to be proactive in implementing quality improvement interventions. NPs are expert clinical thinkers who listen carefully to the stories that their patients tell them. To ensure quality care, primary care NPs can partner with patients and families. Relationships with patients should always be therapeutic. As partnerships deepen, the relationship becomes an even more significant clinical tool. Quality outcome studies are presented later in this chapter.

Practice Inquiry Competencies

Expert clinical thinking and skillful performance are cultivated through repeatedly evaluating similar sets of health and illness scenarios and formulating plans of care based on patient expectations, standards of care, experience, clinical judgment, and current research. Primary NPs continuously synthesize knowledge and experience so that, over time, they acquire practical wisdom, defined by Oberle and Allen (2001) as "knowing when a particular action ought to be taken" (p. 151). Experienced APNs incorporate this practical wisdom into their decision making, taking actions that they might have been unlikely to take as novice practitioners.

An assessment of the chief complaint often unearths a multitude of issues and the patient may not be aware of all of these. The skilled practitioner helps the patient sort through the issues, establish priorities, and understand the interconnectedness of these priorities. Practical wisdom guides the practitioner to use expert clinical thinking and skillful interviewing to develop a prioritized plan of care that is likely to improve health and quality of life and to be carried out by the patient.

Primary care NPs play a critical leadership role in the translation of new knowledge into practice. To shorten the time spent translating bench science to bedside clinical practice, or for dissemination to population-based community interventions, primary care NPs are expected to provide leadership in translating new knowledge into practice and to generate knowledge from clinical practice to improve practice and patient outcomes. Thus, a primary care NP's education should be sufficient to prepare her or him to apply clinical investigative skills to improve health outcomes and lead practice inquiry, individually or in partnership with others. Finally, the primary care NP should be able to disseminate evidence from such inquiry to diverse audiences using a number modalities. Practice inquiry and quality competencies are cross-mapped with the research competency of the APN in Box 15-1.

Technology and Information Literacy Competencies

There is extensive evidence linking information technology with improved patient safety, care quality, access, and efficiency (Fetter, 2009). Primary care NPs must demonstrate competencies in computers, informatics, and information literacy to use information technology for practice, education, and research. In particular, they need to be able to integrate appropriate technologies for knowledge management to improve health care and translate technical and scientific health information appropriate to various users' needs. NPs rely on their technology and information literacy competencies to guide them in their assessments of patient and/or caregiver educational needs, in conjunction with the goal of effective, personalized health care. To serve as an expert primary care provider who coaches patients and caregivers toward positive behavioral change, primary care NPs need to demonstrate the use of information literacy skills in complex decision making. Exemplar 15-3 presents a situation in which technology and the use of the EHR enhance the care of a patient—that is, making timely consultation and referrals and consequently improving the outcomes of care for the patient. Their technology and information literacy competencies also inform NP contributions to the design of clinical information systems that promote safe, quality, and cost-effective care and enable NPs to use technology systems that capture data variables for the purpose of evaluating nursing care.

Policy Competencies

The evolution of advanced nursing practice has been influenced by changes in health care delivery and policy. APNs play an important role in providing direction for policy associated with primary care. Research has shown that nurses' involvement in the decision making of health care organizations is crucial for maximizing positive health outcomes for clients (Mackay, 2002). The development of key leadership skills is essential for primary care NPs to become more critically aware of underlying power structures in the health care system and ultimately to move toward being acknowledged as interdependent health professionals in primary care organizations. To play such a role, primary care NPs need to understand the interdependence of policy and practice. They need to able to advocate for ethical policies that promote access, equity, quality, and affordability. Furthermore, they must analyze the ethical, legal, and social factors that influence policy development and contribute to the development of health policy. Finally, primary care NPs should be able to analyze the implications of health policy across disciplines and evaluate the impact of globalization on health care policy development.

Health Delivery System Competencies

Health care delivery in the United States has often been characterized by fragmentation at the national, state, community, and practice levels. There is no unified entity or set of policies that guide the greater health care system. To keep pace with the complex demands of today's sicker and higher acuity patients, primary care NPs need to be competent within health delivery systems. In particular, they must be able to apply knowledge of organizational practices and complex systems to improve health care delivery. According to the Commonwealth Fund Commission (Davis, 2005), this fragmentation has divided providers' responsibilities among a number of agencies; that is, although providers may practice in the same community and care for the same patients, they often work independently from one another. The fragile primary care system in the United States has been on the verge of collapse. To minimize risk to patients and providers at the individual and systems level, primary care NPs should effect health care change using broad-based skills, including negotiating, consensus building, and partnering. For example, primary care NPs can help patients and families navigate different providers and care settings. They need to facilitate the development of health care systems that address the needs of culturally diverse populations, providers, and other stakeholders.

It is important for the primary care NP to understand that poor communication and lack of patient accountability among multiple providers leads to medical errors, waste, and duplication. Primary care NPs need to able to evaluate the impact of health care delivery on patients, providers, other stakeholders, and the environment. Finally, they should be competent about analyzing organizational structures, functions, and resources to improve the delivery of care.

Ethics Competencies

The primary care NP may encounter patient care concerns that raise ethical issues. This competency is cross-mapped with the APN ethical decision making competency. Examples include reproductive issues, informed consent, individuals excluded from the health insurance market, and conflicting health care goals among family members. NPs have opportunities to engage in preventive ethics by initiating discussions about advance directives and organ donation with patients in a relaxed and thoughtful manner, before they become pressing issues. In addition, NPs identify and address ethical conflicts that arise when clinical goals conflict with institutional goals (American Nurses Association [ANA], 2001; Johnson, 2005; McCaughan, Thompson, Cullum, et al., 2005; Ulrich, Soeken, & Miller, 2003).

Primary care NPs are accountable primarily to their patients and honor patient confidentiality at all times. This professional value has become the focus of more intense government regulation and scrutiny with the implementation of the 1996 Health Insurance Portability and Accountability Act (HIPAA). Primary care NPs must be vigilant in their protection of confidential patient information in whatever form it takes. In an era of managed health care, the primary care clinician's accountability to the health care system in which he or she practices may create tension, especially with the use of resources for patient care. Primary care NPs must always be ethically accountable for their actions, particularly when financial incentives related to resource use are involved (Bodenheimer & Grumbach, 2007).

Text continued on p. 416

 EXEMPLAR 15-1   **Longitudinal Relationship with Patient: Direct Clinical Practice of the Primary Care Nurse Practitioner**

Carol Liang (CL) is an adult primary NP in a university-affiliated internal medicine practice. She has practiced in this setting for 9 years and works with six internists and a variety of specialists from the university medical center. Although her focus is primary care, she has access to several subspecialists for consultation purposes

(APN consultation competency and NP practice inquiry competency). Patient scheduling occurs in several ways. A triage nurse makes a brief telephone assessment of the patient's symptoms and then schedules the patient to see CL or a physician, depending on availability. Educational, counseling, and annual examination visits

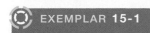

are scheduled with a primary care NP as appropriate (direct clinical practice and NP quality competencies). Physicians refer patients to an NP for follow-up on chronic medical problems such as hypertension, diabetes, and asthma. Assessment of additional problems, counseling, education, and medication management may occur during these visits. Patients are also free to self-schedule appointments with the NP. CL sees some patients on an intermittent basis whereas others see her for most of their primary care needs. Many women in the practice see CL for their annual examination. The following details a sample patient, Kelly Ingersol (KI), and illustrates the range of competencies used by CL, including APN competencies of direct clinical practice, collaboration, and consultation and NP competencies of scientific foundation, leadership, and practice inquiry. These competencies are identified in parentheses.

KI is a 26-year-old woman appearing for her annual examination. CL first met KI when KI's mother, a current patient, brought her daughter in to discuss contraception. At the time of her initial visit, KI was 17 years old and was considering becoming sexually active. During that visit, CL began to develop a trusting rapport with KI that would serve as the foundation of their relationship for subsequent years. The first visit focused on contraception education, emotional readiness to begin a sexual relationship, safe sex, and a brief screening for any type of high-risk behavior. There were no contraindications for hormonal contraception and so KI was given a prescription for a 3-month supply of birth control pills and instructed to return for follow-up after 3 months of use (direct clinical practice and scientific foundation competencies). She was given written instructions about oral contraception, including signs and symptoms of clotting issues related to estrogen use. CL also made herself available via phone and e-mail for any questions that KI may have had (technology and information literacy competency).

During her college years, KI continued to see CL for her annual examination. During those years, KI engaged in some high-risk sexual behavior, some of which was related to excessive alcohol use. CL used each annual visit to continue to raise awareness of the consequences of high-risk sexual behavior and alcohol use and to reaffirm safe sex practices (e.g., condom use). KI kept her annual visit appointment during those tumultuous years. Each visit included screening for chlamydia, gonorrhea, syphilis, and HIV (ethics competency).

KI finished college and took a job teaching kindergarten in a nearby school district. She is now in her fifth year of teaching and has been dating a young man for 3 years. She takes birth control pills and calcium supplements. She had no major concerns during her last visit except a question about a mole on her right leg. KI is satisfied with her teaching job and she and her partner have recently talked about getting married. CL noted during the interview that KI's exposed skin is tanned.

KI's annual examination focused on wellness and prevention issues. She has no current weight issues and reports a negative history for eating disorders. She has no current or remote symptoms of depression. Her dietary intake is adequate and includes a variety of meats, fruits, and vegetables. She does not drink milk, however, and only eats cheese or yogurt about three times a week. She drinks two to four glasses of wine weekly and does not smoke. She does not get any regular exercise according to national guidelines. Now that she has settled in to her teaching position, she has developed an interest in gardening and scrapbooking. She happily reports that her relationship with her boyfriend is steady and mutually loving. She denies any physical or emotional abuse. She and her partner have decided to forego condom use because they are monogamous and eventually plan to be married. KI reports a normal libido and is satisfied with her sex life. A brief overview of newer contraceptive options was given, but KI is satisfied with the oral contraceptive pill that CL prescribed 3 years earlier. KI has no new contraindications for estrogen use and denies any side effects as a result of taking the hormone.

There is no change in KI's family history since her last visit. Significant family history includes her mother's diagnosis of melanoma 5 years ago, for which she has been disease-free for 4 years. KI denies a family history of early heart disease, breast cancer, colon cancer, skin cancer (other than mother's melanoma), or diabetes. She does admit to several bad sunburns as a teenager. Her immunizations are up to date, and she receives an annual flu shot through the school system (practice inquiry and independent practice competencies). Her review of symptoms is negative except for a reported increase in the size of a mole on her right leg. The physical examination includes skin, thyroid, cardiovascular, respiratory, breast, abdominal, and pelvic examinations. Findings are normal except for a 10-mm mole on her right lateral knee, with a slightly irregular border,

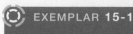 **EXEMPLAR 15-1   Longitudinal Relationship with Patient: Direct Clinical Practice of the Primary Care Nurse Practitioner—cont'd**

and bathing suit tan lines. Thin-layer Pap testing was done, along with chlamydia, gonorrhea, and potassium (KOH) and saline wet prep. Blood glucose and cholesterol test results are normal from the previous year and are not repeated.

The opportunity for teaching and counseling occurs at the conclusion of the visit. KI is offered the opportunity to ask questions, and she expresses interest in the human papillomavirus (HPV) vaccine, Gardasil. CL provides a handout with information about the vaccine. CL explains that the vaccine immunizes a young woman against the strains of HPV that are implicated in cervical cancer. Because of her age, she is eligible for the vaccine. KI indicates that she will check with her insurance company about coverage and consider starting the series (health delivery system competency).

CL reviews the need for adequate calcium and provides a list of calcium-rich foods. Options for exercise that fit with KI's lifestyle are reviewed. The health benefits of exercise are reinforced. Current recommendations for daily sunscreen use are reviewed and a sunscreen handout is provided. The importance of protective clothing, including a hat and sunglasses, is emphasized. CL realizes that a more in-depth discussion of sun-related issues will occur with the dermatologist, so she chooses to limit her counseling at this time.

A referral is made to a nurse practitioner colleague specializing in dermatology. This is the same colleague who has followed KI's mother since her melanoma diagnosis. KI will be notified of her laboratory results in writing in about 2 weeks. Recommended follow-up is in 1 year (leadership competency).

 EXEMPLAR 15-2   Student Health Care in a University Setting*

Larry Mahler (LM) is a 21-year-old college student seen by Roy Lucas (RL), a family NP. LM was referred to RL after multiple meetings with the college nutritionist revealed significant, progressive, and rapid weight loss. LM is an otherwise healthy white man who wanted to lose weight so that he had more energy and endurance for playing soccer. The nutritionist reported that LM lost about 20 pounds by exercising, eating healthier choices, and reducing portion sizes. After successfully losing 20 pounds in 2 months, LM exhibited signs of anxiety (e.g., heart palpitations and sweaty palms) when faced with eating. LM reports that the anxiety is caused by the fear that he will gain the weight back. He reports feeling fatigued but otherwise feels well. LM denies purging or using laxatives or diuretics. His vital signs on initial presentation are as follows: weight, 112 pounds; height, 5'7"; body mass index (BMI), 17.5; blood pressure (BP), 90/60 mm Hg, with no evidence of orthostatic hypotension. He appears pale, has sunken temples, and is very thin for his stature. The rest of his examination is unremarkable. LM is talkative, is well-groomed, and exhibits good eye contact, with a broad affect.

Blood specimens are drawn for basic laboratory studies (complete blood count [CBC], phosphate, magnesium, complete metabolic panel [CMP], thyroid-stimulating hormone [TSH]), and an appointment is made for LM to see university counselors and the student health psychiatrist. LM and RL talk openly and express their concerns and thoughts on his weight loss.

LM reports that he is doing better and that he will not lose more weight if given 1 week more. LM and RL develop a plan as to what he can do this week to ensure that he maintains his weight. LM reports he is agreeable to the plan and is scheduled for follow-up in 1 week. The next visit reveals another 6 pounds of weight loss in 6 days, despite reporting sufficient caloric intake. Clinical examination reveals a cachectic young man with clothes that hang on him, temporal wasting, gaunt features, and a flat affect, with slight psychomotor retardation. The rest of the examination is unremarkable except for bradycardia. Because of LM's physical state and psychomotor retardation from his nutritional deficiencies, it was decided in concert with LM and his psychiatrist, nutritionist, counselor, and family that he needed to be admitted to a local hospital for nutritional supplementation, as well as tests to rule out possible malignant causes of weight loss (signifying leadership competency). Throughout his relationship with LM, RL had tried to use touch, validation, active listening, and encouragement, but LM's physical and mental well-being continued to decline. At this visit, LM pleads and bargains not to go to the hospital, but RL explains that the clinical significance of his weight loss is too profound at this time to wait any longer. The admission would improve his physical status (gain weight, normalize all laboratory values) and mental health status (improve his altered mental status, monitor antianxiety medication).

EXEMPLAR 15-2   **Student Health Care in a University Setting***—*cont'd*

LM's father and girlfriend of 5 years come to the clinic to accompany LM to the hospital. RL and the nutritionist meet with LM's father to explain the urgent medical and psychological situation. They actively listen to his questions and answer them with an open and honest manner. Their intention is to decrease the family's anxiety, stress, and uncertainty regarding the diagnosis of anorexia nervosa and the pending hospital admission (ethics competency). LM and his family are concerned about the impact of a hospitalization on LM's college courses. With the help of the psychiatrist and LM's girlfriend, RL is able to involve LM's professors by writing them a letter explaining his current medical condition. In doing this, LM and his family are able to focus on his physical and mental health instead of worrying about missed classes or falling grades (direct clinical practice, leadership and practice inquiry competencies).

LM's hospital stay lasts several days, during which time the hospital staff rules out other causes of rapid weight loss. LM's diagnosis of anorexia nervosa is confirmed and his health is stabilized. LM and his family decide that inpatient treatment for anorexia nervosa is not appropriate for them at this time. Therefore the university psychiatrist, RL, physician, nutritionist, and university counselor agree to attempt to monitor LM's mental and physical status through an outpatient team approach. LM is involved in developing this plan and he agrees that if his weight decreases or if he misses follow-up appointments, inpatient treatment would become the only option (ethics competency). LM is agreeable to this plan.

It has been 1 year since this crisis for LM and he continues to maintain the weight that he gained. LM continues to see his counselor and psychiatrist on a regular basis. His visits with RL have stopped because he is medically stable, but they can resume at any time. The lines of communication remain open, specifically by e-mail, phone and clinical visits, between LM and his team.

*We gratefully acknowledge Courtney Bickett, FNP, for assistance with this exemplar.

 EXEMPLAR 15-3   **Nurse Practitioner Practice in a Nurse-Managed Health Center**

Juan Gonzales (JG) is a 43-year-old Hispanic man whose primary language is Spanish. He has been in the United States for 3 years. He presents to the NMHC, where Adrian Finch (AF), adult NP, is practicing. JG has usually seen the bilingual NP provider, but he was not available for this same day visit. JG had called for an appointment to be seen as soon as possible because of lower abdominal pain. The NMHC is small, staffed usually by an NP and medical assistant (some of whom are bilingual), and a part-time social worker. Physicians are not on site. Because of state regulations, a physician collaborator is also linked with the NMHC for delegated prescription writing and billing for some third-party payers, including Medicaid and Medicare. JG has a local county health plan that is similar to Medicaid but coverage is not as extensive. He is employed in a fast food restaurant that does not offer health benefits to their employees. He is married, with one child.

The NMHC is owned and operated by a school of nursing but also is linked with the university's health system in terms of their EHR, so that all visit information, laboratory results, consults, and medications are in the database and available to all providers in the health system, including the emergency department and all specialists. Translators are also available by phone through the health system. Because Spanish was his primary language and he was most comfortable communicating in Spanish, we used the translator phone line (our bilingual staff members were not available that day). In terms of NP competencies, use of appropriate technologies was thought to be part of providing safe, quality, ethical care. The use of multiple competencies was evident in this situation.

Mr. Gonzales presented with a history of sudden onset of back pain (rated as a 10/10) radiating to his lower abdomen. Pain lasted about 4 hours. Although the pain began to diminish, he was uncomfortable. His wife thought he should have gone to the emergency room, but he didn't want to. He had not thought to call our on-call number at the time. After obtaining a full history, AF, the NP, was sure that this could be a kidney stone. She explained her thinking and approach to testing through the interpreter (critical member of the team in this case). Appropriate laboratory work was ordered, with an ultrasound scheduled the same day in the health system (competencies of direct clinical practice, scientific foundation, practice inquiry). A referral was made to a urologist in the system as well (consultation

EXEMPLAR 15-3   **Nurse Practitioner Practice in a Nurse-Managed Health Center—*cont'd***

competency). All notes were entered on the EHR and an e-mail notification went to AF's collaborating physician, in case she was called regarding the patient, and to the urologist (use of collaboration and the appropriate team, as well as technology and information literacy). The urologist responded within 1 hour, saying that he would be looking for the patient and all the laboratory results. He agreed that we should start the patient on tamsulosin (Flomax). He also confirmed that all tests needed were ordered. Having an electronic health information system that could be tracked by all providers was most helpful in this situation.

JG left the visit very satisfied with a clear understanding of the diagnosis, where and when all testing would occur, referral visit time, and location. In addition, AF gave him a prescription for pain and advice on using the emergency room if his acute pain recurred before seeing the urologist. The on-call number was also reviewed with him. The patient was able to avoid an emergency room visit because the team in this case communicated clearly and also had an integrated EHR available for all team members to track information and test results.

Ultimately, JG was treated for his kidney stone; he returned to the NMHC for ongoing primary care. In this case, the NP was able to provide the necessary team through the use of a translator on the phone, referral to the necessary specialist, and ordering needed tests that were then entered into the same EHR. In reviewing the APN and NP competencies, most of them were used in this case. Direct clinical practice and consultation from the APN competencies were evident. Additional NP competencies were used for a correct diagnosis, effective collaboration, and communication, with appropriate referral to deliver the care needed. Technology played a significant role in this situation, and the NP was practicing independently, accountable for the quality of her care, but with the appropriate collaboration and referral that any primary care provider would use.

 EXEMPLAR 15-4   **Urban Pediatric Nurse Practitioner Primary Care Practice**

Jane Guttman (JG) is a pediatric NP caring for children in a low-income urban community. This community once thrived as part of a major industrial center but was devastated by factory closings and a declining local economy. Recent health status indicators for this urban area reveal increasing rates of teen pregnancy. Concern is growing in the community about substance abuse, school dropout rates, and community violence.

This setting is a challenging one, but JG believes that by working with children and families through the community child health clinic, she might be able to help them deal with the risks that poverty introduces to their health and wellness (clinical, professional, and systems leadership competencies). The clinic is a public-private venture jointly funded by the local health department, community hospital, and various charitable organizations in the greater metropolitan area. It serves as a source of primary care to many of the community's children, whose health care is subsidized by Medicaid and who are now enrolled in a statewide managed care program. The clinic also provides services to non-Medicaid recipients using a sliding scale fee. JG sees a variety of infants, children, and adolescents who come to the clinic for well-child visits and acute or episodic health problems. Her care entails thorough health assessments using history taking, physical assessment, and appropriate diagnostic studies or screening examinations (direct clinical practice and use of NP scientific foundation and leadership competencies). She then recommends appropriate interventions (pharmacologic and nonpharmacologic) for the child. These are in keeping with established national and clinical guidelines (APN research competency and NP quality and scientific foundation competencies). Much of JG's time is spent discussing normal childhood growth and development, effective parenting skills, nutritional needs, immunizations, and age-specific injury prevention guidelines with the parents. If the child is ill, JG describes ways to monitor the child's health status. JG's days are a busy because she sees children for regularly scheduled well-child visits and manages a variety of episodic health problems during the clinic's walk-in hours.

Collaboration in this practice goes in both directions; at times, JG may consult with the clinic pediatrician about acute health problems or abnormal health screening findings and at other times the pediatrician may consult with JG to discuss management issues of a child and the family situation. For children and families with complex health problems, JG may also consult with other members of the clinic team for further evaluation and management. Public health nurses are available for home assessment and case management services, and the clinic social worker provides additional outreach services. A nutritionist and eligibility worker from the women, infants, and children (WIC) nutrition program are on site to address nutritional needs in depth (leadership that includes use of excellent communication competencies and NP competency of the health care delivery system).

JG also engages with this community outside the walls of the clinic. Involvement with community activities enhances her credibility and acceptance among this low-income population. On occasion, she is asked to assist with health screening examinations for the local Head Start program. Recently, concern has been growing about unmet needs for child health services in the greater urban area. Inappropriate use of local emergency

rooms for episodic health care and a rising incidence of asthma and lead poisoning have contributed to a renewed commitment to pediatric primary care. JG works closely with the school nurses to follow high-risk children and to provide backup for emergency situations. As a respected primary care provider for an underserved community, JG has been asked to serve on a local child health task force. She will work with other health care providers and community leaders to identify ways to use public and private resources more effectively in addressing children's health needs. Together, they hope to promote a healthier future for the community at large. This exemplar again demonstrates a very broad use of the APN and NP competencies and includes a focus on population health and the larger community.

 EXEMPLAR 15-5 Rural Nurse Practitioner Primary Care Practice

With 3 years of experience as a family nurse practitioner (FNP) at the Mountain Breeze Rural Health Center, Dan Ahmad (DA) realized how well he had developed as a primary care provider. He had worked as a public health nurse for 10 years in this coal-mining and industrial community of Appalachia and was familiar with its poverty and limited access to health care. The mountains themselves, with their narrow winding roads, posed one of the major barriers to care in this area—transportation.

Before the long-time local family physician retired, DA had been able to pursue his NP education through a master's degree program offered by the state university satellite program on the community college campus 40 miles away. The 1-hour commute to school seemed long, but that trip was short compared with the additional 300 miles he would have had to travel if teleconferencing with faculty on the main campus was not available. DA was the recipient of a state scholarship for his graduate education and, in return, he agreed to practice in a medically underserved area of the state that had been his home for his entire life.

Anticipating the loss of their beloved physician, the community had worked hard to support the establishment of a rural health center in the area. DA was well known to the local citizens as a public health nurse and they readily accepted him in his new role as an FNP. The nearest hospital, 30 miles away, had recently been engaged in the development of rural health networks and provided physician coverage in the center 3 days per week. The retiring family physician had

been an important professional asset for DA in his first year after graduation as he made the transition to his new role. Now, on the 3 days per week that physicians were on site to collaborate, he could be sure that patients requiring more complex medical management were scheduled. These days also provided an opportunity to review and discuss other patient management issues and to develop skills and knowledge related to the medical issues in his practice (leadership competency, with good use of collaboration and consultation).

DA's days at the center were always full, but never predictable. As an FNP, he provided care for a wide range of episodic health concerns for patients across their life spans. He cared for many adults with chronic health problems, such as diabetes and hypertension. He devoted much of his effort to working with patients and their families on improved nutritional status and implementing other health promotion strategies. One of his diabetic patients had recently started insulin therapy. After teaching him how to monitor his glucose level at home, he was able to adjust his initial insulin therapy over the phone. The phone proved to be a valuable tool for his practice because many families had no regular source of transportation to the clinic or Internet access at home. DA frequently discussed family health problems with them during his visits. He also followed many children from infancy through childhood for well-child and episodic visits (APN direct clinical practice, NP independent practice, scientific foundation, and practice inquiry competencies).

One afternoon a week, DA left the clinic and made rounds to visit patients in the local nursing home. He worked closely with the staff there to identify ways to assist this older adult population in maintaining as much independence as possible. He also enjoyed occasional trips to the local high school to assist with sports physicals. From time to time, he was invited to be a speaker at the employee health seminars held at the nearby packaging plant.

His work was rewarding and many challenges were ahead. He had recently discussed the area's low childhood immunization rates with local leaders. They were now developing a proposal for a mobile health unit to increase access to immunizations and other primary preventive services to remote sections of the tricounty area. DA was asked to describe some of this Appalachian community's health needs to a contingent of state and federal legislators visiting the area. He hoped to make a compelling case for a mobile health unit so that funding for the project could be secured (APN professional and systems leadership, NP policy and health delivery system competencies). This rural practice requires a clinician who is working to the fullest extent of one's preparation and uses all the NP competencies in a very broad sense.

NP Elizabeth McCabe (EM) met George Mill (GM) when she was working as an adult NP in a hospital-affiliated, senior health clinic in a university town. An interdisciplinary health care team composed of a geriatrician, nurse practitioner, social worker, registered nurse, and pharmacist staffs the clinic. The team meets bimonthly to discuss patient cases, blending each professional's unique talents and skills to provide seamless, holistic, patient-centered care. Each team consists of an NP and physician, each with a small panel of patients that they follow more independently and a larger panel of patients that is shared between them, alternating visits with the physician and NP. The NP is responsible for acute and chronic care management and for providing health maintenance care, including annual examinations, health screenings, risk assessments, and education. The team also includes a social worker.

GM is an independent and spirited 81-year old gentleman who had lived in a small farming community several hours north of the lively university town he now calls home. A history of cognitive decline and loss of functional independence, which worsened significantly after a recent fall, prompted his wife to schedule an appointment for a comprehensive geriatric assessment.

The health of older adults is not static but is a dynamic and interactive state, influenced by multidimensional domains, including functional, physical, psychological, and social. The geriatric team in this assessment was used to gather detailed information in each of these domains, identifying salient issues to design an individualized plan of care that helps mitigate or prevent frailty, improve health outcomes and quality of life, and identify short- and long-term care requirements. A geriatrician, social worker and NP (EM) were present for GM's assessment.

GM was accompanied by his wife, and her own declining health was evident by her gray complexion and cachectic appearance. She spoke quietly about her own recent health challenges; her worsening chronic obstructive pulmonary disease (COPD); a constellation of chronic conditions had left her increasingly dependent on her husband. Mrs. Mill became teary-eyed as she chronicled the past several months, beginning with her husband's hospitalization for multiple vertebral fractures with subsequent kyphoplasty, the consequence of a fall, his second this year. His hospital stay was prolonged because of delirium and his symptoms improved initially; however, during his stay in subacute rehabilitation, his memory declined and he became irritable and agitated. According to his wife, GM began experiencing memory problems 10 years ago and underwent a comprehensive evaluation by his former primary care provider (PCP), including magnetic resonance imaging (MRI and laboratory studies, which were unremarkable. His previous PCP generated a referral for neuropsychiatric testing, with results supporting a diagnosis of probable Alzheimer's disease. The neurologist started him on donepezil and there was initial symptom improvement. His past medical history was significant for dementia, dyslipidemia, benign prostatic hyperplasia (BPH), and hypertension.

EM, the physician, and social worker completed a comprehensive medical and social history and medication review. EM inquired into GM's social history, revealing a love for his family, including a son, daughter, and four grandchildren, and passion for the outdoors. He retired as a farmer at age 73, shortly after his diagnosis of Alzheimer's. His history of farming prompted EM to ask GM about exposure to environmental toxins. GM admitted that he had been exposed to pesticides since he began working on the farm at age 10. He and his wife lived in a small apartment near their son. He denies current or former use of tobacco, alcohol, or illicit drugs.

GM reported no symptoms of depression or visual or auditory hallucinations. Although he denied feeling depressed, his body language suggested otherwise; he spent most of the visit looking down at the table, his hands clasped in front of him. When asked how his recent health setbacks and move had affected his emotional and functional status, he acknowledged that leaving his home "up north" has been challenging for him, he missed working in his garden and tinkering around in his work shop. His appetite had been improving since he returned home and he denied any difficulty sleeping, but admitted to frequent naps throughout the day, which he attributed to being bored and old.

After the comprehensive medical and social history and medication review was completed, EM and the social worker met with GM and performed a functional evaluation—Mini–Mental State Examination (MMSE) and geriatric depression scale (GDS)—and GM scored 17/30 and 6/15, respectively. A baseline MMSE score was not available at the time of his assessment. GM showed functional deficits in instrumental activities of daily living (IADLs)—handling finances, driving and taking his own medications.

After a comprehensive medical examination, the team reconvened with GM and his wife. The recommendations, based on the team assessment, included continuing donepezil and adding memantine, given his deteriorating cognition, agitation, and irritability. The team discussed the possibility of a comorbid condition, such as depression or sleep apnea, that may be exacerbating his symptoms but elected to address this at a future visit. GM and his wife were satisfied with that plan. EM and the social worker communicated their concerns about safety, specifically the risk for falling, as well as the need for assistance with IADLs. The possibility of alternative living arrangements, considering the financial implications, was recommended. Although GM was not familiar with the role of the NP, he felt comfortable following up with EM after establishing a relationship of mutual respect. A return visit in 4 weeks to see EM and a same-day appointment with the social worker was made. He and his wife were given contact information, including the clinic phone number, e-mails, and after hours contact information.

At the follow-up visit with EM, GM's demeanor was abrupt. His wife stated that she had not noted any benefit from the meantine. His appetite remained the same; he spent his days watching TV and napping and denied any

recent falls. Further inquiry into sleep patterns revealed a history of snoring for many years with momentary episodes during which he stops breathing. He had never been evaluated for obstructive sleep apnea. He was asked to continue the memantine and was given a referral for a sleep study. He agreed to return in 6 weeks with the physician to discuss the results of his sleep study. His wife had kept in contact in the weeks following his geriatric assessment. After some consideration, GM and his wife were interested in moving to an assisted living facility near the senior health clinic, and their son and daughter were supportive of their decision. In addition, his wife began attending a caregiver support group, run by a social worker and held once a week at the senior health clinic.

GM returned in 6 weeks for a visit with EM and the physician. His sleep study results indicated significant obstructive sleep apnea, one of the worse cases that the physician had ever encountered. GM was asked to follow up in 6 to 8 weeks with EM after beginning continuous positive airway pressure (CPAP) treatment. At follow-up visits over the next few months, GM's symptoms improved dramatically. He continued to experience some mild cognitive impairment, but his memory improved remarkably since treatment for his obstructive sleep apnea.

Over 4 years of care, GM continued to alternate visits with EM and the physician for acute and chronic care follow-up. Over time, a sense of partnership developed among GM, EM, and the physician. He often jokes with the staff when he comes for his follow-up visits. He has required no further hospitalizations. GM has been using his CPAP machine consistently since his diagnosis and the results have been life-changing. The number of medications he is on has been reduced over time with resulting improved stamina. EM recommended referral to physical therapy to restore his strength and endurance. GM now walks daily, weather permitting and, on warm sunny days, he can be seen working outside his assisted living apartment planting flowers and weeding.

The role of the NP in this case demonstrates the importance of a team approach, yet the NP practices independently within a team using additional competencies, including leadership, scientific foundation, practice inquiry, and ethics. Management decisions were made based on the needs of the patient and family so that at some visits, the patient saw only the NP or physician or social worker, and at other times might see two or three members of the team. GM and his wife also knew that they could contact anyone from the team and their concerns would be addressed appropriately.

*We wish to thank Laura Carter, ANP-BC, DNP, for contributing to this exemplar.

Illness can create a range of negative emotions in patients, including anxiety, fear, powerlessness, and vulnerability. In the ever-expanding health care system, primary care NPs increasingly face ethical issues, particularly involving, but not limited to, the allocation of care. How to resolve these ethical issues is becoming an important task for NPs who work in primary care settings. Nursing practice must embrace thoughtful reflection on the meaning of moral concepts in terms of culture and diversity. Moral values are native to a particular culture and influence one's beliefs about health, illness, and how to set health care priorities (Pierce, 1997). Operating with a context-sensitive approach can enable primary care NPs to understand ethical issues in nursing practice more easily and to integrate ethical principles into their decision making (Lützén, 1997). Primary care NPs need to evaluate the ethical consequences of decisions and apply ethically sound solutions to complex issues related to diverse individuals, populations, and systems of care.

Summary

These NP competencies are clearly complementary to the broad APN competencies. They ensure that primary care NPs have sufficient knowledge, skills, and abilities to support independent clinical practice. The exemplars in this section are meant to demonstrate APN and NP competencies across a number of situations and populations.

Models of Primary Care and the Nurse Practitioner Role in Current Primary Care in the United States

Before presenting specific models of primary care, it is important to understand the current definition of primary care used in the United States and how that integrates with NPs. Primary care is the foundation of most international health care systems and seen as the basis for any effective health care system. Although secondary and tertiary care are essential components of health care systems, they are generally viewed as complementary to primary care and not foundational (Starfield, 1992; Starfield et al., 2005). Figure 15-1 illustrates the foundation that primary care holds globally (left pyramid). Health outcomes have been documented to improve when primary care is the foundation of a national health care system (Macinko et al., 2003; Starfield et al., 2005). In the United States, specialty care has had more emphasis and significantly more funding than primary care. The IOM (1996) has defined primary care as "the provision of integrated, accessible health care services by clinicians who are accountable for addressing a large majority of personal health needs, developing a sustained partnership with patients, and practicing in the

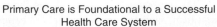

Primary Care is Foundational to a Successful
Health Care System

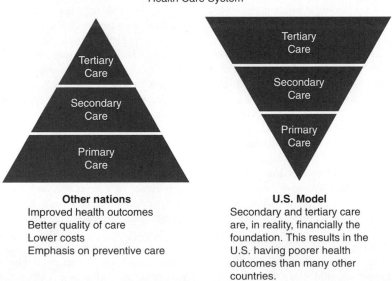

Other nations
Improved health outcomes
Better quality of care
Lower costs
Emphasis on preventive care

U.S. Model
Secondary and tertiary care are, in reality, financially the foundation. This results in the U.S. having poorer health outcomes than many other countries.

FIG 15-1 Models of primary care and the NP role in current primary care in the United States. *(Adapted from Macinko, J., Starfield, B., & Shi, L. [2003]. The contributions of primary care systems to health outcomes within Organization for Economic Cooperation and Development (OECD) countries, 1970-1978. Health Services Research, 38, 831-865.)*

BOX 15-2 **Institute of Medicine Terms Used to Define Primary Care**

Integrated
- Comprehensive, coordinated care throughout the life cycle
- Focused on particular needs of patients
- Clinician continuity
- Effective communication of information
- Patient record continuity

Accessibility
- Ease with which care is attained
- Elimination of geographic, cultural, language, reimbursement, and administrative barriers

Clinician
- Uses recognized scientific knowledge base
- Authority to direct the delivery of care

Accountable
- Clinician and system accountability for services provided

Most Personal Health Care Needs
- Competency to manage most health problems
- Use of consultation or referral as needed
- Sustained partnership
- Relationship between patient and clinician over time

Context of Family and Community
- Understanding of the circumstances and facts surrounding the patient (socioeconomic status, family dynamics, work issues)
- Awareness of public health trends
- Need for specific health promotion and disease prevention strategies

From Institute of Medicine. (1996). *Primary care: America's health in a new era.* Washington, DC: National Academies Press.

context of family and community" (p. 31). Box 15-2 summarizes the defining characteristics of the key terms, which are explained in detail in the IOM report. Within the NP role, there are four population foci of primary care—adult and gerontology, family, pediatric, and women's health (APRN Consensus Work Group, 2008). The IOM definition of primary care encompasses much of the essence of advanced practice nursing and advanced practice registered nurse (APRN) competencies, with its emphasis on accountability, a holistic approach to direct patient care, inclusion of health promotion and disease prevention activities, and description of a patient-clinician relationship "predicated on the development

of mutual trust, respect, and responsibility" (IOM, 1996, p. 37). A primary care NP brings these attributes and activities to the primary care setting. In Chapter 7 the use of a holistic framework and the forming of partnerships with patients are identified as two of the major characteristics of the APN. Through the use of the competencies discussed in this text, and specifically this chapter, an NP can effectively provide primary care. The population of patients for whom the NP is prepared to provide care—such as families, adults, neonates, children, women, and older adults—serves to differentiate the types of primary care NPs practice. The ANA "Scope and Standards of Advanced Practice Registered Nursing" reflects the integration of primary care delivery and the nursing process in this APN role (ANA, 2010).

The concept of integrated, accessible health care services described by the IOM (1996) also underscores the importance of a team approach in primary care delivery. An important APRN competency is collaboration among the professionals providing health services (see Chapter 12). Nursing models of care have emphasized developmental, family, and systems theories in considering human responses to illness (e.g., caring over time or finding deep meaning through illness). Using a holistic approach to assessment and treatment, the primary care NP addresses illness, promotes health, and prevents disease. Developing trusting relationships through strong interpersonal skills, patient and family education, and coaching and guidance is a critical element of practice. APNs integrate elements of care from nursing and medical models in a collaborative approach to clinical practice that enhances the comprehensiveness and quality of the care rendered. Many of the skills and competencies in primary care NP practice are based on the knowledge and skills needed to manage common acute and chronic health problems encountered in primary care settings. By using expert clinical reasoning and diverse management approaches, the NP provides appropriate, cost-effective primary care (see Chapter 7).

Nurse Practitioners as a Disruptive Innovation

In a classic paper in the Harvard Business Review (Christensen, Bohmer, & Kenagy, 2000), disruptive innovations in health care were described as those that are less expensive, more convenient products and services that start by meeting the needs of less demanding customers. The authors continued by saying that NPs are an example of such a phenomenon, which may help save our failing health care system. That is, NPs are a disruptive innovation to the traditional medical model of primary care delivery. It is to be expected that stakeholders who have dominated an industry would resist a disruptive innovator who has the potential to overturn the status quo. Although NPs have worked within the medical system as collaborative partners, more must be done to meet the primary care needs of the nation. Enhancing the supply of APNs, specifically primary care NPs, through removing barriers to practice in every state and expansion of DNP programs will be required. As DNP graduates in primary care stream into the workforce, it is expected that the primary care system will be substantially strengthened with nursing leaders who have the clinical credibility to influence change and create policy that builds a population-based health care system. NPs as disruptive innovators will be likely leaders in new models of the future. The next sections describe examples of models of primary care.

Patient-Centered Medical Home

The patient-centered medical home concept is a model of health care initially introduced in 1967 as the "medical home" by the American Academy of Pediatrics (Sia, Tonniges, Osterhus, et al., 2004). In 1978, the World Health Organization (WHO) met at Alma Ata and further identified the basic tenets of the medical home and its key role in primary care (International Conference on Primary Health Care, 1978). Almost 2 decades later, the IOM published its work on primary care (IOM, 1996) and specifically mentioned "medical home." Soon after the IOM report, the term *medical home* was increasingly evident in the family medicine literature (Robert Graham Center, 2007). The PCMH embraces the patient-provider relationship and the full spectrum of primary care, including standards of accessibility, continuity, comprehensiveness, integrated care, and interdisciplinary care (Robert Graham Center, 2007). Box 15-3 lists the overall criteria for the PCMH as identified by the National Committee on Quality Assessment (NCQA), which sets standards for PCMHs. There is strong emphasis on accessibility to care, patient-provider-staff communication, quality and safe care, and use of technology. There is strong consistency across the PCMH criteria and the APN and NP competencies identified in this text and chapter.

Much of the initial language related to the PCMH concept was physician-centric and presented the physician as the sole leader of the team, despite the increasing shortage of primary care physicians and the evidence that other, probably lower cost, PCPs and models of care are equipped and willing to provide a PCMH—and have been doing so—to diverse populations (Dwyer, Walker, Suchman, et al., 1995; Pohl, Tanner, Barkauskas, et al., 2010). Moreover, the medical home concept is patient-centric and therefore must accommodate patient needs

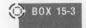 **BOX 15-3**   **What is a Patient-Centered Medical Home?**

PCMH strengthens the clinician-patient relationship by replacing episodic care with the following:
- A personal clinician, coordinated care, and a long-term healing relationship
- A relationship with a primary care clinician who leads a team that takes collective responsibility for patient care, providing for the patient's health care needs and arranging for appropriate care with other qualified clinicians
- A more personalized, coordinated, effective, and efficient model of care
- A high level of accessibility
- Excellent communication among patients, clinicians, and staff
- Full use of the latest information technology to prescribe, communicate, track test results, obtain clinical support information, and monitor performance
- An emphasis on quality and safety

Adapted from National Committee for Quality Assurance (NCQA). (2011). Patient-centered medical home: Health care that revolves around you (http://www.ncqa.org/LinkClick.aspx?fileticket=ycS4coFOGnw%3d&tabid=631).

with expanded and longer hours, including weekends and increased accessibility through technology. Many PCMHs include comprehensive integrated care so that mental and physical health needs are met in one setting through the use of multidisciplinary teams. In 2011, NCQA changed their criteria to include nurse-led PCMHs, such as nurse-managed health care centers. There are now NMHCs across the country who have met various levels of the NCQA's criteria for PCMH.

Nurse-Managed Health Centers

NMHCs are nurse-led, usually primary care, delivery sites that provide family and community-oriented primary care. In these practices, NPs provide much of the care, often in collaboration with other nursing and health care providers, such as nurse midwives, physicians, dentists, and social workers. NMHCs are often associated with academic institutions that provide significant educational settings for undergraduates and graduate students across disciplines (Pohl, Tanner, Barkauskas, et al., 2010). They have been rooted historically in the communities they serve and many use the word *community* in their names (Pohl, Barkauskas, Benkert, et al., 2007). Because there is no national tracking of all NMHCs, the exact number of

NMHCs is unknown, but it is estimated at around 200 to 250 (Lockhart, 1995; Pohl et al., 2007). The centers represent a model of care similar to that of the PCMH and community health centers funded by the U.S. Bureau of Primary Health Care. In many cases, they increase access to care for vulnerable populations and manage common acute problems and chronic diseases, such as diabetes, hypertension, depression, and asthma. Patient satisfaction in NMHCs tends to be exceptionally high (Benkert, Barkauskas, Pohl, et al., 2002) and the centers are successful in managing chronic illnesses based on national benchmarks (Barkauskas, Pohl, Tanner, et al., 2011). Students also report high satisfaction with these centers as sites in which they practice what they learn in the classroom (Tanner, Pohl, Ward, et al., 2003), Ongoing challenges to the NMHCs include reimbursement policies and inconsistent NP state regulation issues that make their sustainability challenging. When compared with federally funded community health centers, cost, diagnoses, and quality outcomes are comparable (Pohl, Tanner, Pilon, et al., 2011).

School-Based Health Centers

School-based health centers (SBHCs) bring essential health care to schools, allowing students to avoid health-related absences and improve success in the classroom. These centers are often directed and staffed by NPs, who provide most of the care (NASBH, 2012). They are located in schools or on school grounds and provide a comprehensive range of services that meet the specific physical and behavioral health needs of the young people in the community. Generally, SBHCs employ a multidisciplinary team of providers, including NPs, RNs, PAs, social workers, physicians, alcohol and drug counselors, and other health professionals. They often have advisory boards consisting of community representatives, parents, youth, and family organizations that provide planning and oversight.

Some SBHCs provide primary care to students and their families, whereas others supplement the care provided by other providers in the community. SBHCs reduce student absenteeism caused by illness, improve the management of chronic illnesses such as asthma, and provide important preventive interventions for physical and mental health issues related to adolescence. Students followed in SBHCs, when compared with those followed in community clinics, were less likely to use the emergency room, more likely to receive health maintenance visits and flu and tetanus vaccines, and less likely to be insured, and made more primary care visits (Allison, Crane, Beaty, et al., 2008).

Approximately 1709 SBHCs exist in the United States (NASBH, 2012). Funding for these centers is derived mainly from local, state, and federal grants. Both NMHCs and SBHCs are challenging to sustain, because they often serve as safety nets, are dependent on grants, and lack effective reimbursement policies for NPs

Convenient Care Clinics

Convenient care clinics, formerly called retail clinics, provide a model of more urgent care than primary care and are often located in pharmacies and grocery chains. As of early 2013, there are over 1400 retail clinics in the United States (Convenient Care Clinic Association, 2013). These clinics do not require appointments and the care that they provide is somewhat limited to common acute diagnoses, such as pharyngitis, otitis, and urinary tract infections using fairly strict protocols. NPs generally provide the care, although the clinics are not owned or managed by NPs. These clinics report high patient satisfaction, with short waiting times and appeal to clientele without insurance or those for whom immediate access is needed and not available. The American Medical Association and American Academy of Pediatrics have expressed concern about the quality of care, potential incentive to overprescribe, and lack of interaction with PCPs and the convenient care clinics. Despite those concerns, studies have shown that care provided at these clinics is cost-efficient for limited diagnoses and that quality is good (Mehrotra, Wang, Lave, et al., 2008).

Care for Homeless and Vulnerable Populations

In 2010, it was estimated that 49.9 million Americans had no health insurance (DeNavas-Walt, Bernadette, & Smith, 2011). The 2010 PPACA (HHS, 2011) expanded the number and capacity of federally qualified health centers to deliver high-quality, lower cost primary care to underserved, specific, and vulnerable populations. Primary care NPs are excellent candidates for providing high quality, lower cost primary care to populations at federally qualified health centers. Research has shown that when primary care NPs have the same authority, responsibilities, productivity and administrative requirements, and patient populations as primary care physicians, patients' outcomes are comparable in terms of their health status, physiologic test results for diabetic and asthmatic patients, and use of health care services after 6 or 12 months (Mundinger et al., 2000).

According to the National Law Center on Homelessness and Poverty more than 3 million people, including 1.3 million children experience homelessness yearly

(2012). From October 2008 to September 2009, there were nearly 1.56 million people who used emergency shelter or a transitional housing program (Cortes, Khadduri, Buron, & Culhane, 2010). Rates of acute and chronic illnesses are high among the homeless. More than 50% of homeless people have a history of mental illness and alcohol and/or substance abuse (Kirst, Frederick, & Erickson, 2011). For many homeless patients, accessing primary care is complicated by competing needs and circumstances. Many rely on the care provided by emergency departments. If primary care settings are available to them, however, their higher rates of hospitalization can be easily prevented (Althaus et al., 2011; Kwan, Ho, Preston, et al., 2008). The lack of primary care access makes this vulnerable population even more susceptible to poor health outcomes and leads to an overuse of emergency departments. Research has shown that tailoring medical care to the specific needs of vulnerable populations can increase primary care use and improve chronic disease monitoring and diabetes management (O'Toole et al., 2011). Using data from the 2003 Health Care for the Homeless (HCH) User Survey, Baggett and colleagues (2010) have found that 73% of 996 homeless respondents using the HCH's federally funded program report at least one unmet health need, such as the inability to obtain needed medical or surgical care (32%), prescription medication (36%), mental health care (21%), eyeglasses (41%), and dental care (41%).

Two successful service models of care for the homeless are the Boston Health Care for the Homeless Program and Glide Health Services, a nurse-managed and federally qualified health care center located in the Tenderloin neighborhood of San Francisco. The Boston Health Care for the Homeless Program provides integrated medical, behavioral, and oral health care and preventive services to more than 11,000 homeless people each year (O'Connell et al., 2010). Primary care NPs play an important role in this service model, which innovatively delivers homeless care in clinics located in two teaching hospitals, 80 shelters and soup kitchens, and a 104-bed medical respite unit. As this model signifies, primary care NPs are in an excellent position to provide care to homeless populations by taking advantage of recent shifts in health care priorities that stress the importance of primary care. The Glide Health Center is also a health care for the homeless program, is nurse-managed, and provides integrated, holistic primary care to an underserved population that has a high rate of homelessness (60%) and poverty (80% under 100% federal poverty level guidelines). They have recorded over 13,000 visits annually and have won awards for their high-quality care and focus on HIV prevention, chronic disease management, and mental health treatment. Outcomes of care are measured and compare favorably with national standards of care.

Veterans Administration

The U.S. Department of Veterans Affairs employs 3344 NPs, the largest employer of NPs in the country. NPs in the VA system work in collaborative interdisciplinary teams and a variety of NP roles have evolved in the VA over the past 36 years (Robinson, 2010). For example, gerontology NPs in the VA have a major role in leading interdisciplinary health care teams that collaboratively manage veterans' care. In addition to primary care roles, the VA has been innovative in their use of models linking practice and management roles, for which the VA is recruiting DNPs (Robinson, 2010). There is an Advanced Practice Nurse Advisory Group (APNAG) in the VA to advise on issues related to APNs and their practice in the VA's many settings.

There are many examples of the use of NPs in the VA. Gerontology NPs are employed extensively in the VA and offer services that include skilled nursing care, rehabilitation, wound care, end-of-life care, respite services, and management of geropsychiatric conditions. In many VA settings, the gerontology NP leads the interdisciplinary team (Robinson, 2010). Other innovations include a program that delivers home-based primary care to frail, chronically ill older veterans in an effort to reduce emergency room visits. These NPs function as the primary care provider and make home visits. Another innovative example of the use of NPs in the VA is with their use of EHRs and creating clinical reminders. Consistent with the NONPF NP competency of technology and literacy information, an NP at the Dubuque, Iowa VA is employed as an information liaison to write clinical reminders that can be used by other NPs and physicians (Robinson, 2010). The VA uses NPs in many roles consistent with the APN and NP competencies presented in this chapter.

Aging Populations and Primary Care

According to the U.S. Census Bureau (Howden & Meyer, 2011), the number of persons 65 years of age and older has increased by 15% from the previous decade to over 40 million, the fastest growing age group in the country. Projections suggest that by 2030, there will be 71 million older adults, representing 20% of the population. The cost of providing health care for this population is three to five times greater than the cost for someone younger than 65 (Centers for Disease Control [CDC], 2007). As a result of these demographic changes, projected health care spending will increase by 25%. Of all seniors, 90% have at least one chronic disease, 77% have two or more chronic diseases, and 85% of Medicare payments go toward treating chronic illness. The burden of preventing and managing chronic diseases in all populations, but especially in older adults, will be an essential component for all PCPs. NPs are an integral part of addressing this need because their approach is holistic, patient-centered, and team-based. NPs success with managing chronic diseases has been well documented (Barkauskas, Pohl, Tanner, et al., 2011; Newhouse et al., 2011). In addition, there is evidence that NPs keep people out of hospitals and help patients and their caregivers manage their environment so that there is a lower risk for exacerbation of chronic illness (see the next section, "Care Transitions and Primary Care"). Whether via leading and other roles in the PCMH and other primary care settings, the NP is well suited to be a cost-effective, high-quality provider. This segment of NP primary care practice offers unlimited opportunity for NPs to engage in community-based care. Exemplar 15-6 presents a team approach, with the NP as a critical member of the team.

Care Transitions and Primary Care

Almost 20% of Medicare patients discharged from the hospital are readmitted within 1 month (Jencks, Williams, & Coleman, 2009). This translates to the rehospitalization of approximately 2.6 million seniors annually, at a cost of over $26 billion every year. Readmission rates are also high for patients covered by Medicaid and/or private insurance. Researchers estimated that Medicare spent $17.4 billion on preventable rehospitalizations (Hennessey & Suter, 2011).

Care transitions refer to the movement of patients from one health care provider or setting to another. Although transitional care is not synonymous with primary care, it focuses on highly vulnerable, chronically ill patients throughout critical transitions in their health care (Wang et al., 2010). As such, it is marked by a shortened hospital stay and restricted duration of transitional service, the specifics of which vary by health insurance policy. Because it is limited in time and duration, transitional care emphasizes the education of patients and their caregivers to anticipate and address root causes of poor outcomes, thereby avoiding preventable rehospitalization. To improve quality of care and cut costs, a systematic literature review of 21 randomized clinical trials of transitional care interventions targeting chronically ill adults has demonstrated the importance of transitional care programs (Naylor, Aiken, Kurtzman, et al., 2011). Effective intervention programs use communal features, specifically those assigning a nurse as the clinical manager or leader of care and incorporating in-person home visits to discharged patients. Naylor and associates (2011) have observed that comprehensive discharge planning, with follow-up interventions that incorporate patient and caregiver goal setting, individualized care planning, education

and behavioral strategies, and clinical management is effective in decreasing readmission. They have also found that interventions that emphasize daily home video (e.g., Skype) or telephone monitoring and transmission of physiologic measurements, self-care instruction, and symptom management are essential components for providing quality transitional care. Thus far, research has demonstrated that APN-directed transitional care is associated with fewer first rehospitalizations or deaths, fewer total number of rehospitalizations, and lower health care costs (Brooten et al., 2002; Brooten, Youngblut, Kutcher, et al., 2004; Naylor et al., 2011). Transitional care programs led by an APN are related to higher functional status as well as satisfaction with care among COPD, heart failure patients, and cognitively impaired older adults and their caregivers (Naylor et al., 2004, 2007; Neff, 2003).

To facilitate the delivery of effective transitional care, primary care NPs need to be equipped with the knowledge and skills to assume expanded roles in the delivery of transitional care. Because of the critical role of family members in the delivery of transitional care, primary care NPs need to prepare and support these informal caregivers.

Quality of Care: Evidence-Based Care

Clinical practice in this age of information offers exciting opportunities and challenges for the primary care NP. Numerous studies over the past 40 years have consistently found that NPs deliver high-quality care and, when compared with national benchmarks and physician outcomes, care is often comparable or exceeds those benchmarks (e.g., Barkauskas et al., 2011; Brown & Grimes, 1995; Horrocks, Anderson, & Sallisbury, 2002; Laurant et al., 2005; Lenz, Mundinger, Hoplins, et al., 2002; Newhouse et al., 2011; Office of Technology Assessment, 1986; Spitzer, Sackett, & Sibley, 1974).

Evidence-based clinical practice guidelines can be used to improve primary care. Practice guidelines are used to reduce costs, standardize practice, and decrease medical liability. NPs can evaluate clinical practice guidelines and work to adopt those that will ensure that best practices are used in primary care delivery. The Agency for Healthcare Research and Quality (AHRQ), Healthcare Effectiveness Data and Information Set (HEDIS), National Guideline Clearinghouse (NGC), and National Quality Measures Clearinghouse are reliable resources for evidence-based clinical guidelines and performance measures (Box 15-4). These guidelines can also be used in conjunction with agency outcomes and performance measures to provide feedback to clinicians about the extent to which best practices are used (Barkauskas et al., 2011; Goolsby, 2004).

BOX 15-4   Useful Websites for Primary Care

Organization	Website	Content
Association of Colleges of Graduate Medical Education	www.acgme.org	Medical education Competencies
Agency for Healthcare Research and Quality	www.ahrq.gov/clinic	Clinical practice guidelines
National Quality Measures Clearinghouse	www.qualitymeasures.ahrq.gov	
Preventive Services	http://www.ahrq.gov/clinic/prevenix.htm	Age-specific screening examination recommendations
National Guideline Clearinghouse	www.guideline.gov	
National Advisory Council on Nurse Education and Practice (NACNEP)	http://bhpr.hrsa.gov/nursing/nursingworkforcereports.html	APRNs in the workforce data
National Organization of Nurse Practitioner Faculties (NONPF)	http://nonpf.org	NP competencies NP education data NPs in the workforce data
American Association of Colleges of Nursing (AACN)	www.aacn.nche.edu	APRNs in the workforce data The Essentials of Master's Education in Nursing
National Sample Survey of Registered Nurses	http://datawarehouse.hrsa.gov/nursingsurvey.aspx	RNs in the workforce data
Healthcare Effectiveness and Data Information Set (HEDIS)	http://www.ncqa.org/tabid/59/Default.aspx	Performance measures for primary care practice
Robert Wood Johnson Foundation	www.rwjf.org	Health policy
Division of Nursing, Bureau of Health Professions, Health Resources and Services Administration, DHHS	http://bhpr.hrsa.gov/nursing/	NP Data on rural and Urban practice
Rural Health Research Center, University of Washington	http://depts.washington.edu/uwrhrc/uploads/RHRC_FR137_Skillman.pdf).	

AHRQ has identified potentially preventable hospitalizations as a critical area of health care quality and has developed indicators for health care problems that afford a high risk for hospitalization. For example, bacterial pneumonia, COPD, and low birth weight fall into this category. These ambulatory care–sensitive outcomes relate directly to quality in primary care in that these are conditions in which a primary care NP can prevent the need for hospitalization.

In the most recent systematic review of the NP literature covering 1990 to 2008, Newhouse and coworkers (2011) again found supporting evidence that NPs and other APRNs "provide effective and high-quality patient care, have an important role in improving the quality of patient care in the United States, and could help to address concerns about whether care provided by APRNs can safely augment the physician supply to support reform efforts aimed at expanding access to care" (p. 18).

In a study using HEDIS national benchmarks, Barkauskas and colleagues (2011) found that NPs in nine NMHCs across the country met and often exceeded national benchmarks for cervical and breast cancer screening and chronic disease outcomes of hypertension, diabetes, and asthma. Unlike previous studies, which included only those patients with insurance, researchers included uninsured and insured patients and found that outcomes met the 50th percentile of HEDIS benchmarks and often approached or exceeded the 90th percentile. The primary care NP must be familiar with national benchmarks, such as HEDIS (NCQA, 2011) performance measures, because these not only serve to incentivize practice, but serve as data to improve practice and protect patients—the ultimate goal (see Box 15-4).

NPs have practiced in various models and settings; the outcomes of their practices have been studied for more than 40 years. Consistently, when quality of care has been assessed in studies that are highly rated on strength of evidence, NP providers have been found to provide high-quality care, meeting and often exceeding national benchmarks and care provided by physicians. It is noteworthy that patient satisfaction is also exceptionally high (e.g., Benkert et al., 2002).

Role of Electronic Health Records in Primary Care

EHRs show enormous promise in improving the quality of care and patient safety for the future of health care, and primary care specifically. The adoption rate of EHRs is still relatively low (Jha et al., 2009), largely because of lack of technology expertise and limited ability to manage complex changes (Dennehy et al., 2011). NPs will need to play a key role in the implementation and use of EHRs in primary care and other settings. The American Recovery and Reinvestment Act (ARRA) of 2009 has placed a prominent focus on incentivizing EHR adoption in smaller and resource-limited primary care settings to help address the issues of low adoption. There is also a nationwide network of health information technology (IT) regional extension centers (RECs) federally funded by Health and Human Services (HHS) and dedicated to assisting smaller practices and practices serving the underserved to purchase and implement EHRs (Torda, Han, & Scholle, 2010). Congress has also aided the health care community via the Health Information Technology for Economic and Clinical Health Act (HITECH) incentive payments through Medicare and Medicaid when they use EHRs privately and securely to achieve specified improvements in care delivery (Blumenthal & Tavenner, 2010). As part of this funding, providers will need to demonstrate meaningful

use, including core measures such as entry of basic data—patients' vital signs and demographics, active medications and allergies, up to date problem lists of current and active diagnoses, and smoking status. Additional objectives include e-prescribing and reporting on quality data. NPs will need to be prepared to use EHRs fully and also provide leadership in regard to the purchase and implementation of products for any setting in which they serve. One example is a group of NMHCs who partnered with a network of federally qualified health centers to implement the same EHR product in six safety net settings to address quality outcomes and patient safety with complex underserved populations (Dennehy et al., 2011). Findings have indicated that implementation can be challenging, but EHRs and health technology can transform practice, and outcomes of care often improve through the use of technology when it is fully embraced.

E-prescribing is part of most EHRs and clearly critical for patient safety. However, in a systematic review, no data were found on NPs and e-prescribing, (Ammenwerth, Schnell-Inderst, Machan, et al., 2008) but e-prescribing was found to reduce the risk of medication errors and adverse drug events significantly among physician users. With meaningful use and the approaching requirement for incentives, NPs will likely be using e-prescribing extensively in primary care settings. Patient portals and personal health records are other ways for patients to be actively involved in their care. These are exciting opportunities already in place in some settings and likely to be increasingly available in primary care settings. Patient portals and personal health records are consistent with a conceptual model of PCMH, in which there is a clear expectation for a partnership between provider and patients. With patient portals, patients have opportunities for more direct communication with their providers and their HER, as well as the larger health care system. Exemplar 15-3 demonstrates use of an integrated EHR and connects all levels of care, from primary to specialty care.

Nurse Practitioners: Challenges and Opportunities

Regulatory Issues and Removing Barriers

Although NPs have made great strides over the past several years in establishing stable independent and collaborative practices, inconsistent state by state regulatory issues create enormous barriers to practice. Many state regulations still require physician involvement in a supervisory or collaborative way. Regulations are often out of date, going back 30 to 40 or more years, when the NP role was new. Regulations are often not based on evidence (Pohl, Hanson, & Newland, 2010; Pohl, Hanson, Newland, et al., 2010). The number of states in which an NP may practice independently has been calculated in various ways. The National Council of State Boards of Nursing (NCSBN, 2012) has reported that 22 states and the District of Columbia defined independent practice as having "no requirements for a written collaborative agreement, no supervision, and no conditions for practice" (https://www.ncsbn.org/2567.htm). Regulations need to protect patients, not professional interests (NCSBN, 2006).

Negotiating the evolving health care marketplace and moving from an invisible provider status to recognized members of provider panels and PCPs of record are major challenges still facing primary care NPs. NPs have long been recognized as providers of cost-effective, high-quality care (see earlier). Key papers and recommendations based on interprofessional discussions are having an important impact on regulation. These include the following: (1) the Josiah Macy Foundation report, *Who Will Provide Primary Care and How Will They Be Trained?* (Cronnenwett & Dzau, 2010); (2) IOM report on *The Future of Nursing* (2011); (3) *The Consensus Document on APRNs* (APRN Consensus Work Group, 2008; Stanley et al., 2009) and (4) the classic work of Safriet on scope of practice (Safriet, 2002, 2011). The Consensus Document brought into alignment the four areas of regulation—licensure, accreditation, certification, and education. That is, the same competencies and requirements are used for accreditation, certification examinations, and educational programs that prepare NPs. The missing link is licensure, in that each state has yet to agree on the same definitions and competencies.

To be accredited, NP programs must prepare their students to practice to their fullest preparation because that is what they will be required to know for certification examinations. However, only 16 states recognize such autonomy through their licensing process. Recommendations from the Josiah Macy Foundation in 2010 (Cronnenwett & Dzau, 2010; Pohl, Hanson, & Newland, 2010) stated that barriers to practice be removed for NPs so that they could "serve as primary care providers and leaders of patient-centered medical homes or other models of primary care delivery" (Cronnenwett & Dzau, p. 4). In another report, which was part of the Macy full report, Pohl and colleagues recommended that barriers be removed so that NPs could work to their fullest educational potential and be accountable for the care they delivered (Pohl, Hanson, & Newland, 2010, Pohl et al., 2010.) The IOM, in their landmark report on *The Future of Nursing* (2011), delivered a similar strong recommendation: "Nurses should practice to the full extent of their

education and training" (p. 9). Safriet's work on scope of practice is the key analysis from a legal perspective on the impact of unnecessarily limiting scope and the impact that this has on patient care.

NPs have demonstrated high-quality, cost-effective care over more than 45 years, and patient satisfaction is exceptionally high. There is evidence that the role of NPs in meeting the primary care needs of the United States is critical, given the physician shortage and redefining of primary care including patient medical homes and ACOs. However, the challenges are substantial and NPs must not only practice but also be willing to be involved when significant decisions are made, whether that is within their practice or health system at the community, state, and/or national levels. We must continue to educate administrators, third-party payers, legislators, and patients about the role of NPs in primary care delivery. Understanding what it takes to have a successful business practice is essential because this represents participating in policy and governance at all levels. The NP core competencies (NONPF, 2012) raise the expectations for professional NP practice. Whether paid by Medicare, Medicaid, and commercial insurers, the primary care NP must be familiar with the reimbursement policies of third-party payers, including documentation and billing guidelines (Buppert, 2012; see Chapter 19). The development of more formal contracting, credentialing, and privileging processes for NPs in a variety of health systems is likely to occur as the health care system evolves. The primary care NP must be familiar with organizational credentialing measures and follow them.

Conclusion

Primary care is the foundation of the evolving U.S. health care system. If access to primary care for all is the goal, while containing costs and focusing on quality outcomes, then NPs will be crucial to achieving these aims. In our current system, there just aren't enough PCPs to meet the need and, with an additional estimated 32 million more people who will be covered and need access to full primary care, based on the PPACA, we will need additional providers more than ever. Physicians are not choosing primary care practice for complex reasons. On the other hand, most NPs choose primary care practice roles (e.g., family, adult, and pediatric NPs) because they enter these programs specifically to provide primary care.

Two areas in particular must be addressed before NPs will be able to contribute fully to primary care delivery nationwide:

1. There must be changes in the outdated state scope of practice laws and regulations of nurse

practitioners. This is because the variation in state regulations on scope of practice and prescribing authority has been a major barrier to using NPs fully and providing increased access to quality, cost-efficient primary care.

2. There must be substantive changes in health professional education to foster true collaboration and teamwork among physicians, NPs, and other health care disciplines in general to obtain the full benefit of diverse competencies inherent in a team. If both of these are addressed, meeting U.S. primary care needs could be significantly affected in a positive way.

Today's NP students and graduates must accept the professional responsibility for being active in the governance of delivery systems and informing and changing policy. There is too much at stake to leave this to a few, or to someone else. The health of the United States population depends on new models of care, on all health care providers practicing to the fullest extent of their education and training, and on strong teams who respect each other and partner with patients. NPs must support their efforts as they take an active role in developing stable health care policy and care delivery systems that allow for patient access to primary care services provided by NPs.

References

Allison, M., Crane, L., Beaty, B., Davidson, A., & Melinkovich, P. (2008). School-based health centers: Improving access and quality of care for low-income adolescents. *Pediatrics, 120,* e887–e894.

Althaus, F., Paroz, S., Hugli, O., Ghali, W. A., Daeppen, J. B., Peytremann-Bridevaux, I., et al. (2011). Effectiveness of interventions targeting frequent users of emergency departments: a systematic review. [Research Support, Non-U.S. Gov't Review]. *Annals of Emergency Medicine, 58,* 41–52. doi: 10.1016/j.annemergmed.2011.03.007.

American Academy of Family Physicians (AAFP). (2011). 2011 Match summary and analysis. http://www.aafp.org/online/en/home/residents/match/summary.html

American Association of Colleges of Nursing (AACN). (2004). *AACN position statement on the practice doctorate in nursing.* Washington, DC: Author.

American Association of Colleges of Nursing. (2006). The essentials of doctoral education for advanced nursing practice (http://www.aacn.nche.edu/dnp/pdf/essentials.pdf).

American Association of Colleges of Nursing (AACN); National Organization of Nurse Practitioner Faculties (NONPF). (2013). *Enrollment and graduation annual survey.* Washington, DC: Authors.

American Nurses Association (ANA). (2001). *Code of ethics for nurses with interpretive statements.* Washington, DC: Author.

American Nurses Association (ANA). (2010). *The scope and standards of practice of advanced practice registered nursing.* Washington, DC: Author.

Ammenwerth, P., Schnell-Inderst, C., Machan, C., & Siebert, U. (2008). The effect of electronic prescribing on medication errors and adverse drug events: A systematic review. *Journal of the American Medical Informatics Association, 15,* 585–590.

APRN Consensus Work Group; National Council of State Boards of Nursing APRN Advisory Committee. (2008). Consensus model for APRN regulation: Licensure, accreditation, certification, and education (http://www.aacn.nche.edu/education/pdf/APRNReport.pdf).

Baggett, T. P., O'Connell, J. J., Singer, D. E., & Rigotti, N. A. (2010). The unmet health care needs of homeless adults: A national study. *American Journal of Public Health, 100,* 1326–1333. doi: 10.2105/ajph.2009.180109.

Barkauskas, V. H., Pohl, J. M., Tanner, C., Onifade, T. J., & Pilon, B. (2011). Quality of care in nurse-managed health centers. *Nursing Administration Quarterly, 25,* 35–41. doi: 10.1097/NAQ.0b013e3182032165.

Benkert, R., Barkauskas, V., Pohl, J. M., Tanner, C., & Nagelkerk, J. (2002). Patient satisfaction outcomes in nurse-managed centers. *Outcomes Management for Nursing Practice, 6,* 174–181.

Blumenthal, D., & Tavenner, M. (2010). The "meaningful use" regulation for electronic health records. *New England Journal of Medicine, 363,* 501–504.

Bodenheimer, T., & Grumbach, K. (2007). *Understanding health policy: A clinical approach.* New York: Lange/McGraw/Hill.

Brooten, D., Naylor, M. D., York, R., Brown, L. P., Munro, B. H., Hollingsworth, A. O., et al. (2002). Lessons learned from testing the quality cost model of advanced practice nursing (APN) transitional care. *Journal of Nursing Scholarship, 34,* 369–375. doi: 10.1111/j.1547-5069.2002.00369.x.

Brooten, D., Youngblut, J. M., Kutcher, J., & Bobo, C. (2004). Quality and the nursing workforce: APNs, patient outcomes and health care costs. *Nursing Outlook, 52,* 45–52. doi: 10.1016/j.outlook.2003.10.009.

Brown, S. A., & Grimes, D. E. (1993). *Nurse practitioners and certified nurse midwives: A meta-analysis of process of care, clinical outcomes, and cost-effectiveness of nurses in primary care roles.* Washington, DC: American Nurses Association.

Brown, S. A., & Grimes, D. E. (1995). A meta-analysis of nurse practitioners and nurse midwives in primary care. *Nursing Research, 44,* 332–339.

Buppert, C. (2012). *Nurse practitioner's business practice and legal guide* (4th ed.). Boston: Jones & Bartlett.

Bureau of Labor Statistics. (2011). Occupational employment and wages, May 2011. 29-1071, physician assistants (http://www.bls.gov/oes/current/oes291071.htm).

Centers for Disease Control (CDC). (2007). The state of aging and health in America (http://www.cdc.gov/Aging/pdf/saha_2007.pdf).

Christensen, C. M., Bohmer, R., & Kenagy, J. (2000). Will disruptive innovations cure health care? (http://hbr.org/web/extras/insight-center/health-care/will-disruptive-innovations-cure-health-care).

Convenient Care Association. (2013). http://www.ccaclinics.org/index.php?option=com_content&view=article&id=4&Itemid=11

Cook, T., & Nolan, W. (1996). A nurse practitioner–led, collaborative, outpatient practice: A case study in outcomes management. Seminars for Nurse Managers, 4, 154–162.

Cortes, A., Khadduri, J., Buron, L., & Culhane, D. P. (2010). The 2009 Annual Homelessness Assessment Report to Congress: US Department of Housing and Urban Development.

Council of State Governments. (2008). Physician shortages and the medically underserved (http://www.csg.org/knowledgecenter/docs/TIA_PhysicianShortage_Final_screen.pdf).

Cowan, M. J., Shapiro, M., Hays, R., Afifi, A., Vazirani, S., Ward, C. R., et al. (2006). The effect of a multidisciplinary hospitalist/physician and advanced practice nurse collaboration on hospital costs. Journal of Nursing Administration, 36, 79–85.

Cronenwett, L., & Dzau, V. J. (2010). Chairman's summary of the conference. In B., Culliton, (Ed.), Who will provide primary care and how will they be trained? Durham, NC: Josiah Macy Jr. Foundation.

Davis, K. (2005). Toward a high-performance health system: The Commonwealth Fund's new commission. Health Affairs, 24, 1356–1360. doi: 10.1377/hlthaff.24.5.1356.

DeNavas-Walt, C., Bernadette, D. P., & Smith, J. C. (2011). Income, poverty, and health insurance coverage in the United States: 2010 (http://www.census.gov/prod/2011pubs/p60-239.pdf).

Dennehy, P., White, M., Hamilton, A., Pohl, J. M., Tanner, C., Onifade, T. J., et al. (2011). A partnership model for implementing electronic health records in resource-limited primary care settings: Experiences from two nurse managed health centers. Journal of the American Informatics Association, I, 820–826. doi: 10.1136/amiajnl-2011-000117.

Dick, K., & Frazier, S. C. (2006). An exploration of nurse practitioner care to homebound frail elders. Journal of the American Academy of Nurse Practitioners, 18, 325–334.

Donaldson, S. K., & Crowley, D. M. (1978). The discipline of nursing. Nursing Outlook, 26, 113–120.

Dwyer, C. M., Walker, P. H., Suchman A., & Coggiola, P., (Eds.). (1995). Nursing centers: The time is now. New York: National League for Nursing.

Fetter, M. S. (2009). Improving information technology competencies: Implications for psychiatric mental health nursing. Issues in Mental Health Nursing, 30, 3–13. doi:10.1080/01612840802555208.

Goolsby, M. J. (2004). Integrating the principles of evidence-based practice into clinical practice. Journal of the American Academy of Nurse Practitioners, 16, 98–105.

Health Resources and Services Administration (HRSA). (2010). The national sample survey of registered nurses (http://bhpr.hrsa.gov/healthworkforce/rnsurveys/rnsurveyfinal.pdf).

Health Resources and Services Administration (HRSA). (2012a). Nurse education, practice, quality and retention (NEPQR) (http://bhpr.hrsa.gov/nursing/grants/nepqr.html).

Health Resources and Services Administration (HRSA). (2012b). Designated health professional shortage areas (HPSA) statistics (http://ersrs.hrsa.gov/ReportServer?/HGDW_Reports/BCD_HPSA/BCD_HPSA_SCR50_Smry&rs:Format=HTML3.2).

Hennessey, B., & Suter, P. (2011). The community-based transitions model: One agency's experience. Home Healthcare Nurse, 29, 218–230. doi: 10.1097/NHH.0b013e318211986d.

Horrocks, S., Anderson, E., & Sallisbury, C. (2002). Systematic review of whether nurse practitioners in primary care can provide equivalent care to doctors. British Medical Journal, 324, 819–823.

Howell, J. D. (2010). Reflections on the past and future of primary care. Health Affairs, 29, 760–765. doi: 10.1377/hlthaff.2010.0014.

Institute of Medicine (IOM). (1996). Primary care: America's health in a new era. Washington, DC: National Academies Press.

Institute of Medicine (IOM). (2011). The future of nursing: Leading change, advancing health. Washington, DC: National Academies Press.

International Conference on Primary Health Care. (1978). Declaration of Alma-Ata. WHO Chronicle, 32, 428–430.

Jencks, S. F., Williams, M. V., & Coleman, E. A. (2009). Rehospitalizations among patients in the Medicare fee-for-service program. New England Journal of Medicine, 361, 311–312. doi:10.1056/NEJMc090911.

Jha, A. K., DesRoches, C. M., Campbell, E. G., Donelan, K., Rao, S. R., Ferris, T. G., et al. (2009). Use of electronic health records in U.S. hospitals. New England Journal of Medicine, 360, 1628–1638.

Johnson, R. (2005). Shifting patterns of practice: Nurse practitioners in a managed care environment. Research Theory in Nursing Practice, 19, 323–340.

Keckley P. H., & Underwood, F. R. (2008). Medical home: Disruptive innovation for a new primary care model. Washington DC: Deloitte Center for Health Solutions.

Kenny, J. W. (2006). Theory-based advanced nursing practice In W. K. Cody (Ed.), Philosophical and theoretical perspectives for advanced nursing practice (pp. 295–310). Sudbury, MA: Jones and Bartlett.

Kirst, M., Frederick, T., & Erickson, P. (2011). Concurrent mental health and substance use problems among street-involved youth. International Journal of Mental Health and Addiction, 9, 543–553. doi: 10.1007/s11469-011-9328-3.

Kwan, L., Ho, C. J., Preston, C., & Le, V. (2008). Puentes clinic: An integrated model for the primary care of vulnerable populations. The Permanente Journal, 12, 10–15.

Laurant, M., Reeves, D., Hermens, R., Braspenning, J., Grol, R., & Sibbald, B. (2005). Substitution of doctors by nurses in primary care. Cochrane Database of Systematic Reviews, 18, CD001271.

Lenz, E. R. (1998). The role of middle-range theory for nursing research and practice. Part 2. Nursing practice. Nursing Leadership Forum, 3, 62–66.

Lenz, E. R., Mundinger, M. O., Hoplins, S. C., Lin, S. X., & Smolowitz, H. (2002). Diabetes care processes and outcomes in patients treated by nurse practitioners or physicians. Diabetes Education, 28, 590–598.

Lockhart, C. A. (1995). Community nursing centers: An analysis of status and needs. In C. M. Dwyer, P. H. Walker, A. Suchman, & P. Coggiola, (Eds.), Nursing centers: The time is now. New York: National League for Nursing.

Lützén, K. (1997). Nursing ethics into the next millennium: A context-sensitive approach for nursing ethics. *Nursing Ethics, 4,* 218–226. doi: 10.1177/096973309700400306.

Macinko, J., Starfield, B., & Shi, L. (2003). The contribution of primary care systems to health outcomes within Organization for Economic Cooperation and Development (OECD) countries 1970 1990. *Health Services Research, 38,* 831–865.

Mackay, B. J. (2002). Leadership development: Supporting nursing in a changing primary health care environment. *Nursing Praxis in New Zealand Inc., 18,* 24–32.

McCaughan, D., Thompson, C., Cullum, N., Sheldon, T., & Raynor, P. (2005). Nurse practitioner and practice nurses' use of research information in clinical decision making: Findings from an exploratory study. *Family Practice, 22,* 490–497.

Mehrotra, A., Wang, M. C., Lave, J. R., Adams, J. L., & McGlynn, E. A. (2008). Retail clinics, primary care physicians, and emergency departments: A comparison of patients' visits. *Health Affairs (Millwood), 27,* 1272–1282.

Mundinger, M. O., Kane, R. L., Lenz, E. R., Totten, A. M., Tsai, W., Cleary, P. D., et al. (2000). Primary care outcomes in patients treated by nurse practitioners or physicians: A randomized trial. *Journal of the American Medical Association, 283,* 59–68.

Murray, M., Davies, M., & Boushon, B. (2007). Panel size: How many patients can one doctor manage? *Family Practice Management, 14,* 44–51.

National Assembly on School-Based Health Care (NASBH). (2012). (http://www.nasbhc.org/site).

National Committee for Quality Assurance. (2012). HEDIS & performance measurement (http://www.ncqa.org/tabid/59/Default.aspx).

National Committee for Quality Assurance (NCQA). (2011). Patient-centered medical home: Healthcare that revolves around you (http://www.ncqa.org/LinkClick.aspx?fileticket=ycS4coFOGnw%3d&tabid=631).

Howden, L. M., & Meyer, J. A. (2011). Age and sex composition:2010 Census Briefs. U.S. Census Bureau. http://www.census.gov/prod/cen2010/briefs/c2010br-03.pdf.

National Council of State Boards of Nursing (NCSBN). (2012). NCSBN's APRN campaign for consensus: State progress toward uniformity (https://www.ncsbn.org/2567.htm).

National Council of State Boards of Nursing (NCSBN), Association of Social Work Boards, Federation of State Boards of Physical Therapy, Federation of State Medical Boards, National Association of Boards of Pharmacy, National Board for Certification in Occupational Therapy (Eds.). (2006). *Changes in healthcare professions' scope of practice: Legislative considerations.* Chicago: National Council of State Boards of Nursing.

National Law Center on Homelessness and Poverty. (2012). Homelessness and poverty in America. (http://www.nlchp.org/hapia.cfm).

National Organization of Nurse Practitioner Faculties (NONPF). (2012). Nurse practitioner core competencies (http://nonpf.org/associations/10789/files/NPCoreCompetenciesFinal2012.pdf).

National Organization of Nurse Practitioner Faculties (NONPF), American Association of College of Nursing (AACN). (2002). *Nurse practitioner primary care competencies in specialty areas: Adult, family, gerontological, pediatric, and women's health.* Washington, DC: Authors.

National Organization of Nurse Practitioner Faculties (NONPF), National Panel for NP Practice Doctorate Competencies. (2006). Practice doctorate nurse practitioner entry level competencies (http://www.nonpf.org/associations/10789/files/DNP%20NP%20competenciesApril2006.pdf).

Naylor, M., Aiken, L., Kurtzman, E., Olds, D., & Hirschman, K. (2011). The importance of transitional care in achieving health reform. *Health Affairs, 30,* 746–754.

Naylor, M. D., Brooten, D. A., Campbell, R. L., Maislin, G., McCauley, K. M., & Schwartz, J. S. (2004). Transitional care of older adults hospitalized with heart failure: A randomized, controlled trial. *Journal of the American Geriatrics Society, 52,* 675–684. doi: 10.1111/j.1532-5415.2004.52202.x.

Naylor, M. D., Hirschman, K. B., Bowles, K. H., Bixby, M. B., Konick-McMahan, J., & Stephens, C. (2007). Care coordination for cognitively impaired older adults and their caregivers. *Home Health Care Services Quarterly, 27,* 57–58.

Naylor, M. D., & Kurtzman, E. T. (2010). The role of nurse practitioners in reinventing primary care. *Health Affairs, 29,* 893–899. doi: 10.1377/hlthaff.2010.0440.

Neff, D. F. (2003). APN directed transitional home care model: Achieving positive outcomes for patients with COPD. *Home Healthcare Nurse, 21,* 543–550.

Newhouse, R. P., Stanik-Hutt, J., White, K. M., Johantgen, M., Bass, E. B., Zangaro, G., et al. (2011). Advanced practice nurse outcomes 1990-2008: A systematic review. *Nursing Economics, 29,* 1–21.

Nutting, P. A., Miller, W. L., Crabtree, B. F., Jaen, C. R., Stewart, E. E., & Stange, K. C. (2009). Initial lessons from the first national demonstration project on practice transformation to a patient-centered medical home. *Annals of Family Medicine, 7,* 254–260.

Oberle, K., & Allen, M. (2001). The nature of advanced practice nursing. *Nursing Outlook, 49,* 148–153.

O'Connell, J. J., Oppenheimer, S. C., Judge, C. M., Taube, R. L., Blanchfield, B. B., Swain, S. E., et al. (2010). The Boston health care for the homeless program: A public health framework. *American Journal of Public Health, 100,* 1400–1408. doi: 10.2105/AJPH.2009.173609.

Office of Technology Assessment. (1986). *Nurse practitioners, physician assistants, and certified nurse midwives: A policy analysis.* Washington DC: U.S. Government Printing Office.

O'Toole, T. P., Pirraglia, P. A., Dosa, D., Bourgault, C., Redihan, S., O'Toole, M. B., et al. (2011). Building care systems to improve access for high-risk and vulnerable veteran populations. *Journal of General Internal Medicine, 26*(Suppl 2), 683–688. doi: 10.1007/s11606-011-1818-2.

Pierce, S. F. (1997). A model for conceptualizing the moral dynamic in health care. *Nursing Ethics, 4,* 483–495. doi: 10.1177/096973309700400605.

Pohl, J. M., Barkauskas, V. H., Benkert, R., Breer, L., & Bostrom, A. (2007). Impact of academic nurse managed centers on communities served. *Journal of the American Academy of Nurse Practitioners, 19,* 268–275.

Pohl, J. M., Hanson, C., & Newland, J. (2010). Nurse practitioners as primary care providers: History, context, and opportunities. Commissioned paper by the Josiah Macy Foundation for their conference on "Primary care: Who will provide it and how will they be trained?" Raleigh, North Carolina, January 8-10, 2010.

Pohl, J. M., Hanson, C., Newland, J., & Cronenwett, L. (2010). Unleashing the full potential of nurse practitioners to deliver primary care and lead health care teams. *Health Affairs, 29,* 900–905.

Pohl, J. M., Sebastian, J. G., Barkauskas, V. H., Breer, L., Williams, C., Stanhope, M., et al. (2007). Characteristics of nursing schools operating academic nurse-managed centers. *Nursing Outlook, 55,* 289–295.

Pohl, J. M., Tanner, C., Barkauskas, V. H., Gans, D., Nagelkerk, J., & Fiandt, K. (2010). Nurse- managed health centers' national survey: Three years of data. *Nursing Outlook, 58,* 97–103.

Pohl, J. M., Tanner, C., Pilon, B., & Benkert, R. (2011). Comparison of nurse-managed health centers with community health centers as safety net providers. *Policy, Politics, & Nursing Practice, 12,* 90–99. doi:10.1177/1527154411417882.

Robert Graham Center (2007). The patient-centered medical home: History, seven core features, evidence and transformational change (http://www.grahamcenter.org/online/etc/medialib/graham/documents/publications/monographs-books/2007/rgcmo-medical-home.Par.0001.File.tmp/rgcmo-medical-home.pdf).

Robinson K. (2010). Roles of nurse practitioners in the U.S. Department of Veterans Affairs. In E. Sullivan-Marx, D. McGivern, & J. Fairman, (Eds.) *Nurse practitioners: Evolution to advanced practice nursing* (5th ed.). New York: Springer.

Safriet, B. J. (2002). Closing the gap between can and may in health care providers' scopes of practice: A primer for policy-makers. *Yale Journal of Regulation, 19,* 301–334.

Safriet, B. J. (2011). Federal options for maximizing the value of advanced practice nurses in providing quality, cost-effective health care. In Institute of Medicine (Ed.), *The future of nursing: Leading change, advancing health.* Washington, DC: National Academies Press.

Sia, C., Tonniges, T. F., Osterhus, E., & Taba, S. (2004). History of the medical home concept. *Pediatrics, 113*(Suppl), 1473–1478.

Spitzer, W. O., Sackett, D. L., Sibley, J. C., Roberts, R. S., Gent, M., Kergin, D. J., et al.(1974). The Burlington randomized trial of the nurse practitioner. *New England Journal of Medicine, 290,* 251–256.

Stanley, J. M., Werner, K. E., & Apple, K. (2009). Positioning advanced practice registered nurses for health care reform: Consensus on APRN regulation. *Journal of Professional Nursing, 24,* 340–348.

Starfield, B. (1992). *Primary care: Concept, evaluation, and policy.* New York: Oxford Press.

Starfield, B., Shi, L., & Macinko, J. (2005). Contribution of primary care to health systems and health. *Milbank Quarterly, 83,* 457–501.

Tanner, C., Pohl, J. M., Ward, S., & Dontje, K. (2003). Education of nurse practitioners in academic nurse-managed centers: Student perspectives. *Journal of Professional Nursing, 19,* 354–363.

Torda, P., Han, E. S., & Scholle, S. H. (2010). Easing the adoption and use of electronic health records in small practices. *Health Affairs (Millwood), 29,* 668–675.

Ulrich, C. M., Soeken, K. L., & Miller, N. (2003). Ethical conflict associated with managed care: Views of nurse practitioners. *Nursing Research, 52,* 168–175.

U.S. Department of Health and Human Services (HHS). (2011). Patient Protection and Affordable Care Act (http://www.healthcare.gov/law/full/index.html).

Wang, E. A., Hong, C. S., Samuels, L., Shavit, S., Sanders, R., & Kushel, M. (2010). Transitions clinic: Creating a community-based model of health care for recently released California prisoners. *Public Health Reports, 125,* 171–177.

The Acute Care Nurse Practitioner

Ruth M. Kleinpell • Marilyn Hravnak • Kathy S. Magdic • Jane Guttendorf

CHAPTER CONTENTS

The purpose of the acute care nurse practitioner (ACNP) is to diagnose and manage disease and promote the health of patients with acute, critical, and complex chronic health conditions across the continuum of acute care services. The ACNP provides comprehensive care in a collaborative model with physicians, staff nurses, and other health care providers, as well as with patients and their families. The ACNP not only shares common functions and skills with the other nurse practitioner (NP) subspecialties, but also applies unique knowledge and skills in caring for very complex and vulnerable patient populations (American Association of Colleges of Nursing [AACN], 2012; American Association of Critical Care Nurses, 2012). The Consensus Model for advanced practice registered nurse (APRN) regulation states that ACNP care includes diagnosing, treating, and managing patients with acute and chronic illnesses and diseases, including the following: ordering, performing, supervising, and interpreting laboratory, diagnostic, and imaging studies;

prescribing medication and durable medical equipment; and making appropriate referrals for patients and families (National Council of State Boards of Nursing [NCSBN], 2008). Practice for the ACNP has been recognized as incorporating the entire spectrum of adults, including young adults, adults, and older adults. New competencies for the adult gerontology acute care NP recognize this evolved focus of care and this chapter will provide a framework for this level of ACNP care (AACN, 2012; Box 16-1). Although all ACNPs share specialty role attributes, there may be intrarole variability based on the nature of the care delivery system, characteristics of a particular position, or location in which they practice (e.g., private practice group versus hospital employee, intensive care unit versus hospital ward or ambulatory care facility) and physiologic specialty (e.g., cardiac, pulmonary, orthopedic, oncology). This chapter presents an overview of the ACNP role, including scope of practice, core and role-specific competencies, issues in practice, and future challenges.

BOX 16-1   Adult Gerontology Acute Care Nurse Practitioner Competencies

I. Health Promotion, Health Protection, Disease Prevention, and Treatment

A. Assessment of Health Status

These competencies describe the role of the adult gerontology acute care NP (ACNP) in terms of assessing the individual's health status, including assessment of the health promotion, health protection, and disease prevention needs of the acute, critical, and chronically ill or injured patient. Activities include risk stratification, disease-specific screening activities, diagnosis, treatment and follow-up of acute illness, and appropriate referral to specialty care.

B. Diagnosis of Health Status

The adult gerontology ACNP is engaged in the diagnosis of health status in patients with physiologic instability or the potential to experience rapid physiologic deterioration or life-threatening instability. This diagnostic process includes critical thinking, differential diagnosis, and the identification, prioritization, interpretation, and synthesis of data from a variety of sources. These competencies describe the role of the adult gerontology ACNP related to the diagnosis of health status.

C. Plan of Care and Implementation of Treatment

The objectives of planning and implementing therapeutic interventions are to return the individual to stability and optimize the individual's health. These competencies describe the adult gerontology ACNP's role in stabilizing the individual, minimizing physical and psychological complications, maximizing the individual's health potential, and assisting with palliative and end-of-life care management.

II. Nurse Practitioner-Patient Relationship

Competencies in this area demonstrate the nurse practitioner-patient collaborative approach, which enhances the adult gerontology ACNP's effectiveness of care. The competencies speak to the critical importance of the interpersonal transaction as it relates to therapeutic patient outcomes considering the cognitive, developmental, physical, mental, and behavioral health status of the patient across the adult lifespan.

III. Teaching-Coaching Function

These competencies describe the adult gerontology ACNP's ability to impart knowledge and associated psychomotor and coping skills to individuals, family, and other caregivers. The coaching function involves the skills of interpreting and individualizing therapies through the activities of advocacy, modeling, and teaching.

IV. Professional Role

These competencies describe the varied role of the adult gerontology ACNP, specifically related to advancing the profession and enhancing direct care and management. The adult gerontology ACNP demonstrates a commitment to the implementation and evolution of the adult gerontology ACNP role. Also, the adult gerontology ACNP implements clinical reasoning and builds collaborative intra- and interprofessional relationships to provide optimal care to patients with complex acute, critical, and chronic illness. The adult gerontology ACNP advocates on behalf of the patient population and profession through active participation in the health policy process.

V. Managing and Negotiating Health Care Delivery Systems

These competencies describe the adult gerontology ACNP role in achieving improved health outcomes for individuals, communities, and systems by overseeing and directing the delivery of clinical services within an integrated system of health care. In addition, the adult gerontology ACNP addresses the development and implementation of system policies affecting services.

VI. Monitoring and Ensuring the Quality of Health Care Practice

These competencies describe the adult gerontology ACNP role in ensuring quality of care through consultation, collaboration, continuing education, certification, and evaluation. The monitoring function of the role is also addressed relative to examining and improving one's own practice and engaging in interdisciplinary peer and colleague reviews.

Adapted from American Association of Colleges of Nursing (AACN). (2012). Adult gerontology acute care nurse practitioner competencies (http://www.aacn.nche.edu/students/nursing-program-search).

Emergence of the Acute Care Nurse Practitioner Role

The role of the ACNP evolved as a result of a number of changes in the delivery of health care including the following: the need for an advanced practitioner to manage hospitalized patients whose clinical presentation was more complex; changes in the regulations of work hour restrictions for medical residents and fellows; and shortages of intensivist physicians. Initially, primary care NPs (family NPs and adult NPs) were recruited to care for adult patients in hospital-based settings, with on the job training to provide secondary and tertiary care skills (an example of advanced practice nurse [APN] evolution is described in Chapter 1). By the late 1980s, NPs were increasingly used in tertiary care centers and it became apparent that a new adult NP specialty was emerging. Education specifically designed to meet the needs of vulnerable adult patients with acute, critical, and complex chronic illness to ensure consistency in the knowledge, training, and quality of care provided by NP graduates in this new specialty was required. Master's-level graduate adult ACNP programs began to emerge in the late 1980s and, in 1995, the first national certification examination for ACNPs was administered. The AACN has identified over 60 adult ACNP educational programs in the United States (AACN, 2012).

Because of these same historical forces, a need for pediatric NPs specifically educated to meet the needs of acutely ill children also emerged. In 2004, the National Association of Pediatric Nurse Associates and Practitioners (NAPNAP) expanded their pediatric nurse practitioner (PNP) scope of practice to reflect the acute care role (NAPNAP, 2010). An acute care pediatric nurse practitioner (PNP-AC) examination from the Pediatric Nursing Certification Board (PNCB) became available in 2005; currently, over 20 PNP-AC programs are in existence (AACN, 2012; NAPNAP, 2010; Reuter-Rice & Bolick 2012).

The National Nurse Practitioner Database of the American Academy of Nurse Practitioners (AANP) indicated that of approximately 135,000 NPs in the United States in 2010, 5.2% were ACNPs (Kleinpell & Goolsby, 2012). National certification for ACNPs began in 1995 and there are now approximately 8,000 ACNPs certified in the United States (American Nurses Credentialing Center, 2012). This NP specialty continues to grow as the continued need for the unique services that ACNPs offer becomes recognized. Furthermore, recent constraints in graduate medical trainee work hour restrictions also provide a growing need for inpatient coverage, a need that can be met by the ACNP (Kleinpell, Buchman, & Boyle, 2012; Lundberg, Wali, Thomas, et al., 2006; Pastores, O'Connor, Kleinpell, et al., 2011). The ACNP role has spread outside the United States and is being implemented to meet the needs of acutely and critically ill patients in the health care systems of other countries (Chang, Mu, & Tsay, 2006; Kilpatrick, 2011; Kilpatrick, Harbman, Carter, et al., 2010; Norris & Melby, 2006; Scherr, Wilson, Wagner, et al., 2012; Schober & Affara, 2006; Sung, Huang, Ong, et al., 2011).

Shaping the Scope of Practice for the Acute Care Nurse Practitioner

The scope of ACNP practice is influenced from five levels: national (professional organizations), state (government), local (health care institution), service-related, and

individual. In common with other APNs, the ACNP's scope of practice is broadly set forth in statements by professional nursing organizations. State governments, as regulatory agencies, further delineate the scope of practice in statutes such as nurse practice acts or title protection statutes. At the national level, the APRN Consensus Model has influenced the further development of the ACNP scope of practice to include adult and gerontology focus areas for the adult ACNP and designating pediatric ACNP as an NP role (NCSBN, 2008). The Consensus Model further clarified that scope of practice for the ACNP is not setting-specific but is determined based on patient's needs for acute care. Because ACNPs frequently provide their services within health care delivery systems, such as hospitals, subacute care facilities, nursing homes, and clinics, their scope may be defined further by policies within these institutions, organizations, and health care entities and even by the needs of a clinically specialized patient population. Finally, individual ACNPs will further define the scope of their practice based on their own talents, strengths, and attributes. How ACNP practice is configured at each of these levels is described in the following sections.

National Level (Professional Organizations)

At the national level, the scope of ACNP practice is influenced by the following: the National Adult Gerontology Acute Care Nurse Practitioner Competencies (AACN, 2012); the *Scope and Standards of Practice of the Adult Gerontology Acute Care Nurse Practitioner* (American Association of Critical-Care Nurses, 2012), which describes expert ACNP role performance; Nurse Practitioner Core Competencies (National Organization of Nurse Practitioner Faculties [NONPF], 2011); and the ACNP national certification examinations.

The *Scope and Standards of Practice for the Acute Care Nurse Practitioner* was initially developed jointly by the American Nurses Association and American Association of Critical-Care Nurses in 1995 and later revised by the American Association of Critical-Care Nurses in 2012 to reflect the focus on adult gerontology acute care practice (American Association of Critical-Care Nurses, 2012). It further describes the scope of practice and standards of clinical and professional performance of the expert ACNP. The population for which the ACNP provides care includes acutely and critically ill patients experiencing episodic illness, stable and/or progressive chronic illness, acute exacerbation of chronic illness, or terminal illness. The ACNP's focus is the provision of curative, rehabilitative, palliative, and maintenance care. Short-term goals include stabilizing the patient for acute and life-threatening conditions, minimizing or preventing complications, attending to comorbidities, and promoting physical and

BOX 16-2 **Standards of Clinical Practice and Professional Performance for the Acute Care Nurse Practitioner**

Standards of Clinical Practice

Standard I: Advanced Assessment
The acute care nurse practitioner (ACNP) independently elicits, selects, and integrates data of acute, critical, and/or complex chronically ill patients.

Standard II: Differential Diagnosis
The ACNP independently analyzes and synthesizes the assessment data in determining differential diagnoses for the patient with acute, critical, and/or complex chronic illness.

Standard III: Outcome Identification
The ACNP identifies individualized goals and outcomes for the patient who has acute, critical, and/or complex chronic illness.

Standard IV: Plan of Care
The ACNP independently develops an outcome-focused plan of care that prescribes interventions for the patient with acute, critical, and/or complex chronic illness.

Standard V: Implementation of Treatment
The ACNP implements the interventions identified in the interprofessional plan of care for the patient with acute, critical, and/or complex chronic illness.

Standard VI: Evaluation
The ACNP evaluates the patient's progress toward the attainment of goals and outcomes.

Standards of Professional Performance

Standard I: Professional Practice
The ACNP evaluates his or her clinical practice in relation to institutional guidelines, professional practice standards, and relevant statutes and regulations.

Standard II: Education
The ACNP acquires and maintains current knowledge in advanced nursing practice.

Standard III: Collaboration
The ACNP collaborates with the patient, family, and other health care providers in patient care.

Standard IV: Ethics
The ACNP integrates ethical considerations into all areas of practice.

Standard V: Systems Thinking
The ACNP develops and participates in organizational systems and processes to promote optimal patient outcomes.

Standard VI: Resource Utilization
The ACNP considers factors related to safety, effectiveness, and cost in planning and delivering patient care.

Standard VII: Leadership
The ACNP provides leadership in the practice setting and the profession.

Standard VIII: Collegiality
The ACNP promotes a healthy work environment for peers, colleagues, and other professionals through the use of effective communication and respect for the unique contributions of individuals.

Standard IX: Quality of Practice
The ACNP systematically evaluates and enhances the quality, safety, and effectiveness of advanced nursing practice and care delivery across the continuum of acute care services.

Standard X: Clinical Inquiry
The ACNP identifies specific research priorities in practice and strives to enhance knowledge and skills through participation in research, translation of scientific evidence, and promotion of evidence-based practice.

Adapted from the American Association of Critical-Care Nurses. (2012). *Scope and standards of practice for the adult gerontology acute care nurse practitioner.* Aliso Viejo, CA: Author.

psychological well-being. Long-term goals include restoring the patient's maximum health potential, providing palliative and end-of-life care, and evaluating risk factors in achieving these outcomes. The practice environment for the ACNP is identified as any inpatient or outpatient setting in which the patient requires complex monitoring and therapies, high-intensity nursing interventions within the range of high-acuity care (American Association of Critical-Care Nurses, 2012). The standards of clinical practice and standards of professional performance, along with measurement criteria examples for the ACNP as specified in this document, are summarized in Box 16-2.

These standards, which are closely aligned with the APN core competencies in Chapter 3, describe a competent level of care and professional performance common to all ACNPs regardless of setting, whereby the quality of expert ACNP practice can be judged. Some common themes in the standards of ACNP clinical practice and professional performance that distinguish the practice of ACNPs from other NP specialties are the dynamic nature of the patient's health and illness status, vulnerability of the patient population, need for continuous assessment and adjustment of the management plan in the face of rapidly changing patient conditions, and complexity of the required monitoring and therapeutics. Additional themes include the collaborative nature of the practice and interactive relationship between the ACNP and the health care system.

Finally, a resource that does not define scope of practice but does specify the knowledge necessary to perform within the specialty scope is the ACNP national certification examination. APN specialty certification serves as a primary criterion for APN practice (see Chapter 21). In addition, Medicare regulations stipulate completion of a national certification examination as a requirement for ACNPs to obtain reimbursement. ACNP certification examinations are offered by the American Nurses Credentialing Center (ANCC, 2012) and the American Association of Critical-Care Nurses (2012). Although it is evident that the content of a certification examination should not drive educational standards or curriculum development, the topics and content for the ACNP certification examinations have been validated by role delineation studies and are consistent with the other documents delineating ACNP practice scope (ANCC, 2009). As such, they serve to further articulate the scope of ACNP practice.

State Level (Government)

Each state's government provides the second mechanism whereby the ACNPs professional scope of practice is defined. The nurse practice statute for each state governs nursing practice. NP practice rules and regulations that are intended to define NP practice vary from state to state (Kleinpell, Hudspeth, Scordo, et al., 2012; NONPF, 2012).

In all states, APN regulation for practice is based on basic nursing licensure, but many states have additional rules and regulations that delineate specific requirements and define and limit who can use a specific advanced practice nursing title with protection (see Chapter 21). Although at the state level it is relatively easy to define limitations in scope of practice based on the age of the patient population, it is more difficult to determine scope based on patient acuity and practice setting. Regulations relative to acuity and setting are not well defined and vary considerably by state (Kleinpell, Hudspeth, Scordo, et al., 2012; NONPF, 2012).

Institutional Level

As noted, most ACNPs provide patient care in health care institutions. Institutions may further delineate the ACNP's scope of practice within that facility by identifying the patient population that the ACNP serves and the process for collaboration with other health care providers in the institution (Kleinpell, Hudspeth, Scordo, et al., 2012; Magdic, Hravnak, & McCartney, 2005).

Further specification of the ACNP's practice scope may be set forth in job descriptions, in hospital policy, or through the health care agency's credentialing and privileging process.

Employers and hospitals have the right to define a specific health care provider's scope of practice within the employment situation. Documentation of initial training and ongoing provider competence in the application of specific skills is needed. This scope of employment may not exceed the scope of practice specified by the state's nurse practice act but may be curtailed based on the needs and mission of the employer. The institutional scope of employment may take the form of a job description, hospital policy, or both. In settings in which the ACNP role is being newly introduced, a job description may not exist. In general, the job description should include ACNP performance standards and responsibilities as they relate to patient care, collaborative relationships, professional conduct, and professional development; these institutional performance standards can provide a template for ACNP performance evaluation.

When providing care within a health care institution, the ACNP will also need to undergo the process of provider credentialing and privileging by the institution whether the ACNP is an employee of the hospital or an employee of a hospital-affiliated or private practice plan (see Chapter 21). The ACNP is required to provide proof of licensure, certification, educational preparation, (generally) malpractice insurance, and skill performance (training, numbers performed, proof of competence). Institutional credentialing is necessary for the ACNP to provide care to patients within the institution, although the ACNP may or may not hold a medical staff appointment.

Once an individual is credentialed, a determination is made regarding the clinical privileges that may be granted and is the process whereby the institution determines which medical procedures may be performed and which conditions may be treated by physician and nonphysician providers (Magdic, Hravnak, & McCartney, 2005). Although an appropriately educated provider may be permitted by statute to perform certain acts or skills, the hospital is not bound to grant the provider this privilege. The clinical privileges of the ACNP are based partly on the ACNP's professional license, certification, and inherent scope of practice, documented training, experience, competence, and health status. For example, the ACNP who has received educational preparation for performing invasive diagnostic procedures (e.g., insertion of central line catheters, endotracheal intubation) may request that these privileges be a part of his or her institutional scope of practice if he or she can provide proof of training and competency along with documentation that the skill is required for the job. An ACNP may periodically request new privileges based on evolving mastery of skills, further training, and changes in services needed by the patient population and institution. ACNPs must understand that although they may be qualified to perform certain procedures, privileges to perform these acts may not necessarily be granted or renewed (usually on a biannual basis) if the patient population that the ACNP serves does not require these skills, or if ongoing application and competency in the skill during the renewal period cannot be documented (Table 16-1). A number of specific institutional examples of ACNP role development, including discussion of formal orientation programs, are available that further outline considerations for competency assessment, credentialing and privileging considerations, and ongoing professional practice evaluation (Bahouth & Esposito, 2009; D'Agostino & Halpern, 2010; Farley & Lathan, 2011; Foster, 2012; Goldschmidt, Rust, Torowicz, et al., 2011; Kapu, Thomson-Smith, & Jones, 2012; Kilpatrick et al., 2010; Kirton, Folcik, Ivy, et al., 2007; Pascual, Holena, Vella, et al., 2011; Shimabukuro, 2011; Yeager, 2010).

Service-Related Level

The functions of the ACNP are also adjusted according to the needs of the specialty patient population served or of the care delivery team (i.e., service) in the organization with which the ACNP is affiliated. This may be inpatient- or outpatient-based. This service-related scope outlines the clinical functions and tasks that may be administered by the ACNP specific to the service team with which the ACNP works and the needs of the specialty patient population served, which may include the following:

- An ACNP working with a cardiology service may initiate treatment for myocardial ischemia or infarction.
- An ACNP working in a pulmonary hypertension clinic may see patients on a regular basis to assess response to vasodilator therapy.
- An ACNP working with an oncology service may perform bone marrow aspirations or order antibiotics for a suspected opportunistic infection.
- An ACNP on a renal medicine service may write orders for hemodialysis and insert central venous dialysis catheters.
- An ACNP with the cardiovascular surgery service may harvest the vein grafts for coronary artery bypass surgery.
- An ACNP in the medical intensive care unit (MICU) may intubate and place arterial and central venous catheters.

Therefore, service-related scope may vary among ACNPs affiliated with various services or specialties within the same institution and even among those who

TABLE 16-1	Procedures Performed as Reported by 962 ACNPs
Procedures Performed in Hospital	**Frequency of Performance of Procedures by NPs (No. of Procedures)**
High Reported Frequency	
Radiologic studies	79.3% (619)
Vasoactive IV drips	67.1% (516)
Resuscitative efforts	67% (516)
Defibrillation	63.4% (512)
Wound care	49.9% (480)
Suture	40.7% (392)
Incisions	40.7% (392)
Ventilation	39.8% (295)
Medium Reported Frequency	
Cardioversion	38.2% (283)
Pacemakers	31.3% (230)
Arterial catheters	25.2% (182)
Central venous catheters	25% (182)
Pulmonary artery catheters	21.7% (157)
Intracardiac catheters	20.3% (165)
Cardiac assistive	18.8% (18.8%)
Endotracheal	17.7% (128)
Chest tubes	15.9% (113)
Lower Reported Frequency*	
Lumbar	16.4% (103)
Surgical first assist	9.5% (91)
Thoracostomy tubes	7.8% (75)
Cutdowns	5.4% (21)
Bladder aspiration	2.8% (16)

*In addition, other procedures that were performed with lower frequencies included bone marrow biopsies ($n = 6$), removing intra-aortic balloon pumps ($n = 4$), paracentesis ($n = 4$), joint aspirations ($n = 3$), and splinting fractures ($n = 3$). Adapted from Kleinpell, R., Goolsby, M. J. (2012). American Academy of Nurse Practitioners National Nurse Practitioner sample survey: Focus on acute care. *Journal of the American Academy of Nurse Practitioners, 24,* 690-694.

function under the same generic job description. The service-related scope outlines a more detailed and specific description of the types of activities that the ACNP will perform as a member of the practice.

In states in which physician collaboration is a requirement, or in cases in which the health care organization has collaborative guidelines, the ACNP's institutional and service-related scope of practice and clinical privileges may be determined collaboratively by the physician and

ACNP and set forth in a written agreement. This written agreement for collaborative practice then provides the source document on which the hospital makes privileging decisions (see Chapters 20 and 21). Written agreements, often formatted as a checklist, are frequently helpful because the detail included in a written agreement cannot be spelled out in a job description. Job descriptions, by their very nature, tend to be more general to cover ACNPs working in a variety of settings within the institution. In addition to outlining the specific activities that the ACNP performs, the agreement might also specify the level of communication or degree of supervision between the ACNP and physician that is required before the performance of a specific function (D'Agostino & Halpern, 2010; Kleinpell, Buchman, & Boyle, 2012). An ACNP with novice skills in central line insertion may require direct supervision for a specified period or number of successful attempts but, as the ACNP approaches expert status, the level of supervision may be decreased to minimal or none. Eventually, as the ACNP's expertise continues to advance, she or he may supervise medical trainees or novice ACNPs in these skills. As skills progress, the written agreement, if required, will also need to be modified. In some cases, the written agreement may be used to communicate the ACNP's scope of employment to other members of the health care team, such as staff nurses and pharmacists.

When negotiating the written agreement, the ACNP and collaborating physicians need to ensure that no function is in conflict with the individual state's nurse practice act and the policies of the particular institution. Nevertheless, the agreement should not serve as a barrier to practice but should be written as broadly as reasonable to allow for practicality, flexibility, and optimization of practice within the context of experience and safety.

Individual Level

The final determinant of scope of practice is role individualization by each ACNP. Experience, specialization, interest, motivation, self-esteem, personal ethics, personality traits, and communication style affect the employment opportunities, clinical specialties, skills, practice arrangements, and degree of autonomy that the ACNP will seek out and/or apply in her or his uniquely personal enactment of the role (Kapu, Thomson-Smith, & Jones, 2012).

Competencies of the Acute Care Nurse Practitioner Role

Most recently, in conjunction with the APRN Consensus Model, the focus of care for the Acute Care Nurse Practitioner has evolved to incorporate adult gerontology because ACNP practice includes the spectrum of adults, including young adults, adults, and older adults. The adult gerontology ACNP provides care to patients who are or may be at risk for physiologic instability. These patients may be encountered across the continuum of care settings because the role is not setting-specific but is dependent on patient care needs. As a result, the practice of the ACNP can span outpatient to hospital settings, urgent care, subacute care and rehabilitation. The central and core competencies for the APN, as explained in Chapter 3, form the foundation of ACNP practice. The central competency for all APNs is direct clinical practice in concert with the other six core competencies of coaching and guidance—consultation, research skills, clinical, professional and systems leadership, collaboration, and ethical decision making skills. The ways in which ACNPs enact these core competencies are consistent with other APN specialties, as discussed in Parts II and III of this text. In addition, ACNPs share common entry-level competencies in accordance with the nurse practitioner core competencies (NONPF, 2012). Although the ACNP may need to use specialty skills and knowledge in the care of acutely, critically and complex chronically ill adults, ACNPs have the following factors in common with the other NP specialties: (1) a generalist nursing foundation, (2) a health promotion basis to their practice, and (3) the development and appreciation of diagnostic reasoning skills. ACNPs prepared at the Doctor of Nursing Practice (DNP) level may have additional knowledge and skills including refined communication, in-depth scientific foundations, analytic skills for evaluating and providing evidence-based practice, advanced knowledge of the health care delivery systems and population-based care, the business aspects of practice, and an emphasis on independent and interprofessional practice (AACN, 2005; National Panel for NP Practice Doctorate Competencies, 2006).

Acute Care Nurse Practitioner Specialty Competencies

In addition to the core APN competencies, each of the NP specialties has unique competencies that differentiate practice. The *Nurse Practitioner Core Competencies* (NONPF, 2011) outline those competencies that are relevant to NP practice, regardless of population focus. ACNP entry-level competencies are illustrated in the AACN national adult gerontology acute care nurse practitioner competencies (AACN, 2012) and the *Scope and Standards of Practice for the Adult Gerontology Acute Care Nurse Practitioner* (American Association of Critical-Care Nurses, 2012). A discussion of how these ACNP competencies are carried out within the framework of the APN core competencies in Chapter 3 follows.

Advanced Practice Nurse Central Competencies of Adult Gerontology Acute Care Nurse Practitioners

Direct Clinical Practice

Direct clinical practice, the central competency of ACNP practice, is the function that consumes the greatest percentage of ACNP practice time. Prior clinical nursing expertise is essential for the ACNP role, because even the novice ACNP cares for acutely and critically ill patients who may precipitously manifest life-threatening conditions that mandate an immediate response. These situations demand a strong clinical practice foundation.

The specialty practice of ACNPs consists of short-term goals (stabilize patients, minimize complications, promote physical and psychological well-being) and long-term goals of care (restore maximum health potential, evaluate risk factors) (AACN, 2012; American Association of Critical-Care Nurses, 2012). ACNPs achieve these specialty practice goals through the performance of cognitive skills common to all APNs, such as patient assessment, critical thinking, diagnostic reasoning, case management, and prescription of therapeutic interventions. Assessing and intervening in complex, urgent, or emergency situations are key components of ACNP specialty competencies.

The central competencies of direct clinical practice as they apply to ACNP specialty practice can be broadly characterized as those related to diagnosing and managing disease and to the promotion and protection of health (see Box 16-1).

Diagnosing and Managing Disease

For ACNPs to achieve the specialty competencies to diagnose and manage disease in their specialty patient population, they must demonstrate mastery of advanced pathophysiology, completion of a prioritized health history and comprehensive and focused physical examinations, rapid assessment of unstable and complex health problems, implementation of diagnostic strategies and therapeutic interventions to stabilize health care problems, demonstration of technical competence with procedures, modification of the plan of care based on a client's changing condition and response to interventions, and collaboration with other care providers to facilitate positive outcomes (AACN, 2012; American Association of Critical Care Nurses, 2012). The varied practice settings of individual ACNPs across the continuum of acute care delivery services result in associated variance in some of the competencies that they perform (Kapu et al., 2012). Most ACNPs practice in acute and critical care settings that include subacute care, emergency care, and intensive care settings. These include but are not limited to acute

and critical care neurology, pulmonology, transplantation, presurgical and perioperative care, emergency care, pain management services, and cardiac surgery (Goolsby, 2011; Kleinpell & Goolsby, 2012). A growing number of ACNPs also practice in specialty-based practice settings, such as clinic, medical rehabilitation, home care, long-term care, sports medicine, holistic medicine, occupational medicine, employee health, mental health services, and medical flight program settings (Goolsby, 2010; Kleinpell, 2005; Kleinpell & Goolsby, 2012). Individual elements of the ACNP role differ, depending on these varied practice settings and on the specialty patient populations served, but the basic elements necessary to function as a generalist ACNP remain.

The performance of patient procedures, some of which are invasive, also constitutes a portion of ACNP's direct clinical practice. Technical procedures most commonly performed by ACNP respondents to the AANP 2008 to 2010 national sample survey are listed in Table 16-1. The literature corroborates ACNP technical skill performance that includes the following: endotracheal intubation, central line placement, pulmonary artery line placement, needle thoracotomy, chest tube insertion and removal, and cricothyrotomy for the trauma critical care focus; nerve block, joint needle aspiration, diagnostic peritoneal lavage, needle decompression of the chest, lumbar puncture, chest tube insertion, cricothyrotomy and tracheostomy, suturing of lacerations and wounds, and splinting of injuries for the emergency care focus; endotracheal and nasotracheal intubation, chest tube insertion and removal, arterial puncture, and insertion of central lines for the critical care focus (Kleinpell & Goolsby, 2012). (Kleinpell, Hravnak, Werner, et al., 2006). A NONPF publication, *Integrating Adult Acute Care Skills and Procedures into Nurse Practitioner Curricula* (NONPF, 2011), outlines a number of advanced procedures performed by ACNPs, including the following: monitoring intracranial pressure; 12-lead electrocardiogram (ECG) interpretation; defibrillation and cardioversion; pacemaker interrogation; hemodynamic monitoring; central venous line insertion; arterial puncture or cannulation; interpretation of a chest radiograph; performing thoracentesis for pleural effusions; chest tube insertion and removal; airway management for the nonanesthesia provider and sedation for procedures; spirometry and peak flow assessment; paracentesis; local anesthesia application; and cutaneous abscess drainage.

It must be understood that procedural skill performance is not limited to the task itself but also includes knowledge of the indications, contraindications, complications, and skill in managing complications. When performing a procedural skill to derive physiologic data, such as mean arterial pressure, pulmonary artery pressure, or

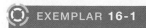 **EXEMPLAR 16-1** Adult Gerontology Acute Care Nurse Practitioner Practice in an Intensive Care Unit

In the cardiothoracic ICU (CTICU), Marie, the ACNP, functions collaboratively with the critical care provider team consisting of the ACNP, attending physician (intensivist), one or two critical care medicine fellows, clinical pharmacist, and other members of the delivery team, including bedside nurses, primary care nurses, and respiratory therapists. The team works in collaboration with the surgeons, surgical fellows, and residents on the cardiac, thoracic, transplant, vascular, and trauma services. As the CTICU ACNP, Marie manages the patient from admission to discharge from the unit.

The day begins with a report from the team members who provided care during the previous night, highlighting changes in patients' conditions and providing information on new patients. Marie participates in dynamic patient-focused rounds, during which each patient is examined at the bedside and interviewed, when possible. A wealth of other data is reviewed, including vital signs, hemodynamic data (pulmonary artery pressures, central venous pressures, cardiac outputs), ventilator settings, and results of previous weaning trials, chest radiographs, diagnostic testing, laboratory and culture data, and a complete list of medications, continuous infusions, and fluid balances. Based on the clinical examination and review of data, and with input from members of the provider and delivery team, a comprehensive plan of care is devised for the patient. Marie assumes varying roles during these patient-focused rounds (e.g., presenting and reviewing data, doing the physical examination, writing orders, calling consultants). During this time, Marie is noting issues to be addressed later, treatment outcomes to be evaluated, planned procedures, culture and diagnostic test results to review, family conferences, and expected admissions and discharges. Once rounds are complete, Marie will begin to address some of the specific issues on her work list.

Marie begins by seeing the four patients who are to be transferred out of the CTICU care unit that morning. She briefly examines each patient and reviews their data to ensure that the patients' responses to interventions are appropriate. She verifies that these patients have been weaned from their vasoactive medicines and removes their chest tubes. Marie reviews each patient's history and physical (H&P) and restarts home medications that are appropriate to the patients' cardiac conditions and comorbidities. She writes transfer orders and collaborates with the bedside nurse to ensure that all patient care issues have been addressed in the orders. One

patient has a history of active smoking, and Marie discusses the relationship between smoking and heart disease with the patient, as well as smoking cessation strategies. One patient needs to maintain a central IV access on the hospital ward. Marie converts the 16-gauge introducer in the patient's right internal jugular vein to a triple-lumen catheter using a rewire technique. One patient has developed an arrhythmia with some hemodynamic instability and Marie initiates appropriate treatment, cancels the patient's transfer to the floor, and informs the intensivist of the change in condition. One patient is being transferred to a subacute care facility. Marie collaborates with the unit case manager to finalize transfer plans, speaks with the patient's family before discharge, and speaks with the receiving team in the subacute care facility to ensure continuity of care. During the course of the day, Marie might perform other invasive procedures, such as inserting arterial lines, central venous lines, dialysis catheters, chest tubes, and nasoduodenal feeding tubes and performing thoracentesis, endotracheal intubation, and removal of intra-aortic balloons. Health promotion and protection assessment and intervention are integral to Marie's role but in different areas than one might expect in the primary care setting. For example, in the CTICU, Marie addresses stress ulcer prophylaxis, preventing complications from immobility, promoting skin integrity, and optimizing nutritional support.

Marie will continuously monitor the patients on the unit throughout the day and provide problem-focused care in response to changing patient needs and condition. She will be contacted by the nurse who is providing bedside care for the patient to address patient problems such as hypotension, hypertension, low cardiac output, low urine output, bleeding, low oxygen saturation, fever, difficulty with ventilation or ventilator changes, agitation and delirium, mental status changes, inadequate pain management, arrhythmias, electrolyte abnormalities, and problems with lines or catheters. She will see patients multiple times throughout the day in response to these concerns, each time assessing possible causes, performing directed physical examinations, formulating a treatment plan, and reassessing clinical findings to evaluate response to therapy. Marie initiates some treatments independently, but other, more complex situations may require her to consult with the intensivist and/or surgeon to review the management options. Marie will communicate with consultants from other teams, such as cardiology, renal

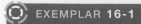

EXEMPLAR 16-1   Adult Gerontology Acute Care Nurse Practitioner Practice in an Intensive Care Unit—*cont'd*

medicine and infectious diseases, to coordinate care and treatment plans.

During the day, Marie also participates in the care of patients newly admitted after surgery. As patients arrive from the operating room, Marie receives a brief report from the anesthesia care provider and surgical fellow. She reviews the chart, examines the patient, and reviews initial laboratory results, electrocardiographic results, and chest radiography results. She reviews the plan of care with the critical care nurse and respiratory therapist, targeting hemodynamic management and ventilator weaning. She documents a progress note, writes orders, and then returns frequently to reassess the patient's status and adjust the plan. One postoperative patient is bleeding severely. Marie alerts the surgeon, orders and reviews a coagulation profile, and ensures that the patient is being rewarmed. She orders blood products to correct the abnormality and monitors the patient to determine whether this therapy is effective or whether the patient will have to return to the operating room for mediastinal exploration.

At the end of the day, the team makes rounds again, seeing the new patients, evaluating the progress of and plans for other patients, and developing a plan for the next 12-hour period. The dynamic environment of the CTICU and the changing CTICU team members require the ACNP to assess and reassess patient conditions frequently, remain flexible and responsive to subtle changes, and to carefully organize and manage time.

As a permanent member of the critical care team, Marie provides needed continuity to care. She is instrumental in developing clinical protocols and communicating care expectations to other members of the team. She is available to interact with social services, case managers, physical and occupational therapists, and nutritional consultants. She is able to participate in discharge planning. She is readily available to the nursing staff for questions or problem solving. She participates in the CTICU's continuous quality improvement activities. She participates in research protocols, screens patients for eligibility criteria, and educates others concerning the research initiatives. Marie plays an important role in communication with patients and families and has a unique opportunity for teaching and reinforcing teaching.

lumbar cerebrospinal fluid pressure, the ACNP must be able to use this information skillfully for patient evaluation. ACNPs are also compelled to collect their individual practice data related to procedure performance, including number and type of complications, and use these data to document ongoing skill competence, to attain positive patient outcomes, and to facilitate patient safety. The practice of an ACNP in a cardiothoracic surgical ICU, which illustrates the integration of technical skills within the context of diagnosis and management of disease, is provided in Exemplar 16-1.

Promoting and Protecting Health and Preventing Disease

In addition to disease diagnosis and management, ACNPs also provide services to promote and protect health and prevent disease (AACN, 2012; American Association of Critical-Care Nurses, 2012). Services include providing anticipatory guidance and counseling to patients and their families. Inevitably, some of the methods that ACNPs use to implement health promotion and protection and disease prevention vary from those used by NPs in the primary care specialties. Variations in application are related to the prioritization of needs during acute and critical illness. In some practice models, the episodic

nature of the relationship between the ACNP and patient and family is limited to a single acute illness event. Hospitalization can also provide a critical window of opportunity for ACNPs to address health promotion and disease prevention with patients.

ACNPs are skilled in a unique form of health promotion and protection and disease prevention—recognizing and modifying health risk factors associated with an inpatient stay. The ACNP is qualified to identify the additional health problems for which the acutely, critically, and complex chronically ill are at risk and to implement strategies to minimize or prevent that risk. This area forms a distinctive health promotion and health protection aspect of ACNP practice. As direct care providers, ACNPs have the ability to activate strategies and systems to implement primary, secondary, or tertiary prevention initiatives related to these unique inpatient risk factors. For example, some of the risk factors imposed by an inpatient stay are physiologic in nature, such as immobility, decreased nutritional intake, fluid and electrolyte imbalance, altered immunocompetence, impairment of self-care ability, existing or developing comorbid disease states, and risks associated with invasive diagnostic and therapeutic interventions. Other risks have a psychological foundation, such as psychological consequences of alterations in the patient's physical abilities and alteration of his or her environment, sleep deprivation, communication impairment, alteration of self-image, role reversal, financial challenges, knowledge deficits, and the consequences of medication administration, including but not limited to delirium and depression. Families are also influenced by many of these risks and require ACNP services.

In addition, there are risk factors related to hospitalization itself and the multiplicity of caregivers, including discontinuity of care, polypharmacy, system inefficiency and redundancy, miscommunication with families, and miscommunication among caregivers (AACN, 2012; American Association of Critical-Care Nurses, 2012). The ACNP is competent to assess patients for these unique risks and implement interventions to prevent their occurrence or minimize their consequences. Although these skills are common to all ACNPs, those prepared at the Doctor of Nursing Practice (DNP) level are equipped to assume leadership roles in developing, implementing, and evaluating evidence-based interventions to address and improve population health and clinical prevention (AACN, 2005).

Advanced Practice Nurse Core Competencies of Adult Gerontology Acute Care Nurse Practitioners

Guidance and Coaching

In addition to direct clinical practice, the ACNP also performs the APN core competencies described in Chapter 3, with specialization unique to the ACNP role. Providing expert guidance and coaching of patients, families, and other health care providers is a core competency that is an essential part of ACNP care. In the primary care area, the plan of care may be mutually determined and fully implemented between the NP and patient-family dyad. In contrast, the process of assessment and diagnosis, care planning, implementation, and evaluation in the acute care setting, although still centering on the ACNP and patient-family dyad, will likely include a number of other individuals, including but not limited to physicians, other nurses, respiratory therapists, dietitians, pharmacists, physical and occupational therapists, social workers, and clergy. In this complex setting, the ACNP's ability to plan, interpret, and explain the plan of care while educating others about disease processes is a valued aspect of the ACNP role. Often, critical illness can require many complex treatments and ACNPs can provide teaching to families, nursing staff, and other members of the health care team to facilitate knowledge of indicated care. The core competency of guidance and coaching is played out at the highest levels when ACNPs prepare patients for discharge after serious illness or when

they assist and prepare family members to care for loved ones who have undergone catastrophic or debilitating health problems. At times, patients (particularly the poor and uninsured) may not have a consistent primary care provider in the outpatient setting. In this case, the ACNP becomes an important source for health information and health promotion and protection interventions during the inpatient encounter. Some patients may be more receptive to health teaching that occurs in proximity to an acute health event (e.g., diet and exercise information after an acute myocardial infarction). ACNPs also provide coaching for experienced and inexperienced nurses in complex care settings.

Consultation and Evidence-Based Care

ACNPs often provide consultation and use, promote, and conduct evidence-based research. The consultative activities of the ACNP may take the form of a formal medical consultation. Sometimes, consultative services by the ACNP are delivered in more informal exchanges regarding the patient's condition and plan of care with other health care providers. This aspect of the ACNP's practice is invaluable in the teaching hospital setting. In this environment, attending physicians and medical trainees rotate on and off the service and staffing patterns may result in inconsistencies in bedside nursing care. As the consistent member of the health care provider team, the ACNP can use consultative skills to keep the team informed of the patient's condition and changing plan of care during the entire length of stay. Evidence-based care competencies may also vary among ACNP providers. All ACNPs use research to deliver evidence-based medical and nursing care, whereas a smaller number of ACNPs may actively participate in or lead research initiatives.

Leadership

All ACNPs provide some form of professional, clinical, and systems leadership in their provider role by serving as mentors and role models for staff nurses, taking on selected administrative responsibilities in the health care agency, and acting as care facilitators and change agents within the health care system. ACNPs prepared at the DNP level perform these activities at an even higher level of specificity and autonomy. ACNPs coordinate care delivery in the health care system; several studies have demonstrated that this aspect of ACNP practice reduces the inpatient length of stay (Burns & Earven, 2002; Russell, Vorder Breugge, & Burns, 2002). Promoting a positive healing environment and espousing assertiveness and conflict negotiation skills are beneficial qualities for ACNPs. ACNPs work to facilitate individual practice and health care system change through their participation in quality assurance or continuous quality improvement

(CQI) initiatives (Elpern et al., 2009; Russell et al., 2002). Participating in the planning and implementation of system-wide cost containment or cost-effective initiatives is also an aspect of the ACNP role.

Collaboration

Collaboration is one of the most frequently practiced core competencies of ACNPs. Collaborative practice in the clinical setting involves working together, with shared responsibilities for clinical decision making for patient care (see Chapter 12). In the acute care setting, patient care delivery is always a collaborative effort of the members of the multidisciplinary health care team. Therefore, the ability to collaborate successfully is one of the critical components of the ACNP role. In a collaborative practice model, the emphasis is on patient outcomes. Each professional should be responsible for providing the care for which he or she is best prepared. A collaborative practice model in acute care focuses on the concept that each patient needs the services of different types of providers simultaneously. The advantage to this model is the ongoing continuity and coordination of care.

Although there has been much support for collaborative practice between nurses and physicians, barriers still exist. Unfortunately, these barriers are created between those for whom collaborative practice should be the focus—other nurses and physicians. However, there is growing recognition that the ACNP role promotes a collaborative model of care (D'Agostino & Halpern, 2010; Kleinpell, Buchman, & Boyle, 2012).

Ethical Practice

Ethical decision making comprises another core competency. ACNPs often find themselves acting as advocates for patients in care dilemmas. Because ACNPs are often involved in planning and implementing end-of-life care, ethical decision making skills are an essential component of ACNP practice (AACN, 2012; American Association of Critical-Care Nurses, 2012). In helping facilitate ethical decision making, ACNPs can be instrumental in resolving moral issues and building ethical practice environments (see Chapter 13).

Profiles of the Adult Gerontology Acute Care Nurse Practitioner Role

Although most ACNPs practice in acute and critical care settings, they have transitioned into a variety of role implementation models in ever-expanding specialty area practice sites (Kleinpell, 2005). One ACNP role implementation model focuses on episodic management of patients in a single clinical specialty unit, one model involves following a caseload of hospitalized patients throughout their hospitalization, and another focuses on managing patients across the entire continuum of acute care services, from hospitalization to home.

The ACNP model focusing on episodic care of patients on a specialty clinical inpatient unit provides the earliest model of ACNP practice (Howie-Esquivel & Fontaine, 2006; Kleinpell & Hravnak, 2005). In this model, the ACNP, in collaboration with a physician specialist, might manage the care of a patient admitted to a specialty inpatient unit with an acutely unstable medical or surgical condition. Once the patient is stabilized, the patient is transferred to another clinical unit under the care of another provider. Under this model, ACNPs confine their practice to episodic care at a defined level of acute care, permitting them to develop their skills and knowledge about specific conditions in a delineated setting (see Exemplar 16-1). The limitation of this model is that it does not allow for continuity of care across the continuum.

In another model of role implementation, the ACNP directly manages the care of a caseload of patients throughout their entire hospitalization, providing individualized ongoing care with continuity to the patient and family. The goal of this model is to facilitate and coordinate a patient's hospital stay to provide high-quality, cost-effective care (Farley & Lathan, 2011; Green & Newcommon, 2006; Landsperger, Williams, Hellervik, et al., 2011; Meyer & Miers, 2005). In this model, the ACNP will, in collaboration with a physician, admit the patient to the hospital, complete the admission history and physical examination, assess the patient's initial clinical status, order and interpret diagnostic and therapeutic tests, perform procedures, evaluate and adjust the plan of care, and prepare the patient for discharge. The ACNP will provide care continuously for patients as they move from high-acuity to lower acuity inpatient care units, facilitate patients' movement through the acute care system, and plan for and implement discharge. Exemplar 16-2 illustrates this model.

In another model of care, the ACNP delivers comprehensive specialty care to a group of patients across the entire continuum of care services. For example, an ACNP member of a heart failure care team may oversee patient management during hospitalization, provide postdischarge clinic follow-up, and ultimately manage home-based infusion therapy. With the growth of specialty-based practices, the number of ACNPs working in this type of model of care is increasing. Exemplar 16-3 illustrates this model with an ACNP in a pulmonary practice who also bills for her services.

Diagnostic reasoning and advanced therapeutic interventions, consultation, and referral to other physicians, nurses, and providers are intrinsic components of this role, as described by the ACNP scope of practice

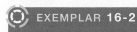

Adult Gerontology Acute Care Nurse Practitioner Practice in an Inpatient Specialty Service

On the inpatient cardiology service of a large university teaching hospital, patients are assigned to the ACNP team or the medical resident team (teaching team). The service covers approximately 50 monitored cardiology beds, including general cardiology patients, interventional cardiology patients, heart failure patients, and electrophysiology patients. Approximately two thirds of the patients are assigned to the ACNP team. In addition, the ACNP team is responsible for seeing outpatients for their preprocedure evaluation in the cardiac catheterization suite. The ACNP team is comprised of 10 full-time positions and is responsible for providing care 7 days a week, from 7 AM until 6 PM, when the service is signed out to night coverage, usually provided by an upper level cardiology fellow.

The day begins when Kate, who is the leader of the four-member ACNP team for the day, receives a sign-out of patients from the cardiology fellow covering the previous night. The fellow reports on the status of the patients on the ACNP team and also adds four new patients to the list who had been admitted overnight. Kate communicates the information to the other three ACNPs on the team and assigns the new patients; she then reviews her nine patients and begins to plan her day. A computer census is generated and she reviews the daily laboratory results, vital signs, intake and output, weight, and current medication list for each patient.

Kate begins to see her patients, starting with the newly admitted patient from the previous night. She reviews this patient's data, reviews the H&P examination findings, and looks at the chest radiograph and ECG. She interviews and examines the patient, validating the H&P findings. This 74-year-old man, with a history of hypertension and non–insulin-dependent type 2 diabetes, was admitted with chest pain and found to be in atrial fibrillation, with a rapid ventricular response. During the night, he was treated with rate-controlling agents and this morning has converted to normal sinus rhythm and does not have chest pain. Kate discusses her plan for ordering an echocardiogram and exercise stress test with imaging with the attending cardiologist and then returns to the patient to inform him of this plan. She describes the two tests, explaining the reasons for doing the studies. After answering his questions, she communicates the plan of care to the nurse. Next, she writes orders

for the studies and carefully reviews the medications, adjusting as needed. She writes a progress note and then notifies the patient's primary care physician of the patient's admission and discusses the planned course of action.

Kate next turns her attention to two patients who are to be discharged. After examining the patients and reviewing the data, she writes discharge orders, completes necessary prescriptions, writes a final progress note, and dictates a discharge summary. In coordination with the nurse, she identifies discharge teaching points and arranges postdischarge follow-up appointments with the cardiologist. One patient will require IV antibiotics for a pacemaker wound infection, so home care and infusion services are also arranged.

Over the remainder of the morning, Kate sees the other six patients in similar detail. One patient has chest pain with new ECG changes and is sent for emergency catheterization. The patient receives a coronary stent and is transferred to the coronary care unit (CCU). Kate will not continue to follow the patient in the CCU but notifies the CCU resident and provides a verbal sign-out. Kate completes the progress notes on her other patients and follows up on the interventions she has ordered throughout the day.

During the day, Kate has fielded multiple calls regarding new admissions to the service and has assigned them to herself or her colleagues accordingly. An H&P is completed and dictated on each newly admitted patient, admission orders written, and a plan of action coordinated with the attending physician. Kate has collaborated with the other ACNP team member who is stationed in the preprocedure area of the cardiac catheterization suite to coordinate the admission of patients to the postprocedure area after their coronary interventions.

At the end of the day, each of the four ACNPs completes a sign-out for the night coverage fellow and a computer-generated census is completed for their reference. The ACNP team updates an electronic database daily that tracks patient volumes, admissions and discharges, and case mix. The ACNPs are also involved in precepting ACNP students, providing formal lecturing and teaching, and enrolling patients in research protocols.

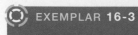

EXEMPLAR 16-3   Adult Gerontology Acute Care Nurse Practitioner Practice Across the Continuum of Acute Care Services

A community-based pulmonary practice consists of three physicians and Suze, an ACNP. Suze has been with the practice for 4 years. When she was hired, Suze applied for her Medicare provider identification number–unique provider identification number (PIN-UPIN). In 2008, she received her Medicare national provider identifier (NPI) number, which replaced the PIN-UPIN as of May 2007. Suze has assigned her NPI number to the practice. This means that when Suze bills for her services, the bill is submitted under her number but payment is made to the practice. Suze's reimbursement rate is at 85% of the physician fee schedule, regardless of whether she bills in the office or in the hospital.

Each member of the practice sees patients in the office and the hospital on a rotating basis. During morning conference, Suze participates with the physicians in reviewing the schedule of that day's office appointments and list of inpatients who need to be followed. Suze sees those patients who have specialized needs relative to learning, treatment adherence, smoking cessation, and caregiver burden or unavailability. Although each one of them has his or her own daily office schedule of patients, the list of inpatients is divided between Suze and the physician assigned to cover inpatients for the week.

Today, Suze will follow up on 15 inpatients—three new overnight admissions and 12 continuing inpatients. On one newly admitted patient, Suze reviews the history and physical examination findings, chest radiograph, and additional diagnostic results. She interviews the patient to confirm and gain additional historical information. She then conducts a physical examination. This particular patient is a 55-year-old man admitted for exacerbation of his chronic obstructive pulmonary disease (COPD) and possible pneumonia. He was treated overnight with broad-spectrum antibiotics, IV steroids, oxygen, and a nebulizer and is currently less dyspneic. Suze discusses with the pulmonologist her plan to order a chest computed tomography (CT) scan because this is the patient's third COPD exacerbation in the past 8 weeks. She is concerned that an underlying condition may be causing the exacerbations. In addition, knowing that he is a current cigarette smoker, she changes the antibiotic to cover organisms more likely to occur in smokers. She discusses smoking cessation with

the patient and they agree to collaborate on developing a smoking cessation strategy at his first office appointment after hospital discharge. Suze and the pulmonologist review the case and treatment plan. He agrees and states that he will also look at the chest radiograph from the office computer but has no need to see the patient that day. Suze writes her progress note and additional orders. At the end of the day, Suze submits her bill for this inpatient under her NPI number to the office manager. Payment will be made to the practice at 85% of the physician fee schedule.

The following day, Suze sees this patient again. She interviews him, performs a physical examination, and reviews the laboratory results and the CT scan. She calls the pulmonologist to tell him that the CT scan is normal. The pulmonologist reviews the CT scan with Suze and visits the patient, asks a few questions related to symptoms, and listens to the patient's lung sounds. He agrees that the chest CT scan is negative, writes a note, which refers to Suze's note and opinion, and documents his H&P examination findings and interpretation of CT scan. Because Suze and the pulmonologist have each seen the patient and performed some part of the service, the total work is combined and Suze submits this day's bill as a shared visit under the physician's number. In this case, the practice will be paid at 100% of the physician fee schedule. Had the pulmonologist not seen the patient and performed and documented a part of the service, the bill would have been submitted only under Suze's NPI number.

The patient is discharged to home on his routine metered-dose inhalers, a steroid taper, and oral antibiotic. He returns in 2 weeks for a follow-up office appointment scheduled with Suze. Suze interviews the patient, who states that he is feeling much better; she performs a physical examination. She finds his lung sounds are much improved. They discuss smoking cessation and the patient agrees to set a stop smoking date. Suze writes a prescription for a drug to help reduce nicotine cravings and also writes refill prescriptions for his inhalers. She documents the events of the visit and later discusses the plan with the pulmonologist. Suze submits the bill under her own NPI number and the practice is reimbursed at 85% of the physician fee schedule.

(AACN, 2012; American Association of Critical-Care Nurses, 2012). Although ACNPs might require some variation in skill sets, depending on the model within which their role is implemented, strong commonalities exist. As with other APN roles, all ACNPs are proficient in advanced physical assessment, clinical decision making (diagnostic reasoning), ordering and interpreting laboratory studies and procedures, and collaborating in the development and implementation of a treatment plan that includes prescribing medication. Using diagnostic reasoning, the ACNP diagnoses the origin of a complex medical problem that develops in an acutely or critically ill patient (see Chapter 7). The skills inherent in effective diagnostic reasoning include the fundamental skills of the ACNP role—history taking, physical examination skills, pattern recognition, ability to analyze and synthesize data, and ability to generate a working diagnosis. A number of factors affect the quality of diagnostic reasoning when applied to the acutely and critically ill, such as multisystem deterioration, hemodynamic instability, depressed level of consciousness, and unavailability of significant others to supply, corroborate, or supplement patient information. All these factors challenge the ACNP's ability to diagnose an acutely or critically ill patient's ever-changing physical condition accurately and expeditiously.

Another inherent portion of the ACNP practice profile is the performance of technical skills, as indicated earlier. Patient needs within a specialty practice ultimately influence the type and level of therapeutic and diagnostic psychomotor skills that an individual ACNP performs (Kapu et al., 2012; Kleinpell & Goolsby, 2012). The ACNP role is one of evidence-based practice, which should be evident in clinical decision making and intervention selection.

Additional skills for continued ACNP role development are based on practice. As ACNP education transitions to the DNP, emphasis on promoting evidence-based practice for patients with acute, critical, and complex chronic illness and the use of information systems and technology for improving health care will actively bring new opportunities for ACNP practice, as well as leadership opportunities focused on systems change and quality improvement.

Comparison with Other Advanced Practice Nurse and Physician Assistant Roles

The ACNP role differs from other APN roles with regard to the type of patient care problems encountered, acuity of the patient's condition, need for rapid and continuous assessment, planning and intervention, and setting in which the care is delivered. For example, the clinical nurse specialist (CNS) enacts the APN role through three spheres of influence—at the patient level, in direct care,

at the nurse level, as with staff development, and at the institutional level, providing oversight for care. In comparison, the ACNP uses clinical assessment skills to assess complex and acutely ill patients through health history taking, physical and mental status examination, performing procedures, and risk appraisal for complications. Both the ACNP and CNS roles are targeted to a patient-centered approach to care for patient populations, but the continuous on-unit presence of the ACNP at the bedside of patients often differentiates the role of the ACNP from the CNS role. Staff education and system change responsibilities represent a larger percentage of the CNS's role than of the ACNP's role. Conversely, CNSs are generally not involved in carrying out many of the procedures and interventions that characterize the ACNP role. Institutional variations in role implementation for CNSs and ACNPs sometimes lack clear-cut differentiation in role responsibilities. However, it is acknowledged that the CNS and NP roles are distinct, with distinct practice foci (Becker, Kaplow, Muenzen, et al., 2006).

Table 16-2 can assist the reader in conceptualizing where the main focus of ACNP practice falls within the health care continuum and where there might be differences or overlap with the primary care NP role. The table presents examples of management strategies for common patient health care problems encountered in the traditional primary, secondary, and tertiary health care settings. With diabetes care, for example, ACNP practice involves predominantly strategies directed toward management of the patient during an acute exacerbation of the diabetes. Because of the severity of symptoms, the patient must be admitted to the hospital, where she or he can be continuously monitored and where management strategies may change from hour to hour (tertiary care). During this same hospitalization, the patient may need to have an infected foot ulcer treated with IV antibiotics (secondary care). Once the crisis is over, but while the patient is still hospitalized, the ACNP may provide discharge teaching on routine foot care (primary care), as well as diabetic diet and glucose monitoring. At this point, the patient may be referred back to his or her primary care provider for further follow-up and management.

In comparison, the primary care NP's practice involves predominantly strategies directed toward management of the patient's diabetes when it is stable (primary care). This would include ongoing surveillance of the patient's self-management of the diabetes, education on diabetic risk factors, and assessment of signs of disease progression and complications. The primary care NP may also assess when the patient's diabetes is not well controlled and requires adjustment of insulin or oral hypoglycemic agents (secondary care). At the point when the patient is not responding or becomes acutely ill, the primary care NP will

TABLE 16-2   **Patient Care Problems and Management Interventions Traditionally Associated with Health Care Delivery Settings**

Delivery Setting	HEALTH PROBLEM AND INTERVENTIONS		
	Diabetes	Hypertension	Pneumonia
Tertiary care management (ICU setting)	Diabetic ketoacidosis management Fluid replacement Electrolyte titration IV insulin	Continuous vasoactive drugs Arterial pressure monitoring Evaluation and management of possible CVA	Mechanical ventilation and artificial airway Pulmonary toilet Culture assessment Sepsis management Continuous monitoring
Secondary care management (inpatient ward)	Diabetic exacerbation management Sliding scale insulin administration and monitoring Hydration Workup of cause(s)	Hypertensive crisis management Additional antihypertensives Adjunct therapy as needed	IV antibiotics Oxygen therapy Advanced assessment CXR, arterial blood gases, SpO_2
Primary care management (outpatient setting)	Initial Dx or stable management Oral antihyperglycemics or subcutaneous insulin Diet Prevention and assessment of associated complications Foot care Risk factor management	Diet Oral agents Lifestyle changes Prevention and assessment of associated complications Risk factor management	Oral or intramuscular antibiotics

CVA, Cerebrovascular accident; *CXR*, chest x-ray; *Dx*, diagnosis; *SpO$_2$*, peripheral arterial oxygen saturation.

recognize the need for the patient to be referred to a setting in which continuous monitoring and management is provided (tertiary care).

Using these examples helps educators and clinicians understand that there is a natural overlap in some areas of knowledge and practice between acute care and primary care NPs. However, each NP specialty also has its own distinct focus. The knowledge base and practice of the ACNP cannot be limited only to unstable conditions requiring complex technologic diagnostic and management strategies for which the acutely or critically ill patient may be admitted to the hospital; the ACNP also needs to be prepared to manage the range of health care problems that accompany the patient. This includes not only the acute illness or exacerbation of chronic illness that requires acute care services, but also the patient's comorbidities, which also must be cared for while in the acute care setting. For example, the hospitalized diabetic patient discussed earlier may also have stable hypertension, stable asthma, osteoarthritis, and an episode of vaginitis. While the patient is hospitalized, the ACNP must simultaneously attend to these stable comorbid health conditions to maintain their quiescence.

APNs, including ACNPs, are different from physician assistants (PAs). The PA role is under the jurisdiction of physician licensure, which is supervisory rather than collaborative and does not allow for independent functions. Some overlap exists between the ACNP and PA in terms of the management of disease; however, the ACNP's direct clinical practice competencies also provide for nursing's holistic perspective, as well as the promotion and protection of health. Whereas PAs are trained in the medical model to focus on providing illness-based care to patients, ACNPs, with their nursing background and practice, bring expertise in patient and family education, communication, collaboration, and health promotion and disease prevention for individuals and populations. A further differentiation is that ACNP practice also incorporates additional APN core competencies around leadership and coaching. A growing number of facilities are integrating PA and ACNP practitioners on hospital-based teams to manage care for hospitalized patients (Moote et al., 2011).

Adult Gerontology Acute Care Nurse Practitioners and Physician Hospitalists

The hospitalist is an internal medicine physician who is responsible for managing the care of hospitalized patients in the same manner that a primary care physician is responsible for managing his or her outpatients. Physicians first described this emerging role in 1996 as a consequence of the explosive growth of the primary care and internist role secondary to managed care. The physician hospitalist role is now being incorporated in many academic teaching centers and community settings, and the ACNP recently has been added as a member of this health care team (Kleinpell, Hanson, & Buchner, 2008; Rosenthal & Guerrasio, 2009). Some ACNPs function as members of the hospitalist team and manage patients independently in collaboration with the physician hospitalist.

A primary care physician refers the patient to the hospitalist team for management during the acute care admission. The team provides care for the patient during hospitalization and refers the patient back to the primary care provider at the time of discharge. The goal of this service is to provide seamless, cost-effective care. This can be an advantage for a primary care physician with busy office hours who may have limited time to make hospital visits and may not be sufficiently familiar with acute care management. The specific role of the ACNP, as a member of the hospitalist team, is similar to the roles previously described, including obtaining an admission history and physical examination, performing daily physical examinations, making rounds with the physician, developing a treatment plan, reviewing laboratory studies and radiographs, and performing procedures. Furthermore, coordinating patient care management when many consultants are involved in decision making is a significant part of the role, as is consultation with the case managers to facilitate discharge planning effectively (Cowan et al., 2006; Howie & Erickson, 2002).

Outcome Studies Related to Acute Care Nurse Practitioner Practice

Measuring outcomes of practice (see Chapters 23 and 24) is an acknowledged component of establishing the value of any APN role (Newhouse et al., 2011). Positive outcomes of ACNP care have been demonstrated in a number of settings, including subacute transitional and rehabilitation care (Casara & Polycarpe, 2004; Green & Edmonds, 2004), emergency care (Cooper, Lindsey, Kinn, et al., 2002), inpatient medical services (Howie & Erickson, 2002), geriatric inpatient care (Lambing, Adams, Fox, et al., 2004), cardiovascular care (Meyer & Miers, 2005), neuroscience care (Green & Newcommon, 2006), respiratory care (Burns & Earven, 2002; Hoffman, Tasota, Scharfenberg, et al., 2002, 2003), intensive care (D'Agostino & Halpern, 2010; Farley & Lathan, 2011; Fleming & Carberry, 2011; Gracias, Sicoutris, Stawicki, et al., 2008; Hoffman, Miller, Zullo, et al., 2006; Kleinpell et al., 2008; Moote et al., 2011; Morse, Warshawsky, Moore, et al., 2006; Nyberg et al., 2007; Shimabukuro, 2011; Sonday &

Grecsek, 2010; Yarema & Judy 2011; Yeager, Shaw, Casavant, et al., 2006), and as rapid response team leaders (Morse, et al., 2006; Rosenthal & Guerrasio, 2009; Sonday & Grecsek, 2010). Research studies have demonstrated the positive impact of ACNP care, including decreased costs, shorter hospital length of stay, decreased use of laboratory tests, lower rates of urinary tract infections and skin breakdown, time savings for house physicians, similar care outcomes compared with physician practices, patient and family satisfaction, and an increased role in discussing patient outcomes with nurses and families.

Although these studies exploring ACNP effectiveness have been conducted in several types of care settings, continued research on the impact of ACNP practice is needed. Most studies on the use and outcomes of ACNPs have focused on comparing ACNP care with physician care, reducing costs, or discussing the impact of ACNP care on a focused area of care (Kleinpell, Hanson, & Buchner, 2008). If ACNPs are to delineate the impact of their care and justify their existence, it is imperative that their worth be supported by careful research (see Chapter 23).

Implementation of the Adult Gerontology Acute Care Nurse Practitioner Role in Other Clinical Practice Settings

The ACNP might participate as a member of a specific clinical specialty or consult service practicing in an acute care setting. Examples might include an ACNP working as part of an internal medicine team, trauma service, surgical service, acute stroke team, emergency department, renal medicine team, pulmonary medicine service, electrophysiology service, preadmission surgical service, oncology service, or medical emergency–rapid response team.

Bone Marrow Transplantation Services

The ACNP working as a member of the bone marrow transplantation service has an autonomous role while functioning as a part of a collaborative practice model; the team may be comprised of a resident, fellow, attending physician, and ACNP. The ACNP provides continuity of care for the service by being the only consistent member of the academic health care team, in which physicians rotate between clinical and research activities. The ACNP carries a caseload of patients and follows them through their hospital stay until discharge. Role responsibilities include carrying out preliminary daily rounds on each patient, performing physical examinations, interpreting laboratory tests (electrolytes and x-ray studies), performing marrow aspirations, and consulting specialists (e.g., gastroenterology, infectious disease, pulmonary

EXEMPLAR 16-4   **Acute Care Nurse Practitioner Practice on a Hospitalist Team**

John is one of three nurse practitioners working on a hospitalist team at a community hospital. He is prepared as an ACNP and his colleagues are prepared as adult NPs. They work with a 10-member hospitalist team to provide care to hospitalized patients. The hospitalist service is the primary admitting service for the hospital and provides medical inpatient consultations. John's role consists of managing a group of patients, following up newly admitted patients, performing a history and physical examination for new admits, discharging patients, and responding to consultation requests. Consultations vary from medical comanagement of surgical patients to the evaluation of acute condition changes (e.g., chest pain, shortness of breath, nausea, vomiting), as well as follow-up of diagnostic tests and needs for changes to the treatment plan. These changes can vary from seeing patients for condition changes, such as alterations in vital signs, onset or worsening of symptoms such as nausea or pain, or laboratory results that require further follow-up for possible order changes (e.g., supplemental potassium).

Because he is prepared as an ACNP, John is also called for consultations in the ICU, or to evaluate patients who might need transfer to the ICU, and works in collaboration with intensivists to manage acute changes in ICU patients. In addition to serving on the code team, he is a member of the rapid response team to assess a patient further who has had an acute change in condition anywhere in the hospital.

John will see patients independently, but has a hospitalist physician in house whom he can further consult for patient care management issues, including generating differential diagnoses, evaluating different treatment options, and discussing care progression in outliers. Often, patients are discussed among the entire team, using the expertise of each member on the hospitalist team.

Other roles of the hospitalist NP include providing patient status updates to family members, explaining the plan of care to clinical nurses, reporting the status of a hospitalized patient to the patient's primary care physician (improving transitions of care communication), planning goals of care for patients being discharged, transferring patients for rehabilitation, ensuring documentation and reporting of core measures (e.g. pneumonia, venous thromboembolism [VTE] prophylaxis), implementing patient satisfaction activities, planning advance directive care, incorporating integrative and complementary therapies (e.g., acupuncture, healing touch, stress reduction interventions), and coordinating care across the spectrum of consultants who are treating the patient.

Working as a hospitalist ACNP requires John to keep current with requirements for documentation and billing, focused professional practice evaluation (FPPE), and ongoing professional practice evaluation (OPPE). He finds that attending the annual national NP conference and the national hospital medicine conference provides him with essential updates for his practice, as well as valuable continuing education. He has negotiated with the hospitalist group to cover travel, registration, hotel costs, and paid time off for these annual conferences. Most recently, John submitted an abstract to present at the national NP conference to speak on the role of the NP on the hospitalist team.

John currently serves on the advanced practice committee, which reviews the applications for medical staff appointment of advanced practice providers within the institution. He also serves on the acute and critical care quality committee, which meets monthly to review quality data, such as infection rates and development of acute care protocols.

Although several physician assistants also serve on the hospitalist team, John's role is different in that in addition to managing patient care, he is also involved in several performance improvement initiatives. As an APN, John brings a strong performance and quality improvement perspective to the team, often identifying opportunities to improve care and care delivery, examining possible solutions, and generating consensus among the interdisciplinary team. One recent initiative is targeting the reduction of unplanned readmissions for heart failure patients at risk for rehospitalization within 30 days by initiating a discharge clinic that will be run by the hospitalist NPs. Building on their educational preparation, ACNPs also promote, mentor, and facilitate the evidence-based practice (EBP) process by identifying clinical issues, critically examining the literature, and disseminating findings to improve EBP, minimize variances among providers, and evaluate clinical and administrative outcomes related to practice changes.

As an ACNP on a hospitalist team, John enjoys the flexibility of the role because he is involved in direct patient care management. He also serves in advanced practice consultation roles for committee work for implementing FPPE and OPPE practice standards and for developing NP-run initiatives, such as the discharge clinic for heart failure patients. John's role represents a growing opportunity for ACNPs as hospitals develop and expand hospitalist services to assist in the management of hospitalized patients.

medicine) to assist in patient management. On the basis of the information gathered, the ACNP collaborates with the other provider team members during daily rounds to develop the daily and long-term treatment plan. In addition, the ACNP teaches the house staff and nursing staff and incorporates health teaching and health promotion and protection activities into his or her practice, especially risks associated with immunosuppression.

Diagnostic and Interventional Services

In preadmission surgical services, the major clinical functions of an ACNP include history taking and physical examinations, performing preprocedure evaluations, providing patient and family education, obtaining and interpreting laboratory, electrocardiographic, and radiologic data, identifying at-risk individuals in need of preadmission discharge planning, initiating contacts with social services, discharge planning, and making management recommendations for patients in the surgical holding area. The ACNP consults with the anesthesiologist and surgeon regarding patient health problems that may affect or preclude anesthesia delivery or surgery. ACNPs may provide services similar to those in the cardiac catheterization suite or the gastrointestinal procedure laboratory.

Alternatively, an ACNP may function as part of a team that provides care in continuity across a spectrum of clinical encounters or settings.

Heart Failure Services

In this example, a team of three ACNPs on the heart failure service in a university medical center collaborate with each other and with physician team members to optimize continuity of care for their patients. Each ACNP has a caseload of patients for whom he or she assumes responsibility in the outpatient area. They see each patient in clinic on a regular basis, examine patients, and adjust the treatment plan. They perform follow-up by phone contact on a weekly basis, helping patients assess their symptoms, follow daily weights, discuss dietary changes, and adjust oral medications as needed. Based on this discussion, the ACNP may have the patient come to the outpatient clinic for further clinical assessment and treatment (e.g., a dose of IV diuretic, adjustment of continuous inotropic medication infusions). When a patient requires admission to the hospital for an acute exacerbation of heart failure, one ACNP (each ACNP team member provides in-hospital coverage on a weekly rotating basis), along with the physician, manages the patient in the hospital setting. They are familiar with the patient's problems and treatment plan, can provide continuity, have established a trusting relationship with the patient and care delivery team, and can

readily facilitate discharge planning and follow-up when the patient is ready for discharge to home.

Orthopedic Services

The role of the ACNP working with patients with orthopedic problems covers a full spectrum of practice settings, including coverage for the emergency room, the orthopedic clinic, and the inpatient orthopedic service. The orthopedic ACNP works closely with the attending physicians, staff nurses, and residents to coordinate care from preadmission testing to discharge. Each of the ACNPs carries a caseload of hospitalized patients and outpatients undergoing short procedures. This role may include perioperative management as first assistant in the operating room.

Rapid Response Team

A more recent role for the ACNP may be as team leader or team member of a hospital medical emergency or rapid response team. When hospitalized patients develop sudden physiologic instability outside of critical care areas, a mismatch between patient needs and available supportive resources occurs. Rapid response teams have been developed to deploy personnel and other resources to meet patient needs in a crisis in any area of the hospital (Devita, Bellomo, Hillman, et al., 2006; Scherr, Wilson, Wagner, et al., 2012). These teams consist of multidisciplinary members such as ACNP, physician, critical care nurse, respiratory therapist, and nursing supervisor. The team might be activated to respond to conditions such as hypotension, acute mental status changes, bleeding, respiratory distress, chest pain, or oliguria. The ACNP may be the team leader, coordinating the assessment, triage, and treatment plan, or she or he may participate as a team member enacting problem-focused response protocols, placing peripheral or central venous lines, assisting with airway management, and coordinating transfer to another level of care, if necessary (Morse, Warshawsky, Moore, et al., 2006; Rosenthal & Guerrasio, 2009; Sonday & Grecsek 2010).

Preparation of Adult Gerontology Acute Care Nurse Practitioners

At present, ACNPs are registered nurses who are prepared at the master's level of graduate nursing education. Programs are being developed to prepare ACNPs with additional knowledge and skills in a clinical practice, awarding the title of DNP. All ACNP programs should provide for program requirements as outlined in the *Criteria for Evaluation of Nurse Practitioner Programs* (National Task Force on Quality Nurse Practitioner Education, 2012).

The ACNP curriculum incorporates the graduate core, advanced practice core, NP specialty curricula, and ACNP subspecialty curricula. Programs that prepare ACNPs at the DNP level do not negate the master's core but, rather, build on it (AACN, 2005). DNP curricula combine foundational or core competencies for all DNP program graduates, as well as ACNP specialty competencies for the practice doctorate.

The ACNP specialty content should focus on the knowledge and skills essential to diagnose and manage the episodic and chronic problems commonly experienced by patients with acute, critical, and complex chronic illness while performing health promotion and protection and disease prevention activities within the context of the continuum of the acute care delivery system (American Association of Critical-Care Nurses, 2012). As illustrated in the conceptual model of care services previously presented in Table 16-2, ACNPs diagnose and manage not only the acute health problems associated with the patient's chief complaint, but also quiescent, stable, comorbid health conditions. Because ACNPs must be prepared to manage health problems across the full continuum of acute health care services, their didactic information and clinical experiences should provide for this broad focus. Similarly, the program should provide didactic and clinical preparation in the competencies delineated in the *Acute Care Nurse Practitioner Competencies* (National Panel for Acute Care Nurse Practitioner Competencies, 2004) and the *Scope and Standards of Practice for the Acute Care Nurse Practitioner* (American Association of Critical-Care Nurses, 2012). Teaching skills in screening and prevention specific to acute care practice are also essential (Heath, Andrews, Thomas, et al., 2002). Because ACNP graduates must be competent in critical incident management, clinical simulation is often used in ACNP education (Hravnak, Beach, & Tuite, 2007; Scherer, Bruce, Graves, et al., 2003). Technical skills training is also commonly incorporated into ACNP programs, as indicated in Table 16-1.

More recently, ACNP education has been transitioning to DNP preparation as entry into ACNP practice or as a post–master's program. These programs prepare ACNPs for the highest levels of leadership in practice and scientific inquiry. Graduates have received additional didactics and experiences to achieve the level of competence indicated in *The Essentials of Doctoral Education for Advanced Practice Nursing* (AACN, 2005). This expansion in direct practice abilities includes advanced communication (interpersonal and technologic), use of an expanded scientific foundation to provide an evidence basis for practice across settings, advanced participation, collaboration and leadership within the health care delivery system and the business of health care, and focus on independent practice (NONPF, 2012). An example of the practice skills of an ACNP who has received practice doctorate education is presented in Exemplar 16-5.

Finally, NPs who have been educated in another NP specialty but who are now working in an acute care setting, in which additional competencies and skills are required, must ensure that their educational preparation is consistent with the focus of their practice (Kleinpell et al., 2005). Neither certification nor licensure grant universal practice rights (Smolenski, 2005), and it is important that NP practice be substantiated by the appropriate education. Individuals with master's preparation in another APN specialty may enroll in a post-master's or DNP ACNP program to ensure that they undergo didactic and supervised clinical practica to prepare adequately for caring for this unique and vulnerable patient population (Kleinpell et al., 2005).

Reimbursement for Acute Care Nurse Practitioners

It is important that ACNPs become knowledgeable about billing and payment mechanisms for professional services, in addition to policy issues, that affect ACNP reimbursement. Obtaining reimbursement for services provided by NPs continues to be a universal challenge for every NP specialty, particularly ACNPs. Some of these challenges include securing admission to provider panels, determining whether a service is covered, billing for critical care time, and deciding which billing option—direct, incident to, or shared (see Chapter 19)—to use. The complexities of how federal and state laws apply to specific practice situations can deter groups from fully using ACNPs (Buppert, 2012). In addition, how an ACNP demonstrates financial productivity affects an employer's decision to hire and/or retain ACNP providers.

Although there are many considerations as to which billing option to use, there are compelling reasons why ACNPs should bill directly under their own number, including the following: (1) recognition of the ACNP's financial worth as a result of produced income; and (2) tangible recognition of the ACNP's professional standing, which in turn leads to professional satisfaction and peer recognition (Magdic, 2006). Direct reimbursement also brings visibility to the quantity and type of care for which an ACNP is compensated. Visibility is accomplished through documentation and monitoring of billed services in the National Claims History file established by the Centers for Medicare & Medicaid Services (CMS; Magdic, 2006; www.cms.gov/research-statistics/). Through evaluation of services billed by ACNPs at the national level, an aggregate profile of ACNP practice with respect to billable direct patient care activities can be developed (Magdic, 2006).

Adult Gerontology Acute Care Nurse Practitioner Role Implementation Following Doctor of Nursing Practice Preparation

Joyce is a DNP-prepared ACNP currently working in a nephrology practice. The practice consists of one ACNP and five physicians. The practice is organized so that each provider has his or her own caseload of patients and follows these patients in the office and in the hospital. In addition, Joyce is responsible for one of the outpatient dialysis clinics, where she sees patients three times per week. This particular dialysis clinic is located in a neighborhood consisting mainly of Hispanics and African Americans. Every month, members of the practice meet for breakfast to discuss issues related to patient care and the logistics of the practice. Her usual schedule consists of daily morning rounds on her hospitalized patients followed by afternoon office hours on Tuesdays and Thursdays and outpatient dialysis clinic patients on Mondays, Wednesdays, and Fridays.

To track her patients, Joyce uses software on her PDA. As she makes her rounds, she enters the patient data and, at the end of the day, uploads the information into her office computer. Having patient data on a PDA or tablet allows Joyce to access patient information quickly when, for example, she admits a patient who was seen in the office a week ago but she herself was not in the office.

Recently, Joyce launched a new set of standard admission orders for patients admitted to the hospital with a diagnosis of chronic renal failure. The standard orders resulted from a series of complications that occurred when new medical residents did not order the appropriate laboratory tests or all the routine medications used to treat renal failure. The result was increased hospital stay and cost. Joyce searched the literature to provide evidence to support orders that she believed necessary and then collaborated with the medical staff, nurses, nutritionist, pharmacist, and manager of the laboratory to develop this order set. Consensus was reached in 6 months and the orders were approved. Joyce then collaborated with the nursing staff to develop a quality assurance project that looked at whether these orders influenced patient outcomes positively.

In addition to seeing clinical patients, every third month Joyce sits on the credentialing and privileging committee at the hospital. She participates in the review of applicants to ensure that they are qualified to provide competent, safe patient care. Joyce's unique role is to provide peer review on the applications of NPs.

At the dialysis clinic, Joyce is the administrator and patient care provider. Physicians from the practice also provide patient care on a rotating basis and are available for consultation. The staff is comprised of registered nurses, nursing assistants, and secretarial support. To maintain optimal patient care, Joyce has implemented policies and evidence-based procedures. A quality assurance committee, led by Joyce, periodically reviews charts for compliance with selected quality indicators. In addition, Joyce coordinates a bimonthly journal club for the clinic's staff as one mechanism to ensure that the staff is current in their practice. Because of the clinic's location, Joyce sits on the local neighborhood board. Her goal is for the clinic to be a good neighbor. Joyce collaborates with the board members to provide culturally appropriate educational opportunities on topics such as hypertension and diabetes in an effort to reduce the incidence of renal failure in that community.

Joyce serves as adjunct faculty at the local university. She lectures to the ACNP students on renal disease and also serves as a clinical preceptor for ACNP students. In addition, she is a member of the ACNP program's local advisory board, which meets annually. The purpose of this board is to provide consultation to the ACNP faculty on ways to recruit and graduate outstanding students who can meet the needs of the community. At the last meeting, Joyce pointed out that students had poor recall of current guidelines related to the management of diabetes, a leading cause of renal disease. Joyce suggested ways to integrate this information into the curriculum. She pointed out that current guidelines on diabetes management can be found on diabetes professional organization websites and can be downloaded into a PDA for easy access in the clinical area.

Almost every encounter between an ACNP and a patient is associated with a payer. The five major categories of payers, each with its own policies and legal structures, are Medicare, Medicaid, indemnity-type insurance, managed care organizations (MCOs), and businesses that contract for certain services (Buppert, 2012; Sample & Dorman, 2011). Reimbursement for ACNP services

within the Medicare framework is a focus of this chapter. Although Medicare serves as the most common form of reimbursement of NP services, other payers may have their own unique variations. If an ACNP understands Medicare regulations, he or she is better equipped to navigate the policies of other payers (Magdic, 2006). New health policy changes in the Patient Protection and

Affordable Care Act (PPACA) will bring new reimbursement configurations for ACNPs (see Chapter 22). Detailed descriptions of third-party payers and related issues are described in Chapters 19 and 22).

At the same time Medicare legislation was enacted in the 1960s, the role of the NP was evolving in the area of pediatrics. Consequently, only limited provisions were made for NPs billing for eldercare services. Medicare regulations specified that NPs could receive direct reimbursement only when they provided care in certain geographic locations, such as skilled nursing facilities and federally designated rural medically underserved areas. The 1997 Balanced Budget Act (BBA) removed the geographic restrictions on the direct option for NPs. However, there are still complex issues in regard to reimbursement and it is important that ACNPs understand the rules surrounding the direct, incident to, and shared billing options. Any or all of these options may be used by the ACNP in certain situations.

Medicare Reimbursement for Acute Care Nurse Practitioners

Office and Nonhospital Clinic Setting

Although ACNPs typically provide services to patients in hospital and hospital-affiliated offices and clinics, a portion of their practice may occur in a non–hospital–affiliated setting, as described earlier in the discussion of ACNP role implementation models. In the office setting, an ACNP must decide whether to bill directly or incident to the physician. Direct billing means that the ACNP provides the evaluation and management (E/M) services and submits the bill under her or his own provider number. Under this option, Medicare will reimburse at 85% of the physician fee schedule. "Incident to" is the part of Medicare law that provides for coverage of services and supplies furnished incident to the professional services of a physician. The decision of which option to use is often a business decision. For more detailed information regarding incident to billing, the reader is referred to the *Medicare Carriers Manual* (CMS, 2012). See Chapter 19.

A third option addresses cases in which the ACNP and the physician share the E/M service in the outpatient setting in which the ACNP performs a portion of an E/M encounter and the physician completes the E/M service. In this situation, the incident to requirements are met and the shared outpatient service should be billed under the physician's number. If the incident to requirements are not met, the shared outpatient service must be reported using the ACNP's number (CMS, 2012). Of note, there is no incident to billing option for ACNPs who provide services to patients in the hospital, emergency department, and hospital-affiliated clinics (CMS, 2012).

Hospital Inpatient, Hospital Outpatient, and Emergency Department Settings

Hospitals and emergency departments are common practice sites for ACNPs. However, billing for ACNP services in these settings can be challenging (Buppert, 2012; Magdic, 2006). Whether an ACNP can bill for services delivered in the hospital depends first on whether the ACNP's salary is listed on the hospital's Medicare cost report. If it is, then the ACNP's services are already paid for under Medicare Part A. A transmittal issued by the CMS, dated January 26, 2007, updated the *Medicare Claims Processing Manual* regarding "Direct Billing and Payment for Non-Physician Practitioner Services Furnished to Hospital Inpatient and Outpatients" (Buppert, 2012; CMS, 2012). According to this transmittal, payments for professional services of the NP (as well as CNS and PA) could be unbundled from the payment to the hospital for hospital services billed under the hospital's cost report. However, the hospital still bills the fiscal intermediary for the facility fee associated with NP, CNS, or PA services (Buppert, 2012; CMS, 2012). Direct payment for the ACNP's professional services furnished to hospital inpatients and outpatients must be made to the ACNP at 85% of the physician fee schedule unless the ACNP reassigns payment to the hospital (CMS, 2012).

Shared billing is another option for ACNPs in the hospital inpatient, outpatient, and emergency department settings (Magdic, 2006). The high patient acuity in these areas fosters a close collaborative relationship with physician colleagues. It is not uncommon for both the ACNP and physician to provide services to the hospitalized patient on the same day. On October 25, 2002, CMS issued a change request (CR) 2321, which updated *Medicare Carriers Manual* §15501 guidelines for E/M services. These guidelines were further clarified by Transmittal 178 in May 2004 (CMS, 2012) and provide direction for billing and reimbursement of E/M services provided by the physician and ACNP when they are in the same group practice and provide services on the same day, either at the same or different times. A shared visit under these circumstances means that the physician has a face to face encounter with the patient, provides some portion of the E/M service, and provides supporting documentation that he or she links to the documentation of the ACNP. For shared billing to occur between the ACNP and physician, the ACNP should be employed by the physician practice, have a contractual relationship between the ACNP and physician, or both should be employed by the same entity (CMS, 2012).

Key issues regarding shared E/M services are as follows (CMS, 2012):

- If the ACNP provides a medically necessary service and there is no face to face encounter between the patient and physician, the service must be billed under the ACNP's provider number. A physician simply reviewing the chart and creating or adding to a note does not constitute a face to face encounter.

- If both the ACNP and physician provide portions of the E/M service on the same day at the same or different times and there is a face to face encounter between the patient and physician, then the physician and ACNP may combine their services and bill for a shared visit under the physician's or ACNP's provider number at the level supported by their combined documentation.

The preceding discussion also applies to billing for ACNP services provided within the hospital outpatient or emergency department. For more information regarding incident to and shared billing, refer to the CMS *Medicare Carriers Manual*—Part 3, Claims Process, Transmittal 1764, and Chapter 12, Section 30.6.4 (CMS, 2012). An example of billing activities of an ACNP in the inpatient setting is provided in Exemplar 16-3, which illustrates the billing practices of an ACNP in a pulmonary specialty practice who sees patients in the hospital and office.

Critical Care Reimbursement for Acute Care Nurse Practitioners

Critical care involves high-complexity decision making to assess, manipulate, and support vital system functions; this often requires extensive interpretation of a number of data sources and application of advanced technology (CMS, 2012). Reimbursement for critical care services can occur in any location in which critical care services are performed, including ICUs, emergency departments, and general medical-surgical floors (CMS, 2012; Vachani, DeLong, & Manaker, 2003). Critical care services are billed according to time-based Current Procedural Terminology (CPT) codes (Sample & Dorman, 2011). The first 30 to 74 minutes of critical care services on a given calendar date are billed under one specific CPT code. For each additional 30 minutes, a second code is used. A physician may not tie into an ACNP's note for either code. The ACNP or the physician, but only one, may provide the initial 30 minutes of critical care time. For each additional 30 minutes, the service is billed by whoever provided the service (Dorman, Loeb, & Sample, 2006). If the total time spent providing critical care services is less than 30 minutes, other E/M codes must be used (American Medical Association, 2012).

It is important to note that rapid changes in health care affecting Medicare, Medicaid, and private payers are occurring at the federal and state levels, especially with the introduction of the PPACA (U.S. Department of Health and Human Services [HHS], 2011). Readers are referred to current Medicare and Medicaid rules and regulations for guidance.

Challenges Specific to the Adult Gerontology Acute Care Nurse Practitioner Role

The role of the ACNP is continuing to evolve and gain recognition. The increased need for ACNPs to manage patient care directly in an expanding health care arena will continue to provide unique practice opportunities. The practice doctorate will provide additional opportunities to expand and increase the emphasis on promoting EBP and organizational and systems leadership (National Panel for NP Practice Doctorate Competencies, 2006). Simultaneously, ACNPs will face challenges to practice that will need to be resolved to establish their role firmly. Practicing ACNPs continue to report that physicians and hospital administrators are unfamiliar with their role and the differences between the ACNP and primary care NP specialties. Also, some physicians feel threatened by the role. Misunderstandings about ACNP practice and labeling of the role as a so-called physician extender have stemmed from the perception that ACNPs are replacements for house staff and function as resident replacements. Many of these perceived threats and misperceptions can be addressed through education. ACNPs can use formal and informal opportunities to educate the professional public about the purpose and practice of ACNPs, providing clear and concrete examples of their use and efficacy. To articulate their role, it is extremely important for ACNPs to frame their practice within the nursing paradigm, one that uses the admitting history and physical examination to develop a plan of care that includes the following: recognizing the patient's holistic problems and the medical diagnosis; addressing these nursing and medical problems throughout the hospital stay; using interventions that not only diagnose and manage disease but also promote and protect health; framing the discharge summary so that patients have a continuum of nursing and medical care as they return to the community; and applying all the ACNP role competencies, not only those related to direct clinical care, to their practice.

Exposure to the comprehensive care that ACNPs provide and the education of the health care team about the role will lead to continued role recognition and acceptance. Educating administrators and other health care professionals can facilitate acceptance of the role, which will in turn provide an opportunity for independent contracting for ACNP professional services. Awareness of worth in terms of billable revenue and the care that ACNPs can provide is imperative for successful contract negotiations and marketing purposes.

In addition to individual efforts, Cummings and colleagues (2003) have suggested five specific recommendations to assist with organizational change when implementing ACNPs on a system-wide level:

- Use a change model to guide the change process and integrate ongoing evaluation for feedback.
- Assign a champion—one or two individuals to support, coordinate, and market the change on both the micro and macro levels within the organization.
- Articulate a vision—clarify and communicate a consistent definition and expectations of the role (including an organization-wide job description that is not service-specific and indicates practice boundaries and reporting lines) and anticipated outcomes of role implementation.
- Establish a forum to facilitate open and ongoing communications among all players.
- Attend to cultural and personality transitions.

Changing employment trends have also affected ACNP practice. Originally, ACNPs were hired predominantly in tertiary medical center settings. ACNPs now report increased employment with physician practice groups, MCOs, accountable care organizations (ACOs), independent subacute care facilities, and even individual contractual relationships. However, these opportunities also bring the challenges of negotiating legal contracts, multiorganizational credentialing and privileging, group practice and MCO and ACO policies, and reimbursement issues (Kleinpell, Buchman, & Boyle 2012; see Chapters 20 and 21).

ACNPs need to continue to develop strong collaborative relationships with physicians and others to provide optimal patient care. The practice doctorate for NPs advocates for advanced interprofessional collaboration for improved health outcomes (AACN, 2005). Working to negotiate a collaborative practice partnership can be a challenge. In working to establish collegial interactions and by sharing successful practice models, ACNPs can promote enhanced collaborative relationships (see Chapter 12).

In the future, ACNPs may practice in multiple settings with individually negotiated contracts. Managing episodes of acute illness or exacerbation of chronic illness in home health care, subacute care, and outpatient settings might be directed by the ACNP, as is already the case in some areas. These areas are natural extensions of acute care services and encompass the scope of ACNP practice, the stabilization of acute and chronic disease. There are myriad opportunities relative to acute and chronic therapeutic management—for example, the management of renal dialysis or ventilator-dependent patients.

Cost reduction in acute care services will continue. Currently, collaborative teams composed of a physician, resident, and ACNP are popular in many practice settings. In the future, certain patient populations may be managed by teams composed of several ACNPs with one physician, as in the heart failure service situation described earlier.

Monitoring the outcomes of ACNP practice remains essential. Although a growing number of utilization and outcome-based studies of ACNP practice have been conducted and published, there is still the need to demonstrate the impact of ACNP care in a growing number of practice arenas. The emphasis on continuous quality improvement will continue to mandate the need for ACNPs to become proactive and involved in measuring the impact of their care.

With all ACNPs holding master's degrees and some holding doctoral degrees, there is an increased potential to apply scientific knowledge to clinical practice and establish and uphold EBP. ACNPs are expected to assume leadership roles in evaluating the scientific literature and applying their findings to change and improve care (see Chapters 10 and 11).

ACNPs must accept the challenge to improve and advance themselves and their profession continually. Strategies for success in the ACNP role include maintaining competency, networking, demonstrating outcomes of practice, and communicating about the role (Kleinpell & Hravnak, 2005). To provide safe, high-quality, and efficient care, the ACNP must persistently pursue ongoing education to be knowledgeable about recent advances in health care and judicious in the application of research findings. ACNPs should not only read the literature but also publish on clinical and role topics. Sharing their clinical expertise and experiences can benefit their peers as those peers seek to develop and enhance their roles. It is important that ACNPs be involved in their NP professional and clinical specialty organizations so that the issues unique to ACNP practice gain recognition by the leaders of the national organizations, and also to ensure that ACNPs have a voice in the legislative and political decision making process. Collaboration with public policymakers to influence legislation issues related to the ACNP role or, on a larger scale, health policy issues is also an imperative for all ACNPs (AACN, 2012; American Association of Critical Care Nurses 2012; see Chapters 12 and 22).

Conclusion

The ACNP role provides an opportunity for NPs to have a significant impact on patient outcomes at a dynamic time in the history of health care delivery. As their role continues to evolve, and as health care systems respond to market forces and economic change, opportunities to develop the ACNP role further will arise. Future development of the ACNP role should be based on the evaluation of the need for the role, understanding the scope of the role, assessment of the practice or organization, and the service needs of the patient population. Ensuring that ACNPs practice to the full scope of their education and training is in alignment with the recommendations of the Institute of Medicine (2011). Because the ACNP role continues to evolve, participation in national organizations to refine consensus regarding role components, program curriculum, marketing, and

role evaluation is necessary. ACNP educators and clinicians must work together to ensure that the preparation and practice of ACNPs is safe, effective, and fully represented as the movement of doctoral APN education evolves. ACNPs must be strong activists in efforts to gain full recognition of their role within their proper scope of practice across acute care settings. In this evolving health care arena, ACNP practice is rapidly expanding and holds unlimited potential. Ongoing challenges include ensuring expansion of the ACNP with a focus on advanced practice nursing, rather than as a physician replacement model of care.

References

American Association of Colleges of Nursing (AACN). (2012). Adult gerontology acute care nurse practitioner competencies. (http://www.aacn.nche.edu/students/nursing-program-search).

American Association of Colleges of Nursing. (2005). *The essentials of doctoral education for advanced practice nursing.* Washington, DC: Author.

American Association of Critical-Care Nurses. (2012). *Scope and standards of practice for the adult gerontology acute care nurse practitioner.* Aliso Viejo, CA: Author.

American Medical Association. (2012). *CPT 2012.* Chicago: American Medical Association Press.

American Nurses Credentialing Center. (2009). Acute care nurse practitioner role delineation study. (http://www.nursecredentialing.org/Documents/Certification/RDS/2008 Surveys/AcuteCareNPRDS2008.aspx).

American Nurses Credentialing Center. (2010). Credentialing statistics. (http://www.nursecredentialing.org/Certification/FacultyEducators/Statistics/2010CertificationStats.aspx).

Bahouth, M. & Esposito-Herr, M. (2009). Orientation program for hospital-based nurse practitioners. *AACN Advanced Critical Care, 20,* 82–90.

Becker, D., Kaplow, R., Muenzen, P. M., & Hartigan, C. (2006). Activities performed by acute and critical care advanced practice nurses: American Association of Critical-Care Nurses study of practice. *American Journal of Critical Care, 15,* 130–168.

Buppert, C. (2012). *The nurse practitioner's business practice and legal guide* (4th ed.). Gaithersburg, MD: Jones & Bartlett.

Burns, S. M. & Earven, S. (2002). Improving outcomes for mechanically ventilated medical intensive care unit patients using advanced practice nurses: A 6-year experience. *Critical Care Nursing Clinics of North America, 16,* 231–243.

Casara, M. & Polycarpe, M. (2004). Caring for the chronically critically ill: Establishing a wound-healing program in a respiratory care unit. *American Journal of Surgery, 188*(Suppl 1A), 18–21.

Centers for Medicare & Medicaid Services (CMS). (2012). Medicare Claims Processing Manual. (http://www.cms.gov/Regulations-and-Guidance/Guidance/Manuals/downloads/clm104c26.pdf). Accessed March 5, 2013.

Chang, W. C., Mu, P. F., & Tsay, S. L. (2006). The experience of role transition in acute care nurse practitioners in Taiwan under the collaborative practice model. *Journal of Nursing Research, 16,* 83–92.

Cooper, A., Lindsey, G. M., Kinn, S., & Swann, I. J. (2002). Evaluating emergency nurse practitioner services: A randomized controlled trial. *Journal of Advanced Nursing, 40,* 721–730.

Cowan, M. J., Shapiro, M., Hays, R. D., Afifi, A., Vazirani, S., Ward, C. R., et al. (2006). The effect of a multidisciplinary hospitalist/ physician and advanced practice nurse collaboration on hospital costs. *Journal of Nursing Administration, 36,* 79–85.

Cummings, G. G., Fraser, K., & Tarlier, D. S. (2003). Implementing advanced nurse practice roles in acute care: An evaluation of organizational change. *Journal of Nursing Administration, 33,* 139–165.

D'Agostino R. D. & Halpern N. A. (2010). Acute care nurse practitioners in oncologic critical care: The Memorial Sloan Kettering Cancer Center experience. *Critical Care Clinics, 26,* 207–217.

Devita, M. A., Bellomo, R., Hillman, K., Kellum, J., Rotondi, A., Teres, D., et al. (2006). Findings of the first consensus conference on medical emergency teams. *Critical Care Medicine, 34,* 2463–2478.

Dorman, T., Loeb, L., & Sample, G. (2006). Evaluation and management codes: From current procedural terminology through relative update commission to Center for Medicare and Medicaid Services. *Critical Care Medicine, 34*(Suppl 3), S71–S77.

Elpern, E. H., Killeen, K., Ketchum, A., Wiley, A., Patel, G. P., & Lateef, O. (2009). Reducing use of indwelling urinary catheters and associated urinary tract infections. *American Journal of Critical Care, 18,* 535–541.

Farley, T. L. & Lathan, G. (2011). Evolution of a critical care nurse practitioner role within a U.S. academic medical center. *ICU Director, 1,* 16–19.

Fleming, E. & Carberry, M. (2011). Steering a course towards advanced nurse practitioner: A critical care perpective. *Nursing in Critical Care, 16,* 67–76.

Foster, S. S. (2012). Core competencies required for the cardiac surgery nurse practitioner. *Journal of the American Academy of Nurse Practitioners, 24,* 472–475.

Goolsby, M. J. (2011). 2009–2010 AANP national nurse practitioner sample survey: An overview. *Journal of the American Academy of Nurse Practitioners, 23*, 266–268.

Goldschmidt, K., Rust, D., Torowicz, D., & Kolb, S. (2011). Onboarding advanced practice nurses: Development of an orientation program in a cardiac center. *Journal of Nursing Administration, 41*, 36–40.

Gracias, V. H., Sicoutris, C. P., Stawicki, S. P., Meredith, D. M., Horan, A. D., Gupta, R., et al. (2008). Critical care nurse practitioners improve compliance with clinical practice guidelines in the surgical intensive care unit. *Journal of Nursing Care Quality, 24*, 338–344.

Green, A. & Edmonds, L. (2004). Bridging the gap between the intensive care unit and general wards: The ICU liaison nurse. *Intensive Critical Care Nursing, 20*, 133–163.

Green, T. & Newcommon, N. (2006). Advancing nursing practice: The role of the nurse practitioner in an acute stroke program. *Journal of Neuroscience Nursing, 38*(Suppl 4), 328–330.

Heath, J., Andrews, J., Thomas, S., Kelley, F. J., & Friedman, E. (2002). Tobacco dependence curricula in acute care nurse practitioner education. *American Journal of Critical Care, 11*(1), 27–32.

Hoffman, L. A., Miller, T. H., Zullo, T. G., & Donahoe, M. P. (2006). Comparison of 2 models for managing tracheotomized patients in a subacute medical intensive care unit. *Respiratory Care, 51*, 1230–1236.

Hoffman, L. A., Tasota, F. J., Scharfenberg, C., Zullo, T. G., & Donahoe, M. P. (2002). Management of ventilator-dependent patients: 5-month comparison of acute care nurse practitioner (ACNP) versus physician in training (PIT). *American Journal of Respiratory and Critical Care Medicine, 165*, A388.

Hoffman, L. A., Tasota, F. J., Scharfenberg, C., Zullo, T. G., & Donahoe, M. P. (2003). Management of patients in the intensive care unit: Comparison via work sampling analysis of an acute care nurse practitioner and physicians in training. *American Journal of Critical Care, 12*, 436–443.

Howie, J. N. & Erickson, M. (2002). Acute care nurse practitioners: Creating and implementing a model of care for an inpatient general medical service. *American Journal of Critical Care, 11*, 448–458.

Howie-Esquivel, J. & Fontaine, D. (2006). The evolving role of the acute care nurse practitioner in critical care. *Current Opinion in Critical Care, 12*, 609–613.

Hravnak, M., Beach, M., & Tuite P. (2007). Simulator technology as a tool for education in cardiac care. *Journal of Cardiovascular Nursing, 22*, 16–24.

Institute of Medicine. (2011). *The future of nursing: Leading change, advancing health*. Washington DC: National Academies Press.

Kapu, A. N., Thompson-Smith, C., & Jones, P. (2012). NPs in the ICU. *Nurse Practitioner, 37*, 46–52.

Kilpatrick, K., Harbman, P., Carter, N., Martin-Misener, R., Bryant-Lukosius, D., Kaasalainen, D. F., et al. (2010). The acute care nurse practitioner role in Canada. *Nursing Leadership, 23*, 114–129.

Kilpatrick, K. (2011). Development and validation of a time and motion tool to measure cardiology acute care nurse practitioner activities. *Canadian Journal of Cardiovascular Nursing, 21*, 18–26.

Kirton, O. C., Folcik, M. A., Ivy, M. E., Calabrese, R., Dobkin, E., Pepe, J., et al. (2007). Midlevel practitioner workforce analysis at a university-affiliated teaching hospital. *Archives of Surgery, 162*, 336–341.

Kleinpell, R., Buchman, T. & Boyle, W. A. (Eds.). (2012). Integrating nurse practitioners and physician assistants in the ICU: Strategies for optimizing contributions to care. Mount Prospect, IL: Society of Critical Care Medicine.

Kleinpell, R. M., Ely, E. W., & Grabenkort, R. (2008). Nurse practitioners and physician assistants in the ICU: An evidence-based review. *Critical Care Medicine, 26*, 2888–2897.

Kleinpell, R. & Goolsby, M. J. (2012). American Academy of Nurse Practitioners National Nurse Practitioner sample survey: Focus on acute care. *Journal of the American Academy of Nurse Practitioners, 24*, 690–694.

Kleinpell, R. M., Hanson, N. A., & Buchner, B. R. (2008). Hospitalist services: An evolving opportunity. *Nurse Practitioner, 33*, 9–10.

Kleinpell, R. M., Hravnak, M., Werner, K., & Guzman, A. (2006). Skills taught in acute care NP programs: A national survey. *Nurse Practitioner, 31*, 7–13.

Kleinpell, R., Hudspeth, R., Scordo, K., & Magdic, K. (2012). Defining NP scope of practice and associated regulations: Focus on acute care. *Journal of the American Academy of Nurse Practitioners, 24*, 11–18.

Kleinpell, R. M. (2005). Acute care nurse practitioner practice: Results of a 5-year longitudinal study. *American Journal of Critical Care, 16*, 211–221.

Kleinpell, R. & Hravnak, M. (2005). Strategies for success in the acute care nurse practitioner role. *Critical Care Nursing Clinics of North America, 17*, 177–181.

Lambing, A. Y., Adams, D. L., Fox, D. H., & Divine, G. (2004). Nurse practitioners' and physicians' care activities and clinical outcomes with an inpatient geriatric population. *Journal of the American Academy of Nurse Practitioners, 8*, 343–352.

Landsperger, J. S., Williams, K. J., Hellervik, S. M., Chassan, C. B., Flemmons, L. N., Davidson, S. R., et al. (2011). Implementation of a medical intensive care unit acute-care nurse practitioner service. *Hospital Practice, 39*, 32–39.

Lundberg, S., Wali, S., Thomas, P., & Cope, D. (2006). Attaining resident duty hours compliance: The acute care nurse practitioner program at Olive View—UCLA Medical Center. *Academic Medicine, 81*, 1021–1025.

Magdic, K. S. (2006). Acute care billing: Shared visits. *Nurse Practitioner, 31*, 9–10.

Magdic, K. S., Hravnak, M., & McCartney, S. (2005). Credentialing for nurse practitioners: An update. *AACN Clinical Issues, 16*, 16–22.

Meyer, S. C. & Miers, L. J. (2005) Cardiovascular surgeon and acute care nurse practitioner: Collaboration on postoperative outcomes. *AACN Clinical Issues, 16*, 169–158.

Morse, K. J., Warshawsky, D., Moore, J. M., & Pecora, D. C. (2006). A new role for the ACNP: The rapid response team leader. *Critical Care Nursing Quarterly, 29*, 137–166.

Moote, M., Krsek, C., Kleinpell, R., & Todd, B. (2011). Physician assistant (PA) and nurse practitioner (NP) utilization in academic medical centers. *American Journal of Medical Quality, 5*, 1–9.

National Council of State Boards of Nursing (NCSBN). (2008). Consensus Model for APRN Regulation: Licensure, accreditation, certification and education (www.ncsbn.org/index.htm).

National Association of Pediatric Nurse Practitioners (NAPNAP). (2010). Position statement on the acute care nurse practitioner. (www.napnap.org).

National Organization of Nurse Practitioner Faculties (NONPF) (2012). *Criteria for evaluation of nurse practitioner programs.* Washington DC: Author.

National Organization of Nurse Practitioner Faculties (NONPF). (2011). *Integrating adult acute care skills and procedures into nurse practitioner curricula.* Washington DC: Author.

National Organization of Nurse Practitioner Faculties (NONPF). (2011). *Nurse practitioner core competencies.* Washington, DC: Author.

National Organization of Nurse Practitioner Faculties (NONPF). (2012). *Statement on acute care and primary care nurse practitioner practice.* Washington DC: Author.

National Panel for Acute Care Nurse Practitioner Competencies (2004). Washington, DC: National Organization of Nurse Practitioner Faculties.

National Panel for NP Practice Doctorate Competencies. (2006). *Practice doctorate nurse practitioner entry-level competencies.* Washington, DC: National Organization of Nurse Practitioner Faculties.

National Task Force on Quality Nurse Practitioner Education. (2012). *Criteria for evaluation of nurse practitioner programs.* Washington, DC: National Organization of Nurse Practitioner Faculties.

Newhouse, R. P., Stanik-Hutt, J., White, K. M., Johantgen, M., Bass, E. B., Zangaro, G., et al. (2011). Advanced practice nursing outcomes 1990–2008: A systematic review. *Nursing Economics, 29*, 230–250.

Norris, T. & Melby, V. (2006). The acute care nurse practitioner: Challenging existing boundaries of emergency nurses in the United Kingdom. *Journal of Clinical Nursing, 15*, 253–263.

Nyberg, S. M., Waswick, W., Wynn, T., & Keuter, K. (2007). Mid-level providers in a Level I trauma service: Experience at Wesley Medical Center. *Journal of Trauma, 63*, 128–134.

Pascual, J. L., Holena, D. N., Vella, M. A., Palmieri, J., Sicoutris, C., Selvan, B., et al. (2011). Short simulation training improves objective skills in established advanced practitioners managing emergencies in the ward and surgical intensive care. *Journal of Trauma, 71*, 330–338.

Pastores, S. M., O'Connor, M. F., Kleinpell, R. M., et al. (2011). The ACGME resident duty-hour new standards: History, changes, and impact on staffing of intensive care units. *Critical Care Medicine, 39*, 2540–2549.

Reuter-Rice, K. & Bolick, B. (2012). *Pediatric acute care: A guide for interprofessional practice.* Burlington MA: Jones & Bartlett.

Rosenthal, L. D. & Guerrasio J. (2009). The acute care nurse practitioner as hospitalist: Role description. *AACN Advanced Critical Care, 20*, 133–136.

Russell, D., Vorder Bruegge, M., & Burns, S. (2002). Effect of an outcomes managed approach to care of neuroscience patients by acute care nurse practitioners. *American Journal of Critical Care, 11*, 353–362.

Sample, G. A. & Dorman, T. (2011). *Coding and billing for critical care: A practice tool* (2nd ed.). Des Plains, IL: Society of Critical Care Medicine.

Scherer, Y. K., Bruce, S. A., Graves, G. T., & Erdley, W. S. (2003). Acute care nurse practitioner education: Enhancing performance through the use of clinical stimulation. *AACN Clinical Issues, 14*, 331–341.

Scherr, K., Wilson, D. M., Wagner, J., & Haughian, M. (2012). Evaluating a new rapid response team: NP-led versus intensivist-led comparisons. *AACN Advanced Critical Care, 23*, 32–42.

Schober, M. & Affara, F. (2006). *Advanced nursing practice.* Oxford: Wiley-Blackwell.

Shimabukuro, D. (2011). Acute care nurse practitioners in an academic multidisciplinary ICU. *ICU Director, 1*, 28–30.

Smolenski, M. C. (2005). Credentialing, certification, and competence: Issues for new and seasoned nurse practitioners. *Journal of the American Academy of Nurse Practitioners, 17*, 201–204.

Sonday, C. & Grecsek, E. (2010). Rapid response teams: NPs lead the way. *Nurse Practitioner, 35*, 40–46.

Sung, S. F., Huang, Y. C., Ong, C. T., Chen, Y. W. (2011). A parallel thrombolysis protocol with nurse practitioners as coordinators minimized door-to-needle time for acute ischemic stroke. *Stroke Research and Treatment, 2011*, 198518. doi:10.4061/2011/198518.

U.S. Department of Health and Human Services (HHS). (2011). Patient Protection and Affordable Care Act. (http://www.healthcare.gov/law/full/index.html).

Vachani, A., DeLong, P., & Manaker, S. (2003). Documentation and coding of critical care professional services. *Clinical Pulmonary Medicine, 10*, 85–92.

Yarema, T. C. & Judy, J. A. (2011). Participation of an acute care nurse practitioner group in a medical-surgical intensive care unit. *ICU Director, 1*, 25–27.

Yeager, S., Shaw, K. D., Casavant, J., & Burns, S. M. (2006). An acute care nurse practitioner model of care for neurosurgical patients. *Critical Care Nurse, 26*, 57–64.

Yeager, S. (2010). Detraumatizing nurse practitioner orientation. *Journal of Trauma Nursing, 17*, 85–101.

The Certified Nurse-Midwife*

Maureen A. Kelley • Jane Mashburn

CHAPTER CONTENTS

Since 2010, the attention of the world has been particularly focused on women and children's health through the platform of the U.N. Millennium Development Goal (MDG) and Global Strategy for Women's and Children's Health; its aim is to save the lives of 16 million women and children by 2015 (U.N. Millennium Development Goals Report, 2010). Midwifery has emerged as a key human resource to help achieve this goal. Internationally, three new reports, *Missing Midwives* (Save the Children, 2011), *State of the World's Midwifery: Delivering Health, Saving Lives* (U.N. Population Fund, 2011), and *Save Lives: Invest in Midwives* (Partnership for Maternal, Newborn and Child Health, 2011) have recommended increasing the number of midwives in the world as one of the best ways to reduce maternal and neonatal mortality. They call on the U.N. and world governments to invest in educating and retaining midwives. These important reports come at the same time as newly released International Confederation for Midwives (ICM) documents, which were

developed and/or updated to "strengthen midwifery worldwide in order to provide high-quality, evidence-based health services for women, newborn, and childbearing families" (ICM, 2013). Collectively, they are the culmination of 3 years of work by global expert task forces to update essential competencies for basic midwifery practice, education, regulation, and association strengthening. As a result, midwives from around the world have a standard against which they can evaluate their profession. The ICM's standards, linked with the three reports and outlining the urgent need for more and better prepared midwives, are a call to action and a blueprint for taking the agenda forward (see Chapter 6).

In the United States, the Institute of Medicine (IOM) released its report on *The Future of Nursing* (IOM, 2011), the impetus of which was the passage of the Patient Protection and Affordable Care Act (PPACA; see Chapter 22). It identified certified nurse-midwives (CNMs) as one of four types of advanced practice registered nurses and called on nurses and midwives to be full partners in redesigning health care in the United States. In a professionally related arena, Childbirth Connections, a national nonprofit organization dedicated to improving maternity care through consumer engagement and health system

*We wish to acknowledge Margaret W. Dorroh, Sheila F. Norton, and Cheryl Sarton for their important contributions to previous editions of this chapter of the textbook. Also, thanks to Michael McCann, ACNM board member, for his consultation.

transformation, sponsored the Transforming Maternity Care Partnership. There was active leadership and participation in this project by CNMs and the professional organization, the American College of Nurse-Midwives (ACNM). The project produced a report, *Blueprint for Action: Steps Toward a High-Quality, High-Value Maternity Care System* (Angood, Armstrong, Ashton, et al., 2010). Although complex, the blueprint called for expanding access to midwives and reducing barriers to midwifery practice, among other system-critical focus areas for improvement. The project has been experiencing exciting growth, and ACNM and Childbirth Connections are partners with the Centers for Medicare and Medicaid Services (CMS) in an initiative entitled *Strong Start,* designed to improve maternity care outcomes through evaluating new models of prenatal care, including group prenatal care, birth center care, and woman and family centered maternity care homes (CMS, 2012). Rima Jolivet, Program Director of the Transforming Maternity Care Symposium, described this as "a time of tremendous momentum ... a tipping point in maternity care quality improvement" (Jolivet, Corry, & Sakala, 2010, p. S52). Hopefully, these global and domestic initiatives will mobilize and intensify worldwide action aimed at transforming the care that is available to all women and children.

Because midwifery and nurse-midwifery in the United States and globally represents different levels of preparation and meaning, we begin by defining the terms internationally and within the U.S. context. The common denominator for all midwives is being with a woman during pregnancy and birth. The ICM definition of a midwife is "a person who has successfully completed a midwifery education program that is duly recognized in the country where it is located and that is based on ICM Essential Competencies and Global Standards for Education; who has acquired the requisite qualifications to be registered and/or legally licensed to practice midwifery and to use the title 'midwife,' and who demonstrates competency in the practice of midwifery" (ICM, 2011). In the United States, there are three groups of professionals who meet the ICM definition of a midwife. CNMs are individuals educated in the two disciplines of nursing and midwifery. "They earn a graduate degree, complete a midwifery education program accredited by the Accreditation Commission for Midwifery Education (ACME) and pass a national certification examination administered by the American Midwifery Certification Board (AMCB) to receive the professional designation CNM" (ACNM, 2012a). Certified midwives (CMs) are individuals educated in the discipline of midwifery. "They earn graduate degrees, meet health and science education requirements, and complete a midwifery education program accredited by ACME. They pass the same national certification examination as CNMs to receive the professional designation CM (ACNM, 2012a).

This direct entry route was developed by ACNM in the mid-1990s in an effort to assert and uphold an equivalent standard among midwives in education, certification, and practice (Fullerton, Schuiling, & Sipe, 2005). A certified professional midwife (CPM) is an individual who is a knowledgeable, skilled, and professional independent midwifery practitioner and who has met the standards of certification set by the North American Registry of Midwives (NARM) and is qualified to provide the midwifery model of care. A CPM is certified via an examination administered by NARM. In addition to CNMs, CMs, and CPMs, there are also direct entry midwives (DEMs), lay midwives (also known as granny midwives, traditional midwives, traditional birth attendants, empirical midwives, and independent midwives), and licensed midwives (Midwives Alliance of North America [MANA], 2012). Some of these practitioners are legally recognized, some have had formal training, and some have had apprenticeship training. In this chapter, we focus only on CNMs who, in 42 states, are practicing in an advanced practice nursing role (Osborne, 2011). We focus on CNMs who are practicing in an advanced nursing role. For the purposes of this text, the terms *midwife* and *CNM* may be used interchangeably and, when issues related to non-nurse midwives are addressed, an attempt is made to clarify that.

Nurse-midwifery in the United States has its roots in nursing and has made many contributions that have paved the way for advanced practice nursing to flourish. By 1970, ACNM had developed functions, qualifications, and midwifery standards of practice; within the next several years, they had also established criteria for the accreditation of midwifery education programs and a national certifying examination. Nurse-midwifery activities have been instrumental in securing prescriptive authority and direct reimbursement by insurers for CNMs. These activities have also had a favorable direct or indirect impact on all advanced practice nurses (APNs). The pioneering efforts of CNMs have helped cultivate a clinical and political climate of acceptance, not only for themselves but also for clinical nurse specialists (CNSs), certified registered nurse anesthetists (CRNAs), and nurse practitioners (NPs) as legitimate and visible providers of care across all settings. The purpose of this chapter is to describe nurse-midwifery practice in the United States so that the reader can appreciate why it can be seen as an advanced practice nursing role and why there are concerns within midwifery if it is seen only as an advanced practice nursing role. As authors, we offer our own perspectives on the issues that prevent full integration of nurse-midwifery into advanced practice nursing. Nurses and CNMs alike have a stake in issues related to this level of professional practice. The reflections presented in this chapter are meant to foster dialogue and understanding as nurses and CNMs work to accomplish their goals related to practice. It is our hope that professional nursing will continue to work productively and collaboratively in activities that promote advanced practice nursing.

Historical Perspective

Midwifery predates nursing and medicine. Throughout time, and in all cultures, the midwife has played an important and respected role. In Biblical times, the midwife assisted a woman in labor, helped birth the baby, and provided for aftercare of the mother and infant. Novice midwives acquired knowledge and skill by apprenticing with experienced midwives and through their own observations and experiences.

In colonial times, midwives were an integral part of community life and were highly respected members of society. In the early 1900s, a number of developments in the United States considerably diminished that respect and led to an ebb in the practice of midwifery. The immigrant population was served by European immigrant midwives and African American women from the South were cared for by traditional African American midwives. These midwives lacked a national organization, methods of communication, access to the health care system, and legal recognition (Burst, 2005). An active campaign to discredit midwives was waged by public health reformers and obstetricians seeking to develop their specialty, even though data demonstrated good care outcomes for these providers (Dawley, 2003). During this same time frame, physicians took over the role of birth attendant and birth moved into the hospital setting. The medicalization of birth did much to eliminate midwifery and continues to influence and regulate the practice of nurse-midwifery.

Although midwifery remained part of mainstream health care in many European, Asian, and African countries, the renaissance of midwifery in the United States did not occur until the 1940s and 1950s. Strong nursing leaders and the childbirth education movement largely shaped the reappearance of midwifery as a nursing role (Dawley, 2003). Like other forms of advanced practice nursing that emerged later, the resurgence of midwifery and the evolution of nurse-midwifery occurred in response to the need for care of the underserved. By the late 1960s, the contributions of nurse-midwives were accepted and recognized. Demand for nurse-midwifery services increased and the profession responded by opening more education programs and more midwifery practices (see Chapter 1).

The Nurse-Midwifery Profession in the United States Today

As of 2012, 12,025 nurse-midwives have been recognized as CNMs by the ACNM and AMCB, and 73 have been recognized as CMs (Smith, 2012). In addition, there are 6,500 active and student members of the ACNM (Hamilton, 2012). Of that number, approximately 6,200 are in clinical practice. In 2009, the most current year for which data are available, CNMs attended 313,516 births, which constituted 11.3% of all vaginal births in the United States (Declercq, 2012). Also, as of 2012, there were 39 ACNM-accredited nurse-midwifery graduate programs in the United States. Thirty-four are located in schools of nursing, one in a school of public health, three in allied health graduate programs, and one is a freestanding institution of higher education Although this is an evolving picture, currently five ACNM accredited programs offer Master of Science (MS) and Doctor of Nursing Practice (DNP) options, and an additional three offer the DNP only (ACNM, 2012e). Based on findings from an analysis of ACNM membership surveys from 2006 to 2008, 82% of CNMs and CMs hold master's degrees and 7% have doctorates.

Approximately 1.4% of CNMs and CMs indicated that they were male (Schuiling, Sipe, & Fullerton, 2010). Nurse-midwifery practice is legal in all 50 states and nurse-midwives have prescriptive authority in 50 states and the District of Columbia (ACNM, 2011e). As with all APRNs, prescriptive authority is regulated by individual state agencies and regulatory boards. As of 2012, 21 states, plus the District of Columbia, had no supervision or contractual agreement required for overall practice, seven states had requirements for prescriptive authority agreements only, and 15 states required various levels of contractual practice agreements for overall practice (ACNM, 2012f). CNMs are also defined as primary care providers under federal law (ACNM, 2012c).

Education and Accreditation

The ACNM established a national mechanism for the accreditation of nurse-midwifery education programs in 1962. Because the organization wanted to have its process subject to peer review and recognition, it applied to the U.S. Department of Education (DOE) for recognition as an accrediting agency. The Accreditation Commission for Midwifery Education (ACME) is the official accrediting body of ACNM and has been recognized by the DOE as a programmatic accrediting agency for certificate, postbaccalaureate, graduate degree, and precertification programs in nurse-midwifery and midwifery. ACME consists of four units, including the Board of Commissioners, Site

Visitor Panel, Board of Review (BOR), and Advisory Committee. The role of the Board of Commissioners is to formulate policy and develop the criteria used by the BOR. The Site Visitor Panel arranges, conducts, and evaluates accreditation visits to midwifery education programs. The BOR reviews the applicant's preaccreditation report or site visit report and determines accreditation status. The Advisory Committee is composed of members representing nursing, medicine, education, public health, and the public and serves to advise in the development of policy and evaluation of ACME. ACNM-accredited programs must receive preaccreditation status before enrolling students and, once the initial accreditation has been granted, the program must be reviewed at least every 10 years (ACNM, 2012I).

Even though the American Association of Colleges of Nursing recommended in 2004 that the DNP be the entry level for clinical practice, neither ACNM nor ACME agrees with that position. ACNM supports a minimum of a master's degree as basic preparation for midwifery practice, and notes inadequate evidence to support the DNP as the entry-level requirement for midwifery education. Midwifery education has always been more broadly based than nursing. Even at the master's level, degrees may be awarded from schools of nursing, midwifery, public health, or allied health. ACNM's Division of Education has developed recommendations for competencies for the practice doctorate in midwifery as one possible option for doctoral preparation for midwives (ACNM, 2011b). There currently is no ACNM or AMCB statement about mandatory doctoral preparation, although the ACNM supports and values the attainment of doctoral degrees for individual CNMs. A 2009 report on the educational level of APRNs found CNMs to have the highest proportion of doctoral degrees among the four advanced practice nursing roles. (Sipe, Fullerton, & Schuiling, 2009).

Certification and Certification Maintenance

A national certification examination for entry into practice was instituted in 1971. At that time, certification rested with the ACNM. In 1991, certification was separated from the professional organization. The AMCB was incorporated as a distinct organization, charged with developing and administering the examination for nurse-midwives and midwives. There are committees within the AMCB charged with keeping the examination content current and appropriate. The Examination Committee works closely with test consultants and annually reviews examination specifications and content outlines. The Research Committee conducts a survey of the face validity of the national certification examination known as the

Task Analysis of Midwifery Practice; the last one was conducted in 2011 (AMCB, 2011).

Certification is time-limited for all CNMs. Mechanisms for certification maintenance, administered by the Certification Maintenance Program (CMP), include completing three modules provided by AMCB plus 20 continuing education units approved by ACNM or the Accreditation Council for Continuing Medical Education (ACCME; AMCB, 2011).

Reentry to Practice

The ACNM has developed guidelines designed to provide a framework for CNMs who are not currently engaged in clinical practice and wish to reenter the practice field. These guidelines are based on how long the CNM has been out of practice—less than 2, 2 to 5, and longer than 5 years. The guidelines have clinical requirements including full-scope practice with a validated clinical preceptor. If the CNM has been out of clinical practice for more than 5 years, the clinical experiences must be precepted through an accredited nurse-midwifery education program. The program may use challenge mechanisms for didactic and/or clinical competency assessment. It is recommended that the needs of each reentering CNM be individually evaluated and a plan for reentry developed on a case by case basis. The ACNM website has a list of schools that offer such reentry programs. The guidelines also recommend checking with state licensing boards and employing institutions, because their requirements would supersede ACNM recommendations (ACNM, 2010b).

Regulation, Reimbursement, and Credentialing

CNMs are regulated on a state by state basis and there are numerous regulatory and reimbursement barriers at the local, state and federal levels regarding the full deployment of all APNs. These barriers are discussed in Chapter 21. Therefore, this chapter will highlight the regulatory, reimbursement, and credentialing considerations that may be distinct to nurse- midwifery. In regard to regulation, currently, CNMs are regulated by boards of nursing in 38 states and recognized as APRNs in 42 states. In the remaining eight states, CNMs are regulated by boards of medicine, health, commerce, and regents (Osborne, 2011).

The Consensus Model for APRN Regulation (APRN Consensus Work Group, 2008) was endorsed by ACNM, which also published recommendations regarding implementation of the Consensus Model specifically related to midwifery practice (ACNM, 2011c). The first recommendation strongly supports the foundational principle that APRNs be licensed as independent practitioners with no regulatory requirements for collaboration, direction, or supervision. The ACNM has given an official statement on independent nurse-midwifery practice (ACNM, 2012d, presented in Box 17-1). Also, the 2011 ACNM–American College of Obstetricians and Gynecologists (ACOG) report, *Joint Statement of Practice Relations Between Obstetricians and Gynecologists and Certified Nurse-Midwives/ Certified Midwives,* is seen as a model document that recognizes each group as licensed independent providers who may collaborate based on the needs of their patients (ACNM, 2011f; Box 17-2). ACNM advocates that nursing boards support separate boards of midwifery or boards of nurse-midwifery. They also recommend that the consensus document clarify that a graduate nursing degree is not required to take the certifying examination, which is an effort to support nurse-midwifery programs accredited and located in other non-nursing departments or separate institutions of higher learning (e.g., public health or allied health programs).

CNMs achieved equitable reimbursement for their services under Medicare, effective January 2011. Their reimbursement rate increased from 65% of the physician's fee to 100% of the Medicare Part B physician fee schedule. This long-awaited provision was part of the PPACA (see Chapter 22). CNMs have not yet been included in the wellness examination provision of the PPACA, but have been working to change this (ACNM, 2012g). Medicaid mandates reimbursement for nurse-midwives in all 50 states; the level of reimbursement ranges from 65% to 100% of physician reimbursement rates (ACNM, 2011e). Thirty-three states mandate private insurance reimbursement for nurse-midwife services and there is the same type of variability in the level of reimbursement as there is for Medicaid (Fulea, 2012).

The effect that this variation in state law and regulation has on nurse-midwifery practice was examined by Declercq and colleagues (1998). They found that when compared with states with low regulatory support for nurse-midwifery practice, states with high regulatory support had a nurse-midwifery workforce three times larger than that in other states, with three times the number of CNM-attended births and twice as many CNM-patient contacts. Similar variation has been observed for APNs, meaning that those states with high regulatory support have higher numbers of APNs, thus exacerbating the current maldistribution of providers (Lugo, O'Grady, Hodnicki, et al., 2007). Some states are regulated by midwifery boards only, but practices in those states are not necessarily more independent for CNMs. For example, Utah's separate midwifery board is more restrictive than New Mexico's regulatory board, which is governed by the Department of Health.

In addition to state regulation, hospitals and health plans have established credentialing requirements for

BOX 17-1 Independent Midwifery Practice

The following represents the position of the American College of Nurse-Midwives (ACNM):

- Midwifery practice is the independent management of women's health care, focusing particularly on common primary care issues, family planning and gynecologic needs of women, pregnancy, childbirth, the postpartum period, and care of the newborn.
- The practice occurs within a health care system that provides for consultation collaborative management and for referral, as indicated by the health status of the woman or newborn.
- Independent midwifery enables CNMs and CMs to use their knowledge, skills, judgment, and authority in the provision of primary health service for women while maintaining accountability for the management of health care in accordance with the ACNM *Standards for the Practice of Midwifery.*

Background

Independent practice is not defined by the place of employment, the employee-employer relationship, requirements for a physician's co-signature, or the method of reimbursement for services. Further, independent practice should not be interpreted to be alone, because there are clinical situations in which any prudent practitioner would seek the assistance of another qualified practitioner.

Collaboration is the process whereby health care professionals jointly manage care. The goal of collaboration is to share authority while providing quality care within each individual's professional scope of practice. Successful collaboration is a way of thinking—a relationship that requires knowledge, open communication, mutual respect, a commitment to providing quality care, trust, and the ability to share responsibility.

From the American College of Nurse-Midwives. (2012). *Position statement: Independent midwifery practice.* Silver Spring, MD: Author.

health care professionals. These credentialing standards determine who may have hospital admitting privileges be employed by health care systems, and be listed on managed care provider panels. An optimum system would create a mechanism consistent with the profession's standards, recognizing nurse-midwifery as distinct from other health care professions and recognizing processes that permit CNMs to build on entry-level competencies within their statutory scope of practice. Credentialing is a particularly thorny issue for CNMs, as revealed in a 2011 online survey

BOX 17-2   College Statement of Policy: Joint Statement of Practice Relations Between Obstetrician-Gynecologists, Certified Nurse-Midwives, and Certified Midwives

The American College of Obstetricians and Gynecologists (the College) and the American College of Nurse-Midwives (ACNM) affirm our shared goal of safe women's health care in the United States through the promotion of evidence-based models provided by obstetrician-gynecologists (OB-GYNs), CNMs, and CMs. The College and ACNM believe that health care is most effective when it occurs in a system that facilitates communication across care settings and among providers. OB-GYNs, CNMs, and CMs are experts in their respective fields of practice and are educated, trained, and licensed independent providers who may collaborate with each other based on the needs of their patients. Quality of care is enhanced by collegial relationships characterized by mutual respect and trust, as well as professional responsibility and accountability.

Recognizing the high level of responsibility that OB-GYNs, CNMs, and CMs assume when providing care to women, the College and ACNM affirm their commitment to promote the highest standards for education, national professional certification, and recertification of their respective members and to support

evidence-based practice. Accredited education and professional certification preceding licensure are essential to ensure skilled providers at all levels of care across the United States.

The College and ACNM recognize the importance of the options and preferences of women in their health care. OB-GYNs, CNMs, and CMs work in a variety of settings, including private practice, community health care facilities, clinics, hospital, and accredited birth centers. The College and ACNM hold different positions on home birth. Establishing sustaining viable practices that can provide broad services to women requires that OB-GYNs, CNMs, and CMs have access to affordable professional liability insurance coverage, hospital privileges, equivalent reimbursement from private payers and under government programs, and support services, including but not limited to laboratory testing, obstetric imaging, and anesthesia. To provide highest quality and seamless care, OB-GYNs, CNMs, and CMs should have access to a system of care that fosters collaboration among licensed, independent providers.

Adapted from the American College of Nurse-Midwives and American College of Obstetricians and Gynecologists. (2011). *Joint statement of practice relations between obstetrician-gynecologists and certified nurse-midwives/certified midwives.* Washington, DC: Authors.

conducted by ACNM. A total of 1893 responses were received; 80% of the CNM respondents stated that they did not have full voting privileges within the medical staffs of their local facilities, almost 50% reported that employment by a physician practice or the hospital was a requirement of privileging, and 65% stated that they had privileges to practice but limitations or supervisory restrictions on scope of practice (Cooney & Johnson, 2012).

The federal government, through CMS exerts a strong influence over hospitals through its conditions of participation (CoP). These are rules with which hospitals are required to comply to maintain eligibility to participate in Medicare and Medicaid programs. In 2012, CMS issued final revisions related to medical staff participation by clarifying that hospitals may grant privileges to physicians and nonphysicians and that regardless of whether they were granted medical privileges, practitioners in the institution are required to adhere to the bylaws and regulations of the institution. The CoP document urges hospitals to use "nonphysician providers" to help them care for the health of the public and requires that an application for credentialing be reviewed by the medical staff and governing body of the hospital. In all, these regulations send a strong signal about the use of CNMs and other APNs in

hospital settings, but fall short of requiring that CNMs be credentialed as members of the medical staff (Cooney & Johnson, 2012).

American College of Nurse-Midwives

During the 1940s, the National Organization of Public Health Nurses (NOPHN) established a section for nurse-midwives. During the reorganization of national nursing organizations, the NOPHN was absorbed into the American Nurses Association (ANA) and National League for Nursing (NLN), but these two organizations did not include a recognizable entity for nurse-midwives. Midwives at the 1954 ANA convention formed the Committee on Organization. This committee approved the definition of a nurse-midwife but the NLN and the ANA could not find a place for the nurse-midwives (for various reasons). Subsequently, at their May 1955 meeting, the Committee on Organization voted to form a separate nurse-midwifery organization—the ACNM (Dawley, 2005; Dawley & Burst, 2005; Varney, Kriebs, & Gegor, 2004).

The growth and development of American nurse-midwifery was fostered by the ACNM, founded in 1955 as the professional organization for certified

---

BOX 17-3   Philosophy of the American College of Nurse-Midwives

We, the midwives of the American College of Nurse-Midwives, affirm the power and strength of women and the importance of their health in the well-being of families, communities, and nations. We believe in the basic human rights of all persons, recognizing that women often incur an undue burden of risk when these rights are violated.

We believe that every person has a right to the following:

- Equitable, ethical, accessible quality health care that promotes healing and health
- Health care that respects human dignity, individuality, and diversity among groups
- Complete and accurate information to make informed health care decisions
- Self-determination and active participation in health care decisions
- Involvement of a woman's designated family members, to the extent desired, in all health care experiences

We believe that the best model of health care for a woman and her family does the following:

- Promotes a continuous and compassionate partnership
- Acknowledge a person's life experiences and knowledge

- Includes individualized methods of care and healing guided by the best evidence available
- Involves the therapeutic use of human presence and skillful communication

We honor the normalcy of women's lifecycle events. We believe in the following:

- Watchful waiting and nonintervention in normal processes
- Appropriate use of interventions and technology for current or potential health problems
- Consultation, collaboration, and referral with other members of the health care team as needed to provide optimal health care

We affirm that midwifery care incorporates these qualities and that women's health care needs are well-served through midwifery care.

Finally, we value formal education, lifelong individual learning, and the development and application of research to guide ethical and competent midwifery practice. These beliefs and values provide the foundation for commitment to individual and collective leadership at the community, state, national, and international levels to improve the health of women and their families worldwide.

Adapted from the American College of Nurse-Midwives. (2004). *Philosophy of the American College of Nurse-Midwives.* Silver Spring, MD: Author.

---

nurse-midwives. The mission of the ACNM is to promote the health and well-being of women and infants within their families and communities through the development and support of professional midwifery. The organization establishes clinical standards, creates liaisons with state and federal agencies and members of Congress, administers and promotes continuing education programs, supports midwifery-relevant research and practice, and supports the accreditation of education programs.

The ACNM philosophy (ACNM, 2004; Box 17-3), code of ethics (ACNM, 2008a; Box 17-4), and standards for practice of midwifery (2011d; Box 17-5) are the core documents that guide the profession and practitioner. ACNM has also seen the recent focus on nurse-midwifery as strategic to women and children's health globally, and maternity care nationally, as a mandate to examine and update their mission and values closely. Specifically, the 2012 vision for the organization is to advance the health and well-being of women and newborns by setting the standards for nurse-midwifery excellence. The mission that follows is to work to establish nurse-midwifery as the standard of care for women, leading the profession

through education, clinical practice, research, and advocacy (ACNM, 2012b). ACNM is also embarking on a public awareness campaign because a 2008 consumer survey revealed that only 11% of women indicated that they had used a midwife for reproductive health care and 48% said it "never occurred" to them to use a midwife for their reproductive health care. If the goal is to have nurse-midwifery be the standard of care for women in the United States, there needs to be substantial work with the public in that direction (ACNM, 2011a).

Implementing Advanced Practice Nursing Competencies

Overview of Advanced Practice Nurse and Certified Nurse-Midwife Competencies

Nurse-midwifery is constantly evolving and has a broader scope of practice now than it did 75 years ago. Nurse-midwifery has six core competencies similar to the APN competencies (see Chapter 3). As with the APN model in Chapter 3, the direct care role is integral to CNM practice

BOX 17-4 **American College of Nurse-Midwives: Code of Ethics**

CNMs and CMs have three ethical mandates in achieving the mission of midwifery to promote the health and well-being of women and newborns within their families and communities. The first mandate is directed toward the individual women and their families for whom the midwives provide care, the second mandate is to a broader audience for the public good for the benefit of all women and their families, and the third mandate is to the profession of midwifery to ensure its integrity, and in turn its ability, to fulfill the mission of midwifery.

Midwives in all aspects of professional relationships will do the following:

- Respect basic human rights and the dignity of all persons.
- Respect their own self-worth, dignity and professional integrity.

Midwives in all aspects of their professional practice will:

- Develop a partnership with the woman in which each shares relevant information that leads to informed decision making, consent to an evolving plan of care, and acceptance of responsibility for the outcome of their choices.
- Act without discrimination based on factors such as age, gender, race, ethnicity, and religion shared without bias, coercion, or deception.

- Provide an environment in which privacy is protected and in which all pertinent information is shared without bias, coercion, or deception.
- Maintain confidentiality, except where disclosure is mandated by law.
- Maintain the necessary knowledge, skills, and behaviors needed for competence.
- Protect women, their families, and colleagues from harmful, unethical, and incompetent practices by taking appropriate action that may include reporting as mandated by law.

Midwives as members of a profession will do the following:

- Promote, advocate for, and strive to protect the rights, health, and well-being of women, families, and communities.
- Promote just distribution of resources and equity in access to quality health care services.
- Promote and support the education of midwifery students and peers, standards of practice, research and policies that enhance the health of women, families, and communities.

Adapted from the American College of Nurse-Midwives. (2008). *Code of ethics. Silver Spring*, MD: Author.

and is well substantiated in both exemplars presented later in this chapter. Consistent with advanced practice nursing, nurse-midwives assume responsibility and accountability for their practice as primary health care providers (ACNM, 2012c). Patient-centered assessment and management are hallmarks of all aspects of CNM care. CNMs have, in common with all APNs, the characteristics of using a holistic, evidence-based perspective. CNMs use research methodologies and ethical decision making to support a caring, low-technology approach to childbirth. ACNM has well-defined position statements on consultation and collaboration in midwifery practice (ACNM, 1997a) that have helped inform APN practice (see Chapters 9 and 12). CNMs have demonstrated leadership in the development of free-standing birth centers, homelike facilities for low-risk women who desire a wellness model of pregnancy and birth. It is informative to take a closer look at the competencies related to advocacy and patient education to understand nurse-midwifery practice further. The ACNM-defined competencies in advocacy and patient education parallel the advanced practice core competencies of ethical

decision making, coaching, and guidance. CNMs enact the seven competencies of advanced practice nursing, as described in the following discussion.

Direct Clinical Practice

CNMs manifest a high level of expertise in the assessment, diagnosis, and treatment of women's life cycle events. They approach these events, such as puberty, pregnancy, birth, and menopause, as physiologic transitions that are best supported by education and midwifery expertise. Nurse-midwives form partnerships with the women that they care for, empowering them to be active participants in their own health care. Nurse-midwives incorporate scientific evidence into clinical practice, are familiar with complementary and alternative therapies, exercise expert clinical thinking and skillful performance, and demonstrate a holistic approach in the care they provide.

The ACNM recently updated its position statement on CNMs as primary care providers and leaders of maternity care homes. Primary care is included as a core competency

BOX 17-5   Standards for the Practice of Midwifery

Midwifery practices, as conducted by CNMs and CMs, is the independent management of women's health care, focusing particularly on pregnancy, childbirth, the postpartum period, care of the newborn, and the family planning and gynecologic needs of women. The CMN and CM practice within a health care system that provides for consultation, collaborative management, or referral, as indicated by the health status of the client. CNMs and CMs practice in accord with the *Standards of the Practice of Midwifery*, as defined by the ACNM.

Standard I

Midwifery care is provided by qualified practitioners. The midwife

- Is certified by the ACNM designated certifying agent.
- Shows evidence of continuing competency as required by the ACNM designate certifying agent.
- Is in compliance with the legal requirements of the jurisdiction in which the midwifery practice occurs.

Standard II

Midwifery care occurs in a safe environment within the context of the family, community, and a system of health care. The midwife

- Demonstrates knowledge of and uses federal and state regulations that apply to the practice environment and infection control.
- Demonstrates a safe mechanism for obtaining medical consultation, collaboration, and referral.
- Uses community services as needed.
- Demonstrates knowledge of the medical, psychosocial, economic, cultural, and family factors that affect care.
- Demonstrates appropriate techniques for emergency management, including arrangements for emergency transportation.
- Promotes involvement of support persons in the practice setting.

Standard III

Midwifery care supports individual rights and self-determination within boundaries of safety. The midwife

- Practices in accord with the philosophy and Code of Ethics of the ACNM
- Provides clients with a description of the scope of midwifery services and information regarding the client's rights and responsibilities.
- Provides clients with information regarding, and/or referral to, other providers and services when requested or when care required is not within the midwife's scope of practice.
- Provide clients with information regarding health care decisions and the state of the science regarding these choices to allow for informed decision making.

Standard IV

Midwifery care is comprised of knowledge, skills, and judgments that foster the delivery of safe, satisfying, and culturally competent care. The midwife

- Collects data, assesses clients, develops and implements an individualized plan of management, and evaluates outcome of care.
- Demonstrates the clinical skills and judgments described.

Standard V

Midwifery care is based on knowledge, skills, and judgments reflected in written practice guidelines and are used to guide the scope of midwifery care and services provided to clients. The midwife

- Maintains written documentation of the parameters of service for independent and collaborative midwifery management and transfer of care when needed.
- Has accessible resources to provide evidence-based clinical practice for each specialty area, which may include, but is not limited to, primary health care of women, care of the childbearing family, and newborn care.

Standard VI

Midwifery care is documented in a format that is accessible and complete. The midwife

- Uses records that facilitate communications of information to clients, consultants, and institutions.
- Provides prompt and complete documentation of evaluation, course of management, and outcome of care.
- Promotes a documentation system that provides for confidentiality and transmissibility of health records.
- Maintains confidentiality in verbal and written communications.

Standard VII

Midwifery care is evaluated according to an established program for quality management that includes a plan to identify and resolve problems. The midwife

BOX 17-5 **Standards for the Practice of Midwifery—*cont'd***

- Participates in a program of quality management for the evaluation of practice within the setting in which it occurs.
- Provides for a systematic collection of practice data as part of a program of quality management.
- Seeks consultation to review problems, including peer review of care.
- Acts to resolve identified problems.

Standard VIII

Midwifery practice may be expanded beyond the ACNM core competencies to incorporate new procedures that improve care for women and their families. The midwife

- Identifies the need for a new procedure taking into consideration consumer demand, standards for safe practice, and availability of other qualified personnel.
- Ensures that there are no institutional, state, or federal statues, regulations, or bylaws that

would constrain the midwife from incorporation of the procedure into practice.
- Demonstrates knowledge and competency, including the following:
   a. Knowledge of risks, benefits, and client selection criteria
   b. Process for acquisition of required skill
   c. Identification and management of complication
   d. Process to evaluate outcomes and maintain competency
- Identifies a mechanism for obtaining medical consultation, collaboration, and referral related to this procedure
- Maintains documentation of the process used to achieve the necessary knowledge, skills and ongoing competency of the expanded or new procedures.

Adapted from the American College of Nurse-Midwives (ACNM). (2011). *ACNM standards for the practice of midwifery.* Silver Spring, MD, Author.

for midwifery practice (ACNM, 2008b); it includes the provision of primary health care for women from the premenarchal through postmenopausal phases, as well as primary care for newborns. This care is provided on a continuous and comprehensive basis by establishing a plan of management with the woman. The maternity care home is a recently developed concept to address women-centered care before, during, and after pregnancy. It is patterned after the patient-centered medical home (see Chapter 15) and aims to reduce the frequency of preterm births in pregnant Medicaid beneficiaries. The approach that will be tested is to expand access to care, improve care coordination, and provide a broader array of health services. ACNM regards midwives as well positioned to lead patient-centered maternity care teams (ACNM, 2012c).

Guidance and Coaching of Patients, Families, and Other Care Providers

Guidance and coaching are APN functions that assist patients through life transitions such as illness, childbearing, and bereavement (see Chapter 8). Nurse-midwives offer skillful communication, guidance, and counseling throughout the nurse-midwifery management process (ACNM, 2008b). Client education is a cornerstone of nurse-midwifery practice. Evidence that nurse-midwives invest time in patient education is supported by Paine (2000), who has reported that nurse-midwives spend

more time during office visits providing patient education and counseling than spent by physicians. For example, when a nurse-midwife counsels a pregnant woman regarding fetal testing, she not only educates the patient about how the test is done but also advises the woman as to what the results might indicate, what further testing would then be offered, and what decisions the woman and her partner may need to make, and offers to provide additional coaching as the process unfolds. In the instance of the quadruple screen, a blood test offered between 15 and 19 weeks' gestation, the woman would learn that it is a blood test conducted on the mother that screens for certain developmental and chromosomal conditions, such as spina bifida or Down syndrome in the fetus. She is informed that it is not diagnostic and that a positive screen means that there is increased risk for the problem, not that the fetus has the problem. A positive result would lead to further decision making on whether to have further testing, such as an amniocentesis or high-level ultrasound. The procedures, risks, and benefits of these tests would then be explained. If the woman opts for further testing and the results indicate a complication, she would then need to decide whether to continue or terminate the pregnancy. This level of guidance requires time, expertise, skill, and commitment.

As noted in Chapter 8, guidance is an interaction between an expert (the nurse-midwife) and the learner (the patient) that enables the learner to develop knowledge and skills within an area of the coach's expertise. Nurse-midwives are expected to apply their knowledge to guide women with regard to pregnancy transitions, birth, breast-feeding, grief and loss, parenthood, changes in family constellation, family planning, and women's health-related issues.

Consultation

Consultation is discussed in detail in Chapter 9. Nurse-midwives use consultation in their practice, both as the consultant and as the consultee. Patients consult with CNMs regarding health care and health promotion. For example, a patient may see a nurse-midwife regarding the desire to quit smoking. She wants to know what is available to help her be successful. The nurse-midwife would then discuss her options, help assess her readiness for change, determine a quit date, and develop strategies to overcome obstacles. Nurse-midwives often provide consultation in the hospital setting. During a labor and birth, nurses and nurse-midwives may consult each other regarding the interpretation of a fetal monitor tracing. Nurse-midwives serve on hospital quality improvement committees, where they can advocate for evidence-based policies and patient-centered care. Physicians often consult nurse-midwives regarding complementary therapies, breast-feeding, and/or alternative birthing options.

Nurse-midwives also consult other professionals. There are many cases in which a nurse-midwife would make use of another's expertise to provide the best care for his or her patients. For example, a CNM caring for a pregnant woman with a low platelet count might consult with the midwife's collaborating physician or a hematologist to decide on the appropriate care and provider for this woman and her fetus. Nurse-midwives frequently consult with lactation consultants to assist women who are having breast-feeding difficulties or with physical therapists to advise on mobility and discomfort problems. Nutritionists, psychologists, chiropractors, acupuncturists, endocrinologists, and cardiologists are other health care providers who may be part of the health care team of an individual pregnant woman.

Collaboration

The ACNM has a series of position statement on collaboration. In the 1997 statement, there is a focus on midwifery management as independent, primarily intended for healthy women; however, in the event of complications, collaborative management or referral to a physician may be an appropriate pathway to ensure a patient's well-being (ACNM, 1997). In the second statement (ACNM, 2011f), the *Joint Statement of Practice*

Relations between Obstetrician-Gynecologists and Certified Nurse-Midwives/Certified Midwives (see Box 17-2), there is shared agreement on high standards of education, certification, and accreditation, mutual support for ensuring that both professions have access to affordable professional liability insurance coverage, hospital privileges, and equivalent reimbursement from private payers, and support services for their work. There is also agreement that these provider groups have access to a system of care that fosters collaboration among licensed independent providers. The 2011 statement also recognized the need for nurse-midwives and physicians to collaborate but stressed the working relationship, respect for each other's abilities and knowledge, and professional responsibility and accountability. A clarifying position statement regarding collaborative agreements has been added to the continuing attempt to delineate the nature of collaboration between physicians and CNMs. This document noted the limitations of collaborative agreements—they do not guarantee effective communication, may wrongly imply that CNMs need supervision, and also may restrict midwives from exercising their full scope of practice (ACNM, 2011f; Box 17-6).

When a complication occurs, the nurse-midwife can continue to be instrumental in the woman's care while benefiting from collaboration with an obstetrician-gynecologist (OB-GYN). This involves the nurse-midwife and physician jointly managing the care of a woman whose case has become medically, gynecologically, or obstetrically complicated. The collaborating physician and nurse-midwife mutually agree on the scope of care that each will provide. If the physician needs to assume the main role in the woman's care, the nurse-midwife will still participate to some degree in the physical care and emotional support and, to a large degree, in counseling, guidance, and teaching. For example, a nurse-midwife caring for a pregnant woman identifies that inadequate fetal growth may be an issue. The nurse-midwife then consults with the collaborating physician and, together, they decide on what further testing and care are required under these circumstances. In this case, the testing does show inadequate growth; therefore, the woman will alternate her prenatal visits between the physician and nurse-midwife so that together they can provide frequent fetal surveillance and the best possible outcome for mother and baby. Effective communication is essential in ongoing collaborative management to maintain an effective working relationship and provide comprehensive care to the individuals under the collaborators' care.

In addition to OB-GYNs, nurse-midwives collaborate with other providers. During labor, nurse-midwives often collaborate with a doula (labor support provider) to provide the laboring woman with the best birth

BOX 17-6 **Position Statement: Collaborative Agreement Between Physicians and Certified Nurse-Midwives and Certified Midwives**

It is the position of the American College of Nurse Midwives (ACNM) that safe, quality health care can best be provided to women and their infants when policymakers develop laws and regulations that permit CNMs and CNs to provide independent midwifery care within their scope of practice while fostering consultation, collaborative management, or seamless referral and transfer of care, when indicated. ACNM affirms the following:

- Requirements for a signed collaborative agreement do not guarantee the effective communication between midwives and physicians that is so critical to successful collaboration:
  - They do not ensure physician availability when needed.
  - There is no evidence that they increase the safety or quality of patient care.
  - In certain circumstances, such as the aftermath of a natural or declared disaster, such requirements have hampered the ability of CNMs and CMs to provide critically necessary emergency relief services.
- Collaborative agreements signed by individual physicians wrongly imply that CNMs and CMs need the supervision of those individuals in all situations. Based on this misconception:

- Professional liability companies have used signed agreements, with their implied requirements for supervision, as the rationale for raising physician premiums, citing increased risk related to such unneeded supervision.
- CNMs and CMs may be restricted from exercising their full scope of practice or from receiving hospital credentials, clinical privileges, or third-party reimbursement for services that fall within the scope of their training and licensure.
- Requirements for signed collaborative agreements can create an unfair economic disadvantage for CNMs and CMs:
  - They have been used to limit the number of midwives who can practice collaboratively with any one physician, effectively barring CNMs and CMs from practice in some cases or restricting the ratio of CNMs and CMs to physicians
  - They allow potential economic competitors to dictate whether or not midwives can practice in a community
  - They restrict access to care and choice or provider for women. This is of particular concern in underserved areas.

Adapted from the American College of Nurse-Midwives. (2011e). Position statement: Collaborative agreement between physicians and certified nurse-midwives and certified midwives. Silver Spring, MD; and American College of Nurse-Midwives. (2004). Philosophy of the American College of Nurse-Midwives. Silver Spring, MD: Author.

experience possible and to meet the goals of her individual birth plan. Nurse-midwives collaborate with nurses and maternity unit managers to develop nursing policies on the optimal care for the pregnant woman and her fetus during the intrapartum and postpartum periods. Nurse-midwives collaborate with other nurse-midwives, labor and delivery nurses, and physician colleagues to develop practice standards and guidelines. These are just a few examples of the myriad ways in which nurse-midwives collaborate in delivering evidence-based practice.

Evidence-Based Practice

Since the early days of the United States, midwives have contributed to knowledge regarding women and infants. Martha Ballard's diary from 1785 to 1812 detailed the care that she gave to women and their families in her rural community; it demonstrated skills, knowledge, outcomes, and political forces that began to control the practice of nurse-midwifery by physicians (Ulrich, 1990). The CNM

evidence-base has grown significantly since Martha Ballard's time.

As an example, Beck has conducted extensive qualitative and quantitative research on postpartum depression (Beck & Gable, 2000, 2001). She then took this understanding and applied it to post-traumatic stress in new mothers and stress on labor room nurses (Beck, Gable, Sakala, 2011; Beck & Gable, 2012). Kennedy is another wonderful example of a CNM researcher who has focused her work on important topics to CNM practice, such as normalizing birth (Kennedy, 2010; Kennedy, Grant, Walton, et al., 2010), group prenatal care (Kennedy, Farrell, Paden, et al., 2009, 2011; Novick, Sadler, Kennedy, et al., 2011; Novick, Sadler, Knafl, et al., 2012), and perinatal safety (Lyndon & Kennedy, 2010).

In addition to distinguished individual midwifery researchers, research is incorporated as a core competency of the ACNM foundation documents. Nurse-midwives are charged with infusing scientific evidence into clinical practice to evaluate, apply, interpret, and collaborate in research (ACNM, 2008b). The ACNM recognizes the importance of building and translating evidence into CNM practice. One of the missions of the ACNM Division of Research (DOR) has been to contribute to knowledge about the health of women, infants, and families and advance the practice of midwifery. The DOR promotes the development, conduction, dissemination, and translation of midwifery research into practice (ACNM, 2010a). The ACNM, through the DOR, has been developing a research agenda that makes a positive difference to women and the midwifery profession (Kennedy, Schuiling, & Murphy, 2007). This agenda promotes research that focuses on policy, evidence-based practice, education, collaboration, visibility and message, and organizational and leadership development (Kennedy, Schuiling, & Murphy, 2007). Nurse-midwifery has its own journal, the *Journal of Midwifery & Women's Health,* a peer-reviewed, clinically focused publication that publishes research pertinent to pregnancy, well-woman gynecology, family planning, primary care of women, and health care policies.

Leadership

Leadership skills are professional responsibilities that are core competencies for nurse-midwives. Not only are nurse-midwives knowledgeable regarding national and international issues and trends in women's health and maternal-infant care, but also they are expected to be leaders in bringing those issues to the forefront. Nurse-midwives are expected to exercise leadership for the benefit of women, infants, and families, the profession of midwifery, and the ACNM. To this end, ACNM has state- and federal-level resource centers aimed at advocacy for issues related to women and children's health, as well as for tracking professional and interprofessional issues. Federal advocacy includes participating in the Coalition for Quality Maternity Care, which endorses legislative initiatives and strengthens outreach to the grassroots level. It also includes work at the federal level to support women's reproductive rights by urging legislators to reject funding cuts that limit access and information to reproductive choice. State advocacy works to enhance the ability of CNMs to function as independent practitioners and has worked to eliminate state requirements for written practice agreements (ACNM, 2011a). ACNM has deepened its leadership and advocacy by representation in external organizations. In 2011, 60 CNMs were ACNM representatives in external organizations, including key partnerships with the ANA, ACOG, ICM, MANA, Childbirth Connections, and the Workgroup on Patient Access to APRN Care and Practice (ACNM, 2011a).

Ethical Decision Making

"The goal of midwifery practice is to promote the health and well-being of women and childbearing families, wherever they reside, raising cultural, value, and ethical concerns that need to be respected and understood before making a final decision on a plan of care or action in the political arena" (Ament, 2007, pp. 280-281). The goal of ethical midwifery practice is to do the right thing for the right reason.

Codes of ethics guide moral behavior and are considered to be part of the criteria that make a practice a profession (Thompson, 2002). The latest edition of the *Code of Ethics* approved by the ACNM Board in 2005 has three mandates (see Box 17-4). The first is directed toward the individual woman and her family. The second is for the benefit of all women and their families. The third is to the profession of midwifery. These mandates are reflected in the core competencies for basic midwifery practice, philosophy of the ACNM (see Box 17-3), and standards for the practice of midwifery (Box 17-5).

Nurse-midwives are faced with ethical decisions in their daily practice, especially in regard to technology, informed consent, and health as a basic right for all (Ament, 2007). Whether and when to use electronic fetal monitoring is an excellent example. It has become a standard of care to monitor the fetal heart rate (FHR) in labor by electronic fetal monitoring. Most places of birth (mainly hospitals) have protocols and guidelines concerning this practice. Many nurse-midwives care for women in hospital settings in which there is are implied and explicit expectations to use routine fetal heart rate monitoring, even though the monitor may be intrusive to the woman and not part of her birth plan. In addition, there is no supporting evidence that electronic FHR monitoring with low-risk women improves outcomes. It is well known that overuse of the fetal monitor has increased the cesarean section rate without improving the health and well-being of mothers or infants (Ament, 2007). Currently, no informed consent accompanies the use of fetal monitoring that addresses any of these issues.

Traditional biomedical ethics developed after the atrocities of World War II. Biomedical ethics is a discipline focused on moral philosophy, normative theory, abstract universal principles, and objective problem solving in dilemmas (Thompson JB, 2002). The medicalization of health care has directed the education and practice of nursing and midwifery and bioethics has guided their codes of ethics. The essence of ethical midwifery practice occurs through human engagement, relationships, and the equilibrium of power within those relationships. In addition, It has been proposed that the ethics of engagement fosters ethical midwifery practice by encouraging practitioners to focus on being with women through human engagement (Thompson FE, 2003).

Advocacy

Client advocacy, as described in the APN model, is a competency that is central to nurse-midwifery practice. Client education and support of clients' rights and self-determination inform every aspect of nurse-midwifery care. These values have been challenged by the burgeoning growth of medical technology over the past 2 decades and the incursion of managed care in the 1990s. The availability of highly technical interventions for many aspects of childbearing—such as infertility, monitoring pregnancies and birth—conflicts with the traditionally low-tech, low-interventionist approach of nurse-midwives. However, by becoming part of key national movements, such as the Transforming Maternity Care Partnership (see earlier) and the Coalition for Quality Maternity Care (national organizations working together to champion federal legislative approaches for improving U.S. maternal and newborn health care), CNMs leverage their ability to ensure that the care being provided to women is woman-centered and evidence-based (ACNM, 2011a). As new structures for care delivery are developed via the PPACA, such as health exchanges and accountable care organizations, it will be crucial for CNMs to be involved in the governance of these entities.

Current Practice of Nurse-Midwifery

Scope of Practice

Nurse-midwifery practice encompasses a full range of primary health care services for women, from adolescence beyond menopause. These services include the independent provision of primary care, gynecologic and family planning services, preconception care, pregnancy care, childbirth and the postpartum period, care of the normal newborn during the first 28 days of life, and treatment of male partners for sexually transmitted infections. CNMs provide initial and ongoing comprehensive assessment, diagnosis, and treatment. They conduct physical examinations, prescribe medications, including controlled substances and contraceptive methods, admit, manage, and discharge patients from birth centers or hospitals, order and interpret laboratory and diagnostic tests, and order the use of medical devices. CNMs' care also includes health promotion, disease prevention, and individualized wellness education and counseling. CNMs must demonstrate that they meet the core competencies for basic midwifery practice of the ACNM (ACNM, 2008b) and must practice in accordance with the ACNM standards for the

practice of midwifery (ACNM, 2011d). With constant changes in health care, CNMs may need to expand their knowledge and skills beyond that of basic CNM practice. Advanced CNM skills, such as level 1 ultrasound or acting as first assistant in surgery, may be incorporated into a CNM's practice as long as the CNM follows the recommendations for acquiring these skills by obtaining formal didactic and clinical training to ensure that the advanced skill is acquired and monitored to ensure patient safety. These steps are outlined in standard VIII of the ACNM standards for practice (ACNM, 2011d; see Box 17-5).

Practice Settings

There are many different settings in which a CNM may practice. A CNM may engage in full-scope practice, which can include care of women from adolescence though the postmenopausal period. She or he may also choose one segment of practice—for example, ambulatory care or hospital care—or work exclusively with a population of interest, such as HIV-positive women or young adolescents. Nurse-midwives practice in urban, suburban, and rural areas. Their practice settings can include private practice (nurse-midwife–owned or physician-owned), hospitals, free-standing birth centers, clinics, or homes. Nurse-midwifery practice can be part of a group practice, with any combination of physicians, nurse-practitioners, physician assistants, or other health care providers, or solo practice. The nurse-midwife's actual practice depends on the needs of the population being served, willingness to undertake a variety of functions or roles, particular requests of patients, availability of physicians and nurse-midwife colleagues for backup and coverage and, finally, personal and philosophical beliefs of the individual midwife (Ament, 2007).

A nurse-midwife–assisted birth can take place in homes, free-standing birth centers, birth centers in hospitals, or traditional hospital settings (community, regional, or tertiary). For nurse-midwives and the women for whom they provide care, the choice of setting may be a matter of philosophy, comfort, convenience, or degree of medical risk, or a combination of these factors. Each setting has unique advantages and disadvantages.

Home births are very family-centered. Risks of iatrogenic and nosocomial infections are minimized. After the birth, the woman can rest or sleep in her own bed, nurse her infant at will, and enjoy the attention and support of her family and friends. A study by Hutton and coworkers (2009) documented the outcomes associated with planned home and planned hospital births in low-risk women attended by midwives in Ontario Canada. The rate of perinatal and neonatal mortality was very low for both groups (0.1%), and no between-group differences in morbidity or mortality were noted. Access to emergency transfer is critical to safe care and good outcomes, as is an integrated maternity care system with excellent communication among providers (Home Birth Consensus Summit, 2011). Analgesia and regional anesthesia are not available in the home setting.

The free-standing birth center has a homelike environment, with some select emergency equipment. Most birth centers do not use analgesics or narcotics. Local anesthesia may be used for perineal repair. Disadvantages are similar to those of a home birth in that emergency transport to a hospital may be necessary if the mother or baby develops complications during labor or birth. Most families are discharged within 6 to 12 hours of birth.

Current U.S. hospital units for labor and birth tend to be dual-purpose rooms; women labor and give birth in the same room, and almost all rooms are private. The room has a rocking chair, pull-out couch, and private bath, with a tub or shower. Although individual and nicely appointed, these rooms are part of the larger medical environment, with fetal monitoring, operating rooms, anesthesia services, and immediate access to neonatal intensive care. The support people available (nurses, physicians) may not hold the same philosophy of birth as a midwife. Even for a low-risk woman, there is more of a tendency to intervene than support a normal physiologic birth. There is a production pressure to keep things moving and a reliance on technology that is palpable in a busy obstetric unit. The traditional hospital labor, delivery, and maternity units are designed to care for several women at a time, making the units easier for staff to function but not necessarily conducive to the normal labor process. These units are well suited for high-risk women and infants who need special care nurseries. However, midwife-attended births in the United States currently occur mostly in a hospital environment. Therefore, it is incumbent on the midwife to help create an atmosphere of normalcy and trust in the midst of a culture of technology.

Certified Nurse-Midwife Practice Summary

Nurse-midwifery care has a unique aspect of continuity as currently practiced in the United States. Nurse-midwives see a designated caseload of pregnant women, attend these women during labor and birth, see them in the postnatal period, and can then become interconceptional or gynecologic care providers for these same women over their life span. Not all U.S. or international practice models function using this form of continuity, but it has been embraced in the United States by women and midwives and is similar to the obstetric model of care. Nurse-midwives, through care provided, scope of practice, management processes, and practice settings, have many opportunities to influence women's health care. Nurse-midwifery care is woman-focused, independent, and collaborative. It offers a woman the opportunity to obtain accessible, understandable, high-quality care that is safe, satisfying, and individualized to her and her family's needs throughout her life and during her reproductive years,.

Exemplars of Nurse-Midwifery Practice

The daily practice of midwifery is similar in all settings. In this section, one of the authors in an earlier edition of this text (Margaret W. Dorroh) describes the practice she established in an autonomous nurse-midwife–owned freestanding birthing center (Exemplar 17-1). Another exemplar is of a regional midwifery practice located in a hospital that serves 17 counties in rural Georgia (Exemplar 17-2). These exemplars illustrate how the components of nurse-midwifery care are enacted in different settings.

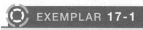 **EXEMPLAR 17-1**   **Nurse-Midwifery Practice in a Birth Center Setting**

The patient education process begins before a patient is accepted into the practice. Orientation sessions are held to provide prospective patients with information to assist them in determining whether they want to have their baby in a birth center. These sessions, conducted by the CNM, are designed to provide information and a tour of the facility. Prospective patients can see firsthand the comfort measures (e.g., the whirlpool tub) and equipment to handle normal deliveries and emergencies. Finances are discussed, because the cost of care in the birth center is approximately half of that for obstetric care in a hospital setting with a physician. Many insurers, Medicaid, and Medicare provide reimbursement.

In an autonomous setting such as this, clinical documentation must be meticulous and an individualized health record ensures that accurate, consistent, and complete information is obtained. Thorough health and family histories are taken, including information about the woman's physical health and her psychological well-being:

- What type of support system does she have in place?
- What resources might she have that are not currently being called on?
- Was the pregnancy planned or a surprise?
- What are her family circumstances?

- Is there a stable relationship?
- Are there other children?

It is important to document positive and negative influences that can have an impact on the patient's health and health of her baby. Once the assessment is complete, risk factors that would prevent us from being able to accept a patient are reviewed; if we cannot accept a patient, we make a referral. If no risk factors are identified, we schedule the patient's first visit.

When patients are accepted into the practice, they are told that they are equal partners in their care. It is the goal of patient education to make this a reality. To be active participants in their care, patients are taught to weigh themselves and do their own urine dipstick tests. They participate in charting the information, thus noting the progress of their pregnancy firsthand. The program of care for pregnant patients at our birth center includes 10 to 15 prenatal visits, childbirth classes, labor and delivery in the birth center, a home visit within 72 hours of birth, and two office follow-up visits for mother and baby, one at 1 week and the other at 6 weeks after birth.

Clinical hours are held daily. The CNMs in the practice share in office visits, teaching classes, and on-call time. Other responsibilities include administration and facility maintenance. We see pregnant patients, postpartum patients with their babies, and gynecologic patients. The amount of time scheduled for a visit is based on need. A first visit for a pregnant patient is 1 hour long. An established gynecologic patient who is coming for her contraceptive medication requires only a few minutes, long enough to establish that she is having no problems.

When a patient is in active labor or her membranes have ruptured, she calls the CNM on duty. She is met at the birth center and examined. Usually, when the woman arrives, she is in active labor. We attribute this largely to the educational process that has taken place. On the rare occasion of false labor or very early labor, we are able to individualize care. If a patient lives far away, we may elect to observe progress for a number of hours. If the woman is sleep-deprived, she and her labor may benefit from some sedation. We remain with our patients in the birth center during labor. An RN is on call for every delivery. If the CNM attending the patient is tiring from having been up for a long labor, or several labors, the RN can be called to come in early to care for the patient while the CNM rests. Sometimes, the RN is not needed until close to time for the birth.

The mother to be helps us accommodate her wishes by preparing a birth plan. As her due date nears, one of her tasks (along with packing a bag to bring to the birth center and readying her home for a baby) is to write a birth plan, which will become part of her record. This allows her to tell us who she wants with her during labor, what she imagines labor will be like, what she hopes labor will be like, and what comfort measures would assist her during labor. We use this tool in several ways. We evaluate the effectiveness of our teaching by reading what the woman thinks labor will be like. Mention of fears not previously revealed gives us an opportunity to resolve any emotional factors that could hinder a successful labor. Knowing the person(s) that the patient wants with her during labor informs us about her support system. The people present during labor are an important factor in enhancing the woman's experience of labor.

The list of comfort measures is mainly a reminder to us, although it is a key contribution from the patient. In the midst of labor, a woman may forget that she was looking forward to the whirlpool tub for relaxation and pain relief. A glance at the birth plan helps us try the things that the patient has already identified as being potentially helpful to her. The birth plan helps emphasize to the patient that this is her labor, with its inherent responsibilities and rights. Her dignity and worth as a human being are of high priority, as are the well-being of mother and baby. We try to nourish the woman's self-esteem and strengths that help in labor, life, and motherhood. The stronger the woman is in every way, the better will be the outcome.

Patients are given ample written material to help with their recall of information covered in classes. (If a patient is unable to read, extra time is spent providing information verbally and making sure that the patient understands it.) To help the patient assume responsibility for herself and her labor, she is expected to bring food and beverages with her to the birth center that she would like to have available during labor and certain supplies, such as perineal pads, bed pads, and diapers. Patients take their babies home dressed in their own clothes and wrapped in their own blankets. They take with them an instructional booklet that they were given in the postpartum class. The booklet describes mother and baby care for the first few days in detail. Because mothers and babies are discharged early, often in 4 to 6 hours, it is imperative that the mother be prepared to check the baby's temperature and respirations, check her own uterus, and be able to recognize signs of complications that require attention. These are all enumerated in the instructions, and there is room for notes and questions.

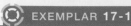

EXEMPLAR 17-1   Nurse-Midwifery Practice in a Birth Center Setting—*cont'd*

Having a reference helps new moms feel more secure. If something needs attention, they can always call the nurse-midwife, but they usually find what they need to know in the booklet. It often confirms what they sensed—that everything was okay or that they need to get in touch with the nurse-midwife. Thus, new mothers start out having faith in their own perceptions regarding their infants reinforced.

Empowering our patients, enhancing their decision making abilities, reinforcing the mind-body connection, and enhancing family life by helping women find their personal power are goals of CNM care at the birth center. When I think of the enormous effects of empowerment, two new moms come to mind.

ML's case is positive proof of the benefits of teaching new mothers to trust their feelings and make decisions based on them. On the third or fourth day after delivery, ML's baby ceased nursing well. He had been nursing vigorously and now was not. Nursing poorly is one of the signs listed in our booklet that requires professional help. ML insisted to her husband that they had to go to the emergency room immediately. They lived a long distance from the birth center and it had been decided earlier that if there should be a problem that seemed serious, she should go to a nearby emergency room rather than try to get to the CNM. Initially, doctors could find nothing wrong, but ML insisted they keep looking. As it turned out, the baby had a congenital heart defect that does not show up on a clinical examination until 3 or 4 days after birth. ML said she was glad she had been given the information at the birth center; it gave her the confidence to trust her feelings that something was seriously wrong. The baby had heart surgery and is doing well.

A woman with confidence and trust in herself can do almost anything, as shown by the case of SJ. SJ was 26 years old and came to the birth center soon after it opened to have her fourth child. She had a high school education and was home with her children, all of whom were younger than 5 years. Her self-esteem was negligible. Her husband came to a few of the prenatal classes but was sullen and unsupportive. SJ seemed to droop, but she was an excellent mother and was an attentive and fast learner regarding everything to do with childbirth, child rearing, and health in general. Her interest and enthusiasm grew as we reinforced her abilities and strengths. By the time she gave birth to her son, she seemed a different person from the withdrawn, self-effacing young woman we had met 7 months earlier. Two years after this baby's birth, SJ visited the birth center. "I just wanted to thank you," she said. "Before I came here, I never felt I was any good at anything. You told me I was a good mother, you noticed how well cared for my children were, and you encouraged me to learn all about birth and even let me borrow books and tapes. Well, I learned I was good—at a lot of things! You all showed me that. And I wanted you to know I'm in nursing school now because I want to be able to do what you do—not just take care of people physically, but help people grow."

EXEMPLAR 17-2   Nurse-Midwifery Practice in a Rural Regional Hospital Setting

In 1976, a southeastern rural regional hospital initiated a nurse-midwifery practice that was sponsored and supported by the hospital, which is still the case. The purpose of the practice was to care for the underserved women in the county in which the hospital was located, as well as the surrounding area. Thus, the practice has always focused on a public health orientation to the care that is being delivered. The practice began with two CNMs and has grown gradually over the years to eight CNMs, one of whom is the director. The practice also has two physicians who work with the midwives and see high-risk women or those who become high risk during pregnancy or labor. Currently, the midwifery practice is attending 700 births per year, and that number is expected to grow.

The nurse-midwives who initiated the practice were committed to a midwifery model of care for these vulnerable women and have successfully maintained that model for over 36 years. For prenatal care, much time is spent in education and ensuring that women have the resources they need to proceed successfully with their pregnancy—women, infants and children (WIC) and social services are part of the array of services available to these women. In the past 8 years, the Centering Pregnancy model has been one of the options offered for prenatal care (see later). For intrapartum care, individuals in the practice believe in a low-intervention privacy, mobility during labor, and position of comfort during birth. The practice has recently begun seeing pregnant women in two outlying counties, where prenatal care is not available due to lack of providers. This outreach has been successful; midwives are now seeing 50 women a month in each office and the numbers are growing. The second clinic serves Hispanic women and has a bilingual CNM delivering care there. Similar to the birth center, the midwives allot 20 minutes for return prenatal visits and 40 minutes for new obstetric visits. They see an average of 15 patients per day, which is a marked contrast to the 25 to 30 patients per day seen in many midwifery and obstetric practices. In its early days, the practice served Medicaid patients only but because of its reputation, now serves public and private insurance patients (30% insurance, 30% Medicaid, and 40% emergency Medicaid, who are mostly Hispanic women). A hallmark of success and respect for this practice in the nursing community is that the hospital nurses seek the care of these practitioners for their birth experience.

As noted, the practice initiated a Centering Pregnancy model of group prenatal care in 2004. This trademarked model uses adult learning theory, group process, and participatory learning to facilitate prenatal care in a group setting. Groups of up to 8 to 12 women at approximately the same gestational age are enrolled and attend group classes from approximately 16 weeks' gestation to birth (10 times over 6 months). Physical assessment by the group provider occurs in the group space and women take responsibility for their weight and blood pressure. Each 2-hour session follows an educational curriculum similar to a childbirth education group, but the care occurs as the same time as the education and sharing. Active sharing and participation is a hallmark of the experience. Women take responsibility for their own learning and share what they discover with their group. The midwives report positive response from their patient population to this enhanced model of prenatal care. The practice director reports that they maintain six groups at any one time, which would represent about one third of their caseload enrolled in this model of care. There is evidence that this model of care can contribute to lower preterm birth rates and higher breast-feeding rates than women receiving individual prenatal visits (Ickovics, Kershaw, Westdahl, et al., 2003).

The practice has excellent outcomes and has maintained a preterm birth rate of 7% throughout its history, compared with a county rate of 13% and a state rate of 13.8%. Recently, the practice joined the national ACNM Benchmarking Project, a national quality management initiative that allows practices to compare their outcomes and care practices with those of other midwifery groups. Over 53,000 births were represented in the 2010 project and 33 benchmarks were identified (ACNM, 2012j). ARMC received a commendation as a "Best Practice" for their very low third- and fourth-degree laceration rates. The director mentioned that participating with a large cohort of midwives in a national program has also allowed them to think about how they might improve their own care processes.

The excellent way in which this practice has listened to women and respected them can be expressed through a case study. A 24-year-old primigravida (SG) presented to the practice at 18 weeks' gestation. She was polite and well educated, and apologetic for coming in relatively late in her pregnancy for her first examination. The father of the baby was not involved in her life. SG talked about being nervous and stated that she had never had a pelvic examination; when it came time for that part of the examination, she was trembling and sweating and clearly not able to be examined. The midwife recognized that this situation might be the result of a previous bad experience with a health care provider, or perhaps SG had a history of sexual abuse. The social worker was brought in and the patient revealed a past long-term history of incest, which she had never revealed. She had never had a truly intimate relationship and this pregnancy was the result of having too much to drink at a party. She delayed care because of shame and fear of being "seen." As a result, the group worked extensively with SG to prepare her for the birth. She did not want an epidural. It was very important to her to feel that she was in control and could move at will. She delivered her baby in a semistanding squat in a low-lit room with only necessary staff present.

SG wrote to the practice several months after her birth and told them how their respect for her situation, listening to her concerns and wishes, and the gentle treatment she received had helped alleviate her fear. She shared that being able to give birth under own power with a midwife who was willing to follow her lead had made her feel differently about her body. She felt powerful and no longer ashamed.

Professional Issues

Image

The image of the nurse-midwife in the United States is not a clear or coherent one. As noted, many practitioners call themselves midwives but there is no single standard for education and practice, which leads to confusion. There is a deeply held belief by many U.S. citizens that being a midwife means that you help women give birth at home, and that a midwife is a practitioner rooted in the past. Our students continue to report this as a response to their announcement to friends and family about becoming a nurse-midwife. In addition to consumer confusion, there has been a fair amount of professional resistance to nurse-midwifery from the medical community. That professional resistance at the organizational level has improved with the recent joint statement of practice relationships between the ACNM and ACOG (ACNM, 2011f). The ACNM has made strategic communication its first priority in its strategic goals and aims to promote the use of midwifery to consumers as a first priority and health care systems as a second priority. They are launching a social media campaign created to unify and mobilize midwifery supporters and create an accurate, positive, and visible image for the practice of midwifery.

Work Life

CNMs provide a full range of primary health care services for women, from adolescence through menopause. There is variety in the way these services can be offered and CNMs are fortunate to have such variety from which to choose. Full-scope women's health care services encompass ambulatory and in-hospital care for a group of women, and usually involve the highest number of hours worked per week. The 2008 National Sample Survey of Registered Nurses did not distinguish the scope of practice, but reported that more than 25% of nurse-midwives worked more than 48 hours per week (U.S. Department of Health and Human Services, Health Resources and Services Administration, 2010). It is not clear in this survey how call hours were calculated.

A 2007 survey of Connecticut CNMs in full-scope practice (antenatal, intrapartum, postpartum, gynecology) reported an average full-time work week of two 24-hour call days, three 7-hour office days, and 2 to 4 hours of education and administration. Thus, the average work week for this group was 77 hours (Holland & Holland, 2007), much higher than reported in the national survey. The national survey also reported that 86.2% of nurse-midwives were moderately or extremely satisfied with their principal position. For nurse-midwives who are in a full-scope midwifery practice, the stress and commitment of on-call time in addition to regular office hours can be daunting. If the practice has several nurse-midwives and the call is shared (e.g., one or two nights of call a week for each midwife), the workload can be manageable. To give their best to their patients, and to stay healthy, nurse-midwives with a heavy on-call schedule need to develop self-care strategies that enable them to balance work with personal responsibilities and relationships. Perhaps more importantly, there is increasing evidence about the relationship between fatigue and medical errors. This has affected the call schedule of medical residents and has prompted numerous organizations to issue alerts and position papers. The National Association of Neonatal Nurses (NANN) has recently issued a position statement that the maximum shift length should be 24 hours, regardless of work setting and patient acuity, and the maximum number of working hours per week should be 60 hours (NANN, 2012). Given the high potential among CNMs for 24- to 72-hour call schedules, it is time that the professional organization becomes more proactive in recommendations about this aspect of quality and safety.

Some nurse-midwives choose a different practice model to enhance their personal interests or maximize work-life balance. They may choose to be a laborist, working shifts, providing maternity services in the hospital, including triage and the management of labor and birth of women whose provider may be unavailable or who have not enrolled with a provider before labor. An ambulatory women's health position is also a possibility and gives the advantage of regular hours, although the intrapartum component would be missing in this position. Some midwives engage in teaching in CNM programs and may also follow an academic research trajectory. Others have positions in medical program education, teaching medical students and obstetric and family medicine residents about preventive health care and normal pregnancy and birth. For those who love it, the satisfaction of providing care to a pregnant woman, following her through her pregnancy, assisting her through the physical and mental demands of labor and birth, anticipating the unpredictability of birth, and seeing the joy of a family greeting their newborn make nurse-midwifery fascinating, exciting, and personally worth the physical and emotional investment of oneself that may be required. It is a privilege to be with families who are experiencing pregnancy and birth. In making this investment, however, midwives struggle to achieve a work-life balance that maintains their personal well-being.

Professional Liability

As noted, physicians sit on hospital credentialing committees, their national and state organizations lobby against being for midwifery and advanced practice legislation, and even their malpractice insurance companies have control over the ability of nurse-midwives to obtain malpractice insurance (Ament, 2007). In general, nurse-midwifery malpractice insurance rates are higher than for other APNs, which reflects the malpractice climate of obstetric care. These rates have been cited as reasons for some midwifery practices to be discontinued. Therefore, the professional organizations and individual nurse-midwives seek to stay abreast of legislative and practice changes that may help reframe the current litigious environment in which health care occurs, especially for practitioners of midwifery and obstetrics.

ACNM, through its state and federal legislative offices, supports tort reform that would cap noneconomic damages, limit the number of years in which a plaintiff can file a health care liability action, place reasonable limits on punitive damages, and expand alternative dispute resolution methods (Kaplan, 2011). In addition to supporting tort reform, ACNM has developed a professional liability resource packet that seeks to keep CNMs updated on these issues. The organization also emphasizes quality and safety in practice and risk management strategies that help prevent adverse events from occurring. Finally, it seeks to ensure that midwives have available a medical malpractice insurance option that has a strong underwriter and national coverage endorsed by the professional organization; such an option currently exists (ACNM, 2012h).

Quality and Safety

Quality and safety issues have become of paramount concern to nurse-midwives. Adverse events in obstetrics have recently been reported, and many of these could be prevented. Approximately 50% of maternal deaths are attributed to substandard care (Mann and Pratt, 2010). The ACNM has increased the activity of its Division of Standards and Practice, which includes committees on clinical practice, quality improvement, and professional liability. A position statement, *Creating a Culture of Safety in Midwifery Care* (ACNM, 2006), outlines the importance of evidence-based practice, interdisciplinary team communication, active involvement of patients in their care, and participation in quality management programs. ACNM also maintains a current website, "Quality Improvement and Patient Safety in Women's Healthcare," which directs midwives to resources, including organizational links of importance to quality and safety for

practitioners. Furthermore, a joint statement, *Quality Patient Care in Labor and Delivery: A Call to Action* (2012), was endorsed by a number of professional societies whose members care for pregnant and laboring women. It is listed as a resource on the ACNM website. In the paper topics such as communications, shared decision making, teamwork, and quality measurement are discussed in the context of quality and safety in labor and delivery.

Nurse-midwifery has a sustained record of reducing disparities among disadvantaged groups, starting in rural Eastern Kentucky where, over a 30-year period, low-birth-weight and maternal mortality rates dropped from levels that were among the highest in the country to those among the lowest. From 1925 to 1958, the maternal mortality rate was 9.1/10,000 for the Frontier Nursing Service and 34/10,000 for the United States (Metropolitan Life Insurance Company, 1960). In view of these outstanding results, numerous studies have continued to document that CNMs have excellent outcomes, usually with less intervention and lower cost (likely from less use of unnecessary technology), and shorter hospital stays. Midwives have been documented to have fewer episiotomies, lacerations, inductions, and epidurals and higher rates of breast-feeding (Hatem, Sandall, Devane, et al., 2008). A recent systematic review (Johantgen et al., 2012) compared labor and delivery care provided by certified nurse-midwives and physicians from 1990 to 2008. Only those articles in which processes or outcomes of care were quantitatively compared were included; 21 articles representing 18 studies were reported. There is moderate to high evidence that CNMs rely less on technology during labor and delivery than physicians and achieve similar or better outcomes.

Conclusion

There have been many recent positive advances in nurse-midwifery and between nurse-midwifery and the broader health care system. The ACNM has been reaching out to professional nursing, midwifery, medical, policy, and public health colleagues nationally and internationally. There has been international recognition of the need for more midwives to reduce maternal and neonatal mortality. In the United States, the IOM report, the *Future of Nursing*, and passage of the PPACA has placed CNMs and other APRNs in a partnership role in redesigning the health care system for the future. From a midwifery perspective, we hope that this system will honor women and offer them support in realizing the power that comes with the choice of a woman-centered health care system.

References

Ament, L. A. (2007). *Professional issues in midwifery*. Sudbury, MA: Jones and Bartlett.

American College of Nurse-Midwives (ACNM). (1997). Collaborative management in midwifery practice for medical, gynecological and obstetrical conditions. (http://www. midwife.org/ACNM/files/ACNMLibraryData/UPLOADFILENAME/000 000000058/ Collaborative%20Mgmt%2005.pdf).

American College of Nurse-Midwives (ACNM). (2004). Philosophy of the American College of Nurse-Midwives. (http://www.midwife.org/index.asp?bid=59&cat=2&button=Search&rec=49).

American College of Nurse-Midwives (ACNM). (2006). Creating a culture of safety in midwifery care. (http://www.midwife.org/ACNM/files/ACNMLibraryData/UPLOADFILENAME/000000000059/Creating%20a%20Culture%20of%20Safety%20in%20Midwifery%20Care%2012.06.pdf).

American College of Nurse-Midwives (ACNM). (2008a). Code of ethics. (http://www.midwife.org/ACNM/files/ACNMLibraryData/UPLOADFILENAME/000000000048/code%20_of_ethics_2008.pdf).

American College of Nurse-Midwives (ACNM). (2008b). Core competencies for basic midwifery practice. (http://www.midwife.org/ACNM/files/ACNMLibraryData/UPLOADFILENAME/000000000050/Core%20Competencies%20June%202012.pdf).

American College of Nurse-Midwives (ACNM). (2010a). Division of research sections. (http://www.midwife.org/DOr-sections).

American College of Nurse-Midwives (ACNM). (2010b). Re-entry guidelines for certified nurse-midwives and certified midwives. (http://www.midwife.org/Re-entry-Guidelines-for-CNMs/CMs).

American College of Nurse-Midwives (ACNM). (2011a). Annual report 2011. (http://www. midwife.org/index.asp?bid=1264#/2).

American College of Nurse-Midwives (ACNM). (2011b). The practice doctorate in midwifery. (http://www.midwife.org/ACNM/files/ACNMLibraryData/UPLOADFILENAME/000000000260/Practice%20Doctorate%20in%20Midwifery%20Sept%202011.pdf).

American College of Nurse-Midwives (ACNM). (2011c). Midwifery in the United States and the consensus model for APRN regulation. (http://www.midwife.org/ACNM/files/ccLibraryFiles/ Filename/000000001458/LACE_White_Paper_2011.pdf).

American College of Nurse-Midwives (ACNM). (2011d). Standards for the practice of midwifery. (http://www.midwife.org/siteFiles/descriptive/Standards_for_Practice_of_Midwifery_12_09_001.pdf).

American College of Nurse-Midwives (ACNM). (2011e). Essential facts about midwives. (http://www.midwife.org/Essential-Facts-about-Midwives).

American College of Nurse-Midwives (ACNM). (2011f). Collaborative agreement between physicians and certified nurse-midwives (CNMs) and certified midwives (CMs). (http://www.midwife.org/ACNM/files/ACNMLibraryData/UPLOADFILENAME/000000000057/Collaborative_Agreement_between_Physicians_and_CNMs_CMs_12_09.pdf).

American College of Nurse-Midwives (ACNM). (2012a). Definition of midwifery and scope of practice of certified nurse-midwives and certified midwives. (http://www.midwife.org/ACNM/files/ACNMLibraryData/UPLOADFILENAME/000000000266/Definition%20of%20Midwifery%20and%20Scope%20of%20Practice%20of%20CNMs%20and%20CMs%20Feb% 202012.pdf).

American College of Nurse-Midwives (ACNM). (2012b). ACNM vision, mission, and core values. (http://www.midwife.org/ACNM/files/ACNMLibraryData/UPLOADFILENAME/000000000269/ACNM%20Vision%20Mission%20Core%20Values%20April%202012.pdf).

American College of Nurse-Midwives (ACNM). (2012c). Midwives are primary care providers and leaders of maternity care homes. (http://www.midwife.org/ACNM/files/ACNMLibraryData/UPLOADFILENAME/000000000273/Primary%20Care%20Position%20Statement%20June%202012.pdf).

American College of Nurse-Midwives (ACNM). (2012d). Independent midwifery practice. (http://www.midwife.org/ACNM/files/ACNMLibraryData/UPLOADFILENAME/000000000073/Independent%20Mid%20Prac%2005.pdf).

American College of Nurse-Midwives (ACNM). (2012e). Midwifery education programs. (http://www.midwife.org/rp/eduprog_all.cfm).

American College of Nurse-Midwives (ACNM). (2012f). Supervisory requirements and contractual agreements. (http://www.midwife.org/index.asp?BVD=1169).

American College of Nurse-Midwives (ACNM). (2012g). Midwives and Medicare after health care reform. (http://www.midwife.org/Midwives-and-Medicare-after-Health-Care-Reform).

American College of Nurse-Midwives. (2012h). Professional liability information. (http://www.midwife.org/Professional-Liability-Information)

American College of Nurse Midwives (ACNM). (2012i). Accreditation commission for midwifery education. (http://www.midwifer.org/ACME).

American College of Nurse-Midwives. (2012j). ACNM 2010 benchmarking project: Selected results summary. (http://www.midwife.org/ACNM/files/ccLibraryFiles/Filename/000000001539/ACNM_BenchmarkingProject_1012.pdf).

American Midwife Certification Board, (AMCB). (2011). American midwifery certification board 2011 annual report. (http://www.amcbmidwife.org/assets/documents/AMCB%20Annual%20Report%202011.pdf).

Angood, P. B., Armstrong, E. M., Ashton, D., Burstin, H., Delbanco, S. F., Fildes, B., et al. (2010). Blueprint for action: Steps toward a high-quality, high-value maternity care system. *Women's Health Issues, 20*, S18–S49.

APRN Consensus Work Group. (2008). Consensus model for APRN regulation: Licensure, accreditation, certification and education. (http://www.aacn.nche.edu/education-resources/APRNReport.pdf).

Beck, C. T. & Gable, R. K. (2000). Postpartum depression screening scale: development and psychometric testing. *Nursing Research, 49*, 272–282.

Beck, C. T. & Gable, R. K. (2001). Further validation of the postpartum depression screening scale. *Nursing Research, 50*, 155–164.

Beck, C. T., Gable, R. K., Sakala, C., & Declercq, E. R. (2011). Posttraumatic stress disorder in new mothers: Results from a two-stage U.S. national survey. *Birth (Berkley, Calif.), 38*, 216–227. doi: 10.1111/j.1523-536X.2011.00475.x.

Beck, C. T. & Gable, R. K. (2012). A mixed methods study of secondary traumatic stress in labor and delivery nurses. *Journal of Obstetric, Gynecologic, and Neonatal Nursing*, Jul 12. doi: 10.1111/j.1552-6909.2012.01386.x.

Burst, H. V. (2005). The history of nurse-midwifery/midwifery education. *Journal of midwifery and Women's Health, 50*, 124–137.

Center for Medicare & Medicaid Innovations (CMS). (2012). Strong start for mothers and newborns: Fact sheet. (http://innovations.cms.gov/initiatives/Strong-Start/StrongStart_FactSheet.html).

Cooney, P. & Johnson, T. (2012). ACNM urges improved access to clinical privileges. *Quickening, 43*(2), 9. *American College of Nurse-Midwives*.

Dawley, K. (2003). Origins of nurse-midwifery in the United States and its expansion in the 1940s. *Journal of Midwifery and Women's Health, 48*, 86–95.

Dawley, K. (2005). Doubling back over roads once traveled: Creating a national organization for nurse-midwifery. *Journal of Midwifery and Women's Health, 50*, 71–82.

Dawley, K. & Burst, H. V. (2005). The American College of Nurse-Midwives and its antecedents: A historic time line. *Journal of Midwifery and Women's Health, 50*, 16–22.

Declercq, E. (2012). Trends in midwife-attended births in the United States, 1989–2009. *Journal of Midwifery and Women's Health, 57*, 321–326.

Fulea, C. C. (2012). Midwifery 101. (http://www.mymidwife.org/Midwifery-101).

Fullerton, J., Schuiling, K. D., & Sipe, T. A. (2005). Presidential priorities: 50 years of wisdom as the basis of an action agenda for the next half-century. *Journal of Midwifery and Women's Health, 50*, 91–101.

Hamilton G. (2012). Personal communication.

Hatem, M., Sandall, J., Devane, D., Soltani, H., & Gates, S. (2008). *Midwife-led versus other models of care for childbearing women* (review). (http://apps.who.int/rhl/reviews/CD004667.pdf).

Holland, M. L. & Holland, E. S. (2007). Survey of Connecticut nurse-midwives. *Women's Health Issues, 52*, 106–115.

Home Birth Consensus Summit. (2011). Common ground statements. (http://www.homebirthsummit.org/outcomes/common-ground-statements).

Hutton, E. K., Reitsma, A. H., & Kaufman, K. (2009). Outcomes associated with planned home and planned hospital births in low-risk women attended by midwives in Ontario, Canada, 2003–2006: A retrospective cohort study. *Birth, 36*, 180–189.

Ickovics, J. R., Kershaw, T. S., Westdahl, C., Rising, S. S., Klima, C., Reyonds, H., et al. (2003). Group prenatal care and preterm birth weight: results from a matched cohort study at public clinics. *Obstetrics and Gynecology, 102* (Pt 1), 1051–1057.

Institute of Medicine (IOM). (2011). *The future of nursing: Leading change, advancing health*. Washington, DC: National Academies Press.

International Confederation of Midwives (ICM). (2011). ICM international definition of the midwife. (http://www.internationalmidwives.org/Portals/5/2011/Definition%20of%20the%20Midwife%20-%202011.pdf).

International Confederation of Midwives (ICM). (2013). ICM Global Standards, Competencies and Tools. Retrieved March 5, 2013.(http://www.internationalmidwives.org/what-we-do/global-standards-competencies-and-tools.html).

Johantgen, M., Fountain, L., Zangaro, G., Newhouse, R., Stanik-Hutt, J., & White, K. (2012). Comparison of labor and delivery care provided by certified nurse-midwives and physicians: A systematic review, 1990–2008. *Journal of Midwifery and Women's Health, 22*, e73–e81.

Jolivet, R. R., Corry, M. P., & Sakala, C. (2010). Transforming maternity care: A high-value proposition: Summary of childbirth connection. 90th Anniversary Symposium proceedings. *Women's Health Issues, 20*(Suppl), S50–S66.

Kaplan, L. K. (2011). Support letter on behalf of American College of Nurse-Midwives. (http://www.midwife.org/ACNM/files/ccLibrryFiles/Filename/000000000922/Support%20Letter%20for%20HR5%20on%20Professional%20Liability%20Reform%202005191l.pdf).

Kennedy, H. P. (2010). The problem of normal birth. *Journal of Midwifery and Women's Health, 55*, 199–201. doi: 10.1016/j.jmwh.2010.02.008.

Kennedy, H. P., Farrell, T., Paden, R., Hill, S., Jolivet, R. R., Cooper, G. A., et al. (2011). A randomized clinical trial of group prenatal care in two military settings. *Military Medicine, 176*, 1169–1177.

Kennedy, H. P., Farrell, T., Paden, R., Hill, S., Jolivet, R., Willetts, J., et al. (2009). "I wasn't alone"—a study of group prenatal care in the military. *Journal of Midwifery and Women's Health, 45*, 176–183.

Kennedy, H. P., Grant, J., Walton, C., Shaw-Battista, J., & Sandall, J. (2010). Normalizing birth in England: A qualitative study. *Journal of Midwifery and Women's Health, 55*, 262–269.

Kennedy, H. P., Schuiling, K. D., & Murphy, P. A. (2007). Developing midwifery knowledge: Setting a research agenda. *Journal of Midwifery and Women's Health, 52*, 95–97.

Lugo, N. R., O'Grady, E. T., Hodnicki, D. R., & Hanson, C. M. (2007). Ranking state NP regulation: Practice environment and consumer healthcare choice. *American Journal for Nurse Practitioners, 11*, 8–24.

Lyndon, A. & Kennedy, H. P. (2010). Perinatal safety: From concept to nursing practice. *Journal of Perinatal and Neonatal Nursing, 24*, 22–31

Mann, S. & Pratt, S. (2010). Role of clinician involvement in patient safety in obstetrics and gynecology. *Clinical Obstetrics and Gynecology, 53*, 559–575.

Metropolitan Life Insurance company. (1960). Summary of the tenth thousand confinement records of the frontier nursing service. *Bulletin of the American College of Nurse-Midwifery, 5, 1*(9).

Midwives Alliance of North America (MANA). (2012). Definitions. (http://mana.org/ definitions.html).

National Association of Neonatal Nurses (NANN). (2012). The impact of advanced practice nurses' shift length and fatigue on patient safety. (http://www.nann.org/uploads/files/Fatigue_and_APRNs.pdf).

Novick, G., Sadler, L. S., Kennedy, H. P., Cohen, S. S., Groce, N. E., & Knafl, K. A. (2011). Women's experience of group prenatal care. *Quantitive Health Research, 21,* 97–116. doi: 10.1177/1049732310378655.

Novick, G., Sadler, L. S., Knafl, K. A., Groce, E., & Kennedy, H. P. (2012). The intersection of everyday life and group prenatal care for women in two urban clinics. *Journal of Health Care for the Poor and Underserved, 23,* 589–603.

Osborne, K. (2011). Regulation of prescriptive authority for certified nurse-midwives and certified midwives: A national overview. *Journal of Midwifery and Women's Health, 56,* 543–556.

Paine, L. L. (2000). Midwife is a metaphor [editorial]. *Journal of Midwifery and Women's Health, 45,* 367.

Partnership for Maternal, Newborn and Child Health (PMNCH). (2011). Analyzing commitments to advance the global strategy for women's and children's health. The PMNCH 2011 report. (http://www.who.int/pmnch/media/press_materials/pr/2011/20110919_ pmnch2011 report_pr/en/index.html).

Quality patient care in labor and delivery: A call to action. [Editorial]. (2012). *Journal of Midwifery & Women's Health, 57,* 112–113.

Save the Children. (2011). Missing midwives. (http://www.savethechildren.org.uk/sites/default/files/docs/Missing_Midwives).

Schuiling, K. D., Sipe, T. A., & Fullerton, J. (2010). Findings from the analysis of the American College of Nurse-Midwives' membership surveys: 2006–2008. *Journal of Midwifery & Women's Health, 55,* 299–307.

Smith D. (2012). Personal communication.

Sipe, T. A., Fullerton, J. T., & Schuiling, K. D. (2009). Demographic profiles of certified nurse-midwives, certified registered nurse anesthetists, and nurse practitioners: Reflections on implications for uniform education and regulation. *Journal of Professional Nursing, 25,* 178–185.

Thompson, F. E. (2003). The practice setting; Site of ethical conflict for some mothers and midwives. *Nursing Ethics, 10,* 588–601.

Thompson, J. B. (2002). Moving from codes of ethics to ethical relationships for midwifery practice. *Nursing Ethics, 9,* 522–536.

U.S. Department of Health and Human Services, Health Resources and Services Administration (HRSA). (2010). The registered nurse population: Findings from the 2008 national sample survey of registered nurses. (http://bhpr.hrsa.gov/healthworkforce/rnsurveys/rnsurveyfinal.pdf).

Ulrich, L. T. (1990). *A midwife's tale: The life of Martha Ballard, based on her diary, 1785–1812.* New York: Knopf/Random House.

United Nations Population Fund. (2011). The state of the world's midwifery: Delivering health, saving lives. (http://www.unfpa.org/sowmy/report/home.html).

United Nations. (2010). The Millennium Development Goals Report. (http://www.un.org/millenniumgoals/pdf/MDG%20Report%202010%20En%20r15%20-low%20res%2020100615%20-.pdf).

Varney, H., Kriebs, J. M., & Gegor, C. L. (2004). *Varney's midwifery* (4th ed.). Sudbury, MA: Jones and Bartlett.

The Certified Registered Nurse Anesthetist

Margaret Faut Callahan • Michael J. Kremer

CHAPTER CONTENTS

Nurse anesthesia is the oldest organized advanced practice nurse (APN) specialty. Standardized postgraduate education, credentialing, and continuing education are all areas pioneered by these APNs. Certified registered nurse anesthetists (CRNAs) were the first nurse specialists to receive direct reimbursement for their services. This chapter discusses professional definitions of nurse anesthesia practice and issues important to this APN specialty. A profile of current CRNA practice is described and challenges and future trends are proposed. The American Association of Nurse Anesthetists (AANA) is described and a model of professional competence for CRNAs is presented. The transition of nurse anesthesia education to the practice doctorate and the associated competencies for CRNAs prepared at the doctoral level will also be reviewed.

Brief History of Certified Registered Nurse Anesthetist Education and Practice

The first organized program in nurse anesthesia education was offered in 1909. However, nurses have provided anesthesia since the American Civil War. There are currently 112 accredited nurse anesthesia programs, with over 2500 clinical sites in the United States and Puerto Rico. These APN educational programs are affiliated with or operated by schools or colleges of nursing, allied health, or other academic entities (Council on Accreditation of Nurse Anesthesia Educational Programs [COA], 2012a). In 1952, AANA established a mechanism for accreditation of nurse anesthesia educational programs that has been recognized by the U.S. Department of Education since 1955.

Nurse anesthetists were among the first APNs to require continuing education. AANA implemented a certification program in 1945 and instituted mandatory recertification in 1978. The CRNA credential came into existence in 1956 (Bankert, 1989). CRNAs currently must be recertified every 2 years, which includes meeting practice requirements and obtaining a minimum of 40 continuing education credits (National Board for Certification and Recertification of Nurse Anesthetists [NBCRNA], 2012).

In 1990, the U.S. Department of Health and Human Services (HHS) published research findings that demonstrated increased demand for nurse anesthetists (Mastropietro, Horton, Ouellette, et al., 2001). Successful efforts to increase the number of nurse anesthesia programs and graduates resulted in programs expanding from 89 in 1994 to 112 in 2012. In 1995, there were 1054 nurse anesthesia graduates. In 2012, 2525 students will complete nurse anesthesia educational programs. Some 45,000 CRNAs currently practice in the United States. The economic downturn of the last several years has caused some practitioners to delay retirement. However, AANA member survey data have indicated that 22% of AANA members plan to retire between 2014 and 2018, and another 20% expect to retire between 2019 and 2022 (AANA 2012a; COA, 2012a). There will continue to be a robust demand for CRNAs in the United States.

Data from the Centers for Disease Control and Prevention (CDC) indicated that 51.4 million surgical and diagnostic procedures were performed in 2010 (CDC, 2010). The number of selected procedures performed is shown in Table 18-1.

CRNAs provide anesthesia for approximately 32 million surgical and diagnostic procedures in the United States each year (AANA, 2012b). The impact of the aging population, coupled with implementation of the Patient Protection and Affordable Care Act (PPACA; HHS, 2011), if operationalized as planned, will result in more surgical and diagnostic procedures being performed.

The Institute of Medicine (IOM) report on the *Future of Nursing* (2010) noted that "transforming the health care system to meet the demand for safe, quality and affordable care will require a fundamental rethinking of the roles of many health care professionals, including nurses. The 2010 Affordable Care Act represents the broadest health care overhaul since the 1965 creation of the Medicare and Medicaid programs, but nurses are unable to fully participate in the resulting evolution of the U.S. health care system" (p. 21). The IOM report expressed concern that physicians challenge expanding scopes of practice for nurses and that "given the great need for more affordable health care, nurses should be playing a larger role in the health care system, both in delivering care and decision making about care" (p. 26). The IOM report concluded that "now is the time to eliminate outdated regulations and organizational and cultural barriers that limit the ability of nurses to practice to the full extent of their education, training and competence. ... Scope of practice regulations in all states should reflect the full of extent of ... each profession's education and training" (IOM, 2010, p. 96).

CRNAs are the predominant anesthesia providers in rural America, enabling health care facilities in these medically underserved areas to provide patient access to surgical, obstetric, pain management, and trauma stabilization services. In some states, these APNs are the sole anesthesia providers in almost 100% of rural hospitals (AANA, 2012a). In addition to providing anesthesia services in rural America, CRNAs have long contributed to the care of medically underserved citizens.

Reports in peer-reviewed journals have continued to document the safety and cost-effectiveness of care provided by CRNAs (Dulisse & Cromwell, 2010; Hogan, Seifert, Moore, et al., 2010; Pine, Holt, & Lou, 2003; Simonson, Ahern, & Hendryx, 2007). Findings reported in these papers demonstrate that there is no difference in the quality of care provided by CRNAs and their physician counterparts.

Legislation passed by Congress in 1986 provided direct billing for CRNAs under Medicare Part B. In 2001, the Centers for Medicare & Medicaid Services (CMS) allowed states to opt out of the reimbursement requirement that a surgeon or anesthesiologist oversee anesthesia services provided by CRNAs. Dulisse and Cromwell (2010) have noted that by 2005, 14 states exercised this option. To date, 17 states have opted out of Medicare Part A CRNA supervision requirements (AANA, 2012c; Table 18-2). An analysis of Medicare data for 1999 to 2005 found no evidence that opting out of the oversight requirement resulted in increased inpatient morbidity or mortality (Dulisse & Cromwell, 2010).

A recent cost-effectiveness analysis of anesthesia providers found that CRNAs are less costly to train than anesthesiologists and can perform the same set of anesthesia services, including relatively rare and difficult procedures such as open heart surgery, organ transplantation, and

TABLE 18-1   Annual Surgical Procedures in the United States (2010)

Procedure	No. Performed
Arteriography and angiocardiography using contrast material	2,400,000
Cardiac catheterization	1,000,000
Small bowel endoscopy (with or without biopsy)	1,100,000
Large bowel endoscopy (with or without biopsy)	499,000
Computerized axial tomography (CAT) scans	497,000
Diagnostic ultrasound	1,000,000
Balloon angioplasty or coronary artery atherectomy	500,000
Hysterectomy	498,000
Cesarean section	1,300,000
Reduction of fracture	671,000
Insertion of coronary artery stent	454,000
Coronary artery bypass graft	395,000
Total knee replacement	719,000
Total hip replacement	332,000

TABLE 18-2 States That Have Opted Out of CRNA Medicare Part A Supervision

State	When Enacted
Iowa	December 2001
Nebraska	February 2002
Idaho	March 2002
Minnesota	April 2002
New Hampshire	June 2002
New Mexico	November 2002
Kansas	March 2003
North Dakota	October 2003
Washington	October 2003
Alaska	October 2003
Oregon	December 2003
Montana	June 2005
South Dakota	March 2005
Wisconsin	July 2005
California	July 2009
Colorado	September 2010 (for critical access hospitals and specified rural hospitals)
Kentucky	April 2012

Adapted from American Association of Nurse Anesthetists. (AANA). (2012c). Federal supervision rule/opt-out information. (http://www.aana.com/advocacy/stategovernmentaffairs/Pages/Federal-Supervision-Rule-Opt-Out-Information.aspx).

pediatric procedures. In concert with the IOM report, the investigators noted that "as the demand for health care continues to grow, increasing the number of CRNAs and permitting them to practice in the most efficient delivery models, will be a key to containing costs while maintaining quality of care" (Hogan et al., 2010, p. 159).

Nurse anesthetists have been the main providers of anesthesia care to U.S. military men and women on the front lines of combat since World War I. Documentation of nurses providing anesthesia to wounded soldiers dates back to the American Civil War. Currently, 3.5% of U.S. nurse anesthetists serve in the military or Veterans Administration (VA) facilities (AANA, 2012d).

Regarding malpractice coverage, insurance rates for self-employed CRNAs have declined significantly since the 1980s (AANA, 2010a). In 2009, the average CRNA malpractice premium was 33% lower than in 1988, or 62% lower when adjusted for inflation. This decline in malpractice premium rate reflects the safe care provided by nurse anesthetists. The rate drop is impressive given inflation, our litigious society, and generally higher jury awards (AANA, 2010a).

Men have historically been more represented in nurse anesthesia compared with nursing as a whole. Approximately 45% of the nation's 45,000 nurse anesthetists and student nurse anesthetists are men, compared with about 8% in the nursing profession. When all employed CRNAs are examined, 45% are men and 55% are women. The gender balance shifts significantly with part-time employees; 77% of part-time CRNAs are women and 23% are men. Currently, more than 90% of U.S. nurse anesthetists are members of the AANA (AANA, 2012a).

Role Differentiation Between Certified Registered Nurse Anesthetists and Anesthesiologists

CRNAs provide anesthesia services in collaboration with surgeons, anesthesiologists, dentists, podiatrists, and other qualified health care professionals. When anesthesia is administered by a nurse anesthetist, it is recognized as the practice of nursing; when administered by an anesthesiologist, it is recognized as the practice of medicine (AANA, 2012e). Regardless of their educational backgrounds, all anesthesia providers adhere to the same standards of care. Nurse anesthetists are APNs who practice in every setting in which anesthesia is delivered—traditional hospital surgical suites and obstetric delivery rooms, critical access hospitals, ambulatory surgical centers, the offices of dentists, podiatrists, ophthalmologists, plastic surgeons, and pain management specialists, endoscopy centers, and U.S. military, public health services, and Department of Veterans Affairs health care facilities.

Profile of the Certified Registered Nurse Anesthetist

A CRNA is a registered nurse who is educationally prepared at the graduate level and certified as competent to engage in practice as a nurse anesthetist, rendering patients insensible to pain with anesthetic agents and related drugs and procedures. Anesthesia services are delivered by anesthesia providers on request, assignment, or referral by the operating physician or other health care provider authorized by law, usually to facilitate diagnostic, therapeutic, or surgical procedures. In addition to general or regional anesthesia techniques, as well as monitored anesthesia care, a referral or request for consultation or assistance may be initiated for the provision of obstetric anesthesia services, ventilator management, or treatment of acute or chronic pain through the performance of selected diagnostic or therapeutic blocks, or other forms of pain management. Education, practice, and research within the specialty of nurse anesthesia promote competent anesthesia care across the life span at all acuity levels. CRNAs practice according to their expertise, state statutes and regulations, and institutional policy (AANA, 2010b). CRNAs work collaboratively with all members of the perioperative team, including nurses, technicians, surgeons, and anesthesiologists.

CRNAs are responsible and accountable for their individual professional practices and are capable of exercising independent judgment within the scope of their education (credentials), demonstrated competence (privileges), and licensure. CRNAs are recognized in all 50 states by state regulatory bodies, primarily boards of registered nursing. Nurse anesthesia is a recognized nursing specialty role and is not a medically delegated act (AANA, 2012e).

Compensation, along with role-related autonomy and responsibility, continue to attract qualified applicants to this advanced practice nursing specialty. The most recent data for full-time CRNAs, excluding those who are self-employed, show a mean salary of $165,571. CRNAs employed by hospitals had higher median annual compensation rates ($171,000) than group employees ($153,000) or military or VA-employed CRNAs ($160,000; AANA, 2012a).

The CRNA practice profile is influenced by the work of the AANA Practice Committee and AANA Professional Practice Department. The Professional Practice Department participates in safety and quality issues, including reduction of needlestick injuries and safe injection practices. AANA is represented at the National Patient Safety Foundation and is involved with the Ambulatory Surgery and Office Surgery Initiative. AANA is a major stakeholder and participant in the National Quality Forum, addressing patient safety issues (AANA, 2012f).

AANA works with accrediting bodies to review standards revisions. There is CRNA representation on The Joint Commission (TJC) Technical Advisory Committees. TJC has created credentialing requirements for all categories of clinicians, a process into which AANA had input. CRNAs are surveyors for the Accreditation Association for Ambulatory Health Care (AAAHC).

Scope and Standards of Practice

The *Scope and Standards of Nurse Anesthesia Practice*, as set forth by the AANA, is comprehensive and includes all aspects of anesthesia care (AANA, 2010b). Regardless of the setting in which CRNAs practice, their role includes meeting the individual anesthesia care needs of patients in the perioperative period, including the following (AANA, 2010b):

- Performing and documenting a preanesthetic assessment and evaluation of the patient, including requesting consultations and diagnostic studies; selecting, obtaining, ordering and administering preanesthetic medications and fluids; and obtaining informed consent for anesthesia
- Developing and implementing an anesthetic plan
- Initiating the anesthetic technique, which may include general, regional, and local anesthesia and sedation
- Selecting, applying, and inserting appropriate non-invasive and invasive monitoring modalities for continuous evaluation of the patient's physical status
- Selecting, obtaining, and administering the anesthetic, adjuvant and accessory drugs, and fluids necessary to manage the anesthetic
- Managing a patient's airway and pulmonary status using current practice modalities
- Facilitating emergence and recovery from anesthesia by selecting, obtaining, ordering, and administering medications, fluids, and ventilator support
- Discharging the patient from a postanesthesia care area and providing anesthesia follow-up evaluation and care
- Implementing acute and chronic pain management modalities
- Responding to emergency situations by providing airway management, administering of emergency fluids and drugs, and using basic or advanced cardiac life support techniques

Additional nurse anesthesia responsibilities delineated in the *Scope and Standards of Nurse Anesthesia Practice*, which are within the expertise of the individual CRNA, include the following:

- Administration and management—scheduling, material and supply management, development of policies and procedures, fiscal management, performance evaluations, preventive maintenance, billing, data management, and supervision of staff, students, or ancillary personnel
- Quality assessment—data collection, reporting mechanisms, trending, compliance, committee meetings, departmental review, problem-focused studies, problem solving, intervention, document and process oversight
- Education—clinical and didactic teaching, basic cardiac life support and advanced cardiac life support instruction, in-service commitment, emergency medical technician training, supervision of residents, and continuing education

- Research—conducting and participating in departmental, hospital-wide, and university-sponsored research projects
- Committee appointments—assignment to committees, committee responsibilities, and coordination of committee activities
- Interdepartmental liaison—interface with other departments such as nursing, surgery, obstetrics, postanesthesia care units (PACUs), outpatient surgery, admissions, administration, laboratory, and pharmacy
- Clinical and administrative oversight of other departments—for example, respiratory therapy, PACU, operating room, surgical intensive care unit (SICU), and pain clinics. (AANA, 2010b)

The *Scope and Standards of Nurse Anesthesia Practice* (AANA, 2010b) addresses the responsibilities associated with anesthesia practice that are performed in collaboration with other qualified health care providers. Collaboration "is a process which involves two or more parties working together, each contributing his or her respective area of expertise. CRNAs are responsible for the quality of services they render" (AANA, 2010b, p. 1).

Anesthesia care is provided by CRNAs in four general categories: (1) preanesthetic evaluation and preparation; (2) anesthesia induction, maintenance, and emergence; (3) postanesthesia care; and (4) perianesthetic and clinical support functions. Parallels between nursing and nurse anesthesia are apparent. CRNAs perform preanesthetic assessment, plan appropriate anesthetic interventions, implement planned anesthetic care, and evaluate patients postoperatively to determine the efficacy of their interventions. CRNAs working independently routinely perform all these aspects of clinical practice. When CRNAs and anesthesiologists work together, a variety of factors, such as billing arrangements and local anesthesia practice patterns, determine to what extent each practitioner is involved in specific anesthesia care areas (AANA, 2010b).

Preoperative evaluation has become more complex with the increasing acuity of surgical patients. Thorough preanesthetic assessments, combined with specialty consultation as needed, are essential activities at which nurse anesthetists must be proficient (AANA, 2010b).

Developing and implementing an anesthetic care plan is another important aspect of CRNA practice. This care plan is formulated with input from the patient, surgeon, and anesthesiologist in those settings in which CRNAs and anesthesiologists work collaboratively. Input from the patient, surgeon, and anesthetist is relevant when making the important decision about which type of anesthetic to administer in a given situation. Compromise and flexibility may be necessary to achieve the goals of surgery

⊙ TABLE 18-3	Techniques Performed by CRNA Survey Respondents
Technique	No. of CRNAs Who Performed This Technique (%)
Monitored anesthesia care (local anesthesia, monitoring by an anesthesia provider, with or without sedation)	99
General anesthesia	99
Arterial catheter insertion	75
IV regional anesthesia	63
Spinal anesthesia	62
Epidural analgesia	53
Fiberoptic intubation	46
Central venous catheter insertion	31
Brachial plexus block	27
Insertion of pulmonary artery catheter	11
Chronic pain management	9
Opthalmologic block	4

Adapted from American Association of Nurse Anesthetists. (AANA). (2012a). AANA member survey data. (http://www.aana.com/myaana/AANABusiness/aanasurveys/Documents/aana-member-survey-data-nov2011.pdf).

and anesthesia to maximize safety and minimize risks during the procedure and postprocedure period.

The scope of practice for CRNAs varies depending on institutional credentialing. Although most CRNAs provide general anesthesia and monitored anesthesia care, survey data show a noticeable decrease in the frequency with which regional anesthesia is performed relative to general anesthesia. Placement of invasive monitoring lines and pain management techniques are less commonly performed by nurse anesthetists. Practice restrictions may not always be imposed via the credentialing process; some providers choose not to perform certain types of procedures. See Table 18-3 for the breakdown of techniques performed by CRNAs who completed AANA member surveys ($N = 5377$) in 2011.

Education, Credentialing, and Certification

To become a CRNA, the following requirements must be met (COA, 2012b):

- Complete a Bachelor's of Science in Nursing degree or other appropriate baccalaureate degree.
- Hold current licensure as a registered nurse (RN).
- Complete at least 1 year as an RN in an acute care setting.

- Graduate from a nurse anesthesia program accredited by the COA or its predecessor.
- Successfully complete the national certification examination offered by the National Board of Certification and Recertification for Nurse Anesthetists for CRNAs or its predecessor.
- Comply with the criteria for biennial recertification as defined by the National Board of Certification and Recertification for Nurse Anesthetists. These criteria include evidence of the following: (1) current licensure as a registered nurse; (2) active practice as a CRNA; (3) appropriate continuing education; and (4) verification of the absence of mental, physical, and other problems that could interfere with the practice of anesthesia.

Nurse anesthesia education occurs in diverse settings. Diversity is demonstrated by the many academic units that house nurse anesthesia educational programs, including nursing, allied health, sciences, and medicine. However, the relative value of this diversity has never been quantified in terms of an academic power base or educational credibility. This diversity exists because the nurse anesthesia educational community values various undergraduate degrees for entrance into nurse anesthesia programs and because of the initial difficulty nurse anesthesia educators met when trying to move certificate nurse anesthesia programs into schools of nursing.

Since 1998, all nurse anesthesia programs have been at the graduate level. However, this requirement does not dictate the movement of programs into one academic discipline. A reason for this may stem from those programs that in the 1970s established relationships with whichever academic unit was open to affiliating with a nurse anesthesia program. Programs that pioneered nurse anesthesia education at the graduate level established relationships with those departments in colleges and universities that were willing to take risks with the small numbers of students in nurse anesthesia programs. This diversified model of nurse anesthesia education has proliferated in the last 20 years, and many of these long-established programs would find it difficult to change their academic affiliations.

In the mid-1970s, over 170 nurse anesthesia educational programs existed. A rapid decline in the numbers of nurse anesthesia programs occurred in the 1980s, a change that was of great concern to the specialty. The closures were attributed variously to physician pressure, declining support, the inability of hospitals to continue support of small programs, and lack of a geographically accessible universities with which a nurse anesthesia program could affiliate (Faut Callahan, 1991). Those who argued that nurse anesthesia programs closed solely because of the graduate degree mandate offered little

evidence to support that claim. One can surmise that if the requirement for graduate education was the only reason for program closures, those programs would have remained open until 1998, when the master's degree was required. Despite the decline in the overall numbers of nurse anesthesia programs, many of which were certificate programs with enrollments of less than five students, the level of educational programs has changed dramatically. After an initial decline in graduates, the newer graduate programs increased their admissions. To accomplish this, programs had to increase the numbers of clinical training sites. This resulted in a strengthened educational system, deeply entrenched in an academic model.

Colleges of nursing now house 57% of nurse anesthesia educational programs in the United States, reflecting increasing collaboration between all APN groups on education, legislative, and policy matters (COA, 2012a). Because AANA founder Agatha Hodgins unsuccessfully sought a place for CRNAs within the American Nurses Association, a separate professional organization (AANA) was formed (Bankert, 1989; Thatcher, 1953). However, rapprochement between nursing and nurse anesthesia has resulted in effective collaboration (Mungia-Biddle, Maree, Klein, et al., 1990). Coalitions of APNs have effectively worked together on the state and federal levels on health reform and other issues for many years. External funding, such as federal traineeships, has helped offset expenses for nurse anesthesia students and helped meet CRNA workforce needs. The AANA closely monitors each proposed federal budget for potential changes in Title VIII funding and has advocated for additional funding in this area. Nurse anesthesia educational programs collectively receive about $3 million each year through the Title VIII Nurse Workforce Development Program.

Programs of Study

Nurse anesthesia educational curricula include time requirements for didactic and clinical activities that reflect minimum standards for entry into practice. Academic content areas are crucial to the preparation of practitioners for beginning-level competence in a highly demanding, rapidly changing specialty. Various colleges and schools that administratively house nurse anesthesia programs may have additional academic requirements. Nurse anesthesia programs in colleges of nursing include core graduate-level courses taken by all graduate-level nursing students. These courses include graduate-level nursing theory, nursing research, advanced physical assessment, pathophysiology, and pharmacology. The mandated content areas for nurse anesthesia programs are listed by the COA by required clock hours (COA, 2012b):

- Pharmacology of anesthetic agents and adjuvant drugs, including concepts in chemistry and biochemistry: 105 hours
- Anatomy, physiology, and pathophysiology: 135 hours
- Professional aspects of nurse anesthesia practice: 45 hours
- Basic and advanced principles of anesthesia practice, including physics, equipment, technology, and pain management: 105 hours
- Research: 30 hours
- Clinical correlation conferences: 45 hours

The clinical component requires that students administer a minimum of 550 anesthetics. An external agency, the National Board of Certification and Recertification for Nurse Anesthetists, requires that students complete given numbers of surgical procedures and anesthetic techniques. For example, all graduates must have administered at least 25 general anesthetics using a mask airway, versus a laryngeal mask or endotracheal intubation, and care for patients across the lifespan. Similarly, required numbers of specific clinical experiences, such as endotracheal intubations or thoracic surgical cases, must be met for nurse anesthesia graduates to be eligible to take the national certification examination. Most programs exceed these minimum requirements. The average student nurse anesthetist logs at least 1694 clinical hours and administers more than 790 anesthetics. In addition, many programs require study in methods of scientific inquiry and statistics, as well active participation in student-generated and faculty-sponsored research (COA, 2012a).

The COA accredits nurse anesthesia educational programs. Council members include nurse anesthesia educators and practitioners, nurse anesthesia students, health care administrators, university representatives, and the public. The COA conducts mandatory, on-site program reviews, with a maximum accreditation period of 10 years. Nurse anesthesia educators and the COA have found that retaining a prescriptive curriculum in terms of hours and types of clinical experiences has helped the survival of educational programs. That is, when documented deviations from established standards for nurse anesthesia educational programs occur, such as physicians restricting clinical access, program administrators can cite COA standards mandating these experiences (COA, 2012a).

Nurse Anesthesia Educational Funding

Despite growth in the national debt, Title VIII funding has continued. The Nurse Anesthetist Traineeship (NAT) program provides support for student registered nurse anesthetists who are enrolled full-time in a master's or doctoral nurse anesthesia program. Traineeship funds may be used to offset costs for tuition, books, fees, and reasonable living expenses for students during the period for which the traineeship is provided. In 2012, the NAT program changed to include first-year nurse anesthesia students, who previously were eligible for traineeship funding under the Advanced Education Nurse Training program. The total NAT funding available for 100 estimated applicants in 2012 is $2,250,000 (Health Resources and Services Administration [HRSA], 2012).

The AANA Division of Federal Government Affairs promotes nurse anesthesia workforce development through legislative advocacy in Congress and through representation before the Health Resources and Services Administration and its Division of Nursing, which administer the Title VIII NAT program. Title VIII funding can lessen the debt load experienced by nurse anesthesia students. Students are not typically encouraged to work as RNs while enrolled in nurse anesthesia programs, because the rigor of these programs usually entails 60 or more hours per week of committed time.

Practice Doctorate

Historically, nurse anesthesia curricular requirements have overloaded the typical master's curriculum. The current required minimum length of nurse anesthesia programs is now 24 months, but that will change by 2025 because all nurse anesthesia programs will be required to be a minimum of 36 months in length, which is required by COA's additional criteria for practice-oriented doctoral degrees (COA, 2012b). The vision of nursing leader Dr. Luther Christman for nurses to be prepared with advanced degrees, both in their discipline and in a basic science, reflects the trend to move to doctoral entry in anesthesia and other advanced practice specialties. At this writing, nurse anesthesia is the only APN specialty to have a timeline requiring the transition of all programs to the practice doctorate level.

Although nurse anesthesia faculty previously described limitations such as time and finances that would interfere with their pursuit of a doctoral degree (Jordan & Shott, 1998), the number of CRNAs prepared at the doctoral level has more than doubled in the recent past, from 1.2% to 3% (AANA, 2012a). Many CRNAs are currently pursuing practice or research doctorates, which bodes well for the future of the specialty and its transition to doctoral education.

Practice doctorates offered in nurse anesthesia programs include the Doctor of Nursing Practice (DNP) and the Doctor of Nurse Anesthesia Practice (DNAP). The DNP is typically offered for programs housed in schools of nursing and the DNAP may be the exit degree for nurse anesthesia programs located in schools of allied health or other academic units. Regardless of the degree offered, nurse anesthesia practice doctorates must comport with the additional criteria for practice-oriented doctoral degrees that are included in the COA *Standards for Accreditation of Nurse Anesthesia Educational Programs*. These criteria include a minimum program length of 36 months, demonstration of adequate numbers of faculty prepared at the doctoral level, and completion of a final scholarly work (COA, 2012b).

Certification

Nurse anesthesia was the first nursing specialty to have mandatory certification. This process began in 1945, when the first certification examination in nurse anesthesia was given (Bankert, 1989). The NBCRNA is separately incorporated from AANA. NBCRNA notes that "certification is a process by which a professional agency or association certified that an individual licensed to practice a profession has met certain standards specified by that profession for specialty practice. The purpose of certification is to assure the public that an individual has mastered a body of knowledge and acquired skills in a particular specialty" (www.NBCRNA.com). NBCRNA uses psychometricians, an academy of test item writers, and computer adaptive testing to assess beginning-level competence in nurse anesthesia practice. A professional practice analysis is performed at regular intervals by the NBCRNA to determine which entry-level competencies are necessary for a new nurse anesthesia graduate.

The AANA Continuing Education Department is responsible for the review and approval of continuing education programs sponsored by the AANA and other organizations, maintenance of attendance records of CE activities, and preparation of CE transcripts and certificates of attendance for AANA-sponsored programs (AANA, 2012g).

In 2012, the NBCRNA announced a Continued Professional Certification (CPC) program that will become operational in 2016. Under this system, the certification period will be 4 years. The continuing education requirements will be 15 assessed continuing education units per year. In addition, 10 professional activity units (developmental activities that do not require assessment) will be required each year. The CPC program will require four self-study modules every 4 years on subjects addressing core competencies in anesthesia, such as airway management techniques, applied clinical pharmacology, physiology, pathophysiology, and anesthesia technology. Continued education credits will be awarded when these modules are completed. A competency examination will be phased into the program over the next 20 years.

Required at 8-year intervals, the first examination will be available in 2020. The examination will be used for diagnostic and developmental purposes. In 2032, all nurse anesthetists will be required to meet a passing standard on the recertification examination at 8 year intervals. Four attempts to pass the test within a 4-year recertification cycle will be allowed (NBCRNA, 2012).

Institutional Credentialing

CRNAs practice according to their expertise, state statutes or regulations, and local institutional policy. Institutional credentialing procedures may require additional evidence of clinical and didactic education in areas such as cardiothoracic or regional anesthesia. State nurse practice acts and practice patterns in the anesthesia community contribute to variability in the scope of nurse anesthesia practice in different settings.

Competence can be partially ensured through institutional credentialing processes. A hospital or other facility may delineate procedures that the CRNA is authorized to perform by the authority of its governing board. Guidelines for granting CRNAs clinical privileges are found in an AANA *Sample Application for Clinical Privileges* (AANA, 2010c). Recommended clinical privileges for CRNAs are in the areas of preanesthetic preparation and evaluation, anesthesia induction, maintenance, and emergence, post-anesthetic care, and perianesthetic and clinical support functions (AANA, 2010c).

COA has required the master's degree as the exit degree for nurse anesthesia programs since 1998. The COA will not approve any new master's degree programs for accreditation beyond 2015. Students accepted into an accredited program on January 1, 2022 and thereafter will need to complete the program with a doctoral degree. COA standards require that program administrators (program administrator and assistant administrator) will be required to have a doctoral degree by 2018; clinical site coordinators will need to have a master's degree by 2014 (COA, 2012b).

Certified Registered Nurse Anesthetist Practice

Workforce Issues

Data that comprise CRNA practice profiles are derived from annual practice surveys completed by CRNAs when they pay their AANA dues. The response rate to these surveys has been as high as 72%, providing a reasonable degree of generalizability. AANA membership has grown by 20,000 from 1996 to 2012, from 25,000 to 45,000 CRNAs. This growth rate bodes well for the future of nurse anesthesia, along with the continued availability of high-quality, cost-effective anesthesia services, especially to citizens in rural and medically underserved areas. This growth reflects the work of the National Commission on Nurse Anesthesia Education (Maree, 1991), which provided the profession with workforce data projections and related strategies to ensure that the market demand for nurse anesthetists will be met. The growth in nurse anesthesia programs and graduates over the last 20 years can be attributed to the advocacy of AANA, through the National Commission on Nurse Anesthesia Education, for the development of new educational programs to meet increasing needs for anesthesia services (Mastropietro, et al., 2001).

The average age of CRNAs reported in the AANA 2011 membership survey was 49.8 years, similar to the average age for registered nurses in the United States. Regarding the duration of time spent in the specialty, 37% of CRNAs who responded to this survey had been in practice longer than 20 years and 23% were in practice for 11 to 20 years. A number of CRNA retirements can be expected between 2014 and 2018, because 22% of survey respondents indicated that they planned to retire during this time frame; another 20% of AANA members believe that they will retire between 2019 and 2022. Given the aging population and the potential impact of the PPACA, with over 30 million additional people covered, it is essential that nurse anesthesia educational programs continue to produce adequate numbers of graduates to meet workforce needs (AANA, 2012a).

A CRNA workforce study conducted 7 years ago showed a CRNA vacancy rate of 12% (Merwin, Stern, & Jordan, 2006). However, the current vacancy rate is much lower. For various reasons, many people in the workforce remain employed beyond the traditional retirement age. CRNA faculty surveyed in 2007 indicated that their timeline to expected retirement was similar to that of clinicians (Merwin, Stern, & Jordan, 2008). Between 2014 and 2022, 42% of CRNA survey respondents plan to retire and, after 2022, 51% plan to retire (AANA, 2012a). The current and future needs of nurse anesthesia programs mandate a faculty cadre to teach the rigorous didactic and clinical portions of nurse anesthesia programs and to manage the transition to the practice doctorate. Faculty survey respondents noted that the salary differential between academic and clinical settings was the biggest barrier to the recruitment of academic faculty.

Projected retirements and increases in health care coverage demand a health care workforce sufficient to deliver patient access to high-quality health care. The PPACA included a 4-year pilot project for Graduate Nursing Education (GNE) intended to support the clinical practice education of APRNs for the growing Medicare patient population. GNE seeks to ensure that the education of advanced practice nurses has funding opportunities similar to those provided for physicians under Graduate Medical Education (GME; CMS, 2012).

AANA membership survey data indicate that 81% of respondents work full time; 15% work part time, 3% are retired, and 1% are unemployed (AANA, 2012a).

Nurse anesthetists have provided most anesthesia services in rural areas since the inception of the specialty. However, most CRNAs reside in urban areas; 81.4% live in urban areas, as defined by Urban Influence Codes 1 and 2, and 18.6% of nurse anesthetists are nonmetropolitan residents, with addresses in Urban Influence Codes 3 to 12. Most CRNAs provide anesthesia services in hospitals with more than 200 beds (AANA, 2012a).

At one time, CRNAs were primarily hospital-employed. However, employment arrangements for CRNAs have changed over time (Table 18-4; AANA, 2012a).

Most nurse anesthetists (96%) are practicing clinicians. Departmental management and administration are listed as primary employment positions by 2% of CRNAs who responded to the AANA 2011 member survey; the remaining 2% of survey respondents were educators. Given the aging CRNA workforce, projected CRNA retirements between 2014 and 2020, and the requirement for movement of nurse anesthesia education programs to the practice doctorate by 2025, more CRNA educators are needed (AANA, 2012a).

Most practicing CRNAs report that they are clinical generalists (82%). Areas of specialty for practicing CRNAs include obstetrics (6%), pediatrics (5%), orthopedics (4%), plastic surgery (3%), gastroenterology (3%), general surgery (3%), ophthalmology (3%), cardiovascular (3%), gynecology (2%), neurosurgery (2%), pain management (2%), urology (2%), geriatrics (2%), and radiology (1%).

TABLE 18-4   Employment Arrangements of CRNAs

Arrangement	No. of CRNAs (%)
Hospital-employed	38
Practice group	34
Independent contractor	13
Other settings	8
Owners or partners in practice groups	4
VA, military	4

Adapted from American Association of Nurse Anesthetists. (AANA). (2012a). AANA member survey data. (http://www.aana.com/myaana/AANABusiness/aanasurveys/Documents/aana-member-survey-data-nov2011.pdf).

Many nurse anesthetists (86%) practice in hospitals, whereas 11% indicate that their primary practice setting is in ambulatory surgery centers, 2% state that they practice in office-based surgical facilities and 1% report "other" as their primary practice setting (AANA, 2012a).

The high demand for nurse anesthetists in clinical and academic settings is not expected to change. The safety, cost-effectiveness, and high quality of nurse anesthesia care, coupled with the advocacy provided by members through the AANA, keep nurse anesthesia at the forefront of the health care workforce.

Practice Settings

CRNAs provide services in conjunction with other health care professionals such as surgeons, dentists, podiatrists, and anesthesiologists in diverse clinical settings. These APNs practice in a variety of clinical environments. Nurse anesthetists provide anesthesia services on a solo basis, in groups, and collaboratively. Some CRNAs have independent contracting arrangements with physicians or hospitals.

Today, most surgery is performed on a same-day admission or outpatient basis. Anesthesia practices have adapted to this change from a predominantly inpatient model for surgery. A number of mechanisms, ranging from preoperative telephone interviews to preanesthesia clinics, are used to conduct preanesthesia assessment and allow anesthesia providers an opportunity to discuss care options, procedures, and risks with patients. However, detailed physical assessment and establishing a rapport between the anesthesia provider and patient often still occurs on the day of surgery.

Access to Health Care

Access to health care remains an ongoing concern across the country, with geographic maldistribution of anesthesia providers and other clinicians being a major factor. U.S. manpower trends in anesthesia have been studied (Kaye, Scibetta, & Grogono, 1999). These investigators suggested that because of changes in GME funding, fewer physicians have pursued anesthesia residencies.

A 2010 anesthesia workforce study conducted by Rand Health (2010) had two major questions:

1. Is there a shortage or surplus of anesthesia providers?
2. What are the demographic patterns, employment arrangements, usages of time across different types of procedures, and working patterns present in the anesthesia provider workforce?

This study, commissioned by the American Society of Anesthesiologists, demonstrated a current shortage of anesthesia providers but estimated a surplus of CRNAs by 2020. The latter finding is inconsistent with AANA member survey data, estimating a significant number of projected retirements between 2014 and 2020 (AANA, 2012a). The Rand study noted that as of 2007, the anesthesiologist vacancy rate was 9.6%, whereas the CRNA vacancy rate was estimated to be 3.8%. Geographic maldistribution of providers was noted, with 95% of anesthesiologists reported to be working in urban locations but only 44% of CRNAs practicing in urban settings. This reinforces the contributions of CRNAs to the care of rural and medically underserved citizens. The Rand study reported the average annual salary for an anesthesiologist to be $337,551, versus $151,380 for a CRNA, reinforcing the cost-effectiveness of nurse anesthetists (Daugherty, Fonseca, Kumar, et al., 2010).

A recent paper (Epstein & Dexter, 2012) has noted that anesthesia groups may wish to decrease the supervision ratio for nontrainee providers (e.g., CRNAs). Because hospitals offer many first-case starts and focus on starting these cases on time, the number of anesthesiologists needed is sensitive to this ratio. The number of operating rooms that an anesthesiologist can supervise concurrently is determined by the probability of multiple, simultaneous, critical portions of cases requiring the presence and availability of cross coverage. The authors conducted a simulation study that demonstrated peak occurrence of critical portions during first cases and frequent supervision lapses. These predictions were tested using actual data from an anesthesia information management system. The practical implication of this research is that it is logistically difficult for anesthesiologists supervising concurrent cases with the same start times to be physically present for the start of those cases. Depending on the billing arrangement, presence of an anesthesiologist for certain portions of a case may not be a requirement.

Using CRNAs to the full extent of their education allows for greater efficiencies in the delivery of safe and cost-effective anesthesia care. A growing body of outcomes research has demonstrated that full implementation of APNs, including CRNAs, is safe and cost-effective (Dulisse & Cromwell, 2010; Hogan et al., 2010).

CRNAs provide 32 million anesthetics annually in the United States (AANA, 2012d). In some rural settings, 100% of anesthesia, trauma stabilization, and obstetric anesthesia services are provided by nurse anesthetists. Without the services of CRNAs in rural communities, many small hospitals would close, leaving few alternatives for health care. Some rural CRNAs have completed additional training in the management of acute and chronic pain and offer services such as pain clinics so that patients do not have to travel to distant centers for pain treatment. CRNAs have traditionally provided anesthesia to rural and medically underserved populations. Academic medical centers and government-operated facilities rely heavily on nurse anesthetists. Many CRNAs practice in the VA hospital system, dealing with high-acuity patients undergoing complex surgical procedures. The military relies heavily on and actively recruits nurse anesthetists. A CRNA may be the only provider on a naval vessel. This essential access to anesthesia care for military men and women is part of nurse anesthesia history, dating back to the Civil War. In combat zones, knowledge of regional anesthesia and the ability to practice autonomously enable the CRNA to respond capably to mass casualty situations, in which many trauma victims require anesthesia simultaneously (AANA, 2012d).

American Association of Nurse Anesthetists

Organization and Structure

The AANA was among the first nursing specialty organizations. At a 1931 regional nurse anesthesia meeting, AANA founder Agatha Hodgins described her vision of the essential elements for a national nurse anesthesia organization (Thatcher, 1953, p. 183):

> Improvement of the present situation is in the hands of the nurse anesthetists themselves. If the work is to be properly safeguarded and hoped-for progress attained, it is necessary that remedies be applied to certain conditions now acknowledged to exist. It would seem that the first step should be the awakening of deeper interest and the development of constructive leadership. Following in logical order would be: self-organization as a special division of hospital service ... educational standards, post-graduate schools of anesthesia ... required to conform to an accepted criterion of education; state registration, putting right the nurse anesthetist to practice her vocation beyond criticism; constant effort toward improving the quality of work by means of study and research, thus affording still greater protection to the patient; [and] dissemination of information gained through proper channels.

Early efforts of nurse anesthetists to affiliate with the American Nurses Association (ANA) were not successful, because each organization had different ideas of what such an affiliation would entail (Gunn, 1991; Thatcher, 1953). With time, the breach between nursing and nurse anesthesia has narrowed considerably. Since its inception as the National Association of Nurse Anesthetists (NANA) in 1931, the AANA has placed its responsibilities to the public above or at the same level as its responsibilities to its membership. The association has produced education

and practice standards, implemented a certification examination for nurse anesthetists in 1945, and developed an accreditation process that was implemented in 1952. The AANA has been a leader in the formation of multidisciplinary councils with public representation to fulfill the autonomous credentialing functions of the profession, including accreditation, certification, and recertification.

When AANA founder Hodgins became ill, Gertrude Fife, who provided anesthesia for pioneering heart surgeon Claude Beck, assumed the role of developing NANA in its early days (Thatcher, 1953). The name of the association was changed to the American Association of Nurse Anesthetists in 1939. Helen Lamb, who served two terms as AANA president (1940-1942), provided anesthesia exclusively for Dr. Evarts Graham, one of the first modern thoracic surgeons (Bankert, 1989). The first anesthetic administered for the correction of tetralogy of Fallot was provided by a nurse anesthetist, Olive Berger, at Johns Hopkins Hospital. Early nurse anesthesia leaders were involved in complex practice settings with surgeons who were also influential in their fields. In addition to the development of a professional identity for nurse anesthesia, early nurse anesthetist leaders developed curricular standards for nurse anesthesia educational programs. These standards initially included a minimum program length of 6 months, with subsequent institution of mandatory certification and recertification policies.

The AANA Board of Directors oversees and governs the association in its efforts to be the pre-eminent association of anesthesia providers by putting patients first and taking a leadership role in policy making, nurse anesthesia education, and research to ensure high-quality, safe anesthesia. A number of committees and task forces support the work of the AANA. Several committees have student representatives.

Mission and Vision

The AANA mission statement is "advancing patient safety and excellence in anesthesia." The accompanying vision statement states that there are "recognized leaders in anesthesia care" (AANA, 2012b). The core values of the profession are integrity, professionalism, advocacy, and quality. The association seeks to support its members and protect patients. Current areas of activity for AANA are the following: safety and quality, including safe injection practices; ensuring that state associations have the necessary resources to meet legislative and regulatory challenges; supporting members who seek to specialize in pain management through post-graduate education; and policy advocacy activities (AANA, 2012a).

Nongovernmental regulation of nurse anesthesia practice is closely monitored by AANA. It is related to the activities of TJC, Accreditation Association for Ambulatory Health Care, and other agencies whose policies may affect nurse anesthesia practice.

Reimbursement issues related to Medicare, Medicaid, and other payers are also closely monitored by AANA, because changes in reimbursement can have a major impact on earnings. An example of this is the proposed 29% reduction in Medicare reimbursement. The AANA also provides members with resources on how to start a business, contracts, reimbursement, practice models, management and staffing, pain management, and disability. Practice trends monitored by the AANA include pain management and scope of practice issues. Provision of sedation and analgesia, including propofol, by nonanesthesia providers, is closely monitored by AANA. Other areas in which the AANA provides support to its members include strategies to address workplace harassment, expert witness identification, development of skills and resources for the possibility of mass casualty events, and bioterrorism situations.

An AANA subsidiary, AANA Insurance Services, provides malpractice coverage for many nurse anesthetists. Trends monitored by this agency include the decreasing number of insurers covering CRNAs and all health care providers. The remaining insurers are being more selective about whom they cover. Consequently, malpractice liability insurance premiums have increased. The principal insurer for CRNAs who need to obtain coverage, as opposed to those who work for self-insured entities, is now CNA Insurance. Applicants must meet underwriting guidelines and criteria.

The AANA closely monitors trends in patient safety and malpractice litigation. There are numerous continuing education meetings across the country that discuss patient safety topics, which is integral to the mission of the association. Reinforcing the 11 standards of care described in the *Scope and Standards for Nurse Anesthesia Practice* (AANA, 2010b), such as performing preanesthesia assessments, routine use of pulse oximetry, and end-tidal carbon dioxide monitoring, is central to these presentations.

Relationships within Nursing

AANA is represented at meetings of many nursing organizations, including the ANA, American Association of Colleges of Nursing (AACN), and National League for Nursing (NLN). CRNAs have played leadership roles in the development of the advanced practice registered nurse (APRN) Consensus Model, which includes state-level determination of the following:

- APRN legal scope of practice
- Recognized roles and titles of APRNs
- Criteria for entry into advanced practice

- Certification examinations for entry-level competence assessment (National Council of State Boards of Nursing [NCSBN], 2012)

Representatives of the AANA, ANA, Association of Perioperative Registered Nurses (AORN), and the International Council of Nurses frequently attend meetings of these nursing organizations, fostering cross-disciplinary collaboration. AANA is a long-time member of the Federation of Specialty Nursing Organizations (Author, 1980). CRNAs were involved in the development of the second edition of the ANA's *Scope and Standards of Practice.*

International Practice Opportunities

The International Federation of Nurse Anesthetists (IFNA) was founded in 1989 by 11 countries in which nurse anesthetists were educated and practiced. IFNA now has over 30 member countries. The IFNA mission "is dedicated to the precept that its members are committed to the advancement of educational standards and practices which will advance the art and science of anesthesiology and thereby support and enhance quality anesthesia care worldwide" (IFNA, 2012). The IFNA establishes and maintains effective cooperation with institutions that have a professional interest in nurse anesthesia. The IFNA vision is to be "the authoritative voice for nurse anesthetists and nurse anesthesia, supporting and enhancing quality anesthesia care worldwide…" (IFNA, 2012). IFNA seeks to "serve as the authoritative voice of nurse anesthesia internationally; to provide a means of communication among nurse anesthetists throughout the world; to promote the independence of the nurse anesthetist as a professional specialist in nursing" (IFNA, 2012). IFNA describes these organizational objectives (IFNA, 2012):

> To promote cooperation between nurse anesthetists internationally; to develop and promote educational standards in the field of nurse anesthesia; to develop and promote standards of practice in the field of nurse anesthesia; to provide opportunities for continuing education in anesthesia; to assist nurse anesthesia associations to improve the standards of nurse anesthesia and the competence of nurse anesthetists; to promote the recognition of nurse anesthesia; to establish and maintain effective cooperation between nurse anesthetists, anesthesiologists and other members of the medical profession, the nursing profession, hospitals and agencies representing a community of interest in nurse anesthesia.

IFNA member countries include European, Scandinavian, African and Asian nations. Since its inception in 1989, IFNA has developed Standards of Education,

Standards of Practice, Standards of Monitoring, and a Code of Ethics for Nurse Anesthetists. Model nurse anesthesia curricula have been developed, along with a recognition process for educational programs. IFNA was initially recognized as a professional resource group by the International Council of Nurses (ICN), and IFNA is currently an affiliate member of the ICN. Research findings have shown that nurse anesthetists participate in 80% of the anesthetics administered worldwide and are sole providers of 60% of the anesthetics (Ouellette & Horton, 2011).

Role Development and Measures of Clinical Competence

Horton (1998) conducted a comprehensive study of the views of CRNAs to determine implicit and explicit ideas about the culture of nurse anesthetists. Dominant rules of behavior were identified. CRNAs identified two major domains of professional activity: (1) remaining active and vigilant in defending and maintaining practice rights; and (2) dedication to patient care. Demonstrating their dedication to patient care, CRNAs note the following as key elements of proactive patient care: individualized care, technology, touch, surveillance, vigilance, and honesty. Horton (1998) found that CRNA dominant values include autonomy, education, continuing education, achievement, group cohesiveness, identity as a CRNA, membership in the AANA, political activism, and technology.

The role of the nurse anesthetist encompasses many facets. Callahan (1994) has described a competency-based model for nurse anesthesia practice that demonstrated areas in which nurse anesthetists must strive to achieve competence. The unifying themes of caring, collaboration, communication, and technology were identified. Many of the characteristics of advanced practice nursing described in Chapter 3 are found in this model. Munguia-Biddle and colleagues (1990) defined components of the model and suggested that the process of care provided by nurse anesthetists uses a problem-solving model that uses assessment, analysis, planning, implementation, and evaluation in the complex decision making and actions that exemplify CRNA practice in the health care environment. They further defined lifelong learning as part of the nurse anesthesia process of care. This essential component reflects the changing nature of nurse anesthesia practice.

The advanced practice of nursing in the specialty of nurse anesthesia has special attributes that speak to the strength and uniqueness of the CRNA role in the provision of anesthesia care in the health environment (Fig. 18-1). Caring for the patient as a holistic being is an important tenet of CRNA professional behavior. CRNAs strive to be altruistic human beings, believing that caring

is essential to one's personal development (Munguia-Biddle, Maree, Klein, et al., 1990).

Collaboration between the nurse anesthetist and other members of the health care team takes place in separate and joined activities and responsibilities directed at attaining mutual goals of excellence in patient care. Communication is sharing information to achieve mutual understanding. Communication skills are a cornerstone of patient interviews, imparting information to other health professionals, documentation of practice, and participation as a contributory member in meeting society's health needs. Technology denotes an area rich in advances and scientific content that requires strengthening and updating throughout the CRNA's professional life. Practitioners have the ability to apply the nursing process to complex problems at a high level of competence (Munguia-Biddle, et al., 1990).

The process of care for nurse anesthetists parallels the nursing process and emphasizes the importance of this approach to comprehensive anesthesia care following the model and its components. CRNA practice is based on the APN competencies found in Chapter 3. Some of these competencies are discussed here and in the three exemplars of CRNA practice.

Direct Clinical Practice

Anesthesia services can facilitate diagnosis, as in the case of the so-called curare test for myasthenia gravis. Anesthesia as a therapeutic modality is seen in the treatment of acute and chronic pain; it is also used in psychiatry for conducting interviews under the influence of ultra–short-acting IV barbiturates and for accelerated detoxification of opioid-dependent patients. However, the most common use of anesthesia resources is for the administration of surgical anesthesia. CRNAs select, obtain, or administer the anesthetics, adjuvant drugs, accessory drugs, and fluids necessary to manage the anesthesia, maintain physiologic homeostasis and correct abnormal responses to anesthesia or surgery (AANA, 2010b). When these APNs perform these activities, they are legally recognized to be providing anesthesia services on request, not to be prescribing as defined by federal law. Since the advent of legislated prescriptive authority for CRNAs and other APNs, these providers can prescribe legend and, in some cases, Schedules II through V controlled substances. However, this authority varies from state to state.

Patient monitoring is another vital area in which CRNAs participate. Nurse anesthetists select, apply, and insert appropriate noninvasive and invasive monitoring modalities for collecting and interpreting physiologic data. These activities are all recognized components of anesthesia services performed on request by CRNAs and

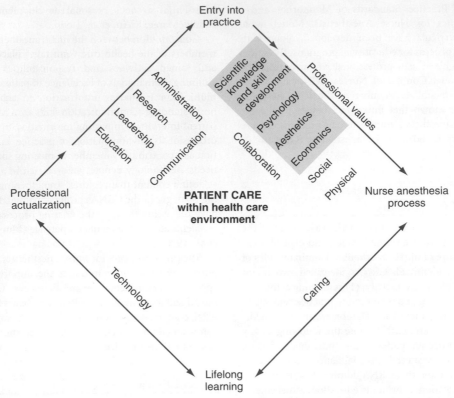

FIG 18-1 Nurse Anesthesia Practice Model. *(From Munguia-Biddle, F., Maree, S., Klein, E., Callahan, L., & Gilles, B. (1990). Nurse anesthesiology competence evaluation: Mechanism for accountability [unpublished document]. Park Ridge, IL: American Association of Nurse Anesthetists.)*

are not prescriptive. Criteria for the use of invasive monitors and who places them vary by institution and geographic region. Professional fees associated with the placement of devices such as pulmonary artery catheters at times leads to conflict over which practitioner—anesthetist or surgeon—will place invasive monitors and receive the associated reimbursement.

Nurse anesthesia practice also includes airway management, with modalities ranging from mask ventilation to placement of laryngeal mask airways or endotracheal intubation. CRNAs are knowledgeable about mechanical ventilation options and the pharmacologic support needed to maintain mechanical ventilation within and outside of the operating room. In some settings, these APNs are the sole providers of ventilator management oversight. A combination of technical skills required for airway management using a variety of instruments (e.g., rigid laryngoscope, fiberoptic bronchoscope, video laryngoscope [Glidescope]), and knowledge of respiratory anatomy and physiology and pharmacology are all important.

Clinicians continue to develop an array of approaches to sedation and analgesia for ventilator-dependent patients. Opportunities exist for collaborative research in this area (Weinert & Calvin, 2007). The expertise that CRNAs can provide in the management of ventilator-dependent patients includes reinforcing the need for appropriate sedation and analgesia when critically ill patients are mechanically ventilated. CRNAs can also help patients and families understand the rationale for procedures and treatments related to mechanical ventilation.

Nurse anesthetists manage emergence and recovery from anesthesia by selecting, obtaining, ordering, or administering medications, fluids, or ventilator support to maintain homeostasis, provide relief from pain and anesthesia side effects, and/or prevent or manage complications (AANA, 2010b). These activities also fall within the scope of providing anesthesia services and are not prescriptive in the traditional sense, such as writing a prescription that is filled by a pharmacist. Releasing or discharging patients from a postanesthesia care area can be performed by the CRNA. Providing postanesthesia follow-up evaluation and care related to anesthetic side effects or complications are other CRNA direct care functions.

Regional anesthesia is used by many CRNAs in the management of surgical anesthesia, labor pain, and postoperative pain. CRNAs are increasingly involved with pain management services. The use of epidural analgesic infusions and patient-controlled analgesia has greatly contributed to the effective treatment of preventable pain. Nurse anesthetists often have a role in the formulation of protocols and staff education when acute pain treatment regimens are introduced.

Anesthesia services are frequently used in obstetrics for providing analgesia and anesthesia to women in labor. Regional anesthesia and applied pharmacology have greatly advanced obstetric anesthesia, which in the past relied on systemic drugs that could cause neonatal depression. Epidural analgesia has become increasingly common for vaginal and cesarean section delivery, often obviating the need for general anesthesia and its attendant risks. In addition to using regional anesthesia in obstetric and postpartum settings, CRNAs have long worked collaboratively with other clinicians in these areas to manage intrapartum and postpartum pain with various pharmacologic and nonpharmacologic modalities (Faut Callahan & Paice, 1990).

Nurse anesthetists respond to emergency situations by providing airway management skills and implementing basic and advanced life support techniques. These APNs can provide leadership in these settings, away from the operating room, reinforcing the need to apply nationally promulgated standards of anesthesia care. An example of one of these standards of care is the measurement of end-tidal carbon dioxide to rule out esophageal intubation (AANA, 2010b). Nurse anesthetists are bound by the standards of practice adopted by their specialty.

Palliative Care

CRNAs possess expert skills in pain and symptom management. Building on experience in acute and critical care nursing, nurse anesthetists have extensive experience with end-of-life care. CRNAs value the close relationship that develops with patients and their families in the critical care environment and may develop close relationships with patients for whom they care during complex surgeries related to serious illness. The knowledge, skills, and experiences of CRNAs have made them uniquely qualified to assist with palliative and end-of-life care (Callahan, Breakwell, & Suhayda, 2011). Not typically a part of CRNA practice, there has been recent interest in exploring this area of care.

There are tremendous gaps in palliative and end-of-life care resources that have been identified by the IOM

(2003), most notably in rural areas. Over the past decade, there have been many efforts to identify gaps and develop strategies to fill them (AACN, 2012; Emanuel, 2012; End of Life/Palliative Education Resource Center [EPERC], 2012; Hospice Association of America, 2012; National Hospice and Palliative Care Organization [NHPCO], 2012). Those in need of palliative and end-of-life care often do not receive adequate care by qualified providers (Hospice Association of America, 2012; NHPCO, 2012). CRNAs are beginning to explore this area of practice.

CRNAs have many skills needed to participate in palliative care but do not typically work in these settings. CRNAs' extensive knowledge in pain and symptom management could enhance existing or new palliative care practices. CRNAs, especially those who have recently entered anesthesia practice and have current critical care knowledge and experience with palliative care, may embrace this additional form of patient care because it provides them an opportunity to develop long-term relationships with patients.

Student registered nurse anesthetists have reported an interest in this type of patient care and noted that they are often asked by families about plans of treatment and resources available to them (Callahan, Breakwell, & Suhayda, 2011). After taking an interdisciplinary palliative care course, student nurse anesthetists demonstrate significant knowledge in all domains of palliative care.

In many rural settings, 100% of anesthesia is delivered by CRNAs. These are the same communities that often do not have palliative and end-of -life services. Recognition of the experience of CRNAs and the knowledge and skills they develop in pain and symptom management may lead to an increase in providers who can assist with the significant gap in palliative care services in the United States.

Collaboration

As with other advanced practice nursing roles, nurse anesthesia practice is based on a collaborative model. Collaboration, one of the seven APN competencies described in Chapter 3, is defined as a dynamic process in which individuals interact with genuine intent to inform each other and solve problems to achieve outcomes. Every day, CRNAs collaborate with other nurses, APNs, physicians, physician assistants, and technicians. Partnerships are formed that provide the best care to patients. Collaborative practice has been described as the practice of forming partnerships to accomplish care for patients. Baggs, (1997) has identified six critical elements in physician-nurse collaborative practice—cooperation, assertiveness, shared decision making, communication, planning together, and coordination. As noted earlier, the IOM report on the *Future of Nursing* (2010) calls for nurses to be full partners with physicians and other health professionals in redesigning health care in the United States. This is a logical extension of collaboration from the bedside to the health care policy level.

Nurse anesthetists first formed collaborative relationships with surgeons in the late nineteenth century. At the request of surgeons, nurses were called on to administer anesthesia because of the then high surgical and anesthetic mortality rates. Today, approximately 80% of nurse anesthetists collaborate with physicians–consultant anesthesiologists in daily practice. There are no statutory requirements for the supervision of nurse anesthetists by anesthesiologists. Therefore, CRNAs also legally collaborate with surgeons, podiatrists, and dentists. There is no increased legal liability for surgeons who collaborate with CRNAs because CRNAs are responsible for their own actions.

CRNAs collaborate with other physicians by sharing their patient assessments and plan for anesthesia care. At the same time, collaboration occurs with the patient, so a mutually agreeable anesthetic plan can be developed; procedures, risks, and benefits associated with the anesthetic are discussed. Nurse anesthesia services are always provided in collaboration with the operating physician, dentist, podiatrist, or consultant anesthesiologist, which has proved to be a beneficial collaborative practice model.

Guidance and Coaching

Because surgery and diagnostic procedures are performed primarily on an outpatient or same-day admission basis, CRNAs are challenged to develop a rapport with their patients rapidly and develop a mutually agreed on plan for anesthesia care. Part of the development of the anesthesia plan involves the CRNA coaching the patient and family. The anesthetic options for the involved surgery or procedure need to be thoroughly discussed, along with the associated risks and benefits. This process can involve teaching the patient and family about postoperative analgesic options and coaching patients to avail themselves of the full benefits of the analgesic regimen, whether the treatment for pain entails patient-controlled epidural or IV analgesia.

Patients who undergo outpatient surgery receive coaching from CRNAs about activity, dietary limitations, and use of postoperative analgesics. Patients and their families in these situations also need coaching about when it may be appropriate for them to contact the office of the surgical or anesthesia provider.

Families of infants and children who undergo surgery and anesthesia need to be coached by the CRNA regarding the assessment and management of pain, postoperative nausea, and vomiting. Parameters for advancing activity and diet need to be clearly conveyed to the family or caregiver as part of this coaching process.

Consultation

Clinical consultations provided by CRNAs include interactions with other clinicians regarding pain management in postoperative patients. In some settings, CRNAs provide guidance in the area of sedation and analgesia for ventilator-dependent patients and management of respiratory care, including ventilator settings, and selection of vasoactive medications for critically ill patients.

In Exemplar 18-1, the CRNA, JR, has a practice focused on the assessment and treatment of acute and chronic pain. In her consultative role, she provides interventional pain management services to a wide array of clients.

CRNAs who serve as clinical managers or administrators of educational programs, frequently consult with colleagues in similar positions. Members of the CRNA educator community often are generous sharing curricular or policy information with colleagues.

Some CRNAs serve as expert witnesses in medical malpractice actions. This consultation activity helps legal counsel determine whether the actions of a defendant CRNA comport with the applicable standards of anesthesia care. CRNAs also serve as editors and editorial reviewers for peer-reviewed journals. In these roles, CRNAs advise colleagues on information ranging from the suitability for publication of an unsolicited manuscript and recommend additions, deletions, or corrections of submitted papers. Also, CRNAs serve as peer reviewers for traineeship grants submitted to the Health Resources and Services Administration. Some CRNAs with active programs of research sit on grant review panels of the National Institutes of Health.

As on-site reviewers for the COA, or other programmatic or institutional accreditation agencies, CRNAs have opportunities to serve as consultant evaluators. Those who have been involved as on-site reviewers frequently express satisfaction with participation in this peer review process.

Evidence-Based Practice

Research is a core APN competency that is valued by CRNAs. Nurse anesthetists have long advocated the use of evidence in their daily practice but, to date, have not accumulated a large body of research-based literature. However, recent outcomes research has confirmed the high quality and reasonable cost of anesthesia services provided by CRNAs (Dulisse & Cromwell, 2010; Hogan et al., 2010). The AANA publishes evidence-based position statements that address practice issues, which can be found in the

AANA *Professional Practice Manual* (AANA, 2010d). This includes the following content:

- Scope and Standards for Nurse Anesthesia Practice
- Standards for Office-Based Anesthesia Practice
- Postanesthesia Care Standards for the Certified Registered Nurse Anesthetist
- Guidelines for Core Privileges for Certified Registered Nurse Anesthetists
- Guidelines for the Management of the Obstetrical Patient for the Certified Registered Nurse Anesthetists
- Guidelines for Expert Witnesses

The *Professional Practice Manual* also contains supporting documents for anesthesia practice, as well as position statements that AANA has promulgated, such as on the administration of sedation for endoscopy procedures and intraoperative use of consciousness monitoring technology:

- Documenting the Standard of Care: The Anesthesia Record
- Informed Consent in Anesthesia
- Infection Control Guide for Certified Registered Nurse Anesthetists
- Latex Allergy Protocol
- Management of Waste Anesthetic Gases

Nurse anesthetists have been adopting the principles of evidence-based practice and teaching advocated by the IOM (Grenier & Knebel, 2003). Nurse anesthesia education and practice reflect patient-centered care, delivered by an interdisciplinary team. Nurse anesthetists are increasingly using the best available evidence when planning and implementing anesthesia care. CRNAs are also committed to quality improvement and the use of data to improve practice and education. Anesthesia practice involves competencies in technology and informatics; CRNAs use these information systems to support and improve patient care. Nurse anesthesia educational programs and continuing education opportunities emphasize the critical evaluation of clinical and research databases that can be used as clinical decision support resources (Kremer, 2011).

CRNAs have written seminal evidence-based texts that provide the foundation for practice. *Nurse Anesthesia*, now in its fourth edition, is a comprehensive compendium of topics ranging from scientific foundations to practice-related technology and intraoperative management (Nagelhout & Plaus, 2010). *Pharmacology for Nurse Anesthesiology*, a text written by CRNAs, is used in many nurse anesthesia programs (Ouellette & Joyce, 2011). *Case Studies in Nurse Anesthesia* (Elisha, 2011) is a valuable resource for students and clinicians. The text of record for professional issues in nurse anesthesia is *A Professional Study and Resource Guide for the CRNA* (Foster & Faut Callahan, 2011). Major content areas in this text include the essence of professionalism, understanding the responsibilities of clinical practice, the health care environment, the politics of health care, and challenges in professional practice.

The *AANA Journal* routinely publishes evidence-based continuing education courses on key topics of importance to the overall mission of promoting patient safety. CRNAs are increasingly making contributions to peer-reviewed literature through case studies, review articles, reports of research findings, and continuing education courses. The common theme is emphasis on continued competency, patient safety, and the development of scholarship, consistent with the values described by Horton (1998). As scholarly publications authored by CRNAs proliferate, useful data-based information is shared that benefits practice.

Accountability and Ethics

CRNAs are legally liable for the quality of the services that they render (Blumenreich, 2007). They make independent judgments and decisions about the appropriateness of their professional services and the probable effects of those services on the patient. A CRNA who believes that the anesthesia care plan for a particular patient is inappropriate should seek consultation for more appropriate direction. CRNAs should be patient advocates and always seek resolution to these and other ethical issues. If reasonable doubt continues, it is the responsibility of the CRNA to consider withdrawal from rendering the service, provided that the well-being of the patient is not jeopardized. The expected behaviors associated with CRNAs are found in the AANA's "Code of Ethics for the Certified Registered Nurse Anesthetist" in the *Professional Practice Manual* (AANA, 2010d).

Bosek (2011) has noted that "ethical situations require CRNAs to consider professional and personal values, think about what is the right thing to do, identify options, and act upon the selected 'right' option" (p. 501). This nurse ethicist believes that nonmaleficence, or to "do no harm," is a fundamental goal that should guide the actions of CRNAs. In concert with the values identified by Horton (1998), Bosek (2011) has indicated that advocating for the welfare of patients is a responsibility that CRNAs must uphold.

Leadership

Nurse anesthesia has grown and prospered as an advanced practice nursing specialty because of the clinical competence and leadership demonstrated by generations of

CRNAs. Despite challenges from organized medicine and initial lack of acceptance by the ANA, CRNAs were undeterred in their forward movement. The leadership provided by nurse anesthetists in the clinical area (see American Association of Nurse Anesthetists above), along with dedication to a rigorous credentialing process and health care policy activism, accounts for achievements such as the attainment of billing rights under Medicare Part B in 1989.

The clinical expertise demonstrated by Alice Magaw at the Mayo Clinic and Agatha Hodgins on the battlefields of France during the World War I resulted in leadership roles for these women, whose anesthetic techniques were taught to physicians and nurses from around the world. Military CRNAs also provided leadership in the development of rigorous, didactically front-loaded curricula that prepared military nurses to provide anesthesia as new graduates in austere environments (Gunn, 1991; Horton, 2007).

CRNA leadership often involves participation in elected and appointed positions at the local, regional, and national levels. At the local level, CRNAs may serve on or chair committees in the clinical and/or academic areas in which they practice. The level of responsibility shouldered by CRNAs in the clinical area provides skills in rapid information processing, and decision making, which may be helpful in governance activities, such as committees. In Exemplar 18-2, CRNA FM demonstrates leadership in his practice group and across the clinical settings for which his anesthesia group provides clinical services.

Exemplars

The following exemplars explain how CRNAs use the APN competencies to enact their APN role. The direct care competency is central to CRNA practice and the exemplars show the importance of the other six supporting competencies for successful implementation of the CRNA APN role.

The CRNAs in these exemplars demonstrate qualities shared by many of their professional predecessors. They are practice-setting leaders, teachers, and risk takers. Their willingness to push conventional practice limits ultimately advances the profession. These exemplars illustrate the implementation of the APN competencies described in Chapter 3 and Part II.

Reimbursement

Reimbursement is one of the most complex aspects of anesthesia practice. From the inception of this specialty through the 1950s, CRNAs were often paid as employees of the surgeon or hospital that employed them. In rural areas, CRNAs often contracted with hospitals to provide services based on fee-for-service structures—that is, a set amount of compensation per case as opposed to a straight salary for hours worked. The advent of private payers such as Blue Cross-Blue Shield has led to the compensation of only physicians and hospitals through these plans. Other health care providers, such as nurse anesthetists, psychologists, and physical therapists, would submit charges to the hospital or treating physician. The hospital or physician would then obtain reimbursement for these services as incident to their own and pass this on to the nonreimbursed provider.

In the 1980s, escalating health care costs caused Medicare to institute a prospective payment system (PPS). This legislation initially affected only Medicare Part A (hospital costs), and subsequently also affected Medicare Part B (physician and nonphysician costs). PPS legislation mandated a fixed payment rate for all hospital care, covering Part A services paid to hospitals based on the diagnosis-related classification group (DRG) of the patient. This fixed rate was to cover all costs associated with hospital admission, including services provided by nonphysician health care providers. CRNAs were in great jeopardy under this system. In their cost-cutting efforts, hospitals had no incentive to hire CRNAs, because the related employment costs would come directly from the hospital DRG payment. Congress inadvertently created reimbursement disincentives for the use of CRNAs while bolstering incentives to use anesthesiologists. AANA lobbying efforts resulted in the Health Care Financing Administration (HCFA), now the Centers for Medicare & Medicaid Services (CMS), rewriting portions of this legislation, enabling all CRNAs to obtain Medicare reimbursement or to sign over their billing rights to their employer (Broadston, 2001).

Historically, anesthesia charges have been based on direct time involvement as a charge for simple time or as a charge based on a combination of time and the complexity of the anesthetic procedure. The resource-based relative value scale (RBRVS), developed in the 1960s, is used to determine anesthesia charges based on the complexity of a surgical procedure. The result is charges for base units, or surgical procedures described by anatomic or functional units. Additional modifier units can be added to base units for factors such as emergency procedures, extremes of age, or anesthetic risk. After adding base and modifier units, time units are calculated at one unit per 15 minutes. The value of time units is determined by the payer, such as Medicare or Blue Cross-Blue Shield, and the market. The total of base, modifier, and time units determines the professional fee for administration of anesthesia. One unit of anesthesia time may be billed at from $15 to more than $70.

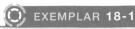

JR has been a practicing CRNA for 17 years. The strongest influences in her professional development are "believing in our profession, my knowledge, skills and competencies, while seizing any and all opportunities for professional advancement that crossed my path."

Her interest in nurse anesthesia was stimulated by early exposure to the CRNA role. Her father was an otolaryngologist who practiced in a Midwestern city with a population of 60,000. At the hospital in which he practiced, there were three anesthesiologists and a CRNA on staff. At that time, the surgeons were allowed to post their cases to the surgery schedule and choose the anesthesia provider. Most of the time, JR's father chose the CRNA to provide anesthesia care for his patients. He stated that the CRNA had excellent skills and was wonderful with pediatric patients.

JR has practiced as a staff CRNA in a large physician-owned anesthesia group with 11 physicians and 26 CRNAs in the Midwest. She has also been a hospital-employed chief CRNA for an obstetric anesthesia practice involving three network hospitals in another Midwestern city. Most recently, her practice has moved into the realm of interventional pain management for a neurosurgical group. Her time currently is divided among direct patient care (80%), teaching (10%), administration (5%), and professional activities (5%). JR acknowledges that working as an employee of a large neurosurgical group in an office-based interventional pain practice is very unique. AANA 2011 member survey data have shown that 2% of responding CRNAs work in pain management (AANA, 2012a). CRNA involvement in this specialty has been contested in multiple states by other providers.

JR's current practice developed following an initial contact by another APN who was employed by the neurosurgical group, demonstrating the value of professional networking. JR was asked to meet with the group to discuss a practice opportunity. The group was interested in hiring a CRNA to reopen an interventional pain clinic that had been closed for over a year. JR was contacted because of her experience with regional anesthesia and her leadership activities in her state nurse anesthesia association. After she met with the physician who championed this effort, she was interested in accepting the challenge. The position "gave me an incredible opportunity for cl... felt this was a perfect example of ... cial in an area outside the tradition... and I strongly setting." ... are beneficial ...

A typical day in JR's practice begins w... ng room review of her schedule and a safety check of equick and medications. Her day usually consists of a mixt... of diagnostic and therapeutic interventional procedu..., such as epidural steroid injections, nerve root block... joint blocks, trigger point injections, and lumbar discography.

"In our pain clinical, a patient checks in at the front desk and an escort assesses his or her vital signs and brings them to an exam room. A nurse will interview the patient, answer questions and obtain informed consent." During that time, JR "reviews the chart, imaging studies, assessment forms, and the order for treatment." She also interviews the patient prior to the procedure to answer questions or obtain additional information pertinent to the treatment plan before deciding on the type and targeted site of injection.

The patient is taken to the fluoroscopic suite and is prepped and draped under sterile technique. JR then performs a diagnostic or therapeutic injection under fluoroscopic guidance. The patient is assessed immediately after the injection and returned to the examination room for 30 minutes for observation. Prior to discharge, the patient is reassessed and information is recorded concerning the type and amount of pain relief provided by the injection. The patient is educated concerning the onset and duration of action of the injected medications and possible complications of the medication and injection and is given discharge and follow-up information.

JR describes the greatest challenges in her practice as "initially … obtaining the necessary knowledge, skills, and competencies to perform the procedures requested by the group that oversees me because there was no other employment situation identical to this practice. Overall, it is dealing with the political environment because there are physicians who feel a CRNA should not be providing pain management care."

JR's story demonstrates the value of professional collaboration, mentoring, networking, and organizational involvement. Her willingness to take risks and improve care elevates the profession.

EXEM... CRNA for 17 years. His initial inter-... ...ion was initiated by a family friend who ...nd who encouraged FM to pursue a career ...e anesthetist. The factors that have most ...ed FM in his professional development are his ...rests in a number of areas, including complex patho-physiology; matching anesthesia techniques to complex patient presentations, pharmacology, and the desire for autonomous practice. FM notes, "I get paid to do anesthesia!" This enthusiasm for his specialty is typical of many practicing CRNAs.

FM was an active duty military CRNA and practiced at several military medical centers. As a civilian CRNA, he moved into a group practice based at a rural critical access hospital and other facilities in the Midwest. He spends 90% of his time in direct patient care. Some of that time he oversees a student rotating through his facility, because he remains with the student and patient at all times. The balance of FM's time is spent "in the business of anesthesia," related to being part owner of his practice.

A typical day in FM's practice includes meeting in the group's office with colleagues for coffee at 6:00 AM. Following that, he prepares for anesthetics that he will administer that day. He then meets, interviews, plans, and administers the anesthetic for the first and subsequent cases of the day until the cases are done. If he is on call, he spends the afternoon in the preoperative clinic performing preoperative assessments and interventions for complex patients who will be coming to the operating room (OR) in the future.

Some of the unique aspects of FM's practice include autonomy and the use of regional anesthesia techniques. He and his practice partners were early adopters of ultrasound-guided regional block techniques, including interscalene and femoral nerve blocks. He enjoys the challenges of caring for high-acuity patients undergoing complex surgical procedures in a small community hospital.

FM describes the greatest challenges in his practice as "autonomy—having to make decisions while caring for very sick and complicated patients with no input from other anesthesia providers [and] the complexity of the patients and the procedures we are performing on them." He also notes that managing a very busy private practice anesthesia group is challenging, "ensuring that we cover all the surgeons and hospitals but at the same time protecting our staff from overwork."

The practice in which FM is a partner evolved from a small hospital-employed group of one anesthesiologist and two CRNAs. As the workload grew and more surgeons were added, the group grew larger. "We eventually ended up with three anesthesiologists and six CRNAs. Unfortunately, several members decided to move closer to family. At this point we decided to take advantage of the turmoil and go independent. We formed our own private practice group, a service corporation. We have been functioning like this for the last 9 years."

FM's military background provided knowledge about infrastructure and resources for personal and professional development that carried over into his later career. His CRNA practice partners are all former military CRNAs and their principal clinical site is a clinical affiliation site for military and civilian nurse anesthesia programs. FM has had extensive involvement with his state and national professional organizations and presents to these groups on clinical and nonclinical topics.

EXEMPLAR 18-3   **A Day in the Life of a Certified Registered Nurse Anesthetist**

KM has been a CRNA for 10 years. Prior to that, he worked as an RN in the emergency department of a busy city hospital in the Midwest, followed by 2 years of medical intensive care unit experience in a tertiary medical center. Since completing his nurse anesthesia program, KM has worked at a level I trauma center in a large Midwestern city. His case mix includes patients across the life span at all acuity levels. KM frequently works with students from a nearby nurse anesthesia program who rotate through his department. His work day is 10 hours a day but, with setup time and other activities, such as postoperative visits, the day can be closer to 12 hours. The CRNAs in this facility are unionized county employees.

KM and his colleagues receive their clinical assignments for the next day by 2 PM the preceding day. Some patients seek care at this public facility because they have no health insurance, but are otherwise healthy. Other patients are of markedly high acuity, with complex comorbid conditions, such as IV drug abuse, reactive airway disease, morbid obesity, and hypertension.

There are 20 operating rooms in this facility. On a given day, KM may do five cases if he is working in an area such as general surgery. If he is the trauma CRNA,

A Day in the Life of a Certified Registered Nurse Anesthetist *cont'd*

he will be assigned to patients from the trauma unit who have experienced blunt and/or penetrating trauma. Skills in airway management, vascular access, and volume resuscitation are essential for anesthesia providers who deal with trauma patients. When assigned to urology cases, KM may do up to 20 cases, mostly under spinal anesthesia, for that surgical service. KM enjoys the ability to provide care to high-acuity patients who undergo complex surgical procedures. He is able to use other regional anesthesia skills, including placement of thoracic epidural blocks and peripheral nerve block catheters. Many of the patients at this facility have challenging airway anatomy, so KM has become skilled at placing endotracheal tubes in sedated using fiberoptic bronchoscopy, a safe technique.

KM values collegial relationships with and other CRNAs with whom he works. Areas would like to see change are the turnover time bhe cases, which is longer than in the private sector, compensation, which lags behind that of private practice. However, the benefits associated with government employment exceed many of those available in the private sector.

KM is also an instructor in a nearby nurse anesthesia program. His day off is spent teaching and mentoring students in this program.

A conversion factor is a dollar amount per unit used to convert the relative value scale intensity measurement into an actual charge for services. Medicare publishes conversion factors annually. Private practices may charge three to four times the Medicare conversion factor. For calendar year 2011, the National Anesthesia Conversion factor determined by CMS was $21.05 (CMS, 2011). The gross charge for services provided is determined by multiplying the total procedure units by the conversion factor (Walker & Broadston, 2011). Many third-party payers, such as Medicare and some Blue Cross insurers, completely ignore the charges of the practitioner and determine payments from their own fee schedules. These payments are often determined by what providers charge on average for their services (Broadston, 2001; Walker & Broadston, 2011).

Medicare Part A provides pass-through funding to eligible rural and critical access hospitals for CRNA services. CRNAs cannot receive direct reimbursement from Medicare Part A. Medicare Part B provides direct reimbursement to CRNAs for anesthesia services. Key differences exist between reimbursement models using medical direction, medical supervision, and nonmedical direction. Many third-party payers, including state Medicaid, private insurers, and others use reimbursement mechanisms similar to those used by Medicare (Walker & Broadston, 2011).

Teaching CRNAs and teaching anesthesiologists have specific reimbursement considerations that influence the education of future anesthesia provides. There is no parity in the reimbursement for teaching cases involving physician residents versus student registered nurse anesthetists (Walker & Broadston, 2011). CRNAs receive national provider identification numbers that are used in the billing process. Billing services are frequently responsible for the generation of anesthesia charges, but anesthesia groups are responsible for ensuring accurate diagnosis and procedural coding on all submitted claims.

CRNAs can valuate their clinical and financial outcomes through data collected, often by billing services, over specified time periods (e.g., monthly, quarterly, or annually). The total number of anesthetics administered during the specified time frame needs to be determined. Then, the total number of relative value units generated is calculated by multiplication of the total number of anesthetics administered by the average number of relative value units per case, which might be 10.5 units. The surgical case mix, payer mix, and breakdown need to be determined—for example, 15% commercial, 35% Medicare, 10% Medicaid. Finally, the specific reimbursement rates per relative value unit per section of the case mix–payer mix are calculated. Payer mix will vary with practice settings; this information is helpful as part of the assessment of a potential new practice setting (Broadston, 2001).

Attempts to control spiraling health care costs and improve access to care have resulted in the development of managed care contracts and resurgent interest in health maintenance organizations (HMOs), with capitated payment schemes. Fee-for-service reimbursement structures may become less common because of the imposition of additional cost containment measures by payers and the national economy. Unfortunately, cost containment in health care does not ensure client access to APNs based on cost-effectiveness. Transition mechanisms in vertical integration strategies, such as combining payers, providers, and a wide spectrum of network services, still focus on physicians and hospitals as the principal health care resources.

There are ongoing efforts by CMS to reduce reimbursement to providers under Medicare. In 2006, Medicare anesthesia reimbursement decreased by 8.6%. Currently,

...ding to decrease Medicare anesthesia ... by 29%. Although that may not be ... a pro... ...amount by which anesthesia reimbursement reim... ...it can be expected that payments will not the... ...the same level.

...ealth care providers receive additional payment ...tives in exchange for reporting quality measures to ...dicare. Providers who report specified quality mea-...sures to Medicare obtain an additional 1.5% incentive payment. These quality measures include the maintenance of perioperative normothermia, appropriate timing of prophylactic preoperative antibiotics, and pain manage-ment planning.

Currently, anesthesiologists can bill for 100% of physi-cian reimbursement on each case when supervising two concurrent cases. In settings in which nonmedically directed CRNAs supervise two nurse anesthesia students concurrently, the nonmedically directed CRNA can also bill for 100% on each case. However, in a scenario that may be more common, if an anesthesiologist is supervis-ing two CRNAs who are in turn each supervising two student registered nurse anesthetists, the anesthesiologist can only bill for 50% on each of the four concurrent cases and the CRNAs would receive only 50% of the anesthesia fee provided (Walker & Broadston, 2011). This creates a disincentive for organizations to support nurse anesthesia education. From a policy perspective, it is desirable that the Medicare anesthesia payment rules treat CRNAs and anesthesiologists similarly.

Future of Reimbursement

There is speculation that changes in anesthesia reimburse-ment, driven by legislation and market economics, may result in payment being limited to the services of one provider. This has generated concern among some in this specialty that graduates of all nurse anesthesia programs will need to have the knowledge, skills, and abilities of a full-service provider, such as one who can work without a collaborating physician when they complete their edu-cational program. Although current accreditation and certification standards do not mandate that graduates of nurse anesthesia programs have the ability to function at this level when they graduate from an accredited program, proposed changes in reimbursement for health care ser-vices, such as the implementation of accountable care organizations (ACOs), need to be monitored so that the education and practice of CRNAs and other APNs adapt to a dynamic market.

ACOs are proposed as a new payment model under Medicare and foster pilot programs to extend the model to private payers and Medicaid. Proponents believe that ACOs will allow providers to work more effectively together to improve quality while decreasing spending.

The success of ACOs will depend on whether the CMS, private payers, and clinicians can collaborate on the development of a tightly linked performance measure-ment and evaluation framework that ensures account-ability to patients and payers and supports timely learning for key participants. A robust, comprehensive, and trans-parent performance measurement system that accurately accounts for the contributions of all clinicians will be necessary to assure the success of ACOs. Studies to date on the cost-effectiveness and safety of services provided by CRNAs should help ensure that CRNAs are represented in ACOs (Fisher & Shortell, 2010).

The proposed differences of ACOs over managed care include more knowledge, additional data, guidelines, and quality metrics, and more interdisciplinary collaboration. In 2012, there was more information available about health care costs than during the managed care era. Almost two thirds of health care costs are concentrated in 10% of patients so, to control costs, the focus will be on these patients, rather than the 50% of the population that is healthier and uses 3% of health care dollars. In the 1990s, managed care plans lacked data on outcomes, utilization, and overall costs. In contrast, it has been estimated that by the end of 2012, more than 40% of practitioners will use electronic health records (EHRs), a significant increase from 12% in 2009. Almost 100% of professionals and health care systems operating in ACOs or risk-based reimbursement models will be using EHRs, enabling smart predictive modeling, patient monitoring, and performance management of the delivery system. In the 1990s, there were few evidence-based guidelines for health care. Today, professional guidelines, pathways, and standards of practice have emerged (Emanuel, 2012).

The incentive for health care providers to implement ACOs successfully is that failure to control health care costs will likely result in Medicare payment reductions by the federal government (see earlier). Under such a sce-nario, providers may try to negotiate higher payment rates from private payers to compensate for lower Medicare rates. Although this scenario does not guarantee success-ful implementation of ACOs, looming, significant price reductions may result in focused efforts to contain costs through increased collaboration in the delivery of health care (Emanuel, 2012).

Continued Challenges

Nurse anesthesia has dealt with challenges since the incep-tion of the specialty. However, the number of CRNAs in the United States is now at an all-time high, which is a tribute to the safe, cost-effective care provided by these clinicians. Nurse anesthesia education has rapidly moved from certificate-level training to degree-granting institutions that initially offered baccalaureate and later master's- and doctorate-level programs.

Reimbursement will continue to be a significant challenge for CRNAs as the health care system continues to evolve. At this writing, proposed decreases of 29.5% to Medicare payments under the sustainable growth rate funding formula have been addressed, with short-term relief by the federal government. Medicare reimbursement is a significant portion of the payer mix in many clinical settings. Population demographics ensure that this trend will continue. In addition to affecting Medicare patients directly, these potential reimbursement reductions also affect all insurance plans whose rates are tied to Medicare, including the TRICARE plan for military personnel and their dependents (AANA, 2012g).

The potential effects of Medicare Part B payment reductions are significant. Although Medicare reimburses most physician services at 80% of market rates, Part B provides reimbursement for anesthesia services at about 45% of market rates. According to AANA member surveys, each CRNA on average provides anesthesia for about 900 cases per year. The potential exists for reductions in compensation for all anesthesia providers if decreases in Medicare reimbursement are enacted (AANA, 2012h).

Conclusion

Nurse anesthesia, the earliest nursing specialty, was also the first nursing specialty to have standardized educational programs, a certification process, mandatory continuing education, and recertification. Nurse anesthetists have been involved in the development of anesthetic techniques along with physicians and engineers. CRNAs have been nursing leaders in obtaining third-party reimbursement for professional services and in coping with challenges such as the prospective payment system, managed care, and physician supervision.

Nurse anesthetists provide surgical and nonsurgical anesthesia services in a variety of settings in the United States and other parts of the world. CRNAs work collaboratively with physicians, as do other APNs, and are capable of providing the full spectrum of anesthesia services.

Activism at the state and federal legislative and regulatory levels is a recognized CRNA activity. Increasing coalition building among nurse anesthetists, other APNs, and nursing educators is congruent with a shared nursing vision. This vision values health care for all Americans, provided in a safe and cost-effective manner by APNs collaborating with other health care professionals.

John F. Garde was a distinguished health care leader who served as AANA Executive Director from 1983 to 2001, and again on an interim basis from February 2009 until his untimely death in July 2009. A statement of his holds true today (Garde, 1998, p. 15):

> The profession has an optimistic future. I point out with pride the commitment that AANA members have toward the future of their profession—a commitment that encompasses being outstanding anesthesia practitioners who belong to their Association. I am reminded, too, what Dick Davidson, President of the American Hospital Association, said when asked about what will remain in health care 100 years from now: 'There will always be personal contact and caring. We will always have hands touching patients. Everything we do is about human need. That's the constant over time.' And, that is the legacy of the nurse anesthesia profession.

References

American Association of Colleges of Nursing (AACN). (2012). End-of-Life Nursing Education Consortium (ELNEC) fact sheet. (http://www.aacn.nche.edu/elnec/about/fact-sheet).

American Association of Nurse Anesthetists. (AANA). (2012a). AANA member survey data. (http://www.aana.com/myaana/AANABusiness/aanasurveys/Documents/aana-member-survey-data-nov2011.pdf).

American Association of Nurse Anesthetists. (AANA). (2012b). Who we are. (http://www.aana.com/aboutus/Pages/Who-We-Are.aspx).

American Association of Nurse Anesthetists. (AANA). (2012c). Federal supervision rule/opt-out information. (http://www.aana.com/advocacy/stategovernmentaffairs/Pages/Federal-Supervision-Rule-Opt-Out-Information.aspx).

American Association of Nurse Anesthetists. (AANA). (2012d). CRNAs and the AANA. (http://www.aana.com/forpatients/Documents/crnas_aana.pdf).

American Association of Nurse Anesthetists. (AANA). (2012e). Anesthesia: Practice of nursing and practice of medicine. (http://www.aana.com/advocacy/stategovernmentaffairs/Pages/Anesthesia-Practice-of-Nursing-and-Practice-of-Medicine.aspx).

American Association of Nurse Anesthetists. (AANA). (2012f). Professional practice division. (http://www.aana.com/myaana/ProfessionalPractice/Pages/default.aspx).

American Association of Nurse Anesthetists. (AANA). (2012g). Continuing education. (http://www.aana.com/ceandeducation/continuingeducation/Pages/default.aspx).

American Association of Nurse Anesthetists. (AANA). (2012h). Impact of proposed Medicare cuts (http://www.aana.com/advocacy/federalgovernmentaffairs/Pages/Medicare-Cuts.aspx).

American Association of Nurse Anesthetists. (AANA). (2010a). Quality of nurse anesthesia practice (http://www.aana.com/aboutus/Documents/qualitynap.pdf).

American Association of Nurse Anesthetists. (AANA). (2010b). Scope and standards for nurse anesthesia practice (http://www.aana.com/resources2/professionalpractice/Documents/PPM%20Scope%20and%20Standards.pdf).

American Association of Nurse Anesthetists. (AANA). (2010c). Sample application for clinical privileges (http://www.aana.com/myaana/ProfessionalPractice/Documents/PPM%20Application%20for%20Clinical%20Privileges.pdf).

American Association of Nurse Anesthetists. (AANA). (2010d). Professional practice manual (http://www.aana.com/myaana/ProfessionalPractice/Documents/PPM%20Table%20of%20Contents.pdf).

Baggs, J., Schmitt, M., Mushlin, A., Eldredge, D., Oakes, D., & Hutson, A. (1997). Nurse-physician collaboration and satisfaction with the decision-making process in three critical care units. American Journal of Critical Care, 6, 393–399.

Bankert, M. (1989). Watchful care: A history of America's nurse anesthetists. New York: Continuum.

Blumenreich, G. (2007). Another article on the surgeon's liability for anesthesia negligence. AANA Journal, 75, 89–93.

Bosek, M. (2011). Ethics and the CRNA. In S. Foster & M. Faut Callahan (Eds.), A professional practice guide for the CRNA. Park Ridge, IL: American Association of Nurse Anesthetists.

Broadston, L. (2001). Reimbursement for CRNA services. In S. Foster & M. Faut Callahan (Eds.), A professional practice guide for the CRNA. (pp. 58–65). Park Ridge, IL: American Association of Nurse Anesthetists.

Callahan, L. (1994). Establishing measures of competence. In S. Foster & L. Jordan (Eds.), Professional aspects of nurse anesthesia practice (pp. 275–290). Philadelphia: F.A. Davis.

Callahan, M. F., Breakwell, S., & Suhayda, R. (2011). Knowledge of palliative and end-of-life care by student registered nurse anesthetists. AANA Journal, 79(Suppl), S15–S20.

Centers for Disease Control and Prevention. (2010). National hospital discharge survey (http://www.cdc.gov/nchs/fastats/insurg.htm).

Centers for Medicare & Medicaid Innovation (2011). Anesthesia reimbursement (http://www.cms.gov/PhysicianFeeSched/downloads/AnesthesiaSharesCY2011.pdf).

Centers for Medicare & Medicaid Innovation. (2012). Graduate nurse education demonstration (http://innovation.cms.gov/initiatives/gne).

Council on Accreditation of Nurse Anesthesia Educational Programs. (COA). Accredited programs. (2012a). (http://home.coa.us.com/accredited-programs/Pages/default.aspx).

Council on Accreditation of Nurse Anesthesia Educational Programs. (COA). (2012b). Standards for accreditation of nurse anesthesia educational programs. (http://home.coa.us.com.).

Daugherty, L., Fonseca, R., Kumar, K., & Michaud, P. (2010). An analysis of the labor markets for anesthesiology. Santa Monica, CA: Rand Corporation.

Dulisse, B., & Cromwell, J. (2010). No harm found when nurse anesthetists work without supervision by physicians. Health Affairs, 29, 1469–1475.

Elisha S., (Ed.). (2011). Case studies in nurse anesthesia. Sudbury, MA: Jones & Bartlett.

Emanuel, E. J. (2012). Why accountable care organizations are not 1990s managed care redux. Journal of the American Medical Association, 307, 2263–2264.

End of Life/Palliative Education Resource Center (EPERC). (2012). Home page (http://www. eperc.mcw.edu/EPERC).

Epstein, R., & Dexter, F. (2012). Influence of supervision ratios by anesthesiologists on first-case starts and critical portions of anesthetics. Anesthesiology, 116, 683–691.

Faut Callahan, M. (1991). Graduate education for nurse anesthetists: Master's versus a clinical doctorate. In National Commission on Nurse Anesthesia Education report (pp. 110–115). Park Ridge, IL: American Association of Nurse Anesthetists.

Faut Callahan, M., & Paice, J. (1990). Post-operative pain control for the parturient. Journal of Perinatal and Neonatal Nursing, 4, 27–41.

Fisher, E., & Shortell, S. (2010). Accountable care organizations: Accountable for what, to whom, and how. Journal of the American Medical Association, 304, 1715–1716.

Foster S., & Faut Callahan M., (Eds.). (2011). A professional study and resource guide for the CRNA (2nd ed.). Park Ridge, IL: American Association of Nurse Anesthetists.

Garde, J. (1998). Annual report of the executive director. AANA News Bulletin, 52, 14–16.

Grenier, A., & Knebel, E. (2003). Health professions education: A bridge to quality. Washington, DC: National Academies Press.

Gunn, I. (1991). The history of nurse anesthesia education: Highlights and influences. In National Commission on Nurse Anesthesia Education Report (pp. 33–41). Park Ridge, IL: American Association of Nurse Anesthetists.

Health Resources and Services Administration (HRSA). (2012). Nursing funding opportunities (http://bhpr.hrsa.gov/nursing/index.html).

Hogan, P., Seifert, R., Moore, C., & Simonson, B. (2010). Cost effectiveness analysis of anesthesia providers. Nursing Economics, 28, 159–169.

Horton, B. (1998). Nurse anesthetists' perspectives on improving the anesthesia care of culturally diverse patients. Journal of Transcultural Nursing, 9, 26–33.

Horton, B. (2007). Upgrading nurse anesthesia educational requirements: Setting standards. AANA Journal, 75, 167–170.

Hospice Association of America. (2012). Directory (http://www.dmoz.org/Health/Medicine/Facilities/Hospice/North_America/United_States).

Institute of Medicine. (2010). The future of nursing: Leading change, advancing health (http://www.iom.edu/Reports/2010/The-Future-of-Nursing-Leading-Change-Advancing-Health.aspx).

Institute of Medicine. (2003). Improving palliative care for cancer: A summary report. (http://www.iom.edu/Reports/2003/Improving-Palliative-Care-for-Cancer-Summary-and-Recommendations.aspx).

International Federation of Nurse Anesthetists (IFNA). (2012). About IFNA. (http://www.ifna-int.org).

Jordan, L., & Shott, S. (1998). Feasibility of a doctoral degree for nurse anesthetists. *AANA Journal*, 66, 287–298.

Kaye, D., Scibetta, W., & Grogono, A. (1999). Anesthesia manpower and recruitment: An update. *Advances in Anesthesia*, 16, 1–27.

Kremer, M. (2011). Evidence-based practice and the CRNA. In S. Foster & M. Faut Callahan (Eds.), *A professional study and resource guide for the CRNA*. Park Ridge, IL: American Association of Nurse Anesthetists.

Maree, S. M. (1991). Report of the National Commission on Nurse Anesthesia Education. An analysis of the cost of nurse anesthesia programs. *AANA Journal*, 59, 577–580.

Mastropietro, C., Horton, B., Ouellette, S., & Faut Callahan, M. (2001). The National Commission on Nurse Anesthesia Education 10 years later. Part 1. The commission years (1989–1994). *AANA Journal*, 69, 379–385.

Merwin, E., Stern, S., & Jordan, L. (2008). Clinical faculty: Major contributors to the education of new CRNAs. *AANA Journal*, 76, 167–171.

Mungia-Biddle, F., Maree, S., Klein, E., Callahan, L., & Gilles, B. (1990). *Nurse anesthesiology competence evaluation: Mechanism for accountability [unpublished document]*. Park Ridge, IL: American Association of Nurse Anesthetists.

Nagelhout J., & Plaus K., (Eds). (2010). Nurse anesthesia. (4th ed.). St. Louis: Saunders Elsevier.

National Board for Certification and Recertification of Nurse Anesthetists (NBCRNA). About us. (2012). (http://www.nbcrna.com/about-us/Pages/Mission-and-Vision.aspx).

National Council of State Boards of Nursing. (2012). APRN consensus model. (http://www.ncbsn.org/aprn.htm).

National Hospice and Palliative Care Organization. (NHPCO). (2012). Position statement (http://www.nhpco.org/i4a/pages/index.cfm?pageid=3253).

On the Federation of Specialty Nursing Organizations and the American Nurses' Association. *AANA Journal*, 48, 113.

Ouellette, R., & Joyce, J. (2011). *Pharmacology for nurse anesthesiology*. Sudbury, MA: Jones & Bartlett.

Ouellette, S., & Horton, B. (2011). Toward globalization of a profession. *AANA Journal*, 79, 12–14.

Pine, M., Holt, K., & Lou, Y. (2003). Surgical mortality and type of anesthesia provider. *AANA Journal*, 71, 109–116.

Rand Health. (2010). Is there a shortage of anesthesia providers in the United States? (http://www.rand.org/pubs/research_briefs/RB9541/index1.html).

Simonson, D., Ahern, M., & Hendryx, M. (2007). Anesthesia staffing and anesthetic complications during cesarean delivery: A retrospective analysis. *Nursing Research*, 56, 9–17.

Thatcher, V. (1953). *History of anesthesia with emphasis on the nurse specialist*. Philadelphia: J.B. Lippincott.

U.S. Department of Health and Human Services (HHS). (2011). Patient Protection and Affordable Care Act. (http://www.healthcare.gov/law/full/index.html).

Walker, J., & Broadston, L. (2011). Reimbursement for CRNA services. In S. Foster, & M. Faut Callahan (Eds.), *A professional practice guide for the CRNA*. (pp 257–274). Park Ridge, IL: American Association of Nurse Anesthetists.

Weinert, C., & Calvin, A. (2007). Epidemiology of sedation and sedation adequacy for mechanically ventilated patients in a medical and surgical intensive care unit. *Critical Care Medicine*, 35, 635–637.

CHAPTER 19

Business Planning and Reimbursement Mechanisms

Charlene M. Hanson • *Sally D. Bennett*

CHAPTER CONTENTS

By virtue of their expanded knowledge and skill set built on a nursing framework, advanced practice nurses (APNs) are uniquely poised as effective alternatives to the traditional physician provider. Several factors in the national health care arena have coalesced to place APNs in an excellent position to offer direct care to their patients. The Institute of Medicine (IOM) report, *The Future of Nursing: Leading Change, Advancing Health* (2011), opened the door to remove barriers that impede APNs from practicing at the full scope of their knowledge and skill. The IOM report, coupled with the nursing and patient initiatives in the Patient Protection and Accountable Care Act (PPACA; U.S. Department of Health and Human Services [HHS], 2011) and the unfolding regulatory changes made possible by the Consensus Model for APRN Regulation (National Council of State Boards of Nursing [NCSBN], 2012), have made it possible for APNs

to practice in more broad-based venues than ever before. Also, doctoral education assists APNs in achieving the direct and indirect goals of care by enhancing their ability to design and deliver effective care (American Association of Colleges of Nursing [AACN], 2006). Enhanced leadership, policymaking, and collaboration skills will augment their ability to make positive change at the system and practice setting levels. The goal of this chapter is to prepare APN graduates for the business components of practice as owners of their own practice or as employees or contractors of service in the health care field.

In today's complex health care environment, communities and families need and demand health services beyond those that have been traditionally available. From the patient's perspective, services must be accessible and affordable. They must reach families who are caught in the web of disparities. From the payer's perspective, services

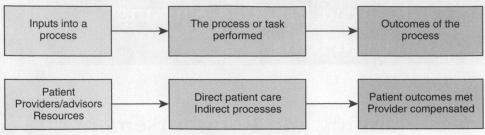

FIG 19-1 Flow charts of processes.

must be cost-effective. Both groups desire and demand high-quality health care services. Thus, the work of the health care system, and consequently the APNs practicing in it is, to give the right care, to the right person, at the right time, and to do this in an increasingly demanding environment. Many different processes contribute to this system, most of which may be classified as those related to direct patient care (with a clinical focus) or those that support the patient care process indirectly (with an administrative focus). Successful APNs develop, implement, and continuously analyze the direct and indirect processes of care used to meet patient outcomes while being cognizant of the other critical environmental elements that affect their practice. Success is measured by the ability of the APN, who uses these existing processes, to attain desired patient outcomes within the constraints of available resources and reimbursement.

One particular innovation in patient care settings that has been successful over time is the conceptualization and organization of the direct and indirect processes of patient care within the context of systems thinking (Colbert & Ogden, 2011; Reel & Abraham, 2007; Solberg, Kottke, Brekke, et al., 2000; Story, 2010). Simply put, any system represents the flow of resources through a process that results in the desired outcomes (Fig. 19-1). The size and complexity of the developed system depends on the number and complexity of processes being used to attain the desired outcome. Evaluation of any system includes assessment and evaluation of the resources used, processes used, and outcomes attained. One recent innovation to assist in this process is the health care dashboard (see later).

This chapter focuses on the process of APN business planning from a systems approach. Although the emphasis is on an APN-managed practice, all APNs, whether employers or employees, need to be aware that patient care delivery is conceptualized as comprising the direct and indirect care processes that ensure that available resources are allocated in a manner that meets desired patient outcomes. Business planning is in itself a process that focuses primarily on the development, implementation, and evaluation of those indirect processes that support patient care. It stands in contrast to a business plan, which is a document used by legal and financial advisors to evaluate the success potential of a particular business venture, such as an individual APN practice. The business plan may be conceptualized as an outcome or product of the business planning process. Reimbursement, as part of overall business planning, is another indirect process supporting patient care and is one of the critical elements affecting APN success. Examples and exemplars are provided to illustrate these essential concepts. It is important to note that much of the information discussed throughout this chapter changes from year to year. Federal, state, and professional websites contain the most current information and should be consulted for the latest changes.

Principles of Practice Management

Designing and Delivering Care to Patients

Success in and satisfaction with one's APN role revolves around the right match between APNs and the work they do and the ability to be flexible and innovative within the scope of that role. APNs' adaptability to the changing health care marketplace is one of their greatest strengths. As noted, APNs participate in direct and indirect care processes in any practice setting. Indirect processes include the steps taken to market the practice, register a patient, and collect demographics, the process of third-party billing, meeting regulatory, safety, and quality imperatives, and the interaction with medical, pharmaceutical, and office supply vendors. Table 19-1 lists examples of clinical and administrative processes and skills. Direct and indirect processes are essential to the successful management of any health care system, whether it is a small, self-contained APN practice, a physician practice, or a large multihospital network.

It is important to note the differences between the direct and indirect care of patients described in Chapter 7 and the discussion here of direct and indirect processes of practice. For example, in this chapter, quality and risk management are included as direct processes, but the management and reporting of these activities are indirect processes.

TABLE 19-1	Examples of Direct and Indirect Processes and Skills

Clinical Direct Processes and Skills	Administrative Processes and Skills
• Disease management • Health promotion, disease prevention • Patient education • Staff education • Wound management • Childbirth education • Lactation consultation • Prenatal, delivery, and postpartum care • Counseling • Pain management • Anesthesia • Patient engagement—group visits, outreach • Minor procedures	• Risk management and assessment • Reporting mechanisms • Support staff supervision • Presenting, teaching, precepting • Grant writing • Computer literacy • Budget development and implementation • Billing for services • Word processing, desktop publishing • Compliance monitoring, HIPAA • Quality, safety monitoring, and reporting

Entrepreneurs and Intrapreneurs

Over an APN's career, the balance between direct and indirect process involvement and the size of the system in which these processes occur may vary. At any given time, such shifts in balance and size of the system may require that APNs adopt an entrepreneurial approach, intrapreneurial approach, or mixture of both (Dayhoff & Moore, 2005; Wilson, Averis, & Walsh (2003). The term *entrepreneur* refers to someone who plans, organizes, finances, operates, and participates in a new health care delivery organization. Entrepreneurs have control over and responsibility for an increased proportion of indirect processes of care in their roles as compared with intrapreneurs. The term *intrapreneur* refers to someone who is generally an employee of an existing health care system, in which many of the indirect processes of the care delivery system may be controlled and managed by other employees or departments. The intrapreneur improves, redesigns, or augments an employer's current direct care processes, with a lesser role in day to day business administrative functions. Entrepreneurs function within the context of the larger, societal health care system. Intrapreneurs function within an institutional health care system—a microcosm of the larger arena. Both entrepreneurs and intrapreneurs are risk takers; however, entrepreneurs are likely to take bigger risks and have a higher tolerance for the accompanying uncertainty. Entrepreneurs and intrapreneurs are individuals who continually search for and are receptive to opportunities and innovation. Innovation comes through the creation of a new process—direct, indirect, or both—or through radical changes to an existing process so that it seems like new.

When embarking on program or practice oversight, the APN needs to understand the balance between direct and indirect processes and the size that the business will have over time. A large portion of time is dedicated to clinical visits and must be financially productive, so there must be a realistic balance between direct and indirect care. The decision about the proportion of one's role to devote to direct care versus indirect processes is based on the professional and personal values and goals of the APN and the needs and demands of the practice.

A self-assessment may assist the APN in clarifying professional and personal values. Types of questions to consider include the following; these are intended to be illustrative only and are not assumed to be exhaustive.

Philosophical and theoretical bases for practice:
- What type of nursing practice or approach to care delivery best describes how I perceive my own nursing practice?
- What do I value most, and how does that value get expressed in my practice?
- Do my options favor this model or some other approach?
- If they favor another approach, how compatible is it with my own beliefs and values? (See Chapter 2.)

Preference for intrapreneurial or entrepreneurial approach:
- Do I thrive on risk taking, like some risk, or prefer situations with a conservative level of risk involved?
- How is a "loss" or being "unsuccessful" defined?
- If I like taking risks, how much of a loss can I afford to take—professionally and personally—if my venture proves to be unsuccessful? (The more risk one is willing to take, the more entrepreneurial one is likely to be.)
- Do I prefer being part of a team or being on my own?
- If I like being on a team, what other team members would I like to be included on this team?
- How big a team am I most comfortable with?
- If I prefer working on my own, how will I interact with my colleagues? (See Chapters 7, 9, and 12.)

Inventory of Skills

A skills inventory can serve as a springboard for the clarification of the APN's professional goals. The extent to which the APN balances the clinical role with administrative demands depends on the APN's skills and preferences and begins with an inventory of those clinical skills and administrative talents that the APN would like to bring, or acquire, in an ideal advanced practice

BOX 19-1   Inventory of Skills

Direct Care Processes

- Can I clearly articulate my existing area of clinical expertise?
- Do I have well-developed advanced clinical skills? If so, what are they?
- What tasks do I particularly enjoy, feel neutral about, and particularly dislike?
- Of those that I dislike but that need to be performed, do mechanisms exist for those tasks to be performed by someone else?
- What processes would I like to do more of or learn more about?
- Does the current situation provide opportunities for me to do them?
- How do I ensure that evidence is infused into practice?
- How do I obtain cultural competence?

Collaboration Style

- Do I get along with peers if a partnership were to form?
- How well do I collaborate?
- Am I comfortable with sharing business decision making and financial loss or gain?

Indirect Care Processes

Internal and External Loci of Support

- Do I have the unflagging support of those closest to me, both personally (e.g., significant other, children, friends) and professionally (e.g., physician collaborators, APN colleagues, financial and legal advisors)?

Basic Management Skills

- Do I have well-honed organizational skills?
- Do I enjoy paying attention to details?
- Am I comfortable in a leadership position?

Financial Management Skills

- Am I familiar with or willing to learn the budgeting cycle and processes of my employer?

- Have I participated in budget preparation and resource allocation in the past?
- Am I comfortable developing a budget for my own practice?

External Regulatory Guidelines Affecting Practice

- What is my plan to review the evidence and translate it into my practice regularly?
- Do I know where to locate copies of the applicable regulations affecting my practice?
- Do I understand the reporting mechanisms that I am required to adhere to for quality and safety?
- Do I understand or do I have access to advisors who understand the specific ramifications of state and federal laws applicable to my practice, such as those pertaining to the Clinical Laboratory Improvement Amendments (CMS, 2012b)?
- Are there any institutional rules and regulations that may limit my ability to practice within the full scope of my role?
- What are the procedures for obtaining approval of the various institutional committees that may be involved?
- Do I understand the participating guidelines of insurance companies and their reporting and auditing mechanisms?

Financial Resources

- Where will funding for the program (capital for start-up expenses) come from?
- Do I have the financial ability to live without a steady income for at least 1 year while the practice is growing or if the grant is not re-funded?

Human Resources Skills and Systems

- Am I willing to be responsible for the work of others and what does that entail?
- Are administrative systems in place for hiring, evaluating, and terminating staff for the duration of the program and practice?

---

role. Box 19-1 lists some questions that may refine one's ideal inventory.

The questions in Box 19-1 are among the many questions to be answered by APNs before deciding how extensive their role will be in the management of their program or practice. Fortunately, several resources help clinicians better understand the indirect processes, or business, of clinical practice. The reader is referred to Buppert (2012a) for an in-depth discussion of nurse practitioner (NP) business and legal concerns. In 2012, the American Medical Association (AMA) launched a new web-based

practice management center (AMA, 2012b) to support physicians in the business management of their practices, which is also useful to APNs.

Entrepreneur and other business magazines provide useful information related to business management and administration. The Small Business Administration (SBA; www.sba.gov) provides general and specific information regarding business management and referral to local supports, including the local office of the Service Corps of Retired Executives (SCORE; www.score.org/business_toolbox.html). There are many other online resources related to business management. Specific websites that may be useful to the development of small businesses include the following:

- www.americanexpress.com (American Express Company, 2012). Go to "Open small business" to find advice about business start-up and community networking.
- www.entrepreneur.com This website offers information about a wide variety of issues regarding financing, technology, and business opportunities.
- www.dol.gov/osbp. The Department of Labor, Office of Small Business Programs, offers good information about minority- and women-owned businesses.
- www.learn.gwumc.edu/hscidist/practice/home/weblinks.htm. This website offers a substantial list of links that support practice business management issues.
- http://barbaracphillips/home/np/promotion. This website offers resources on marketing an APN practice or employment.
- www.health caresuccess.com. This website offers health care success strategies, resources for profitable growth.
- www.score.org/resources. This website offers information about the SCORE association business counseling.
- www.webNPonline.com. This website offers "Practice Management: A Business Guide for Nurse Practitioners."

Direct Processes of Care

Direct Patient Care

Direct care of patients and families is the central competency for APNs (see Chapters 3 and 7). The direct process of care for a given practice or practice population is defined as those patients who will receive direct clinical care by the APN in a practice environment. High-quality care and patient satisfaction sustain any level or configuration of practice over time. The patient population served, components of care and procedures based on the APN role, scope of practice, and mission must be carefully considered before implementing care. Ongoing evaluation with regard to patient outcomes and patient satisfaction is an important tool to maintain high-quality, safe care over time. The therapeutic relationships that are the trademark of APN direct practice provide opportunities for innovative business opportunities (Person & Finch, 2009; Thomas, Finch, Schoenhofer, et al., 2005).

One way to think about practice environments is that they represent small health care systems based on a patient population with identified needs. This patient population is identified through a variety of means, including individual APN expertise and preference based on the role and scope of practice of the individual APN. For certified nurse-midwives (CNMs) and certified registered nurse anesthetists (CRNAs), the patient population is essentially defined by their roles with childbearing women and their families and with patients undergoing surgical anesthesia, respectively. NPs and clinical nurse specialists (CNSs) have a broader population base (e.g., family NP, psychiatric CNS; see Part III). Sometimes, APNs identify patient populations through other modifiers, such as age, health promotion specialty, or disease state specialty (e.g., CNMs who care for adolescent mothers-to-be, CRNAs who specialize in providing anesthesia in pain management centers, and adult NPs or CNSs who specialize in the management of asthma or diabetes). In other cases, it is the geographic location or organizational setting that differentiates one's patient population of interest. Examples of these populations are the rural underserved populations cared for by National Health Service Corps providers, veterans cared for in Veterans Affairs Medical Centers, and those in the newly designated accountable care organizations (ACOs; see Chapter 22). APNs must be able to define the patient populations they are serving in their clinical practice clearly and succinctly.

Mission, Vision, and Values

After the patient population has been identified and the patient care processes have been outlined, the APN will need to formalize this information in a mission and vision statement. This is where APNs differentiate their practices from physician practices using the nursing model of care and nursing attributes. The mission and vision statement describe to patients and prospective funding agencies the APN practice's reason for existence and future direction; this brief statement serves to remind the APN entrepreneur about where the program or practice's priorities should lie. Professional values include those tenets of nursing practice that provide significance and meaning to the APN's practice of nursing (American Nurses Association [ANA], 2001; Sellman, 2011). The mission and goal statements of national APN organizations clearly portray these values as well. One's professional and personal values influence one's comfort with risk taking and preference about the arena in which care is delivered. The written summary of program or practice values may be combined with the mission and vision statement into one document, such as a brochure or program information sheet. This summary is available for review by any interested party and should be given to every patient at the time of the first practice encounter. These values must be held by all staff, especially those who come into direct contact with patients. As a business owner, it is important for the APN to create a culture of caring and holism throughout the organization.

The mission states the goal of the direct processes of care in one sentence—for example, "comprehensive primary care and wellness care for pediatric and adult individuals and families." This can be distilled into a tag line, such as "innovative health care" (see Chapter 20). The vision statement describes the ideal 5-year goal (i.e., what the APN envisions the clinical care to be 5 years from inception). The mission and vision statements should enhance transparency and interdisciplinary collaboration as APNs clearly articulate their values, goals, and vision of patient care to existing and potential colleagues, consultants, and third-party payers. If the APN is functioning through an intrapreneurial approach as an employee, the organization's mission and vision should be carefully examined to ensure that the practice or program fits into the overall goals of the organization and into the APN's personal goals. If the program's mission conflicts with that of the organization, problems may take the form of delays in funding, changes to the program's direct or indirect processes of care, barriers to program implementation, and outright denial of program development. If other providers, individuals, or groups have a stake in the program, the mission and vision statement should be determined through consensus of the group (see Chapter 20 and SCORE [www.score.org/business _toolbox.html]).

The values of a practice or program describe the focus, preferences, and ethical precepts that underlie relationships among the provider, practice, patients, and external groups. They may be related to direct or indirect care processes. Values include core nursing beliefs, that all people have the right to fair and equitable health care within the context of their environment and support system. Some of the ways that these precepts are carried out are described here and are a part of direct and indirect processes of care.

Informed Consent

Informed consent is an ethical and legal mandate that requires providers to obtain a competent patient's fully informed and voluntary consent before any medical or nursing treatment. The APN must describe the general nature of the treatment and any consequences involved, the normal risks and hazards inherent to the treatment, any known side effects or complications that may occur, and any alternative treatments available to the patient. Final informed consent comprises the patient's understanding of this information and the agreement to proceed with treatment. Both the APN's information and the patient's agreement within the informed consent discussion must be documented as part of the patient's medical record.

Compliance with the Health Insurance Portability Accountability Act

Privacy and confidentiality are important ethical issues that require careful consideration. The balance between the patient's right to privacy and society's need to be protected is important. State laws clearly explicate those patient issues, such as sexually transmitted diseases, abuse, or tuberculosis, that are reportable by law. Patient confidentiality is critical to the provider-patient relationship. Other than legal reporting obligations, it is the patient's right to decide which information the APN and all other members of the health care team may share with others. The federal Health Insurance Portability and Accountability Act (HIPAA) became law in 1996. Mandatory compliance with federal regulations began in 2003. HIPAA mandates the proper use and disclosure of personal health information. APN business owners and providers must have policies and trained personnel in place to implement privacy standards (Buppert, 2012b). An APN employee must also be knowledgeable about office policy and all HIPAA compliance regulations. HIPAA guidelines are detailed on the Centers for Medicare & Medicaid Services (CMS) website (2012a). This site provides a good overview of the privacy rule, current updates related to electronic records, and answers to frequently asked questions about implementation.

In addition to the right to confidentiality regarding their health information, patients are entitled to a degree of personal privacy during the clinical encounter. Courtesy demands that the patient's dignity be maintained, including providing the patient with a well-fitting patient gown and cover sheet during the physical examination. Privacy includes careful attention to cross-cultural issues that may be unfamiliar to American APNs. Attention should be paid to the physical layout of the patient encounter area, ensuring that conversations cannot be overheard and that the room is secure from line of gaze through open doors and/or windows.

Quality, Safety and Security

The APN must advocate for measures that improve quality, safety, and security in the office environment and that provide a sense of well-being for staff, patients, and their families. An important component of any health care practice endeavor is a commitment to high-quality care (Barkauskas, Pohl, Tanner, et al., 2011; Johnson, Harper, Hanson, et al., 2007; Muller, Hujcs, Dubendorf, et al., 2010). Measures to ensure quality outcomes should be in place. Title III of the PPACA (HHS, 2011) defines initiatives that pertain to quality health care. Several resources found online (www.ncqa.org; www.naqc.org and www. nationalforum.com) can help APNs set a quality agenda (see Chapters 22 and 24).

Safety policies should clearly articulate how to maintain patient, provider, and staff safety, including provisions for securing a patient's valuables during procedures and for managing hostile persons in the area, including a policy for managing violent and armed persons. The waiting room door should be locked to the patient care area. Adequate lighting, railings, and paved walkways are necessary, as well as adequate parking close to the facility. The level of security needed depends on the APN's practice environment, knowledge of staff about patients' conditions and potential safety issues, and available resources within the facility (see www.qsen.org and Chapters 22 and 24). Each practice must adhere to Occupational Safety and Health Administration (OSHA) guidelines (www.OSHA.gov). One employee should be designated as an OSHA officer.

Risk Management

Ethical clinical practice demands honesty and integrity in all patient interactions. Under the best circumstances, communication lines will be open and the APN and patient will understand each other and feel as if they have been understood. When misunderstandings occur, the APN should manage the issue as if it were a patient complaint, seeking to address the concerns in an objective and timely manner. Risk management policies and protocols must be enacted to ensure that timely and thorough communication is delivered to the patient regarding all visit outcomes, plans of care, and diagnostic test results (Cox, 2010; Hall, 2010). This is of vital importance to the legal and ethical success and safety of the APN practice. Dealing with difficult and noncompliant patients requires a distinct skill set, experience, and understanding. Over time, many issues can be resolved between the patient and caregiver with a skillful APN who is knowledgeable about appropriate interventions for resistance and the stages of change. If termination of the provider-patient relationship is necessary, this may be accomplished in many ways. It is important to provide alternatives for another provider so that the patient does not feel abandoned. Finally, whatever rules the APN practice has set as grounds for termination of this relationship must be in writing, well-documented, and sent to the patient as a certified, return receipt letter.

Resolution of Complaints

Resolving complaints is not usually an ethical issue; however, it is good business practice to monitor patient satisfaction with the clinical experience from the time that the patient enters the waiting room until the final bill for services is paid. Many valid, reliable patient satisfaction tools are available to health care providers to measure patients' responses to how care is delivered (Kleinpell, 2001; Tingle, 2011; see www.qualitymeasures.ahrq.gov). Despite one's best efforts, however, patients may be dissatisfied with some aspect of their experience at some point during an APN's career. It is important that any patient's complaint or sign of dissatisfaction be addressed immediately, preferably at the time of the complaint (Buppert, 2012a). A formal policy related to the management of patient complaints includes how patient complaints are recorded, who investigates and responds to the patient's concerns, and how quickly the complaint is addressed. Specific guidelines for managing patient complaints may be supplemented by risk management information provided by the APN's malpractice carrier.

Clinical Relationships with Other Staff and Providers

Although the APN is assumed to be the primary provider in this discussion, attention must be paid to the development of clinical relationships with other APNs, physicians, pharmacists, and allied health colleagues. (In-depth discussions related to clinical mentorship, consultation, and collaboration are found in Part II.) To be successful, the APN must maintain a collegial relationship with other health care providers (Clausen, Strohshein, Farem, et al., 2012; Horns, Czaplijski, Endelke, et al., 2007; Lindeke, 2005; Young, Siegal, McCormick, et al., 2011). An important legal consideration is defining the parameters of the association with a collaborating physician. In states that require medical collaboration, it may be through the development of a collaborative practice or contracting agreement. Even without a state statute, strong collegial relationships that provide support and coverage for time off are essential to the success of the APN practice. Also, in APN-owned practices, impediments to care can occur when referring to out of area facilities for diagnostic testing. Although less common than in the past, some facilities want a Doctor of Medicine (MD; physician) as the referring provider to be identified on patient orders and correspondence. In some states, if APNs' names are not accepted as the primary provider, patient test results may be sent to the collaborating physician, who is off site and unable to prescribe or otherwise care for patients. APNs must be able to track these results to provide adequate safe care for patients; arrangements in which referral specialists do not communicate directly with the referring APN jeopardize safe and responsible patient care.

APNs need to find consultants and referral sources for patients whose medical problems require additional expertise from a specialist. Locating referrals for indigent or uninsured patients who need specialized medical care or hospitalization may be difficult because of the lack of services or reimbursement for these populations. A list of consultants and referral sources should be generated that outlines the services they offer and their willingness to accept referrals for indigent patients, as well as their participation in third-party payer plans. Consultants are identified through word of mouth recommendations from clinical mentors and colleagues, through the recommendation of lay public support groups who have worked with certain specialty groups, and through direct provider interviews. Over time, the APN develops a referral and consultation base and develops strong relationships with providers who can assist the APN in meeting patients' needs. Once relationships have been established, acknowledging a consultant's assistance and support is equally important. This acknowledgment may be as simple as learning from the consulting registration staff what demographic information they need to schedule the patient, providing the most recent office notes to the consultant in time for the patient's appointment, and sending seasonal cards thanking them for their support.

The numbers and variety of APN providers available in local communities are growing rapidly (see Part III). APN colleagues who can serve as peer consultants to other APNs or serve as potential partners are an added strength that can be fully used to build practice relationships.

APNs must also carefully decide about the support staff that will assist with the direct care of patients. Staff positions include nurses, certified nurse aides, office manager, and clerical staff. Other staff such as respiratory and physical therapists, pharmacists, and nutritionists may be on site on a daily basis. All permanent and part-time staff need to be oriented to the organization and the goals of care, with clear role delineation. Staff should be clearly identified so that the consumer is aware of their role in the provision of care; in particular, non-nursing personnel should not be identified as nurses.

Indirect Processes of Care

Indirect processes support patient care and include administrative and operational structures and functions. Although they require a different set of advisors, staff, and equipment, indirect processes are equally important to a successful APN practice. Business relationships and business structures are necessary to define the context and framework under which clinical practice is performed. Knowledge of the external regulatory bodies that have an impact on APN practice is essential in today's complex and rapidly changing health care arena. This discussion presents an overview of these issues but is not intended to be comprehensive. The APN is referred to business consultants for up to date information reflective of the laws and guidelines in a particular state and practice setting.

It is important to understand that the APN creates a nursing foundation to the care he or she delivers in a self-owned and administered practice or as part of a larger organization. Although business advice and relationships are vitally important, it is the APN who keeps the "nurse" and nursing-focused care as the heart of the practice.

Business Relationships

Hiring Business Experts

Separate from, but as important as, the clinical advisors and resources described earlier are the administrative advisors and resources required to develop and maintain smooth indirect processes to support patient care. An independent practice will need to contract or consult with an accountant, attorney, banker, and insurance agent for specific services (Buppert, 2012a). In addition, the services of a practice management consultant with medical billing expertise should be enlisted (www.learn.gwumc.edu/hscidist/practice/home/weblinks.htm; Reel & Abraham, 2007). The accountant will assist the APN in setting up an accounting system, establishing internal controls, and preparing an operating budget. She or he will set up the practice to ensure that the best tax advantages and flexibility are obtained (Buppert, 2012a; Burman, 2010). Attorneys with expertise in health care law should establish the legal structure of the practice and provide advice on an as-needed basis for special purposes. It would be best if the attorney and accountant have a working relationship so that the legal structure selected provides the best legal, financial, and tax advantages for the providers involved. The banking relationship serves to establish a line of credit or business loan (if needed) and to meet business banking needs. A business insurance agent provides expertise in the areas of health, liability, and Workers' Compensation insurance programs. The practice management consultant serves to develop policies and procedures manuals, billing procedures and fee schedules, and job descriptions for an entrepreneurial enterprise (Buppert, 2012a; Letz, 2002; Reel & Abraham, 2007). A medical billing expert provides guidance for the efficient completion and processing of billing forms to receive third-party reimbursement or capitation payment for the provider's services and for the thorough and accurate completion of any third-party payer's contracting paperwork required for the APN's participation in selected contracts. The APN needs to carefully decide which of these functions can be done by the APN–APN practice staff and which need to be purchased as externally contracted services. It is important for the

APN entrepreneur to ask himself or herself the following questions:

- Is this an area of strength and interest, or is this an area to which I do not want to attend?
- Is this an indirect process of care to which I want to devote time and energy?
- More importantly, is up-front capital sufficient to sustain the practice until it can generate its own income (usually at least 6 to 12 months)?

No matter who the APN hires to implement business procedures, the APN must be available and make the final decisions about how the practice will operate and do business.

Creating an Advisory Board

Community and consumer support is an important adjunct to APN practice. A practice advisory body in which the APN identifies three to five outside professional members (not all in nursing) and a consumer to review the practice and offer ideas for growth or change is necessary. The board should meet at least biannually. It can be as informal as the APN taking the group to dinner or, if profit margins are robust, offers them a stipend in exchange for their review and advice. It is imperative to have consumer involvement in major decision making to meet population and community needs.

Community Outreach

The importance of the APN entrepreneur interacting with the community cannot be underestimated. Offering support groups, such as breast cancer survivorship, hosting teen discussions on adolescent sexuality, and coordinating support groups or community discussions about current community health care concerns (e.g., drug use, current health issues) builds the APN's practice.

Day to Day Administrative Support

The organization of day to day administrative support staff services (separate from the services of business advisors) revolves around the processes of care being delivered and the environment in which services are delivered. Once the APN knows what the direct patient care processes will include, and has identified those indirect processes that will support the patient encounter, additional ancillary personnel may be needed. The APN maintains ultimate responsibility for all operations if she or he owns the practice, even if a practice manager is managing daily operations. APN employees must be aware of their specific responsibilities and understand which belong to them and which belong to the owner. In a community-based primary care setting, the practice may require someone to assist in patient registration and scheduling (the first process box

in Fig. 19-1), assist the clinician in certain elements of patient care (the second box), and collect or process patient fees (the third box). Any additional administrative roles support these primary roles and may include someone to manage patient medical records and new technologies, such as the electronic health record (EHR) and a reporting (see Chapter 24), triage acutely ill patients by telephone, and perform office cleaning functions. Those who fill these roles should have skills and qualifications complementary to those of the APN and should be able to meet practice goals for patient care. An organizational chart and job descriptions of the roles required should be developed, placed in a common personnel manual, and shared among staff members so that everyone is aware of his or her role within the successful functioning of the system. At the end of each day, the APN should ensure that all direct and indirect processes of care have been completed. Some practices are now using dashboards to display their practice metrics in a form that is most useful to project quality, cost, and performance (www.dashboards. com). All these factors provide the patient with the most comprehensive health care and the provider with timely and accurate reporting; support services information is completed and insurance companies' claims for reimbursement are processed.

The administrative structure taken by a particular intrapreneurial program depends on the organization's overall guidelines for program development. For example, a hospital may wish to open a satellite primary care or oncology clinic staffed partially by APNs. The structure of the new clinic would fall under the business structure and plan of the hospital. In hospital-based settings, CRNAs, CNSs, and CNMs often collaborate with the nurse managers of the area in which they practice to obtain the assistance of the unit's support staff and ancillary personnel.

Program and Business Structure

An entrepreneurial program structure is often dictated by the requirements of whichever funding agency has provided the startup and operating capital. The APN developing a practice or program that depends on the guidelines of other organizations is referred to the particular organization participating in program sponsorship. Many grant-funding agencies have criteria for funding and program guidelines (available on the Internet).

APNs may adopt one of several business structures, depending on the organizational context in which the practice is set. Practices may be hospital- or community-based. Hospital-based practices may be inpatient or ambulatory in nature. Community-based practices are often primary care settings, free-standing health centers, birthing centers, nurse-managed clinics, or retail clinics.

They may also be a part of an ACO, health care home, or other payer-based primary care site. Practices may be established on a for-profit or not- for-profit basis. APNs should consult with business advisors to determine the best business structure to match their values and goals.

The three basic ways to structure the practice are a sole proprietorship, a partnership, or a corporation (www.irs.gov/business/small/article; Buppert, 2012a). The primary differences among these structures lie in differing tax restrictions and liability.

The simplest form of business organization is a sole proprietorship, which involves one owner. It is relatively straightforward and inexpensive to establish, and control remains with the sole owner. For tax purposes, the business income is taxed at the personal tax rate. The major disadvantage of the sole proprietorship is the unlimited liability that accompanies the structure. The owner assumes all liability, including that for any negligent acts of employees. Most medical practices are for-profit partnerships. A general partnership may be advantageous for the APN because partnering with another professional may attract venture capital. The unlimited liability for each individual partner remains, as does the personal tax rate on business income. A disadvantage of this structure is the possibility of personality conflicts and disagreements arising between the partners over control and decision making. As noted, the legality of relationships between different professionals is often dictated by state law. For example, CRNAs can join business arrangements as consultants to hospitals and anesthesia groups; CNMs may contract with hospitals for delivery services.

A corporation is a separate legal entity for tax and liability purposes. Incorporation protects the owners from some, but not all, liability because a corporation's liability is limited. Consequently, because the medical professional owners retain a portion of any liability incurred, it is strongly advised that APNs and other providers have an individual liability policy. A general corporation, also known as a C corporation, is the most common corporate structure. A general corporation may have unlimited number of stockholders; consequently, it is usually chosen by those companies with more than 30 stockholders or large public stock offerings. Because a corporation is a separate legal entity, a stockholder's personal liability is usually limited to the amount of investment in the company, and no more. A professional corporation can elect a small business (subchapter S) status, which allows owners to retain the benefit of taxation at the personal rate or, as is sometimes said, to avoid double taxation—first on corporate income and then on shareholder dividends. Other advantages of a corporation include the ability to start pension and profit-sharing plans and the possibility of attracting venture capital investors. The main disadvantage for a corporation not choosing small business status is the higher tax rate incurred by corporations. A corporation may also be more expensive to establish and operate.

A limited liability company (LLC) is not a corporation but offers many of the same advantages. Many small business owners and entrepreneurs prefer an LLC because it combines the limited liability protection of a corporation with pass-through taxations of a sole proprietorship or partnership (www.activefilings.com). See Table 19-2.

Titling the Practice

Most APN practices are eponymous (named after the owner). However, selecting a name for the practice may be an option worth considering in certain situations. For example, a specific practice name may assist in describing the services offered and reflect the business focus (e.g., "Coastal Cardiac Rehabilitation" suggests a geographic location and type of service). Many professionals use their own name to connote a more personalized service and to promote themselves. Most individual states regulate the selection and registration of business names as part of the registration of the business structure process. The process entails registering the business name, conducting a formal state agency search to ensure that the name is not being used by another business, paying a registration fee, and awaiting the receipt of a formal document confirming assignment of the business name to the APN (www.bizfilings.com). Furthermore, the APN may want

---

⬡ TABLE 19-2   Table of Corporations

C Corporation	S Corporation	LLC	Sole Proprietorship/Partnership
• General corporation	• General corporation	• Not a corporation	• Not a corporation
• Most common corporate structure	• Special tax status	• Avoids double taxation	• Individual owned
• >30 stockholders	• Most common small business	• Does not have to be a U.S. citizen	• Owner responsible for all debts and liabilities
• Personal liability limited to amount invested	• Taxed as sole provider	• Similar to sole proprietor	• Owner pays as personal income
	• Avoids double taxation		
	• Limited liability		
	• Must be a U.S. citizen		

www.activefilings.com 2012

to protect his or her business name with a federal service mark or trademark (www.legalzoom.com).

External Regulatory Bodies

An interwoven fabric of regulations and guidelines serves as the basis on which APN professional practice is built and developed (see Chapters 21 and 22 and the individual APN chapters in Part III for an in-depth discussion of APN credentialing and regulation). Federal and state regulations, policies of private insurance companies and, in some cases, local politics determine in which business structures and practice environments an APN may work and obtain reimbursement, and whether this practice is independent or collaborative. Although APN students routinely learn about the importance of the rules and regulations established by many different stakeholders within health care systems, the impact on daily practice may not be appreciated until the student becomes a practicing clinician. The major external regulatory vehicles affecting APN practice include the following:

- State and federal statutes pertaining to regulation and credentialing requirements for advanced practice nursing (www.ncsbn.org or www.ncqa.org, or individual state government websites)
- Guidelines for health care organizations regarding multiple facets of the management, environment, and delivery of health care established by The Joint Commission (TJC; www.jointcommission.org)
- OSHA regulations related to safe working conditions for employees (www.OSHA.gov)
- Clinical Laboratory Improvement Amendments (CLIA) regulations pertaining to laboratory services (http://www.cms.gov/Regulations-and-Guidance/Legislation/CLIA/index. html?redirect=/clia)
- Patient privacy and confidentiality (www.cms.hhs.gov/hipaa)
- CMS regulations pertaining to Medicare and Medicaid reimbursement processes (www.cms.hhs.gov/medicare)
- Guidelines and rules from private payers that reimburse care

Evaluation Processes That Ensure Quality and Safety

A major component of any APNs practice as an independent APN owner or partner or as part of a larger health care organization requires careful attention to evaluation processes. Chapter 24 offers in-depth guidance and tools that support the skills in which APNs need to have competency as direct care providers or as APN administrators to be able to evaluate care and respond to national and state benchmarks.

The use of electronic dashboards as a way to organize data and track measurable indicators of patient care outcomes have positively changed reporting and evaluation techniques in recent years. New systems and processes, almost all electronically driven, allow APNs and others to discern how "fit" their practices are (Richardson, 2008, see Chapter 24). The use of dashboards and other so-called governance score cards make it possible to improve clinical outcomes and patient safety and thus demonstrate the impact of APN care in the hospital (Griffin, Staebler, Muery, et al., 2007; Chandraharan, 2010). Tools such as the Hedis measures are making similar strides in community-based primary care settings (www.ncqa.org).

An excellent resource for quality is the Nursing Alliance for Quality Care (www.naqc.org). Samples of risk management guidelines may be obtained through the malpractice insurance carriers or as described by Buppert (2012a). Also, Buppert publishes *The Gold Sheet*, a monthly newsletter on quality for APNs.

TJC (2012) evaluates a health care organization's system performance in patient-focused (direct) and organizational (indirect) care areas to improve the quality of care provided to the public. Patient-focused functions include patient rights and organizational ethics, assessment of patients, care of patients, education, and continuum of care. Organizational functions include improving organization performance, leadership, management of the environment of care, management of human resources, management of information, and surveillance, prevention, and control of infection. In addition, TJC examines an organization's governance, management, and functions related to medical and nursing staff. Surveys are conducted every 3 years by TJC-employed provider and nonprovider survey teams. An overall score is determined, along with any recommendations for improving scoring deficiencies. Accreditation is based on the organization's compliance with TJC guidelines and implementation of any recommendations to resolve deficiencies (TJC, 2012). Health care safety management and hazard control are proven processes that produce results by preventing accidents, reducing injury rates, and increasing organizational efficiency (www.OSHA.gov). Topics include emergency planning and fire safety, general and physical plant safety, managing hazardous materials, managing biologic waste, safety in patient care areas, and health care support area safety. In terms of external regulators, safety management is carefully scrutinized by both TJC and OSHA. APNs functioning as entrepreneurs or employers must be well-versed in the rules, regulations, and implementation of safety programs governing these areas of safety management and hazard control, especially with respect to the management of biologic waste and OSHA guidelines regarding bloodborne pathogens.

Created as part of the Department of Labor, OSHA was charged by the Occupational Safety and Health Act of 1970 to ensure safe and healthful working conditions for U.S. workers. In 2002, Congress amended OSHA to expand research on the "health and safety of workers who are at risk for bioterrorist threats or attacks in the workplace" (OSHA, 2012).

Diagnostic Services

Any provider or laboratory service planning to collect, prepare, and analyze patient specimens is bound by CLIA rules and regulations (CMS, 2012b). Enacted to safeguard the public, the CLIA established minimum acceptable standards for all categories of laboratory testing in the United States. Providers offering laboratory services must meet the criteria and apply for the appropriate level of CLIA certification. Fees for the certificates are based on the test complexity, number of specimens being processed, and cost of survey or inspection. Four categories of laboratory testing are defined by the CLIA: waived tests, provider-performed microscopy (PPM), moderate-complexity procedures, and high-complexity procedures. If laboratory specimens are going to be tested by the APN, the first two categories of CLIA testing (waived tests and PPM) apply to the usual level of procedures performed. Moderate- and high-complexity procedures are generally performed by independent or hospital-based laboratories.

Waived tests are simple laboratory examinations and procedures cleared by the U.S. Food and Drug Administration (FDA) for home use. They are simple and accurate, which minimizes the likelihood of error, and pose no significant harm to the patient. CLIA-waived tests (CMS, 2012b) include fecal occult blood, nonautomated dipstick or tablet urinalysis, visual color comparison pregnancy urine tests, and qualitative color comparison pH testing of body fluids. The laboratory would apply and pay for a CLIA Certificate of Waiver, allowing the laboratory to perform only waived tests. The certificate is valid for 2 years. Provider-performed microscopy (PPM) is a subcategory of the moderate-complexity level of testing. These examinations may be performed by clinicians during the patient visit on a specimen obtained from the provider's patient or a patient of the group practice (American Academy of Family Physicians, 2012a). Other key criteria related to PPM stipulate the following: (1) that the primary instrument for the test be the microscope; (2) that the specimen must be labile, or a delay in the testing could compromise test accuracy; and (3) that limited specimen handling is required. PPM procedures include wet mounts, including preparation of vaginal, cervical, or skin specimens, all potassium hydroxide (KOH) preparations, pinworm examinations, and nasal smears for eosinophils. The certificate for this level of laboratory service, the Certificate for Provider-Performed Microscopy Procedures, allows the provider to perform waived tests as well (American Academy of Family Physicians, 2012b).

With the new structure at CMS, quality and personnel rules for clinical laboratories have been streamlined and simplified. CLIA information may be obtained at www.cms.hhs.gov/clia and www.aafp.org/pt.

If the APN does not intend to perform laboratory testing in the practice setting, he or she will need to identify providers of diagnostic testing services with appropriate CLIA certification who will accept requisitions for diagnostic tests. In the absence of an in-house laboratory, external laboratory services basically include specimen collection, specimen processing, and reporting of results. Some APN practices choose to collect specimens themselves and then send them to the laboratory for processing and reporting. The APN would set up all business agreements and arrangements with the receiving laboratory for complete processing and reporting of the specimens, including billing and payment practices. For practices that choose to collect and process their own specimens, additional equipment and supplies will be needed, depending on the nature of the tests being performed.

Recent revisions in Medicare regulations have resulted in the heightened enforcement of the policy of medical necessity with respect to diagnostic services. In an attempt to decrease costs related to inappropriate diagnostic testing, certain laboratory and radiologic services have been identified as requiring proof of medical necessity for them to be covered by Medicare, Medicaid, and other carriers. The determination of medical necessity is made by CMS and codified by the International Classification of Diseases (ICD; AMA, 2012c; see later, "ICD Codes"), a list of diagnoses and symptoms that will justify the diagnostic service requested. For example, to have thyroid-stimulating hormone (TSH) testing paid for by Medicare, the patient must have an ICD-9-CM diagnosis (AMA, 2012c) that is on the list of diagnoses for TSH testing, such as goiter (ICD-9-CM codes 240.0-240.9) or acquired hypothyroidism (ICD-9-CM codes 244.0-244.9). ICD-9 codes need to be specific, adding a fifth digit when possible. Those diagnostic tests for which medical necessity has been determined in specific U.S. locales are listed in local Medicare medical policies found through the laboratory service or directly from the local Medicare intermediary newsletter (www.cms.hhs.gov). Most other carriers follow the Medicare medically necessary requirements. It is important to note that CMS uses private companies, termed *fiscal intermediaries,* that contract with Medicare to pay Medicare Part A and some Part B bills. These fiscal intermediaries influence which procedures and tests are covered at the local level.

On January 16, 2009, the HHS published a final rule for the adoption of ICD-10-CM and ICD-10-PCS, with a compliance date of October 1, 2013. The final rule does not allow for the use of ICD-10 codes prior to the compliance date (Innovative Medical Practice Advisors, Consultants, Trainers [IMPACT], 2011). It is imperative that APNs pay close attention to CMS rules and regulations for all coding compliances for reimbursement. If the patient's diagnosis does not comply with CMS guidelines but testing is determined to be necessary by the provider, the patient must be notified, in advance, that the cost of this testing may become the responsibility of the patient. This notification is formalized in the completion of an Advanced Beneficiary Notice (ABN), detailing the test requested and the symptoms or disease state necessitating the testing, and indicates that the patient has been advised that the testing may not meet the guidelines for Medicare reimbursement. The patient signs the ABN and the signature is witnessed by another staff person. Although on the surface this process may seem to limit provider discretion, it serves to deepen the provider's knowledge of appropriate use of diagnostic testing and recognition that diagnostic testing is an expensive and limited resource, with significant financial impact on the health care system. This process also holds true for certain procedures that may be considered cosmetic, such as some lesion removals. The current ABN has been expanded to include any procedures and injections not covered by Medicare (www.cahabagba.com).

Process Resources

Facility, Equipment, and Supplies

Using the paradigm of systems thinking, the processes of care to be delivered and the setting in which these processes occur will determine the tools needed to deliver that care. Choice of facility and office space depends on capital resources and is beyond the scope of this chapter. Equipment and supplies will vary, depending on the population served and the type of facility used. The most effective way to determine what is needed for a program or practice is to visit a site already in full operation and/or use the business planning resources listed in Box 19-2. Inventory lists will need to be made for direct and indirect processes of care, including prices. This approach is the basis for cost-based analysis, which examines the actual costs of the supplies, equipment, and personnel needed to perform a particular care process. Additional expenditures related to overhead, such as air conditioning and billing, are calculated into the final cost, which is then used to determine the charge to the patient for that process

BOX 19-2 **Useful Business Planning Resources for Advanced Practice Nurses**

Centers for Medicare and Medicaid Services
7500 Security Blvd.
Baltimore, MD 21244-1850
1-800-MEDICARE
1-800-633-4227
www.cms.hhs.gov
Drug Enforcement Administration (DEA)
Mailstop AES
8701 Morisette Drive
Springfield, VA 22152
202-307-1000
Medi-Scripts
Franklyn Building
5 Latour Avenue
Plattsburgh, NY 12901
www.medi-scripts-services.com
Counselors to America's Small Business (SCORE)
www.score.org
The Joint Commission
One Renaissance Blvd.
Oakbrook Terrace, IL 60181
630-792-5000
www.jointcommission.org
Pharmaceutical Research/Manufacturers of America (PhRMA)
950 F. Street NW
Washington, DC 20004
202-835-3400
fax 202-835-3414
www.phrma.org
Robert Wood Johnson Foundation
www.rwjf.org
Business Statistics
www.bizstat.com
www.healthcaresuccess.com
www.caqh.org (nonprofit alliance of health plans and trade associations)
Marketing and Promotion (see Chapter 20)
http://barbaracphillips/home/np/promotion

From Active Filings for Corporations. (2012). Business startup. (www.activefilings.com).

of care. The actual charge for each service should be based on the Medicare relative value unit times a conversion factor amount, which not only is necessary for the practice but also is consistent with other services in the area (Reel & Abraham, 2007). By using this system, APNs will be assured that they will not be overcharging or undercharging for clinical services. The charge profile should be reviewed annually.

Additional methods available for identifying needed equipment and supplies include the following:

- Relying on clinical expertise of the APN and her or his familiarity with the items needed to deliver the particular service
- Using evidence-based guidelines that report the needed materials
- Consulting a clinical procedures manual that lists the equipment needed
- Consulting with a collaborating physician
- Interviewing other providers who are performing the same or similar services
- Interviewing support staff to determine what they require to perform their roles
- Referring to standardized equipment listings

After determining the program and practice needs, lists or inventories are generated. Equipment and supply inventories enable the APN to establish an initial budget and timeline for business planning purposes and provide information related to budgetary requests required by lenders and grantors. (These inventories may be included in any business plan, grant application, or office procedure manual, thus eliminating the need to rewrite them for each application.) Inventories and bar coding also help the APN create an initial ordering list, record business assets, establish minimum par levels for an inventory of disposable supplies, and identify the locations in which items are kept in the office to facilitate inventory management.

The initial inventories for medical and office equipment and supplies, such as durable equipment, reusable equipment and supplies, and disposable supplies, follow the same template and could be set up as separate spreadsheets in any commercial office software package. One advantage to this separation is that it enables the program administrator or practice manager to assess quickly how much money is needed to set up the program or practice, as opposed to how much will be needed on an ongoing basis for replenishment of supplies. Durable equipment includes desks, chairs, file cabinets, examination tables, autoclave, electrocardiograph, and computers purchased as a one-time expense. Reusable equipment includes items such as otoscopes, stethoscopes, computer software, and trash containers. Disposable supplies can be separated into two lists, one for office supplies (e.g., pens, paper, staples) and one for medical supplies (e.g., syringes, bandages). These initial inventories will become part of the overall dashboard used to organize the practice.

For accounting and budgeting purposes, request professional advice to separate these items into capital and noncapital expenses. Each list includes the specific name of the equipment or supply needed and the number of units required. Quotes from potential vendors for disposables should be sought on a yearly basis. Once a vendor is identified, the price per unit (unit cost) and a total price for that item (total cost) are added to the inventory template. It is possible to obtain some disposable supplies free of charge from other sources. For example, in primary care, the laboratory analyzing the blood specimens drawn at the practice will often provide alcohol swabs, small gauze pads, Band-Aids, and other supplies used during venipuncture or other specimen collection as part of its service to the practice. Many pharmaceutical representatives are often willing to provide pens, note pads, and clipboards, although these items will have the names of the pharmaceutical company's products on them as part of its marketing plan.

Decisions related to which processes will be performed in house, as opposed to those being contracted externally, will determine the types of equipment and supplies needed. Other indirect processes of care that need to be budgeted include the following:

- Creating a patient database. Several medical office computerized systems of varying complexity and cost are available for the management of patient information. Some of the processes supported by these programs are appointment scheduling, generation of patient encounter forms (superbills), and electronic claims filing. Electronic claims filing is essential to any practice as a way to keep the needed outreach accounts receivable under control and should be HIPAA compliant (Buppert, 2012b). Electronic health records (EHRs) interface with software programs to enable risk management reporting on selected schedules to generate an alert when patients are due for yearly testing and disease-based follow-up testing. They may also be set up to track other parameters, such as group sessions or community outreach.
- EHRs: This software is available from multiple vendors. The Medicare-Medicaid EHR incentive program is a program to receive incentive pay to help offset the cost of EHR. It is necessary to adhere to their reporting guidelines. Medicare's meaningful use has to be interoperable and more than a billing mechanism; it must measure and improve quality as well. Meaningful use is described more fully in Chapter 24.
- Transcription services. For entrepreneurial APNs, transcription services may be available through the larger organization's facilities if they have not transitioned fully to EHR. For independent APNs who have not yet moved to EHRs, the decision to

contract for transcription services should include a review of the available voice to text computer software programs that allow the APN to dictate the patient's progress note (or other printed material) directly into a commercially available word processing or desktop publishing program. Several voice to text programs are available, with different degrees of complexity and adaptability and varying sizes of medical vocabulary lexicons.

- Ensuring staff safety. One staff member should be designated an OSHA officer to maintain OSHA compliance and training for all staff. Medical assistants or other clinical support personnel can be good OSHA officers. All staff must attend OSHA training, which can be done off site, by the OSHA officer or through a program subscription purchased online.
- HIPAA compliance. HIPAA training must take place annually. Delegate the office manager to train and maintain staff in HIPAA compliance. Off site training and online training are available, usually at a higher cost. HIPAA materials for patients need to be posted and readable, with copies available.
- Patient education materials. These are available in a variety of formats, including videotape, interactive computer software, and written brochures or pamphlets. The APN should review the direct patient care processes for which educational materials can be anticipated. Part of the initial planning process includes reviewing available materials that can be incorporated into the APN's practice. Educational material should be evaluated for quality, readability and literacy level, availability in different languages, and cost. Oral presentations to individuals or groups are also an important component of patient education.

Managing Prescriptive Authority and Sample Medications

One process of care that requires particular attention is the use of pharmaceutical agents in direct patient care by APNs with prescriptive privileges. Prescriptive authority involves nonpharmacologic and pharmacologic interventions, but the focus here is on pharmacologic interventions.

- Writing the physical prescription or using e-prescriptions. APNs need to follow the regulating board's rules for prescribing in each state. Prescription pads should include the APN's name and credentials, name of the APN's practice setting and, in several states, name of the collaborating physician.

- Receiving drug samples. A system to track lot numbers, expiration dates, and the patients to whom the drugs were dispensed needs to be developed to address the issue of lot number recalls and to meet certain states' requirements for oversight.
- Prescribing controlled substances. In states in which APNs can prescribe controlled substances, the APN must obtain an individual Drug Enforcement Administration (DEA) number. A completed DEA registration form will be required, with the registration fees paid, before the APN can prescribe controlled substances allowed by statute. The DEA registration is renewable every 3 years. Forms may be requested on the Internet (see Box 19-2). In addition to a DEA number, a locked secure location for storage needs to be established and a procedure for access must be determined before acceptance of a supply if the APN dispenses controlled substances from the office.

Prescription pads are available through MediScripts (See Box 19-2), as well as local printing companies. All prescription pads must comply with tamper-resistant guidelines, be numbered, and have the print of their state pharmacy seal (www.rxsecurityfeatures.com). E-prescriptions are rapidly becoming the fastest, most error-free way to prescribe.

The use of medications, herbals, or homeopathic supplements in a program or practice depends on the nature of the services to be delivered but is also constrained by the scope of practice granted by individual state nurse practice acts. When decisions have been made regarding the use of pharmaceutical agents, a list of anticipated pharmacy supplies, along with cost, vendor, and drug comparison information, may be generated from the same software spreadsheet as the other inventories. When a pharmaceutical inventory is prepared, practices that provide children's services will find enrollment in the state immunization program extremely useful. States provide immunizations free to children who fall within certain eligibility guidelines (e.g., Medicaid recipients, uninsured patients, participants in a federally funded health center). These programs involve practice enrollment, a monthly vaccine use report, and some record keeping regarding recipient eligibility. Some state programs have established an Internet-based system, allowing practices to report monthly usage and reorder vaccines online. The maximum benefit of the Internet-based system is that it allows confirmation of childhood vaccinations to other enrolled practices in a secure and confidential network environment.

When writing prescriptions, the APN must be aware of the patient's financial resources and constraints and know the requirements and procedures for prescribing from insurance companies' formularies or for obtaining prior approval for nonformulary items, when indicated. The uninsured and low-income patients may have access to prescription assistance from the pharmaceutical company available on their websites. In addition, a number of foundations assist underinsured patients to meet their copay expenses.

It is important to note that certain third-party payers, government agencies, and mail order prescription drug companies will not accept prescriptions from APNs. The primary reason for this exclusion is that the state to which the prescription and enrollment forms are sent does not permit APNs to write prescriptions. The second reason for this exclusion is that the parent company is unaware of revisions to state practice acts that allow APNs to write prescriptions in certain states. The solution to the first issue is the development of a prescribing policy whereby the APN's collaborating physician writes the prescription for that patient's medications. The solution to the second issue is continued efforts on the part of APNs to educate and collaborate with pharmaceutical companies to ensure that accurate timely information about current state regulations is being shared. Patients who obtain their prescriptions through the Internet or patients whose insurance prescription plan requires a written prescription may also experience the inconvenience of being told that the APN cannot write their prescriptions.

Business Plan Summary

Once the process of business or program planning has been accomplished, the APN should summarize, in one document, the mission, vision, values, and processes of care and required resources to meet patients' needs. Traditionally, this summary has taken the form of a business plan, which is then distributed to potential sources of financial backing. Even if the program is not seeking external funding, a summary is needed to describe the available services to others. One way of writing this summary is to modify the traditional business plan so that it reflects an APN and systems-thinking approach to patient care. Box 19-3 provides an outline of a program and practice summary. See Reel & Abraham (2007), Buppert (2012a), Letz, (2002), SBA (www.sba.gov), and local business advisors for additional information and advice.

Consideration must be given to the audience for whom the summary is being prepared. As noted, funding agencies have specific guidelines for the compilation of a program's operational documentation. If the summary is written for the community of patients being served, issues related to literacy, language, and emphasis need to be addressed. If the summary is written for potential investors or potential physician colleagues, issues related to capital expenditures, numbers of patients to be served, services to be delivered, and expected revenue need to be emphasized. Consequently, the first step in preparing the summary is to identify the anticipated audience.

A successful business plan describes what the business does, how it does it, and how it evaluates the outcomes achieved (Ettinger & Blondell, 2011; Kleinpell, 2001). A successful APN develops, implements, and evaluates patient care and indirect processes that support outcomes by organizing these tasks as a system. Today's health care consumers demand that patient care delivery be individualized, compassionate, effective, and resource-efficient. A sound knowledge of the system in which care is delivered enables APNs to meet the demands of today's complex environment and the patients that they serve.

Choosing the type of practice to engage in as an APN is a difficult and challenging task, one that the APN will have to live with on a daily basis. Decisions around practice type require careful planning, research, and discussions with other APNs who have entered into various types of practice arrangements. Exemplar 19-1 describes a practice arrangement and illustrates how one APN was able to purchase a turnkey family practice business in a short time and eventually employ a second APN.

Health Care Payment Mechanisms

The process of reimbursement is perhaps the most important and complex indirect process supporting patient care. Figure 19-2 provides an overview of reimbursement. All APNs are involved in the completion of the patient's clinical encounter, documentation of the encounter in the patient's medical record and, frequently, completion of the patient's bill for services. Office managers and billing clerks are key to this process, but APNs must be closely involved in the subsequent steps in the reimbursement process—the actual payment collection from the patient or third-party payer and the posting of the payment to the patient's account in the provider's office. They should be cognizant of the major concepts and issues related to third-party reimbursement and to APN compensation. To ensure profitability, APNs need to check regularly that the reimbursement is consistent with the most recent contracted fee schedules and that monies are collected in a timely manner. Future payment arrangements will be profitable only if the APN is actually improving the patient's health and using fewer resources; this new future must be addressed in health care homes, ACOs, and other innovations. As illustrated in Figure 19-2, reimbursement links payment of the APN with the clinical encounter,

BOX 19-3 Outline of a Program and Practice Summary

I. Introductory Elements
  A. Overview, summary
    1. Mission and vision statements
    2. Overarching program/practice values
  B. Table of contents

II. Description
  A. Background information
  B. Direct processes of care to be delivered
  C. Key factors in the delivery of patient care

III. Market
  A. Description of the patient population to be served
    1. Patient demographics
  B. Analysis of the market
  C. Marketing strategy
    1. Initial
    2. Ongoing
  D. Competition and how this practice is different
  E. Advertising and promotion

IV. Program and Practice Structure
  A. Structure, ownership
  B. Management
  C. Advisory body with consumer input
  D. Clinical advisors and services offered (includes APN)
  E. Business advisors and services offered
  F. Support staff and services offered
  G. Outreach for high-risk and poorly managed patients

V. Resources
  A. Budget
    1. Projected income
      a. Start-up capital—business loans, grants
      b. Ongoing capital—patient revenues, other funding
    2. Projected expenses
      a. Office space and overhead
      b. Durable equipment
      c. Reusable equipment
      d. Disposable items
      e. Provider and staff compensation
      f. Compliance budget
      g. Technology updates
        i. Software for databases
        ii. Subscriptions
        iii. Classification updates
        iv. EHR and e-prescribing
  B. Collaboration community and agency resources

VI. Compliance
  A. Federal and/or state regulations
    1. TJC
    2. OSHA
    3. CMS
    4. CLIA
    5. HIPAA
  B. Other agency regulations
  C. Provider-specific licensing, credentialing, privileging
  D. Risk management

VII. Outcome Evaluation
  A. APN performance measures
  B. System performance measures
  C. Internal review parameters and timeline
  D. External review parameters and timeline

patient's medical record, patient's bill for services, claim submitted to the appropriate third-party payer (if any), and payment of the APN for services delivered. In this section, an overview of documentation is presented, along with a description of the major third-party payment schemes and the patient's financial responsibility for self-pay. Examples are used to illustrate steps in the reimbursement process.

Documentation of Services

Documenting the care given to each patient and maintaining and managing patient records are high-priority tasks for APNs in any type of practice arrangement. Coordinating care across time and various settings and providing continuity for patients with chronic illnesses and multiple comorbidities requires a well-thought-out process, attention to detail, and appropriate documentation for reimbursement purposes. The following discussion presents various approaches to documenting care. Several manuals and classification systems are used to bill for services, including these widely accepted medical classification systems, the *International Classification of Diseases, Ninth Revision, Clinical Modification* (ICD-9-CM) and Current Procedural Terminology (CPT) codes. The ICD-9 code was developed by the World

EXEMPLAR 19-1   **The Entrepreneurial Advanced Practice Nurse**

Sally is a family NP who was employed by an obstetric-gynecologic (OB-GYN) physician to offer family practice services at his busy private practice. This was her first job as an NP. Her experience included 20 years as a critical care registered nurse (RN), with 7 of those years as an internal medicine office manager in a private practice setting. After 1 year of employment as an NP, her employer decided to move out of the area, offering her first refusal on purchasing the practice. This practice would become a family practice business only. Because his move would take place almost immediately, decisions had to be made quickly. Sally had never really thought about owning her own practice; however, this idea was certainly attractive. A quick feasibility study was necessary.

Sally solicited advice from family and peers, who were supportive. She developed a collaborative practice agreement with a local physician to provide backup and referral. Sally's collaborating physician had his own practice at another site and believed strongly that this was a great opportunity for her. She received assistance from her employer in writing a business plan and then reviewed the business plan with a local business owner and an accountant friend for advice. Was this a good, sound business investment or not? After receiving positive feedback on her business plan, Sally met with a local banker to discuss financing. A small business loan for women was compared with a conventional bank loan. The small business loan was possible but very restrictive and required frequent reporting. The conventional bank loan was actually a better idea, with a better interest rate. The president of the bank reviewed Sally and her husband's assets and agreed to the loan, with a line of credit for any start-up expense needed. Sally used the bank's attorney for all legal advice. He advised her to establish a subchapter S-type corporation, set this up for her, and prepared the closing papers and all documents

necessary to complete the transaction. Sally's accountant friend agreed to be the business accountant and set up all computer programs for her. He also became her business advisor and a most valuable asset to the success of her practice.

From the time Sally was approached by her employer in May 2000, the entire process was completed in 8 weeks. Although this went from start to finish quickly, several things were in place to make this happen. Because this was a turnkey business, all staff, equipment, supplies, medical software, vendor accounts, payroll services, medical records, patients, and accounts receivable were already established. All direct and indirect processes of care were established, with the cost and budget known at time of purchase. Because she was already credentialed with insurance companies under her employer's name, a change of business name and new tax identification number for reimbursement were all that were required. There was no interruption in service to the patients being served by the practice. After 4 years of business success, Sally was able to employ another family NP. Beverly was hired as an employee the first year and then was able to become incorporated and work as an independent contractor to Sally's business in the second year of her employment. Today, Sally and Beverly operate one of the most successful practices in the region. Sally attributes much of her success to the attention that the practice pays to each patient and the focus on open lines of communication among staff, patients, and families. Because the practice is NP-owned and not governed by a larger entity (a hospital or corporate physician affiliates), time is flexible and each patient is allowed the amount of time necessary to ensure that a holistic approach based on the nursing paradigm is achieved in completing their visit. This NP model of health care has provided these two NPs with a flourishing, popular, highly productive practice.

Health Organization (WHO) in Geneva, Switzerland; the ICD-9-CM is the U.S. version of ICD-9. ICD-9-CM is continuously updated and contains one more level (decimal) than the original ICD (www.cdc.gov). The evaluation and management (E/M) services guidelines (CMS, 2012c) were developed to compensate providers for clinical and cognitive effort rather than time expended. On January 16, 2009, HHS, Centers for Disease Control and Prevention (CDC), published a final rule for the

adoption of the ICD-10-CM and ICD-10-PCS, with a compliance date of October 1, 2013 (CDC, 2012). The ICD-10 is so different and complex compared with the ICD-9 that a learning curve to adopt these new coding guidelines will take time to implement. Applying computer software for compliance with billing and coding and training for learning these new codes must have been done prior to the universal adoption of the ICD-10 in 2013.

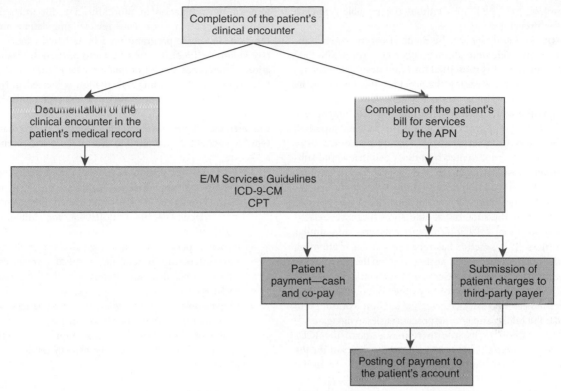

FIG 19-2 Overview of reimbursement.

Medical and Nursing Classification Systems

International Classification of Diseases

ICD-9-CM Codes

The ICD-9-CM codes are diagnostic codes that identify the diagnosis, symptom, or condition to be treated. Their purpose is to aid in standardizing coding practices across the United States (AMA, 2012c), as directed by the CMS. The CMS has prepared guidelines for use of the ICD-9-CM codes in the area of medical billing. These guidelines are available online at the CMS website (www.cms.hhs.gov) and from Medicare's local fiscal intermediaries. The codes are published each year in two volumes that are combined into one spiral-bound text for ease of use. Volume 1 contains the *Tabular List of Diseases,* based on the ICD-9-CM code attached to the diagnosis, symptom, or condition of concern. Volume 2 contains the *Alphabetic Index to Diseases* (Buck, 2013). To identify the appropriate code for a particular symptom, a clinician would begin the search in volume 2 under the alphabetical listing. Once the code is obtained, the clinician then turns to the tabular listing of the code itself to determine any additional modifiers necessary to clarify the entity being coded. For example, if an NP diagnoses otitis media, volume 2 indicates that "Otitis" is coded as 382.9. Volume 2 also indicates that additional information is needed to determine which code best matches the type of otitis media that the patient has, such as acute (382.9), with effusion (381.00), allergic (381.04), serous (381.01), and with spontaneous rupture of ear drum (382.01). A listing of common ICD-9-CM codes used in family practice may be found on the American Academy of Family Practice website (www.aafp.org).

The primary function of the ICD-9-CM is to facilitate medical billing. Therefore, it is sometimes used at the point of care to classify the patient's diagnosis (or diagnoses) on the patient's billing form, or superbill. The superbill is so-named because all subsequent forms generated for that encounter are based on this first bill, completed at the time of service. The superbill may have a listing of frequently seen diagnoses or symptoms accompanied by the appropriate ICD-9-CM code for the provider to check off. This practice is discouraged by CMS because of a concern that diagnostic bias may be introduced by the presence of preprinted diagnoses. The CMS would prefer that the provider write the diagnosis or symptom independently, without the possible influence of the preprinted list.

The billing coder for the medical practice then transcribes this code onto a uniform billing form (CMS-1500 claim form) that is submitted for reimbursement, preferably by electronic means. If the provider does not know the code assigned to his or her assessment findings, the coder assigns the code based on the diagnosis (or diagnoses), sign(s), or symptom(s) written on the patient's superbill. In addition, each service or procedure performed for a client must be represented by a diagnosis that would substantiate those particular services or procedures. In other words, the procedure performed must match the diagnosis coded. For example, if a urine dipstick test is performed in the office, the superbill should show diagnoses related to urinary tract infection, polyuria, dysuria, and similar disorders. This practice has received particular attention in the realm of diagnostic testing through the use of ABNs (see earlier, "Diagnostic Services") for services that may not fall within Medicare or any other insurer's guidelines for medical necessity. Electronic support continues to make the billing and coding process easier to navigate.

In addition to its role in reimbursement, the ICD-9-CM serves as a guide to the practicing clinician for the classifications of diseases and symptoms. It is a useful tool for the evaluation of morbidity data for indexing medical records, medical care review, ambulatory and other medical care programs, and basic health statistics (see Exemplar 19-2). This tool can also be used for evaluation of outcomes as part of quality improvement initiatives. Supplemental coding information is located in the ICD-9-CM to capture those patient encounters with the health care system that may not entail a disease or injury classified elsewhere in the manual. There are three main types of encounters that fall into this category and receive a V code:

- When a well person encounters the health care system for some specific purpose (e.g., organ or tissue donation [V42.0 for kidney recipient], prophylactic vaccination [V04.8 for influenza vaccination])
- When a person with a known disease or illness encounters the system for a specific treatment related to that disease or illness (e.g., chemotherapy [V58.1])
- When some circumstance exists that influences the person's health status but is not in itself a current illness or injury (e.g., inadequate housing [V60.1], no other household member able to render care [V60.4]).

⊙ EXEMPLAR 19-2   **Analysis of ICD-9-CM Codes to Determine Practice Performance**

LM, a CNM and adult NP, wants to improve the outcomes of care that she is offering to patients in her rural health clinic. In this rural women's health practice, in addition to maternity patients, LM sees many women for primary health care needs. She knows that as she moves her business to incorporate EHRs, and as reporting mechanisms become more stringent through value-based purchasing directives, she will need to be able to track the success of her diagnoses and management, as well as screening requirements for her primary care patients. LM wants to know which nonobstetric symptoms or diagnoses are most common in her practice. Collaborating with her medical billing administrator, LM defines a sort of the administrative billing database by ICD-9-CM code. The sort tallies the numbers of patient encounters associated with each code. The resulting list captures the most frequent diagnoses seen in her practice.

Among the top five ICD-9-CM codes represented, hypertension, unspecified (401.9) and type 2 diabetes mellitus, uncontrolled (250.22), rank numbers 1 and 2. Based on this information, LM commits to implementing the Seventh Report of the Joint National Committee on Prevention, Detection, Evaluation, and Treatment of High Blood Pressure (JNC 7: Complete Report, 2003), for the management of hypertension, and the American Diabetes Association (2012) guidelines for the management of diabetes. Flow sheets for blood pressure readings, urinalysis results, glycosylated hemoglobin testing, and scheduled referrals to specialists and routine follow-ups are developed and placed on LM's dashboard for easy reference. Through this method, she is able to keep a current inventory of the processes she is using to care for patients and the quality of the care she is providing. Next, LM commits to evaluating what percentage of patients with hypertension are reaching the goal of systolic blood pressure lower than 140 mm Hg and diastolic blood pressure lower than 90 mm Hg and what percentage of patients with diabetes are reaching the goal of a glycosylated hemoglobin level below 7 g/dL. New electronic tools accessed from the Internet make the work easy to accomplish. She has asked a Doctor of Nursing Practice (DNP) student who is precepting with her to help with the project and to consider a new project that would help her track women's health information easily for her teenage patients and women who are approaching menopause.

For example, the practice should be able to determine their immunization rates with a few keystrokes; this allows for quality measurement. Environmental events, circumstances, and conditions that are the cause of injury (e.g., motor vehicle accidents), poisoning, fire, and/or other adverse effects are assigned an E code.

ICD-10 and ICD-10-PCS

The ICD-10 (diagnoses) and ICD-10 PCS (procedures) are expected to contain the broadest scope of any diagnosis coding revision. The ICD-10 incorporates much greater specificity and detail of clinical information, which results in an improved ability to measure health care in greater accuracy in communicating a patient's condition and to provide more detail in electronic transactions (IMPACT, 2011).

Current Procedural Terminology Codes

CPT codes are those listed in the *Current Procedural Terminology* manual published annually by the AMA; this text is a listing of the descriptive terms and identifying codes for reporting medical services and procedures (AMA, 2012a). As with the ICD-9-CM, the CPT manual serves to provide a uniform language that accurately describes medical, surgical, and diagnostic services. The CPT codes for reimbursement should accurately reflect the services or procedures performed for those ICD-9-CM codes assigned to the patient's diagnosis (or diagnoses) or symptom(s). All services or procedures are assigned a five-digit code and represent procedures consistent with contemporary medical practice and performance by many providers in multiple locations. The CPT manual is divided into several sections—evaluation and management (see earlier), anesthesiology, surgery, radiology, pathology and laboratory, and medicine. Medicare and state Medicaid carriers are required by law to use CPT codes for the payment of health insurance claims; all insurance carriers recognize and use CPT codes. Although a CPT code may describe a current medical procedure, a particular insurance carrier may deny reimbursement for that specific procedure.

Occasionally, modifiers are used to indicate that a service or procedure has been performed and has not changed in its description or code but has been altered by some specific or extenuating circumstance. The use of modifiers attached to the end of CPT codes eliminates the need for separate procedure codes in these instances. Understanding the proper use of modifiers substantially affects insurance claim reimbursement. The reader is referred to the CPT manual for an in-depth explanation of the use of modifier codes. CPT codes are available in paper, disk, and CD-ROM formats from the AMA (AMAc, 2012).

E/M Services Guidelines

The E/M services guidelines (CMS, 2012c) are available online at the CMS website (www.cms.hhs.gov) or through the local Medicare intermediary. There are seven components of E/M services, with the first four bearing the most weight:

- Nature of the presenting problem. The reason or need for the client's office visit.
- History. The client's chief concern, brief history of the present issue or illness, and related systems review. A family and/or social history is included.
- Physical examination. May be focused, addressing only the affected body area or organ system, or comprehensive, addressing a complete examination of a single system of concern, or a multiple system physical examination.
- Medical decision making. Refers to the complexity in establishing a diagnosis and selecting a certain management strategy. It includes the differential diagnoses and management options, analysis of medical records, all diagnostic tests, and other information analyzed to make a competent decision.
- Counseling. Includes discussions or meetings with client, family, caregivers, and nursing staff (as in long-term care). Counseling can include discussions about disease process, results of diagnostic tests, prognosis, education and instructions on management, and treatment options.
- Coordination of care. Refers to time spent working with other health care providers and agencies to direct care. This process must be well documented in the client's medical record if it is intended to denote the type of service or care delivered because other providers may be billing for direct care of the patient.
- Time. In the case of encounters that predominantly consist of counseling or coordination of care, time is the key component used to determine the level of E/M services provided. Time is defined as face to face time in the office, time spent reviewing records and tests and arranging further services, or time spent with staff, such as in the nursing home. Time should be averaged in minutes and recorded in the client's medical record. Time is considered only when coordination, chart review, and counseling services represent more than 50% of the visit.

As noted, the major elements used to determine the level of service provided under the E/M system are the patient history, physical examination, and complexity of medical decision making required to manage the patient. Elements of at least these three components must have been performed and consequently documented in the patient's medical record. The documentation guidelines provide minimum assessment data points within each component that will support a particular level of E/M service. Each level of service is assigned a separate five-digit CPT code. The codes vary for new patients and established patients, even if the same level of service has been provided (Box 19-4).

Nursing Classification Systems

Clinically excellent, holistic patient care delivered by APNs includes nursing and medical diagnoses, interventions, and outcomes. Nursing diagnoses provide the basis for the selection of nursing interventions that achieve the identified patient outcomes for which the nurse is accountable (Guler, Eser, Khorshid, et al., 2012; McCloskey &

 BOX 19-4   Example of Implementing Documentation Guidelines: Subjective, Objective, Assessment, Plan, Evaluation

Subjective

RM is an 82-year-old woman brought to the office by her daughter. She is an established patient. RM reports uncontrolled blood sugars since her recent hospitalization for a myocardial infarction (MI). She was started on insulin in the hospital and her daughter is checking her sugars and administering insulin at night. Prior to her MI, RM's glucose was well controlled on oral medications. Now her fasting glucose reading is in the mid-100s and her random glucose readings are greater than 200. Both RM and her daughter do not understand what to do, because RM's diet has not changed. RM denies chest pain, shortness of breath, visual changes, or other associated symptom changes. She does complain that her feet tingle and are burning more over the past month.

RM's current medical problem list consists of DM-II with neuropathy (ICD-9-CM 250.62), HTN (ICD-9-CM 401.9), CHF (ICD-9-CM 428.0), NSTEMI (ICD-9-CM 410.7), and newly diagnosed metastatic lung cancer (ICD-9-CM 518.89).

RM'S only new medications are Lantus insulin, 10 units at bedtime, and Coreg, 6.25 mg bid.

SH: RM quit smoking 1 month ago. She continues to drive and live independently.

Objective

GEN: Alert, well-developed, well-nourished, 82 y/o female in no acute distress. VS: T-98.4, BP 118/72, HR-68, RR, 14, Wt, 157 lbs, HT 5 ft 2 in. HEENT: Fundoscopic exam WNL, PERRLA, TM's clear bilaterally, oropharynx without erythema, tonsils absent, buccal mucosa pink, moist, dentition in good repair. CVS: Heart R,R,R w/o M,R,G; apical rate 68. NO JVD, pulses 2+ bilaterally X4, no CCE. RESP: Lungs CTAP, Abdomen soft, nontender, +BSX4, skin warm, with good turgor, including bilateral foot exam. Neuro: CN II-XII intact. Vibratory sense to all toes slightly diminished. Urinalysis dipstick without microscopy WNL (CPT 81002). Lab

review form fasting labs drawn 2 days prior to visit. HgbA1C 7.6. Comprehensive metabolic panel WNL except glucose of 126. Total cholesterol 175, triglycerides 122, HDL-C 58, LDL-C 102.

Assessment, Plan

Diabetes mellitus type 2 uncontrolled with complication of neuropathy ICD-9 250.62. Increase Lantus insulin to 20 units at dinnertime. Increase Neurontin to 300 mg tid. Diet diary reviewed and changes suggested.

Hypertension ICD-9 401.9. No treatment plan changes.

Non-ST elevation myocardial infarction ICD-9 410.7. Medication management only, by cardiology. Follow-up visits scheduled.

Metastatic lung cancer ICD-9 518.89. Tissue pathology results pending. Will follow with oncology next week for treatment plan.

Congestive heart failure (ICD-9 428.0)—resolved.

Evaluation

Diabetic education with regard to blood sugar increasing during illness, injury and stress on the body. Reviewed times to check glucose and continue to keep a diary. Reviewed all medications with patient and daughter and coordinated insulin administration to best fit their lifestyle. Discussed new cancer diagnosis; oncology's opinion needed on next course of treatment. Discussed RM's continued independence, agrees to quit driving, and is agreeable to have assistance in the home when needed. Follow-up visit in 1 month to review blood sugar diary.

Meeting with all three daughters, without patient present, scheduled after pathology report completed to help them best determine treatment care plan for their mother.

Evaluation and Management

99214 Detailed (not expanded) visit, established patient.

CPT, Current procedural terminology; *ENT,* ears, nose, and throat; *GEN,* general; *HR,* heart rate; *ICD-9-CM, International Classification of Diseases, Ninth Revision, Clinical Modification; NC,* noncontributory; *NIC,* nursing interventions classification; *RR,* respiratory rate; *STREP,* streptococcus; *T,* temperature; *VS,* vital signs; *Wt,* weight.

Bulechek, 2000; NANDA International [NAANDA-I], 2012). Thus, documentation by an APN on the patient record would reasonably include a combination of nursing and medical diagnoses, interventions, and outcomes languages. APNs, such as CNSs, work in settings in which documentation standards are based on a nursing taxonomy, such as NANDA-I. However, in many settings, third-party reimbursement requires that medically oriented information be recorded in chronologic order in the patient record. Such information includes reason for the visit, health history (including past and present illnesses), physical examination findings, test results, treatments, and outcomes (CMS, 2012c). Therefore, APN students precepted by APNs in these settings are not routinely prepared to continue the use of the nursing-sensitive language that they learned in their undergraduate nursing education. One likely reason may be economically driven because reimbursement policies are based on medical language. In general, APNs are unable to bill third-party payers or be reimbursed for nursing diagnoses or interventions unless the diagnosis or intervention is also recognized as a medical one. In the future, direct financial compensation may be paid for nursing diagnoses and interventions that are independent of a medical model counterpart, but they have not gained a foothold to date.

The current strategic goals of NANDA-I including a new NANDA-I taxonomy for 2012-2014 is available, and plans to incorporate NANDA-I diagnoses in standardized language systems and health care databases and research can be found at www.nanda.org. The Iowa Intervention Project has developed an evolving codified taxonomy of nursing interventions, the Nursing Interventions Classification (NIC), to list the treatments that nurses perform, assist practitioners in documenting their care, and facilitate the evaluation of nurse-sensitive patient outcomes (McCloskey & Bulechek, 2000). The Nursing Outcomes Classification (NOC) codifies a standardized language of nursing-sensitive patient outcomes (Iowa Intervention Project, 1997). Familiarity with these standardized languages, which capture the nursing care provided by APNs and their consistent use in clinical practice and documentation, provides APNs with valuable tools in support of APN practice, now and in the future.

Health Care Payment Mechanisms Summary

Familiarity with the guidelines and external regulations that govern reimbursement programs for health care enables the APN to obtain health care reimbursement through existing reimbursement classification structures and demonstrates to third-party payers that the APN is a viable and important participant in health care. This degree of professional accountability may reduce barriers to full APN participation as providers of record in their own right and expand the inclusion of nursing care within the realm of reimbursed elements of patient care. Recent incentives in the PPACA (HHS, 2011) open the door for APNs to function as full providers of care.

All services submitted for reimbursement must be supported by appropriate documentation in the patient's medical record. Explanation of unusual services or extenuating circumstances must be clear and unambiguous. From a financial standpoint, insurance carriers will frequently limit or deny reimbursement for services because of insufficient documentation. In addition, they may request refunds from the provider if audited medical records do not substantiate the reported services. To bill for services, many insurance carriers require the use of specific medical documentation guidelines, classifications, reimbursement codes, and ongoing evidence of APN credentials. Documentation guidelines provide standardization and structure for the clinical encounter record. The various classifications available provide a standard language used by insurance carriers and health care providers to provide a uniform interpretation of medical conditions and identify the billable services of the provider.

Reimbursement for Advanced Practice Nurses

At the conclusion of the patient encounter, two parallel processes occur (Fig. 19-3). The APN documents the clinical encounter in the patient's record and completes the patient's superbill. Ideally, the medical record should provide data in support of the level of service selected, ICD-9-CM diagnoses used, and CPT codes used. As noted, it is anticipated that the record will also document nursing diagnoses and interventions appropriate to the clinical scenario. Both medical and nursing outcomes and plans for evaluating the efficacy of the plan of care are expected to be included. Viewed through the lens of process improvement and innovation, the implementation of these external resources allows APNs to improve the existing processes of care while establishing baseline information for reimbursement. Improvement may be accomplished by the use of guidelines to support the appropriate level of third-party reimbursement and include key elements of patient care. The key to improvement in the quality of care is for APNs to capture the full range of nursing and medical interventions. In this way, APNs can be reimbursed for the full range of interventions that they provide. Guidelines can be adapted by individual APNs to create encounter forms incorporating the anticipated elements of the patient's history, physical examination, and diagnostic testing for any particular APN practice. Today's health care economic landscape presents several obstacles to the inclusion of APNs in reimbursement strategies, from the barriers related to scope of

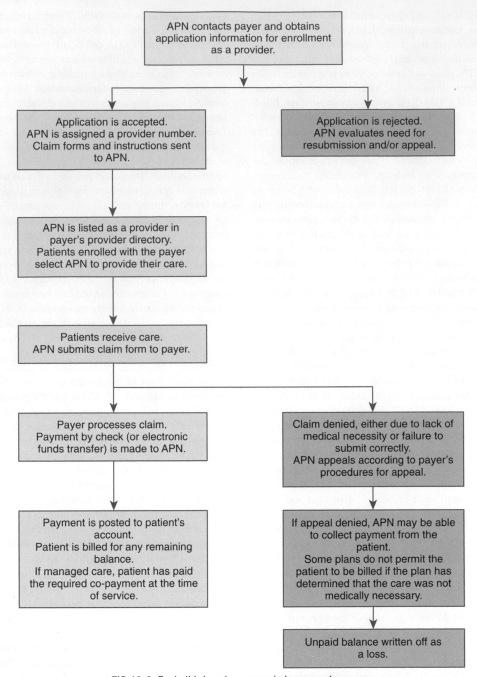

FIG 19-3 Basic third-party payer reimbursement process.

practice (see Chapter 21) to the lack of recognition of nursing diagnoses and interventions for monetary compensation. From a systems thinking approach, APNs must continue efforts to rectify these inequities through an understanding of, active participation in, and knowledge-based improvement of, the current processes of reimbursement. An overview of direct patient payer and third-party payer reimbursement strategies is presented here. The reader is referred to the individual programs described for the most recent legislation and information affecting APN participation or enrollment.

Fostering Patient Responsibility

Patients need to assume some level of self-care and financial responsibility for their health care. Self-care measures include active participation in the development and implementation of the plan of care for wellness maintenance and/or illness management. This could include establishing wellness goals, such as a normal body mass index (BMI) and hemoglobin A1c (HbA1c) levels in the normal range. Patients must make every effort to alter their lifestyle to mitigate the effects of chronic illness. Financial responsibility includes recognition of the valuable services provided by the APN and subsequent compensation of the APN for those services. Patients should be familiar with their insurance programs, particularly with regard to understanding that many programs do not provide the blanket insurance elements that were common in the past. Patients without insurance should expect to pay for the services rendered at the time of their delivery, unless prior arrangements have been made with the APN. Most practices offer sliding scale and financial hardship discounts for self-pay. Many hospitals have indigent care policies for diagnostic testing based on income or ability to pay.

Financial Responsibility Statement

The billing process includes the development of clear and concise written procedures and policies that will enhance the efficiency of the practice, allow review of individual patient bills to ensure accuracy, and accurately communicate to clients where their responsibilities for payment lie. A clearly written patient financial responsibility statement, specifically describing payment expectations, should be provided to and signed by each client on entry into the APN's practice. These expectations not only include what is expected from the patient, but also describe what the patient may expect from the APN's billing procedures and staff. It is required that the APN obtain a signed insurance claim form allowing the assignment of insurance benefits directly to the APN as part of the financial responsibility statement if the provider participates with the insurance company. This release expedites the processing of insurance claims when the patient's signature is required and should be renewed annually. Annual renewal of financial responsibility not only complies with most insurance payers, but also acts as a reminder to the patient of her or his responsibility. It is extremely important to check the patient's insurance card at every visit, because one release form does not carry over to another company. Payment guidelines should be posted in the patient waiting room stating; for example, "Co-pay required at time of service" and "You must have a valid insurance card and picture ID to be seen, if you have insurance." Self- pay patients have individualized payment plan options determined by the office manager and provider based on the patient's ability to pay. In these cases, financial hardship forms are signed.

Installment Plans

In the event that the uninsured or self-pay client is unable to pay for services when they are rendered, offering alternative payment plans provides financial flexibility while supporting the patient's financial responsibility to pay for the care delivered. These alternatives should be negotiated and documented before the patient's appointment. The agreed-on payment should then be collected at the time of service. Based on systems developed by consumer lenders, installment payment plans enable patients to pay their bills in regularly scheduled partial payments. These plans are negotiated between the APN's practice and patient on a case by case basis according to predetermined policies established by the practice. Interest is not added to the installment payment because the payment is not considered a financial loan per se; however, a service charge may be added.

Sliding Fee Scales

Sliding fee scale programs set up by the business using state and federal guidelines may be offered to eligible applicants who have been denied Medicaid because they exceed that program's income guidelines. Practices offering sliding fee scales require that the patient apply for and be refused other forms of medical financial aid before applying for the practice's program. From a patient's perspective, the information needed to complete the application for sliding fee scale is often identical to that used for a state Medicaid application. Consequently, it is possible for the patient to have to compile the mandatory financial information only once while applying to two different funding programs.

Failure to Pay

Consequences for failure to meet the agreed-on payments under practice-based aid programs may result in collection services being initiated against the patient and/or the decision by the provider to not offer services to the patient any longer. As noted, issues related to denial of care must be clearly documented before the provider takes any action and must include providing the patient with an opportunity to secure the services of another provider.

Reimbursement Mechanisms

There are as many different payment mechanisms as there are different health insurance companies. Each company has its own process for becoming a recognized provider and providing reimbursement for care delivered to its beneficiaries. The unstable health care environment means that the information for each plan can change quickly from month to month and varies from state to state. However, the need for uniformity is ever-present as health care reimbursement becomes more difficult and costly to obtain. The basic process involved in reimbursement, as an independent provider, is illustrated in Figure 19-3. APNs should be familiar with and participate in the major programs that are the mainstay of U.S. health care.

Medicare

Since its authorization by Title XVIII of the Social Security Act in 1965, Medicare has provided access to care to individuals 65 years of age and older. In 1972, Medicare coverage was extended to include those individuals younger than 65 years with long-term disability (of at least 2 years' duration and eligible for Social Security disability insurance) and those with end-stage renal disease. In 1982, the Tax Equity and Fiscal Responsibility Act introduced a risk-based option, facilitating the involvement of health maintenance organizations (HMOs). In 1983, the inpatient hospital prospective payment system (PPS) was adopted. This system replaced cost-based payments with a plan in which a predetermined rate was paid based on a patient's diagnosis. The Balanced Budget Act of 1997 included the most extensive legislative changes for Medicare since its inception. Among these changes were the expansion of covered preventive benefits and the establishment of Part C, which created new managed care and other health plan choices for beneficiaries (www.cms.hhs.gov/medicare). The Medicare Advantage Plan is offered by private insurance companies approved by Medicare.

Medicare coverage consists of two parts. Hospital insurance (Part A) covers inpatient hospital services, short-term care in skilled nursing facilities, postinstitutional home health care, and hospice care. Those individuals eligible for Social Security are automatically enrolled in Part A. Other qualified beneficiaries need to initiate the enrollment process. Supplementary medical insurance (Part B) covers physician services, outpatient hospital services, home health care not covered by Part A, and other medical services, such as diagnostic testing, durable medical equipment, and ambulance costs. Enrollment in Part B is voluntary to beneficiaries receiving Part A. Medicare Part A is funded primarily through payroll taxes, although beneficiary cost sharing in the form of deductibles and co-insurance also funds the program. Beneficiaries participating in Part B pay into the system through monthly premiums that are established yearly based on system expenses and through deductibles and co-insurance programs for various services. Medicare (Part C) benefits are available through participation in coordinated care or private fee-for-service plans and medical savings accounts (www.cms.hhs.gov/medicare). Beginning January 1, 2006, Medicare Part D prescription drug coverage became available to all people with Medicare. (www.cms.hhs.gov/prescriptiondrug) (see Table 19-3).

Providers are not required to participate in Medicare. For participating providers, the Medicare fee schedule for physicians' professional services, services and supplies provided incident to physicians' professional services (e.g., certain medications and biologic agents), and patient physical and occupational therapy services, diagnostic tests, and radiology services is 5% higher than for nonparticipants (National Heritage Insurance Company [NHIC], 2012). At present, NPs, CNSs, CNMs, and CRNAs are permitted to bill Medicare as individual providers in some settings. Payments are set at 85% of the physician's fee schedule for NPS, CNSs, and CRNAs. As of 2011, CNMs are reimbursed at 100%. APNs who are being reimbursed

TABLE 19-3	**Medicare Coverage**		
Part A	Part B	Part C	Part D
Inpatient hospital services	Provider services	Medicare Advantage Plan	Prescription drug coverage
Skilled nursing facility	Outpatient coverage	Offered by private companies approved by Medicare	Voluntary participation
Hospice and home health care	Diagnostics, durable medical equipment	Monthly premium	
Social Security eligible automatically enrolled	Voluntary enrollment	Coverage the same as Part B	
Premium-free	Monthly premium		

"incident to" the physician provider are reimbursed at 100% of the physician amount (see Chapter 22 and also see www.cms.hhs.gov/provider for the current year physician fee schedule).

APNs who are Medicare providers must be participating providers, which means that they will accept, on "assignment," the allowable charge determined by Medicare. As of May 2007, APNs needed the following qualifications to be a Medicare provider:

- State RN and APRN license
- National certification in an advanced nursing specialty
- Master's degree in nursing
- National provider identifier (NPI) number

The unique provider identification number (UPIN) and all former legacy numbers used to identify APNs with Medicare were replaced by the NPI number. On May 23, 2007, the NPI became the only way used by Medicare to recognize APNs in all standard transactions. The NPI also replaced the numbers that APNs use in communicating with other payers (NPI information can be found at https://nppes.cms.hhs.gov; see Chapter 21).

Medicaid

Medicaid provides health insurance benefits and other assistance for eligible low-income individuals and families. Medicaid is a jointly funded state and federal insurance program. Coverage varies by state according to federal requirements that stipulate eligibility and basic services covered. Payment is usually lower than that which is available through other insurance groups. Privatization has occurred in some states because states have contracted with private HMO companies to administer previously state-funded Medicaid plans. In 1989, Congress mandated that state Medicaid agencies provide direct reimbursement to family NPs, pediatric NPs, and CNMs. Some states cover the services of other APNs; however, the resulting inconsistencies have caused significant confusion. The Medicaid site (www.cms.hhs. gov/medicaid) offers links to individual states and their Medicaid rules and regulations. A change in Title XXI of the Social Security Act offers services for children through the State Children's Health Insurance Program (SCHIP; see Chapter 22 and www.cms.hhs.gov/schip for detailed information about this payment mechanism for APN services).

A service offered through CMS is especially helpful to APNs. Regularly scheduled "Open Door Forums" are accessible by phone, on the Internet, or on site, in which APN participants may discuss current issues and concerns about Medicare, Medicaid, and other federal reimbursement programs. To access this resource, go to www.cms.hhs.gov, click on "Open Door Forums," and then proceed to the nursing and allied health section to

schedule admission to the forum or read current and recent minutes.

Federal Employee Health Benefit Program

The Federal Employee Health Benefit Program (FEHBP) is the health insurance plan for the approximately 3 million federal employees (in 2010) and their dependents. This is a voluntary contributory program open to all employees of the federal government. Contracts are held with private health insurance carriers to offer health insurance plans to federal employees. Public Law 101-509, enacted in 1990, allows federal employees enrolled in the FEHBP direct access to NPs, CNSs, and CNMs, thus enabling direct reimbursement for APN services. Under this provision, insurance carriers for federal plans must make payment directly to APNs if their services are covered under the plan. Collaboration with or supervision by a physician or any other health care provider is not required. The payment level is determined by the individual health insurance plan. Additional information is available at the Office of Personnel Management website under federal employee insurance programs (www.opm.gov/insure).

Private Health Insurance—Fee-for-Service Plans

Private health insurance plans include carriers such as Blue Cross-Blue Shield, Aetna, Prudential, and Metropolitan. Because of health care reform, many of these carriers are seeking system-wide changes and efficiencies. These traditional fee-for-service plans reimburse providers for patient charges according to the usual and customary charges for that local area. An insurance policy does not explicitly need to include the coverage of nursing services for APNs to be reimbursed for their services. APNs' direct reimbursement by private insurance carriers varies from state to state (Pearson, 2011). When considering application for third-party reimbursement, the nurse needs to be familiar with the state's nurse practice act, state insurance laws and codes (including reimbursement amendments), judicial decisions, and opinions by the attorney general.

State health insurance laws do not necessarily prohibit third-party reimbursement to nurses. In Florida and Maine, for example, direct third-party reimbursement is essentially a 1:1 process. The individual APN applies to the third-party insurer and requests provider status. If reimbursement is rejected, familiarity with the state's nursing practice act and the state's health insurance laws can assist the nurse in appealing the decision. Some third-party payers reimburse under the APN's collaborating physician's name. APNs should contact each insurance company directly for credentialing and reimbursement protocols. When choosing to become a participating provider with a third-party insurance company, reimbursement is from a negotiated fee schedule. The APN or practice manager has the ability to negotiate for the best fee possible.

Managed Care Contracts

Managed care contracts encompass various prepaid group practice arrangements. These programs usually offer health care services to members enrolled in the plan for a predetermined, prepaid, or discounted fee. Prepaid means that the organization receives a fixed payment or premium to care for members of a certain population and that the organization bears the financial risk for the care that members receive. Participating providers are required to provide services for contracted reimbursement amounts. This reimbursement can range from a discounted fee for service to a lump sum for all services required.

Cash and Credit Card

Some patients pay cash for the care that they receive or pay a copayment out of pocket. Cash payment requires that the practice site have the ability to make change for patients who pay cash or who meet sliding scale requirements on a cash basis. The APN provider may choose to honor major credit cards to facilitate payment. Finally, a practice owner needs to decide whether to extend credit options with the additional billing procedures to their customers.

Reimbursement Summary

Reimbursement is an indirect process supporting patient care that provides a vehicle for APN compensation for the services rendered to patients. The process begins with the appointment for the patient's clinical encounter and ends with the posting of the patient's payment through patient payment or third-party reimbursement. The level to which the APN is involved in a practice setting's administrative procedures depends on whether the APN has chosen to practice in an entrepreneurial or intrapreneurial manner. Usually, the process of reimbursement is and should be delegated to an individual familiar with medical billing who can dedicate the time and effort required to become expert in this level of practice management. If the APN decides to become directly involved in reimbursement procedures, it is strongly urged that a professional billing advisor be contracted or hired; this is just as important as consulting with an attorney and accountant during business planning. The advisor serves to provide the APN with the latest and most accurate information regarding this vital process to ensure the APN's financial viability.

The reality of health care economics is that reimbursement varies considerably over time, depending on the payer mix—specifically, on the percentage of Medicare,

Medicaid, and other payments to be received—and the amount charged to patients. The average expectation is 50% to 55% of billable charges. Medicaid usually pays a lower proportion of billed charges than Medicare pays, based on the local Medicare fee structure. Managed care contracts can result in financial losses if enrolled beneficiaries use the health care system more frequently than the anticipated risk calculation had allocated.

During the business planning phase, the APN should become intimately familiar with the reimbursement rates in the local area, anticipated mix of the patient population to be served, and available resources and personnel to design and implement a reimbursement process that meets the APN's financial expectations. APNs should never allow one payer to dominate their practice and should set goals based on the percentage of each payer for their practice. As with any system, the reimbursement process should undergo periodic evaluation to determine where improvements may be made, including electronic claims submission, tighter internal audit controls, and efficient cross-training of staff to ensure consistency during staff absences.

Value-Based Purchasing

There has been a move by payers to link quality and payment for services. *Value-based purchasing* is the current term that many APNs have known as pay for performance (P4P). Many APN's are reimbursed under a value-based purchasing plan. Individual states and private sectors have established guidelines linking quality of care and improved outcomes with payment; the Minnesota Department of Human Services (2012), in August 2008, implemented a P4P program for fee-for-services providers. This program awards $250 up to two payments in 12 months when physicians or APNs render optimal chronic disease care to their qualified Minnesota Health Care Programs (MHCP) recipients with cardiovascular disease and diabetes. Clinical results and treatment measures are used for determining eligibility of payment through reporting and documentation measures (www.dhs.state.mn.us/main):

- September 7, 2011. As part of health care reform, the federal government has been testing different ways to reward physicians for the quality, not quantity, of their services, all in the hope of improving care. Health care homes and ACO demonstration projects are showing enhanced quality and cost reductions (see http://www.pcpcc.net/content/pcmh-outcome-evidence-quality).
- January 1, 2012. Blue Cross Blue Shield of Georgia (BCBSGA) adopted a Quality-In-Sights Primary Care Incentive Program Pay for Performance

Amendment. This program rewards physicians for meeting or exceeding established targets related to quality, patient safety, applicable external recognition programs, and adoption of technology. EHRs are a requirement for participation. To date, APNs are not included in the BCBSGA program (see Chapter 22).

Evaluation of Patient Care Services

Information technology (IT) is an APN responsibility that is steadily increasing in importance. Proficiency in the evaluation and use of IT is essential for APNs to achieve direct care, leadership, and research (evidence-based practice) competencies. From a business point of view, there are a number of ways that information systems drive the success of APN practice, whether the APN owns and manages the business, is an employee, or is in a contract service arrangement (Crosson, Stroebel, Scott, et al., 2005). In a health care system in which patients see several providers and have many comorbidities, electronic documentation on interoperable systems is essential to facilitate prompt and efficient communication. New interactive systems make it possible for providers to share important information and findings across settings and from home. Electronic budgeting assists APNs in planning and managing costs and in running a business from day to day. The ability to understand budget constraints is accommodated if APNs who work for others can access budget information to use resources wisely.

Electronic billing and coding is a most useful application of IT. The ability to track reimbursement and interface with payers electronically is exceedingly time advantageous and cost-effective (Miniclier, 2007). From a patient care standpoint, the ability to develop and access Internet-based patient and staff education is important to APNs in all types of business and practice arrangements. Exciting new models of interactive education targeted to individual patients make it possible for the APN to implement care that is personal and time-efficient. Also, the opportunity to join with other colleagues to develop, implement, and publish research initiatives is greatly enhanced by electronic communication.

APN competencies identified for the DNP place a high priority on the need for IT skills at the highest level of expertise (AACN, 2006). Health care services will increasingly depend on electronic systems to manage the business and patient care aspects of practice. It is incumbent on APNs to be able to select vendors appropriately for integrated clinical, administrative, and database software products that are useful to their practice settings. APN providers will need to continually augment their IT competencies and strive to learn new measures to enhance

their ability to communicate and share data electronically. There is also incentive pay for providers that use EHRs (PPACA; HHS, 2011). Telehealth or remote monitoring technology is a way for APNs to monitor their community-based patients and reduce visits to the office or house calls without decreasing patient contact. With newer technologies that make it possible to connect disparate systems, telehealth is a promising information technology for consultation that offers opportunities for improving quality of care while controlling costs (see Chapter 7).

Evolving Business Opportunities for Advanced Practice Nurses

Business opportunities abound, and in health care practice businesses continue to flourish as APNs respond to the needs of patients and communities in a complex and mobile society. The current health care environment is ripe for innovation. Nurses have led the way in strategies that make care more accessible to individuals who have busy lifestyles and to those populations who are vulnerable. Both entrepreneur and intrapreneur APNs can take advantage of new arenas of health care to carve out rewarding businesses such as the ones described below.

Managed Care Organizations

Although managed care is a vital part of the payment system, the trend is moving to pay for performance, pay for reporting, and provide incentive pay. It denotes a spectrum of arrangements that entail some connection between financing and delivery of care, usually with cost containment (Bodenheimer & Grumbach, 2012). In a managed care organization (MCO), the financial risk associated with health care delivery is shared among the payers, contracted providers, and enrolled beneficiaries. Risk is lessened for payers by the exclusive enrollment of beneficiaries with a particular health status profile. Risk is lessened for any one provider by the addition of providers to a pool of providers sharing the care for a particular population of patients. Risk is lessened for the beneficiaries through the use of providers who are within the contracted pool, or network, of providers. MCOs offer unlimited possibilities for APNs.

Accountable Care Organizations

ACOs are also a pay for performance strategy. An accountable health care system provides patient-centered, integrated health care across all settings (e.g., home, office, hospital). Care is offered from prevention through rehabilitation by a variety of health care providers. Accountable coordinated care models are structured to ensure optimal outcomes of care. A well-configured ACO must have a panel of at least 5000 patients and ensure that all the providers know the patient's condition and preferences and work together to optimize tests, procedure referrals, and education; to coordinate care plans to provide safe and efficient care, and be accountable for their care (National Academies of Practice, 2009). There are over 65 reportable measures for ACOs, and EHRs must be in place. The PPACA (HHS, 2011) offers many opportunities for APNS to work collaboratively with colleagues in ACO configurations.

The Medical Home

Many new configurations exist to support complex patients with multiple chronic conditions. The Medicare Improvement and Extension Act of 2006 provided for initiation of the Medicare Medical Home. Demonstrations to reward primary care physicians (PCPs)—initially physicians only—for coordinating chronic care were established. On July 8, 2008, the Medicare language was read into the Congressional record to include NPs. NP-led, patient-centered medical home practices can be reimbursed for coordinating chronic care, specifically for those complex patients with multiple chronic conditions (Schram, 2010). There are also several variations of the medical home in the private sector that may or may not include NP providers.

Nurse-Managed Health Centers

Nurse-managed health centers (NMHCs) have cared for chronically ill patients over the years; they have served as an excellent component of the medical home concept. However, until recently, they were restricted by state, federal, and reimbursement barriers that limited the APN's full scope of practice (Pohl, Hanson, Newland, & Cronenwett, 2010). Financial incentives and new collaborative models of care written into the PPACA (HHS, 2011), coupled with the enhanced scope of practice recommended by the IOM (2010), make nurse-managed clinics a viable reality, with many new opportunities for APNs. NMHCs are a desirable option for entrepreneur APNs wishing to open their own practice or for intrapreneurs who wish to work with a nursing-based model of care.

Other Opportunities

Traveler Health Services

An exciting opportunity for entrepreneurial APNs exists in the area of international travel health. Individuals and families have been travelling globally for business and pleasure with increasing frequency. Although prevention and planning can avert travel-related health problems and protect the traveler and society in general, little has been done to incorporate travel-related services into routine health care (Lugo, 2007). Newer models of traveler health services offer business opportunities for knowledgeable NPs, CNMs, and CNSs to offer their patients education about infectious disease, immunizations, and counseling about comorbidities, before traveling and after they return. Several APN journals carry columns related to travel health.

Pain Management Clinics

Pain management clinics are not a new phenomenon. However, because pain continues to be undertreated and remains a major public health problem (www.painfoundation.org), numerous business opportunities exist for APNs, especially CRNAs and CNSs. Community-based, free-standing pain clinics have been rapidly expanding and APNs' skill in assessing and managing pain is a sought-after commodity. CRNA entrepreneurs are expanding their practices in this area with good success.

Retail Clinics

The trend toward APN-delivered health care offered in retail locations has been growing rapidly because of the need for accessible, affordable, and convenient care. These clinics are appearing faster than they can be regulated, so it is extremely important for APNs to provide high-quality, safe care that will set the standard for this type of patient encounter. Retail giants such as Walgreens, CVS, and Target have primary care clinics staffed by NPs who, in addition to providing affordable, episodic care in a convenient, community-based environment, are providing education and important introductions to other health-related services (Ahmed & Fincham, 2011; Kaissi, 2010; Klein, 2006). Corporations who are entering the market have little experience with NP care; this offers expanding opportunities for APNs to be at the ground-breaking level to set up a new model of APN-focused care.

Hospitalist Services

APNs are entering the market as important collaborators in hospitalist care. Physician-APN teams are achieving positive results with patients (e.g., fewer readmissions) and have reduced costs. APN competencies in bridging the gap between hospital and community-based care offer an excellent niche for practice that is worth exploring (Cowan, Shapiro, Hays, et al., 2006; Kleinpell, Hanson, Buchner, et al., 2008; Kleinpell, 2006; Kleinpell, Hudspeth, Scordo, et al., 2012; see Chapter 16). A hospitalist is an employee of the hospital or part of a contracted group to the hospital. Two models of reimbursement are contract billing with the group and hospital at a flat rate, with incentive pay for positive outcomes, and split billing, in which the hospital and group bill separately for services.

These examples are just a few of the many business ventures open to APNs who may want to explore setting up their own practice, contracting their services, and/or expanding their existing practice. All require careful exploration of needs for services, funding, and capitalization in the short term and the potential for professional satisfaction, financial remuneration, and return on investment over the long term.

Conclusion

Through the development of innovative programs and practices grounded in a systems-thinking approach, APNs define, demonstrate, document, and thereby claim their contributions to patient care. Business planning establishes a clear picture of how the APN will function on a daily basis, as well as how midrange and long-term goals are to be met. Knowledge of the processes involved in care delivery increases the sharing of information among APNs and their patients, other health care providers, and colleagues. Reimbursement is identified as the major indirect process of care that has a direct impact on the success of the APN's business planning efforts. Equally important to success is the APN's candid self-evaluation and determination of whether an entrepreneurial or intrapreneurial approach is the most appropriate model under which to deliver patient care. The emergence of clinically focused DNP education for APNs enhances their ability to recognize and implement new practice models and innovate within existing organizations. The recognition that others in the greater health care system (e.g., other APNs, physicians, attorneys, practice managers) have skills and expertise to offer provides the APN with a safety net of advisors who can play an active role in the actualization of advanced practice nursing. Above all, the success of the APN is grounded in the professional recognition of and active participation in the larger system to ensure that the needs of patients are met through the delivery of clinically excellent, holistic health care.

References

Active Filings for Corporations. (2012). Business startup. (www.activefilings.com).

Ahmed, A., & Fincham, J. E. (2011). Patients' view of retail clinics as a source of primary care: Boon for nurse practitioners? *Journal of the American Academy of Nurse Practitioners, 23,* 193–199.

American Academy of Family Physicians. (2012a). CLIA and other regulatory information. (www.aafp.org).

American Academy of Family Physicians. (2012b). Provider-performed microscopy. (www.aafp.org/PPM).

American Association of Colleges of Nursing (AACN). (2006). *Essentials of doctoral education for advanced practice nurses.* Washington, DC: Author.

American Diabetes Association. (2012). Standards of Medical Care for Diabetes-2012. (www.care.diabetesjournals.org/content/35/supplement_1/S11.full).

American Express Company. (2012). Small business exchange: Creating an effective business plan. (www.americanexpress.com/smallbusiness/resources/starting/bizplan).

American Medical Association (AMA). (2012a). *CPT 2012.* Chicago: Author.

American Medical Association. (2012b). Practice management center. (www.AMA-assn.org/go/pmc).

American Medical Association (AMA). (2012c). *International classification of diseases, 9th revision, clinical modification (ICD-9 CM 2012).* (Vols 1 and 2). Chicago: Author.

American Nurses Association (ANA). (2001). *Code of ethics for nurses with interpretive statements.* Washington, DC: Author.

Barkauskas, V., Pohl, J., Tanner, C., Onifade, T., & Pilon, B. (2011). Quality of care in nurse managed health centers. *Nursing Administration Quarterly, 35,* 34–43.

Bodenheimer, T., & Grumbach, K. (2012). *Understanding health policy: A clinical approach.* New York: Lange/McGraw/Hill.

Buck, C. J. (2013). 2013 *ICD-9-CM, Volumes 1 and 2.* St Louis: Elsevier and American Medical Association.

Buppert, C. (2012a). *The nurse practitioner's business practice and legal guide.* (4th ed.). Boston: Jones & Bartlett.

Buppert, C. (2012b). HIPAA patient privacy. In *The nurse practitioner's business practice and legal guide* (pp. 157–159; 4th ed.). Boston: Jones & Bartlett.

Burman, N. (2010). Choosing an accountant. *Australasian Dental Practice,* Mar-Apr, 52.

Centers for Disease Control and Prevention (CDC). (2012). International classification of diseases, tenth revision, clinical modification (ICD-10-CM). (www.cdc.gov/nchs/ icd/icd10cm.htm#10update).

Centers for Medicare & Medicaid Services (CMS). (2012a). HIPAA—general information. (http://www.cms.gov/Regulations-and-Guidance/HIPAA-Administrative-Simplification/HIPAAGenInfo/index.html).

Centers for Medicare & Medicaid Services (CMS). (2012b). CLIA: General program description. (www.cms.hhs.gov/clia).

Centers for Medicare & Medicaid Services (CMS). (2012c). Evaluation and management documentation guidelines. (www.cms.hhs.gov).

Chandraharan, E. (2010). Clinical dashboards: Do they actually work in practice? Three-year experience with the maternity dashboard. *Clinical Risk*, *16*, 176–182.

Cox, C. (2010). Legal responsibility and accountability. *Nursing Management*, *17*, 18–20.

Colbert, C. Y., & Ogden, P. E. (2011). Systems-based practice in graduate medical education: Systems thinking as the missing foundational construct. *Teaching and Learning in Medicine*, *23*, 179–185.

Cowan, M. J., Shapiro, M., Hays, R. D., Afifi, A., Vazirani, S., Ward, C. R., et al. (2006). The effect of a multidisciplinary hospitalist/physician and advanced practice nurse collaboration on hospital costs. *Journal of Nursing Administration*, *36*, 79–85.

Clausen, C., Strohshein, F., Farem, S., Bateman, D., Posel, N., & Fleiszer, D. (2012). Developing an interprofessional care plan for an older adult woman with breast cancer: From multiple voices to a shared vision. *Clinical Journal of Oncology Nursing*, *16*, 18–25.

Crosson, J., Stroebel, C., Scott, J., Stello, B., & Crabtree, B. (2005). Implementing an electronic medical record in a family medicine practice: Communication, decision making and conflict. *Annals of Family Medicine*, *3*, 307–311.

Dayhoff, N. E., & Moore, P. S. (2005). CNS entrepreneurs: Innovators in patient care. *Nurse Practitioner*, *30*(Suppl 1), 6–8.

Ettinger, A. B., & Blondell, C. (2011). The clinician's guide to composing effective business plans. *Journal of Medical Practice Management*, *26*, 348–356.

Griffin, E., Staebler, S., Muery, K., McCorstin, P., & Harrington, L. (2007). Dashboards: A tool to demonstrate the impact of the advanced practice nurse in the hospital setting. *Oncology Nursing Forum*, *34*, 572.

Guler, E. K., Eser, I., Khorshid, L., & Yucel, S. C. (2012). Nursing diagnosis in elderly residents of a nursing home: A case in Turkey. *Nursing Outlook*, *60*, 21–28.

Hall, J. (2010). Assessing the quality of nurse prescribing. *Nurse Prescribing*, *8*, 547–550.

Horns, P. N., Czaplijski, T. J., Endelke, M. K., Marshburn, D., McAullife, M., & Baker, S. (2007). Leading through collaboration: A regional academic/service partnership that works. *Nursing Outlook*, *55*, 74–78.

Innovative Medical Practice Advisors, Consultants, Trainers (IMPACT). (2011). *Update on ICD-10-CM and ICD-10-PCS* (pp. 127–132). Marietta, GA: IMPACT.

Institute of Medicine (IOM). (2011). *The future of nursing: Leading change, advancing health*. Washington DC: National Academies Press.

Iowa Intervention Project, M. Johnson & M. Maas (Eds.). (1997). *Nursing outcomes classification*. St. Louis: Mosby.

Johnson, J., Harper, D., Hanson, C., & Dawson, E. (2007). Forging a quality agenda. *American Journal for Nurse Practitioners*, *11*, 10–19.

Kaissi, A. (2010). The future of retail clinics in a volatile health care environment. *Health Care Manager*, *29*, 223–229.

Klein, T. A. (2006). Working in a retail clinic: What nurse practitioners need to ask. *Topics in Advanced Practice Nursing eJournal*, posted 9/20/06.

Kleinpell, R. M. (2001). *Outcome assessment in advanced practice nursing*. New York: Springer.

Kleinpell, R. M. (2006). Expanding opportunities in ACNP practice. *Nurse Practitioner*, *Spring* (Suppl), 8–9.

Kleinpell, R. M., Hanson, N. A., Buchner, B. R., Winters, R., Wilson, M. J., & Keck, A. C. (2008). Acute care advisor. Hospitalist services: An evolving opportunity. *Nurse Practitioner*, *33*, 9–10.

Kleinpell, R., Hudspeth, R., Scordo, K., & Magdic, K. (2012). Defining NP scope of practice and associated regulations: Focus on acute care. *Journal of the American Academy of Nurse Practitioners*, *24*, 11–18.

Letz, K. (2002). *Business essentials for nurse practitioners: Essential knowledge for building your practice*. Fort Wayne, IN: Previcare.

Lindeke, L. L. (2005). Nurse-physician workplace collaboration. *Online Journal Issues in Nursing*, *10*, 1–7.

Lugo, N. R. (2007). International traveler health: A national prevention opportunity: A white paper by the Nurse Practitioner Health Care Foundation. *American Journal for Nurse Practitioners*, *11*, 51–56.

McCloskey J. C., & Bulechek G. M., (Eds.). (2000). Nursing interventions classification. (3rd ed.). St. Louis: Mosby.

Minnesota Department of Human Services. (2012). Program for fee for service providers. (www.mn.gov/dhs/search).

Miniclier, P. (2007). Credentialing, reimbursement, and billing for nurse practitioners. (www.medscape.com/viewarticle/425419).

Muller, A. C., Hujcs, M., Dubendorf, P., & Harrington, P. T. (2010). Sustaining excellence: Clinical nurse specialist practice and magnet designation. *Clinical Nurse Specialist*, *24*, 252–259.

NANDA International (NANDA-I). (2012). NANDA international taxonomy II. (www.nanda.org/searchresults.aspx?Search=Taxonomy+II).

National Academies of Practice. (2009). *Models of accountable, coordinated health care: A policy paper of the National Academies of Practice*. Edgewood, MD: Author.

National Council of State Boards of Nursing (NCSBN). (2012). APRN Consensus Model toolkit. (https://www.ncsbn.org/2276.htm).

National Heritage Insurance Company. (2012). Medicare physical fee schedule database. (www.medicarenhic.com).

Occupational Safety and Health Administration. (OSHA). (2012). (www.OSHA.gov).

Pearson, L. (2011). The Pearson report: A national overview of nurse practitioner legislation and health care issues. *American Journal for Nurse Practitioners*, *9*, 9–135.

Person, A., & Finch, L. (2009). Bedside manner: Concept analysis and impact on advanced practice nursing. (http://www.ispub.com/journal/the-internet-journal-of-advanced-nursing-practice/volume-10-number-1/bedside-manner-concept-analysis-and-impact-on-advanced-nursing-practice.html).

Pohl, J. M., Hanson, C. M., Newland, J. A., & Cronenwett, L. (2010). Unleashing nurse practitioners' potential to deliver primary care and lead teams. *Health Affairs*, *29*, 900–905.

Reel, S. J., & Abraham, I. L. (2007). *Business and legal essentials for nurse practitioners: From negotiating your first job through owning a practice.* St Louis: Mosby.

Richardson, M. (2008). *How fit is your business? A complete checkup and prescription for better business health.* Charleston, SC: Elevate.

Schram A. P. (2010). Medicare medical home demonstration project. *Journal for Nurse Practitioners, 6,* 132–139.

Sellman, D. (2011). Professional values and nursing. *Medicine, Health Care and Philosophy, 14,* 203–208.

Seventh Report of the Joint National Committee on Prevention, Detection, Evaluation, and Treatment of High Blood Pressure (JNC 7: Complete Report). (2003) (www.nhlbi.nih.gov/guidelines/hypertension/jnc7full.htm).

Solberg, L. I., Kottke, T. E., Brekke, M. L., & Magnan, S. (2000). Improving prevention is difficult. (www.acponline.org/journals/ecp/mayjune2000/solberg_2.htm).

Story, P. (2010). Systems thinking for better health care delivery. *Hospitals and Health Networks, 84,* 46.

The Joint Commission (TJC). (2012). Joint Commission requirements. (www.joint commission.org).

Tingle, J. (2011). Ensuring safe health care and dealing appropriately with patient complaints. *British Journal of Nursing, 20,* 1386–1387.

Thomas, J. D., Finch, L. P., Schoenhofer, S., & Green, A. (2005). The caring relationship created by nurse practitioners and the ones nursed: Implications for practice. (www.medscape.com/viewarticle/496420).

U.S. Department of Health and Human Services (HHS). (2011). Patient Protection and Affordable Care Act (PPACA). (http://www.healthcare.gov/law/full/index.html).

Wilson, A., Averis, A., & Walsh, K. (2003). The influence on and experiences of becoming nurse entrepreneurs: A delphi study. *International Journal of Nursing Practice, 9,* 236–245.

Young, H., Siegal, E., McCormick, W., Fulmer, T., Harootyan, L., & Dorr, D. (2011) Interdisciplinary collaboration in geriatrics: Advancing health for older adults. *Nursing Outlook, 59,* 243–251.

Marketing and Negotiation

Charlene M. Hanson • Barbara C. Phillips

CHAPTER CONTENTS

The current changes in the health care environment for advanced practice nurses (APNs) brought about by the Institute of Medicine (IOM) report, *The Future of Nursing* (2010), the Patient Protection and Affordable Care Act (PPACA; U.S. Department of Health and Human Services [HHS], 2011) and the changes in regulation based on the Consensus Model for APRN Regulation (National Council of State Boards of Nursing [NCSBN], 2008), all affect how advanced practice nurses (APNs) market themselves and negotiate practice contracts. Marketing is an important way for APNs to achieve stature as principal players in the health care arena during these unsettled times.

To market themselves successfully, it is essential that APNs integrate clinical expertise, leadership, collaboration, other APN competencies, and business skills. In addition to understanding reimbursement payment mechanisms discussed in Chapter 19 and regulatory and credentialing requirements discussed in Chapter 21, all APNs—new graduates, seasoned professionals and those APNs striving to develop and maintain their own independent practices—must understand marketing and contracting. This chapter will focus on marketing the role of the APN as new graduates and experienced clinicians and marketing APN practice. It includes contracting skills and strategies for all APNs. Basic marketing concepts that any APN can easily use will be discussed.

Health Care Marketing: Yesterday and Today

Although the idea of health care marketing is widely accepted, there is still APN reluctance about marketing and how to market oneself ethically so as not to be associated with the dubious distinction of being regarded as a used car salesman. For many APNs, the notion of marketing oneself is seen as painful and fraught with a mother's warning of not to brag about yourself. Much of the confusion and mystery of marketing for health care providers comes from the early AMA Code of Ethics ("It's not right to sell health care") and Health Insurance Portability and Accountability Act (HIPAA) regulations ("I cannot use my patient's name in my testimonial").

Although nursing has been consistently rated as the most trusted professional in terms of honesty and ethical standards for the 10th time in 11 years (Gallup Poll, 2010), health care has had its share of individuals who were labeled as charlatans or quacks, those who dealt in secret remedies, dubious procedures, and patented medicines. In an effort to distance themselves from these unsavory health care providers, the American Medical Association (AMA) created a Code of Ethics when it was founded in 1847 to address this issue. Chapter 2, Article 1, Section 3 of that document states (AMA, 2012a, p. 18):

It is derogatory to the dignity of the profession, to resort to public advertisements or private cards or handbills, inviting the attention of individuals affected with particular diseases—publicly offering advice and medicine to the poor gratis, or promising radical cures or to publish cases and operations in the daily prints or suffer such publications to be made; to invite laymen to be present at operations, to boast of cures and remedies, to adduce certificates of skill and success, or to perform any other similar acts. These are the ordinary practices of empirics, and are highly reprehensible in a regular physician.

This policy continued into the 1903 revision, which stated that "It is incompatible with honorable standing in the profession to resort to public advertisements or private cards inviting the attention of persons affected with particular disease" (AMA, 2012b, p. 3). In 1922, the AMA Judicial Council amended its Principles of Medical Ethics and outlawed the solicitation or marketing of patients by physicians. This particular policy remained in effect until 1980.

This historic prohibition must be addressed, corrected, and appropriately applied so that APN services can be made known to the public. Health care marketing is an evolving science. APNs, whether new graduates or experienced clinicians, have often relied exclusively on referrals, recommendations, and word of mouth to market themselves and their practice. Today, although marketing continues to include these venues, there is a trend toward specific marketing strategies and the socialization of health care marketing (e.g., via social media), which is changing the way marketing of any business or product will be done for years to come (Kingma, 1998; Segbers, 2010; Somers, Finch, & Birnbaum, 2010).

Two Types of Advanced Practice Nurse Marketing

APN marketing can be divided into two separate and distinct areas. First, new APN graduates must market themselves as they prepare to embark on their positions as APN providers. In this case, the APN is focused on preparing a portfolio that describes credentials, skills, and competencies that will induce a future employer to offer an interview, subsequent employment, and a contract. The portfolio allows the new APN to explore practice venues and to be as competitive as possible in the marketplace. The second form of marketing occurs when an APN chooses to embark on a business venture. This type of APN marketing is more complex and includes marketing to the community, populations of interest, and other health care providers. Both types of APN marketing will be discussed in detail throughout this chapter. Chapter 19

offers APN entrepreneurs further guidance in marketing strategies.

Definition of Marketing

Marketing has many definitions. In the broadest sense, marketing is promotion and education. When APNs adequately educate and promote healthy habits, for example, their goal is for the patient to buy in to the idea of wellness and adopt healthy behaviors.

According to Kotler (2011), marketing is "The process by which companies create value for customers and build strong relationships to capture value from customers in return." That definition can easily be applied to APNs by rewording it as "the process whereby APNs create value for their patients and build strong relationships with them to meet goals and to capture value from them in return." In other words APNs create the value by caring for patients and families and achieving better outcomes; in return, they are reimbursed for their work, more clients come to see them, and patients have improved health.

One author's working definition for marketing is broader: "Marketing is everything you, an APN, does, everyday to promote your practice, your ideas, your profession and you, the APN" (Phillips, AANP CE Center, 2010). Any health care–related business should be an ethical one. This implies that everyone—clients [patients], community, and APN—will win, getting what they need and want. So, this actually does include everything that the APN does to promote the practice, business, and advanced practice nursing.

Marketing Frameworks and Concepts

Although the previous definition makes marketing look rather simple, in reality it is a science that is based on psychology, neurology, sociology, and biology. Marketing aims to see how people are influenced by what they experience—see, hear, smell, taste and touch. People receive 3,000 to 20,000 images daily, which includes walking down an urban street, but more accurate research suggests that individuals visualize or take in an average of 247 messages a day (http://www. fluiddrive media.com/advertising/marketing-messages).

Therefore, it is becoming more and more difficult for people to see and act on any message in front of them. Marketing experts are constantly looking to scientists to see what makes people see and respond to these messages.

The Four Ps of Marketing

The four classic concepts of marketing, often termed the *4Ps*—product, price, place, and promotion—are the hallmarks of marketing (Chang, Pfoutz, & Price, 2001;

Letz, 2002). Each of these categories provides opportunities to expand APN practice in diverse areas. A fifth concept, "partnering," has become important as health care providers collaborate to provide better outcomes for patients. Many believe that the most important P is people, who are the recipients of the product being marketed (Reel & Abraham, 2007).

Product

The product is the entity that is offered to the market, such as a book or service, that is for sale. For the APN, the product is the APN and the services that APNs provide, regardless of the setting. Although professionals are not in the habit of thinking of themselves as products, doing so helps establish the value of APNs to the consumer when they offer high-level, nurse-driven care. Box 20-1 provides examples of the many types of products that APNs provide.

Price

Price is the amount of money that an individual will be asked to pay for the product being offered. Myriad factors contribute to the price for a product, including the cost of providing the product or service, practice or business overhead (e.g., salaries, malpractice insurance, business overhead expenses, utilities, regulatory costs, third-party

---

> ### ⊚ BOX 20-1 | Product Categories
>
> Goods—direct care, health care applications, supplements, books
>
> Services—health care practice in APN's specialty, health and wellness coaching, teaching patients and students
>
> Events—Continuing education conferences, other educational events, health fairs
>
> Persons—providing a service (e.g., motivational speaker, researcher, consultant)
>
> Places—healing centers, adolescent pregnancy clinics, professional offices, event, service
>
> Properties—Not always connected to health care, but a property can also be considered (e.g., clinics, hospitals, community) or intellectual (e.g., research, technology)
>
> Ideas—can lead to breakthroughs in research and other products that enhance practice and outcomes
>
> Information—educational materials provided to patients, students, and professionals for basic and continuing education; includes books, CDs, DVDs
>
> Organizations—national, international, specialty professional associations and organizations; universities

---

payers). APNs are often viewed as cost-effective health care providers who focus on preventive strategies to help the chronically ill stay out of the hospital. In today's cost-conscious environment, this is often used as a marketing strategy. For the APN seeking a position, it is important to understand the position of the potential employer with regard to patient care and the value placed on the APN.

Place

Place refers to the accessibility and various tasks necessary to make the product available to the market (Chang et al., 2001). Places can be real or they can be virtual. In the past, patients, clients, and employers accessed APN services from a real place, such as a hospital, clinic, professional office, operating room, conference hall, or classroom. Today, and well into the future, APNs will find themselves using more technology and providing many of their products and services in a virtual space.

Promotion

Promotion encompasses activities that communicate the value of the product to the market (Chang et al. 2001). The terms *marketing* and *promotion* are often used interchangeably. On one hand, promoting (marketing) is educating patients, clients, and employers to increase their awareness of the service that the APN provides. Another use of promotion is an event or specific campaign within the overall marketing plan. In both cases, the desired outcome is to increase awareness and sell the product or service. Several strategies used to promote or market APN services will be described later in the chapter.

Marketing Influence

One scientist frequently referred to in marketing circles is Dr. Robert Cialdini, who explored the concepts of influence and persuasion. Cialdini (2009) has studied how influence, persuasion, and compliance affect human behavior. He outlined six major factors that affect how individuals behave and how persuasion and compliance influence our buying patterns.

- **Reciprocation.** Reciprocation has to do with give and take. For the purposes of marketing, the APN marketer gives something away or does something kind for someone else. In return, people have a strong overpowering urge to want to reciprocate. This phenomenon is frequently observed in fundraising (for example, receiving address labels along with a letter requesting a donation), free samples, and political lobbying (dinner with a celebrity).
- **Commitment and Consistency.** Most people have a strong desire to look and be consistent in terms of their words, beliefs, attitudes, and deeds. They not only want to be seen as respected and highly

valued in society, but they realize that consistent behavior benefits them in daily life. Consistency provides guidelines that allow people to streamline the process of living. In other words, people can make assumptions and rely on prior procedures without having to think each step through. An example would be preparing a meal or getting ready for work each day. Commitment is equally important; committing to daily exercise or committing to a life partner. In health care, APNs understand that getting people to commit to an idea (e.g., quitting smoking) is a large part of the battle in changing behavior. Once patients have made the commitment to change this behavior, they are far more likely to follow through.

- **Social Proof.** Social proof is experienced in almost every aspect of one's life. We may ask our friends which restaurant they would recommend. We ask our colleagues which Doctor of Nursing Practice (DNP) program we should look into. Also, our patients ask which health care provider they see and what they think of that individual. We usually are more comfortable with referrals and recommendations than we are with striking out on our own or paying attention to the marketing of others. This is why social media has become so important in marketing and will continue to play an important role in the future.

- **Liking.** Liking is self-explanatory. Everyone likes to be around and say "yes" to people they know and like. Factors that influence liking are physical attractiveness, talent, kindness, intelligence, similarity, and familiarity. Liking can directly affect marketing efforts, regardless of the product. Social media has taken this to a new level. Patients, clients, and health care policymakers are more likely to do business with or champion a cause of the APN who they know, like, and trust.

- **Authority.** Studies referenced by Cialdini (2009) paint an almost chilling picture of how the idea of authority exerts influence over people. It seems that humans feel a strong pressure to listen and defer to authority. This has been played out numerous times, including studies done showing how nurses in the past almost blindly deferred to physicians. Today, in many circles, APNs are recognized as authority figures for their expertise and trustworthiness. This promises that APNs can have a great deal of influence in their marketing efforts.

- **Scarcity.** Scarcity is another center of influence that has been experienced by people worldwide. According to Cialdini (2009, p. 200), "opportunities seem more valuable to us when they are less available." One example is the limited launch of a product such as an iPad or Nike shoes, or having limited quantities of influenza immunizations. The limited availability of these products caused some stores to put up crowd control barricades and have police on hand. People seem to give more value to an item or opportunity that is less available. APNs can observe this in employment and educational opportunities. Patients may experience this in the possible limited availability of a favorite health care provider.

Preparing for an Advanced Practice Nurse Position

Whereas understanding these principles and other considerations that are important to beginning the process of marketing, there are several basic tasks to which APNs must attend as they begin their careers or change positions. For new graduates, the type of practice, location, population served, and support available for novice APNs are important considerations. Basic components of an APN's portfolio, such as the query letter, resumé, and/or curriculum vitae, must be addressed. Then, attention must be given to the interview itself. Attending to these important components gives the APN applicant confidence to go into the marketing process ready to be successful.

Resumé Versus the Curriculum Vitae

Resumés and curriculum vitae (CV) are often regarded as being one and the same. However, they have different structures and serve different purposes. Both reflect an APN's professional life; the more extensive his or her nursing experience and accomplishments, the stronger will be the CV and resumé. The curriculum vita has been described as the so-called whole cloth of an APN's experience and is a complete array of all her or his achievements over time. CVs are standard in format and content, are concise and organized, and content is added throughout a career. Usually, CVs are used for academic employment. On the other hand, the resumé is tailored to a particular job; it is marketing oneself to a prospective employer. The goal of a resumé is a visually clear and interesting representation of accomplishments. The average resumé receives about 20 seconds of review but may make the difference in getting a face to face interview with a potential employer. Table 20-1 lists the content categories for the CV and resumé. It is important to think through salary needs clearly prior to an interview, but past or current salary requirements should not be included in a CV or a resumé. Finally, and most important, is the need to proofread the document. Spelling errors, typos, poor grammar, and misleading data are certain avenues to failure. Exemplar 20-1 provides an example

EXEMPLAR 20-1   **Applying for an Advanced Practice Nurse Position**

Jack is an acute care nurse practitioner (ACNP) who has just graduated from his graduate program in nursing. His goal is to be hired as an ACNP in the intensive care unit (ICU) at a local medical center. The medical center is a teaching hospital and Jack is excited about being able to care for patients, gain experience and, in time, be able to teach and precept ACNP students as part of his role. The position is highly sought after, and Jack knows he will have competition for the job. The base salary starts at $95,000 annually so Jack wants to be sure that he becomes the choice candidate for this position.

To accomplish this goal, Jack considers his career goals and why this job is important to fulfilling his dreams of an ideal practice environment. First, he prepares a letter of inquiry that opens the door for an interview (Box 20-2). He updates the design of his resumé

and CV so it is crisp and professional. He creates a portfolio highlighting his ACNP graduate education, volunteer work with community-based programs, and his emergency medical technician (EMT) experience. Also, he works with a faculty mentor to practice his interviewing skills to ensure that his presentation will be polished. He thinks carefully about what questions he might be asked, how he would answer them, and what questions he might have. He writes down important points that he wants to be sure to include if he is asked. Jack requests letters from faculty and patients who have benefited from his care as an ACNP DNP student. He looks forward to this exciting opportunity to fulfill his dream of practicing as an ACNP and teaching in a major medical center.

 TABLE 20-1   **Content Categories for Curriculum Vitae and Resumé**

Curriculum Vitae	Resumé
Education	Career goals
National certification	Professional accomplishments
Professional experience	Education and certification
Honors	Targeted professional experience
Publications	Community, leadership activities
Research and grants	Other pertinent CV items related to the position
Presentations	
Consultations	
Workshop, conference attendance	
Professional memberships	
Activities and committees	
Community involvement	

of an APN applying for a position as an acute care nurse practitioner (ACNP).

Query Letter

Query letters are a marketing tool used to explore or create a need in a potential area of practice. They are personalized in the first sentence or two through the name of the referrer or through interest or ties to the clinical or geographic area. It is important to emphasize experiences that

particularly qualify the person for the job. Query letters are short, longer than a paragraph but not a full page. They should be written as a business letter and carefully proofread before they are sent (see Box 20-2).

Interview Process

New graduate APNs are often unsure of themselves when interviewing for positions. Being as prepared as possible may include having a resumé or CV professionally edited and formatted, or hiring a coach to improve interviewing skills, as Jack did. How much the APN will want to do and how much to invest is up to the individual. The SBA published guidelines about 3% to 5% of gross or projected revenues (www.sba.gov) is likely much more than most APNs will want or even need to spend, unless they are doing a major marketing effort to launch a practice (see next section).

Successful interviews require careful preparation (Reel & Abraham, 2007). It is useful first to think about what APNs bring to the table. Asking these questions of yourself will build confidence:

- Why are you the "ideal" APN provider in this case?
- Why are you the person they should choose for the job?
- Have you packed your portfolio with a current resumé, CV, credentials, and other information that this employer may want to see or that you want to present (e.g., example of a presentation, successful grant, community honor received)?

Finally, ask yourself what questions a prospective employer might ask so that you can be prepared. Here are some questions to consider:

BOX 20-2 Sample Query Letter

February 15, 2013

John Andrews, Director of Clinical Services
First Coast Medical Center
1111 Twin Forks Avenue
Los Angeles, California 19475

Dear Mr. Andrews:

I recently graduated with a Doctor of Nursing Practice degree, with an acute care nurse practitioner (ACNP) concentration, from St. Peter's University School of Nursing. I have successfully passed national certification and have my license as an ACNP. I did most of my student clinical work at First Coast Medical Center and I am most interested in staying in the Los Angeles area. I am writing to apply for your advertised ACNP position in the ICU. Having worked with the nurses and physicians at FCMC, I know that your hospital has the collaborative team orientation and holistic perspective that match what I am looking for in a practice environment.

In addition to my graduate studies, I have worked with underserved populations locally through a church-based clinic in your area for the past 4 years. Since high school, and throughout my nursing education, I have worked as an Emergency Medical Technician with the Hospital Ambulance Service.

I have attached a resumé with more details regarding my education and experience. I can be easily reached by e-mail or by phone. I look forward to talking with you about the position.

Sincerely,
Jack Rogers, MSN, ACNP-BC
123 North Street
Los Angeles, CA 19475
800-222-1222
Rogjdnp@google.com

- "Tell me about a time when you had to make a decision that you were unsure of."
- "How would you respond if you were facing 'push-back' from a physician?"
- "So, why community-based primary care after all these years in acute care nursing?"
- "How do you organize your day to get your work done?"
- "We practice according to guidelines. What would you do if you thought it was not in the best interest of the patient to follow the guideline?"
- "What, specifically, is your clinical experience?"

Health Care as a Business

An important concept for APNs to understand is that the service they offer as an employee or through their own private practice is a business (see Chapter 21). Practice generates revenue for the APN and/or employer. Although all APNs may not seem to generate revenue directly, all save money by preventing complications, improving outcomes, assisting others to do a better job, or educating patients to be healthier. This is particularly true if APNs are allowed to function to the full scope of their education and training as recommended by the IOM *Future of Nursing* report (IOM, 2010) and the PPACA (HHS, 2011).

APNs who do not think of themselves as a business may not recognize that they have customers and clients who have different needs and require a myriad of services. Box 20-3 shows the people and entities considered to be potential customers and clients for APNs.

As APNs become more experienced, particularly in primary care settings, they begin to explore marketing their services directly to the public. The next section focuses on these APNs, although the principles and techniques can be useful to all APNs, regardless of setting. For example, a clinical nurse specialist (CNS) or ACNP in a tertiary care hospital, or a certified registered nurse anesthetist (CRNA) or certified nurse-midwife (CNM) who is contracting across several hospitals, could use these principles and techniques to market their services internally to administrators.

Preparing to Market Advanced Practice Nurse Services

Understanding these marketing concepts is key to success. However, there is still more work that must be done before APNs can carry out marketing. In this section, the legal and ethical questions that APNs have about marketing, as well as some precautions, are presented. The first step is to identify clearly exactly what is being marketed and who are the intended recipients.

What is your Product?

Every business, whether an individual or a company, has a product—that is, something they are selling. For many APNs, that product will be themselves and their services (Box 20-1 lists other product categories). Note that several products can actually belong to more than one category, depending on how they are marketed.

If you are unclear about your product, consider the core competencies that define APNs and their particular niche. Perhaps an APN's expertise is education, research, clinical practice, or leadership. APNs must understand

BOX 20-3   Advanced Practice Nurse Marketing Niches and Services

Setting	Service
Acute care hospital	Adolescent specialist
Assisted living facility	Brokering advocacy for specific populations
Birthing center	Cardiovascular care
College, university	Chronic illness management
Convenient care clinic	Daycare consultant
Correctional health care	Diabetes management
Government agency	Disaster preparation
Homeless shelter	Employee health care
Insurance company	Gerontology
Multidisciplinary clinical practice	First-assistant surgery service
Mobile health service	Fitness, exercise consultant
Pediatrics, school health clinic	Health policy consultant
Retirement center	Health, wellness coaching
Same-day surgery center	HIV-AIDS care
Urgent care facility	Lactation consultant
Women's health center	Mammography, breast health counseling
	Pain management
	Palliative care
	Population-focused program of care (e.g., heart failure clinic)
	Psychiatric care and counseling
	Risk management consultant
	Special population (e.g., lesbian, gay, immigrant health)

what it is they do and how that translates into benefit for clients.

Who is the Ideal Client/Patient?

Two common terms, *ideal client (patient)* and *target market,* are used to identify who it is that may have the greatest interest in the product of an APN. It is a way of segmenting the population so that the message is heard by those who are most interested. The target market or ideal client can be a patient, employer, potential business or research partner, educational organization, or company.

Identifying the ideal client or employer does several things. It allows the APN to create a message aimed directly to the client or employer in a way that they can hear above all the marketing noise. Being able to identify these ideal clients will allow the APN to be most effective, making their work more satisfying for all involved.

There are several steps involved in identifying the ideal client, beginning with understanding your objective. This decision usually requires deep reflection. For example, is the objective to get a first job after graduation or is it to grow a new independent practice? The next question may be "who do I want to work with?" Taking this a step further, it is vital that each APN understand that he or she works better with certain clients and patients than others. For example, the family nurse practitioner (FNP) who has

been educated to work with patients of all ages may find she or he works best with a younger or older population. Who, what, when, where, and how do you do your best work most enjoyably?

As the picture of an ideal client emerges, the next step is identifying the behaviors of this ideal client.

- If the client is a patient, how do they like to access health care, including days, time, location, and method?
- Where does he or she spend time?
- What activities do they like to do?
- What publications or books do they read?
- What are their learning styles?

For an organization in which you hope to gain employment, consider the location, mission, and values of the organization, community activities, and education offerings for staff and the public.

The process of identifying the ideal client will create a clear picture of the client. Marketing experts often recommend creating an actual picture and name for that one ideal person because it helps in improving marketing skills when talking to one individual as opposed to the general population. Identifying an ideal client and creating a message that resonates with this client will greatly increase the odds that the ideal client (or employer) will receive, hear, and act on the APN's message.

EXEMPLAR 20-2   A CNS-Led Clinic Influences System-Wide Policy Change

A DNP-prepared CNS, Clara, employed in a health system, found a great deal of satisfaction establishing a nurse-managed center for patients with cardiovascular disease. The establishment of the clinic was feasible only after careful research and discovering that the number of patients who were being rehospitalized for the same cardiovascular problems was increasing. After analyzing the evidence-based literature, Clara thought that a clinic would promote patient self-care and improve understanding of how lifestyle behaviors could enhance quality of life. She convinced the system administrators that a clinic in which patients' status could be monitored regularly using technology (e.g., via e-mail, phone contacts, video camera, smartphone) would eventually decrease system costs because of decreased readmissions. Clara marketed the concept to the hospital administrators and implemented the clinic. Marketed through community brochures, speaking opportunities, and distribution of flyers to local physicians and clinics, she was able to change system-wide policy with the development of the first APN-directed clinic for the system. Patient outcomes improved and rehospitalizations for cardiac patients decreased. The clinic became an excellent revenue source and marketing tool for the hospital.

The next step involves research to explore the characteristics of the patients with whom the APN most enjoys working. An APN may look at age, gender, educational level, occupation, financial income, and geographic location. If the objective is employment, specific information is necessary, including the benefits that the APN hopes to gain (e.g., salary, continued professional development, education opportunities, research and publication, advancement opportunities).

Depending on the objective, the APN may also want to consider psychodemographics. This may include the interest, mission, values, and ethics of the individuals and companies. Baum and Henkel (2010) have suggested that attention to patients' needs drives effective, ethically sound, marketing practices for health care. APNs interested in wellness-based practice will likely want to target individuals and organizations who value health, wellness, and prevention.

Features Versus Benefits of Marketing

It is critical for APNs to be clear on what it is that they actually do for their client as opposed to what their product has or does. This is the difference between benefits and features; benefits focus on outcomes whereas features focus on activities. This distinction is often misunderstood. For example, the statement "I help women move through breast cancer journeys" is a benefit to emphasize rather than "I provide oncology care", a feature of APN practice.

As an APN offering services to a local clinic, these features may include credentials, availability, competencies, and experience. The benefit for that clinic is that the APN will ease the burden on other providers; patients of the clinic will have better outcomes and increased satisfaction, which in turn will allow the clinic continued growth and success.

Identifying features of a product is often much easier than identifying the benefits of that product. One way for APNs to do this is to ask "What do I really do for my patients?" and "What do my patients really get out of being cared for by me?" (Phillips, 2011a). Most important is "What difference do I make to my patients' outcomes?" If the APN is unsure, one excellent way to find out is to question the patient and listen for feedback. Exemplars 20-2 and 20-3 exemplify the benefits APNs bring to patients.

Message

Understanding the problems faced by clients and the benefits that clients will receive through APN care allows the APN to create a message that will speak directly to them. The marketing message is a fluid one. It is a succinct message that sums up the benefits that an ideal client will receive when cared for by an APN. This message can then be encapsulated to create a tag line (five to nine words) or expanded to various lengths for advertisements, Internet copy, brochures, and more. It can be regarded as an accordion that can be expanded and contracted as necessary, but the core message remains intact.

Famous brands are often the easiest to reference. Consider this one: "Just Do It." Many people will recognize this tag line as belonging to Nike. It is directed at individuals who want to exercise and have many excuses not to exercise; they just need to do it. This message is repeated again in the company's product line, websites, stores, and events. Everything Nike does is focused on those three words. Although not as widely recognized as Nike or FedEx, medical centers also often have a tag line. For example, the University of Washington Medical Center uses the tag line, "Empowering people to live healthier lives here and around the globe through exceptional patient care, research, and education." Individuals, businesses, and

EXEMPLAR 20-3   A Certified Nurse Midwife (CNM) Builds a Home Birthing Practice

Marie is a CNM who provides home birthing services in a small Midwestern community. To market her business and practice, she has developed a marketing campaign that focuses on the benefits that her services provide to families.

Marie realizes that the *features* of her CNM prenatal and delivery care services are certainly important, but it is the *benefits of her care* that convince patients and their families to try her services. For example, features include the fact that she or a colleague is available 24 hours a day to come to a family's home for midwifery services and that backup emergency services, if needed, are readily available at the hospital 24/7. Another feature is that her services are covered by most insurance plans and are cost-effective.

The CNM understands that the benefits of the services that she provides are what is most important to the family. For example, families using her services have found that the home birthing environment is a perfect setting for welcoming a new family member. It is less stressful on the child and promotes a stronger family bond for all in attendance. In addition, because pregnant mothers are carefully screened prior to planning a home birth, home births have fewer complications and infections and are more comfortable for the baby and mother (more information can be found at www.birthcenters.org).

By being able to articulate the features and benefits of her services, Marie was able to market and build her practice in her small community successfully.

 BOX 20-4   Advanced Practice Nurse Tag Lines

Nurse	Tag Line
Theresa Hill, FNP: Walk-in Clinic	Health Care on Your Schedule
Cheryl Winter, RD, FNP; DiabeteStepsRx	Simplifying Diabetes Remedies
Nan Sprouse, FNP, Seasons of Farragut, TN	Balance Your Body, Balance Your Life
Karen Swift, CNM, WomanCare	Care for Women of All Ages in All Stages
Elena Schjavland, NP, Keys2Mem♥ry	Putting the Heart First in Neuro-Cognitive Disease Care

practices deserve a tag line. Some examples of APN tag lines can be found in Box 20-4.

As can be seen, each of these APN-owned businesses uses a tag line to tell potential clients what they do and how they do it. It drives their marketing and the philosophy of their business.

Marketing Avenues, Media, and Technology

It is important to understand that not all marketing channels, sometimes referred to as marketing venues, are appropriate for everyone. This is the prime reason why it is important for APNs to understand the ideal patient, client, and employer. In today's health care arena, all APNs must be able to assist with marketing, whether they are employees or entrepreneurs. For example, as

day surgery moves to the private community-based office, the APN may be the person who is given the task of preparing marketing materials. With greater understanding, the APN will recognize which channels will provide the best chance of getting the marketing message to the desired client. It is vital to understand that one venue is rarely enough; multiple marketing channels are generally required.

It has been estimated that people are exposed to a large number of marketing messages every day. With all that noise, it is hard to hear the message. Marketing experts agree that to ensure that the client hears the message, they need to be exposed to it at least seven to ten times over a 3-month period. Thus, multiple (ideal) channels and multiple exposures of the correct message are needed.

Marketing can be accomplished both online and offline and these lines may be blurred. It is vital for APNs to use a combination of media. Health care consumers and clients of APN services are becoming more technology savvy and will be using online searches and similar methods to locate services, learn about providers and health care conditions, obtain references and, in general, look for the evidence that a particular APN is the provider that they need.

Offline Marketing

Offline channels are associated with traditional marketing. Some have called these channels old-fashioned and ignore them. Although online marketing is newer, millions of people still read paper mail, newspapers, and listen to the radio. It is important for APNs to understand how the channel they are using fits their market and how they can use it creatively.

Print media include items that can be given out, as well as anything printed in the traditional sense. Printed business cards and brochures are still a mainstay for APN marketing. Business cards have a variety of uses. Many people advocate for putting messages on the back, but leaving the back blank may be even better. The person who is receiving the card can then use it for notes and reminders. Many APNs make recommendations to patients about obtaining a book or other item, their next appointment, or a place to write down their blood pressure.

Some experts have suggested that printed brochures are becoming unnecessary now that consumers can access that information online in the form of websites and downloadable PDF documents. However, our personal experience and that of colleagues has suggested that brochures are essential. Patients may hold on to brochures for a long time before calling for an appointment or pass them on to their friends, who may eventually come in to be seen.

Whatever print form is used, it must be professional, distinctive, and readable. It is important to avoid too much information and essential to include: name, business name (as appropriate), how to be contacted, website, and tag line. Brochures should include information about the practice, services being offered, the provider(s), and anything else that is essential. An APN employed by a practice that does not have a brochure may want to help them to craft one.

Written Word

Printed material is not limited to business cards and similar items. Perhaps writing a health- related column in the local newspaper or magazine on a regular or semi-regular basis is a possibility. An amazing thing seems to happen when an author is published; suddenly she or he is seen as the expert and the "go to" person among health care consumers in the community.

Other forms of the written word include flyers. These can be placed on bulletin boards in locations that clients frequent, inserted into bags at the pharmacy or grocery store, or even inserted into the local paper.

Direct mail includes sending a letter, brochure, or post-card directly to the patient or potential client. There is a whole science behind direct mail; readers who are interested in this approach might want to begin their search at the Direct Marketing Association (www.the-dma.org).

Air Waves

Being on the air is not something that is limited to large companies with large budgets. It is an excellent way to get the word out about APN care, the practice, and what services are offered. Consider local radio stations. All have some version of a morning talk show and many are looking for guest experts to talk about something that is in the news or is important to the health care community. Local television is often the same, although it is more difficult to get on the air; a more accessible route is the local cable access channel. In many communities with local access, it may be possible to create a TV spot, focusing on an APN niche topic for a nominal fee.

Networking

There are many types of networking and almost all of them can bring in clients, directly or indirectly. When networking, it is important to understand that you are not there to sell your products and services but to build relationships. This is true with direct face to face networking and online networking. People generally purchase care or hire a health care provider from someone they know, like, and trust. Thus, networking is about building relationships.

Prepare ahead of time and have an elevator speech ready. An elevator speech is being able to answer the question, "So what do you do?" in the time it takes to go up or down in an elevator, in many cases in less than 30 seconds and occasionally up to 2 minutes, although shorter is better. The purpose is to give enough information in a clear and concise manner that is benefit-driven. Done correctly, an ideal client will ask for more information, so it will be important to have that prepared as well. APNs will want to practice the speech so it can be delivered confidently and competently and to practice on colleagues to get their feedback.

Word of Mouth

Word of mouth marketing is important, so much so that it has its own association dedicated to helping its members build their brand by word of mouth, the Word of Mouth Marketing Association (www.womma.org). Simply put, it is people talking to one another, making recommendations to like a product (APNs) and do business with them or not; it is a powerful but often undervalued marketing technique (Clay, 2011; Gombeski, Britt, Wray, et al., 2011). Word of mouth (positive or negative) recommendations are often subjective; they can make or break a practice or ruin or elevates one's reputation. The buzz created is often emotional and may or may not be factual.

Unfortunately, people talk about the negative far more often than the positive. When health care providers have an unhappy client, they are likely to express their displeasure to friends, family, and colleagues, and perhaps go even further. Alternatively, in professional situations, the same thing may occur but without any verbal action. For example, a former employer or colleague may decline to give a recommendation. In such cases, the adage "silence speaks louder than words" holds true. APNs can, however, be proactive with patients and colleagues by encouraging them to spread the word when they are pleased with the care provided. An APN may want to request something written or in electronic format that defines a service well done.

Community Involvement

Getting involved in the local community is a powerful way for APNs to give back and build positive awareness about themselves and their practice. This is an excellent way for potential clients to meet and feel comfortable coming in to see APNs. Other venues for community involvement include local health fairs, community fundraisers, especially those focusing on health and health care, local chamber of commerce, or volunteering to be on hand for first-aid service at a sporting event.

Online Marketing

The term *online marketing* refers to tools, techniques, and strategies found online. The Pew Research Center (http://pewresearch.org/) has been tracking trends around the world and characterizing them for years. One of their projects examines health care trends, offline and online. Although much of their research is U.S.-based, they are now looking at global attitudes.

According to Pew, 78% of U.S. adults use the Internet and 83% of adults own a cell phone; smartphones can now access the Internet. Of adult Internet users, almost 60% look up health care information. In one author's (BCP) own practice over a 5-year period, a large majority of new patients came from two sources, the Internet and word of mouth. Searching the Internet also allows the patient to find out which providers are covered in their network.

These days, and in the future, whether APNs are looking for a job, growing a practice, or communicating with clients, using the Internet is a major tool. Harnessing its power, regardless of where they are in the world, will allow APNs to have a greater and faster reach than by using strictly offline marketing channels.

Websites

Despite the prevalence of the Internet in everything clinicians do, the question as to whether a website is necessary is often asked. The answer is an unequivocal and enthusiastic "yes!" Setting up a website is a fairly simple process and low-cost tools are available to do it personally or locate outlets where competent individuals can create a site at a reasonable cost.

Although it is very easy to get online today, APNs should take caution in regard to what they publish. First and foremost, a website needs to be current and updated regularly. A website, name plate site, or social media profile should say something about the APN, the practice or business and, if applicable, what opportunities the APN is interested in. However, it is vital that APNs do not publish any information anywhere that they do not want to be public, in any online venue, ever.

Audio and Video

Another area to consider is producing audio and video files. This is relatively easy and can be done for free. When looking for an APN position that involves teaching, speaking, and working with the general public, a potential employer would benefit from seeing and hearing the APN in public. If an APN is marketing a business or practice, potential patients and clients would also enjoy seeing this up front to determine whether the APN is the type of person with whom they wish to work. Some people even produce regular shows (audio or video) and have their own channels, for example, using YouTube or Skype. All one needs is interesting content, a microphone, and a webcam (or smartphone) to be a producer.

Advertising

There are many places for APNs to advertise themselves or their business online. One just needs to browse using Google or another search engine to see thousands of ads. The APN can go directly to the websites used by ideal clients and see if they can advertise directly on their website. Perhaps they publish an electronic newsletter where they can place an ad. Also, it is important, not to forget all the social media sites that are now available. Again, APNs will want to find the places that their ideal client frequents to target advertising efforts.

Teleclasses and Webinars

Online presentations can have a global reach, so if the desired outcome is not limited by geography, APNs should consider learning how to create and participate in teleclasses and/or webinars. This venue is similar to doing a talk in the community to teach and build a practice. In this case, instead of face to face, it is done through the telephone or, in the case of a webinar, through software in which an APN might share a slide presentation of himself or herself live via webcam.

Local Online Searches

APNs with a business or practice in a specific location will want to be listed on popular search engines such as Google, Yahoo, and Bing. According to the Pew Commission Report (Fox, 2011) more patients are finding their health care provider not only online with computers but with smartphones. By doing a bit of research, it is possible to see what is popular for locating businesses in a desired area and how to find out how to get listed. In many cases, these listings are free.

Mixed Marketing

Marketing channels most often include a mix of online and offline venues; many venues are now a combination of online and offline (Cockrum, 2011). For example, one service that is available to all is called HARO, "Help A Reporter Out" (http://www.helpareporter.com/). It is an online service in which reporters and/or publishers request that an individual with experience in some field answer some questions or be interviewed for a print or online publication. There is even a health category. This is a fantastic opportunity for APNs to be mentioned or even interviewed as an expert. Expert status helps APNs market themselves and their practice.

Emerging Channels: Mobile Devices

Mobile devices (e.g., smartphones, tablets) are now outpacing computer sales worldwide. According to the World Bank, at the time of this writing, 6 billion people worldwide have mobile devices (www.worldbank.org/category/tags/mobilephones). People can use them to conduct business, receive their paychecks, and even check to see whether their medication is counterfeit. Several of the techniques mentioned in this section can be used in a mobile environment. There are many ways that an APN can direct marketing outreach to mobile devices.

Social Media Marketing

Although websites may come and go, the popularity and effectiveness of social media are undeniable. And while one sees them as "social," they are really much more. Obviously, the most popular social media site at the time of this writing is Facebook. Currently, it has more than 1 billion users worldwide, more than half using Facebook on a mobile device (https://en.wikipedia.org/wiki/Facebook). To put this statistic into perspective, it is said that if Facebook were a country, it would be the third most populated country in the world.

Many professionals want to know why social media sites such as Facebook are important marketing sites. Simply, it is because the APN's ideal clients and patients are there. It is imperative that APNs claim their own identity and that APN practices and businesses be present on these sites. Not having a social media marketing (SMM) presence is like not being listed in the phone book.

The pull of social media for many is that the content generated, regardless of the site, is user-generated. Because of this, APNs will want to set up a means to generate a presence and then monitor what is being said. It would be unwise to think that an SSM site is only for patients. An employer (or potential employer), university, malpractice insurance carrier, graduate school, publisher, and more will be searching for what is being generated by and said about an individual (Porterfield, Khare, & Vahl, 2011).

Understanding Legal and Ethical Considerations

One of the most important aspects of being online, particularly social media sites, is remembering that everything that goes online stays there forever. Even more important to APNs is the fact that online communication, including websites, forums, and social media sites, are subject to the legal process of discovery should they be named in an investigation. The following are some extremely important key principles when marketing professional services online:

1. Create professional identities across several venues. Upload one or more professional photographs.
2. Create a biosketch to add to these sites and keep it current.
3. Never, ever talk about patients, their families, clients, or even personnel at work, even if their identity is not revealed. Friends, families, and patients can read themselves or their loved ones into comments.
4. Do not publish anything online at any time that would be of concern if seen by a judge, administrator, or family member.
5. Always err on the side of caution. If in doubt, do not share it online.

Ethical Concerns

A key competency for APNs is ethical decision making (see Chapter 13). Although there are many theoretical approaches, when it comes to marketing, the principle of veracity, which means the duty to tell the truth and not to deceive others, is key. The principle of veracity appears to be absent in some marketing practices today. One needs to look no further than the advertisements by pharmaceutical companies direct to consumers, weight loss aids, and products marketed to boost one's athletic performance.

APNs who hold a DNP have been criticized by some in organized medicine that using the title "Doctor" will confuse health care consumers, legislatures, and employers. However, the APN who follows the rule of not to deceive will avoid this particular ethical and perhaps legal issue by ensuring that he or she is clearly stating their APN credentials in addition to the title "Doctor." Some may seek to prevent APNs from using their doctoral title, citing patient confusion, but there are already rules and regulations via the U.S. Federal Trade Commission to ensure truth in advertising.

A common question asked by APNs is how to use the reviews or testimonials that patients and clients bestow on them. Many worry about the legality of using testimonials citing privacy and HIPAA regulations (HHS, 2012; see Chapter 19). Testimonials can be used with written permission from patients and clients, including whether or not they want their name used. The issue is the patient's willingness to be identified. When it comes to websites, patients are free to identify themselves without worry on the part of the clinician.

Marketing Plan

In 1866, *Alice in Wonderland* author Lewis Carroll wrote, "If you don't know where you are going, any road will get you there." When considering marketing and promotion, these words ring true. Anyone can begin to promote themselves, but if they don't have clear goals and a strategic plan, they will still get results, but they may not be the results that are desired. For most APNs, a simple marketing framework (Table 20-2), called W5HE—W5 (who,

what, when, where, why), H (how), E (evaluate)—will work (Phillips, 2011b).

With this information, the APN can move forward to plan and create various campaigns. Because the public is bombarded with marketing messages, as noted earlier, one message will need to be repeated from seven to ten times before it is heard. In other words, do not expect great results from a onetime marketing effort.

A marketing campaign is where the APN identifies the goal and implements action steps that will achieve that goal or objective. An example of a marketing campaign for a diabetes clinic is shown in Table 20-3.

The APN's marketing plan will depend on the objectives, clients, time frame, theme, and budget (Luther, 2011). It's helpful to plan and schedule marketing activities on a quarterly or even annual basis. Keeping marketing messages fresh is a universal challenge. It helps to include marketing efforts with something that is already in the minds of the clients, such as community and

TABLE 20-2   W5HE Marketing Plan Framework

Why	Why are you marketing? What is your goal, your objective? What is the anticipated outcome from this activity?
Who	Who are you marketing to? Who is your ideal client, patient or family?
What	What is the care or service you want to offer? What is the budget you are working with? What is your strategy?
When	When will you market yourself? What is the best timing? What is your strategy? How often will you repeat this process?
Where	Where will you be marketing? What are the best venues for your ideal clients, patients?
How	How will you carry this plan out? Will you have assistance or be doing all of the work yourself? What systems will you need to have in place to ensure that it gets done?
Evaluate	What results did you achieve? Do you need to adjust and repeat the process? What is your return on investment?

Adapted from Phillips, B. C. (2011a). Marketing—your other full-time job (part 1 of 2) (http://www.nppracticemgt.com/articles/article_details/marketingyour-other-full-time-job-part-1-of-2); and Phillips, B. C. (2011b). Marketing—your other full-time job (part 2 of 2) (http://www.nppracticemgt.com/ currentissue/currentissue_details/marketingyour-other-full-time-job-part-2-of-2).

TABLE 20-3   Example of Marketing Plan for a Diabetes Clinic

Why	Objective, goal: Bring 20 new patients into the diabetes clinic in June 2013.
Who	Individuals 21 years and older with type 2 diabetes who are interested in holistic diabetic treatment in addition to medication
What	The APN practice is a diabetes specialty practice that works closely with patients to achieve their goals using lifestyle modifications, including diet, exercise. and appropriate medications as necessary. Event: Open House on June 2, 2013, with follow-up appointments throughout the month Budget: $300.00 for the June campaign
When	Begin in May and continue throughout June.
Where	Event location: 123 Main Street, Anywhere, USA Marketing locations: Health food stores, Facebook page and ads, announcements at the hospital diabetes class, pharmacies; consider door prize to increase interest.
How	Word of mouth: Invite current patients and encourage them to invite others. Local health food stores, gym, diabetes mellitus class, pharmacies: talk with staff, post announcement, perhaps insert flyer in the bags. Facebook: Announcement on clinic page, Facebook ads targeting specific criteria Announcement on clinic website and in e-newsletter
Evaluate	How many people came to the open house? How many new patients booked evaluations? Calculate the return on investment.

TABLE 20-4	**Spreadsheet Example**								
							COST		
Dates	Objective	How Long?	Media	Who	Copy Due	Estimated	Actual	Results
Every Wednesday in October	Breast cancer screening	4 wk	Newspaper display ad	Sue	9/15	$300	$315	$600 for six new patients
11/1 and 11/15	Diabetes clinic	2 issues	Practice e-newsletter	Bob	10/25	$0	Time	10 patient appointments; diabetes primary care
11/10	Diabetes clinic	30 min	Local radio station talk radio guest	Jane	N/A	$0	Time	Three inquiries for initial patient visits

sporting events or holidays. As health care professionals, another tool is the health observances calendar that is updated annually. For example, February is Heart Health Month. There are also specific days and weeks set aside for World AIDS Day, Poison Awareness Week, Brain Health Week, and Hepatitis Awareness Month. At the time of this writing, the list is available at http://healthfinder.gov/nho/nho.asp, or do a search for "Health Observances Calendar."

One consideration is using a spreadsheet or a calendar that can be shared with those who may be helping to keep track of plans throughout the year. The spreadsheet will not only help track marketing efforts, but will also help track results. There are several free tools online, such as Google Docs, that will help make this process easier. See Table 20-4.

Return on Investment

What is return on investment (ROI)? This simply indicates whether the results and benefits of the marketing campaign outweighed the cost in terms of time, effort, and dollars spent.

APNs commonly ask how much should be budgeted for marketing. Unfortunately, there is no easy answer to this question. Although the SBA (www.sba.org) recommends anywhere from 2% to 10% of gross revenues, this figure is variable for health care business ventures.

Regardless of how the marketing budget is determined, it is important to realize that APNs in many practices must invest in marketing, whether they are marketing themselves or their practice. It is imperative that they track marketing efforts subsequent to revenue results and make adjustments accordingly.

Negotiating and Contracting

Knowledge of contracts is an important component of the APN's employment process. A contract is a legally binding agreement between two or more parties. Contracts can be verbal but usually are written. They define who is involved, what is agreed on, including all the terms, and how the contract may be terminated. Contracts are used in a variety of situations, from buying a house to getting a job. APNs are exposed to several different types of contracts throughout their careers—independent contractor contracts, employment agreements or contracts, contracts with third-party payers, vendors, and sometimes with clients. In addition, many APNs are required by their state and local statues to have what are termed *collaborative practice agreements*, a form of contract with physician preceptors to practice. This section will focus on contracts that APNs commonly use during their day to day work, including employment and independent and agreements with collaborating physicians. Third-party payer contracts are discussed in Chapters 19 and 21.

Importance of Contracts

It is important to understand why contracts are essential to practice. As a whole, nurses and APNs are a trusting group and often prefer to use a verbal agreement rather than a business formality. However, contracts are protective for the individual APN and employer or business with whom they are contracting. The best case scenario is a contract that provides for a win-win situation for all parties involved.

Contracts provide clarity in the terms of agreement and responsibilities; they force negotiation of issues between the parties and reduce the chance for misunderstanding. When written, they provide a reference for parties to refresh their memory of the agreement. Also, if necessary, contracts provide for legal enforcement if the situation warrants it. Contracts have little to do with trust, mistrust, or liking or not liking the individuals involved; they are about doing business in a professional manner.

Independent Contractor Contract

One way that APNs can contract for their services is through an independent contractor (IC) contract with a health care facility. CRNAs and CNMs often use this type of contract when working with a hospital or other facility in which they are not full-time employees. Before an APN can venture out as an independent contractor, it is essential to have an understanding of what constitutes an IC. In the United States, the Internal Revenue Service (IRS) defines an IC. Misrepresentation and misunderstanding of the IC can cause difficulty for the business that is doing the contracting and the individual APN.

According to the IRS (2013):

People such as doctors, dentists, veterinarians, lawyers, accountants, contractors, subcontractors, public stenographers, or auctioneers who are in an independent trade, business, or profession in which they offer their services to the general public are generally independent contractors. However, whether these people are independent contractors or employees depends on the facts in each case. The general rule is that an individual is an independent contractor if the payer has the right to control or direct only the result of the work and not what will be done and how it will be done. The earnings of a person who is working as an independent contractor are subject to Self-Employment Tax.

You are not an independent contractor if you perform services that can be controlled by an employer (what will be done and how it will be done). This applies even if you are given freedom of action. What matters is that the employer has the legal right to control the details of how the services are performed.

In general, to be considered an IC, APNs control how and what they do (employers control and/or direct the results), are free to offer services to others, have the potential for profit or loss from the professional relationship (Buzogany, 2010), do not receive any benefits from the employer, and are given an IRS 1099 form at the end of the year for tax purposes (see Exemplar 20-4).

When drafting an IC contract, it is wise to consult an attorney who is knowledgeable about APN practice, needs and local laws. In general, an IC contact should define the following:

- General information
- Who the contract is between: the APN (name, credential, professional designation, licensure) and the business or agency (name, location, purpose as related to the contract)
- Dates that the contract will be in effect
- Services being provided by the business or agency and services being provided by the APN

- Business or agency responsibilities
- Operations and facilities as they relate to the APN
- Location, physical support
- Clinical services support, including medical records, physician collaboration if needed, medical equipment
- Billing services (if this is what is being proposed; in some cases, APNs may bill for their services; in others, the agency bills)
- APN responsibilities for services
  - Pays for licensure, certification, and malpractice insurance
  - Provides own tools to perform services (e.g., examination instruments, personal digital assistant)
  - Sets hours within parameters for the business with on-call coverage if agreed on
  - Adheres to standard of care and practice for the work
- Joint responsibilities of the parties
  - Working together to meet compliance and regulatory issues
  - Achieving positive patient outcomes
- Contract term and termination should address the following:
  - What is the term?
  - How can the contract be terminated?
  - What is cause for immediate termination on behalf of either party?
  - Termination notice?
  - End of term—what happens?
  - What options are available for continuation, if any?
  - Legal or administrative matters
  - Payment

Employment Contract

Although many APNs work at will, many are now asking for contracts or employers are offering contracts. Each state has employment laws and most provide for what is known as at will employment. This means that an individual's employment will continue as long as both parties agree—that is, the APN (the employee) wants to remain employed, and the employer that hired the APN (e.g., hospital, agency, physician group practice) wants to continue to have the APN working for them. Either party can terminate at any given time, for any reason. There is no legal right to the position. As an employee, the only legal protection has to do with laws prohibiting discrimination.

On the other hand, a contract will provide the APN and employer with some legal protection and define various aspects of the agreement. A contract can be

EXEMPLAR 20-4 **A CRNA as an Independent Contractor**

Jillian is a CRNA working as an independent contractor in a rural section of the state where she provides anesthesia services to three small rural hospitals and one outpatient surgical center. She is not a hospital employee. Jill provides preanesthesia care prior to surgical procedures, administers anesthesia, and cares for patients in recovery room and postanesthesia care areas. She rotates one day each week in the three hospitals and outpatient surgical center.

Prior to setting herself up as an IC, Jill researched each hospital so that she clearly understood their policies and what the job entailed. She reviewed the standards of care and practice for the work. She also reviewed her credentials and prepared a list of questions she wanted to ask, including hours of work, on-call requirements, payment, and terms of termination. She carefully thought out the terms she needed in an IC contract to provide the best anesthesia service possible at each place of service and also to protect her own interests.

To protect herself, she set herself up as a business by incorporating as a limited liability company (LLC) (see Chapter 19). She carefully calculated her costs, including her tax obligation, malpractice insurance, continuing education, and health insurance. Because the facilities were billing for her services, she did not have to provide billing services. She took these factors into account when calculating her asking fee.

To be prepared for these contracts, and any future contracts, Jillian keeps copies of all contracts, required documents to prove her qualifications, and notes on any negotiation done, in one central location. In the case of her current facilities, each had their own standard contract that is used for ICs. Jillian carefully evaluated the contract, made requests for changes, and had her attorney review the contract.

---

considered preventive because it puts issues on the table where they can be addressed before they become a problem (Letz, 2002; Roberts, 2010).

Employment contracts are similar to the contract for an IC, with some critical differences. Employment contracts define the role that will be filled, the legal issues around the terms of employment, and issues around compensation. Employment contracts are specific to the hospital or agency involved and should be carefully reviewed before signing.

Role and Position

There are several issues surrounding role or position:
- What is the specific service that the APN will be providing during employment?
- Does it include on-call responsibilities?
- Is it clinical or perhaps split among clinical care, education, research, mentoring of students, and more?
- Are there provisions for assistance to carry out the APN role? For example, as a provider seeing patients in a clinic setting, will there be an assistant to help the APN?
- Is staying current in the specialty essential for any clinical provider?
- Will tools and resources, such as memberships, subscriptions and continuing education, be provided?
- Are there office hours or is there time for administrative duties?

These and other factors are extremely important for APNs to fulfill their roles in a chosen practice environment. It is also imperative that legal issues be addressed:
- What is the length of the contract?
- How can or will this contract be adjusted or updated?
- What happens when it is time for the contract to be renewed?
- Is there a noncompete clause, sometimes called a restrictive covenant (Box 20-5)?
- Are issues addressed for legal requirements for practice, such as a collaborating physician if necessary?
- Are termination of employment issues addressed—both for the employer and the APN?

In regard to reimbursement, the following must be considered:
- How will you be compensated?
- Is it hourly wage or salary?
- Is your compensation tied to productivity?
- If so, how? What is the formula?
- Are there bonuses and how are they calculated?
- What happens if you do not meet productivity benchmarks?
- If payment is via an hourly wage, is the overtime or on-call process clearly stated?

Other benefits, such as health care coverage, continuing education (with time off to attend courses), vacation, retirement, and disability insurance are all important items for consideration. Professional APNs are required to

BOX 20-5   Restrictive Covenant

A restrictive covenant, also known as a noncompete clause, is often put into employment agreements by employers. The clause restricts the employee from working for another organization within a set distance for a set amount of time after the APN leaves that employer. The basic reason for such a clause is to prevent patients from leaving the current facility and moving with the APN to another facility.

BOX 20-6   Items to include in Collaborative Practice Agreement

- Delineate the responsibilities of the collaborating physician and the APN according to state and local requirements.
- Include the date the agreement starts and when it will need to be updated or renegotiated.
- Include time commitments, chart reviews, and on-site requirements.
- Address the method and frequency of communication, as required.
- Identify any written protocols or reference material as required by regulation.

maintain licenses and certification, so it should be determined beforehand whether these fees are also part of the benefit package. A clothing allowance (e.g., scrubs, laboratory coats) should also be considered.

Collaborative Practice Agreement

Collaborative practice agreements (CPAs) outline the agreement between a physician and APN as required by state and local law in some states (see Chapter 21). In the United States, requirements vary from state to state, with some states eliminating them altogether whereas others mandate that APNs have written CPA agreements. APNs in states that require a CPA should look to the state's board of nursing to find out what is required and whether there have been recent changes in state rules. See Chapter 21 for a detailed discussion of new changes in state law proposed by the Consensus Model for APRN Regulation (NCSBN, 2008).

A CPA is much like any other contract; it is a proactive document that allows issues to be discussed up front. It outlines expectations and responsibilities of the parties involved and defines the terms of the agreement. In many cases, the APN who is employed by a physician or organization will have this document as part of her or his employment. Before drafting a CPA, it is essential that the APN fully understand what the state law requires and the responsibility of the collaborating physician. For example, in one state, the APN may find that all that is needed is a document that states you will contact Dr. Jane Doe should you have questions about a patient or if you need consultation. Dr. Doe would sign, stating that she will be available. Other states may have limitations on the number of APNs with whom collaborators can work, specialty of the collaborating physician, rules regarding signing off on charts, collaborating physician's name on prescriptions, and geographic location. In a worst case scenario, the APN would have specific protocols to follow, although this is becoming much less common in today's environment.

As in other contacts and agreements, it is important to include information identifying who the contract is between, time frame, responsibilities of both parties, and a contingency plan if the collaborating physician is not available for a length of time. Box 20-6 outlines items that could be included in the agreement. Many states or locations may have a suggested or mandatory outline or form to be used and several states have collaborative agreements available online to download. In most cases, a CPA is a simple agreement defining the collaboration between the physician and APN. There are many examples of CPAs available for download on the Internet.

Contract Negotiation

Negotiation is something that most people do every day, even if they do not realize it. People are uncomfortable with the words and what they mean, especially regarding negotiating employment contracts. There are numerous reasons for this, including understanding one's own individual worth and what one brings to the workplace, power issues, and self-esteem. Many books, multimedia courses, and live seminars are available that can help APNs strengthen their negotiation skills (Buppert, 2012; Fisher, Ury, & Patton, 2011). Although contract negotiation may seem overwhelming to the average clinician, there are some strategies that can be taken to improve one's negotiation skills (Dahring, 2012).

The first thing an APN must do is to identify personal goals. Some important questions for the APN to ask include: Why am I entering into this negotiation, and exactly what do I hope to achieve? A complete list of key requirements is important. For a new position, items on the list may include working hours, on-call requirements, salary and benefits, continuing education, restrictive covenants (see Box 20-5), collaboration, and administrative time. Later, it will be necessary to come back and revise the list based on more knowledge about the position. Lastly, the APN should prioritize what is most important

BOX 20-7 | **Contract Negotiation Tips**

- Do your homework first.
- Ask many questions.
- Create a list of negotiable and non-negotiable items.
- Use silence, a powerful tool.
- Don't rush the process.
- Remember, it's about business.

and what is a deal breaker versus the points which may be open for compromise.

It is important to go into negotiation as thoroughly prepared as possible. If it is a first or new position, explore information about the facility, the people that work there, salaries in the surrounding community, working conditions, benefit packages and other perks that may come with this position. What is the reputation of the facility? Have there been any legal complaints about the facility or providers?

Being as prepared as possible provides the APN insight into those with whom they will be negotiating. This preparation allows them to adjust the initial list of desired items as necessary. Determine which items on the list are not essential and will allow some room for negotiation. Remember that there is always some give and take. Box 20-7 offers tips to successful negotiation

A point that is often of most concern to both parties is salary. Buppert (2012) has suggested that it is important to ask for the reasonable salary that you need and one that you deserve for the service provided, based on what other APNs are getting for the same service.

It is important to have an established price point from which to negotiate. Use national APN salary surveys from the Internet. Do not give the lowest salary option or a salary that offers a range (e.g., between $90,000,000 and $130,000). Choose an amount that is reasonable, on the upper end of the scale based on research, and verbalize it.

This number gives the applicant room for negotiation. If the APN were to give a range, it is likely that an employer will start them at the bottom of that range. It is also important for the APN to have a minimal salary in mind as they begin salary negotiations, below which they will not accept the position.

Take time to listen to what the other party wants. Listening allows one to hear that schedule is more important than salary, which may be something to negotiate. For some APNs, alternative working hours are an important benefit to accommodate child care. Silence is a strong and often effective negotiating tool.

As ethical providers with growing business acumen, APNs need to find what works for them in a particular situation. Just remember the definition of negotiate: "to confer with another so as to reach an agreement on some matter" (Merriam-Webster, 2012).

Conclusion

Marketing and contracting can seem overwhelming, especially when first starting out as a new APN or even seasoned APNs who have not considered the long term impact that their skills can have on their careers. Marketing is a critical skill for APNs to develop as they embark on a career or when they decide to start their own practice. The role of the APN has never been more important. It is essential that all APNs realize that marketing is not just about growing a practice or getting a job, but includes promotion for the entire profession.

Marketing oneself and one's services is critical to the survival of APNs. As the health care environment changes, clients are becoming more sophisticated about what they need and want in a health care provider. APNs must become familiar with marketing concepts and be flexible enough to meet client's needs. As a result of successful marketing strategies, clients will specifically request APNs and demand their services, recognizing the value they provide in the ever-expanding and complex health care marketplace.

References

American Association of Birth Centers. (www.birthcenters.org)

American Medical Association. (2012a). *Code of Medical Ethics of the American Medical Association*, 1847 edition (http://www.ama-assn.org/resources/doc/ethics/1847code.pdf).

American Medical Assoication. (2012b). 1903 Principles of Ethics (http://www.ama-assn.org/resources/doc/ama-history/1903 principalsofethi.pdf).

Baum, N., & Henkel, G. (2010). *Marketing your clinical practice: Ethically, effectively, economically*. Sudbury, MA: Jones & Bartlett.

Buppert, C. (2012). *Nurse practitioner's business practice and legal guide* (4th ed.). Sudbury, MA: Jones & Bartlett.

Buzogany, W. A. (2010). Independent contractors versus employees: The costs and benefits for your practice. *Journal of Practice Management. 25*, 332–334.

Chang, C. F., Ploutz, S. K., & Price, S. A. (2001). *Economics and nursing: Critical professional issues*. Philadelphia: FA Davis.

Cialdini, R. B. (2009). *Influence: Science and practice* (5th ed.). Boston: Pearson Education.

Clay, C. (2011). Building a brand—one patient at a time. *Marketing Health Services, 31*, 5–7.

Cockrum, J. (2011). *Free marketing: 101 low cost and no-cost ways to grow your business online and off.* New York: Wiley.

Dahring, R. (2012). Contract negotiation:don't be afraid (http://www.ftc.gov/bcp/menus/resources/guidance/adv.shtm).

Fox, S. (2011). Pew Internet: Health (http://www.pewinternet.org/Commentary/2011/November/Pew-Internet-Health.aspx).

Fisher, R., Ury, W., & Patton, B. (2011). *Getting to yes: Negotiating agreement without giving in* (3rd ed.). New York: Penguin.

Gallup Poll. (2010). (http://www.gallup.com/video/145199/Nurses-Top-Ethic-List-Lobbyists-Bottom.aspx).

Gombeski, W. J., Britt, J., Wray, T., Taylor, J., Adkins, W., & Riggs, K. (2011). Spread the word. Word of mouth is a powerful, but often undervalued, marketing strategy—here's how to harness it. *Marketing Health Services , 31*, 22–25.

HARO (Help a Reporter Out). (http://www.helpareporter.com).

Institute of Medicine (IOM). (2011). *The future of nursing: Leading change, advancing health.* Washington DC: The National Academies Press.

Internal Revenue Service (IRS). (2013). Independent contractor defined. (www.irs.gov/Businesses/Small-Businesses-&-self-employed/Independent-Contractor-Defined).

Kingma, M. (1998). Marketing and nursing in a competitive environment. *International Nursing Review. 45*, 45–49.

Kotler, P. A. (2011). *Marketing management* (14th ed.). Upper Saddle River, NJ: Prentice Hall.

Letz, K. K. (2002). *Business essentials for nurse practitioners.* Fort Wayne, IN: PreviCare.

Luther, W. M. (2011). *The marketing plan: How to prepare and implement it* (4th ed.). New York: AMACOM.

Merriam-Webster Dictionary. (2012). Negotiate (http://www.merriam-webster.com/dictionary/negotiate).

National Council of State Boards of Nursing (NCSBN). (2008). Consensus model for APRN regulation: Licensure, accreditation, certification and education (www.ncsbn.org/index.htm).

Phillips, B. C. (2010). Presentation: Marketing for APNs. www.cecenter.aanp.org

Phillips, B. C. (2011a). Marketing—your other full-time job (part 1 of 2) (http://www.nppracticemgt.com/articles/article_details/marketingyour-other-full-time-job-part-1-of-2).

Phillips, B. C. (2011b). Marketing—your other full-time job (part 2 of 2) (http://www.nppracticemgt.com/currentissue/currentissue_details/marketingyour-other-full-time-job-part-2-of-2).

Porterfield, A., Khare, P., & Vahl, A. (2011). *Facebook marketing all-in-one for dummies.* New York: Wiley.

Reel, S. & Abraham, I.(2007). *Business and legal essentials for nurse practitioners: From negotiating your first job through owning a practice.* St. Louis: Elsevier/Mosby.

Roberts, M. J. (2010). Legal file: Plain talk about employment contracts. *Nurse Practitioner; 35*, 12–13.

Segbers, R. (2010). Go where the customers are. Marketing (and managing) your patient experience with social media. *Marketing Health Services, 30*, 22–25.

Somers, M. J., Finch, L., & Birnbaum, D. (2010). Marketing nursing as a profession: Integrated marketing strategies to address the nursing shortage. *Health Marketing Quarterly, 27*, 291–306.

University of Washington Medical Center. (www.UWMC.org).

U.S. Department of Health and Human Services (HHS). (2011). Patient Protection and Affordable Care Act (http://www.healthcare.gov/law/full/index.html).

U.S. Department of Health and Human Services (HHS). (2012). Health information privacy (www.hhs.gov/ocr/privacy).

Understanding Regulatory, Legal, and Credentialing Requirements

Charlene M. Hanson

CHAPTER CONTENTS

It is important to note at the beginning of this chapter that the term *APRN* will be used throughout as this is the term used to describe advanced practice nurses in a regulatory context. The term *advanced practice nurse* as described in chapter 3 is an expansive, powerful idea, not a physician substitute or a narrow set of skills or credentials. The highest level of nursing practice cannot be reduced to a regulatory definition. The regulation of APRNs is more narrow as it guides state boards of nursing on how to consistently regulate APRNs across the United States. The APN concept is far larger than that and APRNs contribute to the health of the nation far beyond the regulatory requirements discussed in this chapter. So, the regulatory term, APRN is used to align with the principals of LACE in this chapter only, and is in no way intended to be reductionist to the larger idea of advanced practice nursing.

Current Issues

The current health care environment requires that any discussion of regulatory issues be fluid, dynamic, and subject to rapid change. Three national events have coalesced to bring about important effects on the regulation of advanced practice registered nurses (APRNs). First, in our last edition, work concerning the *Consensus Model for Regulation: Licensure, Accreditation, Certification and Education* was in its early stages. Today, this important regulatory change is being implemented across 50 states (www.aacn.nche.org/education-resources/aprnreport/pdf; www.ncsbn.org/aprn.htm).

At the same time, two other events have resulted in a careful evaluation of APRN education and practice and, more specifically, APRN regulation. In 2010, the broadest health reform legislation since the enactment of Medicare in 1965 was passed. The role of APRNs in the Patient Protection and Affordability Care Act (PPACA; U.S. Department of Health & Human Services [HHS], 2011) as primary care providers, members of accountable care organizations (ACOs), medical home configurations, and providers in nurse-managed clinics drives the need to ensure the highest levels of education and effective regulation. Finally, the Institute of Medicine (IOM, 2011) *Future of Nursing* report recommendation that APRNs "should be educated and practice to the fullest extent of their scope of practice" (p. 4-6) affects the state by state regulation of APRNs.

At this time, APRNs must influence health policy at the national and grassroots levels to ensure regulatory configurations that allow for successful APRN practice and reimbursement. This activity may be as simple as interpreting APRN regulatory decisions to patients, administrators, and coworkers locally or as complex as negotiating equitable regulatory decisions about reimbursement with the Centers for Medicare & Medicaid Services (CMS; www.cms.org; see Chapter 22).

Issues involving education, including advanced practice nurse competencies, competencies from APRN organizations and masters and doctoral essentials, scope of practice, reimbursement, and prescriptive authority are all embedded in regulatory language. The complexity of regulatory issues and the multiplicity of stakeholders require ongoing monitoring, reevaluating and updating. In 1998, the Pew Health Professions Commission recommended that national policy initiatives were urgently needed to research, develop, and publish national scopes of practice and continuing competency standards for state legislatures to implement (O'Neil & Pew Health Professions Commission, 1998). This work is ongoing today and continues to be vitally important, with continuous and careful input from APRNs.

This chapter will describe credentialing and regulation, provide an update on the status of the Consensus Model, the Nursing Model Act and Rules National Council State Boards of Nursing (NCSBN, 2011), and its implications and implementation. The purpose of this chapter is to help the reader understand the multiple steps in the process of licensure as an APRN.

Titling of Advanced Practice Registered Nurses

The issues surrounding the titling and credentialing of APRNs have been difficult since the inception of APRN roles. At the state regulatory level, the preference is to use the title "advanced practice registered nurse." The Consensus Model makes this preference a permanent change. Advanced practice nursing has evolved in differing ways over time, with multiple titles, which confuse

policymakers, patients, and the profession. Currently, there are four APRN roles. Certified registered nurses anesthetist (CRNA) and certified nurse-midwife (CNM) certification and credentialing are the most clearly uniform and standardized based on their longevity, singleness of purpose, and specialty. The credentialing and oversight of nurse practitioners (CNPs) and clinical nurse specialists (CNSs) is less clear because of the multiplicity of programs, areas of increasing specialty practice, and continuing need to develop certification examinations in some areas (see next section and Part III). Credentialing is furnishing the documentation necessary to be authorized by a regulatory body or institution to engage in certain activities and to use a certain title. Currently, not all states recognize all advanced practice roles for title protection. As new APRN roles evolve, the problems around credentialing and titling become increasingly acute.

As noted, this chapter describes basic national and state regulatory and credentialing realities and discusses the critical elements of regulation and credentialing that currently affect APRNs. For specific questions about up to the minute, current APRN rules and regulations, especially those that pertain to specific state statutes regarding licensing of APRNs, prescriptive authority, and reimbursement, the reader should refer to individual state regulatory bodies for practice requirements.

The skills required for successful policy activism and advocacy, which are crucial to negotiating regulatory mechanisms, are part of the APRN core competencies of clinical, professional, health policy, and systems leadership and collaboration. These concepts and skills, outlined in Chapters 11 and 12, are crucial to the role APRNs play in shaping credentialing and regulatory policy mechanisms and should be considered as this chapter is read.

Consensus Model for Advanced Practice Registered Nurse Regulation: Licensure, Accreditation, Certification, and Education

Before a discussion of regulation can take place, it is important to understand the progress to date surrounding the Consensus Model and the Nursing Model Act and Rules for APRN licensure (NCSBN, 2011). Credentialing for APRNs is composed of four components—licensure, accreditation, certification, and education (LACE). Several years ago, the NCSBN's Advanced Practice Committee created a vision paper that spoke to the recommendations of the Quality Chasm report (Committee on Quality of Health Care in America, IOM, 2001) and the concerns surrounding multiple roles and specialties for APRNs. At about the same time that the NCSBN began its work (March, 2004), various stakeholders, including leaders from the American Association of Colleges of Nursing

(AACN; NCSBN, 2008), National Organization of Nurse Practitioner Faculties (NONPF), National Association of Clinical Nurse Specialists (NACNS), American Association of Nurse Anesthetists (AANA), American College of Nurse-Midwives (ACNM), and several APRN certifying bodies, accreditors, and regulators met to establish a process that would result in a consensus statement on the credentialing of APRNs. Both groups worked toward consensus about a regulatory model that would establish a model of education, certification accreditation, and licensure to strengthen and standardize the public and private regulatory scene. The IOM reports of 2000 and 2001 suggested that the various regulatory bodies needed to develop models of regulation that were most beneficial to patients. Several recommendations in these important reports heightened the need for collaboration, transparency, evidence-based decision making, and information exchange (O'Sullivan, Carter, Marion, et al., 2005). The vision was to implement one national regulatory scheme that would be most beneficial to patients and that allowed APRNs to be innovative and meet patient needs (NCSBN, 2008).

Since that time, many years of work by a Joint Dialogue Committee, made up of the major APRN leaders and stakeholders, crafted the Consensus Model (NCSBN, 2008). The collaborative work of this committee is currently endorsed by 48 national nursing organizations, including all the major APRN organizations. A new model for APRN regulation is now a reality and is synchronized with the credentialing stakeholders. Based on this important work, the Consensus Model is currently being implemented across the United States. It is important that readers access the Consensus Model documentation and familiarize themselves with the new changes (www.aacn.nche.org; www.ncsbn.org). The reader must understand that although the target date is 2015 for implementation, transition to the new regulation will take years to fully implement in some states (Williams, 2010; Yoder-Wise, 2010).

Unfortunately, at the current time, vast differences exist regarding rules and regulations and the credentialing process across states. Making change to this legislative process is and will be difficult, at best. State regulatory data can be reviewed in the references for this chapter (Kaplan, Brown, & Simonson, 2011; NCSBN, 2012a; Osborne, 2011; Pearson, 2012). Lugo, O'Grady, Hodnicki, et al. (2007) have demonstrated wide variations across states, which indicate that APRNs are not able to reach their full practice potential in many states. This same study analyzed the data from the perspective of patient access to NPs and NP services, again finding wide variations from state to state, which indicates lack of uniform regulations of APRNs.

Implementation of Consensus Model Regulation

LACE organizations have continued to meet regularly to move the process of implementation forward, keep lines of communication open, maintain transparency, and identify and strategize about important and ongoing issues. The LACE network is a virtual social networking configuration. A platform is in place whereby LACE member organizations pay a membership fee to belong to the working group that sustains the core components of the Consensus Model. A public site for updates is also available free at http://aprnlace.org.

All four LACE groups are working to meet new requirements and assist with state implementation. NCSBN has launched the Campaign for Consensus (www.ncsbn.org/4214.htm) to help individual states implement the new regulatory process by offering administrative and technical support. Access maps showing states' progress can be found at www.ncsbn.org/aprn.htm. Also, the American Nurses Credentialing Center has information on their website regarding changes in APRN certification offerings (www.nursecredentialing.org). See other APRN websites for updated changes in any LACE category for a particular role.

Definitions Associated with the Regulation of APRNs

It is important for APRNs to understand the language and terms used to describe the credentialing process. Credentialing, including education, national certification, and licensure, involves several steps before one has full authority to practice as an APRN. To complicate matters, as noted, the credentialing procedures and requirements vary somewhat among states and practice settings. Definitions for the major components of APRN credentialing are presented in Box 21-1.

State Licensure and Recognition

Individual state nurse practice acts define the practice of nursing for registered nurses (RNs) throughout the 50 states and territories. State laws overseeing APRN's are divided into two forms: (1) statutes as defined by the nurse practice act are enacted by the state legislature; and (2) rules and regulations are explicated by state agencies under the jurisdiction of the executive branch of state government. Historically, under Title X of the U.S. Constitution, states have the broad authority to regulate activities that affect the health, safety, and welfare of their citizens, including the practice of the healing arts within their borders. Licensure stems from this history, grounded in public protection, whereby each state creates standards to ensure basic levels of public safety. In 27 states, the state

BOX 21-1   Advanced Practice Registered Nurse Credentialing Definitions

Accreditation. The voluntary process whereby schools of nursing are reviewed by external nursing educational agencies for the purpose of determining the quality of a nursing and/or APRN program.

Certification. A formal process (usually an examination, but may be a portfolio) used by a certifying agency to validate, based on predetermined standards, an individual's knowledge, skills, and abilities. Certification provides validation of the APRN's knowledge in a particular specialty. It is used by most states as one component of second licensure for APRN practice.

Credentialing (institutional level). The process that an individual institution uses to permit an APRN to practice in an APRN position within the institution. Generally, APRNs submit particular documentation to an institutional credentialing committee, which reviews and authorizes the APRN's practice.

Credentialing (state level). The requirements that a state uses to assess minimum standards of competency for APRNs to be authorized to practice in an APRN role. The purpose of credentialing is to protect the health and safety of the public. These requirements include an unencumbered RN license, graduate education transcripts, national certification in one of six population foci.

Legal authority. The authority assigned to a state or agency with administrative powers to enforce laws, rules, and policies.

Licensure. The process whereby an agency of state government grants authorization to an individual to engage in a given profession. For nursing, licensure is usually based on two criteria—the applicant attaining the essential education and degree of competency necessary to perform a unique scope of practice and passing a national examination. APRNs are licensed first as RNs and second as APRNs.

Regulations. The rules and policies that operationalize the laws and policies that recognize APRNs and credential them for practice in an APRN role.

board of nursing has sole authority over advanced practice nursing; in others, there is joint authority with the board of medicine, board of pharmacy, or both (NCSBN, 2012; Pearson, 2012). The states require that all APRNs carry current licensure as RNs. *Authority to practice as an APRN is tied to scope of practice and varies from state to state*, depending on the degree of practice autonomy that the APRN is granted. The current status of advanced practice nurse licensure and scope of practice and application

information in a particular state can be easily obtained by accessing the NCSBN website (www.ncsbn.org), which has a link to each individual state board of nursing.

Some states require a temporary permit for a new graduate to practice as an APRN while awaiting national certification results (Pearson, 2012) or other requirements, such as an internship or added pharmacology hours for prescriptive authority. New graduates should contact their state board of nursing and submit the required application for a temporary advanced practice nursing permit if the state allows this practice. With the advent of electronic testing, the time lapse between testing and obtaining results for licensure is minimal and markedly reduces the need for a temporary permit. When the Consensus Model takes effect, states will have removed the need for a temporary license option.

Prescriptive Authority

Credentialing and licensure for prescriptive authority also occur at the state level. Pharmacology requirements vary among states although, currently, most states require a core advanced pharmacotherapeutics course (a requirement of the Consensus Model) during the graduate APRN educational program and some states require yearly continuing education (CE) credits thereafter to maintain prescriptive privilege. Prescriptive authority may be regulated solely by the board of nursing, as it is in several states, jointly by the board of nursing and board of pharmacy, as it is in several others, or by a triad of boards of nursing, medicine, and pharmacy (NCSBN, 2012; Pearson, 2012). It is incumbent on the APRN to understand the mechanism of prescriptive authority regulation clearly in his or her state and to understand whether ongoing continuing education is required (Armstrong, 2011; Lovatt, 2010).

As prescriptive authority has evolved over the past several years, certain basic requirements have become fairly standard for APRN prescribers (Box 21-2). These requirements vary among states but provide a core regulatory process for prescriptive authority (Buppert, 2012; Pearson, 2012).

As noted, state boards of nursing should clearly document the numbers of hours of pharmacology required for an APRN to receive and maintain prescriptive privilege in terms of the APRN educational program and annual CE. APRN programs that previously integrated pharmacologic content in clinical management courses are required to have a stand-alone advanced pharmacotherapeutics course to comply with state requirements and accreditation standards (www.aacn.nche.edu/Accreditation). Pharmacology content should be taught by faculty pharmacists or a nurse-pharmacist faculty team who have an in-depth knowledge of therapeutic prescribing. Some states are

BOX 21-2 | **Requirements for Advanced Practice Registered Nurse Prescribers**

- Graduation from an approved masters- or doctoral-level APRN program
- Licensure and recognition in good standing as an APRN
- National certification in an APRN population focus area
- Recent pharmacotherapeutics course of at least 3 credit hours (45 contact hours)
- Evidence of a collaborative practice arrangement (in some states)
- Ongoing CE hours in pharmacotherapeutics to maintain prescribing status (in some states)
- State prescribing and national DEA numbers (in some cases)

requiring that APRN nursing programs verify specific course and content hours that can be used in a board of nursing application for prescriptive authority. Furthermore, several states require documentation of the number of hours of CE for pharmacology per year or per cycle. The direction is clearly to require APRNs to attend ongoing CE in pharmacology to maintain prescriptive privileges, although APRNs should update their knowledge in this changing area whether or not their state requires it. Timely CE offerings and distance learning modalities (e.g., podcasts, Internet-based offerings) are available to meet the needs of busy clinicians. Over time, the states will likely move in the direction of interdisciplinary pharmacology education for nurses and physicians. Technologic advances, including handheld smartphones and tablets, offer clinicians on-site information about prescribing modalities and state of the art drug information. These represent a positive response to the increasing evidence of medication prescribing errors (Committee on Quality of Health Care in America et al., 2000; www.Epocrates.com).

Drug Enforcement Administration Number

In addition to prescriptive authority, APRNs who plan to prescribe or dispense controlled substances will need to apply for a Drug Enforcement Administration (DEA) number, as required by federal and state policy (www.deadiversion.usdoj.gov). DEA numbers are site specific; therefore, APRNs practicing at more than one site will need to obtain an additional DEA number for each site (Buppert, 2012; Reel & Abraham, 2007).

Scope of Practice for Advanced Practice Nurses

By definition, the term *scope of practice* describes practice limits and sets the parameters within which nurses in the various advanced practice nursing specialties may legally practice. Scope statements define what APRNs can do for and with patients, what they can delegate, and when collaboration with others is required. Scope of practice statements tell APRNs what is actually beyond the limits of their nursing practice (American Nurses Association [ANA], 2003, 2012; Buppert, 2012; Kleinpell, Hudspeth, Scordo, et al., 2012). The scope of practice for each of the four APRN roles differs (see Part III). Scope of practice statements are key to the debate about how the U.S. health care system uses APRNs as health care providers; scope is inextricably linked with barriers to advanced practice nursing. CRNAs, who administer general anesthesia, have a scope of practice markedly different from that of the primary care nurse practitioner (NP), for example, although both have their roots in basic nursing.

In addition, it is important to understand that scope of practice differs among states and is based on state laws promulgated by the various state nurse practice acts and rules and regulations for APRNs (Lugo, O'Grady, Hodnicki, et al., 2007, 2009; NCSBN, 2012; Pearson, 2012). On the Internet, scope of practice statements can be found by searching state government websites in the areas of licensing boards, nursing, and advanced practice nursing rules and regulations, or by visiting the NCSBN site (www.ncsbn.org). Recent federal policy initiatives, including the IOM *Future of Nursing* Report, (2011). the PPACA (HHS, 2011), and the Josiah Macy Foundation (Cronenwett & Dzau, 2010) have all issued recommendations with important implications for expanding the scope of practice for APRNs. The National Health Policy Forum (http://www.nhpf.org/library/background-papers/BP76_SOP_07-06-2010.pdf) and Citizen Advocacy Center (https://www.ncsbn.org/ReformingScopesofPractice-WhitePaper.pdf) reports state firmly that current scope of practice adjudication is far too technical, subject to political pressure, and therefore not appropriate in the legislative sphere. There must be a more powerful forum so that the public can enter into the dialogue (see Chapter 22).

As scope of practice expands, accountability becomes a crucial factor as APRNs obtain more authority over their own practices. First, it is important that scope of practice statements identify the legal parameters of each APRN role. Furthermore, it is crucial that scope of practice statements presented by national certifying entities are carried through in language in state statutes (Buppert, 2012). Our society is highly mobile and APRNs must recognize that their scope of practice will vary among states; in a worst case scenario, one can be an APRN in one state but not meet the criteria in another state (Minnesota Nursing, 2011; Taylor, 2006). This is discussed more fully later in the chapter.

APRNs owe Barbara Safriet, former Associate Dean at Yale Law School, a debt of gratitude for her vision and clarity in helping APRNs understand and think strategically about scope of practice and regulatory issues. In her landmark 1992 monograph, Safriet noted that APRNs are unique in that there is a multiprofessional approach to their regulation based on ignorance and on the fallacy that medicine is all-knowing, particularly about advanced practice nursing (Safriet, 1992).

As Safriet has implied, restraints on advanced practice nursing result from ignorance about APRNs' abilities, rigid notions about professional roles, and turf protection. She cited reforms in scope of practice laws in Colorado that encouraged solutions to long-time tensions over control of practice between organized medicine and nursing. Their new provision defines the term *practice authority* in terms of ability and thus redirects the regulatory focus from providers' status to the APRN's training and skills (Safriet 2002, 2010). This example and the imminent move to Consensus Model regulation offers hope that in the future, policies can be formulated to close the gap between what APRNs can do and what they are allowed to do by scope of practice statutes. Scope of practice is hampered in many states where APRN practice is carved out of the medical practice act as a medically delegated act that precludes reasonable autonomy for the APRN. The ability to diagnose disease and treat patients, inherent in the role of the APRN, is fluid and evolving and is often tied to the collaborative relationships that APRNs have with physician colleagues. It is important to note that although APRNs desire autonomous licensure through the state boards of nursing, the need to work interprofessionally as colleagues and team members is essential to attaining high-level patient outcomes (Interprofessional Education Collaborative [IPEC], 2011; HHS, 2011).

Benchmarks of Advanced Practice Nursing and Education

Three components of APRN education and practice are related to scope of practice and provide additional important benchmarks—APRN competencies, professional APRN competencies, and master's and Doctor of Nursing Practice (DNP) essentials These three benchmarks form the foundation on which boards of nursing develop APRN statutes. It is important to mention here that in the Consensus Model, six designations for practice for NPs and CNSs have been identified—adult-gerontology, pediatric,

family (primary care and acute), psychiatric–mental health, neonatal, and women's health–gender-related. In the new model, APRNs are licensed within a population focus. Specialty areas such as palliative care, oncology, and orthopedics are additional certifications above the population focus at which APRNs are licensed.

Advanced Practice Nurse Competencies

Underpinning scope of practice statements are termed *APRN competencies,* which are carefully outlined in Part II of this text. They form the core that distinguishes APRN practice. Scope is directly linked to the APRN competencies of direct clinical practice and coaching and guidance. These two interact with other core competencies to make up the quality care spectrum that APRN providers offer to their patients. These competencies are mirrored in the master's and doctoral essential competencies described here.

Professional Advanced Practice Registered Nurse Competencies

In addition, professional organizations such as the NONPF, NACNS, ACNM, and American Association of Nurse Anesthetists (AANA) support each role and population focus with their own set of competencies. These more specific competencies provide benchmarks particular to the role and population focus (see Chapters 14 to 18 for examples and sources for these competencies).

Master's and Doctor of Nursing Practice Essentials

The AACN has promulgated the *Essentials* of masters and doctoral education for advanced practice nursing (AACN, 2006a, 2011; NONPF, 2006). These documents support scope of practice for APRNs by providing the requirements for graduate core content and APRN core advanced physical assessment and diagnosis, pathophysiology, and pharmacotherapeutics. At the DNP level, a stronger foundation in population-based care, organizational leadership, collaboration, public policy, and information systems enhances APRN roles (AACN, 2006a).

Standards of Practice and Care for Advanced Practice Nurses

Standards of practice for nursing are defined by the profession nationally and help explicate and delineate scope of practice further. Standards are overarching authoritative statements that the nursing profession uses to describe the responsibilities for which its members are accountable (ANA, 2012; www.nursingworld.org). As such, they complement and enable the APRN core, population focus, and specialty competencies. APRNs are held to the standards of practice promulgated by the nursing profession and to standards of the various APRN specialties. At both levels, standards of practice describe the basic competency levels for safe and competent practice (e.g., see Chapters 14 through 18 for the standards of practice for NPs, CNS, CNMs, and CRNAs). Professional standards of practice match closely with the core competencies for APRNs, outlined in Chapter 3, which undergird advanced practice nursing.

Standards of care differ from the standards of practice set forth by the nursing profession. These standards are often termed *practice guidelines*. Practice guidelines provide a foundation for health care providers to administer care to patients. Ideally, these guidelines cross-cut the health professions' disciplines and provide the framework whereby basic safety and competent care are measured. For APRNs, this means that the standard used to evaluate advanced practice is often the same as the standard used to review medical practice. Clinical guidelines are used as the standard of care in legal decisions; therefore, it is essential for APRNs to be part of the team developing new guidelines.

Standards of care are derived from evidence-based practice and are continuously evolving. At the federal policy level, the Agency for Healthcare Research and Quality (AHRQ) has responsibility for conducting the research needed to evaluate clinical practice guidelines that define a standard of appropriate care in specific areas (AHRQ, 2012 [www.AHRQ.gov]; Buppert, 2012). The Centers for Disease Control and Prevention (CDC) and professional medical and nursing specialty organizations also promulgate guidelines for practice (www.aafp.org). It is important that APRNs be part of interdisciplinary teams that develop and test practice guidelines for care. The ability of APRNs to download cutting edge practice guidelines onto electronic devices such as tablets, smartphones, and PDAs for use in clinical settings and at the bedside is a major step toward competent and safe practice.

Components of Advanced Practice Nurse Credentialing and Regulation

Credentialing used to ensure that APRNs meet competency and safety standards to protect the public has developed rather haphazardly. The Consensus Model of regulation that embraces all credentialing stakeholders is a major step forward. Two credentialing changes have or will occur as states move to the new regulation. First, titling will require that APRNs legally represent themselves as an APRN first and then by their role (CRNA, CNM, CNP, CNS). Many states already use this title, but some do not (NCSBN, 2011). Second, APRNs will need to have a second license. Second licensure means that an APRN must meet certain criteria established by a state board of nursing to receive an additional license or

recognition to be authorized to practice at an advanced level of nursing practice. The notion of second licensure is unprecedented among the health professions and is onerous to some nurses but, given the various routes of entry into the nursing profession, it seems the only way to ensure a minimum set of competencies or requirements. The issue of titling and second licensure is an important issue for all APRNs and one to which individual APRNs must pay attention to protect their ability to practice, prescribe, and be reimbursed for their services.

Elements of Regulation

Several important steps lead the way to state licensure as an APRN. The regulatory process begins when a student is admitted to a university-based, accredited APRN program and proceeds through national certification in a population focus and then to second licensure and prescriptive authority. As APRNs become more mobile across state and international boundaries, and as communications allow for increased interaction, it is important that credentialing and regulatory parameters be well understood. Box 21-3 lists the elements of regulation for APRNs.

Credentialing

Credentialing is an umbrella term that refers to the regulatory mechanisms that can be applied to individuals, programs, or organizations (Styles, 1998). Credentialing can be defined as getting your ducks in a row for the purpose of meeting standards, protecting the public, and improving quality. For the purposes of this text, credentialing (as it relates to APRNs) is defined as follows: credentialing is furnishing the documentation necessary to be authorized by a regulatory body or institution to engage in certain activities and use a certain title. Credentialing occurs at a state level in terms of applying for a second

> **BOX 21-3   Elements of Regulation for Advanced Practice Registered Nurses (LACE)**
>
> **Licensure**
> - Prescriptive authority (see Box 21-2)
>
> **Accreditation of APRN Programs**
>
> **Certification (National)**
> - Recertification
>
> **Education**
> - Master's
> - Post-master's
> - Doctoral

license as an APRN. The term can also apply to a local institutional process that requires certain documentation from an APRN before the individual is allowed to practice and use an APRN title within the institution or facility. Credentialing in health care is used to ensure the public that the individual meets proposed standards and is prepared to perform the duties implied by the credential. National certification is only one part of credentialing and is used by many states as a vehicle to ensure a basic level of competence to practice; education is the other one. Certification alone does not provide a credential to practice as an APRN. Regulatory groups commonly request evidence of the primary criteria of graduate education, national certification, and patient-focused practice (see Chapter 3).

Credentialing may be mandatory, as in state second licensure, or voluntary, as with some states that only register APRN providers in the state (very few of these states remain). State boards of nursing and others that regulate APRNs to ensure public safety recognize voluntary credentialing bodies, such as national nursing certification organizations, as part of their mandatory state credentialing mechanism.

APRN program accreditation and approval, scope of practice, standards of practice, practice guidelines, and collaborative practice agreements all have important implications for APRNs in terms of proper credentialing and interactions with the judicial system. The documents specified in Box 21-3 create the standard whereby advanced practice nursing is monitored and regulated and deemed safe or unsafe, and whereby APRNs are disciplined from state to state. The components of advanced practice nursing education and practice are described in the following section.

Advanced Practice Nurse Master's and Doctoral Education

The first criterion that any new APRN must meet is successful graduation from an approved, accredited APRN program. Educational programs for APRNs must be at the graduate nursing level (Master of Science in Nursing [MSN] or DNP); many programs are transitioning from master's to DNP education. The recommendation by the AACN is that at least until 2015, and most likely beyond this writing, the master's degree will be the level at which APRNs are credentialed (AACN, 2006b). The Consensus Model and Nursing Model Acts and Rules do not establish a timeline for the move to doctoral education for APRNs in the foreseeable future. Eligibility to sit for national certification and obtain APRN licensure or recognition by the state requires a transcript showing successful completion of a graduate degree from an accredited university that specifies the role and population focus of the graduate

(NCSBN, 2008). This is the norm for APRN licensure or recognition in all states.

Advanced Practice Nurse Program Accreditation

For a graduate nursing program (master's or DNP) preparing APRNs, credentialing has a somewhat different meaning. Program credentialing includes accreditation for the educational program by the Commission on Collegiate Nursing Education (CCNE) or National League for Nursing Accreditation Center (NLNAC), regional and state university boards and commissions, or groups such as the ACNM or the AANA accreditation bodies. For an institution (e.g., hospital, clinic), credentialing includes adhering to The Joint Commission (TJC) and Occupational Safety and Health Administration (OSHA) guidelines.

Graduate programs in nursing and related fields that prepare APRNs must be accredited as educationally sound, with appropriate content for the population focus or specialty and adequate clinical hours of supervised experience. As noted, the NLNAC and CCNE accredit graduate programs in the nursing major (CCNE, 2009). The accreditation process provides an overall evaluation of the graduate nursing and APRN programs. Oversight of APRN education occurs through the use of several different models. The clearest models are those administered by the ACNM and the AANA, which oversee and review their educational programs. These bodies provide a process to review and regulate CRNA and CNM programs nationwide that is separate from the overall graduate nursing accreditation processes of the CCNE and NLNAC. The National Task Force Criteria for Nurse Practitioner Education and the competencies developed by the National Task Force for Quality Nurse Practitioner Education (2012) and NACNS (2011) provide guidance to CCNA and NLNAC for the accreditation of NP and CNS programs.

Certifying agencies such as the ANCC and American Academy of Nurse Practitioners Certification Program (AANPCP) review programs, to some degree, to sanction eligibility for APRN graduates to sit for national APRN certification examinations. A change based on the work of the NCSBN and consensus groups that was suggested by Hanson and Hamric (2002) has been adopted by the accreditors. Preaccreditation procedures before the start of new programs is now the norm. Preaccreditation will ensure that all new programs are well developed with appropriate curricula in place before students are admitted and that the program prepare graduates who can be licensed as APRNs. The use of grandfathering mechanisms to protect APRNs during transition periods of standardization provides leeway for positive change to occur (NCSBN, 2008). For example, students who are in educational programs that are phasing out or phasing into new configurations will be allowed to graduate, sit for certification, and be credentialed until the transition period is complete.

The review and monitoring of NP and CNS education at the population focus level is more complex than for CRNAs and CNMs because of the multiplicity of program foci. The NONPF, National Certification Board of Pediatric Nurse Practitioners and Nurses (NCBPNP/N), NACNS, and other similar bodies provide curriculum guidelines, program standards, and competencies to assist APRN programs with curriculum planning. In 1997, 2002 and 2008, the National Task Force on Quality Nurse Practitioner Education established national criteria by which to monitor and evaluate NP programs according to broad-based criteria in six overarching areas—organization/administration, students, curriculum, resource facilities and services, faculty and faculty organizations, and evaluation. In 2012, the National Task Force (NTF) Criteria for Quality NP Education were updated and revised; these guidelines are scheduled for ongoing revision every 5 years (www.nonpf.org). The NTF criteria were developed and endorsed by a consortium of NP education and practice associations, NP regulators, and NP national certifiers and accreditors. The criteria evaluate the APRN program in the above-mentioned areas to ensure that APRN competencies are being met. The AACN's *Essentials of Master's Education for Advanced Practice Nursing* (2011) and *Essentials of Doctoral Education for Advanced Nursing Practice* (2006a) define graduate nursing core and advanced practice nursing core (advanced pathophysiology, physical assessment, and pharmacology) curriculum requirements. These three documents provide needed structure and guidance for NP nursing education.

The CNS community is working toward clear structure and progression of CNS specialty education to ensure compliance with credentialing and regulation as APRN providers. Core CNS competencies and doctoral level CNS competencies have been implemented (NACNS, 2010).

Postgraduate Education

The number of postgraduate APRN programs targeted to students who have already attained a graduate degree in nursing but who wish to add an additional population focus is common practice. However, many individuals who choose to return to school now pursue DNP education. Post–master's APRN education is often tailored to meet the individual needs of post–master's students. The Consensus Model requires that post–master's education programs obtain formal graduate nursing accreditation. It is important that master's-prepared nurses who aspire to do postgraduate work to acquire a new or additional APRN credential identify programs that offer curricula that meet the standards of eligibility for national certification and state licensure for the particular APRN role that they seek to attain.

Dual Role Education

Some programs and tracks for APRNs are dual programs, preparing the APRN for more than one population focus or specialty area. These programs require careful consideration of content and meaningful clinical experiences to ensure mastery of basic advanced practice nursing competencies and clinical experiences in both focus areas. Dual programs are, by necessity, longer and require more clinical experiences and hours. Many APRNs are dually prepared and therefore must sit for more than one national certification and meet the eligibility requirements for both foci. Today's complex health care system makes this a viable option for many APRNs who are functioning in diverse settings. Also, the practice doctorate offers a new educational path that allows practicing APRNs to attain new knowledge and skills, which can lead to additional APRN certification and licensure.

Advanced Practice Registered Nurse Certification

National certification for APRNs is a primary vehicle used by state boards of nursing to ensure a basic measure of competence. Advanced practice nursing certification is national in scope and it is a mandatory requirement for APRNs to obtain and maintain credentialing in most states (NCSBN, 2012; Pearson, 2012). Multiple stakeholders for certification such as the American Nurses Association Credentialing Center (ANCC, 2012), faculty groups (e.g., NONPF), specialty organizations (e.g., AANPCP, AANA, NACNS, NONPF), and many others have worked to accomplish the multifaceted tasks needed for successful advanced practice nursing certification. These efforts have resulted in a broad range of certification and credentialing requirements. Typically, certification mechanisms develop when a role delineation study is undertaken to define the competencies that provide the framework for appropriate testing within the APRN population focus or specialty. CRNAs were credited with the first national certification in 1945, with other APRN specialties following suit, although few standards for certification were in place early on (see Chapter 1 and Part II). A perceived weakness of APRN certification is the multiplicity of certification configurations for advanced practice nursing, although the work leading to the new regulatory model and the move to a broader base for APRNs through population focus areas rather than specialties has reduced the number of certification options significantly.

Much work is being done to enhance transparency between the NCSBN, individual state boards of nursing,

BOX 21-4   ## Websites for National Advanced Practice Nursing Accreditation, Regulation, and Certification

American Academy of Nurse Practitioners Certification Program (AANPCP)—www.aanpcert.org

American Association of Colleges of Nurses (AACN) and Commission on Collegiate Nursing Education (CCNE)—www.aacn.nche.edu (links to CCNE)

American Association of Nurse Anesthetists (AANA)—www.nursecredentialing.org

American College of Nurse-Midwives (ACNM)—www.acnm.org

American Midwifery Certification Board (AMCB)—www.amcbmidwife.org

American Nurses Credentialing Center (ANCC)—www.nursecredentialing.org

Pediatric Nursing Certification Board (PNCB)—www.pncb.org

National Certification Corporation (NCC) for obstetric, gynecologic, and neonatal nursing specialties—www.nccwebsite.org

National Council of State Boards of Nursing (NCSBN)—www.ncsbn.org

National League for Nursing (NLN) and National League for Nursing Accreditation Corporation (NLNAC)—www.nln.org/nlnac

National Association of Nurse Practitioners in Women's Health (NPWH)—www.npwh.org

Data from National Task Force on Quality Nurse Practitioner Education (NTF). Criteria for evaluation of nurse practitioner programs (www.nonpf.org).

and APRN certifiers. The groups are striving for a better way to regulate all APRNs who diagnose and prescribe and are reimbursed for services. The situation creates challenges for graduate programs as they develop and revise curricula to prepare students who are eligible to sit for particular advanced practice nursing certifying examinations. The certification websites listed in Box 21-4 identify the criteria for eligibility, test outlines, and recertification and practice requirements.

Continued Competency Measured Through Recertification

Overall, APRNs must fulfill CE and practice requirements to maintain their national certification successfully, although requirements differ according to role. Each advanced practice nursing certification entity clearly lays out the requirements and time frame for recertification. Generally, national certification lasts from 5 to 8 years and requires that the candidate be retested unless the

established didactic and clinical parameters are met. There continues to be controversy around retesting versus recertifying through CE and practice mechanisms. Many other professions retest throughout the individual's career to determine competence. Simulations and other electronic innovations are also showing promise.

Mandatory Continuing Education Requirements

CE requirements differ as to the type and amount of CE needed to maintain current national certification in a particular population foci. Each role and focus area sets the parameters for the number of hours required for successful recertification. CE should be in the area of the APRN specialty, although it may be interdisciplinary. For example, CRNAs may choose to attend a conference with collaborating anesthesiologists, or family NPs may attend a conference with family practice physicians. It is encouraging to note that more conferences are offering interdisciplinary speakers and panels at specialty-specific conferences. APRN expert clinicians are serving as conference faculty for medical CE, and vice versa. Ongoing CE hours can be met by attending CE courses and workshops, working toward degree requirements, completing journal CE offerings, writing for publication, and completing online offerings, simulations, audiotape, and CD-ROM materials. Many nursing and medical journals offer CE credit to subscribers. The move to interdisciplinary offerings has broadened the scope of information available.

Mandatory Practice Requirements

Most APRN specialties have specific requirements built in for an adequate number of clinical practice hours between the years of recertification to ensure that APRNs remain clinically current and competent through regular practice. Each certification process clearly spells out the clinical hour practice requirement for the specialty. If individuals are not maintaining an APRN practice, they should not represent themselves as APRNs (see Chapter 3). APRNs who do not meet stipulated CE and practice requirements must retake the national certifying examination to continue to practice, if that is an option. With the transition to the new regulatory model, some certification examinations will no longer be available, so the need to keep certification current is critical. Certification is one way to ensure that competent APRNs provide needed health care to patients and families. Therefore, standardization of APRN certification and recertification processes is paramount to ensuring the credibility of advanced practice nursing (NCSBN, 2008).

Institutional Credentialing

The need for hospital privileges for APRNs varies according to the nurse's practice. For example, CNMs and many rural NPs cannot care for patients properly without the ability to admit patients to the hospital should the need arise. Conversely, many CNSs are employed by hospitals and have no need for admitting privileges. It has not been necessary for CRNAs and some NPs to admit patients to the hospital independently to give comprehensive care, but they may need to see patients in the emergency room.

The rules for practice as part of the hospital staff are even more specific and variable than those for state regulation; they are bound to the local hospital or medical facility and medical staff of the granting institution. Unfortunately, most of the criteria and guidelines are written exclusively for medical practitioners and therefore are not compatible with the APRN's education and supporting credentials (Buppert, 2012). In many hospitals, professional privileges are granted by a committee made up of physicians and administrators. However, more committees are adding APRN members to physician privileging committees or are setting up nurse privileging committees as APRNs gain stature in hospital settings.

The first step for APRNs seeking hospital privileges is to ask the top-level nurse administrator how the credentials committee is organized, who makes up the membership, and what support there is for nonphysician applicants. Is there a process for nurses or others to petition for privileges? Nursing administrators are often members of these committees and the APRN should meet with nurse colleagues for advice and support before the application process. A second step is to obtain the application package and begin to collect the necessary documents, which include, for example, licenses and certifications, transcripts, letters of support, and provider numbers. Support from collaborating physicians is key; in some committee structures, a collaborating physician may serve as the petitioner for a nurse colleague. Dialogue among the hospital administration, physician staff, and other stakeholders (e.g., APRN colleagues and other team members) is necessary if admitting privileges are required for the desired practice role. Alliances with consumers often add support to the application. Some hospitals have specific guidelines and protocols for all nonphysician providers; others do not.

Determination of the specific privileges desired is critical to the process. For example, is it necessary to be able to admit or discharge patients, write orders, perform particular procedures, visit in-hospital patients, or take emergency room call? Many hospitals have different levels of hospital privileges, ranging from full privileges to associate privileges for specific functions (Buppert, 2012; Reel & Abraham, 2007). Asking for full privileges may not be prudent or useful in a particular setting. A good rule is to ask for what is needed, establish a solid track record, and expand privileges later as the need arises. In today's

 BOX 21-5 Organization and Timeline for APRN Education, Certification, Licensure, and Practice

1. Final Semester in Graduate School—Graduate—Get Transcript
2. Application for Certification from Approved Certifying Organization
3. Application for Licensure from State Board of Nursing (www.ncbsn.org/boards.htm)
4. Apply, Interview, and Obtain Practice Position as APRN
5. Develop Practice Agreement with Precepting Physician (if needed)
6. Apply for Prescriptive Authority from Board of Nursing (if needed)
7. Apply for DEA Number
8. Apply for NPI Number
9. Obtain Malpractice Insurance
10. Apply for Institutional Practice Privileges

market, professional turf issues are losing ground and opportunities for hospital privileges are opening the door for new APRN practice alternatives (Box 21-5).

Issues Affecting APRN Credentialing and Regulation

The definition of an APRN requires that the four established APRN roles be clinically focused and that the APRN provide direct clinical care to patients (Hamric, 2005, 2009). The definition developed in this text goes beyond this requirement and is discussed further in Chapter 3. From a legal and regulatory perspective, inclusion in the designation of what constitutes an APRN is driven primarily by three factors: (1) the diagnosis and management of patients at an advanced level of nursing expertise; (2) the ability of APRNs to be directly reimbursed; and (3) the degree to which nurses wish to hold prescriptive and hospital admitting privileges. Although this may seem restrictive to some, there must be a well-defined and efficacious way for state boards, insurers, prescribing entities, and similar groups to monitor the scope of practice, prescribing, and reimbursement patterns of APRNs. These groups need clear criteria that can be validated to ensure patient safety and monitor proper certification and credentialing.

The multiplicity of titles and roles for APRNs is a problem from policy and regulatory viewpoints. The primary reason is that it is confusing to policymakers and regulators, especially at agencies such as the CMS, where major designations for Medicare and Medicaid reimbursement set the standard for all APRN reimbursement nationwide. In addition, discrepancies in the advanced practice nursing definition and licensing criteria across states make mobility difficult for APRNs in terms of prescriptive authority and reimbursement. The Consensus Model has mitigated some of these problems by restricting specialty advanced practice to six population foci (NCSBN, 2008).

APRNs are responsible primarily to and are disciplined by individual state boards of nursing. One of the licensing and credentialing difficulties faced by APRNs is the variance in board regulations among states. In some states, advanced practice nursing is governed only by the board of nursing; in others, it is jointly administered by the boards of nursing and medicine; and in still others, it is governed by the boards of nursing and pharmacy. In many states, CNMs are answerable to nurse-midwifery boards attached to boards of medicine. Although restrictive statements delegating only medical acts approved by the board of medicine and cosigned by a physician preceptor are not as prevalent as they were in the 1980s, they are still the norm in some states, predominantly in the South (NCSBN, 2012; Pearson, 2012). Currently, states that have delegated medical authority for APRNs often require what are termed *collaborative agreements* for APRNs who diagnose diseases, manage treatment, and prescribe medications for patients. As implied, collaborative agreements provide a written description of the professional relationship between an APRN and a collaborating physician that defines the parameters whereby the APRN can perform delegated medical acts.

Collaborative Practice Arrangements

The general term *practice guidelines* can be confusing to the APRN in that it is used in several different contexts. First, as defined earlier, it is an evidence-based standard of care. Practice guidelines are used by health care clinicians and provide interdisciplinary support for state of the art practice. However, the term may sometimes be used to refer to a collegial agreement between an APRN and physician to define parameters of practice for the APRN. Many states require this as part of APRN licensure (Buppert, 2012; Lugo et al., 2007; NCSBN, 2012). A collaborative agreement or arrangement may take many forms, from a one-page written agreement defining consultation and referral patterns to a more exact, prescribed protocol for specific functions, based on state statutes for advanced practice nursing. Collaborative agreements need to be written as broadly as possible to allow for practice variations and new innovations. Examples of sample collaborative practice agreements can be found on the Internet.

The term *protocol* in relation to advanced practice nursing was common several years ago as a physician-directed, specified guideline for the medical aspects of practice that defined each patient problem and the treatment approach. Some states used this so-called cookbook approach to NP practice as a way to oversee prescriptive and other treatment modalities. For the most part, specific protocols for care are no longer used in most settings because it is difficult to update and tailor them to the individual needs of patients and practices. More important, advanced practice nursing has evolved. As APRNs have proven their ability to provide competent care with positive outcomes, protocols have been replaced by evidence-based practice guidelines and collaborative practice agreements. However, it is important to note that the specificity of the collaborative arrangement is usually based on trust and respect between the collaborating APRN and physician colleague. For example, a newly graduated APRN might have a more tightly drawn collaborative agreement than a more experienced one in a new practice arrangement. APRNs must often show that they are competent health care providers in the medical world before they are granted more autonomous practice. Although it should not be this way, physicians are assumed to be competent in the workplace, whereas APRNs need to prove their worth (Fagin, 1992).

The norm today in APRN regulation is shifting toward loosely configured collaborative relationships that offer support to all parties and protect the safety of patients. In any case, to achieve compliance with state regulations for practice, the collaborative agreement, if required in a given state, must be updated annually, have current signatures, and provide relevant and up to date information. Collaborative relationships vary widely among advanced practice nursing roles. APRNs who expand their scope in a practice (e.g., from pediatric to family NP) must update their collaborative practice agreement accordingly. The chapters in Part III of this text help explain the differences in collaborative structures for APRNs.

Identifier Numbers

National Provider Identifier Number

In addition to prescriber and DEA registration, APRNs will need to apply for a national provider identifier (NPI) number. The administrative simplification provisions of the Health Insurance Portability and Accountability Act (HIPAA) of 1996 mandated the adoption of a standard unique identifier for health care providers. The National Plan and Provider Enumeration System (NPPES) collects identifying information on health care providers and assigns each provider a unique NPI (CMS, 2012). Every APRN should go to https://nppes.cms.hhs.gov for further information or to apply for an NPI enumerator. NPI numbers are important for APRN prescribers because many drugs are on insurance company formularies and prescriptions are billed via the NPPES system.

Medicare and Medicaid Provider Numbers

The new NPI number for APRNs will eventually replace Medicare billing numbers, but currently APRNs still need to register with the state for a Medicaid provider and a State Children's Health Insurance Plan (SCHIP) number. See www.cms.org/Medicaid and individual state Medicaid websites for instructions.

Reimbursement

On a par with the need to be able to prescribe medications for patients is the need to be appropriately paid for services delivered and reimbursed for care. Clearly, APRNs should be paid for services rendered for health care whether they work independently, share a joint practice with a physician colleague, or are employed in an institution or provider network. Although the insurance industry is regulated by the individual states, many of the private pay insurance standards used to set payment mechanisms are modeled after federal Medicare and Medicaid policy (www.cms.gov). Federal mandates that encourage direct payment of nonphysician health care providers are often blocked at the state level by discriminating rules and regulations. The terms *nonphysician provider* and *midlevel provider* both denote caregivers who are not prepared as medical doctors. This category includes NPs, CNSs, CNMs, CRNAs, physician assistants (PAs), psychologists, and other reimbursable providers of care. Most third-party payers, including some major insurance companies, are now reimbursing APRNs and other nonphysician providers directly, but others are not. As states move more directly into reimbursement models for APRNs in the private and public sectors, and into large ACOs, in which APRNs are providing care as part of interdisciplinary teams, reimbursement is becoming more readily available. (See Chapter 19 for a more detailed discussion of APRN reimbursement.) However, tensions remain with regard to provider status and membership on patient panels. From a credentialing standpoint, attention to CMS rules, Medicare and Medicaid provider numbers, Clinical Laboratory Improvement Amendments (http://www.cms.gov/Regulations-and-Guidance/Legislation/CLIA/index.html?redirect=/clia/) regulations, and provider requirements are extremely important to ensure that APRNs are reimbursed. How APRNs fit into reimbursement systems is a critical issue for nurses. It is important for APRNs to know how to contract for their services at the individual level as they negotiate employment

packages but, even more importantly, they need to be present at the negotiating table as members of executive management teams who are setting the policies for provider services where the rules for payment are made. Exemplars 21-1 and 21-2 describe the many credentialing requirements needed to begin practice as an APRN.

It is important that APRNs differentiate and clearly articulate the differences between their practices and those of physicians. The argument continues about whether nurses should be paid the same fee for service as a physician or be paid only a percentage of the physician payment. Payment by private insurers is contract-specific and varies with each state's insurance commission. Both the ACNM and AANA vigilantly monitor reimbursement to stay on the cutting edge of payment schemes for APRNs. The ACNM recently was successful in moving nurse midwives to 100% of physician reimbursement (see Chapter 17). Equal payment and comparable worth are difficult issues. On the one hand, there is a comparable worth issue in that treating a urinary tract infection costs the same whether it is done by an NP or physician; on the other, the cost savings of using a less expensive provider are rarely passed on to the patient. There is no clear path forward on this comparable worth versus cost savings issues for APRNs.

It is critical that APRNs position themselves to sit on policymaking boards for private enterprise. To accomplish this, APRNs must have visibility with local, state, and national entities that make the important decisions for health care.

Policy issues surrounding the reimbursement of APRNs require careful reflection before strategies to remove constraints to payment are undertaken. For all health care providers, outcomes of care will take precedence in reimbursement over all other issues, so attention to quality of care is a paramount consideration. Several other important questions should be considered when policy is being shaped, such as the following:

- For what services do APRNs want to be paid?
- Are they different from physician services or the same?
- Are there specific nursing services that need to be reimbursed?
- Is direct payment the issue, or does it matter who gets the payment?
- Will the payment level be the same as or lower than what physicians receive for equivalent service?

These are important questions because, in most states, APRNs historically have been reimbursed indirectly, incident to physicians, and at a considerably lower rate (Buppert, 2012; CMS, 2012; Reel & Abraham, 2007).

As noted, *incident- to billing* is a difficult issue and hinders APRN efforts to overcome invisibility. An NP can

EXEMPLAR 21-1   **Meeting the Requirements for Credentialing and Regulation**

Jeni is in the final semester of her master's family nurse practitioner (FNP) program at a state university. She is in the process of negotiating a contract with a provider network of physicians and APRNs in a satellite health maintenance organization (HMO) practice. Jeni knows that she must begin the process of acquiring the necessary credentials to be able to practice in her state. When she applied to her FNP program, she made sure that the university and graduate program were accredited in good standing. Now that she is ready to leave, she must prepare for a new and challenging professional life.

In her seminar class, Jeni received the application to sit for national certification the month after she graduates and has sent the application forward to register the date for her examination. Her next step is to download the advanced practice nursing rules and regulations for her state, as well as the application materials. Jeni reviews these documents carefully so that she fully understands the application process, materials, and fee that she will need to submit to the state licensing board.

Jeni carefully notes in the advanced practice nursing rules and regulations that to be able to prescribe in her state, she must show proof that she has completed a 45–contact hour, state-approved graduate nursing course in pharmacotherapeutics. Also, she must complete 6 hours of CE in pharmacotherapeutics each year to maintain her status as a prescriber. She makes a note to request the transcript and syllabus for her

pharmacotherapeutics course to attach to her application for her APRN license.

The HMO in which Jeni plans to practice has sent her several documents that she must complete to be able to practice. First, on signing her contract, she will need to negotiate a written collaborative arrangement with the precepting physician colleague, who will see the patients who are beyond her scope of practice. Second, she needs a Medicaid provider number to see children in the Medicaid program. She will need to apply for her NPI and DEA numbers. In addition, this health care system requires that Jeni apply to the local hospital and nursing home privileging committees so that she can see patients on rounds, do admitting and discharge planning, and follow nursing home patients on a regular basis.

As part of her package, Jeni has negotiated for the employer to pay the premium on her malpractice insurance as an APRN. She also negotiates $3000 per year for CE. She needs to call her insurance carrier to discuss the transfer of her student policy to a full policy to cover her as a certified APRN with the appropriate scope of practice that she will need in her new position. She knows that she wants to purchase an occurrence type of policy. Jeni uses the support of her colleagues and mentors as she works through this important process of preparing her credentials to practice as an APRN (see Box 21-5).

charge the full physician rate if billing is incident to the physician provider but only 85% if billing is done directly by the NP, an unfortunate disincentive for physician practices to let APRNs bill independently. Most physicians want to bill for APRN services under their own Medicare number to receive the highest rate of reimbursement. On the other hand, APRNs want and need to bill independently to be viewed as the caregivers of record. Many rules are associated with incident-to billing, including the need for the physician to be on the premises. The CMS (www.cms.gov) is currently studying incident to billing to understand the prevalence of APRN care better and the cost to the system for billing APRN services through the physician for a higher fee for service. It is advantageous for APRNs who are planning to practice clinically, no matter what the setting or physician relationship, to seek counsel about the reimbursement realities in their state and in their particular practice setting(s) before beginning to care for patients.

In particular, it is important to identify the third-party payers of most patients for whom the APRN will be caring and to learn their requirements for reimbursement of APRNs. Only then are APRNs in an appropriate position to seek status as reimbursable providers with Medicare, Medicaid, and the many private payers (see Chapter 19). There are several areas in which reimbursement schemes directly affect the regulation of advanced practice nursing. Although private payment by the patient is gaining strength, Medicare and Medicaid, commercial insurers, ACOs, and HMOs cover most health care costs in today's market. These entities build networks of providers by hiring, purchasing services from, or contracting with physicians and APRNs, hospitals, and others to provide health care services to patients. When APRNs join a provider network, they must meet all the requirements, regulations, and standards of care established by the plan. For example, a primary care NP applying for a position in an HMO would need to meet all the criteria listed in Box 21-2 and obtain appropriate Medicare and Medicaid provider status, as well as malpractice history and coverage. It is incumbent on the APRN to have all credentials and regulatory documentation in good and accessible order when preparing to practice, because third-party payers are often located in and governed by reimbursement administrators in a distant state.

Risk Management, Malpractice, and Negligence

Although malpractice suits involving APRNs are rare, malpractice issues are ever-present for all providers of health care, regardless of credential or setting. In an unstable health care environment, patients look to the tort system to ease the apprehension and anxiety about the care that they receive. Patients are more likely to seek redress if they mistrust their provider or believe that they have been harmed by the system. First and foremost, APRNs need to understand clearly what constitutes negligent practice and grounds for malpractice and to put safeguards in place so they do not have to confront the legal system.

By definition, negligence is the failure to act in a reasonable way as a health care clinician. Negligence may lead to malpractice and legal action. The following four factors must be present for a malpractice suit to be valid (Buppert, 2012):

- A duty of care must be owed to the injured party, through direct office or hospital care or through phone or e-mail advice, and a patient-nurse relationship must be established.
- The accepted standard of care was breached.
- The patient must have damage or sustained an injury.
- There must be direct causation demonstrated—that is, the patient suffered an injury that was caused by the APRN clinician. (Often, there are multiple causative factors based on care by several caregivers over time.)

Within the judicial system, care is evaluated by preset criteria in the form of medical and advanced practice nursing standards. National professional organizations set the standards for appropriate care. APRNs are often held to the medical standard of care as advanced practice nursing standards continue to be developed. There is much blurring between medical and nursing standards, creating a dire need for interdisciplinary standards of care that will hold care providers to the same standards as their peers (Buppert, 2012; IPEC, 2011; Letz, 2002). There are several ways that legal standards of care are established in a particular case. The most common is through expert testimony offered by a person who is qualified by education, experience, knowledge, and skill level to judge the actions of the providers in the case. Other mechanisms include review of professional literature, manufacturers' package inserts, and documented professional standards of care. Letz (2002) has suggested four ways to prevent malpractice events: establish a good rapport with patients over time; follow an established standard of care to ensure competence; document accurately and completely; and take a course in risk management.

APNs can use several risk management techniques to mitigate against malpractice occurrences. First and foremost, APNs should offer patients and family members the level of care and outcomes they would want to receive for themselves. It is important to document well and to audit charts frequently for mistakes and omissions. Engaging in regular chart peer review is a good practice whenever possible. Further, Reel and Abraham (2007) advise APNs against altering the medical record in any way, referencing an incident report, or venting emotions in the record. Also, APNs must be careful when asked to give advice, diagnose, or treat patients (or family) outside of the practice setting. In such instances, treat as an office visit and fully document the event on the patient's record.

Omissions in follow-up for laboratory and x-ray results are common mistakes by health care providers. Electronic records offer useful tools and tracking devices (such as "jelly beans" at the top of the computer screen) to alert the APN about phone messages or laboratory testing and can prompt the APN to follow through in a busy hospital or community-based practice. Buppert (2010) offers good advice in two other important areas. She counsels APNs to order only what the patient needs and no more when prescribing; and the APN must refer the patient when it is not possible to make a clear diagnosis in a reasonable length of time.

Many risk management resources to assist APRNs are available through professional advanced practice nursing organizations and public and private entities. Malpractice carriers offer discounts to APRNS who take risk management courses. Visit the professional websites suggested throughout this text to find comprehensive risk management tools and a current discussion of legal questions confronting APRNs.

Malpractice Insurance

APRNs need a thorough understanding of liability insurance coverage, types of policies, and extent of coverage required. It is important to understand the difference between the two most common types of professional liability insurance plans, *claims-made* and *occurrence*. A claims-made insurance policy covers claims made against the APRN only while the policy is in effect. Coverage must be continued indefinitely to ensure coverage for claims filed in the future for actions that occurred in the past. A claims-made policy can be extended through the purchase of a tail. Conversely, with an occurrence policy, the APRN is covered for alleged acts of negligence that occurred during the time that the policy was in effect. The benefit of occurrence coverage is that even if the policy is cancelled at some future date, coverage for events that occurred while the policy was in effect will be honored. For more information about advanced practice nursing liability insurance, visit websites for the major malpractice insurance carriers. Each APRN must understand the extent of coverage per incident and how personal legal costs are covered in the policy. The amount of insurance needed is governed by the type of practice in which the APRN is engaged; CRNAs and CNMs, who are under more risk, need more coverage.

It is important that APRNs carry their own individual liability coverage, even if they are covered by an employer group practice. Employer-based insurance contracts are geared to protect the institution or practice as a whole and are not targeted to the individual APRN. The comfort of having your own council during litigation far outweighs the cost of individual liability insurance. Conferences, workshops, and Internet offerings are available to assist APRNs in choosing the appropriate insurance carrier and plan.

As APRNs move in and out of what is considered the domain of medicine, serious thought must be given to the standard whereby APRNs will be judged if they are deemed to have made an error. Although not many documented cases have cited APRNs who have injured patients by wrongful action, the question about whether APRNs should be tried by the courts according to medical or nursing standards is important and needs to be clarified. It is incumbent on APRNs to set clear standards for practice that are based on clinical competency.

Privacy Issues

Health Insurance Portability and Accountability Act

The federal Health Insurance Portability and Accountability Act became law in 1996. Legal requirements were finalized by HHS in 2002 and mandatory compliance with federal regulations was required by April 14, 2003. Visit www.hhs.HIPAA.gov to view the ruling and its latest amendments and documentation.

HIPAA mandates implementation of statewide, uniform, minimum patient privacy standards. The main goal of HIPAA is to protect the privacy of a patient's identifiable health information that is maintained or transmitted by health care providers and insurers (HHS, 2012). This includes any information that would identify

the patient, patient's problem, plan of care, and how care is paid for. The regulations for privacy established by HIPAA have placed a new level of legal responsibility on health providers, including APRNs. If APRNs accept third-party reimbursement or transmit any health information in any form, they are required to comply with HIPAA regulations.

Providers and facilities need to adhere to several operating standards to comply with HIPAA regulations. The rules state that providers are required to train all their staff members regarding HIPAA rules and on-site procedures. Facilities and providers can design their own policies and procedures to meet the needs and scope of their practice, but these policies must adhere to all the standards included in the operating standards of HIPAA (Buppert, 2012). Penalties are severe and include civil monetary fines and, in some cases, felony criminal penalties (www.hhs.gov/ocr/hipaa/privacy.html).

Telehealth and Telepractice

Federal and state legislation change daily as new and better ways to connect through virtual innovations emerge. Regulatory issues surrounding the changes in the way health care providers practice based on electronic capabilities will continue to challenge policymakers and APRNs well into the twenty-first century. A model described as mutual recognition allows an APRN licensed in a home state to be recognized as licensed in another state. The mutual recognition model would hold the APRN accountable for the laws and regulations in the state in which the APRN provides the health care but would rely on reciprocity licensure from the home state (Minnesota Nursing, 2011; NCSBN, 2008, 2012b). This model has been in place successfully for decades with RNs working in the United States and worldwide in the U.S. military. Exemplar 21-2 illustrates an interstate practice.

It is interesting to note that new technologies and a system of virtual practice, as described in Exemplar 21-2, focuses attention on pervasive barriers that have plagued APRNs for many years (Safriet, 2002, 2010). Although implementation of a mutual recognition system is well underway for RNs, the same type of recognition is lagging behind for APRNs because of the lack of stability and standardization of regulatory schemes from state to state with regard to scope of practice, prescriptive authority, and reimbursement. Based on the Comprehensive Telehealth Act of 1997 (Govtrak, 2012) and the implementation of Consensus Model regulation in the current environment, physicians and other health care providers, including nurses, fall within the boundaries of electronic practice and all require regulation. Enabling telehealth legislation and reform could provide the catalyst needed

EXEMPLAR 21-2   **Interstate Practice**

As a pediatric CNS in private practice caring for children with chronic illnesses, Alice has been comanaging, with Dr. Pete Johnson, the health care of 4-year-old David in North Carolina. Alice and Dr. Johnson have taken care of David, a child with insulin-dependent diabetes mellitus, since he was born. . The child and his mother have grown to trust and depend on Alice's care for David over time.

While on vacation at Disneyland in Florida, David develops diarrhea and vomiting. His mother chooses to e-mail Alice for advice rather than take David to an unfamiliar emergency room and provider. Alice responds to the mother with directions about management of the gastroenteritis and potential changes in David's insulin dosage, if needed. In providing this guidance, Alice has cared for David in a state (Florida) other than the one in which she is licensed (North Carolina) and recognized as an APRN. This situation places Alice in a highly vulnerable position, even though she is giving high-quality, patient-centered care, which is presently illegal.

As geography becomes less relevant in care provision, these state geographic boundaries will become irrational in a high-value care delivery system. A system of mutual regulatory recognition (multistate licensure) between Florida and North Carolina would allow Alice to care for David using her North Carolina APRN credentials. Without modernizing to a system of mutual recognition between states, Alice is practicing in Florida without a license. Alice hopes that the work being done by national and state leaders to promote multistate licensure for APRNs will be successful. She considers volunteering with the coalition in her state to help with this issue.

---

to ensure that all states recognize and authorize key elements of scopes of practice for APRNs (e.g., prescriptive authority).

It will be important for APRNs to monitor the development of practice across state boundaries carefully and work closely with advanced practice nursing associations to effect regulatory change that removes barriers and augments practice. From a legal and regulatory standpoint, clear statutes are needed that offer broad practice standards to allow for mobility across state lines. This change will require national standards of practice and certification and credentialing requirements that can satisfy many different jurisdictions and APRN stakeholders, not an easy task. These standards will require diligent collaboration among educators, state boards of nursing, professional associations, and all practicing APRNs (AACN, 2008; NCSBN, 2008). Part of the professional agenda that APRNs must address is the need for accountability and responsibility for competence in practice. As a professional group, APRNs must build strong national standards of practice, scope, and skills to create enabling telehealth reform legislation.

Safety and Cost Containment Initiatives

Although more work is needed to collect the data needed to substantiate the positive outcomes by APRN providers, research has shown that APRNs are safe and cost-effective alternatives to physician-based health care (see Chapter 23). This increased visibility makes it imperative that APRNs monitor the competencies of their own practices and clearly understand the costs of providing care to patients. If APRNs want to be providers of record, they must show positive and safe outcomes of their work to justify Medicare reimbursement.

Acts of Congress since the events of 9/11, economic downturns, and federal budget crises have cut programs for the poor. These factors, plus the increase in the number of older adults with chronic illness, will augment the need for APRNs, even while funds to pay for this care are reduced, causing increased stress on underserved populations with health problems. Language in the PPACA also calls for increased numbers of APRN primary care providers, nurse-managed clinics, and ACO configurations, such as medical or health care homes (PPACA, 2011). Bodenheimer and Grumbach (2012) have suggested several alternatives to painful cost controls that APRNs can implement. Initiating simple policies, such as the judicious use of supplies and prudent choice of diagnostic tests and procedures, is a first step. Physician groups have moved quickly to fill the quality gap because they recognize the potential relationship of quality to payment issues, which is now a fact of practice through value-based purchasing. APRNs need to engage and participate in value-based purchasing projects fully as a way to ensure the visibility, quality, and cost-effectiveness of their practice (www.ahrq.gov; CMS, 2012; Johnson, Harper, Hanson, et al., 2007; see Chapter 22).

Institute of Medicine (IOM) reports, such as *To Err is Human* (2000) and *Crossing the Quality Chasm* (2001) have focused on human factors that influence patient safety. In addition to a healing environment for patients, initiatives that enhance patient safety, such as enlarging the safety knowledge base of caregivers and providing technologic assistance in the form of PDAs, smartphones, and tablets are useful tools. The initiation and resources of nurse-driven initiatives, such as the Quality and Safety Education of Nurses (QSEN, 2012) and Nursing Alliance for Quality Care (NAQC, 2012) are excellent examples of progress toward quality and safer care for patients. Funding opportunities and demonstration projects for APRNs to improve safety outcomes and decrease errors are clearly evident in the national agenda (HHS, 2011).

Influencing the Regulatory Process

APRNs can directly influence the regulatory process in several ways, including using political strategies. At all levels, regulators are eager to find practicing APRNs and advanced practice nursing educators who will take an active role in assisting them to develop and implement sound regulatory policies and procedures. The information explosion has brought the ability to communicate and connect with others at a moment's notice, which makes it easier for APRNs to influence the system directly. Chapters 11 and 22 provide in-depth discussions of skills needed for leadership and political advocacy. This section presents some additional ways for novice and expert APRNs to engage actively in any regulatory process that affects their practice.

Novice and Advanced Practice Nurses

Participate in professional organizations and become involved in regulatory activities, such as educating lawmakers, providing public comment on APRN issues, writing letters, and being part of campaign activities:

- Monitor current APRN legislation and legislation that affects patients.
- Offer to participate in test-writing committees for national certification examinations as item writers and/or reviewers.
- Respond to offers to review, edit, and provide feedback about circulated draft regulatory policies that directly affect advanced practice nursing education and practice.

Experienced and Expert Advanced Practice Nurses

- Seek out a gubernatorial appointment to the board of nursing or advanced practice committee that advises the board of nursing in your state.
- Seek membership as the APRN or consumer member of the advisory council for the state medical board or state board of pharmacy.

- Seek appointment to CMS panels on which Medicare and Medicaid provider issues are decided.
- Seek appointment to hospital privileging committees and ensure that privileging materials are appropriate for APRNs.
- Seek appointment on advisory committees and task forces that are advising the NCSBN and other regulatory and credentialing bodies.
- Provide public comment on draft legislation regarding health care and health care providers.
- Offer testimony at state and national hearings at which proposed regulatory changes in advanced practice nursing regulation, prescriptive authority, and reimbursement schemes will be discussed.

To accomplish these activities, APRNs need to use research data, a powerful tool for shaping health policy (Hamric, 1998). By actively participating in the regulatory process, APRNs ensure themselves of a strong voice in regulatory and credentialing processes. At the very least, it is incumbent on the practicing APRN to monitor the process carefully through websites and newsletters to stay informed.

Current Practice Climate for Advanced Practice Nurses

The current practice environment is a positive one for APRNs in all venues. Population growth, health reform, new technologies and modes of delivery of services, and growing APRN collaborative and autonomous practice are creating new opportunities for exploration. Change is noted in media awareness as APRNs are finally approaching a juncture at which their roles are visible and part of the health care agenda (Cronenwett & Dzau, 2010; IOM, 2011; Pohl et al., 2010; PPACA, 2011, Knowledge@ Wharton, 2013).

The continued preference of physicians for specialty practice and away from primary care practice is important for APRNs to consider. Currently, the combined health care needs of an aging population and a period of economic retrenchment offer opportunities for APRNs, whether as employees, members of health care teams, or owners of practice venues. Community-based health care systems that rely on interdisciplinary health care team approaches have positively benefited from APRNs but, in some cases, have heightened tensions between the disciplines of medicine and nursing. Health policy issues surround APRN practice parameters, reimbursement, and patients' abilities to choose APRN providers. All these environmental factors have a direct or indirect impact on the credentialing and regulatory policies that govern advanced practice nursing.

Need for True Collaboration

Complex health care systems and patient population needs that require a multifaceted approach to multiple problems demand effective interdisciplinary team building. Parallel play, or working side by side, is not enough; a true blending of nursing and medical models to offer a comprehensive health care approach is needed. Larger teams of health care providers must collaborate fully to provide comprehensive care to families and communities (IPEC, 2011). To be able to move forward as full-fledged team members in cooperation with other interprofessional health care providers, APRNs need to shift their practice ideal from one of complete autonomy to a truly collegial interdisciplinary paradigm. This change in practice stance is necessary and long overdue. APRNs struggle to answer questions such as the following:

- Does any health care professional, including the most renowned vascular surgeon, practice with full independence?
- Or, does this surgeon call on the internist, APRN, and physical therapist to assist with providing competent, evidenced-based, expert care?
- Will APRNs do themselves a disservice if they maintain an isolationist stance based on barriers and professional turf issues?
- Have APRNs reached a point in their evolution at which they can feel comfortable as peers and colleagues with providers in other disciplines?

Moving Out of the Shadows and Into the Light

When APRNs seek to change statutes and regulations, it is not because they see themselves as needing to practice in a vacuum of independence apart from the rest of the health care team, but to be a valued part of a health care team. It is a hard fact that APRNs must have authority over their own practices and the decisions they make about patient care. They must be able to defend their actions within the legal system based on nursing-driven standards and regulation. Only in this way can an APRN move out of the darkness of being a shadow provider (Wilcox, 1995). Issues related to being a shadow provider are best exemplified by incident-to billing by NPs using the physician's Medicare number. Advanced practice nursing care is invisible to regulators and reimbursers with this type of billing procedure.

This is one example of the challenges for APRNs across the United States who are working to clarify statutory policies within state boards of nursing. It may be that APRNs will feel comfortable only when their position in the health care community is fully secure in all states; this will require focused and coordinated political and legislative work related to credentialing and regulatory issues.

Visioning for Advanced Practice

Impressive strides have been made over time in the areas of credentialing and regulation of APRNs. The health care provided by APRNs has had far-reaching effects on all members of society; thus, the evolution of advanced practice nursing in the United States is a source of pride to nurses. The positive excitement of the IOM's 2011 recommendations, Josiah Macy Foundation's recommendations, and PPACA language is countered with the responsibility for higher accountability and the need for more standardized ways to credential, certify, regulate, and sanction competent practice for a growing number of APRNs (IOM, 2011; Cronenwett & Dzeu, 2010). The vision for advanced practice nursing should include an APRN interstate compact with a national regulatory model consistent across states, so that each APRN would apply for only one license in the state in which he or she resides and have reciprocity in other states (www.ncsbn.org/nlc.htm).

Forces within health care, as well as needs within the regulatory and educational climate of advanced practice nursing, have set the stage for an era of progressive change. The pressing health care needs in the United States have serious implications for education, practice, and regulation of APRNs. Advancing technologies, enhanced mobility of APRNs across state lines, and diversity among state regulatory mechanisms have brought together APRN leaders and stakeholders to craft a new vision for the future of advanced practice nursing.

Future Regulatory Challenges Facing Advanced Practice Nurses

Health professions reports published over the past decade have continued to recommend the need for generic benchmarks and standards for health care education and practice for all health care professions (AACN, 2006b; IOM, 2011, 2001; Johnson et al., 2007; NCSBN, 2008; O'Neil & the Pew Health Professions Commission, 1998).

The future requires that APRNs promulgate clear, broad-based, competency-based standards for education and practice to allow for growth and movement across state lines. It is important that APRNs accomplish this work in preparation for the next phase—interdisciplinary credentialing and regulation based on defined patient outcomes—because this is becoming a reality in some specialties, such as advanced diabetes management (see Chapter 5). The wave of the future is to move to interdisciplinary regulation whereby, for example, family practice physicians, family NPs, and CNMs caring for menopausal women would all be held to a like standard of education and practice. In another example, the American Association of Diabetic Educators (AADE) allows multiple disciplines to take their examination and all are held to the same standards. Burroughs and colleagues (2007) and Safriet (2002, 2010) have suggested that regulation for the health professions will require a new approach that dispels notions of exclusivity, exclusion, or independence from other disciplines. This move toward overarching regulation for the health professions, when and if it comes to pass, will require much higher levels of collaboration among the disciplines and specialties than now exist (IPEC, 2011; see Chapter 12) and, most importantly, broad-based standards and regulations for advanced practice nursing. New models of regulation will require strong leadership and increased involvement by practicing APRNs, as exemplified in the current master's and DNP essentials, and dynamic, cutting-edge competencies put forth by APRN organizations.

Conclusion

At no time has it been more important for APRNs to understand and value the important relationships among groups that control the complex processes and systems that regulate practice. New models of health care and varying configurations of how APRNs practice in interdisciplinary teams have escalated the importance of regulatory considerations.

The growth of virtual health care delivery makes the picture even more complex. APRNs will need to provide leadership and clear direction to policymakers to ensure the development of broad-based practice standards that will satisfy state statutes and make sense in all areas of advanced practice nursing. The implementation of the Consensus Model that is currently being implemented across the United States places APRNs in an excellent position of leadership for the future. The need for APRNs to move into key roles as health care providers in the next decade requires careful vigilance with regard to the LACE components of credentialing and regulation.

References

Agency for Healthcare Research and Quality (AHRQ). (2012). Clinical guidelines (www.ahrq.gov/clinic).

American Academy of Nurse Practitioners Certification Program. www.aanpcert.org.

American Association of Colleges of Nursing. (2006a). The essentials of doctoral education for advanced nursing practice (www.aacn.nche.edu/pdf/essentials).

American Association of Colleges of Nursing (AACN). (2006b). DNP roadmap task force report. Washington, DC: Author.

American Association of Colleges of Nursing. (2008). Consensus Model for APRN Regulation: Licensure, accreditation, certification and education (www.aacn.nche.org/education-resources/aprnreport.pdf).

American Association of Colleges of Nursing. (2011). The essentials of master's education in nursing (www.aacn.nche.edu/education-resources/MastersEssentials.pdf).

American Association of Family Physicians (AAFP). Practice guidelines (http://www.aafp.org/online/en/home/policy/policies/c/clinicalpractguidelines.html).

American Association of Nurse Anesthetists. (2012). Council on Accreditation of Nurse Anesthesia Educational Programs (http://www.aana.com/Style%20Library/AANA/i/aana-logo.png).

American Midwifery Certification Board. (2013). Requirements for nurse-midwife certification. (www.amcbmidwife.org).

American Nurses Association (ANA). (2003). Nursing's social policy statement. (2nd ed.). Washington, DC: Author.

American Nurses Association (ANA). (2012). Scope and standards of advanced nursing practice. Washington, DC: Author.

American Nurses Credentialing Center (ANCC). (2012). Advanced practice certification exams (http://www.nursecredentialing.org/Certification.aspx).

Armstrong, A. (2011). Legal considerations for nurse prescribers. Nurse Prescribing, 9, 603–607.

Bodenheimer, T. S., & Grumbach, K. (2012). Understanding health policy: A clinical approach (6th ed.). New York: McGraw-Hill/Appleton & Lange.

Buppert, C. (2010). Avoiding malpractice: 10 rules, 5 systems, 20 cases (3rd ed.). Annapolis, MD: Law Office of Carolyn Buppert (www.buppert.com).

Buppert, C. (2012). Nurse practitioner's business practice and legal guide (4th ed.). Boston: Jones & Bartlett.

Burroughs, R., Dmytrow, B., & Lewis, H. (2007). Trends in nurse practitioner professional liability: An analysis of claims with risk management recommendations. Journal of Nursing Law, 11, 53–60.

Centers for Medicare & Medicaid Services (CMS). (2012). Medicare and Medicaid reimbursement (www.hhs.cms.gov).

Centers for Medicare & Medicaid Services (CMS). (2012). National plan and provider enumeration system (NPPES) (https://nppes.cms.hhs.gov/NPPES).

Commission on Collegiate Nursing Education (CCNE). (2009). CCNE Standards and professional nursing guidelines (http://www.aacn.nche.edu/leading-initiatives).

Committee on Quality of Health Care in America, Institute of Medicine (IOM); Kohn, L. T., Corrigan, J. M., & Donaldson, M. S. (Eds.). (2000). To err is human: Building a safer health system. Washington, DC: National Academies Press.

Committee on Quality of Health Care in America, Institute of Medicine (IOM). (2001). *Crossing the quality chasm: A new health system for the 21st century.* Washington, DC: National Academies Press.

Cronenwett, L., & Dzau, V. (2010). In B. Culliton & S. Russell, (Eds)., *Who will provide primary care and how will they be trained? Proceedings of a conference sponsored by the Josiah Macy Jr. Foundation.* Durham, NC: Josiah Macy, Jr. Foundation.

Drug Enforcement Administration (DEA). (2012). Application for DEA provider number (www.deadiversion.usdoj.gov).

Fagin, C. (1992). Collaboration between nurses and physicians: No longer a choice. *Nursing and Health Care, 13,* 354–363.

Govtrak. (2012). S. 385 (105th): Comprehensive Telehealth Act of 1997 (www.govtrack.us/congress/bills/105/s385).

Hamric, A. B. (1998). Using research to influence the regulatory process. *Advanced Practice Nursing Quarterly, 4,* 44–50.

Hamric, A. B. (2005). A definition of advanced practice nursing. In A. B. Hamric, J. A. Spross, & C. M. Hanson (Eds.), *Advanced practice nursing: An integrative approach* (pp. 85–108; 3rd ed.). Philadelphia: Saunders.

Hamric, A. B. (2009). A definition of advanced practice nursing. In A. B. Hamric, J. A. Spross, & C. M. Hanson (Eds.), *Advanced practice nursing: An integrative approach* (pp. 75–94; 4th ed.). St. Louis: Elsevier.

Hanson, C. M., & Hamric, A. B. (2002). Reflections on the continuing evolution of advanced practiced nursing. *Nursing Outlook, 51,* 203–211.

Interprofessional Education Collaborative (IPEC). (2011). Core competencies of interprofessional collaborative practice (www.aacn.nche.edu/education/pdf/IPECreport.pdf).

Institute of Medicine (IOM). (2011). *The future of nursing: Leading change, advancing health.* Washington DC: National Academies Press.

Johnson, J., Harper, D., Hanson, C., & Dawson, E. (2007). Forging a quality agenda. *American Journal of Nurse Practitioners, 11,* 10–19.

Kaplan, L., Brown, M., & Simonson, D. (2011). CRNA prescribing practices: The Washington state experience. *AANA Journal, 79,* 24–29.

Kleinpell, R., Hudspeth, R., Scordo, K., & Magdic, K. (2012). Defining NP scope of practice and associated regulations: Focus on acute care. *Journal of the American Academy of Nurse Practitioners, 24,* 11–18.

Knowledge@Wharton (2013). Nurse practitioners are in—and why you may be seeing more of them. Knowledge@Wharton, February 13, 2013. www.knowledge.wharton.upenn.edu/article.cfm?articleid=3183.

Letz, K. (2002). *Business essentials for nurse practitioners: Essential knowledge for building your practice.* Fort Wayne, IN: Previcare.

Lovatt, P. (2010). Legal and ethical implications of non-medical prescribers. *Nurse Prescribing, 8,* 340–342.

Lugo, N. R., O'Grady, E., Hodnicki, D., & Hanson, C. (2007). Ranking state NP regulation: Practice environment and consumer healthcare choice. *American Journal for Nurse Practitioners, 11,* 8–24.

Lugo, N. R., O'Grady, E., Hodnicki, D., & Hanson, C. (2009). Are regulations more consumer-friendly when boards of nursing are the sole regulators of nurse practitioners? *Journal of Professional Nursing, 26,* 29–34.

Minnesota Nursing Accent. (2011). *Interstate nurse licensure compact passes key committee.* St. Paul, MN: Author.

National Association of Clinical Nurse Specialists (NACNS). (2011). (www.NACNS.org).

National Association of Clinical Nurse Specialists Competencies Task Force. (2010). *Clinical Nurse Specialist Core Competencies.* Philadelphia: National Association of Clinical Nurse Specialists. (www.nacns.org/docs/CNSCoreCompetencies).

National Council of State Boards of Nursing (NCSBN). (2008). Consensus Model for APRN Regulation: Licensure, accreditation, certification and education (www.ncsbn.org/index.htm).

National Council of State Boards of Nursing (NCSBN). (2011). Nursing model act and rules (www.ncsbn.org/1455.htm).

National Council of State Boards of Nursing (NCSBN). (2012a). Campaign for consensus maps. (www.ncsbn.org/2567.htm).

National Council of State Boards of Nursing (NCSBN). (2012b). Interstate compact (www.ncsbn.org/nlc.htm).

National Organization of Nurse Practitioner Faculties (NONPF), Practice Doctorate Task Force. (2003). The practice doctorate in nursing: Future or fringe. *Topics in Advanced Practice Nursing Journal, 3.*

National Organization of Nurse Practitioner Faculties (NONPF), National Panel for NP Practice Doctorate Competencies. (2006). Practice doctorate nurse practitioner entry level competencies. (www.nonpf.org/NONPF2005/PracticeDoctorateResourceCenter/PDresource.htm).

National Task Force on Quality Nurse Practitioner Education. (1997). *Criteria for evaluation of nurse practitioner programs.* Washington, DC: Author.

National Task Force on Quality Nurse Practitioner Education. (2002). *Criteria for evaluation of nurse practitioner programs.* (2nd ed.). Washington, DC: Author.

National Task Force on Quality Nurse Practitioner Education. (2008). *Criteria for evaluation of nurse practitioner programs.* (3rd ed.). Washington, DC: Author.

National Task Force on Quality Nurse Practitioner Education. (2012). *Criteria for evaluation of nurse practitioner programs* (4th ed.). Washington, DC: Author.

Nursing Alliance for Quality Care (NAQC). (2012). (www.gwumc.edu/healthsci/departments/nursing/naqc).

O'Neil, E. H.; Pew Health Professions Commission. (1998). *Recreating health professional practice for a new century.* San Francisco: Pew Health Professions Commission.

Osborne, K. (2011). Regulation of prescriptive authority for certified nurse-midwives and certified midwives: A national overview. *Journal of Midwifery and Women's Health, 56,* 543–556.

O'Sullivan, A., Carter, M., Marion, L., Pohl, J., & Werner, K. (2005). Moving forward together: The practice doctorate in nursing (http://nursingworld.org/MainMenuCategories/ANAMarketplace/ANAPeriodicals/OJIN/TableofContents/Volume102005/No3Sept05/tpc28_416028.aspx).

Pearson, L. (2012). The Pearson report (http://www.pearsonreport.com).

Pohl, J. M., Hanson, C. M., Newland, J. A., & Cronenwett, L. (2010). Analysis & commentary. Unleashing nurse practitioners' potential to deliver primary care and lead teams. *Health Affairs, 29,* 900–905.

Quality and Safety Education for Nurses (QSEN). (2012). (www.qsen.org).

Reel, S. J., & Abraham, I. L. (2007). *Business and legal essentials for nurse practitioners: From negotiating your first job through owning a practice.* St. Louis: Mosby.

Safriet, B. (1992). Health care dollars and regulatory sense: The role of advanced practice nursing. *Yale Journal of Regulation, 9,* 417–487.

Safriet, B. (2002). Closing the gap between can and may in health care providers' scopes of practice: A primer for policymakers. *Yale Journal of Regulation, 19,* 301–334.

Safriet, B. (2010). Federal options for maximizing the value of advanced practice nurses in providing quality cost effective health care (www.webNPonline.com).

Styles, M. M. (1998). An international perspective: APRN credentialing. *Advanced Practice Nursing Quarterly, 4,* 1–5.

Taylor, C. L. (2006). State controlled licensure and interstate mobility: Questions from Katrina. *Communication Disorders Quarterly, 27,* 232–239.

U.S. Department of Health and Human Services (HHS). (2011). Patient Protection and Affordable Care Act (http://www.healthcare.gov/law/full/index.html).

U.S. Department of Health & Human Services (HHS). (2012). Summary of the HIPAA privacy rule (http://www.hhs.gov/ocr/privacy/hipaa/understanding/summary).

Wilcox, P. (1995). Advanced practice model response to needs of women at risk for female malignancies. Abstract presented at the Oncology Nurses Society National Conference, Anaheim, CA.

Williams, D. (2010). Consensus model for advanced practice nurse regulation: Implications for midwives. *Journal of Midwifery and Women's Health, 55,* 415–419.

Yoder-Wise, P. (2010). LACE: The consensus model and implications beyond advanced practice. *Journal of Continuing Education in Nursing, 41,* 291.

Health Policy Issues in Changing Environments

Eileen T. O'Grady • Jean Johnson

CHAPTER CONTENTS

Powerful advanced practice nurse (APN) clinical experiences, when effectively communicated, serve to deepen policymakers' understanding of health-related issues. APN practice experiences are poignant stories that enlighten policy issues by providing a human context while bringing nursing's value to the health policy arena. Most APNs in practice today have experienced the effects of ill-conceived policies that lead to needless suffering, poor resource use, and poorly coordinated, fragmented health care. This practice experience, coupled with the ability to analyze the policy process, provides a strong foundation to propel APNs into politically competent action and advocacy. The purposes of this chapter are to (1) familiarize the APN with the U.S. health care policy process to help APNs be more effective in influencing policy makers, (2) provide information about specific current and emerging U.S. health care policy issues that are the focus of policymaking, and (3) demonstrate policy and political competence through exemplars.

Engaging in policymaking is a core element of leadership to be cultivated by all APNs (see Chapter 11). In 2014, major health reform legislation, the Patient Protection and Affordable Care Act (PPACA; U.S. Department of Health and Human Services [HHS], 2011a), mandated health insurance coverage which will sweep an additional 50 million people into the U.S. health care delivery system. The system must accommodate this new surge in demand while raising the quality of care and lowering costs. Meeting these goals poses significant challenges. The Institute of Medicine (IOM) report on the *Future of*

Nursing (2010) has determined that nurses must be central to an improved U.S. health care system of the future. Of the eight specific IOM recommendations, three are highly pertinent to APNs engaging in policymaking:

- Recommendation 1. Removal of scope of practice barriers so that nurses can function at the highest level of their education and training will require persistence and a strong degree of political competency because approximately 50% of the states have outdated nurse practice acts that do not reflect modern APN practice or national licensing standards. It will take a significant degree of political organizational networking, coalition building, campaigning, and educating the public to modernize the nation's nurse practice acts.
- Recommendation 7. Preparing and enabling nurses to lead change to advance health will require APNs to develop leadership skills, which include shaping and influencing policymaking at all levels. This recommendation will require APNs to become insightful knowledge sources on translational research and best practices, coupled with highly developed political competence. This recommendation emphasizes that nurses must be in key leadership positions across decision making bodies in the government and private sector.
- Recommendation 8. Building an infrastructure for the collection and analysis of interprofessional health care workforce data requires nurses to be involved in improving the research enterprise

around the U.S. nursing and health care workforce. This requires expertise in research methods and interprofessional collaboration skills so that nursing workforce data can better inform policymaking.

Policy Process

Policy: Historic Core Function in Nursing

Florence Nightingale spent much of her career in the halls of Parliament promoting policy change to improve quality, dignity, and equity, first for the Crimean war soldiers and later for the poor of London. Her 3 years of clinical practice gave her clinical expertise and credibility to assume the role of policymaker. She embraced that role because of her high degree of internal distress and concern about needless suffering and premature death of her patients (McDonald, 2006). Empowered by her clinical practice during the Crimean war, she used data that she had collected systematically to persuade Parliament to make needed military and civic law reforms that promoted health. In 1858, Nightingale became the first woman elected as a member of the Royal Statistical Society and later became an honorary member of the American Statistical Association (Gill & Gill, 2005). Her work and prestige were Victorian era validations of the importance of using evidence to inform policy. Nightingale's activism presaged the APN as patient advocate and policy shaper. She leveraged statistics and clinical expertise to become an effective advocate for influencing policy. She expected nurses to have a high degree of social interest and to be involved in the policymaking process.

This historic covenant with the public must be strengthened. APNs must deepen their commitment to and become masterful at critiquing, formulating, and influencing policies that interfere with human wholeness and health. Most APNs in practice today have experienced the effects of polices that lead directly to poor health care. We must substantively weave policy into the core APN roles so that those experiences move APNs into leadership roles and they become advocates for change.

Overview of the Health Policy Process: Politics Versus Policy

Health Policy

All policy involves decisions that influence the daily life of citizens. Longest (2010) has defined health policy as the authoritative decisions pertaining to health or health care, made in the legislative, executive, or judicial branches of government, that are intended to direct or influence the actions, behaviors, or decisions of citizens.

Although there are many definitions of policy and politics, policy generally refers to decisions resulting in a law or regulation. Politics refers to power relationships. It is the responsibility of a multitude of policymakers, whether mayors, county supervisors, government employees, legislators, governors, or presidents, to make health policy. Overall responsibility generally places authority with the legislative branch to crafts laws, the executive branch crafts rules to implement the laws, and the judicial branch interprets conflicts among the spheres of government, citizens, and a public or private entity. The federal government plays a substantial role in setting health policy, although to a far lesser degree than Canada or Great Britain, where policymakers have integrated, centralized, government-run health care systems. The federal government is a provider of health services via the prison system and Veterans Administration. However, for the most part, health care delivery is still largely under private sector control, making U.S. health policy development incremental, fragmented, and decentralized.

Politics

Politics is the process used to influence those who are making health policy. Politics introduces nonrational, divisive, and self-interested approaches to policymaking, often along ideological lines. Any political maneuvering to enhance one's power or status within a group may be described as politics. Politics is largely associated with a struggle for ascendancy among groups having different priorities and power relationships. Preferences and interests of stakeholders and political bargaining (favor swapping) are important and extremely influential political factors that overlie the policymaking process. The self-interest paradigm suggests that human motives are not any different in political arenas than they are in the private marketplace. This behavioral assumption implies that it is rational for people and organizations to use the power of government to achieve what they cannot accomplish on their own. Ideally, elected officials seek office to serve the public interest, not their own. However, to be successful in the electoral process, they need electoral support through financial contributions, rendering them beholden to fundraising and funders (Feldstein, 2006). Highly politicized decisions may often create outcomes that have little to do with efficient use of scarce resources and what is best for the general public. These forces, which may or may not be based on evidence, contribute to the lack of coordination among health policies in the United States, making policy formulation highly complex and exceedingly interesting.

APN's must engage in the political process to influence public policy and resource allocation decisions within political, economic, and social systems and institutions. APN political advocacy facilitates civic engagement and collective action, which may be motivated by patient-centered moral or ethical principles or simply to protect what has already been allocated. Advocacy can include many activities undertaken by a person or organization, such as media campaigns, public speaking, commissioning and publishing policy-relevant research or polls, and filing an *amicus curiae* (friend of the court) briefs. Lobbying as a political advocacy tool is only effective if a relationship between the lobbyist and legislator influences or shapes a policy issue. Social media for political advocacy is playing an increasingly significant role in modern politics (Non-Profit Action, 2012).

United States Differs from the International Community

The U.S. health system and political process for creating health care policy is unique in that the system is decentralized. In the United States, there is no single entity responsible for health care delivery, payment, or policymaking. There are many spheres of policymaking with overlapping authority involving a wide diversity of people, cultures, traditions, and illness patterns. Although the federal government may create broad guidelines, states, for the most part, have the autonomy to create policies that best serve their citizenry—hence, the large patchwork of public, private, local, state and federal entities. These can be operating as governmental, nonprofit, or for-profit entities, all of which are creating policies and/or delivering care. For most of the rest of the world, and in countries such as China, Switzerland, and the Netherlands, there is a highly centralized health authority for policymaking and care

delivery. These nations, with centralized systems of care, are able to track the impact of their policy decisions more closely and build more tightly controlled surveillance systems to follow epidemics, immunization rates, spending, workforce, and other important markers of a strong health care system. Moreover, centralized health care systems limit the number of policymakers that need to be influenced, which can be a great advantage. Although there are a smaller number of people to influence, if those policymakers are strongly opposed to expanded APN practice or patient-centered care, centralization becomes disadvantageous. The unique U.S. public-private, federal-state, nonprofit and for-profit arrangements make it difficult to transport programs that are effective in other nations into the United States.

In a review of published literature, Docteur and Berenson (2009) tried to determine how the quality of U.S. health care compares internationally. Compared with other developed nations, life expectancy is shorter and rates of death from treatable conditions such as asthma and diabetes are higher in the United States. Their findings suggested no support for the oft-repeated claim that U.S. health care is the best in the world. The United States does relatively well in some areas, including cancer care, and less well in others, including chronic conditions amenable to prevention and coordinated management. The United States ranks below other nations in patient safety. The authors concluded that health reform is needed and will not diminish the areas of health care that are excellent (Docteur & Berenson, 2009). Exemplar 22-1 depicts the experience of nurse practitioners (NPs) who practice across the boundaries of two countries' health care systems, Canada and the United States.

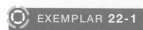 **EXEMPLAR 22-1**   **A Tale of Two Countries, Two Nurse Practitioners, and Two Different Health Care Systems***

A husband and wife NP team, Nancy Brew and Mark Schultz, had been living and practicing in Alaska for over 20 years when they emigrated to British Columbia, Canada, in 2006. Nancy had worked as a family nurse practitioner (FNP) in Alaska for many years. She experienced increasing moral distress[†] (see Chapter 13) from trying to provide equitable and quality care to uninsured and underinsured patients in the expensive, private-payer U.S. health care system.

When Nancy and Mark met, they were drawn to the concept of health care access for all, so the idea of working in a country in which everyone had access to health care and no one had to fear bankruptcy or

losing their home if medical disaster struck, was very appealing. NP-authorizing legislation is now present in all 10 Canadian provinces and three territories, and there are over 2000 NPs licensed and practicing in Canada.

In Canada, the health care system is chiefly administered via provincial and territorial regional governments. Each regional government determines how to fund APN practice. In the province of British Columbia (BC), almost all primary care is still provided by small physician group practices in a fee-for-service model. In this model, each patient visit is individually billed to BC's Medical Services Plan (MSP), the main primary

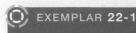 **EXEMPLAR 22-1**   **A Tale of Two Countries, Two Nurse Practitioners, and Two Different Health Care Systems*—cont'd**

care funding stream, for reimbursement. To date, BC NPs and certified nurse-midwives (CNMs) are not authorized to bill MSP; thus, APNs in BC are unable to open their own practices or join existing physician practices, even in the most underserved rural areas, because there is no designated funding mechanism to support their employment. A limited number of salaried positions were created for BC NPs, but many of these were in specialty areas with considerable primary care physician resistance. Hence, Mark has worked predominantly in acute care settings of cardiology and orthopedics since becoming an NP, although he was trained in family practice. This is ironic because the NP role in BC was initially legislated to improve access to primary care. There is a great need for primary care providers in BC, with a significant number of patients unable to find one. NPs could be doing more to address the Canadian primary care shortage but Canada, as a single-payer, government-run system, does not have a market-based approach to workforce shortages.

Nancy and Mark found it interesting to have worked in health care on both sides of the border during the 2010 American health care reform debate. The Canadian health care system was held up as a cautionary tale, that the Canadian system was an egregious example of poor care, long waits, and unaccountable all-empowering bureaucracy that ran health care into the Canadian ground. Although it is true there can be months' long wait times to see specialists for non-urgent conditions, appropriate specialty referrals are given rather freely. Non-urgent CT scans can occur in a week, non-urgent MRIs may take a few months, and the wait times for hip and knee replacements can approach 6 months.

Since emigrating to Canada, Mark and Nancy have become more aware of the U.S. concept that suspects that anything obtained for free must be second rate. Canadian colleagues and patients would ask them, "Is our Canadian health care system really that bad compared with the United States?" They would answer, "If you are in a tertiary care, highly specialized, well-known center, undergoing a high-risk procedure, the care will be second to none." The couple has found that in Canada,

visits are shorter and charting is more concise, but Canadian health care is similarly evidence-based and equal in quality. In contrast to the United States, all Canadian residents and citizens have full access to inpatient and outpatient health care. Canadians are only responsible for the cost of outpatient prescriptions, which are priced on a sliding fee scale.

As they reflect on 5 years on Canadian practice, with summers in temporary jobs in rural villages in Alaska, they have seen first-hand the strengths in each system and how the different health care policies play out. In the United States, they see poor care as a result of an individual's inability to pay and cite the example of an uninsured man from a rural fishing village with advanced heart failure. He cannot afford the ferry ride to the clinic and cuts his pills in half or runs out of them altogether. If he were in the Canadian system with his presenting symptoms, he would likely be hospitalized to be medically managed, followed more closely, provided prescriptions, and offered a transportation solution. On the Canadian side, the NPs have experienced the moral hazard[‡] of getting something for nothing.

They cite the example of a patient who presented to the ER with a 1-cm uninfected paper cut. It was easier for her to present to the emergency room for a Band-Aid than it was to drive to the store. So, they occasionally see the Canadian sense of entitlement, using resources that are not necessary.

What has been so interesting to this couple is the role that the lack of insurance coverage plays in the lives of Americans juxtaposed with the sense of entitlement in the Canadian system. Both these problems are policy-driven and have enormous impact on the lives of their citizens. Although they recognize the grass is not greener in Canada for APN practice authority, they are grateful overall to live and work in Canada for its all-inclusive health care system, provided at a per capita cost that is considerably less than in the United States. There are times when they wish they could take the best parts of both systems and combine them to decrease the moral distress in the United States and the moral hazard in Canada.

*Nancy Brew and Mark Schultz are gratefully acknowledged for writing this exemplar.
[†]Moral distress—when one knows the right thing to do, but institutional constraints make it almost impossible to pursue the right course of action (Jameton, 1984; Hamric, 2009).
[‡]Moral hazard –when a party insulated from risk behaves differently than [he or she] would behave if [he or she] were fully exposed to the risk (Jameton, 1984).

Policy Frameworks and Key Concepts

Longest Model

Longest (2010) has conceptualized policymaking as an interdependent process. The Longest model defines a policy formulation phase, implementation phase, and a modification phase (Fig. 22-1). This has immense usefulness for nursing because it illustrates the incremental and cyclical nature of policymaking, two of the most important features of the U.S. health care policymaking process. Essentially, all health care policy decisions are subject to modification because policymaking in the United States involves making decisions that are revisited when circumstances shift. Our system is not designed for big bold reform. Rather, it considers intended or unintended consequences of existing policy and tweaks changes (Longest, 2010).

Federalism

The locus of responsibility between the states and federal government is highly relevant to most health care programs, such as Medicare, Medicaid, the State Children's Health Insurance Program (SCHIP) and the creation of an interoperable health information system. Federalism refers to the allocation of governing responsibility between the states and federal government. The states and federal government have a complex relationship governing health policy, which explains a large part of our chaotic and fragmented approach to health care in place today. Passage of the PPACA in 2010 requires states to expand access, enhance quality, and lower costs, albeit with a great degree of flexibility. The PPACA has amplified the tensions between federal mandates and states' rights, to the degree that the Supreme Court had to clarify the constitutionality of the federal government's powers in requiring individuals to purchase health insurance.

The Constitution unambiguously gives the federal government absolute power to preempt state laws when it chooses to do so. However, the states are also granted unfettered authority, such as regulation of health care professionals and health insurance plans (Bodenheimer & Grumbach, 2012). Ambiguity between state and federal authority allows states to experiment with policy

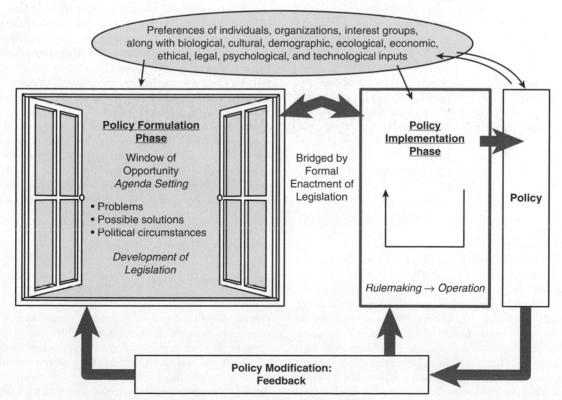

FIG 22-1 The Longest model. *(From Longest, B. [2010]. Health policymaking in the United States (5th ed.). Chicago: Health Administration Press.)*

solutions. The "states as learning laboratory" concept has grown out of local health policy problems and enables states to experiment with innovative policy solutions that could not be done on a national level. Moreover, states have local health care problems, requiring local, flexible, and humane solutions. Many federal health policy decisions are devolving decision making to the states, as evidenced by the increase in block grants (a large sum of money granted by the federal government to a state, with only general provisions as to the way it is to be spent, contrasted with a categoric grant, which has stricter and more specific provisions) and Medicaid waivers. Because much of health care is experienced at the local level, APNs must be aware of the overlapping state and federal spheres of government and the tension between their authorities.

Incrementalism

Although the policymaking process is a continuous inter-related cycle, most efforts to change policy stem from the negative effects of an existing policy. The modification phase creates a feedback loop to the agenda-setting process. This concept of continuous, often modest modification of existing polices is termed *incrementalism*. Major reforms of health policy are seen rarely, usually one in a generation, such as Medicare and Medicaid in 1965 and the PPACA in 2010. Minor changes of existing policies play out slowly over time and are therefore more predictable. Incrementalism promotes stability and stakeholder compromise. A good example of incrementalism is the gradual increase in federal spending for biomedical research from $300 in 1887 to more than $31 billion in 2013, going to NIH's 27 institutes and centers. Within that structure, the National Center for Nursing Research was created in 1985 by a congressional override of a presidential veto as a result of the influence of strong nurse leaders. In 1993, the Center for Nursing Research was elevated to the Institute for Nursing Research and funded with $50 million; funding levels in 2013 will exceed $145 million.

The Kingdon Model

Agenda setting is a major component of the Longest policy formulation phase. With so many health policy problems in this country, why do some problems get attention and others languish at the bottom of the policy agenda for decades? Kingdon (1995) conceptualized an open policy window, with three conditions streaming through the open window at once. First, the problem must come to the attention of the policymaker; second, it must have a menu of possible policy solutions that have the potential actually to solve the problem; and third, it must have the right political circumstances. If all three of these conditions occur simultaneously, the policy window

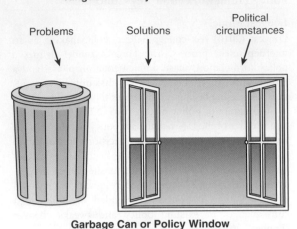

Kingdon's Policy Streams Model

Problems   Solutions   Political circumstances

Garbage Can or Policy Window

FIG 22-2 Kingdon's policy streams model.

opens and progress can be made on the issue (Fig. 22-2). Conversely, once shut, this policy window (opportunity) may never open again.

Policy problems come to the attention of policymakers in a number of ways, including constituents, litigation, research findings, market forces, fiscal environment, crisis, special interest groups, and the media, singly or collectively. Wakefield (2008) has identified policy dynamics particular to agenda setting (Table 22-1). Additional dynamics have been added and each dynamic has one or more so-called accelerators, which drives the agenda setting or triggers policymakers to take action on an issue. The political circumstances that push problems onto the agenda must have a high degree of public importance and low degree of stakeholder conflict surrounding the policy solution. If there is a great deal of stakeholder disagreement, there may be competing proposals put forth, weakening the likelihood that the problem will be addressed. Strong health services research can provide the evidence base to help policymakers specify and therefore accelerate agenda setting (Longest, 2010).

Federal Budget Cycle

Entitlement Versus Discretionary Spending

Federal spending has two categories. People who are entitled to benefits must meet eligibility rules (age, income); the three largest entitlement programs are Medicare, Medicaid, and Social Security. These three programs consume two thirds of federal spending and do not go through the appropriations process because they are permanently enacted. These large programs are expected to consume progressively more of the federal budget as the

TABLE 22-1 Policy Dynamics Influence on Agenda Setting

Dynamic	Activator	Examples
Constituents	The constituent can have enormous impact on agenda setting. When members of Congress learn from their constituents about deeply moving tragedies that could have been prevented or lessened, the member is moved to introduce legislation.	An automobile accident in a remote area killed three members of a family and seriously injured two. A senator knew the family, which prompted introduction of the Wakefield Act, designed to improve pediatric emergency response in rural areas and honor the family. It became public law, the Wakefield Emergency Medical Services for Children.
Litigation	Court decisions play an increasingly prominent role in setting health policy.	Stringent control of tobacco products stems from a long history of 46 states suing the tobacco industry for tobacco-related health care costs. The courts decide that certain tobacco marketing practices must stop and that tobacco companies must pay the states, in perpetuity, to compensate them for some of the medical costs of caring for persons on Medicaid with smoking-related illnesses. The first 25 years will total payments of $206 billion.
Research findings	Research on care transitions and coordination by nurses reduces hospitalizations and emergency room use and greatly reduces costs. The IOM report, *The Future of Nursing: Leading Change. Advancing Health,* provides a compelling evidence base to strengthen the nation's nursing workforce (IOM, 2011).	Elements of managing care transitions are embedded in the PPACA (HHS, 2011a) by way of ACOs, in which the delivery system takes full responsibility for the care of patients as they transition home and to other care settings. The PPACA's many provisions to expand access, reduce cost, and improve quality of care can only be accomplished by the inclusion and expansion of APNs. This will accelerate removing state and federal barriers to APN practice so that new innovation delivery models can be developed.
Market forces	The fractured health care delivery system creates opportunities for highly profitable businesses.	The CEOs of insurance companies earn enormous salaries. The PPACA includes the "Medical Loss Ratio" provision, in which insurers must spend 85% of premiums dollars on direct health care. The other 15% can go to marketing and salaries, greatly capping the multimillion dollar CEO salaries.
Fiscal environment	Very different budget decisions are made when the government is addressing deficit rather than surplus spending. Deficit spending restricts budgets to a pay as you go policy	Deficit financing forces budgetary restrictions in fiscal year 2013. The Centers for Disease Control and Prevention budget gets a $600 million cut during a deficit crisis. Many other health programs get budget cuts or receive level funding.
Special interest groups	Well-organized special interest groups with a clear message can have an enormous impact on government action or inaction.	The autism advocacy community frames the increase in autism spectrum disorders as a public health emergency, motivating Congress to pass legislation spanning a wide range of provisions for those with autism, including research, treatment and services (www.autismvotes.org).
Crises	Crises can promote rapid response policy changes, usually centered on quality and access.	World Trade Center first responders in New York endure debilitating diseases, sickened from the toxic dust. A program is passed into law to provide federal reparatory and remedial compensation; $300 million is proposed.
Political ideology	The majority party (Democrats versus Republicans) has a large impact on agenda setting. The divide centers on what role the government should play in U.S. society.	The newly installed 112th Republican-controlled House of Representatives introduced the second bill of the session in January 2011, the Repealing the Job-Killing Health Care Law Act, a failed attempt to repeal the PPACA.
Media	The lay press, reporting on policy issues or crises, often compel policymakers to take action.	Major news outlet reported that millions of unencrypted personal health care records were stolen or mistakenly made public. Tensions rise between added reporting requirements and privacy. Legislation is introduced on strategies to enforce the Health Insurance Portability and Accountability Act (HIPAA) and mandate encryption.

Continued

TABLE 22-1	Policy Dynamics Influence on Agenda Setting—*cont'd*	
Dynamic	Activator	Examples
U.S. president with a high degree of commitment	When the occupant of the White House sets health reform as a major domestic policy agenda by linking unsustainable health care costs to the health of the macroeconomy, the power of that office becomes evident.	In March 2010, President Obama signs the historic PPACA, despite a 2-year debate, town hall meetings across the nation, and multiple national speeches explaining to the public why reform is necessary.

Adapted from Wakefield, M. K. (2008). Government response: Legislation. In Milstead, J. (Ed.), *Health policy and politics: A nurse's guide.* (pp. 65–88; 3rd ed.). Sudbury, MA: Jones & Bartlett.

demographic shifts to an older population. However, most of the debate and discourse regarding federal health spending is centered around the more modest discretionary programs. Discretionary spending includes almost every other government service, including the military, post office, education, national parks, and health care workforce (e.g., nursing). Once a program is authorized through legislation, Congress will then assign a funding amount, an entirely different procedure, termed *appropriations*, or spending legislation. All discretionary programs, such as the Nurse Reinvestment Act, must have their funding renewed each year to continue operating and almost all health programs (other than Medicare and Medicaid) are discretionary. Discretionary programs make up one third of all federal spending and the President's budget spells out how much funding is recommended for each discretionary program.

The federal budget process is not linear, in part because of the influence of stakeholders. Throughout the process, lobbyists and interest groups are vying to keep their funding cycle level or increased, depending on the fiscal and political circumstances.

Budget Cycle

The budget process begins with the President's State of the Union Address (before the first Monday in February) to highlight the Executive Branch's spending priorities for the upcoming fiscal year. The President's budget guides the activities of the Office of Management and Budget (OMB) staff, appointed by the President to do the following: create the budget; communicate to Congress the President's overall federal fiscal priorities; and propose specific spending recommendations for individual federal programs. The President's budget is merely a suggestion until acted on by Congress. In February and March of each year, the House and Senate budget committees hold hearings on the proposed budget and these joint conference committees hammer out differences. On April 15, Congress passes a House-Senate budget resolution and no other spending bill can be considered until the budget resolution is adopted. Finally, the House and Senate

appropriates or subdivides their allocations among the 13 appropriations subcommittees that have jurisdiction over specific spending legislation. If the appropriations process is not completed by October 1, Congress must adopt a continuing resolution to provide stop-gap funding (Congressional Research Service, 2011).

The budget resolution is not an ordinary bill, and therefore does not go to the President for his or her signature or veto. It requires only a majority vote to pass and is one of the few pieces of legislation that cannot be filibustered in the Senate.

Policy Formulation: How a Bill Becomes Law

Figure 22-3 illustrates a linear process for federal legislation; however, it is more of a choreographed effort than a stepwise process. Only when each step in the process is completed can legislation be passed. Therefore, very few legislative proposals introduced are ever enacted. For example, in the 110th Congress, 14,000 pieces of legislation were introduced and 449 became law (a 3.3% passage rate). Of those 449 laws passed, 144 (32%) were purely ceremonial, such as naming post offices (Singer, 2008). Counting the number of bills dropped or passed in Congress is not an accurate measure of its productivity because it does not consider the impact that the bill has on the larger society. Omnibus bills are on the rise, which role dozens of bills into a single packaged bill, making the total number smaller, but the legislation more ambitious.

The process begins with the introduction of a bill that is the result of legislators trying to address a policy problem. Getting involved in the process or policy solution at this conceptual phase, rather than responding to legislation already crafted, is extremely important, because it maximizes APN influence. A number of reimbursement bills pertaining to APNs are generally initiated by APN organizations working closely with a member of Congress. The Nursing Workforce Development programs, authorized under Title VIII of the Public Health Service Act (42 U.S.C. 296 et seq.), and the legislation creating the

The Path of Legislation

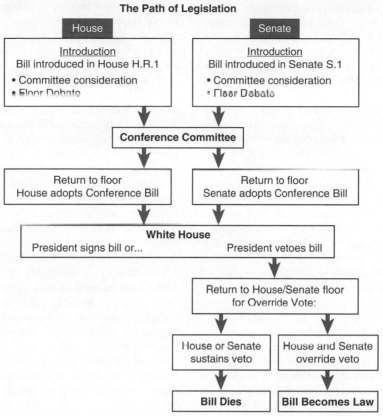

FIG 22-3 The path of federal legislation. *H.R.1,* House of Representatives introduced; *S.1,* Senate introduced.

National Institute of Nursing Research are examples of nursing organizations shaping legislation. Although these examples are not specific to APNs, they significantly benefit APNs, the larger nursing community, and the patients they serve.

Any member of Congress can introduce legislation, which is assigned a number and posted (Box 22-1). The legislation gets referred to the committee of jurisdiction, referred to more than one committee, or split so that parts are sent to different committees.

Congressional Committees

There are over 200 Congressional committees and subcommittees, which are functionally structured to gather information, compare and evaluate highly specific legislative alternatives, identify policy problems and propose solutions, select, determine, and report measures for full chamber consideration, provide oversight to the executive branch, and investigate allegations of wrongdoing. Committee membership enables members of Congress to develop in-depth knowledge of the matters under their jurisdiction. There are more than 13 committees and

BOX 22-1   How to Find a Legislative Bill and Determine Bipartisan Support

To find a federal bill, go to the Library of Congress website, http://thomas.loc.gov/home/ thomas.php. Search keywords or enter the bill number. Once you get to the bill summary, do an analysis to determine whether the bill has any chance of passing by going to the list of cosponsors. The Library of Congress does not list political affiliation next to the cosponsor's name, which requires looking up each member to find out to which party they belong. Be sure that members of Congress from each party are cosponsoring the bill in equivalent numbers. If it is only one party sponsoring the bill, you may conclude that the bill is largely partisan, with a small chance of passage. A politically competent APN will always look for bipartisan cosponsorship of bills, which have the highest chance of actually becoming law. The same method will work for each state legislature (found on each state government website).

subcommittees with jurisdiction over health care. In 1885, Woodrow Wilson said, "Congress in its committee rooms is Congress at work," which still rings true today (Wilson, 1913).

The very first action that a committee can perform on a piece of legislation is not to take any action, which is equivalent to killing it. If the committee chair chooses to act on the legislation, the federal agency that would be affected by the legislation is queried for its opinions on the bill's merit. The bill is assigned to a subcommittee and hearings may be held. Politically astute APN organizations will have developed relationships with committee staffers and seek invitations to testify before the committee. It is critical that the testimony has accurate data, is not purely self-serving, and attempts to solve the problem at hand. Subcommittees report their findings to the full committee, which holds a mark-up, session during which it will make revisions and additions. The House and Senate chambers must approve, change, or reject all committee amendments before conducting a final passage vote.

House or Senate Floor Action

The legislation is sent back to the entire House or Senate chamber for a vote and, if passed, is then sent to the other (House or Senate) chamber unless that chamber already has a similar measure under consideration. If either chamber does not pass the bill, it dies. If the House and Senate pass the same bill, it is sent to the President. If the House and Senate pass a different bill, which is more often the case, the bill goes to a conference committee. Members from the Senate and House form conference committees to work out the differences, with each chamber trying to maintain their version of the bill. Once the conference committee reaches a compromise, it prepares a written conference report, which must be voted on by both the House and the Senate and then signed into law by the President.

Presidential Action

A bill becomes law if signed by the President or if not signed within 10 days of receipt and Congress is in session. If Congress adjourns before the 10 days and the President has not signed the bill, it does not become law (termed a *pocket veto*). If the President vetoes the bill, it is sent back to Congress with a note listing her or his reasons. The chamber that originated the legislation can attempt to override the veto by a vote of two thirds of those present. If the veto is overridden in both chambers, it becomes law. Once a bill is signed by the President or his or her veto is overridden by both houses, it becomes a law and is assigned an official number with "PL" (public law) preceding it.

Interpretative Function of Rulemaking: Policy Implementation

Once the bill becomes public law, legislative activities shift to policy implementation in the executive branch. Rulemaking launches the formal regulatory process to operationalize fully what Congress has formulated. The executive agency responsible for implementing the law must make clear who is responsible for implementation and how it will be financed. These operational decisions are an important dimension of health policy and can have an enormous impact on health care. Regulations can be added, deleted, or modified at any time, making rulemaking a continuous process. Each federal agency has a number of public advisory bodies that inform the agency on rulemaking and policy. Serving on advisory bodies and engaging in the rulemaking process are key venues for APNs to influence policy. For example, the National Advisory Council on Nurse Education and Practice (NACNEP) of the Health Resources and Services Administration (HRSA) is an advisory body that advises the Secretary of the HHS and Congress on policy issues related to the Title VIII programs (nurse workforce supply, education, and practice improvement); HRSA's National Advisory Council on Primary Care and Dentistry now requires the appointment of a nurse. Other important boards for APNs to serve on are each state's highly influential board of nursing.

Congressional Advisory Bodies

Congress has created alternative bodies outside the executive branch to assist with complex, high-conflict rulemaking or oversight. For example, Medicare is essentially undergoing constant rulemaking revisions, so Congress created MedPAC, a free-standing advisory body to Congress on Medicare policy. Congress has developed its own information source by creating the Government Accountability Office and Congressional Budget Office. Their sole purpose is to help Congress make informed decisions through detailed reports.

Policy Modification

Our system is based on continuous policy modification of a few policies initiated earlier. Almost every policy results in some form of unintended consequence, which is only learned through implementation of a prior policy. Policies that are appropriate and relevant at one point in time become highly inappropriate as time passes and economic, social, demographic, and commercial circumstances shift. Policy consequences are the reason that stakeholders and policymakers seek to modify policy continually. These policy changes can be driven by stakeholders when a policy negatively affects a group or driven by members of Congress or rule makers when policy does not meet their objective. Understanding the process of policy modification and amendment of earlier polices is a key to mastering political competency.

Role of Public Comment

Public laws do not contain specific language about how the policy or program is to be carried out. For health-related issues, the executive branch agency, usually the HHS, must publish its proposed rules in the daily *Federal Register* seeking public comment. The public comment opportunity is usually limited to 60 days; however, stakeholder groups can exert an enormous degree of influence in the rulemaking process during this limited period. This public comment stems from two important American principles: (1) that democracy can only work if its citizenry is informed and participates; and (2) the federal government does not hold all the expertise, but must solicit comment from experts involved in the issue to alert the agency to unforeseen options or consequences (Regulations.gov, 2012). APN organizations can powerfully influence rulemaking by submitting evidence-based public comment and by activating the APN grassroots to launch a public comment campaign. The *Federal Register* will tally the number of responses received and report how many were in favor or opposed to the proposed rule. Thoughtful, well- crafted public comments submitted by an APN organization have been directly incorporated into final rules, rendering submission of public comments and the rulemaking process crucially important activities for APNs. For example, when the *Federal Register* published rules removing Medicare payment restrictions for APNs, excerpts of a letter submitted by the American College of Nurse Practitioners were quoted and used as an evidence source to support the payment expansions.

Current and Emerging Health Policy Issues Relevant to Advanced Practice Nurses

Context for Framing APN Policy Issues: Cost, Quality, and Access

The cost-quality-access triad (Fig. 22-4) is considered the framework for health policy, whether it is at the international, national, state, local, community, institutional, or corporate level. All health care policy issues and solutions can be considered in terms of increasing access to health care, improving health care quality, and/or decreasing health care costs. These principal health policy drivers overlap and are inherently interdependent; a shift in one inevitably affects the others. For example, the current increase in the cost of health insurance causes it to be too expensive to be offered by small businesses to employees

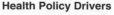

Health Policy Drivers

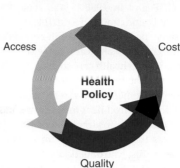

Access   Cost

Health Policy

Quality

FIG 22-4 Cost-quality-access schema.

or for individuals to purchase, thus creating barriers to access. Cost, quality, and access issues are not tangential problems to our health care challenges—they are the challenge.

Cost

The total amount spent on health care in the United States in 2010 was $2.6 trillion compared with $2.5 trillion in 2009 and $2 trillion in 2005 (Centers for Medicare & Medicaid Services [CMS], 2011). The increase in health care costs slowed in 2009 and 2010, although still is increasing at a rate faster than inflation, mainly because the economic recession created less demand for health services. The effect of the economy is also seen in the growth of health care compared with the growth of the economy, as measured by gross domestic product (GDP), which is the value of all the goods and services produced in the United States. The growth in health care costs for 2010 increased at 3.9% and GDP increased at 3.8% (CMS, 2011). In the past, the growth of health care costs outpaced the growth of GDP, with health care consuming ever-larger portions of the economy. Although health care remained a fairly robust part of the economy at the beginning of the recession, businesses were less able to manage the increasing costs to provide health insurance to employees as more people lost jobs and as contracts between insurers and businesses came up for renewal. However, CMS (2011b) has projected that overall average health spending increases through 2020 will average 5.8% and outpace the increase in the overall economy by 1.1%. Health care spending is currently 17.6% of the GDP (CMS, 2011). By 2020, it is projected to be 19.8% of GDP (CMS, 2011). The proportion of the country's GDP expended on health care is vital to the future of the United States because every dollar spent on health care is a dollar less spent on education, transportation, housing, food, and other essentials. In comparison with the current percent of GDP, the cost of health care in 1960 was about 6% of the GDP and in 1980 it was about 9% of GDP (Kaiser Family Foundation [KFF], 2011).

Policymakers have a large stake in continuing policies to control the cost of health care. Government programs account for 45% of all health care spending, with this share projected to increase to 50% by 2020 (CMS, 2011). This expansion of government costs is a result of the Medicaid program, increased enrollment in Medicare, and subsidies provided for the health insurance exchanges. Past efforts to control costs included the implementation of health plans in the 1970s, introduction of diagnosis-related groups in the 1980s, and instituting competition in the health care market in the 1990s. Efforts in the 2000s were marked by cost control through price regulation and in the 2010s by linking payment to quality and continuing price controls. Even with the varied attempts to control costs, they have had limited impact.

The decade of 2010 to 2020 will be marked by the advent of accountable care organizations (ACOs), which shifts the responsibility of care coordination and cost savings onto delivery systems and therefore to providers. ACOs are integrated systems that bring together hospitals, outpatient clinics, and specialty services to deliver better care coordination and quality of service. ACOs are a vehicle to implement the intent of the PPACA by creating more integrated systems that can coordinate care better, thus improving quality and managing costs more effectively.

Quality

Attention to quality became a national issue following the IOM series of reports in the late 1990s and early 2000s focusing on the problems in the health care system leading to poor care (IOM, 1999, 2001). Linking quality to payment has been how government and private companies try to ensure that quality of care is not compromised because of cost-saving measures. Linking quality to cost control was initially referred to as pay for performance. This concept is more currently referred to as value-based purchasing. As part of value-based purchasing, in 2006 CMS identified 26 so-called *never* events and established a policy that hospitals would not get paid for taking care of patients experiencing an event that should never happen, such as wrong site surgery and any stage 3 or 4 or unstageable pressure ulcers acquired after admission or presentation to a health care setting. "Never" events are now referred to as serious reportable events (SREs); the National Quality Forum (NQF) recognizes 29 SREs. Most SREs occur not only in hospitals, but also in office-based surgery centers, ambulatory practice settings, and long-term care or skilled nursing facilities (NQF, 2011). APNs are expected to know these SREs and work to ensure that they do not occur. A compilation of SREs can be found online (http://www.qualityforum.org/Topics/SREs/Serious_Reportable_Events.aspx).

As part of nursing's effort to improve quality of care, the Nursing Alliance for Quality of Care (NAQC) was initiated in 2009 and funded through the Robert Wood Johnson Foundation. The NAQC was modeled after other alliances that primarily focused on improving the quality of care. The Hospital Quality Alliance, founded in 2002, was the first quality alliance formed, bringing together numerous stakeholders supported by CMS and the American Hospital Association, primarily to get hospitals on board to report quality measures. In the past decade, several more alliances have emerged that focus on the review and/or development of quality measures.

Nursing had no alliance to bring together stakeholders and there was concern that nursing would not address the critical issues surrounding care (NAQC, 2010). The NAQC is comprised of nursing organizations and consumer groups. Policymakers recognize the contributions of nurses in advancing consumer-centered, high-quality health care. APNs can obtain information about alliances through monitoring websites, advancing nursing quality by becoming a member of NAQC and, in general, being aware of the work being done in quality improvement.

Access

Access to health care has been linked to health insurance, which has been dependent on employment for decades. With economic downturns and loss of jobs the numbers of uninsured always increase such as with the recession of 2007. Coupled with economic changes, health insurance premiums have continued to increase to the point that fewer small business owners can afford to offer health insurance coverage to their workers. In 2001, the cost for a family insurance policy was, on average, $7,061, with employers contributing $5,290 and workers $1,787 (KFF, 2011). By 2011, the total cost had increased to $15,073, with employers paying $10,944 and workers $4,129. In addition, workers now pay a higher deductible than before, with the average annual deductible being $1,000 or more. These costs put health insurance out of the financial range for many workers. In addition, people must now choose lower cost options, which leave many of them underinsured. In 2008, it was estimated that more than 50% of the underinsured postponed treatment or did not take medications, and almost 50% had trouble paying their health care bills, with many being plagued by collection agencies and having to take out loans to pay their bills (Commonwealth Fund, 2008).

Although the recession has exacerbated the problems of those who are uninsured, there has been a trend of increasing numbers of uninsured since 2000 (Holahan &

Chen, 2011). The latest report released by the Census Bureau has indicated that 50 million people, 16.3% of the U.S. population, were without health insurance (DeNavas-Walt, Proctor, & Smith, 2011) compared with 46.6 million people (15.6% of the population) in 2005. There is agreement that the cost of health care will continue to increase, including higher coinsurance payments, deductibles, and employee contribution to health insurance. A hazard for the uninsured is that they are often charged the full price for health services (Families USA, 2007). Insurance companies negotiate payment levels–often 40% to 60% discounted from established prices—but uninsured individuals do not have the same benefit. Several states have passed laws requiring hospitals to charge the same price to all patients and have established limits on what can be done by collection agencies. However, this remains a problem in many states, with those least able to pay being charged the most for health care.

Policy Initiatives in Health Reform

The PPACA of 2010, and the Health Care and Education Reconciliation Act of 2010, which amended some provisions in the PPACA, represent the most far-reaching legislation enacted since the passage of Medicare and Medicaid in 1965 (Fig. 22-5). Major elements of the PPACA include the creation of a high-value health care system through payment reform mechanisms, such as bundled payment, requiring reporting on quality measures for informing the public and as a basis for payment, strengthening the primary care system, controlling costs through better coordination of services, especially for individuals with multiple chronic illnesses, and increasing access to health care. Many requirements in the PPACA overlap the cost, quality, and access policy issues.

Cost and Quality

Newer systems of care, ACOs, are being developed that link patient care outcomes to costs incurred in treatment to create a high-value health care system (Fig. 22-6). An ACO is a system that integrates care across a continuum and includes at a minimum primary care providers, specialists, and a hospital. Examples of ACOs include the Geisinger Health System, Kaiser Permanente, and Mayo Clinic. ACOs are responsible for providing high-quality care to Medicare enrollees while controlling costs. Instead of insurers being responsible for controlling cost, providers will be responsible. Based on reduced costs of care, savings are then shared with the providers. Although there have been previous attempts to create coordinated care systems, a new requirement—that ACOs must report quality measures—is transformational.

Measures that need to be reported fall into five categories—patient and caregiver experience of care, patient safety, preventive health, care coordination, and at risk-populations, frail individuals, and older adult health. As ACOs evolve, advanced practice registered nurses (APNs) will be part of these organizations. CMS (2011a) is also exploring the concept of bundled payments, in which payment for care is based on an episode of care rather than on an individual visit, procedure, or service. By 2013, a pilot program will establish payment

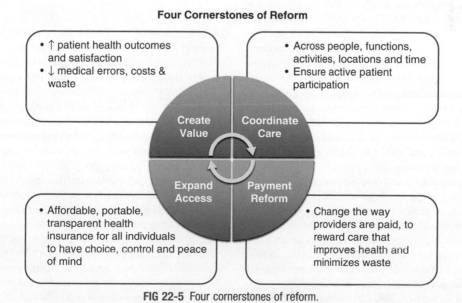

Four Cornerstones of Reform

- ↑ patient health outcomes and satisfaction
- ↓ medical errors, costs & waste

- Across people, functions, activities, locations and time
- Ensure active patient participation

Create Value

Coordinate Care

Expand Access

Payment Reform

- Affordable, portable, transparent health insurance for all individuals to have choice, control and peace of mind

- Change the way providers are paid, to reward care that improves health and minimizes waste

FIG 22-5 Four cornerstones of reform.

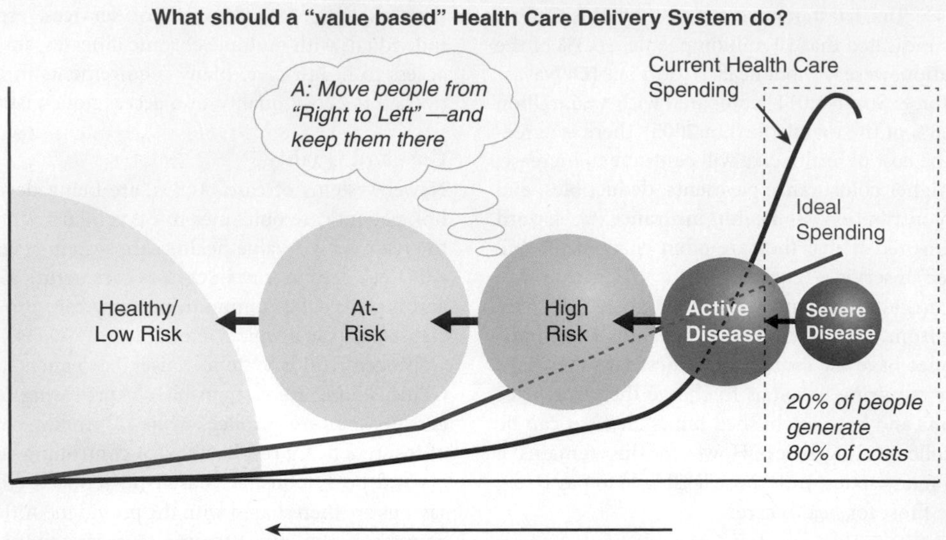

What should a "value based" Health Care Delivery System do?

FIG 22-6 Value-based health care delivery system. *(Adapted from Nursing Alliance for Quality Care. [2010]. Strategic policy and advocacy roadmap [http://www.gwumc.edu/healthsci/departments/nursing/naqc/documents/Roadmap.pdf].)*

rates for care that includes a hospitalization and other services, such as primary care, nursing home, and rehabilitation, which are necessary to manage a specific health problem (e.g., hip fracture). Coincident with efforts to provide better coordination through bundled payments, PPACA also specifies a program to reduce readmission. Hospitals will be required to report on all readmissions over a specific time period and the readmission rates will be posted on Hospital Compare (http://www.hospitalcompare.hhs.gov/), a website available to the public and supported by the CMS (HHS, 2011b). In addition, a 5-year transitional care program has been established to provide care coordination to Medicare enrollees through the Community Care Transitions program to improve care and reduce costs. APNs will be important providers in this program and will need to look at possible entrepreneurial opportunities. Future work of CMS will include costs for specific services on the Hospital Compare website. Currently, health care is one of the only markets in which individuals buy a service without knowing the costs.

As another cost and quality requirement to understand the effectiveness of specific, high-use interventions better, there are new programs in addition to the work of the Agency for Health Care Research and Quality. One is the Patient-Centered Outcomes Research Institute (PCORI), which was established as part of the PPACA to conduct and fund research related to testing health care interventions, with the goal of identifying those interventions that truly make a difference. There is nursing representation on the PCORI board. In addition, in 2012, the Center for Medicare and Medicaid Innovations released $1 billion to support pilot innovative projects in care delivery that increase quality and decrease cost. The projects funded will need to address payments and practice reform, management of individuals with multiple chronic illnesses who are unable to do activities of daily living, coordination of care of those with chronic illnesses, establishment of community-based teams, and patient engagement.

Access

Access to health care is emphasized in the PPACA through many policy mechanisms. A controversial section of the PPACA is the requirement for individuals to purchase health insurance, known as the individual mandate. Anyone not covered by an employer or government program must purchase health insurance or pay a penalty. Twenty-six states challenged this requirement in court, with two decisions stating that Congress has the authority to require this and one court decision finding it unconstitutional (Taylor, 2011). On June 28, 2012, the Supreme Court issued a historic decision that upheld the individual mandate by considering it a tax that was within the power of the federal government to levy. The ruling was masterful in bridging different philosophic views among the justices and many different political agendas. To make the required insurance affordable to those who are not covered through employment or a government program, health insurance exchanges are being established by states. These will provide information about costs and benefits so that individuals can choose the best plan. All insurance plans are required to offer essential benefits, as established by the HHS.

In addition, the PPACA required an expansion of the Medicaid program to all individuals younger than 65 years with incomes up to 133% of the poverty level. This part of the PPACA significantly expanded coverage that had previously been limited primarily to pregnant women, children, and other select groups. The bill was written to require that states participate in this expansion or lose all Medicaid funding from the federal government. The Supreme Court decision said that states could opt out of the expansion and not lose federal funding for programs already in existence, thus finding a middle ground.

Additional PPACA requirements address access by making insurance affordable and available. These requirements include the following:

- Dependents can remain on their parent's health insurance until age 26 years.
- Insurers cannot exclude individuals because of pre-existing conditions.
- The same premium must be offered, regardless of area of the country, age, or preexisting condition.
- Insurance companies can no longer drop coverage if an individual gets sick, which is termed *rescission*.
- Annual spending caps on health insurance and lifetime limits will not be allowed.
- Insurance companies cannot require a copay or deductible for preventive care that meets specific requirements in terms of effectiveness, such as well-child visits and vaccinations.
  - Nonprofit insurance companies must have a spending-to-income ratio of 85% to be eligible for tax benefits; if this amount is not met, companies must give a rebate to customers.
  - Insurance companies also have to make public specific information about executive pay and administrative costs.

A promising and expanding opportunity for APNs to increase access to care is working for or developing nurse-managed clinics (NMCs). The PPACA provides funds to help support expansion of the NMCs. There are currently over 250 NMCs with most clinics being part of a school of nursing. Expanding this capacity will be essential for meeting the additional demand for services in 2014, when it is expected that almost 50 million additional people will have health insurance and need primary care services. NMCs can become a recognized, patient-centered health home approved through the National Committee for Quality Improvement (Kennedy, Caselli, & Berry, 2011). To be recognized, a clinic must comply with all the quality reporting requirements and have electronic health records. (See Chapter 15).

A home demonstration program that brings primary care services to the home-bound will be implemented that "will test a service delivery model that utilizes physician and nurse practitioner directed primary care teams to provide services to high-cost, chronically ill Medicare beneficiaries in their homes" (HHS, 2011b). This demonstration program will open an important door for nurse practitioners to gain a significant niche in the primary care home–based delivery market.

Emerging Advanced Practice Nurse Policy Issues

Payment Issues

There are continued challenges for APNs related to payment rates. Medicare has had a policy of paying APNs 85% of the physician rate, unless services are billed as "incident-to" physician care, in which case billing can be at the 100% rate (see Chapter 19). As of 2011, nurse-midwives receive 100% of the physician fee schedule. Certified registered nurse anesthetists (CRNAs) have a specific fee schedule established by Medicare that defines payment for specific services that are modified by the level of independence of practice, ranging from supervision by a physician to no supervision by a physician. There has been considerable discussion about the 85% rate, with many APNs advocating for same pay for the same service. Others have argued that having reduced payment makes APNs a cost-effective solution to high health care costs. From a policy perspective, the looming cost increases from PPACA-mandated changes to the Medicare program, coupled with pressures to reduce the national deficit, have created a difficult policy situation. Legislators have shied away from reining in the Medicare program and have referred to it as the third rail, meaning that tackling this would likely end political careers. A yearly report to Congress by the Trustees of the Social Security and Medicare trust funds has projected an earlier than expected time frame for Social Security and Medicare trust funds to run out of money (Social Security and Medicare Boards of Trustees, 2011). The report emphasized that the current cost projections for Medicare cannot be sustained and that the Medicare Hospital Insurance trust funds that pay for most hospital-based services will run out of funds by 2024. The Supplemental Medical Insurance (SMI) trust that funds Part B of Medicare, which pays for outpatient care and physician and APN charges, is not projected to run out of funds, primarily because 75% of the cost of SMI is paid for through general revenues (tax income). However, the projected cost of SMI, particularly because it is funded through tax revenue, is also not sustainable.

A tool to control Medicare costs of physicians, APNs, and other services has been the sustainable growth rate (SGR). The SGR is a target set for spending that links payment per Medicare enrollee to increases in the GDP. Because health costs have traditionally increased faster than GDP, this is a way to limit the growth of Medicare expenses. The Medicare Payment Advisory Commission (MedPAC) has reported that the cuts associated with the SGR are steep and not realistic, and that the more patients that a provider sees (volume), the more income generated, rather than rewarding high-quality care and efficiency (Social Security and Medicare Boards of Trustees, 2011). The medical community has lobbied extensively to prevent the SGR from being implemented; for years, Congress has voted to not implement the SGRs. Currently, about 30% of family physicians are not accepting new Medicare enrollees (MacKinney, Xu, & Mueller, 2011). Caring for Medicare patients is a role that APNs, particularly NPs and clinical nurse specialists (CNSs), need to explore, using nurse-managed clinics as a vehicle for care.

Payment by private insurers continues to be challenging in many states. Because insurers are regulated at the state level, approval of APNs as part of a network has to be done state by state. However, there are examples of private insurers cutting payment rates to nonphysicians. An example of this is in Oregon, where insurers cut payment rates to nonphysicians for mental health care. Subsequently, NPs in primary care have received notices of payment cuts (Nurse Practitioners of Oregon, 2012). The Nurse Practitioner Payment Parity bill has been introduced, but with no action taken as of this writing. Cuts by private insurers will need to be monitored and addressed continually.

The cost reduction benefits of APNs have been elusive. Even though APNs usually make about 50% or less of the comparable physician salary, this benefit has not accrued to the system, but has accrued to organizations by increasing their profit margins. Rand (2009) conducted a study in Massachusetts to determine what the most powerful levers would be to control costs in that state. Expanded use of NPs and physician assistance was estimated to result in a $4.2 to $8.4 billion savings, relative to the status quo; NPs are the fastest growing primary care providers, with an estimated 83,000 NPs providing primary care services, accounting for 27% of the primary care workforce (Eibner, Hussey, Ridgely, et al., 2009).

Retail Clinics

In addition, retail clinics represent an alternative to traditional models of care by providing a set of defined services offered within large retail businesses, such as Wal-Mart or CVS pharmacies. Services are usually offered by NPs.

Although retail clinics are still relatively new, there are aggressive plans for building additional clinics. Studies of retail clinics have indicated that they provide safe, effective, and timely care (Cross, 2011; Schleiter, 2010; Weinick, Burns, & Mehrotra, 2010; Wilson et al., 2010). In an attempt to expand services, community health centers have explored providing services through retail clinics (Scott, 2010). However, many physician groups are concerned about the proliferation of retail clinics. This concern is based on quality and economic issues; the quality issue is one of coordination of care. Models are emerging in which medical records from the retail clinic are shared with the person providing the regular source of care. The economic concern is that healthier people will go to the retail clinics because they are more likely to experience the type of problems seen at retail clinics and that physicians' groups will be left with the more expensive, sicker patients. A report in 2009 had projected continued gradual expansion of retail clinics (Deloitte, 2009). It is likely that there will be innovative linkages of these clinics to ACOs, outpatient clinics, and group practices, and an expansion of the types of care delivered, such as chronic care.

Data

Data about the U.S. nursing workforce has been critical to formulating rational policies related to APNs. Lack of data has been a major issue in defining the benefits of APNs. The primary source of valid and reliable data has been through HRSA, which has conducted a national survey of nurses every 4 years. The report, *National Sample Survey of the Registered Nurse Population,* has been the source of information about the profession for many years. There has been a subset of APNs included in the report that has provided an estimate of numbers of each of the APN roles and information about practice, salaries, and education. HRSA has made a decision to discontinue doing the survey and to work with state boards of nursing to develop a unified database that can be used in place of the national survey. This will require an identifier that can track nurses from the beginning of their nursing education through their entire education and practice history. Ultimately, this will be a useful source of data if the data from each state board are aggregated, but until all state boards of nursing implement a robust unified database, having sufficient data for policy formulation will be challenging.

There are data available on nursing through the Department of Labor (Bureau of Labor Statistics, Department of Labor, 2012). This database includes numbers, geographic data, and practice settings and salaries for CRNAs, NPs, and CNMs, but excludes CNSs. The information related to APNs is limited but there are discussions about expanding this database to include more information about APNs. The only sources of data that will be available until then will be through nursing organizations, current NCSBN national data, and some state nursing workforce centers. The quality of data from these sources is variable.

A policy issue to which APNs will need to pay considerable attention is data collection and reporting related to practice. It is difficult to know how well APNs are doing in the quality measures that have been established, particularly when NP services are billed "incident-to" the physician services. Although much focus has been on collecting data from physicians, a model for data collection for APNs is nurse-managed clinics. Some nurse-managed clinics have already established effective data collecting and reporting systems and have been recognized by the National Committee for Quality Assurance as patient-centered medical homes.

Workforce Policy

One of the most important policy issues for APNs is that of workforce development. Significant attention has been paid to primary care as a way to provide higher quality and lower cost of overall health care. The current shortage of primary care providers highlights the importance of APNs. NPs have been the fastest growing primary care providers, with an estimated 83,000 NPs providing primary care services, accounting for 27% of the primary care workforce (American Academy of Nurse Practitioners, 2010). There is concern about having enough primary care providers to take care of the additional 50 million new patients mandated to purchase insurance. HRSA plays a critical role in workforce monitoring, development, and deployment. There is mandatory funding in the PPACA to fund more National Health Service Corps loan repayment recipients and scholars, with a required payback to practice in health professions shortage areas for which APNs are eligible. Title VIII of the Public Health Service Act also supports nursing through the Nursing Education Loan Repayment Program (NELRP), in which qualifying portions of educational loans will be paid in exchange for service. Recently, nursing faculty going back to school for advanced degrees were made eligible for funding.

The Graduate Nurse Education Demonstration Program was included in the PPACA. The demonstration has funded five hospitals partnered with schools of nursing with total funding for the project at $200 million. The funding is modeled after graduate medical education and includes stipends for students and costs of clinical education. At least 50% of the education has to take place in a community-based setting (American Association of Colleges of Nursing, 2011).

Political Competence in the Policy Arena

Health Policymaking: A Requisite Skill For Individual Advanced Practice Nurses

Early APNs prepared in continuing education, which evolved to master's programs created a strong foundation for the necessity of APN involvement in policy. The move to doctoral education raises this standard to a higher level. Policy competence is clearly emphasized in the clinical practice doctorate (Doctor of Nursing Practice [DNP]) competencies (5. Health care policy for advocacy in health care) and is embedded in all of the other DNP competencies, requiring APNs to incorporate policy strategies continuously among the practice, research, and policy nexus in all practice settings (Table 22-2). As APNs move through DNP programs, policy analysis must be integrated into every course, content area, and project so that the DNP graduate has the ability to assume a broad leadership role on behalf of the public and nursing profession. The solutions to today's social injustices, perverse financing, and uneven quality in the health care system are difficult. APNs are well positioned with clinical credibility to inform, design, and influence policy solutions, but this will happen only if they expand their arena of influence beyond the clinical setting.

Political Competence

Politically competent APNs serve as content experts with policymakers and their staff. Often, policymakers are generalists who have to command expertise in a broad range of topics, such as transportation, energy, agriculture, and tax policy. Serving as a resource to policymakers with evidence-based information and helpful suggestions that are in the public interest is crucial. When serving in this capacity, it is important to avoid a self-serving posture. To influence or participate meaningfully and effectively in policy development, APNs must be aware of the policymaking process, from conception to implementation, and the open windows of political opportunity. Furthermore, intentionally developing and maintaining strong relationships with policymakers and other health care interest groups are important APN activities. Heeding the U.S. policy process, policymakers seek advisement on highly specific policy modifications, rather than major reform recommendations. Elected officials turn over at a far higher rate than civil servants who make careers out of formulating and implementing health policy. Because of the longevity of their careers, the strong trustworthy relationships APNs make with the policymaker's staff members is important.

TABLE 22-2   Doctor of Nursing Practice Competencies* for Health Policy and Politics

DNP Essential†	Requisite Policy Skill
1. Scientific underpinnings for practice	Analyze policy and the practice of politics, political systems, and political behavior with nursing science to effect policy level change.
2. Organizational and systems leadership for quality improvement and systems thinking	Create and sustain coalitions on health care quality and access via an orientation to policy development, whether at an institutional, community, corporate, regional, national or international level.
3. Clinical scholarship and analytic methods for evidence-based practice	Participate in design, translation, or dissemination of APN practice inquiry within the context of health services research. Use research best practices to inform policymakers about APN practice and quality.
4. Information systems and patient care technology for the improvement and transformation of health care	Overcome APN invisibility by ensuring the inclusion of nursing and APNs in all administrative and clinical databases. Provide policy leadership to link meaningful data on nursing activity electronically to cost, quality, and health outcomes.
5. Health care policy for advocacy in health care	Engage in political activism and policy development, mentor activism, and participate on boards that affect health policies.
6. Interprofessional collaboration for improving patient and population health outcomes	Build interdisciplinary coalitions as a powerful advocacy tool to promote positive change in the health care delivery system. Communicate across disciplines to build common ground.
7. Clinical prevention and population health for improving the nation's health	Promote the financing and delivery of evidence- based clinical preventive and population health services in all health policy arenas.
8. Advanced nursing practice	Function as a content expert and policy change leader as an advanced practice nurse.

*Relevant to all APNs.
†Adapted from American Association of Colleges of Nursing. (2006). The essentials of doctoral education for advanced nursing practice (http://www.aacn.nche.edu/publications/position/ DNPEssentials.pdf).

Individual Skills

The value of APNs is an important idea but, to be heard effectively, a great degree of maturity, discipline, humility, restraint, and respect for self and others must be practiced. Most political careers are created with small steps; when the person is effective, they are elevated into larger and larger spheres of influence. The politically competent APN will have a long history of developing strong relationships with individuals inside and outside of nursing. For the most part, the APN must be held in high regard and be extremely knowledgeable, highly competent, and authentic, with solid integrity and a great degree of personal warmth. The APN must have the trust of others to serve from a universal posture of problem solving and not make decisions solely to elevate the nursing discipline (effective use of power). The locus of responsibility for a politically competent APN must be far broader than just nursing interests (see Exemplar 22-2 and Box 22-3). There must be a commitment to practical problem solving to increase access to care, lower costs, and improve quality of care. This requires the APN to be careful about burning bridges so that there are no constituents who want to see the APN fail.

BOX 22-2   Op-Ed Suggestions

Op-eds are not formulaic, but some general guidelines may enhance the potential for publication. Op-eds and letters to the editor are both unsolicited, but letters to the editor are usually shorter and in direct response to a story or article that has previously been published. Op-eds are longer opinion pieces (generally opposite the editorial page) that are usually related to some current event or news story. A strong 750-word op-ed piece starts with the credentials and experience of the author. The policy problem is hooked to a leading current problem or news story. Add a specific poignant story to describe how the problem affects people. Offer policy solution(s) backed up by three points of evidence. Add a "to-be-sure" segment, which anticipates and counters opponents' views and inoculates against those stakeholders who oppose your ideas. Finally, a conclusion with possible action items for members of the public (e.g., call or write legislator, support a bill). Ask at least five people with strong writing skills to critique the piece prior to submission.

BOX 22-3   Three Ways to Build and Stay Current with Health Policy Knowledge

1. News Feeds

The best way to stay informed about current and emerging news is to subscribe to a few news feeds that come directly into your e-mail box from reputable, bipartisan policy sources. Glance at the headlines and read only what is of interest. APNs must be aware of the larger context of health care delivery and develop telescoping skills, in which one hooks smaller institutional policy issues into what is happening in the larger world. Having knowledge of the larger policy world positions the APN's capacity to participate more powerfully in institutional policy. Subscribe to three of the following (free) news feeds from the list below:

- Agency for Healthcare Research and Quality (AHRQ)—https://subscriptions.ahrq.gov/.../multi_subscribe.html?code=USAHRQ
- Institute of Medicine news—www.iom.edu/Global/Media%20Room/News.aspx
- Commonwealth Fund—www.commonwealthfund.org/
- Robert Wood Johnson Foundation news digests—www.rwjf.org/en/about-rwjf/program-areas/quality.../newshtml
- Center for Studying Health System Change—www.hschange.com/

- Kaiser Family Foundation—http://www.kff.org
- Rand—www.rand.org/
- Medicare Payment Advisory Commission—www.medpac.gov

2. Watch the PBS News Hour

See local listings for your TV station (http://www.pbs.org/newshour). This hour-long program is usually on twice an evening (repeated). It differs from network news in that there are long conversations with policy experts and the viewpoint is balanced and of the highest quality. It avoids news by sound bites and there is frequent emphasis on health policy issues. Moreover, listening to the conversations with experts in the field, with a high degree of civility, on topics related to the economy or politics will assist the APN to become a more informed citizen and raise the level of political competency. This is an easy way to stay informed and experience depth behind the issues.

3. Read and Glance at Newspapers

Newspaper articles may seem old-fashioned, whether print or online, but almost every daily regional print outlet has at least one current health policy article. Often, these are found in the business or opinion sections. Read the Sunday opinion pages and the health section of your regional news source.

A great degree of humility is required; one effective way to embody humility is to seek out respected individuals with expertise (content experts), including those whose political agenda may be different from one's own agenda. Consulting experts along the way to gain insight and knowledge builds trust because the seeker of expertise does not presume to be an expert in all matters related to health care. The APN must integrate all sides of an issue (stakeholder analysis) and then make a determination about how and whether to use that expertise.

Content expertise is not the only skill set required to be effective in influencing policy in an interdisciplinary arena. The APN must be always extremely mindful of process and carefully measure how one participates in discussions to maximize being heard (political antennae). Developing political antennae can be strengthened by engaging stakeholders who may oppose or support an action that the APN may want to take. This stakeholder analysis, done privately before issues become public (or before a meeting), is an effective way to learn about all the issues, especially the opposition viewpoint, so that a creative strategy can be developed to inoculate the opposing ideas with an evidence base. By learning others' opinions

about contentious issues, the APN can carefully garner support.

In terms of public meetings and how APNs conducts themselves, impromptu remarks should be avoided because they could be used against the person, nursing profession, or other interests in the future. It is important to continuously gauge the other stakeholders at the meeting; if, for example, a physician has made a point about nursing that the APN wanted to make, let that external validation stand as a comment that is supportive of nursing, rather than repeating the point. It is important to show restraint in meetings, waiting until everyone else has spoken before contributing to the discussion, so that the APN can consider their comments and respond. To be successful, the APN must keep cool, responding factually and avoiding rhetorical inflammatory comments, which might diminish other disciplines. By participating in meetings with this respectful approach, deep content expertise, and a focus on process, the APN is well positioned to encourage others to support nursing issues.

Another essential responsibility for APNs is to inform and contribute to the public discourse on important health policy issues because APN interests and public

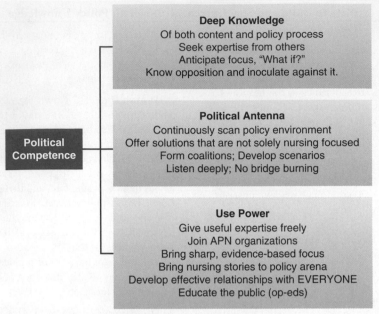

FIG 22-7 Political competence.

interests are not at odds. Gaining public support and influencing public opinion can help get the attention of policymakers or propel issues onto the policy agenda. Submitting an op-ed (meaning "opposite the editorial page" in the publication) to major news outlets is a powerful way to do this (see Box 22-2). This requires writing that links the issues to the community, uses poignant stories to bring the problem to life, and incorporates evidence to build a strong case about why a policy change is needed. APNs must also seek media invitations to news programs to inform the public about the APN's expertise on major issues of the day. APNs must use their professional credentials and expertise with a sense of responsibility toward educating the public and not be hesitant to act as advocates based on their knowledge and experience.

There are numerous opportunities for APNs to serve on federal, corporate, and health-related advisory boards, which are crucial to integrating APNs into policymaking. Although the opportunities to serve directly in this capacity are limited to a few, it is possible to influence a board's policy recommendations. This can be done by meeting with the agency staff, seeking invitations to testify before advisory boards, and meeting with board members. Often, APNs are appointed because they have strong working relationships with people who happen to be on boards and are familiar with the APN as a compelling knowledge source who is effective in groups. A definite set of behaviors is required to serve on national advisory or corporate

boards and a high degree of mastery is necessary to be reappointed or invited back (Fig. 22-7).

Barriers to Political Competence

Using Force Versus Power

Power accomplishes with ease what force, even with extreme effort, cannot accomplish. On the interpersonal front, it is important for APNs to avoid using force in advancing their positions in the policy arena. Doing so can diminish one's power. This is commonly done by nurses who participate in interdisciplinary policy or problem-solving meetings. The twin approaches of being judgmental and parochial can quickly compromise effectiveness. Judgmentalism, criticizing other people or disciplines, distracts from effective problem solving and, in the process, can reflect poorly on the person who judges, greatly diminishing the power to influence. Diminishing others or the work they do can provoke defensiveness and consequently limit the capacity to influence others meaningfully. Nursing parochialism occurs when nurses present a narrow restricted scope or outlook in which only nursing and nursing's interests are offered as solutions. These postures in the policy arena (or any other setting) do not build wide-based support or strong relationships. The value of APNs and their potential impact on cost, quality, and access, if fully unleashed, is an enormously powerful solution to some of today's most significant health care problems. Power is characterized by humility and truth, which needs no defense or rhetoric; it is self-evident. Force is divisive and exploits people for individual or personal gain (Hawkins, 2002).

Behavior at Meetings

We all have seen nurses and other leaders who become shrill and consistently present positions that reflect pure self-interest in public arenas, whereby each person in the room knows what she or he will say before they speak.

This is a posture of parochialism that APNs must work hard to avoid. To be effective in interdisciplinary and influential arenas, and to pursue larger roles, APNs must build strong relationships built on trust and respect. In policy-related meetings, APNs must demonstrate that nurses can solve problems in the health care system, not just for nurses' sake. APNs will be most effective when they bring a broader perspective to all of health care, not just nursing.

 EXEMPLAR 22-2   **From Registered Nurse Diploma to Elected Official: What Pulled Gale Adcock into Public Office**

Gale Adcock

It has been said, "If you are not at the table, then you are on the menu."

Gale Adcock graduated from nursing school with her nursing diploma. How did this small town Virginia girl, a first-generation college graduate raised in an apolitical family, evolve into a state and nationally recognized APN thought leader, director of a primary care practice for a global corporation, and an elected official? In 1980, the North Carolina Nursing Practice Act was preparing to sunset (expire at a predetermined date). A statewide call to action was made for nurses to partner with a member of the General Assembly, acting as their conduit of information and influence as the bill made its way (successfully) through the General Assembly. Gale jumped with both feet into this effort and was immediately very interested in the process. She sought out a position on the North Carolina Nurses Association (NCNA) Board of Directors and was its vice president by 1983, its president-elect in 1987, and its president in 1989. She accepted opportunities to chair the North Carolina Center for Nursing, the NCNA Council of Nurse Practitioners, the American College of Nurse Practitioners Public Policy Committee, and a 7-year term on the North Carolina Board of Nursing. She was part of the successful lobbying effort for direct third-party reimbursement to North Carolina APNs in 1993.

In the mid-1990s, Gale was the sole nurse appointed by the governor to the North Carolina Health Planning Commission and, as a spin-off the following year, she co-chaired the Preventive Services Task Force. In 2009, she was again the sole nurse appointee (the governor's only appointment, representing business, no less) to the Blue Ribbon Task Force on the State Health Plan for Teachers and State Employees. She was elbow to elbow with the state's business leaders, insurers, and legislators who made up most of the task force members.

Over the last decade, Gale was urged by many in her community to run for political office. Her road map included getting involved with her local party, attending precinct meetings and political fundraisers, working on high-profile state and national campaigns, serving as a board member of her local political party women's club, and completing a fellowship in the North Carolina Institute of Political Leadership, a candidate training program. In 2007, when her local town council seat was vacated by a two-term incumbent, she was recruited to run by a group of determined supporters.

Gale won her first race against two opponents, with 55% of the vote. In 2011, she ran for reelection to the Cary Town Council against a single opponent and won handily, with 66% of the vote. Immediately after being sworn in for her second 4-year term, she was unanimously elected as the town's Mayor Pro-Tem (she stands in for the mayor when the mayor is unavailable).

Municipal officials have immediate and sustained influence on the overall quality of life of the 140,000 citizens in Cary, North Carolina. "Local government is where the rubber really meets the road," declared Adcock. "We may not get the headlines that state and national officials do, but people in Cary know who to call when they don't want the traffic impacts of a shopping center in their neighborhood, when they want a safe way to ride their bikes to work, when they want their kids to have a park within walking distance of their home and school, and when they want their water quality protected. We are their first stop—they recognize us and know us by name much more often than their state House or Senate member."

Gale firmly believes that every level of elected office offers opportunities to make decisions that affect health care and that raise the profile of APNs as informed and decisive policymakers with a broad range of interests. No longer can or should APNs be content to see themselves as players on only one field.

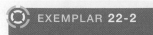 **EXEMPLAR 22-2**   From Registered Nurse Diploma to Elected Official: What Pulled Gale Adcock into Public Office—*cont'd*

From Gale's Playbook: Fail-Safe behaviors

After more than 30 years working up and down the health policy pipeline, from diploma nurse to elected official, Gale has learned to serve with the following skill sets:

A Content Expert

Get to know the APN statutes and rules in your state. Be unshakable in your understanding of APN authority to practice. Question every incidence of misinterpretation of APN authority to practice, regardless of intention. It is astonishing how often others are misinformed about APN practice. On at least this issue, strive always to be the expert in the room.

A Student of Process

Know how things actually get done in your state legislature—the committee structure, unwritten norms, and other operational nuances. Learn the faces and names of those with influential power. Become familiar with parliamentary procedure and read the local political pundits.

A Trusted Partner

There is no place for partisanship at any table you join. Do not make assumptions about motivation. Give everyone the benefit of the doubt and form partnerships with everyone possible. Party affiliation does not tell you about what an individual actually believes or how she or he will operate.

A Well-Rounded Advocate

Seek out and use new venues to share the APN message of wellness, primary prevention, and unencumbered access to health care. Consider running for a local elected office, such as the following: school board (making decisions about cafeteria meals, how much gym time is included in the school day, health curriculum, presence of vending machines); county commission (funding for the local health department, substance abuse programs, mental health services, schools); town or city council (greenways, bike lanes, parks, walkable communities, air and water quality.

Organizational Skills

There are numerous ways for APN organizations to exert influence continuously on the policymaking process. Forming coalitions with other APNs and other nursing, health care, and consumer groups strengthens political effectiveness. Although there is a rich diversity of nursing organizations (more than 120 nationally and scores of state and regional organizations), none has a membership base that is more than a fraction of the more than 3 million nurses. Forming coalitions and strategic plans around policy reforms is necessary to maximize impact. APN organizational leaders can play a role in defining health policy problems and designing possible solutions. The APN movement has advanced tremendously, but a greater degree of policy solidarity would significantly strengthen the political effectiveness of APN groups. APNs are characteristically pioneers, blazing new trails that have pushed the role and boundaries of nursing forward. As the total number of APNs and those with DNPs continue to grow exponentially, their political influence will also grow.

Longest (2010) has asserted that organizations that form policy communities (build coalitions) can exert enormous influence on the policy process. Policy communities are comprised of loosely structured, heterogeneous networks defined by the level of investment that each group has around the issue. There is an enormous difference between sharing an investment in health policy issues and reaching concordance on policy positions. Reaching concordance in the development of policy positions is what adds great power to policy communities and is the organizational challenge for APN groups. Table 22-3 depicts the policy process and the requisite political competency skills that can be deployed throughout the process.

Moving Advanced Practice Nurses Forward in Health Policy

Communicating Findings

Findings on APN research must be published in journals outside of nursing to reach a broader policymaking and public audience. Key policymakers and the public must be made more aware of the contributions that APNs make in reducing health care costs and improving access and quality of care. Achieving broader recognition, reducing APN invisibility, and removing barriers to APN practice will be contingent on APNs communicating methodologically sound APN research, which produces results that are generalizable to the larger delivery system. Moreover, APNs must expand publications to journals outside of nursing, which have a much broader readership. Below is an abstract exemplar of APNs publishing in the highly

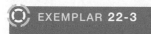

TABLE 22-3   Influencing Health Policy Throughout the Process

Policy Area	Skill	Examples
Formulation	Agenda setting	Defining and documenting problems Develop and evaluate solutions Influencing political circumstances by lobbying or court decisions Educating the public (o.g., writing op ods)
	Legislation development	Participating in drafting legislation Testifying at hearings Activating the grassroots Forming coalitions
Implementation	Rule making	Making formal comments about draft rules Providing input to rulemaking advisory bodies
	Policy operation	Interact with policy implementers
Modification	Unintended consequences	Creating a case for modification through evaluation and evidence Educating the public about need for change

Adapted from Longest, B. (2010). *Health policymaking in the United States.* (5th ed.). Chicago: Health Administration Press.

EXEMPLAR 22-3   Organizational Political Competency—The Power of Coalitions: American College of Nurse Midwives and Medicare Equity

Debbie Jessup

When the PPACA became law in March 2010, one of its provisions deleted a long-standing regulation that limited Medicare reimbursement of CNMs to 65% of what a physician would be paid for the same service. For the American College of Nurse Midwives (ACNM), this marked the culmination of a 19-year effort to attain equitable Medicare reimbursement for its members. The story of ACNM's effort illustrates the growth of a small and predominantly female professional association into a politically competent organization.

CNMs were first recognized as providers under Medicare when the Omnibus Budget Reconciliation Act (OBRA) of 1987 included a provision that established direct Medicare payments for CNM services, limited to the maternity cycle, at 65% of prevailing charges for the same service when performed by a physician. Initially, 65% of the physician fee was deemed adequate, especially given the small numbers of Medicare patients who were eligible for maternity benefits. However, passage of OBRA 1989 lowered CNM reimbursement using the resource-based relative value scale (RBRVS). When the Physician Payment Review Commission elected to extend the 65% nonphysician reimbursement levels to this new scale, ACNM resolved to find a legislative solution to the problem.

The first legislation to address Medicare reimbursement for CNMs was introduced in 1991, which included a 97% reimbursement rate for CNMs, NP, and CNSs.

CNMs worked with other APN groups to promote this legislation, but those in the other APN roles were pushing APNs to earn a Master of Science in Nursing (MSN) degree as the entry requirement for advanced practice nursing. This was a problem for ACNM, which still supported the certificate route to midwifery, and they fully supported non-nurses entering midwifery. Therefore, when APNs pushed to increase the rate to 85% reimbursement, ACNM decided to withdraw from the coalition and pursue solo legislation. It proved to be a fateful decision. The Primary Care Health Practitioner Act of 1995 and 1997 did not include CNMs and, when the bill passed as part of the 1997 Balanced Budget Act, NPs and CNSs received 85% reimbursement under Medicare and nurse-midwives remained at 65%.

The first solo CNM Medicare bill was introduced in 1998. ACNM was certifying a non nurse pathway to midwifery, so the Certified Nurse Midwife Medicare Services Act set reimbursement at 95% for CNMs and certified midwives (CMs) who are not nurses (currently, there are approximately 70 certified midwives in the United States who are not nurses). Throughout all this, the ACNM worked tirelessly to find champions and cosponsors. Finally, in 2000, both chambers had ACNM companion bills. Medicare equity for CNMs seemed elusive because everything changed politically on September 11th, when terrorist-hijacked planes bombed the Pentagon and brought down the Twin Towers in New York. A month, later the United States went to war, and all subsequent political efforts focused on

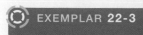 EXEMPLAR 22-3   Organizational Political Competency—The Power of Coalitions:
                                             American College of Nurse Midwives and Medicare Equity—*cont'd*

recovery from the attacks, defense efforts, and homeland security. The congressional champions receded and Congress' session ended in 2003, with no action taken on midwife reimbursement.

The ACNM was developing and maturing in its understanding of the political process. It replicated the Harvard study that developed the RBRVS system and found that the only difference between CNMs, CMs, and physicians was a slight variation in malpractice costs. The ACNM hired an actuarial firm to conduct a cost analysis, began efforts to have the Congressional Budget Office (CBO) take up the bill for scoring, and hired a legislative consultant to begin efforts to attach the bill to a larger vehicle. Also, the ACNM formed a political action committee (PAC), hired a marketing firm, and held intensive lobbying days with their members. Next, they reintroduced a simplified midwife bill and hired a CNM fellow to work full-time for 6 months on promoting bipartisan cosponsors. However, despite a record number of cosponsors for the House bill, they were unable to secure a Senate companion bill. The Medicare Modernization Act was signed into law in 2003 without the CNM Medicare reimbursement provision.

Again, ACNM decided to change how it conducted its legislative efforts and hired an established lobbyist in Washington, DC, to make passage of the Medicare bill its number one priority. The new message was to drop the confusing 95% concept and instead advocate for equal pay for equal work. Thus, the Improving Access to Nurse-Midwife Care Act of 2005 was introduced in both chambers, with 100% reimbursement for CNMs and CMs. Although the American College of Obstetricians and Gynecologists (ACOG) spoke out publicly for the first time against the legislation, 23 national nursing organizations lent their support to the midwife bill. At

their annual meeting in Washington, DC, over 500 midwives visited 300 members of Congress asking them to support Medicare equity for midwives. Once again the political climate changed, however, when Hurricane Katrina ravaged the city of New Orleans in September 2005. All major legislative efforts focused on Gulf Coast support and restoration.

ACNM's Government Affairs Committee mobilized an unprecedented advocacy effort to promote Medicare equity for CNMs in the Children's Health and Medicare Protection Act of 2007, which passed the House with the midwife reimbursement piece included, but the Senate was not as successful in moving the legislation. Later, when the Senate passed its Medicare vehicle, they pushed to reduce the midwife provision to 85%. Midwives rejected this proposal and the final Medicare update passed as a stripped down bill that did not include the midwife provision.

This was a huge blow to midwives, who had thought they were finally at the finish line, but the 2008 election opened the window of opportunity that midwives had been waiting for—a president with an ambitious health reform agenda. The entire nursing community formed a coalition to develop an agenda for health reform that including midwife equity. ACOG, in collaboration with ACNM to promote a women's health home, also spoke out in support of midwife reimbursement.

The House and Senate both introduced bills that contained 100% equity for CNMs, although a last minute compromise excluded CMs. The rest of the story is history. PPACA passed the House in October 2009, was amended and passed the Senate in December 2009, and the final bill passed in the House on March 21, 2010. After 19 years, midwives had finally achieved Medicare equity.

---

regarded journal, *Health Affairs.* This journal reaches a wide and highly influential audience. It is read by and used as a reliable knowledge source by health policymakers.

Advanced Practice Nurse Policy Research Agenda

If APNs unite through organizations committed to policy solidarity, a more robust APN policy research agenda could be realized. This could build on the NAQC to create a more comprehensive and strategic APN research and policy agenda. There are a number of policy

initiatives that would strengthen patient care quality, enhance access, and add to a more robust data collection system, which could positively impact health care delivery overall. Table 22-4 shows policy initiatives that APN groups could undertake.

Conclusion

The health care policy environment is rapidly changing and comprehensive health care reform will be implemented over the next decade, and beyond. APNs must play a larger role in shaping how health care gets delivered

TABLE 22-4 Advanced Practice Nurse Research Policy Agenda

Area of Inquiry	Issues to Be Addressed
How APNs create value for payers to improve the quality of health care	• Are APNs a competitive advantage in the health care marketplace? • Does APN practice demonstrate cost-effectiveness, reduction of errors, and misuse or overuse of services? • What is the added value an APN brings to an organization and how can measures be developed and tracked to make this contribution visible? • How is APN practice most economically efficient and effective (specify sectors [acute care, palliative care] or content areas [obesity, cardiac disease] in which APNs are most effective)? • Explore the most effective health care team composition for acute care, primary care, and palliative care. • Explore how to build an evidence base on interdisciplinary approaches or "collaboratories" to function as incubators and disseminators of team-delivered care. • Explore best practice on patient engagement. • Explore strategies for the cost savings of APN practice to be passed onto consumers, Medicare, ACOs, health care homes, and other payers. • Identify the impact of APNs on vulnerable segments of the population, including the uninsured, older adults, children, and those living in rural areas, and create a safety net to close the health care disparities gap. • What is the role of APNs in care transition? • How should the population be segmented for APN care transition services?
Best practices for modernizing all 50 state nurse practice acts to align with licensure, accreditation, certification, and education (LACE) standards	• Identify how access and quality of care are affected once a state has adopted the National Council of State Boards of Nursing (NCSBN) regulatory vision for APN practice, which eliminates regulatory barriers to APN practice. • Is there a road map for states to apply universally to modernize the state practice acts regardless of political context? • Are there federal or other levers that could accelerate modernization of U.S. nurse practice acts? • How might APNs shape or be included in state health exchanges?
Creation of stronger methods to study the impact of APN interventions to align with principles of health services research	• Identify the most reliable, valid, and feasible approach(es) to measure quality of care delivered by APNs. • Identify the outcomes of APN interventions targeted at changing patients' behavior or lifestyle. Do APNs uniquely or qualitatively use effective strategies to prevent disease?
Dismantling exclusion and invisibility of APNs in the larger delivery system	• Discover levers to eliminate all APN "incident-to" billing via Medicare. • Include political competency evaluation in APN programs on the same par as physical assessment skills to ensure that the APN workforce is politically astute. • Create an action plan for highly qualified APNs to serve on policymaking boards, including retail health, health insurance, delivery system, and key federal and state health advisory boards. • Encourage all U.S. APNs to be identifiable and included in some quality measurement process in their practices (e.g., Healthcare Effectiveness Data and Information Set [HEDIS]). • Develop a plan to include APNs in all health care quality initiatives, including CMS demonstrations on pay for performance, such as ACO and health care homes, the development of National Quality Forum quality measures (NQF, 2011), and private sector initiatives. • Create a prominent award for APNs who serve as exemplars in health care quality. The alliance could award organizations or individual nurses who have had a major impact on quality improvement.

because they have a social covenant with the public to serve as patient advocates in the broadest sense. Policymakers are looking for solutions to escalating costs and continued patient safety problems. To be able to do this, APNs must resist the pull of the familiar and overcome invisibility and passivity. Political competency needs to be part of every APN's professional role. Membership in professional organizations that advance issues critical to APN practice and the health of the United States is vital to the continued viability of APNs. The first step to being involved in policy formulation is to be knowledgeable about the policy process and the current and emerging

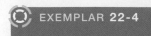

EXEMPLAR 22-4   **Advanced Practice Nurses Publish in Widely Read and Influential Journals Outside of Nursing**

Joanne M. Pohl; Charlene Hanson; Jamesetta A. Newland; Linda Cronenwett

Unleashing Nurse Practitioners' Potential to Deliver Primary Care and Lead Teams
Abstract

Highly skilled primary care is a hallmark of high-performing health care systems. We examine nurse practitioners' role in delivering primary care and the effects of current restrictions on their ability to practice. By resolving differences between states' individual scope of practice regulations, we can fully benefit from the skills of advanced-practice nurses in all 50 states. We recommend substantive changes in the way health care professionals in all disciplines are trained, and in their roles, so that patients can receive appropriate and cost-effective care from skilled and fully functional health care teams (Pohl, Hanson, Newland, et al., 2010).

EXEMPLAR 22-5   **Nurse-Led Research and the Patient Protection and Affordable Care Act**

Mary D. Naylor, RN, PhD, observed in clinical practice that frail older people with chronic conditions must navigate a care system that is ill-equipped to meet their needs, resulting in a devastating human and economic toll. One in five Medicare patients gets readmitted to the hospital within 1 month. As a nurse-researcher, she set out to find promising solutions to address the care needs of chronically ill people. As a result of this clinical experience, she built on the earlier work of Brooten and colleagues (1988) and further developed the transition care model, an innovative approach to the care of high-risk, chronically ill older adults and their family caregivers. Her research is highly relevant to the policy arena because it developed knowledge around an intractable, expensive problem—the frail older adult's transitions after hospital discharge. Her approach used rigorous methods in interdisciplinary science and shines a spotlight on the compelling and unique contribution of nurses working with the health care team to improve the outcomes of vulnerable, chronically ill adults who are making the difficult transition from hospital to home. Her findings have broad relevance to all stakeholders in health care policy who are interested in improving patient safety, lowering cost, and addressing the unacceptably high hospital readmission rate.

Building on the earlier work of Brooten, Youngblut, and associates (1988, 2001, 2002), Dr. Naylor demonstrated the effectiveness of making a nurse accountable as a transitional care nurse, who conducts a comprehensive assessment of patient and family caregiver needs, coordinates the patient's discharge plan with the family and hospital provider team, implements the plan in the patient's home, assists the patient with management of her or his care needs, and facilitates communication and the transition to community providers and services. This nurse is available to the patient 7 days a week through home visits and telephone access for 1 to 3 months of home follow-up. Naylor's research team has partnered with a major insurance organization and health care plan to translate this model into clinical practice and promote its widespread adoption; then the model has been adopted by the University of Pennsylvania Health System, with local insurers providing transition care reimbursement for their members served.

Under the PPACA (HHS, 2011a), a variety of transitional care programs, born directly from Dr. Naylor's research, have been established to improve and help hospitalized patients with complex chronic conditions, who are often the most vulnerable patients, transfer in a safe and timely manner from one level of care to another or from one type of care setting to another. APNs are critical caregivers in this arena. The research has identified specific interventions that prevent avoidable hospital readmissions, a core priority under health care reform. The Community-Based Care Transitions Program is a provision in the PPACA that authorizes $500 million of funding, from 2011 to 2015, to health care systems that provide care transition interventions to high-risk Medicare beneficiaries. There are several other vehicles in the PPACA that support care transitions, such as ACOs and health care homes, which must address how they intend to keep frail older adults healthy, whether in their homes or across care settings (Naylor, Aiken, Kurtzman, et al., 2011). CMS has estimated that if every high-risk Medicare patient were provided with transition care, it could save $12 billion annually (CMS, 2013). Based on these findings, Dr. Naylor and her colleagues have developed

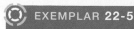 **EXEMPLAR 22-5**   **Nurse-Led Research and the Patient Protection and Affordable Care Act—*cont'd***

and deepened the knowledge describing the crucial roles that nurses and APNs will play in these emerging bundled payment arrangements. The level of rigor, its interdisciplinary approach, and its highly relevant policy problem converge to create a policy imperative to move

care transition services to the mainstream. Dr. Naylor and her coworkers have embodied policy and political competence through advancing the nursing profession in a very public way so that the research findings could shape health reform.

TABLE 22-5   **Selected Health Policy Experiences for Advanced Practice Nurses**

Policy Experience, Internship, Fellowship Opportunity	Contact
Academy Health	www.Academyhealth.org
Nurse in Washington Internship	www.nursing-alliance.org
Robert Wood Johnson Executive Nurse Fellowship	www.enfp-info.org
Robert Wood Johnson Health Policy Fellowship	http://www.healthpolicyfellows.org/home.php
White House Fellows Program	www.whitehouse.gov/fellows
AARP–American Academy of Nursing Joint Fellowship	www.aannet.org

For an expanded list of opportunities see Mason, D., Leavitt, J. & Chafee, M. (2012) Policy and politics in nursing and health care, (6th ed.). St. Louis, Missouri: Elsevier-Saunders. Pp 741-9.

issues relevant to APNs. To be involved, APNs need to understand the details related to funding issues, measures of quality, how they reflect APN practice, and specific programs designed to improve access (Table 22-5). The important lesson for APNs and policy is that a single

person, with deep understanding of an issue, along with highly developed political skills, can make a difference. An individual backed by organizational strength, particularly by coalitions of organizations, can make an even more significant difference.

References

American Academy of Nurse Practitioners. (2010). 2009-2010 AANP national sample survey: An overview. (http://www.aanp.org/images/documents/research/2009-10_Overview_Compensation.pdf).

American Association of Colleges of Nursing. (2006). The essentials of doctoral education for advanced nursing practice (http://www.aacn.nche.edu/publications/position/DNPEssentials.pdf).

American Association of Colleges of Nursing. (2011). Preparing for the Medicare graduate nursing education program (http://www.aacn.nche.edu/membership/members-only/GNEUpdate.pdf).

Bodenheimer, T. & Grumbach, K. (2012). *Understanding health policy: A clinical approach* (6th ed.). New York: McGraw-Hill.

Brooten, D., Brown, L., Munro, B., York, R., Cohen S., Roncoli, M., et al. (1988). Early discharge and specialist transitional care. *Image: The Journal of Nursing Scholarship, 20*, 64–68.

Brooten, D., Youngblut, J. M., Brown, L., Finkler, S. A., Neff, D. F., & Madigan, E. (2001). A randomized trial of nurse specialist home care for women with high risk pregnancies: Outcomes and costs. *American Journal of Managed Care, 7*, 793–803.

Bureau of Labor Statistics, Department of Labor. (2012). *Occupational handbook, 2010-2011 edition: Registered nurses.* Washington, DC: Department of Labor.

Centers for Medicare & Medicaid Services (CMS). (2011a). Medicare program; Medicare shared savings program; accountable

care organizations final rule (https://www.federalregister.gov/articles/2011/11/02/2011-27461/medicare-program-medicare-shared-savings-program-accountable-care-organizations).

Centers for Medicare & Medicaid Services (CMS). (2011b). National health expenditure projection 2010-2020 (https://www.cms.gov/NationalHealthExpendData/downloads/proj2010.pdf).

Centers for Medicare & Medicaid Services (CMS). (2013). Innovation Center. Community-based care transition program. (http://innovation.cms.gov/initiatives/CCTP/).

Congressional Research Service. (2011). Duration of continuing resoultions in recent years (http://assets.opencrs.com/rpts/RL32614_20110322.pdf).

Cross, M. (2011). Retail clinics expand in numbers, services. *Managed Care (Langhorne, Pa), 20*, 37–38.

Deloitte Center for Health Solutions. (2009). Health care retail clinics continue gradual expansion through 2012 (http://www.deloitte.com/view/en_US/us/Industries/US-federal-government/center-for-health-solutions/6fa41d3b16de4210VgnVCM10).

DeNavas-Walt, C., Proctor, B., & Smith, J. (2011). *Income, poverty, and health insurance coverage in the United States, 2010 (Current Population Reports, P60-239).* Washington, DC: U.S. Census Bureau.

Docteur, E. & Berenson, R. (2009). How does the quality of U.S. health care compare internationally? Timely analysis of immediate policy issues (http://www.urban.org/UploadedPDF/411947_ushealth care_quality.pdf).

Eibner, C., Hussey, P., Ridgely, M., & McGlynn, E. (2009). Controlling health care spending in Massachusetts: An analysis of options (www.rand.org/pubs/technical_reports/TR733.html).

Families USA. (2007). A pound of flesh: Hospital billing, debt collections, patients rights. (http://www.familiesusa.org/assets/pdfs/medical-debt.pdf).

Feldstein, P. (2006). *The politics of health legislation: An economic perspective* (3rd ed.). Chicago: Health Administration Press.

Gill, C. & Gill, G. (2005). Nightingale in Scutari: Her legend re-examined. *Clinical Infectious Diseases, 40*, 1799–1805.

Hamilton, M. S., Brooten, D., & Youngblut, J. M. (2002). High-risk pregnancy: Postpartum rehospitalization. *Journal of Perinatology, 22*, 566–571.

Hamric, A. (2009). Ethical decision-making. In Hamric, A. B., Spross, J. A., & Hanson, C. M. (Eds.). *Advanced practice nursing. An integrative approach* (pp.315–345; 4th ed.). St. Louis: Saunders.

Hawkins, D. (2002). *Power vs. force: The hidden determinants of human behavior*. Alexandria NSW, Australia: Hay House.

Holahan, J., & Chen, V. (2011). Changes in health insurance coverage in the great recession, 2007-2010 (http://www.kff.org/uninsured/upload/8264.pdf).

Institute of Medicine. (1999). *To err is human: Building a safer health system*. Washington, DC: National Academies Press.

Institute of Medicine. (2001). *Crossing the quality chasm: A new health system for the 21st century*. Washington, DC: National Academies Press.

Institute of Medicine (IOM). (2011). *The future of nursing: Leading change, advancing health*. Washington, DC: National Academies Press.

Jameton, A. (1984). *Nursing practice: The ethical issues*. Englewood Cliffs, NJ: Prentice Hall.

Kaiser Family Foundation (KFF). (2011). Employer health benefits: 2011 summary of findings (http://ehbs.kff.org).

Kennedy, D. M., Caselli, R. J., & Berry, L. L. (2011). A roadmap for improving health care service quality. *Journal of Health Care Management/American College of Health Care Executives, 56*, 385–400.

Kingdon, J. (1995). *Agendas, alternatives, and public policies* (2nd ed.). New York: Harper Collins College.

Longest, B. (2010). *Health policymaking in the United States* (5th ed.). Chicago: Health Administration Press.

MacKinney, C., Xu, L., & Mueller, K. (2011). *Medicare beneficiary access to primary care physicians—better in rural, but still worrisome*. Iowa City, IA: RUPRI Center for Health Policy Analysis.

McDonald, L. (2006). Florence Nightingale and public health policy: Theory, activism and public administration (http://www.uoguelph.ca/~cwfn/nursing/theory.html).

National Quality Forum (NQF). (2011). NQF releases serious reportable events (www.qualityforum.org/News_And_Resources/Press_Releases/2011/NQF_Releases_Updated_Serious_Reportable_Events.aspx).

Naylor, M., Aiken, L., Kurtzman, E., Olds, D. & Hirschman, K. (2011). The care span: The importance of transitional care in achieving health reform. *Health Affairs, 30*, 4746–4754.

Non-Profit Action. (2012). A resource for non-profit organizations to engage in advocacy (http://www.npaction.org/article/archive/225).

Nurse Practitioners of Oregon. (2012). NP parity action center (http://www.nursepractitionersoforegon.org/displaycommon.cfm?an=1&subarticlenbr=94).

Nursing Alliance for Quality Care. (2010). Strategic policy and advocacy roadmap (http://www.gwumc.edu/healthsci/departments/nursing/naqc/documents/Roadmap.pdf).

Pohl, J. M., Hanson, C., Newland, J. A., & Cronenwett, L. (2010). Analysis & commentary. Unleashing nurse practitioners' potential to deliver primary care and lead teams. *Health Affairs (Millwood), 29*, 900–905.

Regulations.gov. (2012). Fact sheet: Public comments make a difference (http://www.regulations.gov/docs/FactSheet_Public_Comments_Make_a_Difference.pdf).

Schleiter, K. E. (2010). Retail medical clinics: Increasing access to low cost medical care amongst a developing legal environment. *Annals of Health Law, 19*, 527–575.

Schoen, C., Collins, S. R., Kriss, J. L., & Doty, M. M. (2008), How many are underinsured? Trends among U.S. adults, 2003 and 2007 (http://www.commonwealthfund.org/Publications/In-the-Literature/2008/Jun/How-Many-Are-Underinsured–Trends-Among-U-S–Adults–2003-and-2007.aspx).

Scott, M. (2010). Establishing retail clinics among community health centers: Notes from the field (http://www.chcf.org/publications/2010/09/establishing-retail-clinics-among-community-health-centers-notes-from-the-field).

Singer, P. l. (2008). Members offered many bills, but passed few (http://www.rollcall.com/issues/54_61/-30466-1.html).

Social Security and Medicare Boards of Trustees. (2011). Status of the Social Security and Medicare programs (http://www.ssa.gov/OACT/TRSUM).

Taylor, S. (2011). Keys to the supreme court's health law review (http://www.kaiserhealthnews.org/Stories/2011/November/14/stuart-taylor-supreme-court-health-law-hearing-analysis.aspx).

U.S. Department of Health and Human Services (HHS). (2011a). Patient Protection and Affordable Care Act (PPACA). (http://www.healthcare.gov/law/full/index.html).

U.S. Department of Health and Human Services (HHS). (2011b). Medicare program; independence at home demonstration program (https://www.federalregister.gov/articles/2011/12/21/2011-32568/medicare-program-independence-at-home-demonstration-program).

Wakefield, M. K. (2008). Government response: Legislation. In Milstead, J. (Ed.), *Health policy and politics: A nurse's guide*. (pp. 65–88; 3rd ed.). Sudbury, MA: Jones & Bartlett.

Weinick, R. M., Burns, R. M., & Mehrotra, A. (2010). Many emergency department visits could be managed at urgent care centers and retail clinics. *Health Affairs, 29*, 1630–1636.

Wilson, A. R., Zhou, X. T., Shi, W., Rodin, H., Bargman, E. P., Garrett, N. A., et al. (2010). Retail clinic versus office setting: Do patients choose appropriate providers? *American Journal of Managed Care, 16*, 753–759.

Wilson, W. (1913). *Congressional government*. Boston: Houghton Mifflin [originally published in 1885].

Integrative Review of Outcomes and Performance Improvement Research on Advanced Practice Nursing

Ruth Kleinpell • Anne W. Alexandrov

CHAPTER CONTENTS

A number of factors have led to the current focus on outcomes of care in health care, including increased emphasis on providing quality care and promoting patient safety, regulatory requirements for health care entities to demonstrate care effectiveness, increased health system accountability and changes in the organization, delivery, and financing of health care. Advanced practice nurses (APNs) are affecting patient and system outcomes in a number of ways, but too often these outcomes are not quantified or attributed to advanced practice nursing. Employers, consumers, insurers, and others are calling for APNs to justify their contribution to health care and to demonstrate the value that they add to the system. The Institute of Medicine (IOM) report on the future of nursing has highlighted the importance of promoting the ability of APNs to practice to the full extent of their education and training and to identify further nurses' contributions to delivering high-quality care (IOM, 2010). Verifying APN contributions requires an assessment of the structures, processes, and outcomes associated with APN performance and the care delivery systems in which they practice.

Assessment of individual APN impact occurs at multiple levels, with supporting evidence collected during annual performance reviews, outcomes measurement activities, process improvement analyses, program evaluations, and small- and large-scale clinical, health systems,

and outcomes research. At the least, individual performance review and outcomes measurement are required of all APNs, regardless of practice setting, population served, or APN role and position responsibilities.

Outcomes evaluation and ongoing performance assessment are essential to the survival and success of advanced practice nursing. The importance of this dimension of advanced practice is highlighted repeatedly in the American Association of Colleges of Nursing (AACN) *The Essentials of Doctoral Education for Advanced Nursing Practice.* Incorporated within each essential competency is a discussion of the need to evaluate the effect of APN action and decision making on care delivery outcome (AACN, 2006). A key rationale supporting the development of the Doctor of Nursing Practice (DNP) degree has included industry demand for APNs capable of gauging baseline clinical outcomes, determining gaps in the use of evidence-based practice (EBP), masterfully leading change that is scientifically sound, and measuring the impact of their interventions.

This chapter focuses on measuring and monitoring the quality of care delivered and the outcomes achieved by APNs. Performance indicators are discussed at two levels—the aggregate level, at which evidence addresses APN role impact and the individual level, with activities directed at the outcomes of a single APN's practice. This chapter defines key terms and describes frameworks for quality and outcomes assessment. APN outcomes research is reviewed extensively and recommendations are made for further study. Strategies for identifying and assessing APN-sensitive outcome indicators are highlighted.

Review of Terms

Numerous interrelated terms are used to define and describe the components of performance appraisal and outcomes assessment. The principal terms used in this chapter are listed alphabetically and defined as follows:

- *Benchmark.* A point of reference for comparison. Benchmarking is the process used to compare an individual's (or organization's) outcomes with those of high performers. It requires an assessment of the processes used by high-performing practitioners or organizations to achieve their outcomes, as well as the strategies and systems used to attain and then sustain performance excellence (Mathaisel, Cathcart, & Comm, 2004). Four phases are involved in the benchmarking process for APNs: (1) the conduct of a comprehensive self-assessment of current processes and outcomes of care, including comparisons of performance across internal departments and documentation of baseline data; (2) the identification of comparable providers whose outcomes are superior to those of the benchmarking APN; (3) an analysis of the differences between the processes used by the high performers and the benchmarking APN, with the establishment of goals for improved performance by the benchmarking practitioner; and (4) the implementation of best practice processes and the monitoring of results over time (DeLise & Leasure, 2001).
- A *performance benchmark* is defined in health care as an ideal practice standard target that has been achieved by some group or organization known for its quality of services. This process-focused benchmark serves as the gold standard against which others are compared. Some evaluators also use this term to denote achievement of an intermediate outcome (e.g., attainment of desired best practice performance).
- *Comparative effectiveness research.* Research evidence generated from studies that compare drugs, medical devices, tests, or ways to deliver health care. It is designed to inform health care decisions by providing evidence on the effectiveness, benefits, and harms of different treatment options (Agency for Healthcare Research and Quality [AHRQ], 2012).
- *Dashboard.* A visual representation of data to enable the review, analysis, and tracking of data trends. The dashboard is like a score card because it allows for the visualization of performance and outcome information (U.S. Agency for International Development, 2010; U.S. Department of Education, 2011).
- *Disease management.* An organized process focusing on the patient's disease as the target of interest, with improvements in outcome seen as a result of attention to the attributes or characteristics of the disease. The intent is similar to *outcomes management,* which implements interventions to achieve a desired effect. The principal difference is the focus, with disease management directed at comprehensive monitoring and management of the patient's underlying condition and outcomes management focused on measurement of the observed effects of treatment (Wojner, 2001).

Quality indicators endorsed and adopted by federal and private health plans commonly target adherence to evidence-based processes that are expected to affect disease management. Program compliance with expected process performance is increasingly tied to pay for performance because of evidence demonstrating improved disease outcomes and cost containment. The medical home concept is tied closely to disease management principles and practice imperatives for the use of standardized evidence-based processes. The primary aim of medical homes is to oversee all health needs from prevention to disease management in one practice setting, thereby ensuring consistency of health strategies, accessibility to knowledgeable practitioners, and provision of seamless health services. Interestingly, reports of outcomes associated with medical homes are limited in the literature, although this model has been widely advocated as a method to improve and prevent disease (Grumbach & Grundy 2010).

- *Effectiveness.* Extent to which interventions or actions taken in clinical settings perform as expected with defined populations (Armenian & Shapiro, 1998). Effectiveness assumes the generalizability of evidence-supported processes, suggesting that these methods may be replicated in clinical practice and will achieve the same results as demonstrated in clinical trials. The principle of effectiveness supports the adoption of standardized health care processes forming the basis for pay for performance core measures, because it assumes that widespread use of evidence-based methods will reduce disease and complication incidence, thus ultimately reducing health care costs. *Program effectiveness* refers to the measurement of the results attained through the systematic adoption of evidence-based structures (e.g., systems such as equipment, manpower) and standardized processes, whereas *intervention effectiveness* refers to the measurement of results in line with implementation of a specific EBP. Ultimately, effectiveness may translate into health care cost savings, but these savings may be remote from the systems and processes implemented.

- *Efficiency.* The effects achieved by some intervention in relation to the effort expended in terms of money, resources, and time. In outcomes assessment, efficiency measures are used to compare two equally effective interventions (Hargreaves, Shumway, Hu, et al., 1998) and, for care providers, often include productivity considerations. In such cases, costs of care, treatment patterns, service volumes, and time required are usually compared (Armenian & Shapiro, 1998).

- *Evidence-based practice.* Integration of research findings (evidence) into clinical decision making and care delivery processes. *Best evidence* for clinical practice is derived from methodologically sound research that is theory-derived, consistent with patient needs and preferences (Ingersoll, 2000), and clinically relevant to the population of interest. The findings of these investigations support and enhance the clinician's clinical expertise; they do not replace it. This is particularly true for decisions concerning individual patients, in whom personal characteristics and circumstances may differ from those of the populations studied. When available, evidence-based information should be used in the selection of process of care measures (e.g., percentage of eligible acute myocardial infarction patients receiving aspirin at time of arrival to hospital). Evidence-based data are also useful in the development of *practice guidelines,* which are used to assist practitioners and patient decisions about appropriate health care for specific clinical care situations (Joanna Briggs Institute, 2012). Practice guidelines are systematically developed recommendations, strategies, or other information to assist health care decision making in specific clinical circumstances (AHRQ, 2010). The shift to pay for performance, based on the systematic implementation of EBP, provides an example of the power of scientifically sound processes and is driving practitioner viability in the health care market.

- *Impact measurement.* An analysis of the difference in a targeted outcome measure and growth of practice systems resulting from use of the outcomes management process (Alexandrov & Brewer, 2010). Impact measurement enables APNs to showcase the effectiveness of programs implemented to improve patient outcomes. Analyzing the impact of an outcomes management process can help identify key aspects of a process that led to changes in an outcome (U.S. Department of Health and Human Services [HSS], Administration for Children and Families, 2010).

- *Metric.* Also described as a measure or indicator, a metric defines parameters for structure, process, or outcome, depending on their level. For example, a metric for rate-based measures would define population numerators and denominators to ensure that each party using the metric measures the same population (validity) in the same way each time (reliability). The National Quality Forum (NQF) has defined criteria that should support all metrics to be submitted for endorsement by their agency, thereby making them eligible for pay for performance adoption by the Centers for Medicare & Medicaid Services (CMS) and other third-party payers. These criteria include the following: (1) the importance of studying the measures and publicly reporting findings; (2) the scientific acceptability of measure properties—that they measure validity and reliability; (3) usability, the extent to which payers, providers, and consumers can understand results and use them for health care decision making; and (4) feasibility, the extent to which the required data are available or could be captured without undue burden (NQF, 2012).

- *Outcome.* The results of an intervention; changes in the recipient of an intervention. Measurement of outcomes will vary according to the intended recipient. For example, recipients may be patients, families, students, other care providers, communities and, in some cases, organizations (if the organization as a whole is the recipient of the intervention). Outcomes may be intended or unintended and reflect positive or untoward results, such as complications. Because of this, measurement plans must be cautiously developed to capture all outcomes (positive or negative) that theoretically align with the planned intervention, including the likelihood of no change in preintervention status (Alexandrov, 2008; Doran, 2011; Wojner, 2001).

Most definitions of outcome have evolved from the original writings of Donabedian (1966, 1980), who defined an outcome as a change in a patient's physiologic health state (i.e., morbidity and mortality). Later authors incorporated psychosocial changes (e.g., patient satisfaction, anxiety), acquisition of health-related knowledge, and health-related behavioral change as additional outcome dimensions (Bloch, 1975). This patient-centered understanding of outcomes is particularly relevant to APNs, whose actions directly or indirectly affect patients and families.

- *Outcome(s) assessment.* An evaluation of the observed results of some action or intervention for recipients of services. Outcome assessments provide the data needed to support or refute the perceived beneficial effect of some clinical decision, care delivery process, or targeted action.

- *Outcome indicators, metrics, or measures.* The results of interventions, including the use of new structures or processes on service recipients. Outcome indicators are derived from systematic determination of all potential results that could occur from a specific intervention or program; these measures should be clearly defined in terms of their measurement properties to ensure validity and reliability, with consideration of their temporal association to the intervention. For example, measure developers must consider whether an outcome should be measured immediately after an intervention, within 24 hours of an intervention, or more remotely, at several months postintervention. Often, surrogate intermediate outcomes that are theoretically in line with a targeted long-term outcome can be appropriately identified for measurement (Wojner, 2001). For example, arterial recannulization with IV tissue plasminogen activator (tPA) in acute ischemic stroke is a surrogate intermediate outcome for disability reduction at 3 months (long-term outcome measure). Today, a variety of well-defined, tested, and endorsed outcome measures are available for use in outcome and disease management programs. Because the development of sound process and outcome measures requires extensive expertise and testing, APNs are encouraged to select NQF-endorsed measures to support many of their projects, because these are thoroughly established. This approach ensures consistency in the methods used to study and improve phenomena of interest.

Outcome measures may be cross-cutting (applicable to any population or care delivery environment) or population-specific. Also, outcomes can be generic (applied to assess general concepts such as health status), or condition-specific, which are used to provide more accurate assessments related to a specific state, such as the impact of congestive heart failure on activity levels. APNs must make their contribution to health care improvement associated with selected outcome measures visible through their leadership of EBP projects and dissemination of their work.

Intermediate outcome indicators are surrogate measures that are theoretically similar and measured proximally to a definitive target outcome (Wojner, 2001). These indicators may alert investigators to the likelihood of meeting a defined outcome target by demonstrating movement toward or away from outcome achievement. Intermediate indicators are most useful when the desired outcome is measured distal to an intervention or is multidimensional, such as outcomes associated with consecutive or cumulative protocols.

Because APNs often influence patient outcomes through indirect means, intermediate outcome indicators may be a useful way for measuring progress toward an overall goal of improving patient care. For example, many APN role responsibilities include the mentoring of other nursing staff or the management of interdisciplinary teams. As a result, changes in team member behavior or staff nurse performance may be an indication of APN effect. However, intermediate outcomes are only valid if they are theoretically in line with the subsequent targeted patient outcome.

- *Outcome(s) management.* Enhancement of outcomes, through development, implementation, and ongoing study of the impact of the interventions, actions, or process changes (Alexandrov, 2008; Wojner, 2001). According to the classic work of Ellwood (1988), a comprehensive outcomes management program does the following: (1) emphasizes the use of standards to select appropriate interventions; (2) measures a broad array of outcomes, including disease-specific, behavioral, functional, and perception of care outcomes; (3) pools outcomes data for groups of like patients in relation to processes of care and patient characteristics; and (4) analyzes and disseminates findings to stakeholders (patients, payers, providers) to inform decision making. The goal is to improve care to aggregate populations.

- *Outcome(s) measurement.* The collection, analysis and reporting of reliable and valid outcome indicators.

- *Outcome(s) research* or *patient-centered outcomes research* (PCOR). The use of the scientific method to measure the result of interventions on targeted patient health outcomes (Alexandrov & Brewer, 2010; Clancy & Collins, 2010). Outcomes research methods target examination of aggregate results in relation to changes in structure and processes. Comparative effectiveness research is the most rigorous form of PCOR, using rigorous randomized clinical trial designs to determine differences in treatment options; these studies provide the basis for fully informed patient decision making.

- *Performance (process) improvement.* Activities designed to increase the quality of services provided. The focus of attention shifts to the actions taken by the provider rather than the outcomes achieved. Although outcomes may be monitored to determine whether the change in process produces a desired effect, primary attention is on the interventions (care delivery processes) delivered. Clearly linked with these actions is outcomes evaluation, which focuses on the impact of care delivery processes and the identification of areas of needed improvement.

Subsumed within performance improvement activities are those associated with quality improvement initiatives, also described by some as *continuous quality improvement* (CQI) or *total quality management* (TQM). Although subtle distinctions are assigned to each of these terms, the focus and the intent are the same—to ensure the delivery of care that is appropriate, safe, competent, and timely and to maximize the potential for favorable patient outcomes. In most cases, the measurement of performance is guided by the use of established indicators of best practice, such as national guidelines for care. These performance indicators may be internally derived or externally developed by expert panels who use existing evidence to specify which indicators are most reasonable and which targets are most desirable for achievement.

- Performance evaluation (assessment). Assessment of individual achievement and the attainment of personal, professional, and organizational goals. Performance assessment activities for APNs include those associated with evaluating and improving day to day interactions with individual patients and health care colleagues and those involving the measurement of APN impact on populations, organizations, and communities. During these self-assessment and peer- or supervisor-initiated reviews, areas for improvement are defined. These performance improvement activities may be directed toward technical skills enhancement, interpersonal style, productivity specifications, professional development, or other individual APN actions linked to improved processes of care or care delivery outcome. In this case, the focus is on the APN's behaviors, with specific goals for improved performance identified for the upcoming quarter or year.

- *Process indicator, measure.* A measure of visible behavior or action that a care provider undertakes to deliver care. Process indicators measure what care providers provide during their interactions with patients and are necessary for demonstrating a cause-and-effect relationship between intervention and outcome. The NQF has halted endorsement of process indicators defined purely by documentation of services provided, such as documentation of provision of smoking cessation counseling. APNs are encouraged to consider more robust measures, such as achievement of smoking cessation (an outcome measure), because documentation does not necessarily guarantee performance of a standardized service.

- *Program evaluation.* Assessment of the quality of structure and processes within a system of care designed to serve a specific patient population. In most cases, program evaluations are designed to provide stakeholders with information about the overall costs in relation to program structure and processes, as well as the outcomes achieved from program services. Because APNs play an integral role in supporting programs, well-articulated APN services and visible APN leadership of program systems may be causally associated with program outcomes.

Well-conducted program evaluation requires significant patience, because the appropriate measurement time point may be years after program creation. A thorough assessment of baseline performance measures must be conducted to ensure the meaningfulness of longitudinal outcome changes.

- *Proxy indicators.* An indirect measure of some anticipated outcome used when a direct measure cannot be obtained or when an accurate indicator has not been identified. An example of a proxy indicator is the collection of self-report data from parents or spouses when patients are unable to respond to questions about perceptions of care or previous health. In the acute care hospital setting, case mix index, patient age, and comorbidity often are used as proxy indicators of risk adjustment for given clinical populations, simply because more direct indicators are not readily accessible. Length of stay has been a commonly measured proxy outcome but there are limitations to its use, because many factors can affect length of stay.

- *Quality of care.* The degree to which health services for individuals and populations increase the likelihood of desired health outcomes and are consistent with professional knowledge (IOM, 2001, p. 232). Quality of care is a dimension of the process and structure of care; it is not an outcome. Outcomes should be assessed in evaluating quality of care to provide an indication of the worthiness of health care structures and services.

- *Risk and severity adjustment.* A process used to standardize groups according to characteristics that might unduly influence an outcome. For example, a past medical history of stroke may alter the ability to achieve a functional outcome in a group of patients when compared with patients with no history of stroke. Severity adjustment is typically disease-specific and based on physiologic findings that are specific to the disease entity (Wojner, 2001). An example of severity adjustment would involve standardizing a patient cohort according to their New York Heart Association Functional Classification in heart failure, which may affect resource use, cost of care, rehospitalization, functional status, and even mortality. The aim of risk and severity adjustment is to level the field among all patients in a sample, so that outcomes associated with interventions may be measured more accurately.

- *Standards.* A profession's authoritative statements that describe the responsibilities of its practitioners (American Nurses Association [ANA], 2010. Standards define the boundaries and essential elements of practice and link practitioners' care, quality, and competence through their delineation of required elements of practice (Dozier, 1998). They also serve as a criterion for the establishment of practice-related rules, conditions, and performance requirements. Standards focus on the processes of care delivery.

- *Structural indicators.* Measures of human, technical, and other resources used in the process of delivering care. These structures focus on the characteristics of the setting, system, or care providers and include such elements as numbers and types of providers, provider qualifications, agency policies and procedures, characteristics of patients served, and payment sources. Examples of structural indicators are the ratio of registered nurses (RNs) or APNs to total nursing staff, nurse-to-patient ratio, nursing care hours per patient day, nursing injury rates, and attrition rates. The assumption underlying these measures is that the provision of adequate structures results in adequate outcomes. Although structural indicators provide important information about the impact of APN practice, they cannot stand alone.

Conceptual Models of Care Delivery Impact

Because APNs usually work with other health professionals, their influence on care delivery outcomes can be

difficult to assess. They may have a direct effect through their interactions with patients and families and/or they may have an indirect effect through their enhancement of the performance of others. Moreover, a number of factors influence APN practice irrespective of their direct or indirect efforts.

Measurement of the full range of APN effect also may be hampered by the organizational or clinician's philosophy underlying the care delivery process. For example, Murphy and Fullerton (2001) have noted that a hallmark of midwifery practice is the "advocacy of non-intervention in the absence of complications" (p. 274). Measuring this advocacy process is difficult and relating it to observed care delivery outcomes is even harder. Similarly, linking noninterventions to outcomes is also a challenge.

Models for Evaluating Outcomes Achieved by Advanced Practice Nurses

Much of the difficulty associated with measuring APN impact can be minimized through the use of a conceptual model to guide assessment and monitoring activities. A number of outcomes measurement and role impact models have been proposed, with several of these evolving from an original quality of care framework proposed by Donabedian (1966, 1980). Donabedian posited that quality is a function of the structural elements of the setting in which care is provided, processes used by care providers, and changes to the recipients of care (i.e., the outcomes). Applying these concepts to APN practice, structural variables relate to the components of a system of care. Process variables pertain to the behavior or actions of the APN or the activities of an APN-directed educational or care delivery program. Interactions among structures and processes result in outcomes. Structure, process, and outcome variables can be studied independently or as a model for overall APN practice. The more complete the model (e.g., the inclusion of all or at least two of the components), the more likely is the successful identification of the APN's impact on care delivery outcome. Two models will be described.

Outcomes Evaluation Model

This Donabedian-guided model, a classic outcomes evaluation model, was designed by Holzemer (1994) and adapted by others (Cohen, Saylor, Holzemer, et al., 2000; Radwin, 2002; Wong, Stewart, & Gilliss, 2000). The value of this model is its program planning structure, which helps identify essential components of any outcomes evaluation plan (Table 23-1). In Holzemer's model, essential outcomes measurement components are defined in a table

TABLE 23-1   Advanced Practice Nurse Outcomes Planning Grid*

	Inputs, Context (Structure)	Processes	Outcomes
Patient	Age Gender Ethnicity Marital status, social supports Educational background Health status (current and past) Previous experience with health system Special needs (e.g., visual, literacy, hearing) Expectations of provider and health system Access to care Insurance coverage	Performance of self-care behaviors Ability Willingness Family involvement in care delivery process Use of alternative or complementary therapies	**Generic** • Physical health • Mental health • Symptom control • Functional status • Perceived well-being • Satisfaction with care • Adherence to treatment regimen • Knowledge of condition, treatment program, and expected outcomes **Specific (dependent on patient condition and need; representative examples)** • Serum glucose level • Birth weight • Reinfarction rate • Transplant rejection rate • Smoking quit rate • Length of stay • Ventilator days • Wound closure, wound healing
APN provider	Educational preparation Specialty focus Years of experience Level of self-esteem Resourcefulness Assertiveness	Expert practice Collaboration Communication patterns Interactions with other care providers & staff Expert coaching Consultation Clinical and professional leadership Ethical decision making Evidence-based practice Case management Care delivery according to practice standards Documentation	Productivity
Setting	Geographic location (rural, urban, mixed) Type of facility (academic health center, acute care, clinic, industry) Diagnostic equipment Organizational culture and philosophy Administrative structure State regulations on advanced practice Policies and procedures Patient mix Type of care delivery model Availability of other services in vicinity Credentialing agency requirements State health department regulations Annual goals Annual budget	Care provider credentialing process Quality improvement process Communication patterns Governance process Care provider documentation process Annual performance review process Provider credentialing process	Length of stay Staff turnover rate Cost of services New program development Revenue generated Community satisfaction Provider satisfaction Staff satisfaction

*Components are not exhaustive of APN-related outcomes planning but serve as a guide for planning activities.
Adapted from Holzemer, W.L. (1994). The impact of nursing care in Latin America and the Caribbean: A focus on outcomes. *Journal of Advanced Nursing, 20,* 5–12.

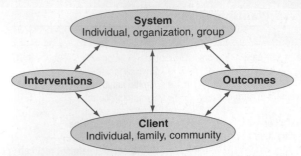

FIG 23-1 Quality health outcomes model (QHOM). This model proposes two-direction relationships among components, with interventions always acting through characteristics of the system and patient. *(From Mitchell, P. H., Ferketich, S., & Jennings, B. M. [1998]. Quality health outcomes model. American Academy of Nursing Expert Panel on Quality Health Care. Image: Journal of Nursing Scholarship, 30, 43–46.)*

consisting of inputs-context (structure), processes, and outcomes, which are identified along the horizontal axis.

For the APN, the patient is any recipient of APN services (e.g., patients, families). The provider is the person (APN) or interdisciplinary group providing the service and potentially could include trained community laypersons who assist with the provision of services. The setting is the local environment in which the services are delivered and includes the resources available to provide care. Table 23-1 contains an application of Holzemer's (1994) model to APN outcomes assessment planning. Included in the table are potential variables that may facilitate assessment of the APN's impact. Additional variables would be selected based on specialty service, population specifics, and additional characteristics of the provider, patient, or environment.

For APNs involved in quality improvement, the quality health outcomes model (QHOM; Fig. 23-1) is particularly relevant (Mitchell, Ferketich, & Jennings, 1998). This model provides a structure for studying complex relationships among patient, provider, and system level variables. As a result, studies guided by the model may better inform our understanding of patient outcomes. It focuses on the individual, organizational, and group dimensions of the health care system that influence and are influenced by care delivery interventions and outcomes and defines the patient as the individual, family, or community receiving the care provider's services.

Mitchell and colleagues' model (1998) extended Holzemer's work (1994) by suggesting that the relationships between model components are reciprocal and that interventions never affect outcomes directly but do so through their interactions with the system and patient. Thus, all assessments of APN impact must include information about the system and individual targeted for the intervention. By proposing a model that allows for multiple inputs at the level of patient, personnel, and system, the authors suggested that the model allows evaluators to analyze the contribution of specific variables to patient outcomes. Because the model incorporates organizational and system level influences, it can guide studies of system level interventions such as program initiatives or reimbursement changes, the results of which can be used to influence health policy.

Nurse Practitioner Role Effectiveness Model

Sidani and Irvine (1999) have proposed a conceptual model designed to facilitate the evaluation of the acute care nurse practitioner (ACNP) role in acute care settings (Fig. 23-2). Developed in Canada, this model was adapted from a nursing role effectiveness model and is also a derivative of Donabedian's framework, with components focusing on structure (patient, ACNP, and organization), process (ACNP role components, role enactment, and role functions) and outcome (goals and expectations of the ACNP role). A concern with this model is the use of the term *goals and expectations* for outcome and the focus on quality of care, which is a dimension of care delivery process rather than outcome. Four processes (mechanisms) within the ACNP direct care component are expected to achieve patient and cost outcomes: (1) providing comprehensive care; (2) ensuring continuity of care; (3) coordinating services; and (4) providing care in a timely way (Sidani & Irvine, 1999). According to this model, the selection of outcome indicators is guided by the role and functions assumed by the ACNP, how the role is enacted, and the ACNP's particular practice model. Like the models before it, the usefulness of this framework for determining APN impact is limited by its virtual absence of testing in clinical settings.

Evidence to Date

A review of the literature suggests that increased attention is being given to the assessment of APN performance. Several recent synthesis reviews highlighted that a number of studies had been conducted that focused on the evaluation of APN roles and on the outcomes of APN care (Hatem, Sandall, Devane, et al., 2009; Newhouse, Weiner, Stanik-Hutt, et al., 2011; Reeves, Hermens, Braspenning, et al., 2009). These focused on all APN roles, including nurse practitioner (NP), clinical nurse specialist (CNS), certified registered nurse anesthetist (CRNA), and certified nurse midwife (CNM) care and included two *Cochrane Database* reviews on the impact of primary care NPs (Reeves et al., 2009) and CNM care (Hatem et al., 2009).

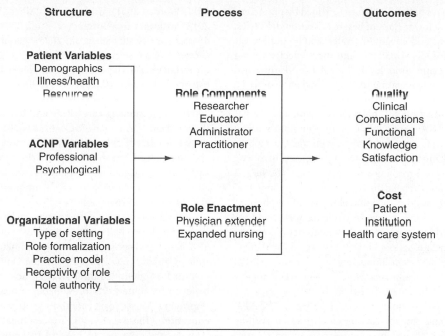

FIG 23-2 Nursing role effectiveness model (NREM) for acute care nurse practitioners. *(From Sidani, S., & Irvine, D. [1999]. A conceptual framework for evaluating the nurse practitioner role in acute care settings.* Journal of Advanced Nursing, *30, 58–66.)*

Before the 1990s, most reports of APN performance were descriptive in nature, with limited use of the experimental or quasi-experimental designs that allow for comparisons across studies. In a meta-analysis of nurse practitioner (NP) and CNM performance in primary care, Brown and Grimes (1995) identified 210 studies pertaining to NPs and CNMs. Of this number, only 53 met study inclusion criteria, which required evidence of NP or CNM intervention, data from patients in the United States or Canada, presence of a control group, measures pertaining to the process of care or clinical outcome, use of an experimental or quasi-experimental design, and data availability to support the calculation of effect size to determine the magnitude of the effect. Outcome indicators varied across studies and cause-and-effect relationships between type of care provider (APN or physician) and outcomes observed were not substantiated.

Outcomes measured for NPs reflected more generic indicators of provider impact (e.g., patient compliance, patient satisfaction, functional status, use of the emergency department [ED]), whereas CNM outcomes were more reflective of specialized practice and included number of cesarean sections, spontaneous vaginal deliveries, incidence of fetal distress, birth weight, and 1-minute Apgar scores. Findings suggested that NPs requested more laboratory testing than physicians and had more favorable

outcomes pertaining to patient satisfaction, health promotion behaviors, time spent with patients, and number of hospitalizations. CNMs used less anesthesia, analgesia, IV fluids, and fetal monitoring and performed fewer episiotomies, forceps deliveries, and amniotomies. Their patients also were more likely to have spontaneous vaginal deliveries, although these were accompanied by an increased number of perineal lacerations. A recent systematic review of 11 studies comparing care provided by midwives found that women who had midwife-led models of care were less likely to experience adverse events, including antenatal hospitalization, regional analgesia episiotomy, and instrumental delivery, and were more likely to experience spontaneous vaginal birth and initiate breast-feeding, among other findings (Hatem et al., 2009).

Most recently, a synthesis review of the research conducted between 1990 and 2008 on the outcomes of APN care focused on comparing APN care with that of other providers (e.g., physicians, teams with APNs); this study identified that care provided by APNs has been demonstrated to affect outcomes positively (Newhouse et al., 2011). Of 107 studies focused on APN care in NP, CNS, CNM, and CRNA roles, substantial evidence demonstrated that APNs provide effective and high-quality care. The results of the review noted that care provided by NPs and CNMs in collaboration with physicians were similar, and in some ways better, than care provided by physicians alone, including lower rates of cesarean section deliveries, less epidural use and episiotomy rates, and higher breast-feeding rates for CNM patients and more effective blood glucose and serum lipid level control for NP-managed patients. The studies relating to CNS care demonstrated a decrease in length of stay and costs of care and high ratings of satisfaction for hospitalized patients. Studies relating to CRNA care, although few in number and observational in design, did suggest equivalent complication rates and mortality when comparing care involving CRNAs with care involving only physicians. The largest number of studies related to NP care; these included 37 studies with 14 randomized control trials and 23 observational studies. A high degree of evidence was found for NP care related to improving patient satisfaction, patient self-assessed health status, blood pressure control, duration of mechanical ventilation, and similar rates of ED visits and hospital readmissions in NP and MD comparison groups (Newhouse et al., 2011).

Studies related to the outcomes of APN care and APN performance and impact can be categorized according to whether they focus on role descriptions or practice characteristics, care delivery processes, process (or performance) improvement activities, program evaluation, disease management activities, outcomes management programs, or outcomes research.

Role Description Studies

Role description studies focus on defining and describing role components and job attributes of APNs. These foundational studies assist in identifying the direct and indirect APN actions that potentially influence care delivery outcome. As such, they provide information about the structure or process components of Donabedian's model (1966, 1980). Without information about the outcomes associated with the characteristics and role behaviors identified in these studies, however, little can be said about their impact on patient care. What these studies provide is evidence to guide the development of theories about which characteristics of APN practice or aspects of the APN role contribute to care delivery outcome. For example, does the APN's expert coaching or collaboration processes contribute to more favorable outcomes when compared with care providers whose use of these processes is less apparent?

Role description studies have explored the role and patient characteristics of APN practices in a variety of specialty-based roles, including psychiatric mental health (Hanrahan et al., 2011), acute pain services (Musclow, Sawhney, & Watt-Watson, 2002), neurovascular care (Alexandrov et al., 2009, 2010; Sung et al.,

2011; Wojner, 2001), urology care (Albers-Heitner et al., 2012), asthma care (Borgmeyer et al., 2008), Alzheimer's disease care (Callahan et al., 2006), geriatric care management (Counsell et al., 2007; Kane et al., 2004), cardiovascular care (Gawlinski et al., 2009; Lowery 2012), osteoporosis care (Greene & Dell, 2010), colorectal care (MacFarlane et al., 2011), oncology care (Cooper, 2009), cystic fibrosis care (Rideout, 2007), eczema care (Schuttelaar, Vermeulen, & Coenraads 2011), and nurse-managed clinics (Pohl et al., 2011), among others. APN activities have been directed primarily toward the oversight and management of patients' needs, followed by administration, teaching, research, program development, and process improvement.

APN roles also have been explored in a grounded theory study by Ball and Cox (2003), who interviewed 39 CNSs, NPs, consultants, and coordinators from Australia, Canada, New Zealand, and the United States. The investigators identified three strategic activities that APNs believe contribute to restoring patients' health, defined as improving patient care, continuity of care, and patient education. These activities, in combination with one another, are expected to prepare patients for transition (to home or independence) to produce high levels of satisfaction with service and enable independence through a clear understanding of illness and health-promoting behaviors.

Role Perception and Acceptance Studies

Studies examining the acceptance of APNs have been conducted since the various roles were introduced and generally involve surveys of staff nurses, administrators, patients, and other care providers. The contribution of role perception studies to the assessment of APN impact lies with their potential for clarifying which contextual (structural) factors influence an APN's ability to perform maximally. If the environment in which an APN practices does not support the APN's delivery of services, or if colleagues view the APN's performance as unsatisfactory or unacceptable, outcomes may be affected. These studies identify potential confounding factors that may need to be controlled when measuring APN effect.

Overall perception of APN performance has been favorable, with most care providers and patients rating the performance and contribution of APNs highly (Allen & Fabri, 2005; Gooden & Jackson, 2004; Johantgen et al., 2012; Mitchell, Dixon, Freeman, et al., 2001; Newhouse et al., 2011). Hardie and Leary (2010) have explored patient perceptions of the value of a CNS in a breast cancer clinic. A questionnaire was given to 50 patients over a 6-week period in May 2007 (pre-CNS survey) and 1 year later (post-CNS survey) to 32 of the original patients. The survey results demonstrated that the CNS improved respondents' experience and satisfaction with the breast cancer service.

APN role receptivity studies also have explored physician acceptance of specialized diagnostic screening and invasive interventions by APNs. In a study of skin cancer screening, from 60% to 70% of family physicians and internists were supportive of NP screening (Oliveria, Altman, Christos, et al., 2002). Similar findings were noted for the acceptance of NP and CNM involvement in medical abortions (Beckman, Harvey, & Satre, 2002).

A phenomenologic design was used to assess families' perceptions of the essence of neonatal NP (NNP) care (Beal & Quinn, 2002). Themes identified included being positive and reassuring, being present, caring, translating information, and making parents feel at ease. In this same study, expert practitioner ability was identified as an expectation that families had of all care providers, regardless of background (medical or nursing) or level of practice (staff nurse or APN). Expectations for the NNP focused on interpersonal style and effectiveness of interactions with families. An important pragmatic implication of this study's findings is the potential difficulty in placing a dollar amount on APN behavior. Because much of health care practice is reimbursement-driven, intangible provider attributes such as interpersonal competence often go unrecognized or are disregarded in provider payment decisions. This is a serious concern because patient and family perceptions of intangible processes often influence overall impressions of care delivery experience and may contribute to more tangible outcomes.

A caution with each of these studies is the potential for respondent bias, with persons unfamiliar with the particular role less likely to respond. In addition, many of the investigations are site-specific, making them more useful for individual performance improvement activities than for global indication of APN acceptance.

Care Delivery Process Studies

Studies evaluating care delivery processes often occur in combination with role definition research. The distinction between these studies and role definition explorations is their attention to what APNs do as part of their roles. Examples include the delivery of preventive services (Becker et al., 2005; Carroll, Robinson, Buselli, et al., 2001; Counsell et al., 2007; Johnson, 2000; Sheahan, 2000; Windorski & Kalb, 2002; Zapka et al., 2000), inclusion of alternative treatments in care delivery processes (Sohn & Cook, 2002), management of ED patients (Lamirel et al., 2011), ordering of antibiotics (Goolsby, 2007), diagnostic tests, and invasive and noninvasive procedures (Cole &

Ramirez, 2000; Sole, Hunkar-Huie, Schiller, et al., 2001; Venning, Durie, Roland, et al., 2000), inclusion of physical activity and physical fitness counseling in primary care practices (Buchholz & Purath, 2007), and the use of collaboration in caring for high-risk patients (Brooten et al., 2005). In these descriptive studies, information is provided about the direct and indirect actions taken by APNs during the delivery of care. No statements can be made about the relationships between any of these processes and care delivery outcomes, however, although some hypotheses can be proposed based on study findings. As a result, these studies are useful as a preliminary step toward outcomes assessment.

In some studies, APN care delivery processes were compared with those of physicians and other care providers. These studies generally examined NP care and have found that NPs are more likely than physicians and other community health providers to spend more time with patients (Seale, Anderson, & Kinnersley, 2005; Venning et al., 2000), nursing staff, and other disciplines (Hoffman, Tasota, Scharfenberg, et al., 2003); informally manage patient care needs (Sidani et al., 2006a, 2006b); discuss treatment options (Seale, Anderson, & Kinnersley, 2006); and discuss and encourage smoking cessation (Sheahan, 2000; Zapka et al., 2000), although this prevention-focused activity may not extend to other health risks (Sheahan, 2000). No differences were seen for the treatment of febrile infants (Badger, Lookinland, Tiedeman, et al., 2002) or the timing and initiation of collaborative action to discuss patient concerns (Brooten et al., 2005). In one study, NPs were more likely to provide structural support for the emergency management of closed musculoskeletal injuries, although other interventions were similar to those of physician providers (Ball, Walton, & Hawes, 2007). In another study, residents spent significantly more time on coordination of care than NPs (Sidani et al., 2006a, 2006b). It is interesting to note that despite this difference, patients managed by NPs reported higher levels of coordination than those overseen by residents.

Other process-focused studies have focused on CNM visit scheduling (Walker et al., 2002) and communication styles between CNMs and physicians, with both groups using informational styles during interactions with patients (Lawson, 2002). Intra-individual differences were noted for the CNM providers, however, suggesting that they changed to a more controlling communication style with certain patients. Contrary to the researcher's expectations, communication style was not related to patient-perceived support for autonomy or patient satisfaction.

Process-focused studies also have explored APNs' use of clinical practice guidelines during the management of symptoms in oncology patients (Cunningham, 2006), NP health counseling behaviors (Lin, Gebbie, Fullilove, et al.,

2004), and prescriptive writing patterns (Shell, 2001). Older studies provide clear evidence to counter early concerns about the potential for NPs to overprescribe (Campbell, Musil, & Zauszniewski, 1998; Hamric, Lindebak, Worley, et al., 1998). In one study of mental health NPs, however, an analysis of prescribing patterns for managing depression suggested that the NPs overused drugs considered less desirable, discontinued medications prematurely, and minimized important patient characteristics such as age when prescribing (Shell, 2001). Other studies have examined clinical practice guideline use, demonstrating increased compliance of NP-led initiatives (Gracias, Sicoutris, Stawicki, et al., 2008).

These process-focused investigations highlight some of the APN activities that are expected to contribute to care delivery outcome. Because most of the studies did not assess the relationship between process of care and any specific outcome, however, little is known about the actual impact of these actions on recipients of care. Qualitative-focused work examining the processes of care have helped identify some characteristics of APN care, including the impact on care coordination and patient and family knowledge (Fry, 2011). In a qualitative study describing barriers and facilitators to implementing a transitional care intervention for cognitively impaired older adults and their caregivers led by APNs, identified themes included patients and caregivers having the necessary information and knowledge, care coordination, and caregiver experience (Bradway, Trotta, Bixby, et al., 2012). Additional studies are needed to highlight the impact of APN-led care that is unique to various APN roles to demonstrate further the unique features of APN care that affect patient and health care outcomes.

Brooten's Advanced Practice Nurse Transitional Care Model

Information about the relationship between APN care and patient outcomes has been demonstrated through a series of studies using a model of comprehensive discharge planning, early discharge, and home follow-up provided by APNs, as described by Brooten and colleagues (Brooten, et al., 2002a; Brooten, et al., 2002b; Brooten, et al., 2003; Brooten, et al., 2005). (Most of these studies used CNSs, although later reports by these authors used the generic term *APN.*) This care delivery model has been tested with high-risk, childbearing women (York, et al., 1997), older postsurgical cancer patients (McCorkle, et al., 2000), and older adults (Naylor, Brooten, Campbell, et al., 1999). In each of these studies, a randomized controlled clinical trial design was used to compare CNS outcomes with those seen with usual care. In all cases, outcomes were superior for the CNS intervention groups. McCorkle and

colleagues' study (2000) was particularly noteworthy because of the finding that the APN-led intervention significantly improved patient survival as compared with the control group receiving usual care.

Cost of care for CNS-directed services was 44% less than for standard care (York, et al., 1997). Most of the cost savings for the older adult group were the result of a significant reduction in the number of readmissions for APN-managed patients (Naylor & Kirtzman, 2010; Naylor, Bowles, McCauley, et al., 2011), very-low-birthweight infants (Brooten, Gennaro, Knapp, et al., 2002a), women with unplanned cesarean birth, high-risk pregnancy, and hysterectomy, and older adults with cardiac diagnoses (Brooten, Youngblut, Deatrick, et al., 2003). During each of these studies, protocols were used to guide APN care delivery; APNs also recorded what was done during their interventions, the number of patient contacts made, the time spent during contacts, patient outcomes, and health care costs. In the study of mothers and infants, most of the APNs' time was spent on assessment activities (69%), with the remaining time devoted to interventions (Brooten, Gennaro, Knapp, et al., 2002a). Assessments of infants focused on physical status, whereas assessments of mothers were directed at coping, health care, availability of support systems, and home environment. Assessments of mothers also addressed caretaking skills, understanding of procedures and medications, knowledge of infant growth and development, and recognition and prevention of infection. Intervention activities were devoted primarily to teaching, followed by liaison or consultation and encouragement of self- or infant care.

In the combined analysis, surveillance was identified as the most common intervention, with APNs spending the greatest amount of time on monitoring signs and symptoms of physical problems (Brooten, et al., 2003). An important finding of this second analysis was the relationship between the magnitude of APN interaction and improvement in patient and cost outcomes. The longer the time spent by the APN, the better the outcomes. A second important finding was the difference in outcomes seen and the amount of APN involvement required across patient populations. This finding reinforces the importance of carefully describing the makeup of the patient population and care delivery setting (both of which are contextual or structural components of the quality of care framework), and the processes of care when measuring APN impact. Without this information, Brooten and colleagues (Brooten, et al., 2003; Brooten, et al., 2005) might have erroneously concluded that some APNs performed better than others, when in fact the differences were the result of patient condition and need.

The APN transitional care model is a well-acknowledged framework; the significant research that has resulted on the impact of APN transitional care is a frequently cited body of work (Naylor & Kirtzman, 2010; Naylor, Bowles, McCauley, et al., 2011). Although no conclusion can be made about which of the APNs' activities contributed specifically to the favorable outcomes seen, the inclusion of a process assessment component provides a preliminary indication of a cause and effect relationship between APN practice and patient outcome. Ongoing research on the model continues because additional research is needed to determine whether selected aspects of the process are more important or if favorable outcomes are achieved only through a combination of APN actions.

Process as Outcome Studies

Among the process as outcome studies reported in the literature are a few that have explored whether the availability of clinical guidelines improves primary care provider documentation of preventive and screening services (Gray, 1998; Windorski & Kalb, 2002). Several studies have focused on improving compliance with EBP and have demonstrated the benefit of APN-led initiatives targeting hospitalized patients (Gracias, et al., 2008; Russell, et al., 2002), as well as primary care practice related to specialty care such as urinary incontinence (Albers-Heitner et al., 2012, cardiovascular risk reduction (Becker et al., 2005), osteoporosis management (Greene & Dell, 2010), and management of depression (Swindel, et al., 2003).

Studies that focus exclusively on processes as indicators of outcome have rarely been published. Usually, investigators mistakenly report some process as an outcome—that is, as an indication of intervention effect. For example, a report by Kinnersley and associates (2000) has described secondary outcomes of a comparison between NP and general practitioner consultations, such as length of consultation, information provided, resources used (prescriptions, investigations, referrals), and follow-up consultations, all of which are structure (e.g., resources used) and process indicators (e.g., information given, referrals made). However, these researchers did collect information about patient satisfaction, resolution of symptoms and concerns, and patients' intentions to deal with future similar illnesses, which constitute reasonable clinical outcome indicators. The ability to measure patients' intentions to deal with future similar illnesses accurately is questionable, however, and the authors provided no information about how they did this.

An example of a case in which all the indicators described as outcomes were actually process-focused involved a retrospective medical record review of ACNP versus resident performance on patients admitted for cardiac catheterization (Reigle, Molnar, Howell, et al.,

2006). In this study, outcome indicators were defined as documentation of education and counseling for risk factors and discharge prescribing practices. Both these measures are indicators of care provider performance (process) rather than patient outcome. Findings demonstrated that ACNPs provided more education and counseling concerning dyslipidemia, exercise, and diabetes; counseling for hypertension and smoking was comparable for both groups. The ACNPs also provided more appropriate medication prescriptions for management of heart disease postdischarge. Other studies comparing NP care with that of medical residents have demonstrated comparable medical management skills and improved staff and family satisfaction (Gershengorn, et al., 2011; Lakhan & Laird, 2009; Pioro, et al., 2001; Pinkerton & Bush, 2000).

Performance (Process) Improvement Activities

The focus on improving process or performance improvement activities is one aspect of outcomes assessment that focuses on the value-added complement to medical care provided by APNs. O'Grady (2008) has highlighted the potential to demonstrate APN importance by evaluating the impact of process improvement initiatives, including the focus on quality of care and patient safety. Several studies have focused on specific APN role components that affected outcomes. The impact of a home-based APN intervention for patients with psychiatric illness and HIV was evaluated in a 4-year randomized control trial that studied 238 community residents. Over a 12-month period, those receiving the APN intervention, which focused on case management and process improvements in the delivery of medical and mental health care, demonstrated improvements in depression and health-related quality of life compared with a control group that received usual care (Hanrahan, Wu, Kelly, et al., 2011).

The use of interdisciplinary rounds as a process improvement approach was described by Halm and coworkers (2003). In this case, a CNS oversaw the shift of unit-based patient rounds to an interdisciplinary approach that involved all disciplines in the review and discussion of care delivery decisions. No information was provided about the impact of this change at the hospital involved. Instead, the authors reported the findings of an Internet survey of APNs who summarized the processes that they used to measure the impact of interdisciplinary rounds on patient outcomes and the outcomes that APNs recommended for measurement of effect. However, several of the outcome indicators suggested were measures of process rather than outcome (e.g., case finding, consults and referrals, accomplishment of plan for patient, continuity of care, ethical issues addressed, quality initiatives for population, evidence-based protocols). Although these may be useful indicators of improved processes of care and the potential for better care delivery outcomes, they should not be labeled as patient or family outcome indicators.

In a third study, an NP-managed performance improvement intervention model achieved improved outcomes through a process designed to facilitate compliance with community-acquired pneumonia (CAP) guidelines (Gross, et al., 2004). Quarterly performance measurement data demonstrated improvements in each of the performance measures for the prevention of CAP. The program also resulted in a reduction in patient length of stay and cost of care. Another study focusing on APN-led rapid response teams demonstrated process improvements for early detection of patient compromise and changes in patient outcomes (Morse, Warshawsky, Moore, et al., 2006). Many newer reports of APN-led programs have been including patient outcomes resulting from the program and process improvements, making a stronger case for the impact of APNs. Table 23-2 outlines examples of APN-directed program evaluations. The focus area of the evaluation, target population, and brief study findings are outlined.

Disease Management Activities

There have traditionally been few formal reports of the APN's role in disease management initiatives. The failure to identify disease management analyses may be, in part, because of their close linkages with other intervention and assessment activities. Recent studies have demonstrated improved disease management from NP care, including care for hypertension, cardiovascular disease, and diabetes (Newhouse et al., 2011) and specialty-based care such as Alzheimer disease management (Callahan, et al., 2006), urology care (Albers-Heitner, et al., 2012), cancer care (Cooper, et al., 2009), and congestive heart failure (Case, et al., 2010; Lowery, et al., 2011). In a recent study assessing the quality of health care provided at a pediatric nurse-managed clinic, NP care to 500 clients was found to improve childhood immunization rates, treatment for children with upper respiratory infection, and increased children's access to primary care providers (Coddington, Sands, Edwards, et al., 2012). It is noteworthy that recent studies have focused on demonstrating the impact of APN care in specialty-based care. This focus has implications to showcase further the impact of APNs in a wide range of specialties.

A description of an APN-directed work site disease management program also has been published (Carioti, Lavigne, Stone, et al., 2001). In this study, 54 employees were surveyed about their perceptions of disease control,

behavioral change, and understanding of disease condition after program completion. Most respondents (who were primarily educated white men managed for hypertension, dyslipidemia, and diabetes) reported behavioral changes as a result of the program. Those who were managed for dyslipidemia and hypertension also reported greater understanding of their disorders. Participants with asthma reported no change in their level of understanding or initiation of behavioral change. Overall, participants were highly satisfied with the program. Because the outcome indicators were self-reports of perceived changes that were measured postintervention only, caution is required when considering the impact of this intervention. Additional indicators, including those that could validate self-reports, are desirable. Moreover, the collection of data before the intervention and at longer intervals after program completion would help ensure that the behavioral and perceptual changes did occur and that the impact was sustained long enough to achieve a true outcome effect. Blood pressure, lipid levels, pulmonary function, medication intake, blood glucose level, and other quantifiable measures collected longitudinally would assist with the validation of self-reports.

Outcomes Management Activities

There are also few reports of APN-directed outcomes management programs. The effectiveness of multidisciplinary NP-coordinated team group visits to medically underserved patients with type 2 diabetes has demonstrated improvement in blood glucose and glycated hemoglobin levels, greater knowledge, and improved self-efficacy (Jesse & Rutledge, 2012). In a study focusing on APN care in psychiatry, admission rates to inpatient psychiatric facilities, visits to the emergency room (ER), referral to rehabilitative services, occupational status, adherence to yearly routine blood tests and medications, and patient satisfaction were found to improve with APN consultations (Cheng, 2012).

The results of an outcomes management approach using ACNPs as outcomes managers was assessed with a population of hospitalized neuroscience patients. The impact of the model was evaluated through a retrospective medical record review of outcomes directly linked to daily management by and interventions of the APNs. A significant reduction in length of hospital stay was seen for patients at risk. Reductions in intensive care unit (ICU) length of stay and incidence of urinary tract infection and skin breakdown also were evident, with overall cost savings approaching $2.5 million for a 1-year period (Russell, VorderBruegge, & Burns, 2002). This outcomes management approach was applied to the care of ICU

TABLE 23-2 Advanced Practice Nurse–Directed Program Evaluations

Study (Year)	Focus of Evaluation	Target Population	Findings
Albers-Heitner et al. (2012)	Urinary incontinence care	Primary care	Improved quality of life; improvement in incontinence severity; more cost- effective care
Allen & Fabri (2005)	Perceptions about impact of role	Older patients and their care providers	Themes focused on holistic health assessment, patient and caregiver values, symptom management, assistance with supplies, education, advocacy, collaboration
Anetzberger et al. (2006)	Achievement of program goals—service to at-risk groups and improved outcomes	High-risk older adults	Completed >1600 visits to targeted population; number of referrals doubled; patients highly satisfied with service
Bissonnette (2011)	APN-led program for kidney transplant patients	Kidney transplant patients	APN-led interprofessional collaborative care model; improved care for patients with chronic kidney disease awaiting kidney transplantation
Brandon et al. (2009)	Telephone follow-up program for heart failure patients	Primary care patients with heart failure	Reduced rates of rehospitalization and improved patient self-care behaviors
Brown et al. (2001)	Diabetes care delivery	Primary care patients	Mean hemoglobin A1c (HbA1c) levels declined significantly; weight declined significantly; patient satisfaction high
Callahan et al. (2006)	Collaborative care model for Alzheimer's disease	Primary care patient	Improved behavioral and psychological symptoms; less caregiver distress
Capezuti et al. (2007)	Consultation and educational services regarding siderail use	Long-term care nursing staff and patients	Reduction in siderail use varied by site; falls significantly reduced for site with reduced use of rails
Carioti et al. (2001)	Work site disease management program	Employees	Significant self-reported change in behaviors related to hypertension, dyslipidemia, and diabetes; employees highly satisfied with program
Cheung et al. (2011)	CNM-led normal birth unit	Obstetrical patients undergoing childbirth	Significant differences in vaginal deliveries, rates of episiotomies, amniotomies (all decreased) and increased postdelivery mobility
Cibulka et al. (2011)	NP-directed oral care program	Low income pregnant women	Improved oral care, including improved frequency of brushing and flossing teeth, dental checkups, and marked reduction in intake of high-sugar drinks
Dahl & Penque (2001)	Service delivery and cost of care	Inpatients with diagnosis of heart failure	Significant reduction in length of stay, mortality, and 30-day readmission rate
DeJong & Veltman (2004)	Screening program with smoking cessation counseling	Persons with chronic obstructive pulmonary disease	Significant reduction in smoking frequency
Dickerson et al. (2006)	Support groups	Patients receiving implantable cardioverter defibrillators	No difference in quality of life scores for support group attendees
Greene & Dell (2010)	Disease management program	Patients with osteoporosis	Increased treatment of osteoporosis; decrease in hip fractures
Gross et al. (2002)	Use of telemetry resources	Inpatients receiving telemetry monitoring	Significant reduction in hours of telemetry use, with no increase in adverse effects

Continued

TABLE 23-2   Advanced Practice Nurse–Directed Program Evaluations—*cont'd*

Study (Year)	Focus of Evaluation	Target Population	Findings
Gross et al. (2004)	Quality improvement program	Inpatients with community-acquired pneumonia	Increased compliance with vaccine screening procedures; reduced length of stay; reduced readmission rate; reduced cost per case
Hamilton & Hawley (2006)	Outpatient management of anemia	Patients with chronic renal disease	Significant improvement in quality of life
Intili & Laws (2003)	Urgent care clinic	Hotel employees	Reduced cost of services
Krichbaum et al. (2005)	Two-tiered care delivery model	Long-term care patients	Significant reductions in depression and improvements in outlook
Kutzleb & Reiner (2006)	Patient education program	Patients with heart failure	Significant improvement in quality of life
Lowery et al. (2012)	Disease management model	Patients with chronic heart failure	Significantly fewer congestive heart failure and all-cause admissions at 1-year follow-up, lower mortality at both 1- and 2-year follow-ups
McCorkle et al. (2009)	Postsurgical care for gynecologic cancer	Women who had undergone gynecological cancer surgery	Improved functional status, less symptom distress, less uncertainty
McMullen et al. (2001)	NP-attending physician collaboration	Inpatient medical patients	Significantly better physical health scores; staff and physician satisfaction high
Morse et al. (2006)	Assessment of NP-led rapid response team	Hospitalized patients	Significant decrease in in-hospital cardiac arrests, decrease in mortality rates
Rideout (2007)	Care coordination	Hospitalized children with cystic fibrosis	Timeliness of nutrition and social work consultation improved significantly; length of stay declined by 1.35 days
Scherr et al. (2012)	Comparison of NP-led program for rapid response teams compared with physician care	Hospitalized patients	No differences in number of cardiac arrests or mortality rates; nurses reported confidence in knowledge of NP team
Stolee et al. (2006)	Role of NP	Long-term care nursing employees	Perception of positive impact; most staff reported improved skill levels
Sung et al. (2011)	NPs as coordinators of acute stroke team	Hospitalized patients with acute stroke onset	Time to CT scan, time to neurology evaluation, and time to initiate thrombolytic therapy significantly improved
Wagner et al. (2007)	Consultation and educational services regarding siderail use	Long-term care patients	Five (median) recommendations per resident; median cost of intervention per resident was $135

patients requiring mechanical ventilation for longer than 3 days (Burns & Earvin, 2002; Burns, et al., 2003). In this study, four ACNPs managed and monitored care delivery using evidence-based weaning trial and sedation withdrawal guidelines. The number of ventilator days, ICU and hospital lengths of stay, and mortality rates all declined significantly after the outcomes management process was implemented. In addition, total costs attributed to this population declined by $3 million during the first year of the ACNP outcomes management intervention.

An NP-directed outcomes management program for patients with coronary heart disease also resulted in favorable outcomes (Allen, et al., 2002). In this comparison of NP-managed care with usual care plus feedback about lipid levels, NP-managed patients achieved low-density lipoprotein (LDL) cholesterol levels that were significantly better than for patients in the usual care group.

NPs achieved these outcomes through the management of patients' lipid levels, provision of individualized lifestyle modifications, and oversight of lipid-reducing medication use for 1 year after hospital discharge. These studies highlight the focus on outcomes management activities, which is an acknowledged aspect of APN care. Conducting evaluations of the impact of APNs on outcomes management is an additional strategy to demonstrate APN outcomes.

Outcomes Research

In the last decade, an increasing number of studies examining the effect of APN practice on patient and systems outcomes have been conducted. Table 23-3 organizes these studies by outcome indicator. The next sections summarize recent outcomes research. Research has investigated care delivery outcomes across providers and among different APN types. In most cases, physician groups (including medical residents) have been used for comparison. As noted, this process is a concern because it implies that physician practice is the gold standard for APNs and that it encompasses the full range of APN activity. Actually, physician practice overlaps in some respects and diverges in others. In the process studies reviewed earlier, APNs routinely used strategies that were not considered by physicians or were not incorporated to the extent evident in APN practice. Ideally, attention should be directed at indicators that accurately measure all care providers' impact and those that can serve as benchmarks for APN practice alone.

In a study to investigate which outcome indicators APNs routinely used or would recommend using for measurement of APN impact, Ingersoll and colleagues (2000) used a Delphi survey method with 177 APNs in Tennessee. The top 10 APN-sensitive outcome indicators selected (in descending order) were as follows: satisfaction with care; symptom reduction or resolution; perception of being well cared for; compliance/adherence with treatment plan; knowledge level of patients and families; trust of care provider; collaboration among care providers; care provider recommendation according to need; frequency and type of procedures ordered; and quality of life. Of note in this listing is the inclusion of three process indicators (collaboration, care provider recommendation, and procedures ordered), which would not reflect the APN's impact on outcomes. However, this list mirrors the core competencies of APN practice (e.g., guidance and coaching, holistic direct care practice, and collaboration). Continued development of process and outcome indicators that focus on the unique contribution of APNs to outcomes is needed to strengthen APN marketability and ability to enact advanced nursing rather than substitute for medical practice.

In this section, studies published in the last decade that measured the actual effect of APN practice on outcomes are reviewed. These studies are further divided into those that compare APN outcomes with outcomes of other provider groups (e.g., physician), those that compare APN outcomes with outcomes of usual care, and those without comparison groups that measure outcomes before and after the introduction of an APN. This section includes representative reports highlighting the indicators measured in outcomes studies, limitations evident in some of the research, and findings described.

Studies Comparing Advanced Practice Nurse and Physician and Other Provider Outcomes

Studies comparing APNs with medical practitioners have been reported in the United States, Canada, the British Isles, Europe, Australia, the Middle East, and elsewhere. As noted, a synthesis review of U.S. APN roles has demonstrated that APN care is equivalent to physician care and, for some outcomes, such as patient satisfaction, APN care was rated higher (Newhouse et al., 2011). A number of studies comparing APN care with physician care internationally have also demonstrated similar results (Albers-Heitner et al., 2012; Scherr et al., 2012) and improved care in outcomes such as rates of vaginal deliveries and episiotomies (Cheung et al., 2011), eczema care (Schuttelaar et al., 2011), skill procedures such as thoracostomy tube insertion (Bevis et al. 2008), and ophthalmic examination techniques in the ED (Lamirel et al., 2011). Alexandrov and colleagues (2009, 2011a, 2011b) have demonstrated that APNs provided with postgraduate academic fellowship education and training in acute neurovascular care were able to diagnose acute ischemic stroke accurately through a combination of clinical localization and neuroimaging (multimodal computed tomography [CT] and magnetic resonance imaging [MRI]) interpretation, and make safe and effective tPA treatment decisions while also increasing the absolute number of tPA-treated stroke patients at their facility.

Nurse Practitioner Outcomes

The trend to focus on NP outcomes by comparing NP care with physician, physician assistant (PA), or medical residents and fellows was popular in earlier years. A recent *Cochrane Database* systematic review on the impact of primary care NPs of studies published between 1996 and 2002 has identified 16 studies that examined a number of outcomes related to patient care management, as well as resource use and costs (Reeves et al., 2009). The impact on physician workload and direct costs of care were variable. In four of the studies, NPs took responsibility for the

Text continued on p. 630

TABLE 23-3   Advanced Practice Nurse–Sensitive Outcome Indicators Tested in Practice*

Outcome Indicator	Study (Year)	Study Design	Focus of Indicator	Findings
Activities of daily living (ADL)	Counsell et al. (2007)	Randomized control trial	Population-generic	Significantly improved
	Krichbaum (2007)	Randomized control trial	Population-generic	Significantly improved over control group
	Neff et al. (2003)	Quasi-experimental comparison		Significantly improved over control group
Adverse events, unplanned incidents, including drug reactions	Simonson et al. (2007)	Retrospective comparison		Comparable to anesthesiologists
Amniotomy rates	Cheung et al. (2011)	Randomized control trial	Population-specific	Significant decreased rates compared with usual care
Anxiety, depression; mental health status; emotional state	Corner et al. (2003)	Case study	Population-generic	Decreased over time
	Krichbaum et al. (2005)	Quasi-experimental repeated measures		Significantly better than control group
	Lenz et al. (2004)	Longitudinal follow-up study		Comparable to physicians
	McCorkle et al. (2007)	Secondary data analysis		Comparable to control group
	McMullen et al. (2001)	Program evaluation		Comparable to physician service
	Moore et al. (2002)	Randomized controlled trial		Significantly better than physicians
	Neff et al. (2003)	Quasi-experimental comparison		Significantly better (depression) than control group
	Ritz et al. (2000)	Randomized controlled trial		Significantly better than control group
	Ryden et al. (2000)	Quasi-experimental comparison		Comparable to control group
Anemia clinical practice guideline compliance	Gracias et al. (2003)	Quasi-experimental comparison	Population-generic	Significantly better than control
Asthma control	Borgmeyer et al. (2008)	Observational	Population-specific	Significantly improved
Autonomous decision making (patient-perceived)	Lawson (2002)	Survey	Population-generic	Comparable to physicians
Blood pressure	Krein et al. (2004)	Randomized controlled trial	Population-generic	Comparable to control group
	Lenz et al. (2004)	Longitudinal follow-up study		Comparable to physicians
	Litaker et al. (2003)	Randomized controlled trial		Comparable to control group
	Scisney-Matlock et al. (2004)	Randomized controlled trial		Comparable to physicians
Cardiac arrest rates after rapid response team call	Morse et al. (2006)	Observational	Population-generic	Significantly decreased
	Scherr et al. (2012)	Retrospective	Population-generic	Significantly decreased
Caregiver psychosocial status	Dellasega & Zerbe (2002)	Randomized controlled trial	Population-generic	Significantly better than control group
Cesarean delivery	Cragin & Kennedy (2006)	Prospective descriptive cohort	Population-specific	Significantly lower than physician group

TABLE 23-3 Advanced Practice Nurse–Sensitive Outcome Indicators Tested in Practice—*cont'd*

Outcome Indicator	Study (Year)	Study Design	Focus of Indicator	Findings
Cholesterol level	Paez & Allen (2006)	Randomized controlled trial	Population-generic	Significantly better than usual care group
	Becker et al. (2005)	Randomized control trial	Population-generic	Significantly better than usual care group
	Krein et al. (2004)	Randomized controlled trial		Comparable to control group
	Allen et al. (2002)	Randomized controlled trial	Population-generic	Significantly better than usual care group
Cost of care	Aigner et al. (2004)	Medical record review	Population-generic	NP-physician team comparable to physicians alone
	Albers-Heitner et al. (2012)	Pre- and postcomparison		NP care cost-effective for managing care for urinary incontinence
	Burns et al. (2003)	Pre- and postcomparison[†]		Significantly reduced with APN outcomes management
	Cromwell & Snyder (2000)	Case study cost comparison		Significantly less with CRNA team model
	Cowen et al. (2006)	Quasi-experimental comparison	Population-generic	Significantly improved compared with control
	Karlowicz & McMurray (2000)	Medical record review		Comparable to residents
	Lambing et al. (2004)	Descriptive comparison		Significantly more than physicians overall; less for charges per patient day
	Naylor et al. (2011)	Randomized controlled trial		Significantly less than control group
	Paez & Allen (2006)	Randomized controlled trial		Incremental costs offset by improved outcome
	Roblin et al. (2004)	Predictive modeling		Significantly less than for physicians
	Russell et al. (2002)	Outcomes management program		Average cost per patient day reduced
	Stone et al. (2000)	Cost estimation		Less than physicians when adjusted for productivity
Depression management	Hanrahan et al. (2011)	Randomized controlled trial		Significantly improved
	Swindle et al. (2003)	Observational	Population-specific	Significantly improved
Discharge disposition	Hoffman et al. (2005)	Quasi-experimental longitudinal comparison	Organizational	Comparable to physicians
Disease activity	Tijhuis et al. (2003)	Randomized controlled trial	Population-generic	Comparable to multidisciplinary teams
Door to needle time for thrombolytic therapy for acute stroke patients	Sung et al. (2011)	Parallel comparison	Population-specific	Significantly better than physician control group

Continued

TABLE 23-3   Advanced Practice Nurse–Sensitive Outcome Indicators Tested in Practice—*cont'd*

Outcome Indicator	Study (Year)	Study Design	Focus of Indicator	Findings
Emergency department use	Aigner et al. (2004)	Medical record review	Population-generic	NP-physician team comparable to physicians alone
	Lenz et al. (2004)	Longitudinal follow-up study		Comparable to physicians
Episiotomy rates	Cheung et al. (2011)	Randomized control trial	Population-specific	Decreased rates with CNM care
Eczema flare-ups	Chuttelaar et al. (2011)	Randomized control trial	Population-specific	Significantly less rates than physician comparison group
Functional status, ability	Lenz et al. (2004)	Longitudinal follow-up study		Comparable to physicians
	McCorkle et al. (2009)	Randomized controlled trial	Population-specific	Significantly improved
	Tijhuis et al. (2003)	Randomized controlled trial	Population-specific	Comparable to multidisciplinary teams
Glucose level, serum	Brown et al. (2001)	Program evaluation	Population-specific	Significantly improved over time
Health state	Dellasega & Zerbe (2002)	Randomized controlled trial	Population-generic	Comparable to control group
	Tijhuis et al. (2003)	Randomized controlled trial		Comparable to multidisciplinary teams
Hemoglobin A1c (HbA1c)	Lenz et al. (2004)	Longitudinal follow-up study	Population-specific	Comparable to physicians
	Litaker et al. (2003)	Randomized controlled trial		Comparable to control group
Hip fracture rate	Krichbaum (2007)	Care coordination program evaluation	Population-specific	Significantly decreased rate of fractures
Hip fractures with osteoporosis screening and treatment	Greene & Dell (2010)	Disease management program evaluation	Population-specific	Significantly decreased rate of fractures, increased rate of osteoporosis treatment
Hospitalizations, including readmissions	Brandon et al. (2009)	Quasi-experimental comparison		Decreased readmissions, improved self-care behaviors
	Brandon et al. (2009)	Telehealth program evaluation	Population-specific	Decreased readmission rates, improved patient self- care behaviors
	Kane et al. (2003)	Quasi-experimental comparison		Significantly fewer than controls
	Lambing et al. (2004)	Descriptive comparison		Comparable to physicians
	Lenz et al. (2004)	Longitudinal follow-up study		Comparable to physicians
	Neff et al. (2003)	Quasi-experimental comparison		Significantly fewer than control group
Incontinence, control of	Ryden et al. (2000)	Quasi-experimental comparison	Population-specific	Significantly better than control group
Length of stay	Aigner et al. (2004)	Medical record review	Population-generic, organizational	NP-physician team comparable to physicians alone
	Burns et al. (2003)	Pre- and postcomparison		Significantly shorter with APN outcomes management

TABLE 23-3   Advanced Practice Nurse–Sensitive Outcome Indicators Tested in Practice—*cont'd*

Outcome Indicator	Study (Year)	Study Design	Focus of Indicator	Findings
	Dahl & Penque (2001)	Program evaluation		Significantly shorter than before program (overall)
	Fanta et al. (2006)	Randomized controlled trial		Significantly shorter than for residents
	Gershengorn et al. (2011)	Retrospective review		No difference in hospital mortality, length of stay (ICU, hospital), and posthospital discharge destination for NP compared with physician care
	Gross et al. (2004)	Pre- and postcomparison		Significant reduction over time
	Karlowicz & McMurray (2000)	Medical record review		Comparable to residents
	Lambing et al. (2004)	Descriptive comparison		Significantly longer than physicians
	Neff et al. (2003)	Quasiexperimental comparison		Significantly shorter than control group
	Rideout (2007)	Pre- and postcomparison		No difference pre to post
	Riegle et al. (2006)	Comparative study		Significantly reduced
	Russell et al. (2002)	Outcomes management program		Significantly reduced
Mechanical ventilation duration and weaning	Burns et al. (2003)	Pre- and postcomparison	Population-specific	Significantly reduced with APN outcomes management
	Hoffman et al. (2005)	Quasi-experimental longitudinal comparison		Comparable to physicians
Mortality	Aubrey & Yoxall (2001)	Medical record review	Population-generic, organizational	Comparable to residents
	Burns et al. (2003)	Pre- and postcomparison		Significantly reduced with APN outcomes management
	Dahl & Penque (2001)	Program evaluation		Significantly less than before program
	Hoffman et al. (2005)	Quasi-experimental longitudinal comparison		Comparable to physicians
	Lambing et al. (2004)	Descriptive comparison		Comparable to physicians
	Morse et al. (2006)	Observational	Population-generic	Significantly lower
	Pine et al. (2003)	Medicare database review		Comparable to anesthesiologists
	Scherr et al., (2011)	Retrospective	Population-generic	Significantly decreased
Nurse satisfaction	Simonson et al. (2007)	Medical record review		Comparable to anesthesiologists
	McMullen et al. (2001)	Program evaluation	Population-specific, organizational	Highly satisfied

Continued

TABLE 23-3   Advanced Practice Nurse–Sensitive Outcome Indicators Tested in Practice—*cont'd*

Outcome Indicator	Study (Year)	Study Design	Focus of Indicator	Findings
	Rideout (2007)	Pre- and postcomparison		Highly satisfied postintervention (no preintervention data)
	Shebesta et al. (2006)	Survey		Highly satisfied
	Stolee et al. (2006)	Survey		Comparable to, significantly greater than residents
Optimality of services[†]	Cragin & Kennedy (2006)	Descriptive cohort study	Population-specific	Significantly greater than physicians
Patient, family satisfaction	Benkert et al. (2002)	Survey	Population-generic	Scores influenced by number of visits, type of contact, and respondent characteristics
	Bryant & Graham (2002)	Survey		Highly satisfied
	Fanta et al. (2006)	Survey		Comparable to or significantly greater than residents
	Green & Davis (2005)	Randomized controlled trial		Highly satisfied
	Krein et al. (2004)	Randomized controlled trial		Significantly greater than controls
	Lenz et al. (2004)	Longitudinal follow-up study		Comparable to physicians
	Litaker et al. (2003)	Randomized controlled trial		Significantly greater than controls
	McMullen et al. (2001)	Program evaluation		Significantly greater for communication rate than physician services
	Moore et al. (2002)	Randomized controlled trial		Significantly greater than physicians
	Roblin et al. (2004)	Survey		Significantly greater than physicians
	Scisney-Matlock et al. (2004)	Quasi-experimental comparison		Significantly greater than physicians
	Sidani et al. (2006a, 2006b)	Cross-sectional comparison		Significantly greater than residents
	Varughese et al. (2006)	Observational	Population-generic	Significantly improved
	Venning et al. (2000)	Randomized controlled trial		Significantly greater than general practitioners
Physician satisfaction, perception of APN performance	Brown et al. (2001)	Program evaluation	Organizational	Highly satisfied
	McMullen et al. (2001)	Program evaluation		Highly satisfied
	Rideout (2007)	Pre- and postcomparison		Highly satisfied postcomparison (no precomparison data)
Pressure ulcers, skin breakdown	Russell et al. (2002)	Outcomes management program	Population-specific	Significantly reduced
	Ryden et al. (2000)	Quasi-experimental comparison		Significantly less than control group
Pulmonary function	Lenz et al. (2004)	Longitudinal follow-up study	Population-specific	Comparable to physicians
	Rideout (2007)	Pre- and postcomparison		No difference in pre- and postcomparison

TABLE 23-3 Advanced Practice Nurse–Sensitive Outcome Indicators Tested in Practice—cont'd

Outcome Indicator	Study (Year)	Study Design	Focus of Indicator	Findings
Quality of life	Corner et al. (2003)	Case study	Population-generic	Initial improvement, with decline by end of study
	Hamilton & Hawley (2006)	Retrospective review		Significant improvement over time
	Kutzleb & Reiner (2006)	Quasi-experimental comparison		Significantly better than control group
	McCorkle et al. (2009)	Randomized controlled trial	Populatio Specific	Significantly improved
	Moore et al. (2002)	Randomized controlled trial		Comparable to physicians
	Ritz et al. (2000)	Randomized controlled trial		Significantly better than control group (for some dimensions)
	Tijhuis et al. (2003)	Randomized controlled trial		Comparable to multidisciplinary teams
Readmission	Hoffman et al. (2005)	Quasi-experimental longitudinal comparison	Organizational	ICU readmissions comparable to physicians
	Lowery et al. (2011)	Pre- and postcomparison		Decreased heart failure readmissions
Symptom control	Corner et al. (2003)	Case study	Population-generic	No change over time
	Moore et al. (2002)	Randomized controlled trial	Population-specific (depending on symptom)	Comparable to physicians; neuropathy significantly less
Time to service delivery	Reigle et al. (2006)	Medical record review	Population-generic, organizational	Significantly less than physicians
Urinary tract infection	Elpern et al. (2009)	Retrospective	Population-generic	Significantly reduced
Urinary tract infection	Russell et al. (2002)	Outcomes management program	Population-generic	Significantly reduced
Vaginal delivery rates	Cheung et al. (2011)	Randomized controlled trial	Population-specific	Significantly reduced
Ventilator-associated pneumonia	Quenot et al. (2007).	Observational	Population-generic	Significantly decreased rates of pneumonia
Weight	Rideout (2007)	Pre- and postcomparison	Population-generic	No difference pre- and postcomparison

NOTE: Some indicators that were used with specific populations in studies have been labeled as generic because they can be applied to multiple patient groups. The outcome measures listed here are not uniformly consistent with the measure properties of similar indicators endorsed by the National Quality Forum.

*Published studies since 2000.

†Constitute both a process (action by provider) and an outcome (condition or response in patient).

Definition of terms for the focus of the indicator:

    Population-generic—indicators that could be used with any patient population.

    Population-specific—indicators that are relevant to specific populations only.

ongoing management of patients with particular chronic conditions, including diabetes and heart disease. A limitation was that the outcomes investigated varied across studies, limiting the opportunity for data synthesis. The study findings highlighted that in general, no appreciable differences were found between NP and physician care on health outcomes for patients, processes of care, resource use as assessed by frequency and length of consultations, return visits, prescriptions, tests and referrals to other services, and direct or indirect costs. However, patient satisfaction was higher when NPs provided care for persons seeking urgent care (Reeves, et al., 2009).

In an earlier systematic review of research conducted between 1966 and 2001 comparing NPs with primary care physicians, randomized controlled trials and studies with prospective experimental designs were reviewed if they included patient satisfaction, health status, health service costs, or process of care measures (Horrocks, Anderson, & Salisbury, 2002). Of 119 potential studies, 35 met review inclusion criteria, although none included sufficient information to compare health care costs. Overall, the research demonstrated that patient satisfaction with care provider was significantly greater for NPs. No differences were seen for health status or quality of life. Process indicators suggested that NPs spent more time with patients, identified physical abnormalities more often, communicated more effectively, and recorded in the medical record more completely than physicians. Ordering and the interpreting of x-ray films were comparable across groups. Evident from this review is the need for additional rigorous research concerning APN impact. Only 29.4% of studies comparing NP with primary care physician outcomes were sufficiently designed to meet the review's inclusion criteria. Without this level of comparison, few recommendations can be made about which indicators are most reflective of and sensitive to APN practice.

Studies also have compared NP performance with that of medical residents, with findings consistently reporting equivalent or better outcomes. In one descriptive comparison study, however, lengths of stay and total costs were higher for the NP group (Lambing et al., 2004). Information about the calculations used to compute cost is limited. In addition, the patient mix for the NPs was sicker, which may have contributed to the differences seen. The investigators noted that differences were likely the result of the NPs consulting more often with other providers, resulting in additional care provider charges. Laboratory and radiology costs were comparable and, when the costs were reported as mean (average) charge per patient day, the costs were less for NPs.

Several studies also have compared physician practice alone with physician practice in collaboration with an NP. In a retrospective review of the outcomes of cardiovascular surgeon alone versus cardiovascular surgeon plus ACNP, postoperative lengths of stay were shorter for the collaborating group (Meyer & Miers, 2005). Collaborative care also resulted in lower cost of care, with organizational savings estimated at over $3 million annually. A second study found similarly favorable findings for NP-physician teams overseeing patients with hypertension and diabetes mellitus (DM; Litaker et al., 2003). A third study comparing outcomes of physician-only care with outcomes of NP-physician care for nursing home residents demonstrated equivalent findings for both groups. ED visits, ED and hospital costs, lengths of stay, and number of hospitalizations all were comparable. The sole difference pertained to the frequency of acute visits, which were higher for the NP-physician group (Aigner, Drew, & Phipps, 2004). Because the increased acute visit frequency was solely related to NP inpatient oversight (with no charges incurred per visit), however, no differences in cost were seen. Had the NP visits resulted in a charge per visit, the costs between the groups might have differed considerably, although the authors suggested that the lower salary costs of the NPs (compared with physician visit) would have offset this rise. Recently, a synthesis review by Newhouse and associates (2011) has confirmed the positive outcomes from NP care in comparison to physician care. However, this focus of comparing NP outcomes with those of other care providers is probably no longer indicated, because demonstrating the impact of the unique aspects of APN care is more valuable.

Acute Care Nurse Practitioner Outcomes

Comparable outcomes between physician care and ACNP care were seen in a study conducted in a subacute ICU (Hoffman, Tasota, Zullo, et al., 2005). In this study, workload, demographic, and medical conditions of patients were comparable for APN–attending physician and resident–attending physician teams. Readmissions to ICU, mortality rates, duration of mechanical ventilation, and weaning status at discharge were comparable. The reintubation rate was higher for patients cared for by the physician group, even though patient acuity was comparable for both groups. A review of studies focusing on ACNP care demonstrated that of 20 studies, most included ER, trauma care, and management of patients with specific acute care conditions, such as stroke, pneumonia, and congestive heart failure (Kleinpell, et al., 2008). Other recent studies related to ACNP care have demonstrated the benefit of specific role components such as NP-led rapid response teams (Morse, et al., 2006; Scherr, et al., 2012).

Clinical Nurse Specialist Outcomes

A number of studies have explored outcomes related to CNS care and CNS productivity (Urden & Stacy, 2012).

Recently, Fulton (2012) reported on validating CNS core practice outcomes. In a survey of 427 CNSs using an international CNS list serve, the most frequently monitored outcomes related to APN nursing interventions (68%, patient sphere; EBP, 87%; 86%, nurse and organizational spheres respectively). The least monitored outcomes related to diagnosing (range, 54% to 57%) and cost and revenue (range 36% to 55%). Other studies have focused on exploring outcomes related to specialty areas of care. Favorable outcomes have been seen for cancer patients managed by CNSs in outpatient settings (Dayhoff & Lyons, 2009; McCorkle et al., 1989; Moore et al., 2002). In the study by Moore and colleagues (2002), CNSs managed patient care in nurse-led clinics and then contacted patients by phone for follow up assessment. CNS-managed patients with a diagnosis of lung cancer had significantly better levels of emotional functioning and less peripheral neuropathy than patients managed by physicians. CNS-managed patients also were significantly more likely to die at home than were patients treated by physicians. Costs of care were comparable for both groups.

In a classic study conducted by McCorkle and coworkers (1989), patients with lung cancer were randomly assigned to one of three treatment groups. The first group received specialized home care provided by CNSs, the second received standard home care consisting of service delivery from an interdisciplinary team, and the third received care provided at a medical provider's office. Patients managed in physicians' offices had significantly more symptom distress and became more dependent earlier in their treatment period than either of the home care groups (standard or specialized). Patients managed by the CNSs had significantly fewer hospitalizations and, although not significant, had shorter lengths of stay. Patients managed by the standard approach and during physician office visits had lengths of hospital stay averaging 73 days longer than patients overseen by CNSs. Other studies related to CNS outcomes in acute care have demonstrated reductions in hospitalization length of stay and costs (Dayhoff & Lyons, 2009; Newhouse et al., 2011).

The outcomes of CNS care have also been investigated in international models of care. Recently, Begely and colleagues (2011) assessed the impact of the CNS and midwifery roles in Ireland. APNs, including CNSs and nurse-midwives, were found to improve service delivery by leading the development of new clinical services, taking responsibility for guideline development, implementation, and evaluation, and positively influencing quality patient care through formal and informal education.

Certified Nurse-Midwife Outcomes

A number of outcome studies have focused on the outcomes of CNM care and have demonstrated significant impact on vaginal delivery rates, decreased rates of episiotomies and amniotomies, less use of pain medication, and high satisfaction ratings, among other outcomes (Arthur, Marfell, & Ulrich, 2009; Chueng, et al., 2011; Johantgen, et al., 2012; Mulloy, et al., 2010). A study of CNM outcomes used an optimality index (OI) to compare midwifery and physician practices according to the extent of preexisting conditions at the time of treatment (Cragin & Kennedy, 2006). The OI contained a list of 40 care delivery processes and outcome measures pertaining to pregnancy, parturition, neonatal condition, and maternal postpartum condition, which were scored according to level of optimality (0 = nonoptimal; 1 – optimal). Women cared for by physicians were 1.7 times as likely as those cared for by CNMs to have a cesarean section during delivery. Women seen by physicians in this study had a significantly greater proportion of chronic illness and drug abuse, although these differences did not explain the higher rate of cesarean section for the group.

A Cochrane Database systematic review comparing midwife-led care with other models of care examined 11 clinical trials and found that midwife-led models of care resulted in patients being less likely to experience antenatal hospitalization, regional analgesia, and episiotomy or instrumental delivery. Patients were more likely to experience no intrapartum analgesia or anesthesia, have spontaneous vaginal births, and initiate breast-feeding. There were no statistically significant differences between groups for caesarean births, but women who were randomized to receive midwife-led care were less likely to experience fetal loss before 24 weeks' gestation and hospital length of stays were shorter (Hatem, et al., 2009).

Certified Registered Nurse Anesthetist Outcomes

A number of studies related to CRNA care have showcased the impact on outcomes (Kremer & Faut-Callahan, 2009). Several recent studies have demonstrated the impact of CRNA care on various outcomes, including cost-effectiveness (Dulisse & Cromwell 2010; Hogan, Seifert, Moore, et al., 2010). Several studies of CRNA impact compared CRNA outcomes with those of anesthesiologists. One of these estimated costs was based on cases from four anesthesia services at four different hospitals—a large academic medical center, large community hospital, medium-sized community hospital, and small community hospital (Cromwell & Snyder, 2000). Labor cost projections for 10,000 anesthetics delivered annually demonstrated that an all–CRNA care delivery model cost less than 50% of an all-anesthesiologist model. The cost savings for a mixed model composed of anesthesiologists and CRNAs in ratios of 1:1 to 1:4 ranged from 33% to 41% of the total costs for an all-anesthesiologist model.

In another study, risk-adjusted mortality rates of patients undergoing carotid endarterectomy, cholecystectomy, herniorrhaphy, hysterectomy, knee replacement, laminectomy, mastectomy, or prostatectomy were compared for CRNAs and anesthesiologists (Pine, Holt, & Lou, 2003). Medicare data were analyzed for a 3-year period, with no differences seen for the type of anesthesia provider. The third study examined obstetric care anesthesia outcomes among hospitals using CRNAs only and those using anesthesiologists only (Simonson, Ahern, & Hendryx, 2007). Although the investigators of this study stressed that the focus of the comparison was on the differences between hospitals rather than care providers, the findings are relevant to the discussion of APN outcomes. Hospitals with CRNA-only staffs had significantly fewer complications, although this difference disappeared when the complication rates were risk-adjusted. This risk adjustment process included examining information about the impact of comorbid conditions, hospital size, teaching status, and patient transfers on the development of complications. The demonstration of equivalent outcomes for CRNAs and anesthesiologists provides additional evidence concerning the quality of care provided by APNs.

Neonatal Nurse Practitioner Outcomes

Studies related to NNP care have focused on comparison of NP care with that of other providers. In a mixed method study combining a retrospective examination and quality assessment of nursing and medical records, the quality of care and clinical outcomes for premature birth babies cared for by a NNP compared with a medical practitioner during the first 6 to 12 hours following admission to a neonatal ICU (NICU) was conducted with a review of a random sample of 61 sets of records. The analysis of the patient outcome data and quality assessment of nursing and medical records revealed that there was no statistical difference in the standard and quality of care provided between the NNP and medical staff (Wood, 2006). In England, the Ashington project, which was implemented in the Ashington Northumberland Health District, was an innovative neonatal service run entirely by NNPs. Evaluation of the model of care demonstrated comparable outcomes for the NNP service with care provided by physician providers with respect to quality of resuscitation at birth, newborn screening for congenital heart disease, incidence of neonatal encephalopathy, congenital hip dysplasia, neonatal readmission, mortality rates, and parent satisfaction rates (Hall & Wilkinson, 2005).

Another study compared NNP outcomes with those of other care providers, including PAs and resident physicians. In this study, chart reviews assessing care delivery outcomes found comparable morbidity and mortality rates, costs of care, and lengths of stay in the NICU and the hospital as a whole (Karlowicz & McMurray, 2000).

Favorable outcomes also were seen for pediatric nurse practitioners (PNPs) when compared with those of trauma service residents (Fanta, et al., 2006). Patients overseen by the PNP group had significantly shorter lengths of stay and reported significantly higher levels of satisfaction.

Studies Comparing Advanced Practice Nurse and Physician Productivity

One of the most difficult and contentious elements of APN outcomes measurement is the assessment of APN productivity, which is an organizational rather than a patient outcome. Productivity is an indication of care provider efficiency rather than skill or capability and, as such, does not provide any guarantee of quality patient care. The issue with productivity is that reimbursement practices and the income generated by care providers are directly tied to productivity levels. Because APNs have historically spent more time with patients, their overall productivity levels may result in changes in potential income for the organization or practice. Until reimbursement decisions are shifted to a care delivery outcomes approach, this will continue to be a problem for APNs.

Relative Work Value of Advanced Practice Nurses

Payment for services provided to Medicare patients is based on a resource-based relative value (RBRV) scale methodology, which incorporates an estimate for the amount of work, practice expense, and professional liability insurance associated with various procedures. The total relative value of each procedure is multiplied by a standard dollar conversion factor to determine the allowable service charge care providers that may request for reimbursement of services (Sullivan-Marx & Maislin, 2000). Until 1994, all RBRVs were calculated solely on physician data. Since then, NP data have been used to adjust the RBRVs for some payment codes, although considerable work is needed to clarify how NPs' work values differ from those of physicians (Sullivan-Marx, 2008).

In this work, quantifying the time required, NPs estimated preservice, intraservice, and postservice time in minutes. Complexity was measured by assessing mental effort, technical skill, and physical effort and the psychological stress associated with an iatrogenic event related to the current procedural technology (CPT) code associated with the situation. In all cases, NPs estimated relative work values were comparable to those established for physician practice, suggesting that their practice patterns were similar for the scenarios described (Sullivan-Marx, 2008). Because the CPT codes and descriptors were designed with physicians in mind, however, other activities by APNs may not have been included in the estimation process. Until these are well defined and marketed by APNs, this process will potentially continue to underrepresent the APN's actual relative value in the delivery of care. Tracking productive and the work value of APN care using productivity tools to capture outcomes has also been advocated (Steuer & Kopan, 2011). Other studies have continued to demonstrate comparable outcomes of APN with physician care (Gershengorn, et al., 2011; Newhouse, et al., 2011).

Several studies have focused on the costs of physician care related to APN care. Two comprehensive cost analyses of APN-managed care facilities were identified in the literature. One study focused on the delivery of services to low-risk pregnant women with CNM provider costs in a free-standing clinic compared with physician costs for care delivered in a hospital setting (Stone, Zwanziger, Walker, et al., 2000). In both cases, costs were estimated according to maternity episode, with direct prenatal and childbirth costs calculated from institutional reports, census reports, office profit and loss statements, and billing records. A sensitivity analysis was performed to determine the effect of patient volume on cost of care. The costs of the CNMs' prenatal services were significantly higher than the physicians' costs; childbirth costs were significantly less. When combined over the episode of care, costs were comparable for both provider types.

Another study focused on cost of care for inpatients managed by physicians compared with that of NP-physician provider teams; the study examined direct care costs and costs associated with services provided outside the inpatient admission (Ettner et al., 2006). These indirect costs included hospitalizations other than the investigational one in the study, nursing home stays, ED visits, primary care physician visits, other care provider visits, and formal home care services. The additional costs associated with NP involvement in inpatient care were more than offset by savings in indirect costs. The NP-physician model of care resulted in approximately $975 saved per patient (Ettner et al., 2006). In a companion article based on the same study, the NP-physician model also resulted in significant reductions in lengths of stay and comparable readmission rates and mortality outcomes (Cowan et al., 2006).

Studies Comparing Advanced Practice Nurse and Usual Practice Outcomes

Some of the strongest APN outcomes research has focused on the impact of early hospital discharge using a CNS-directed discharge planning and home follow-up intervention of Brooten and colleagues, reviewed earlier (Brooten, Naylor, York, et al., 2002b). Other studies comparing APN outcomes with those of standard care have been conducted. A workload analysis of a CNS role in a specialty lung cancer practicefound that the role was primarily used to support processes and administrative components. Restructuring the role to implement standardized

care based on national practice guidelines led to proactive case management that resulted in a decrease in admissions for nonacute health care problems from four to a mean of 0.3/month (Baxter & Leary, 2011). A study of postoperative patients with hypercholesterolemia involved a randomized clinical trial designed to compare the cost-effectiveness of services provided by an NP with that of usual care enhanced by feedback to a primary care provider (Paez & Allen, 2006). The incremental costs associated with the oversight of the NP included the costs of the NP's time and of the lipid-lowering medications and laboratory monitoring activities of the NP. At 12 months after surgery, the incremental costs of the NP-managed group were $26/mg/dL of cholesterol outcome and $39 per percentage reduction in mg/dL of lipid level. NP management was most intensive during the first 6 months of the year and medication costs were highest during this period, when NPs titrated dosages to achieve maximum effect. Although more costly during this initial period than for the usual care group, the ultimate outcome of achieving better lipid management offset the extra cost.

Internationally, the number of studies focusing on APN outcomes has been increasing as APN roles expand worldwide. Partiprajak (2012) has followed 100 type 2 DM patients in Thailand to assess the impact of an APN-led support group ($n = 44$) compared with a comparison group ($n = 56$). The results indicated that the APN-led support group patients had lower systolic blood pressure, higher self-care abilities, increased quality of life and satisfaction with care compared with the comparison group. Other international studies have demonstrated outcomes related to NP care (Ball, Walton, & Hawes 2007), CNS care (Baxter & Leary, 2011; Begley, et al., 2010; Oliver & Leary, 2010), and CNM care (Wood, 2007).

Studies Using Noncomparison Groups

A number of studies have compared care delivery outcomes before and after the APN's introduction into clinical practice. In many of these studies, a preintervention and postintervention approach was used to test for differences. A weakness of these studies is the frequent reliance on retrospective reviews of medical records for evidence of outcomes before the APN's arrival. The absence of a comparison group also makes confirmation of the relationship between APN and outcome difficult. Nevertheless, the studies provide useful information for further exploration in controlled trials and should be viewed as preliminary indications of possible effect. Oliver and Leary (2010) used an interrelational Structured Query Language (SQL) database to examine the impact of CNS care in the specialty area of rheumatology in the England; they studied day to day activities and qualitative narrative data. Income generation activity, patient safety, and efficiency were also explored. The study findings indicated that the CNS used proactive case management, including the use of vigilance, rescue work, and brokering to achieve a cost savings (in pounds) of 175,168 to the employing NHS Trust. The authors noted that this figure is likely to be an underestimation, because calculations on reduction in bed days in hospital were not included. A study examining the impact of the CNS in providing lung cancer care in England used a workload analysis to demonstrate that the CNS role directly affected patient care through proactive case management; this was based on the use of national care standards for lung cancer and resulted in a decrease in admissions for nonacute problems from four to a mean of 0.3/month, representing a significant saving in bed days (Baxter & Leary, 2011).

Several other studies have focused solely on patient or staff satisfaction with APN practice as an indicator of care provider effect (Benkert et al., 2002; Bryant & Graham, 2002; Knudtson, 2000). In many cases, these studies used questionnaires with limited reliability and validity estimates and included single-site samples of patients. In most cases, no comparison groups were available. Because of the methodologic issues associated with the measurement of satisfaction, reliance on this outcome indicator alone is generally not sufficient for assessing APN impact. Patient satisfaction data are often skewed, with only the most satisfied or dissatisfied patients responding. In addition, general satisfaction measures may not be sufficiently sensitive to detect differences across APN providers. However, their use should not be completely avoided because they do offer one indication of care provider impact. When serious problems with delivery of services occur, satisfaction levels drop. In stable environments, the variation may not be sufficient to detect differences across care providers.

As noted, Table 23-3 provides a comprehensive summary of APN outcome studies organized by outcome indicators. As outlined in the table, an impressive number of studies have been conducted that examine a number of specific outcomes. Most of the studies have demonstrated improved outcomes as a result of APN care and/or comparable outcomes with other health care providers. As APN roles continue to expand to different practice settings and to specialty-based practices, continued evaluation of the impact of APN care is warranted to identify APN contributions to care.

Summary of Advanced Practice Nursing Outcomes Research

The evidence of APNs' impact on individual patient and organizational outcomes suggests that the quality of care that APNs deliver is comparable or superior to that of other care providers in the specialty. Various studies have explored the direct and indirect processes that APNs use to manage patient care and the outcomes achieved. All have determined that APN practice overlaps that of other care providers in some respects and differs in others. These distinctions, and their potential to confound comparisons with other care providers, contribute to the complexity inherent in measuring the effect of APNs. Moreover, the limited research linking specific APN processes to care delivery outcomes makes it difficult to determine which role components achieved the effect. Difficult or not, a clear distinction is needed if APNs are ever to receive the recognition they deserve or the financial reimbursement they are due.

This review of APN outcomes research suggests that the quality and quantity of research pertaining to APN outcomes has improved over time, with initial studies focusing primarily on role description and acceptance issues and more recent studies addressing performance and outcome considerations between APN and other provider groups. A variety of research designs are now being used to measure APN impact, with an increasing number of investigators using prospective designs and including comparison groups. Although medical record reviews continue to provide much of the data for these comparison studies, methods to control for differences in patient populations and the use of more sophisticated data analysis techniques are providing more reliable, replicable, and generalizable information.

Despite these improvements, intensive work is needed in several areas. The first of these involves the consistent use of a set of core outcome indicators relevant and sensitive to differences in APN practice. An important step in this direction relates to the work performed by the NQF to establish a list of endorsed measures, many of which are applicable to the work of APNs. National leadership groups should assume responsibility for measure development and testing using the methods outlined by the NQF to guide their work; such a process would increase the number of measures in the domain of APN practice and would ultimately facilitate standardized approaches to the evaluation of APN effect and public reporting. Collaborations between APNs and nurse researchers and the development of outcomes consortia also will facilitate this process. Bringing together clinical practice and research design and measurement experts from multiple locations and specialties is the best approach for the development and subsequent testing of reliable and valid indicators of the effect of APN-directed and APN-delivered care. Networks of APN groups and institutions in which APNs practice should also play an active role in the collection of data for measure testing to further development of APN-sensitive measures. An understanding of the important role that the NQF plays in relation to endorsing measures recognized by CMS is essential, given the fact that other pathways to widespread measure adoption are lacking, particularly in regard to publicly reported measures. As noted, Table 23-3 lists examples of the various APN-sensitive outcome indicators that have been used in previous studies; however, the conformity of these measures with the NQF- endorsed measures for use by CMS, third-party payers, and public reporting is inconsistent.

Second, there is an urgent need to reexamine reimbursement practices that reinforce productivity levels according to physician performance, especially with implementation of the Patient Protection and Affordable Care Act (Wakefield, 2010). Process-focused and cost-effectiveness studies have demonstrated that APNs take more time with patients and, as such, are at risk for failing to meet organizational or group practice productivity standards based on the medical model. Because research has not compared different types of productivity estimations, the true magnitude and impact of APN efficiency is unknown. A shift in focus from time spent during individual patient interaction to one that considers total time spent during episode of care (as was done by Ettner et al., 2006, and Stone et al., 2000) might be more realistic for measuring and comparing APN practice. In the episode of care approach, total time and resources used per episode are preferable indicators of productivity. In this case, the extra time spent by APNs and the number of interactions with patients at the outset of service may eliminate the need for longer term, sustained interactions that occur when patients and families are not sufficiently prepared to manage their health care needs. In addition, the increased time spent in education and counseling in the initial phase may eliminate the need for more costly care over the course of the episode. At this time, the evidence is insufficient to determine whether this or alternative approaches to productivity measurement more accurately assess the efficiency and benefits of APN practice.

Closely linked with this issue is the third need, which is to determine whether the increased patient and family satisfaction evident when APNs spend extra time also contributes to improvements in longer-term care delivery outcomes. Because APNs have traditionally spent more time with patients and provide additional teaching and healthy behaviors counseling, their impact may be most evident in the long-term prevention of diseases and the adverse outcomes commonly associated with poor health behaviors. Studies thus far have followed patient outcomes for relatively short periods, usually 6 to 12 months post-APN intervention. Additional longitudinal studies are needed to determine the true long-term impact of these early outcomes on overall lifestyle, quality of life, and health.

Fourth, a predominance of research has focused on comparing APNs with other providers, particularly physicians, medical residents, or PAs. Although these studies are useful, they do not address the unique contributions of APN care nor identify which outcome indicators are most sensitive to differences in APN practices. The focus of outcomes assessment research needs to turn to the value of APN care on patient and population outcomes, rather than comparison of care with other health care providers.

Fifth, this review makes evident the pressing need to explore the value-added impact of APNs in collaborative practice with physicians and other care providers. Although the recent work of Newhouse and associates (2011) has highlighted that an impressive number of studies have been conducted that demonstrate outcomes of APN care, additional research is needed as APN roles continue to expand and as roles in novel practice areas develop. Because APNs and physicians bring different perspectives about care and demonstrate distinct but complementary behaviors, studies are needed to determine how these combined practices reinforce and maximize the beneficial effects of one another. These studies may generate the data needed to demonstrate the value-added benefits of combining APN and physician practices. By documenting favorable outcomes when a collaborative APN-physician approach is used, the profession can more effectively argue for altered reimbursement procedures and reveal the contributions of APNs to the public.

The literature also highlights the difficulties evident in generating widespread interest in measuring care delivery outcomes. Many APNs view the ongoing assessment of care delivery impact as an additional burden to an already full agenda. This problem was highlighted in a survey of oncology APNs who identified critical issues that warranted planning for future nursing society projects (Lynch, Cope, & Murphy-Ende, 2001). Only 2% of respondents included outcomes management as important content for APN programs. At the same time, outcomes documentation was identified as one of the top five priority issues for oncology APNs. Clearly, the foundational work pertaining to outcomes assessment needs to begin during graduate education. Because APN outcome measurement activities begin immediately when an APN is hired, preparation for identifying target outcomes, collecting data, and managing and reporting findings is the minimum information required in graduate programs. In addition to clinically focused outcomes content, several individuals and groups have recommended including content on health care financing, health care information systems, database query, and statistics, particularly in DNP education for APNs (AACN, 2006).

Conclusion

APN care has been cited as being valuable but often invisible because APNs traditionally have not focused on highlighting the impact of their care. This invisibility in the health care system further threatens the recognition of APNs as viable and important providers of health care services. The current emphasis on quality of care and care effectiveness mandates that APNs demonstrate their impact on patient care, health care outcomes, and systems of care. It is apparent that the need for well-designed, longitudinal assessments of APN impact has never been greater. Assessing the outcomes of APN care has become a necessary rather than an optional endeavor. It is only through demonstrating the outcomes of APN care for patients, providers, and health care systems that the value of this care can be defined.

In addition, focusing on APN-sensitive outcome indicators is important for highlighting the unique contributions of APNs. Addressing APN-sensitive outcome indicators will require focused attention on the continued development of electronic information systems that support the identification and tracking of process and outcome data in line with APN contributions. An important component in this process is national agreement on a core set of outcome indicators relevant to APNs, the initiation of standards that support the collection of APN-sensitive data, testing of these core measures, and ultimately measure endorsement by the NQF.

This chapter has presented a review of concepts related to APN outcomes and several frameworks for measuring and monitoring APN practice. Other approaches are also available; the APN should begin the process by selecting one and refining it to meet her or his individual and organizational needs. The best approach is to begin small and expand activities over time. Networking with other APNs is useful for identifying beneficial outcomes and sharing personal experiences about what does and does not work when integrating outcomes measurement into busy practices. Publishing and presenting on outcome evaluation initiatives are imperative to disseminating successful methods for assessing APN outcomes and highlighting exemplars for replication.

Effective outcomes measurement requires APNs to work collaboratively with others, plan and organize processes of care and assessment of quality in highly complex health services environments, and expose their individual practices to the scrutiny of others. Experience with organizational change behaviors and a willingness to seek information and assistance from others will help with this process. In the end, the quality and value of care will improve, as will the community's recognition of the APN's positive impact on outcomes of care.

Acknowledgment

We acknowledge the work of the late Gail Ingersoll, EdD, RN, FAAN, FNAP, in advancing the focus on advanced practice nursing outcomes. In addition to writing on APN outcomes in the previous editions of this book and elsewhere, Dr. Ingersoll was involved in research related to APN care; her contributions to the state of the science of advanced practice nursing outcomes have been significant.

References

Agency for Healthcare Research and Quality (AHRQ). (2010). What criteria must guidelines meet? (http://www.ahrq.gov/clinic/ngcfact.htm).

Agency for Healthcare Research and Quality (AHRQ). (2012). What is comparative effectiveness research? (http://effectivehealthcare.ahrq.gov/index.cfm/what-is-comparative-effectiveness-research1).

Aigner, M. J., Drew, S., & Phipps, J. (2004). A comparative study of nursing home resident outcomes between care provided by nurse practitioners/physicians versus physicians only. *Journal of the American Medical Directors Association, 5*, 16–23.

Albers-Heitner, C. P., Joore, M. A., Winkens, R. A., Lagro-Janssen, A. L. M., Severns, J. L., & Berghmans L. C. (2012). Cost-effectiveness of involving nurse specialists for adult patients with urinary incontinence in primary care compared with care as usual: An economic evaluation alongside a pragmatic randomized controlled trial. *Neurology and Urodynamics, 31*, 526–534. doi 10.1002/nau21.204.

Alexandrov, A. W., Baca, T., Albright, K. C., DiBiase, S., Alexandrov, A. V.; NET SMART Faculty and Fellows. (2011a). Post-graduate academic neurovascular fellowship for advanced practice nurses and physician assistants significantly increases tPA treatment rates: Results from the first graduating class of the NET SMART program. *Stroke, 42*, e206.

Alexandrov, A. W., Baca, T., Brewer, B. B., et al.; NET SMART Faculty and Fellows. (2011b). Post-graduate academic neurovascular fellowship education for APNs and PAs: Impact on first-year graduates and sponsoring physicians. *Stroke, 43*, e352–e353.

Alexandrov, A. W., & Brewer, B. B. (2010). The role of outcomes in evaluating practice change. In B. Melnyk & E. Finout-Overholt (Eds.), *Evidence-based practice in nursing and health. A guide for translating research evidence into practice* (pp. 226–237; 2nd ed.). Philadelphia: Wolters Kluwer, Lippincott Williams & Wilkins.

Alexandrov, A. W., Brethour, M., Cudlip, F., Swatzell, V., Biby, S., Reiner, D., et al. (2009). Post-graduate fellowship education and training for nurses: The NET SMART experience. *Critical Care Nursing Clinics of North America, 21*, 435–449.

Alexandrov, A. W. (2008). Outcomes management. In H. R. Feldman, M. Jaffe-Ruiz, M. J. Greenberg, & T. D. Smith (Eds.), *Nursing leadership: A concise encyclopedia.* New York: Springer.

Allen, J. K., Blumenthal, R. S., Margolis, S., Young, D. R., Miller, E. R., & Kelly, K. (2002). Nurse case management of hypercholesterolemia in patients with coronary heart disease: Results of a randomized clinical trial. *American Heart Journal, 144,* 678–686.

Allen, J., & Fabri, A. M. (2005). An evaluation of a community aged care nurse practitioner service. *Journal of Clinical Nursing, 14,* 1202–1209.

American Association of Colleges of Nursing (AACN). (2006). *The essentials of doctoral education for advanced nursing practice.* Washington, DC: Author.

American Nurses Association (ANA). (2010). *Nursing: Scope and standards of practice* (2nd ed.). Silver Spring, MD: Author.

Anetzberger, G. J., Stricklin, M. L., Gaunter, D., Banozic, R., & Laurie, R. (2006). VNA Housecalls of Greater Cleveland, Ohio: Development and pilot evaluation of a program for high-risk older adults offering primary medical care in the home. *Home Health Services Quarterly, 25,* 155–166.

Arthur, R., Marfell, J., & Ulrich, S. (2009). Outcomes measurement in nurse-midwifery practice. In R. M. Kleinpell (Ed.), *Outcome assessment in advanced practice nursing* (pp. 229–254). New York: Springer.

Aubrey, W. R., & Yoxall, C. S. (2001). Evaluation of the role of the neonatal nurse practitioner in resuscitation of preterm infants at birth. *Archives of Disease in Childhood: Fetal and Neonatal Edition, 28*(2), F96–F99.

Badger, M. J., Lookinland, S., Tiedeman, M., Anderson, V., & Eggett, D. (2002). Nurse practitioners' treatment of febrile infants in Utah: Comparison to physician practice nationally. *Journal of the American Academy of Nurse Practitioners, 14,* 540–553.

Ball, C., & Cox, C. L. (2003). Restoring patients to health: Outcomes and indicators of advanced nursing practice in adult critical care. Part 1. *International Journal of Nursing Practice, 9,* 356–367.

Ball, S. T. E., Walton, K., & Hawes, S. (2007). Do emergency department physiotherapy practitioners, emergency nurse practitioners and doctors investigate, treat and refer patients with closed musculoskeletal injuries differently? *Emergency Medicine Journal, 24,* 185–188.

Barton, A. J., Baramee, J., Sowers, D., & Robertson, K. J. (2003). Articulating the value-added dimension of NP care. *Nurse Practitioner, 28,* 34–40.

Baxter, J., & Leary, A. (2011). Productivity gains by specialist nurses. *Nursing Times. 107,* 15–17.

Beal, J. A., & Quinn, M. (2002). The nurse practitioner role in the NICU as perceived by parents. *MCN, The American Journal of Maternal Child Nursing, 27,* 183–188.

Begley, C., Murphy, K., Higgins, A., Elliot, J., et al. (2010). *Evaluation of clinical nurse and midwife practitioner roles in Ireland (SCAPE): Final report.* Dublin: National Council for the Professional Development of Nursing and Midwifery in Ireland.

Becker, D., Kaplow, R., Muenzen, P. M., & Hartigan, C. (2006). Activities performed by acute and critical care advanced practice nurses: American Association of Critical-Care Nurses study of practice. *American Journal of Critical Care, 15,* 130–148.

Becker, D. M., Yanek, L. R., Johnson, W. R., Jr., Garrett, D., Moy, T. F., Reynolds, S. S., et al. (2005). Impact of a community-based multiple risk factor intervention on cardiovascular risk in black families with a history of premature coronary disease. *Circulation, 111,* 1298–1304.

Beckman, L. J., Harvey, S. M., & Satre, S. J. (2002). The delivery of medical abortion services: The views of experienced providers. *Women's Health Issues, 12,* 103–112.

Benkert, R., Barkauskas, V., Pohl, J., Corser, W., Tanner, C., Wells, M., et al. (2002). Patient satisfaction outcomes in nurse-managed centers. *Outcomes Management, 6,* 174–181.

Bevis, L. C., Berg-Copas, G. M., Thomas, B. W., Vasquez, D. G., Wetta-Hall, R., Brake, D., et al. (2008). Outcomes of tube thoracostomies performed by advanced practice providers vs. trauma surgeons. *American Journal of Critical Care, 17,* 357–363.

Bloch, D. (1975). Evaluation of nursing care in terms of process and outcome: Issues in research and quality assurance. *Nursing Research, 24,* 256–263.

Bissonnette, J. (2011). Evaluation of an advanced practice nurse led inter-professional collaborative chronic care approach for kidney transplant patients: The TARGET study (http://www.ruor.uottawa.ca/en/handle/10393/19975).

Borgmeyer, A., Gyr, P. M., Jamerson, P. A., & Henry, L. D. (2008). Evaluation of the role of the pediatric nurse practitioner in an inpatient asthma program. *Journal of Pediatric Health Care, 22,* 273–281.

Brady, M. A., & Neal, J. A. (2000). Role delineation study of pediatric nurse practitioners: A national study of practice and responsibilities and trends in role functions. *Journal of Pediatric Health Care, 14,* 149–159.

Bradway, C., Trotta, R., Bixby, M. B., McPartland, E., Wollman, M. C., Kapustka, H., et al. (2012). A qualitative analysis of an advanced practice nurse-directed transitional care model intervention. *Gerontologist, 52,* 394–407.

Brandon, A. F., Schuessler, J. B., Ellison, K. J., & Lazenby, R. B. (2009). The effects of an advanced practice nurse led telephone intervention on outcomes of patients with heart failure. *Applied Nursing Research 22,* e1–e7.

Brent, N. J. (2001). Are ignoring best practice changes putting your agency at legal and financial risk? *Home Healthcare Nurse, 19,* 721–724.

Briggs, L. A., Heath, J., & Kelley, J. (2005). Peer review for advanced practice nurses. What does it really mean? *AACN Clinical Issues, 16,* 3–15.

Brooten, D., Gennaro, S., Knapp, H., Jovene, N., Brown, L., & York, R. (2002a). Functions of the CNS in early discharge and home follow-up of very low birthweight infants. *Clinical Nurse Specialist, 16,* 85–90.

Brooten, D., Naylor, M. D., York, R., Brown, L. P., Munro, B. H., Hollingsworth, A. O., et al. (2002b). *Lessons learned from testing the quality cost model of advanced practice nursing (APN) transitional care.* Image: Journal of Nursing Scholarship, 34, 369–375.

Brooten, D., Youngblut, J., Blais, K., Donahue, D., Cruz, I., & Lightbourne, M. (2005). APN-physician collaboration in caring for women with high-risk pregnancies. *Image: Journal of Nursing Scholarship, 37,* 178–184.

Brooten, D., Youngblut, J. M., Deatrick, J., Naylor, M., & York, R. (2003). Patient problems, advanced practice nurse (APN) interventions, time and contacts among five patient groups. *Image: Journal of Nursing Scholarship, 35*, 73–79.

Brown, A. W., Wolff, K. L., Elasy, T. A., & Graber, A. L. (2001). The role of advanced practice nurses in a shared care diabetes practice model. *Diabetes Educator, 27*, 492–500.

Brown, S. A., & Grimes, D. E. (1995). A meta-analysis of nurse practitioners and nurse midwives in primary care. *Nursing Research, 44*, 332–339.

Bryant, R., & Graham, M. C. (2002). Advanced practice nurses: A study of client satisfaction. *Journal of American Academy of Nurse Practitioners, 14*, 88–92.

Bryant-Lukosius, D., & DiCenso, A. (2004). A framework for the introduction and evaluation of advanced practice nursing roles. *Journal of Advanced Nursing, 48*, 530–540.

Bryant-Lukosius, D., DiCenso, A., Browne, G., & Pinelli, J. (2004). Advanced practice nursing roles: Development, implementation and evaluation. *Journal of Advanced Nursing, 48*, 519–529.

Buchholz, S. W., & Purath, J. (2007). Physical activity and physical fitness counseling patterns of adult nurse practitioners. *Journal of the American Academy of Nurse Practitioners, 19*, 86–92.

Burns, S. M., & Earvin, S. (2002). Improving outcomes for mechanically ventilated medical intensive care unit patients using advanced practice nurses: A 6-year experience. *Critical Care Nursing Clinics of North America, 14*, 231–243.

Burns, S. M., Earven, S., Fisher, C., Lewis, R., Merrell, P., Schubart, J. R., et al. (2003). Implementation of an institutional program to improve clinical and financial outcomes of mechanically ventilated patients: One-year outcomes and lessons learned. *Critical Care Medicine, 31*, 2752–2763.

Callahan, C. M., Boustani, M. A., Unverzagt, F. W., Austrom, M. G., Damush, T. M., Perkins, A. J., et al. (2006). Effectiveness of collaborative care for older adults with Alzheimer disease in primary care: A randomized controlled trial. *Journal of the American Medical Association, 295*, 2148–2157.

Campbell, C. D., Musil, C. M., & Zauszniewski, J. A. (1998). Practice patterns of advanced practice psychiatric nurses. *Journal of American Psychiatric Nurses Association, 4*, 111–120.

Capezuti, E., Wagner, L. M., Brush, B. L., Boltz, M., Renz, S., & Talerico, K. A. (2007). Consequences of an intervention to reduce restrictive siderail use in nursing homes. *Journal of the American Geriatrics Society, 55*, 334–341.

Carioti, C. A., Lavigne, J. E., Stone, P., Tortoretti, D. M., & Chiverton, P. (2001). Work site disease management outcomes: Expanding the role of the APN. *Outcomes Management for Nursing Practice, 5*, 179–184.

Carroll, D. L., Robinson, E., Buselli, E., Berry, D., & Rankin, S. H. (2001). Activities of the APN to enhance unpartnered elders self-efficacy after myocardial infarction. *Clinical Nurse Specialist, 15*, 60–66.

Case, R., Haynes, D., Holaday, B., Parker, V. G. (2010). Evidence-based nursing: The role of the advanced practice registered nurse in the management of heart failure patients in the outpatient setting. *Dimensions of Critical Care Nursing, 29*, 57–62.

Chen, D., McNeese-Smith, D., Cowan, M., Upenieks, V., Afifi, A. (2009). Evaluation of a nurse practitioner-led case management model in reducing inpatient drug utilization and cost. *Nursing Economics, 27*, 160–168.

Cheng, C. (2012). The impact of an APN-led clinic on patients with psychosis. Presented at the 7th Annual International Nurse Practitioner/Advanced Practice Nursing Network Conference. London, August 20-22, 2012.

Cheung, N. F., Mander, R., Wang, X., Fu, W., Zhou, H., & Zhang, L. (2011). Clinical outcomes of the first midwife-led normal birth unit in China: A retrospective cohort study. *Midwifery, 27*, 582–587.

Cibulka, N. J., Forney, S., Goodwin, K., Lazaroff, P., & Sarabia, R. (2011) Improving oral health in low-income pregnant women with a nurse practitioner-directed oral care program. *Journal of the American Academy of Nurse Practitioners 23*, 249–257.

Clancy, C. & Collins, F. S.; Agency for Health care Research and Quality. (2010). Patient-centered outcome research institute: The intersection of science and health care. *Science and Translational Medicine, 2*, 18–37.

Coddington, J., Sands, L., Edwards, N., Kirkpatrick, J., & Chen, S. (2012). Quality of health care provided at a pediatric nurse-managed clinic. *Journal of the American Academy of Nurse Practitioners 23*, 674–680.

Cohen, J., Saylor, C., Holzemer, W. L., & Gorenberg, B. (2000). Linking nursing care interventions with client outcomes: A community-based application of an outcomes model. *Journal of Nursing Care Quality, 15*, 22–31.

Cole, F. L., & Ramirez, E. (2000). Activities and procedures performed by nurse practitioners in emergency care settings. *Journal of Emergency Nursing, 26*, 455–463.

Cooper, J. M., Loeb, S., & Smith, C. A. (2009). The primary care nurse practitioner and cancer survivorship care. *Journal of the American Academy of Nurse Practitioners 22*, 394–402.

Corner, J., Halliday, D., Haviland, J., Douglas, H. R., Bath, P., Clark, D., et al. (2003). Exploring nursing outcomes for patients with advanced cancer following intervention by Macmillan specialist palliative care nurses. *Journal of Advanced Nursing, 41*, 561–574.

Counsell, S. R., Callahan, C. M., Clark, D. O., Tu, W., Buttar, A. B., Stump, T. E., et al. (2007). Geriatric care management for low-income seniors: A randomized controlled trial. *Journal of the American Medical Association, 298*, 2623–2633.

Cowan, M. J., Shapiro, M., Hays, R. D., Afifi, A., Vazirani, S., Ward, C. R., et al. (2006). The effect of a multidisciplinary hospitalist/physician and advanced practice nurse collaboration on hospital costs. *Journal of Nursing Administration, 36*, 79–85.

Cragin, L., & Kennedy, H. P. (2006). Linking obstetric and midwifery practice with optimal outcomes. *Journal of Obstetric, Gynecologic, and Neonatal Nursing, 35*, 779–785.

Cromwell, J., & Snyder, K. (2000). Alternate cost-effective anesthesia care teams. *Nursing Economic$, 18*, 185–193.

Cunningham, R. S. (2006). Clinical practice guideline use by oncology advanced practice nurses. *Applied Nursing Research, 19*, 126–133.

Dahl, J., & Penque, S. (2001). The effects of an advanced practice nurse–directed heart failure program. *Dimensions of Critical Care Nursing, 20,* 20–28.

Darmody, J. V. (2005). Observing the work of the clinical nurse specialist: A pilot study. *Clinical Nurse Specialist, 19,* 260–268.

Dayhoff, N. & Lyons, B. (2009). Assessing outcomes of clinical nurse specialist practice. In R. M. Kleinpell (Ed.), *Outcome assessment in advanced practice nursing.* (pp. 201–228) New York: Springer.

DeJong, S. R., & Veltman, R. H. (2004). The effectiveness of a CNS-led community-based COPD screening and intervention program. *Clinical Nurse Specialist, 18,* 72–79.

Dellasega, C., & Zerbe, T. M. (2002). Caregivers of frail rural older adults: Effects of an advanced practice nursing intervention. *Journal of Gerontological Nursing, 28*(10), 40–49.

DeLise, D., & Leasure, A. (2001). Benchmarking: Measuring the outcomes of evidence-based practice. *Outcomes Management for Nursing Practice, 5*(2), 70–74.

Dick, K., & Frazier, S. C. (2005). An exploration of nurse practitioner care to homebound frail elders. *Journal of American Academy of Nurse Practitioners, 18,* 325–334.

Dickerson, S. S., Wu, Y. W. B., & Kennedy, M. C. (2006). A CNS-facilitated ICD support group: A clinical project evaluation. *Clinical Nurse Specialist, 20,* 146–153.

Dierick-van Daele, A. T. M., Metsemakers, J. F. M., Derckx, E. W., Spreeuwenberg, C., & Vrijhoef, H. J. (2009). Nurse practitioners substituting for general practitioners: Randomized control trial. *Journal of Advanced Nursing 65,* 391–401.

Donabedian, A. (1966). Evaluating the quality of medical care. *Milbank Quarterly, 44,* 166–206.

Donabedian, A. (1980). *Explorations in quality assessment and monitoring: The definition of quality and approaches to its assessment.* Ann Arbor, MI: Health Administration Press.

Doran, D. (2011). *Nursing outcomes: The state of the science* (2nd ed.). Sudbury, MA: Jones & Bartlett.

Dulisse, B., & Cromwell, J. (2010). No harm found when nurse anesthetists work without supervision by physicians. *Health Affairs, 29,* 1469–1475.

Edwards, J. B., Oppewal, S., & Logan, C. L. (2003). Nurse-managed primary care: Outcomes of a faculty practice network. *Journal of American Academy of Nurse Practitioners, 12,* 563–569.

Ellwood, P. M. (1988). Outcomes management. A technology of patient experience. *New England Journal of Medicine, 318,* 1549–1556.

Elpern, E. H., Killeen, K., Ketchem, A., Wiley, A., Patel, G., & Lateef, O. (2009). Reducing use of indwelling urinary catheters and associated urinary tract infections. *American Journal of Critical Care, 18,* 535–541.

Esperat, M. C., Hanson-Turton, T., Richardson, M., Debisette, A. T., Rupinta, C. (2012). Nurse-managed health centers: Safety-net care through advanced practice nursing. *Journal of the American Academy of Nurse Practitioners, 24,* 24–31.

Ettner, S. L., Kotlerman, J., Abdelmonem, A., Vazirani, S., Hays, R. D., Shapiro, M., et al. (2006). An alternative approach to reducing the costs of patient care? A controlled trial of the multi-disciplinary doctor-nurse practitioner (MDNP) model. *Medical Decision Making, 26,* 9–17.

Fanta, K., Cook, B., Falcone R. A., Jr., Rickets, C., Schweer, L., Brown, R. L., et al. (2006). Pediatric trauma nurse practitioners provide excellent care with superior patient satisfaction for injured children. *Journal of Pediatric Surgery, 41,* 277–281.

Freed, G. L., & Stockman, J. A. (2009). Oversimplifying primary care supply and shortages. *Journal of the American Medical Association, 301,* 1920–1922.

Fry, M. (2011). Literature review of the impact of nurse practitioners in critical care services. *Nursing in Critical Care. 16,* 58–66.

Fulton, J. (2012). Validation of clinical nurse specialist core practice outcomes. Presented at the 7th Annual International Nurse Practitioner/Advanced Practice Nursing Network Conference. London, August 20-22, 2012.

Gawlinski, A., McCloy, K., Jesurum, J. (2009). Measuring outcomes in cardiovascular APN practice. In Kleinpell R. (Ed.), *Outcome assessment in advanced practice nursing* (pp. 131–188). New York: Springer.

Gershengorn, H. B., Wunsch, H., Wahab, R., et al. (2011). Impact of non-physician staffing on outcomes in a medical ICU. *Chest, 139,* 1347–1353.

Gooden, J. M., & Jackson, E. (2004). Attitudes of registered nurses toward nurse practitioners. *Journal of American Academy of Nurse Practitioners, 16,* 360–364.

Goolsby, M. J. (2007). Antibiotic-prescribing habits of nurse practitioners treating adult patients: Antibiotic use and guidelines survey adult. *Journal of the American Academy of Nurse Practitioners, 19,* 212–214.

Goolsby, M. J. (2009). Ambulatory NP outcomes. In R. Kleinpell (Ed.), *Outcome assessment in advanced practice nursing* (pp. 187–200). New York: Springer.

Gracias, V. H., Sicoutris, C. P., Meredith, D. M., Haut, E, et al. (2003). Critical care nurse practitioners improve compliance with clinical practice guidelines in the surgical intensive care unit. *Critiical Care Medicine, 31*(12), A93.

Gracias, V. H., Sicoutris, C. P., Stawicki, S. P., Meredith, D. M., Horan, A. D., Gupta, R., et al. (2008). Critical care nurse practitioners improve compliance with clinical practice guidelines in "semiclosed" surgical intensive care unit. *Journal of Nursing Care Quality, 23,* 338–344.

Gray, M. (1998). The impact of the "Put Prevention into Practice" initiative on pediatric nurse practitioner practices. *Journal of Pediatric Health Care, 12,* 171–175.

Green, A., & Davis, S. (2005). Toward a predictive model of patient satisfaction with nurse practitioner care. *Journal of American Academy of Nurse Practitioners, 17,* 139–148.

Greene, D. & Dell, R. M. (2010). Outcomes of an osterporosis disease-management program managed by nurse practitioners. *Journal of the American Academy of Nurse Practitioners. 22,* 326–329.

Gross, P. A., Aho, L., Ashtyani, H., Levine, J., McGee, M., Moran, S., et al. (2004). Extending the nurse practitioner concurrent intervention model to community-acquired pneumonia and chronic obstructive pulmonary disease. *Joint Commission Journal on Quality and Safety, 30,* 377–386.

Gross, P. A., Patricio, D., McGuire, K., Skurnick, J., & Teichholz, L. E. (2002). A nurse practitioner intervention model to maximize efficient use of telemetry resources. *Joint Commission Journal on Quality Improvement, 28,* 566–573.

Grumbach, K., & Grundy P. (2010). Outcomes of implementing patient-centered medical home interventions: A review of the evidence from prospective evaluation studies in the United States   (http://www.pcpcc.net/files/evidence_outcomes_in_pcmh.pdf).

Hall, D., & Wilkinson, A. R. (2005). Quality of care by neonatal nurse practitioners: A review of the Ashington experiment. *Archives of Disease in Childhood. Fetal and Neonatal Edition, 90,* F195–F200.

Halm, M. A., Gagner, S., Goering, M., Sabo, J., Smith, M., & Zaccagnini, M. (2003). Interdisciplinary rounds. Impact on patients, families, and staff. *Clinical Nurse Specialist, 17,* 133–142.

Hamilton, R., & Hawley, S. (2006). Quality of life outcomes related to anemia management of patients with chronic renal failure. *Clinical Nurse Specialist, 20,* 139–143.

Hamric, A. B., Lindebak, S., Worley, D., & Jaubert, S. (1998). Outcomes associated with advanced nursing practice prescriptive authority. *Journal of the American Academy of Nurse Practitioners, 10,* 113–118.

Hanrahan, M. P., Wu, E., Kelly, D., Aiken, L. H., & Blank, M. B. (2011). Randomized clinical trial of the effectiveness of a home-based advanced practice psychiatric nurse intervention: Outcomes for individuals with serious mental illness and HIV. Nursing Research and Practice; 1-10. doi:10.1155/2011/840248.

Hardie, H., Leary, A. (2010) Value to patients of a breast cancer clinical nurse specialist. *Nursing Standard 24,* 42–48.

Hargreaves, W. A., Shumway, M., Hu, T. W., & Cuffel, B. (1998). *Cost-outcome methods for mental health.* New York: Academic Press.

Hatem, M., Sandall, J., Devane, D., Soltani, H., & Gates, S. (2009). Midwife-led versus other models of care for childbearing women. *Cochrane Database of Systematic Reviews,* (4), CD004667.

Hillier, A. (2001). The advanced practice nurse in gastroenterology: Identifying and comparing care interactions of nurse practitioners and clinical nurse specialists. *Gastroenterology Nursing, 24,* 239–245.

Hoffman, L. A., Tasota, F. J., Scharfenberg, C., Zullo, T. G., & Donahoe, M. P. (2003). Management of patients in the intensive care unit: Comparison via work sampling analysis of an acute care nurse practitioner and physicians in training. *American Journal of Critical Care, 12,* 436–443.

Hoffman, L. A., Tasota, F. J., Zullo, T. G., Scharfenberg, C., & Donahoe, M. P. (2005). Outcomes of care managed by an acute care nurse practitioner/attending physician team in a subacute medical intensive care unit. *American Journal of Critical Care, 14,* 121–132.

Hogan, P., Seifert, R., Moore, C., & Simonson, B. (2010). Cost-effectiveness analysis of anesthesia providers. *Nursing Economics, 28,* 159–169.

Holcomb, L. O. (2000). A Delphi survey to identify activities of nurse practitioners in primary care. *Clinical Excellence in Nursing Practice, 4,* 163–172.

Holzemer, W. L. (1994). The impact of nursing care in Latin America and the Caribbean: A focus on outcomes. *Journal of Advanced Nursing, 20,* 5–12.

Horrocks, S., Anderson, E., & Salisbury, C. (2002). Systematic review of whether nurse practitioners working in primary care can provide equivalent care to doctors. *British Medical Journal, 324,* 819–823.

Howie, J. N. & Erickson, M. (2002). Acute care nurse practitioners: Creating and implementing a model of care for an inpatient general medical unit. *American Journal of Critical Care. 11,* 448–458.

Hughes, W. J. (2000). Health department nurse practitioners as comprehensive primary care providers. *Family & Community Health, 23,* 50–65.

Ingersoll, G. L. (2000). Evidence based nursing: What it is and what it isn't. *Nursing Outlook, 48,* 151–152.

Ingersoll, G. L., McIntosh, E., & Williams, M. (2000). Nurse-sensitive outcomes of advanced practice. *Journal of Advanced Nursing, 32,* 1272–1281.

Institute of Medicine (IOM). (2001). *Crossing the quality chasm: A new health system for the 21st century.* Washington, DC: National Academies Press.

Institute of Medicine (IOM). (2010). *The future of nursing. Leading change, advancing health.* Washington DC: National Academies.

Intili, H., & Laws, C. (2003). Delivering health care in a large urban hospital. *AAOHN Journal, 51,* 306–309.

Irvine, D., Sidani, S., Porter, H., O'Brien-Pallas, L., Simpson, B., Hall, L. M., et al. (2000). Organizational factors influencing nurse practitioners' role implementation in acute care settings. *Canadian Journal of Nursing Leadership, 13,* 28–35.

Jackson, P. L., Kennedy, C., Sadler, L. S., Kenney, K. M., Lindeke, L. L., Sperhac, A. M., et al. (2001). Professional practice of pediatric nurse practitioners: Implications for education and training of PNPs. *Journal of Pediatric Health Care, 15,* 291–298.

Jackson, D. J., Lang, J. M., Ecker, J., Swartz, W. H., & Heeren, T. (2003). Impact of collaborative manage ment and early admission in labor on method of delivery. *Journal of Obstetric, Gynecologic, and Neonatal Nursing, 32,* 147–157.

Jackson, D. J., Lang, J. M., Swartz, W. H., Ganiats, T. G., Fullerton, J., Ecker, J., et al. (2003). Outcomes, safety, and resource utilization in a collaborative care birth center program compared with traditional physician-based perinatal care. *American Journal of Public Health, 93,* 999–1006.

Jessee, B. T. & Rutledge, C. M. (2012). Effectiveness of nurse practitioner–coordinated team group visits for type 2 diabetes in medically underserved Appalachia. *Journal of the American Academy of Nurse Practitioners, 24,* 735–743. doi: 10.1111/j.1745-7599.2012.00764.x.

Joanna Briggs Institute. (2012). Using evidence-based practice (http://www.joannabriggs.edu.au).

Johantgen, M., Fountain, L., Zangaro, G., Newhouse, R., Stanik-Hutt, J., & White, K. (2012). Comparison of labor and delivery care provided by certified nurse midwives and physicians: A systematic review, 1990-2008. *Woman's Health Issues, 22,* e73–e81.

Johnson, J. E. (2000). Assessment of older urban drivers by nurse practitioners. *Journal of Community Health Nursing, 17,* 107–114.

Johnson, K. C., & Daviss, B. A. (2005). Outcomes of planned home births with certified professional midwives: Large prospective study in North America. *British Medical Journal, 330,* 1416–1422.

Kane, R. L., Flood, S., Keckhafer, G., & Rockwood, T. (2001). How EverCare nurse practitioners spend their time. *Journal of American Geriatrics Society, 49,* 1530–1534.

Kane, R. L., Flood, S., Bershadsky, B., & Keckhafer, G. (2004). Effect of an innovative medicare managed care program on the quality of care for nursing home residents. *Gerontologist, 44,* 95–103.

Kane, R. L., Keckhafer, G., Flood, S., Bershadsky, B., & Siadaty, M. S. (2003). The effect of EverCare on hospital use. *Journal of the American Geriatrics Society, 51,* 1427–1434.

Kannusamy, P. (2006). A longitudinal study of advanced practice nursing in Singapore. *Critical Care Nursing Clinics of North America, 18,* 545–551.

Karlowicz, M. G., & McMurray, J. L. (2000). Comparison of neonatal nurse practitioners' and pediatric residents' care of extremely low birth weight infants. *Archives of Pediatrics & Adolescent Medicine, 154,* 1123–1126.

Kleinpell, R. (2011). Assessing outcomes of nurse practitioners and physicians assistants in the ICU. In R. Kleinpell, T. Buchman, & W. Boyle (Eds.), *Integrating nurse practitioners and physician assistants in the ICU* (pp. 73–86). Chicago: Society of Critical Care Medicine.

Kleinpell, R., & Gawlinski, A. (2005). Assessing outcomes in advanced practice nursing practice: The use of quality indicators and evidence-based practice. *AACN Clinical Issues.16,* 43–57.

Kleinpell, R. M. (2005). Acute care nurse practitioner practice: Results of a 5-year longitudinal study. *American Journal of Critical Care, 14,* 211–221.

Kleinpell, R. M. (Ed.). (2009). *Outcome assessment in advanced practice nursing.* New York: Springer.

Kleinpell, R. M., Ely, E. W., & Grabenkort, R. (2008). Nurse practitioners and physician assistants in the ICU: An evidence-based review. *Critical Care Medicine 26,* 2888–2897.

Knudtson, N. (2000). Patient satisfaction with nurse practitioner service in a rural setting. *Journal of American Academy of Nurse Practitioners, 12,* 405–412.

Krein, S. L., Klamerus, M. L., Vijan, S., Lee, J. L., Fitzgerald, J. T., Pawlow, A., et al. (2004). Case management for patients with poorly controlled diabetes: A randomized trial. *American Journal of Medicine, 116,* 732–739.

Kremer, M. J., Faut-Callahan, M. (2009). Outcome assessment in nurse anesthesia. In Kleinpell R. (Ed.), *Outcome assessment in advanced practice nursing.* (pp. 255–276). New York: Springer.

Krichbaum, K., Pearson, V., Savik, K., & Mueller, C. (2005). Improving resident outcomes with GAPN organization level interventions. *Western Journal of Nursing Research, 27,* 322–337.

Krichbaum, K. (2007). GAPRN postacute care coordination improves hip fracture outcomes. *Western Journal of Nursing Research, 29,* 523–544.

Kutzleb, J., & Reiner, D. (2006). The impact of nurse directed patient education on quality of life and functional capacity in people with heart failure. *Journal of American Academy of Nurse Practitioners, 18,* 116–123.

Lakhan, S. E., & Laird, C. (2009). Addressing the primary care physician shortage in an evolving medical workforce. *International Archives of Medicine, 2,* 14.

Lambing, A. Y., Adams, D. L. C., Fox, D. H., & Divine, G. (2004). Nurse practitioners' and physicians' care activities and clinical outcomes with an inpatient geriatric population. *Journal of American Academy of Nurse Practitioners, 16,* 343–352.

Lamirel, C., Bruce, B. B., Wright, D. W., Delaney, K. P., Newman, N. J., & Biousse, V. (2011). Quality of nonmydriatic digital fundus photography obtained by nurse practitioners in the emergency department: The FOTO-ED Study. *Ophthalmology. 119,* 617–624.

Laurant, M., Reeves, D., Hermens, R., Braspenning, J., Grol, R., & Sibbald, B. (2005). Substitution of doctors by nurses in primary care. *Cochrane Database of Systematic Reviews,* (2), CD001271.

Lawson, M. T. (2002). Nurse practitioner and physician communication styles. *Applied Nursing Research, 15,* 60–66.

Lenz, E. R., Mundinger, M. O., Hopkins, S. C., Lin, S. X., & Smolowitz, J. L. (2002). Diabetes care processes and outcomes in patients treated by nurse practitioners or physicians. *Diabetes Educator, 28,* 590–598.

Lenz, E. R., Mundinger, M. O., Kane, R. L., Hopkins, S. C., & Lin, S. X. (2004). Primary care outcomes in patients treated by nurse practitioners or physicians: Two-year follow-up. *Medical Care Research and Review, 61,* 332–351.

Lin, S. X., Gebbie, K. M., Fullilove, R. E., & Arons, R. R. (2004). Do nurse practitioners make a difference in provision of health counseling in hospital outpatient departments? *Journal of American Academy of Nurse Practitioners, 16,* 462–466.

Lin, S. X., Hooker, R. S., Lenz, E. R., & Hopkins, S. C. (2002). Nurse practitioners and physician assistants in hospital outpatient departments, 1997-1999. *Nursing Economic$, 20,* 174–179.

Lincoln, P. E. (2000). Comparing CNS and NP role activities: A replication. *Clinical Nurse Specialist, 14,* 269–277.

Lind, P. (2001). Disease management: Applying systems thinking to quality patient care delivery. In E. Cohen & T. Cesta (Eds.), *Nursing case management: From essentials to advanced practice applications* (pp. 37–48; 3rd ed.). St. Louis: Mosby.

Litaker, D., Mion, L. C., Planavsky, L., Kippes, C., Mehta, N., & Frolkis, J. (2003). Physician-nurse practitioner teams in chronic disease management: The impact on costs, clinical effectiveness, and patients' perceptions of care. *Journal of Interprofessional Care, 17,* 223–237.

Low, L. K., Seng, J. S., Murtland, T. L., & Oakley, D. (2000). Clinician-specific episiotomy rates: Impact on perineal outcomes. *Journal of Midwifery and Women's Health, 45,* 87–93.

Lowery, J., Subramanian, U., Witala, W., et al. (2012). Evaluation of nurse practitioner disease-management model for chronic heart failure: a multi-site implementation study. *Congestive Heart Failure 18*, 64–71.

Lynch, M. P., Cope, D. G., & Murphy-Ende, K. (2001). Advanced practice issues: Results of the ONS advanced practice nursing survey. *Oncology Nursing Forum, 28*, 1521–1530.

MacFarlane, K., Dixon, L., Wakeman, C. J., Robertson, G. M., Eglinton T. W., & Frizelle, F. A. (2011). The process and outcomes of a nurse-led colorectal cancer follow-up clinic. *Colorectal Disease, 14*, e245–e249. doi 10.1111/j.1463-1318.2011.02923.x.

Mahn, V., & Zazworsky, D. (2000). The advanced practice nurse case manager. In A. B. Hamric, J. A. Spross, & C. M. Hanson (Eds.), *Advanced nursing practice: An integrative approach* (pp. 549–606; 2nd ed.). Philadelphia: WB Saunders.

Malloy, M. H. (2010). Infant outcomes of certified nurse midwife–attended home births: United States: 2000-2004. *Journal of Perinatology 30*, 622–627.

Mathaisel, D. F. X., Cathcart, T. P., & Comm, C. L. (2004). A framework for benchmarking, classifying, and implementing best sustainment practices. *Benchmarking: An International Journal, 11*, 403–411.

McCorkle, R., Benoliel, J. Q., Donaldson, G., Georgiadou, F., Moinpour, C., & Goodell, B. (1989). A randomized clinical trial of home nursing care for lung cancer patients. *Cancer, 64*, 1375–1382.

McCorkle, R., Dowd, M. F., Ercolano, E., Schulman-Green, D., Williams, A. L., Siefert, M. L., et al. (2009). Effects of a nursing intervention on quality of life outcomes in post surgical women with gynecological cancer. *Psycho-Oncology 18*, 62–70.

McCorkle, R., Dowd, M. F., Pickett, M., Siefert, M. L., & Robinson, J. P. (2007). Effects of advanced practice nursing on patient and spouse depressive symptoms, sexual function, and marital interaction after radical prostatectomy. *Urologic Nursing, 27*, 65–77.

McCorkle, R., Strumpf, N. E., Nuamah, I. F., Adler, D. C., Cooley, M. E., Jepson, C., et al. (2000). A specialized home care intervention improves survival among older post-surgical cancer pagients. *Journal of the American Geriatric Society, 48*, 1707–1713.

McGlynn, E. A., Asch, S. M., Adams, J., Keesey, J., Hicks, J., DeCristofaro, A., et al. (2003). The quality of health care delivered to adults in the United States. *New England Journal of Medicine, 348*, 2635–2645.

McMullen, M., Alexander, M. K., Bourgeois, A., & Goodman, L. (2001). Evaluating a nurse practitioner service. *Dimensions of Critical Care Nursing, 20*, 30–34.

Meyer, S. C., & Miers, L. J. (2005). Cardiovascular surgeon and acute care nurse practitioner: Collaboration on postoperative outcomes. *AACN Clinical Issues, 16*, 149–158.

Mick, D. J., & Ackerman, M. H. (2000). Advanced practice nursing role delineation in acute and critical care: Application of the Strong model of advanced practice. *Heart & Lung, 29*, 210–221.

Mills, A. C., & McSweeney, M. (2002). Nurse practitioners and physician assistants revisited: Do their practice patterns differ in ambulatory care? *Journal of Professional Nursing, 18*, 36–46.

Mitchell, J., Dixon, H. L., Freeman, T., & Grindrod, A. (2001). Public perceptions of and comfort level with nurse practitioners in family practice. *Canadian Nurse, 97*, 21–26.

Mitchell, P. H., Ferketich, S., & Jennings, B. M. (1998). Quality health outcomes model. American Academy of Nursing Expert Panel on Quality Health Care. *Image: Journal of Nursing Scholarship, 30*, 43–46.

Moore, S., Corner, J., Haviland, J., Wells, M., Salmon, E., Normand, C., et al. (2002). Nurse-led follow-up and conventional medical follow-up in management of patients with lung cancer: Randomized trial. *British Medical Journal, 325*, 1145–1147.

Morse, K. J., Warshawsky, D., Moore, J. M., & Pecora, D. C. (2006). A new role for the ACNP: The rapid response team leader. *Critical Care Nursing Quarterly 29*, 137–146.

Moote, M., Krsek, C., Kleinpell, R., & Todd, B. (2011). Physician assistant and nurse practitioner utilization in academic medical centers. *American Journal of Medical Quality 26*, 452–460.

Murphy, P. A., & Fullerton, J. T. (2001). Measuring outcomes of midwifery care: Development of an instrument to assess optimality. *Journal of Midwifery & Women's Health, 46*, 274–284.

Musclow, S. L., Sawhney, M., & Watt-Watson, J. (2002). The emerging role of advanced nursing practice in acute pain management throughout Canada. *Clinical Nurse Specialist, 16*, 63–67.

National Association of Pediatric Nurse Practitioners. (2004). Scope and standards of practice (www.napnap.org/Docs/FinalScope2-25.pdf).

National Quality Forum. (2012). ABCs of measurement (http://www.qualityforum.org/Measuring_Performance/ABCs_of_Measurement.aspx).

Naylor, M. D., Brooten, D., Campbell, R., Jacobsen, B. S., Mezey, M. D., Pauly, M. V., et al. (1999). Comprehensive discharge planning and home follow-up of hospitalized elders: A randomized controlled trial. *Journal of the American Medical Association, 281*, 613–620.

Naylor, M. D., Bowles, K. H., McCauley, K. M., Maccoy, M. C., Maislin, G., Pauly, M. V., et al. (2011). High-value transitional care: Translation of research into practice. *Journal of Evaluation in Clinical Practice*. doi: 10.1111/j.1365-2753.2011.01659.x.

Naylor, M. D., & Kurtzman, E. T. (2010). The role of nurse practitioners in reinventing primary care. *Health Affairs, 29*, 893–899.

Neff, D. F., Madigan, E., & Narsavage, G. (2003). APN-directed transitional home care model: Achieving positive outcomes for patients with COPD. *Home Health care Nurse, 21*, 543–550.

Newhouse, R. P., Weiner, J. P., Stanik-Hutt, J., White, K. M., Johantgen, M., Steinwachs, D., et al. (2011). Advanced practice outcomes 1990-2008: A systematic review. *Nursing Economics, 29*, 230–250.

O'Grady, E. (2008). Advanced practice registered nurses: The impact on patient safety and quality (http://www.ahrq.gov/qual/nurseshdbk/docs/O'GradyE_APRN.pdf).

Oliver, S., & Leary, A. (2010). Return on investment: Workload, complexity and value of the CNS. *British Journal of Nursing, 21*, 32, 34–37.

Oliveria, S. A., Altman, J. F., Christos, P. J., & Halpern, A. C. (2002). Use of nonphysician health care providers for skin cancer screening in the primary care setting. *Preventive Medicine, 34*, 374–379.

Oncology Nursing Society (ONS). (2003). *Statement on the scope and standards of advanced practice nursing in oncology* (3rd ed.). Pittsburgh: Author.

Partiprajak, S. (2012). *Outcomes of advanced practice nurse–led type 2 diabetes support group.* Presented at the 7th Annual International Nurse Practitioner/Advanced Practice Nursing Network Conference. London, August 20–22, 2012.

Paez, K. A., & Allen, J. K. (2006). Cost-effectiveness of nurse practitioner management of hypercholesterolemia following coronary revascularization. *Journal of the American Academy of Nurse Practitioners, 18,* 436–444.

Pine, M., Holt, K. D., & Lou, Y. B. (2003). Surgical mortality and type of anesthesia provider. *AANA Journal, 71,* 109–116.

Pioro, M. H., Landefeld, C. S., Brennan, P. F., Daly, B., Fortinsky, R. H., Kim, U., et al. (2001). Outcomes-based trial of an inpatient nurse practitioner service for general medical patients. *Journal of Evaluation in Clinical Practice, 7,* 21–33.

Pohl, J., Tanner, C., & Benkert, R. (2011). Comparison of nurse-managed health centers with federally qualified health centers as safety net providers. *Policy, Politics and Nursing Practice, 12,* 90–99.

Quenot, J. P., Ladoire, S., Devoucoux, F., Doise, J. M., Cailliod, R., Cunin, N., et al. (2007). Effect of a nurse-implemented sedation protocol on the incidence of ventilator-associated pneumonia. *Critical Care Medicine. 35,* 2031–2036.

Radwin, L. (2002). Refining the quality health outcomes model: Differentiating between client trait and state characteristics. *Nursing Outlook, 50,* 168–169.

Reavis, C. (2004). Nurse practitioner–delivered primary health care in urban ambulatory care settings. *American Journal for Nurse Practitioners, 8,* 41–49.

Reeves, L. M., Hermens, D., Braspenning, J., Grol, R., & Sibbald, B. (2009). Substitution of doctors by nurses in primary care. *Cochrane Database of Systematic Reviews,* (2), CD001271.

Reigle, J., Molnar, H. M., Howell, C., & Dumont, C. (2006). Evaluation of in-patient interventional cardiology. *Critical Care Nursing Clinics of North America, 18,* 523–529.

Rideout, K. (2007). Evaluation of a PNP care coordinator model for hospitalized children, adolescents, and young adults with cystic fibrosis. *Pediatric Nursing, 33,* 29–34, 48.

Roblin, D. W., Becker, E. R., Adams, K. E., Howard, D. H., & Roberts, M. H. (2004). Patient satisfaction with primary care: Does type of practitioner matter? *Medical Care, 42,* 579–590.

Roblin, D. W., Howard, D. H., Becker, E. R., Adams, E. K., & Roberts, M. H. (2004). Use of midlevel practitioners to achieve labor cost savings in the primary care practice of an MCO. *Health Services Research, 39,* 607–625.

Rosenfeld, P., McEvoy, M. D., & Glassman, K. (2003). Measuring practice patterns among acute care nurse practitioners. *Journal of Nursing Administration, 33,* 159–165.

Ruiz, R. J., Brown, C. E., Peters, M. T., & Johnson, A. B. (2001). Specialized care for twin gestations: Improving newborn outcomes and reducing costs. *Journal of Obstetric, Gynecologic and Neonatal Nursing, 30,* 52–60.

Russell, D., VorderBruegge, M., & Burns, S. M. (2002). Effect of an outcomes-managed approach to care of neuroscience patients by acute care nurse practitioners. *American Journal of Critical Care, 11,* 353–364.

Scherr, K., Wilson, D. M., Wagner, J., Haughian, M. (2012). Evaluating a new rapid response team: NP-led versus intensivist-led comparisons. *AACN Advanced Critical Care 23,* 32–43.

Schuttelaar, M. L. A., Vermeulen, K. M., Coenraads, P. J. (2011). Costs and cost effectiveness analysis of treatment in children with eczema by nurse practitioner vs dermatologist: Results of a randomized, controlled trial and a review of international costs. *British Journal of Dermatology. 165,* 600–611.

Scisney-Matlock, M., Makos, G., Saunders, T., Jackson, F., & Steigerwalt, S. (2004). Comparison of quality-of-hypertension care for groups treated by physician versus groups treated by physician-nurse team. *Journal of the American Academy of Nurse Practitioners, 16,* 17–23.

Seale, C., Anderson, E., & Kinnersley, P. (2005). Comparison of GP and nurse practitioner consultations: An observational study. *British Journal of General Practice, 521,* 938–943.

Seale, C., Anderson, E., & Kinnersley, P. (2006). Treatment advice in primary care: A comparative study of nurse practitioners and general practitioners. *Journal of Advanced Nursing, 54,* 534–541.

Shebesta, K. F., Cook, B., Rickets, C., Schweer, L., Brown, R. L., Garcia, V. F., et al. (2006). Pediatric trauma nurse practitioners increase bedside nurses' satisfaction with pediatric trauma patient care. *Journal of Trauma Nursing, 13,* 66–69.

Shell, R. C. (2001). Antidepressant prescribing practices of nurse practitioners. *Nurse Practitioner, 26,* 42–47.

Sidani, S., Doran, D., Porter, H., LeFort, S., O'Brien-Pallas, L. L., Zahn, C., et al. (2006a). Outcomes of nurse practitioners in acute care: An exploration (http://www.ispub.com/journal/the-internet-journal-of-advanced-nursing-practice/volume-8-number-1/outcomes-of-nurse-practitioners-in-acute-care-an-exploration.html).

Sidani, S., Doran, D., Porter, H., LeFort, S., O'Brien-Pallas, L. L., Zahn, C., et al. (2006b). Processes of care: Comparison between nurse practitioners and physician residents in acute care. *Nursing Leadership, 19,* 69–85.

Sidani, S., & Irvine, D. (1999). A conceptual framework for evaluating the nurse practitioner role in acute care settings. *Journal of Advanced Nursing, 30,* 58–66.

Sidani, S., Irvine, D., Porter, H., O'Brien-Pallas, L., Simpson, B., McGillis-Hall, L., et al. (2000). Practice patterns of acute care nurse practitioners. *Canadian Journal of Nursing Leadership, 13,* 6–12.

Simonson, D. C., Ahern, M. M., & Hendryx, M. S. (2007). Anesthesia staffing and anesthetic complications during cesarean delivery: A retrospective analysis. *Nursing Research, 56,* 9–17.

Smolenski, M. C. (2005). Credentialing, certification, and competence: Issue for new and seasoned nurse practitioners. *Journal of American Academy of Nurse Practitioners, 17,* 201–204.

Sohn, P. M., & Cook, C. A. L. (2002). Nurse practitioner knowledge of complementary alternative health care: Foundation for practice. *Journal of Advanced Nursing, 39,* 9–16.

Steuer, J., & Kopan, K. (2011). Productivity tool serves as outcome measurement for NPs in acute care practice. *Nurse Practitioner, 36,* 6–7.

Stolee, P., Hillier, L. M., Esbaugh, J., Griffiths, N., & Borrie, M. J. (2006). Examining the nurse practitioner role in long-term care. *Journal of Gerontological Nursing, 32*, 28–36.

Stone, P. W., Zwanziger, J., Walker, P. H., & Buenting, J. (2000). Economic analysis of two models of low-risk maternity care: A freestanding birth center compared with traditional care. *Research in Nursing & Health, 23*, 279–289.

Stuart, D., & Oshio, S. (2002). Primary care in nurse-midwifery practice: A national survey. *Journal of Midwifery & Women's Health, 47*, 104–109.

Sullivan-Marx, E. M. (2008). Lessons learned from advanced practice nursing payment. *Policy, Politics and Nursing Practice. 9*, 121–126.

Sullivan-Marx, E. M., Happ, M. B., Bradley, K. J., & Maislin, G. (2000). Nurse practitioner services: Content and relative work value. *Nursing Outlook, 48*, 269–275.

Sullivan-Marx, E. M., & Maislin, G. (2000). Comparison of nurse practitioner and family physician relative work values. *Journal of Nursing Scholarship, 32*, 71–76.

Sung, S. F., Huang, Y. C., Ong, C. T., Chen, Y. W. (2011). A parallel thrombolysis protocol with nurse practitioners as coordinators minimizing door-to-needle time for acute ischemic stroke. *Stroke Research and Treatment.* Doi:10.4061/2011/198518.

Swindle, R. W., Rao, J. K., Helmy, A., Plue, L., Zhou, X. H., Eckert, G. J., et al. (2003). Integrating clinical nurse specialists into the treatment of primary care patients with depression. *The International Journal of Psychiatry in Medicine, 33*, 17–37.

Sze, E. H., Ciarleglio, M., & Hobbs, G. (2008). Risk factors associated with anal sphincter tear difference among midwife, private obstetrician, and resident deliveries. *International Urogynecology Journal, 19*, 1141–1144.

Tijhuis, G. J., Zwinderman, A. H., Hazes, J. M. W., Breedveld, F. C., & Vlieland, P. M. T. (2003). Two-year follow-up of a randomized controlled trial of a clinical nurse specialist intervention, inpatient, and day patient team care in rheumatoid arthritis. *Journal of Advanced Nursing, 41*, 34–43.

U.S. Agency for International Development (2010). Dashboards and data use. Online forum 2010. (http://www.cpc.unc.edu/measure/networks/datausenet/dashboards-and-data-use-forum-may-2010/dashboards-and-data-use-forum-online-may-2010).

U.S. Department of Education. (2011). United States education dashboard (http://dashboard.ed.gov/about.aspx).

U.S. Department of Health and Human Services (HHS), Administration for Children and Families. (2010). Measuring outcomes guidebook (http://www.acf.hhs.gov/programs/ocs/ccf/ccf_resources/measuring_outcomes.pdf).

Urden, L., Stacy, K. (2012). *Clinical nurse specialist productivity and outcomes.* Presented at the 7th Annual International Nurse Practitioner/Advanced Practice Nursing Network Conference. London, August 20-22, 2012.

Varughese, A. M., Byczkowski, T. L., Wittkugel, E. P., Kotagal, U., & Dean, K. (2006). Impact of a nurse practitioner–assisted preoperative assessment program on quality. *Pediatric Anesthesia, 16*, 723–733.

Wagner, L. M., Capezuti, E., Brush, B., Boltz, M., Renz, S., & Talerico, K. A. (2007). Description of an advanced practice nursing consultative model to reduce restrictive siderail use in nursing homes. *Research in Nursing & Health, 30*, 131–140.

Wakefield, M. K. (2010). Nurses and the Affordable Care Act. *American Journal of Nursing, 110*, 9–11.

Walker, D. S., Day, S., Diroff, C., Lirette, H., McCully, L., Mooney-Hescott, C., et al. (2002). Reduced frequency prenatal visits in midwifery practice: Attitudes and use. *Journal of Midwifery & Women's Health, 47*, 269–277.

Way, D., Jones, L., Baskerville, B., & Busing, N. (2001). Primary health care services by nurse practitioners and family physicians in shared practice. *Canadian Medical Association Journal, 165*, 1210–1214.

Williams, D., & Sidani, S. (2001). An analysis of the nurse practitioner role in palliative care. *Canadian Journal of Nursing Leadership, 14*, 13–19.

Windorski, S. K., & Kalb, K. A. (2002). Educating NPs to educate patients: Cholesterol screening in pediatric primary care. *Journal of Pediatric Health Care, 16*, 60–66.

Wojner, A. W. (2001). *Outcomes management: Application to clinical practice.* St. Louis: Mosby.

Wong, S. T., Stewart, A. L., & Gilliss, C. L. (2000). Evaluating advanced practice nursing through use of a heuristic framework. *Journal of Nursing Care Quality, 14*, 21–32.

Woods, L. (2006). Evaluating the clinical effectiveness of neonatal nurse practitioners: An exploratory study. *Journal of Clinical Nursing 15*, 35–44.

Yeager, S., Shaw, K. D., Casaant, J., & Burns, S. M. (2006). An acute care nurse practitioner model of care for neurosurgical patients. *Critical Care Nurse, 26*, 2657–2664.

Using Health Care Information Technology to Evaluate and Improve Performance and Patient Outcomes

Vicky A. Mahn-DiNicola

CHAPTER CONTENTS

The health care reform debate of this decade has generated countless hours of discussion on what the U.S. health care system will look like and how it will be paid for. Even with major steps forward, such as the Patient Protection and Affordable Care Act (PPACA; U.S. Department of Health and Human Services [HHS], 2011) and the creation of the Center for Medicare & Medicaid Services (CMS) Innovation, which is designed to stimulate new ways to pay for and deliver care (http://innovations.cms.gov), there is little agreement on which health care models will best achieve measureable progress on the challenges of cost and quality. Innovating health care systems, such as Kaiser Permanente, Intermountain Health Care, the Mayo Clinic, Geisinger Health System, and Bellin Health, are already taking action to achieve what the Institute for Healthcare Improvement (IHI) calls the Triple Aim. These three imperatives aim to do the following: (1) provide effective, safe, and reliable care to individuals; (2) improve the health of populations by focusing on prevention, wellness, and improved management of chronic disease; and (3) decrease per capita costs. (For an informative discussion on health care system innovation strategies in the United States, the reader is referred to Bisognano & Kenney, 2012).

Among the many options available to promote these goals, one stands out—wider deployment of and expanded practice parameters for advanced practice nurses (APNs). There is a fundamental fit between these national imperatives and the skills and expertise of each APN role. However, there are impediments in the regulatory environment that may place barriers to the full deployment of APNs. In a recent white paper published by the Institute of Medicine (IOM, 2011), *The Future of Nursing: Leading Change, Advancing Health,* Safriet (2011) noted that there are "conflicting and restrictive state provisions governing [APNs] scope of practice and prescriptive authority … as well as the fragmented and parsimonious state and federal standards for their reimbursement" (p. 2). Numerous examples are cited, in which APNs may not examine and certify patients for worker's compensation, order treatment for long-term care, or even make declarations of death. Extreme limitations in prescriptive authority exist in many states, as well as constraints for ordering durable medical equipment, physical therapy, or laboratory tests. Although Safriet (2011) has provided a comprehensive review of the many restrictions and limitations on APN practice and offers an array of arguments for reforming these regulatory restrictions, expanding APN practice autonomy and allowing for direct reimbursement, one thing is clear—the ability to demonstrate in a reliable and quantifiable manner that quality and cost-effective care can be consistently delivered by APNs is essential. Not only is this information needed to reform regulatory restrictions, it is needed by health care organizations to promote broader adoption and optimization of APN professional services in their emerging health care delivery models. Finally, this information is needed by the public to help raise awareness that APNs can deliver quality care in cost-effective ways. This means that it is every APN's responsibility to engage fully in meaningful evaluative activities that will inform all stakeholders, including other APNs, about their effectiveness.

This chapter will introduce basic to intermediate skills for using health care information technology and information management for the purposes of evaluating and improving practice and evaluating and improving outcomes for the patient populations served by APNs. For our purposes here, the terms *outcome evaluation* and *performance improvement* will be used interchangeably and may refer to three levels of outcome evaluation: (1) activities that evaluate individual APN practice, such as peer review; (2) activities that evaluate the collective value of all APNs to an organization or population, such as a research or demonstration project; or (3) outcomes in clinical populations served by all providers, including APNs, in an organization or population. Depending on the nature of the outcome evaluation activity and metrics used to monitor performance, these activities may at times overlap and are not always mutually exclusive. For example, a performance indicator that examines the percentage of patients with diabetes who are evaluated annually to determine their hemoglobin A1c (HbA1c) level may be used to evaluate an individual APN's compliance to a standard of care, or it could be used to illustrate that populations managed by APNs have an acceptable rate of compliance compared to medical providers. This same indicator could also be what may be referred to as provider-agnostic, and used by a health care organization to report compliance to this best practice standard to a broader audience to demonstrate their ability to monitor high-risk populations appropriately in their community or region. Regardless of whether APNs engage in activities to monitor their own practice or the practice of other individual APNs in their organization, it is likely that APNs will also be engaged in the evaluation of quality and financial outcomes for broader populations, such as for a given payer (e.g., the Medicare population). The focus of the chapter will be on the competencies needed to perform outcome evaluation and manage health information using systems that are developing in the United States, although there are many resources used internationally that are also identified. This is an exceedingly complex landscape, with terminology unfamiliar to most clinicians, but it is critical to APN success in the current health care climate.

Regulatory Reporting Initiatives that Drive Performance Improvement

In addition to the regulatory environment that affects APN practice, there is also a dynamic and ever-changing regulatory environment to which health care organizations must respond. In the United States, legislative requirements are being released by the CMS or HHS and posted in the *Federal Registry* numerous times each year. With each new posting, expanding reporting requirements are imposed on almost every point of service across the health care continuum. Although these reporting requirements are generally presented in the spirit of improving quality and patient safety, requirements for reporting quality data are increasingly being tied to financial reimbursement. Reimbursement for Medicare and Medicaid claims can be reduced for excessive readmissions, hospital-acquired infections and complications, substandard performance in evidence-based best practices, and decreased patient satisfaction scores. In postacute care settings there are emerging reporting requirements to monitor worsening of pressure ulcers, catheter-acquired urinary tract infections (CAUTIs), central line–associated blood stream infections (CLABSIs), and vaccination of health care personnel for influenza. The United States has truly evolved from a pay for reporting culture to one of pay for performance. Table 24-1 provides a summary of these reporting programs, along with a brief description of their impact on Medicare reimbursement.

Because many CMS reporting initiatives reuse the same measures, it is possible for substandard performance in even a single measure to have a number of financial impacts across a health care organization. For example, one measure that looks at the delivery of percutaneous coronary intervention (PCI) within 90 minutes of hospital arrival for acute myocardial infarction (AMI) is used in three reporting programs, including the CMS Hospital Inpatient Quality Program (HIQR), CMS Value-Based Purchasing (VBP) program, and CMS Stage 2 Meaningful Use of the electronic health record (EHR) program for hospitals and critical access hospitals. Failure to collect accurate and complete data, report it to the CMS by designated time frames, and achieve acceptable results in performance for even one required measure can result in sizeable reduction in payment to the hospital from the CMS.

Some measures, such as CLABSI, not only apply to multiple quality reporting programs in a single health care facility, they also apply to multiple care settings across the continuum, including acute care hospitals, cancer care hospitals, ambulatory surgery centers, and long-term care facilities. Thus, failure to comply with reporting

TABLE 24-1 Summary of Center for Medicare & Medicaid Services Quality Reporting Programs Affecting Financial Reimbursement in the United States

Program	Description	Measures Reported in 2013-2014	Web Resource
VBP program	Hospitals contribute 1% in fiscal year (FY) 2013, progressing to 2% of their total annual Medicare revenue by 2017; have the opportunity to earn back up to 1.8 times their annual contribution based on their performance ranking compared with approximately 3092 U.S. hospitals in the 2012 VBP program.	• 12 clinical process of care metrics for AMI, heart failure, pneumonia, and surgical care improvement program (SCIP) • Hospital Consumer Assessment of Healthcare Providers and Systems (HCAHPS) survey • One AHRQ patient safety composite measure • CLABSI • Medicare spending per beneficiary	• http://www.cms.gov/Medicare/ Quality-Initiatives-Patient-Assessment-Instruments/ hospital-value based-purchasing/ index.html?redirect=/Hospital-Value-Based-Purchasing/
Hospital readmission reduction program	Hospitals with readmission rates > national median will be financially penalized by calculating the excess readmission ratio for AMI, HF, and pneumonia, which is a measure of a hospital's readmission performance compared with the national average for the hospital's set of patients with that applicable condition.	Risk-adjusted, 30-day readmissions for the following: • Acute MI • HF • Pneumonia • Total knee arthroplasty (beginning October 1, 2014) • Total hip arthroplasty (beginning October 1, 2014) • All cause inpatient unplanned 30-day readmissions (reported but not tied to payment adjustments; beginning October 1, 2014)	• http://www.cms.gov/Medicare/ Medicare-Fee-for-Service-Payment/AcuteInpatientPPS/ Readmissions-Reduction-Program.html
Hospital inpatient quality reporting program	Hospitals can lose 2% of their Medicare annual market basket update for failing to report data for all the required measures.	• Clinical process measures for AMI (four), HF (three), pneumonia (two), SCIP (eight) • ED throughput (two), global immunization (two), stroke (eight), venous thromboembolism (VTE; six), perinatal care (one) • HCAHPS survey • Structure of care (four measures in 2013, safe surgery checklist use to be added in 2014) • Medicare mortality (three measures) • Medicare readmission (five measures) • AHRQ patient safety composite measure • AHRQ death among surgical inpatients with serious treatable complications • Cost efficiency (one) • Surgical complications (one) • Hospital-acquired infection measures (six)	• http://www.cms.gov/Medicare/ Quality-Initiatives-Patient-Assessment-Instruments/ HospitalQualityInits/ HospitalRHQDAPU.html
Physician quality reporting system (PQRS)	PQRS uses incentives and up to a 0.5% payment adjustment to encourage reporting of quality data for covered services provided to Medicare Part B fee-for-service beneficiaries. Beginning in 2015, providers will incur penalties in the form of payment adjustments if they do not report data on these measures. PAs, NPs, CNSs, CRNAs, CNMs, clinical social workers, clinical psychologists, audiologists, physical therapists, occupational therapists, speech-language pathologists and registered dieticians are all eligible to participate in this program; highly applicable to APNs practicing in ambulatory settings.	• There are 196 PQRS measures, organized into 14 measure groups (asthma, back pain, coronary artery bypass graft, coronary artery disease, community-acquired pneumonia, chronic kidney disease, diabetes, hepatitis C, heart failure, HIV-AIDS, ischemic vascular disease, perioperative care, preventive care, rheumatoid arthritis). Of these, 56 measures can only be reported through a registry. Each group contains four to 10 individual measures. • An eligible provider can choose to report a minimum of three individual measures or all the measures in a single measure group. • The threshold for successful PQRS participation is at least 30 eligible patient encounters for measure group reporting or on 80% of all eligible Medicare Part B fee-for-service patients over a 12-mo time frame. • Measures are updated annually.	• http://www.medicare.gov/ find-a-doctor (S(qsuddyukjiazx5243zyxyv55))/ staticpages/data/pqrs/ physician-quality-reporting-system.aspx ?AspxAutoDetectCookieSupport=1

Continued

TABLE 24-1 Summary of Center for Medicare & Medicaid Services Quality Reporting Programs Affecting Financial Reimbursement in the United States—cont'd

Program	Description	Measures Reported in 2013-2014	Web Resource
Hospital outpatient quality reporting program	Hospitals lose 2% of their annual payment rate (APU) if they do not meet the administrative, data collection, submission, validation, and publication requirements of the outpatient prospective payment system.	• 24 outpatient measures (13 chart-abstracted measures for AMI, chest pain, and SCIP) • Seven imaging efficiency measures computed from CMS claims data for Medicare patients only • Four structure of care measures	• http://www.cms.gov/Medicare/Quality-Initiatives-Patient-Assessment-Instruments/HospitalQualityInits/HospitalOutpatientQualityReportingProgram.html
Ambulatory surgery center quality reporting program	A VBP incentive program; hospitals have the potential to earn an additional 1% in 2013 (increasing to 2% in 2017) depending on their performance on these measures relative to the national benchmarks.	• Five ambulatory surgical care measures for 2014 • Increasing to seven measures in 2015, with the addition of two structure of care indicators	• http://www.cms.gov/Medicare/Medicare-Fee-for-Service-Payment/ASCPayment/Downloads/C_ASC_RTC-2011.pdf • http://www.gpo.gov/fdsys/pkg/FR-2012-05-11/pdf/2012-9985.pdf
Long-term care hospital quality program	Effective for the 2014 payment update, hospitals will lose 2% of their APU for failing to report the required measures.	• Pressure ulcers • CAUTIs for ICU patients • CLABSIs for ICU and high-risk nursery patients	• http://www.cms.gov/Medicare/Quality-Initiatives-Patient-Assessment-Instruments/LTCH-Quality-Reporting/index.html • http://www.gpo.gov/fdsys/pkg/FR-2012-05-11/pdf/2012-9985.pdf
Inpatient psychiatric facility quality reporting	Beginning in 2014, inpatient psychiatric facilities must report the required measures to receive 2% of their Medicare payment.	• Six hospital-based inpatient psychiatric service (HBIPS) measures, including restraints, seclusions, medication management, and care transitioning	• http://www.cms.gov/Medicare/Quality-Initiatives-Patient-Assessment-Instruments/HospitalQualityInits/HospitalHighlights.html
Home health quality reporting program	Home health agencies will be required to report the required measures to avoid a 2% reduction in their market basket payment.	• Submission of the outcome and assessment information set (OASIS) measures • Five home HCAHPS measures	• http://www.gpo.gov/fdsys/pkg/FR-2012-07-13/pdf/2012-16836.pdf
Hospice quality reporting program	Beginning in 2014, hospice facilities will be required to submit required quality data to avoid a 2% reduction in their market basket increase.	Proposed rule for 2013: • Structure measure to assess if hospice collects at least three or more quality indicators • One pain management measure	• http://www.gpo.gov/fdsys/pkg/BILLS-111hr3590enr/pdf/BILLS-111hr3590enr.pdf
Prospective Payment System (PPS)-exempt cancer hospital quality reporting program	PPS-exempt cancer hospitals are required to report quality data. However, there are currently no financial incentives for doing so.	• Two National Healthcare Safety Network (NHSN) hospital-acquired infection measures • Three chemotherapy and hormonal therapy measures	• http://www.cms.gov/Medicare/Quality-Initiatives-Patient-Assessment-Instruments/HospitalQualityInits/HospitalHighlights.html

NOTE: The reader is encouraged to review the measures for each program annually, because legislation and health care reform result in frequent modifications to the reporting requirements of each program.

BOX 24-1 Shared Savings Program for Accountable Care Organizations Quality Measures

Patient and Caregiver Experience (CAHPS)*

- Getting Timely Care, Appointments, and Information
- How Well Your Doctors Communicate
- Patients' Rating of Doctor
- Access to Specialists
- Health Promotion and Education
- Shared Decision Making
- Health Status/Functional Status

Care Coordination and Patient Safety

- Ambulatory-sensitive conditions admissions—COPD and CHF (AHRQ prevention quality indicator)
- Number of primary care providers (PCPs; %) who successfully qualify for an EHR incentive program payment
- Medication reconciliation after discharge from an inpatient facility
- Screening for fall risk

Preventive Health

- Influenza immunization
- Pneumococcal vaccination
- Adult weight screening and follow-up
- Tobacco use assessment and tobacco cessation intervention
- Depression screening
- Colorectal cancer screening
- Mammography screening
- Proportion of adults ≥18 yr who had their blood pressure measured within the preceding 2 yr

At-Risk Populations

- Diabetes composite (all or nothing scoring)—nonuse of tobacco, aspirin use
- Diabetes mellitus—HbA1c poor control (>9%)
- Hypertension—blood pressure control
- Ischemic vascular disease—complete lipid profile and LDL control < 100 mg/dL, use of aspirin or another antithrombotic
- Heart failure—beta blocker therapy for left ventricular systolic dysfunction (LVSD)
- Coronary artery disease composite (all or nothing scoring)—angiotensin-converting enzyme (ACE) inhibitor or angiotensin receptor blocker (ARB) therapy for patients with CAD and diabetes and/or LVSD

Adapted from Center for Medicare & Medicaid Services (CMS). (2011). Medicare program; Medicare shared savings program: Accountable care organizations (https://www.federalregister.gov/articles/2011/11/02/2011-27461/medicare-program-medicare-shared-savings-program-accountable-care-organizations#h-68).

COPD, Chronic obstructive pulmonary disease.

*CAHPS asks patients to report on their experiences with a range of health care services at multiple levels of the delivery system. The survey asks about experiences with ambulatory care providers (e.g., health plans, physician offices, home care programs, mental health plans). The survey used to ask about experiences with care delivered in facilities such as hospitals and nursing homes, referred to as the HCAHPS survey. Although similar in nature, CAHPS and HCAHPS use slightly different questions and require specific protocols for survey administration. For additional information, see http://www.cahps.ahrq.gov/surveysguidance.htm.

requirements has the potential to affect reimbursement across an entire health care system. Additional measurement and reporting requirements for specialized services and health care systems also exist. Box 24-1 illustrates a recent set of measures that are required for health care systems reorganizing as accountable care organizations (ACOs). These measures focus on ambulatory populations and may overlap with several other reporting programs that exist simultaneously across an integrated health care organization, such as the measures required by the Health Resources and Services Administration (HRSA) for federal qualified health centers (see Box 24-2) or those required by providers who care for patients within selected payer niches, such as the Medicaid Adult Quality Measures Program (Box 24-3).

In addition to payer-mandated reporting programs, health care organizations also have specific reporting requirements to their accreditation bodies, including The Joint Commission (TJC), Healthcare Facilities Accreditation Program (HFAP), and Det Norske Veritas Healthcare

(DNV). It is not unusual for many of the measures required for accreditation to overlap with those reported to the CMS, although these measures typically reflect an all-payer population. What is important to note is that although many of these measures are similar across reporting programs, each program has its own specific requirements for data collection, data quality, and data submission, which must be strictly adhered to in order to ensure proper accreditation, achieve financial incentives, or avoid financial penalties. APNs should become familiar with the regulatory reporting requirements in their organization, recognizing that some measures may merit higher degrees of APN engagement and stewardship to create and sustain optimal results. The National Quality Forum (NQF) Community Tool to Align Measurement is a useful tool for the APN to review so he or she can become familiar with the measures required for his or her practice setting. This tool organizes NQF-endorsed clinical quality measures associated with major national and state reporting initiatives for all practice

BOX 24-2   Health Resources & Services Administration (HRSA) Uniform Data Set for Clinical and Financial Performance Measures*

Outreach and Quality of Care (%)

- Pregnant women beginning prenatal care in the first trimester
- Children age 2 yr during measurement year, with appropriate immunizations
- Women 21-64 yr of age who received one or more tests to screen for cervical cancer
- Patients 2-17 yr of age who had BMI percentile documentation, counseling for nutrition, and counseling for physical activity during the measurement year
- Patients ≥18 yr of age who had BMI calculated at last visit or within last 6 mo and, if overweight or underweight, had follow-up plan documented
- Patients ≥18 yr of age who were queried about tobacco use one or more times within 24 mo
- Patients ≥18 yr of age who are tobacco users and who received advice to quit smoking or tobacco use
- Patients 5-40 yr of age with a diagnosis of persistent asthma who were prescribed the

preferred long-term control medication or an acceptable alternative pharmacologic therapy during the current year

Health Outcomes and Disparities (%)

- Diabetic patients whose HbA1c levels are less than 7 percent, less than 8 percent, less than or equal to 9 percent or greater than 9 percent.
- Adult patients with diagnosed hypertension whose most recent blood pressure was less than 140/90
- Newborns weighing < 2500 g born to health center patients

Financial Viability and Cost

- Total cost per patient
- Medical cost per medical visit
- Change in net assets–to–expense ratio
- Working capital–to–monthly expenses ratio
- Long-term debt–to–equity ratio

Adapted from Health Resources and Services Administration (HRSA). (2011). Clinical and financial performance measures (http://bphc.hrsa.gov/policiesregulationsperformancemeasures/index.html).
*Required for federally qualified health centers.

settings into a single spreadsheet, which can then be sorted by various programs of interest. Hyperlinks are embedded in the spreadsheet so that it is easy to access the Quality Positioning System on the NQF website, on which measure definitions for each metric are maintained (http://www.qualityforum.org/AlignmentTool).

Traditionally, many reporting requirements required manual chart abstraction efforts, along with an element of clinical judgment to determine the correct response to questions about whether or not a particular standard of evidence-based best practice was met. Questions such as "Did the patient get smoking advice or cessation prior to discharge?" are typically abstracted by a review of patient education documentation in the medical record. However, some questions, such as "Was the patient eligible for ACE inhibitors at discharge?" may require a review and synthesis of multiple sources of information in the record, including the history and physical examination, cardiac imaging tests, or medical provider progress notes, before a determination can be made. These types of activities can be time-consuming and often are called into question about their reliability. APNs may be engaged in many aspects of the data collection and analysis activities

associated with chart-abstracted measures and should be mindful to avoid data collection activities that are strictly clerical in nature. Additional considerations about the APN role in data abstraction activities will be presented later, in the section on foundational competencies.

Finally, additional regulatory reporting requirements are beginning to emerge in the areas of patient safety, an area in which APNs will likely become engaged. The Patient Safety and Quality Improvement Act of 2005 established a voluntary patient safety event reporting system and guidelines for the establishment of patient safety organizations (Agency for Healthcare Research and Quality [AHRQ], 2005). This act called for the standardization of data used for event reporting based on the common formats established and maintained by AHRQ. Some of the initial risk events being reported include medication errors, patient falls, central line infections, and pressure ulcers. At the time of this writing, the NQF is proposing to include the reporting of readmissions data into patient safety organizations (PSOs) for purposes of shared learning across organizations. Although these emerging reporting requirements have not yet been adopted internationally, they are originally based on an

BOX 24-3   CMS Medicaid Adult Quality Reporting Quality Measures

Prevention and Health Promotion

- Flu shots for adults ages 50-64 yr (collected as part of HEDIS CAHPS supplemental survey)
- Adult BMI assessment
- Breast cancer screening
- Cervical cancer screening
- Medical assistance with smoking and tobacco use cessation (collected as part of HEDIS CAHPS supplemental survey)
- Screening for clinical depression and follow-up plan
- Plan all-cause readmission
- Diabetes, short term complications admission rate
- Chronic obstructive pulmonary disease admission rate
- Congestive heart failure admission rate
- Adult asthma admission rate
- Chlamydia screening in women ages 21-24 yr

Management of Acute Conditions

- Follow-up after hospitalization for mental illness
- Elective delivery
- Antenatal steroids

Management of Chronic Conditions

- Annual HIV-AIDS medical visit
- Controlling high blood pressure
- Comprehensive diabetes care—LDL cholesterol screening, HbA1c testing
- Antidepressant medication management
- Adherence to antipsychotics for individuals with schizophrenia
- Annual monitoring for patients on persistent medications

Family Experiences of Care

- HCAHPS health plan survey v. 4.0—adult questionnaire with CAHPS health plan survey v. 4.0, H-NCQA supplemental

Care Coordination

- Care transition record transmitted to health care professional

Availability

- Initiation and engagement of alcohol and other drug dependence treatment
- Prenatal and postpartum care—postpartum care rate

Adapted from Center for Medicare & Medicaid Services (CMS). (2012). Medicaid program: Initial core set of health care quality measures for Medicaid-eligible adults (https://www.federalregister.gov/articles/2012/01/04/2011-33756/medicaid-program-initial-core-set-of-health-care-quality-measures-for-medicaid-eligible-adults#h-17).

international movement through the World Health Organization (WHO), which adopted a framework for an International Classification for Patient Safety to compare patient safety across disciplines and organizations and examine the roles of system and human factors in patient safety (WHO, 2009). The longitudinal work of the WHO is to develop an international classification system of codes that can be used to track patient safety events and the contributing factors leading up to the adverse event. APNs can play a critical role in identifying potential safety issues and developing priorities and safety solutions across all care delivery settings.

Relevance of Regulatory Reporting to Advanced Practice Nursing Outcomes

The national quality, patient safety, and accreditation reporting requirements are relevant to APN outcome evaluation for several reasons. First, they are of critical interest to the organizations that employ APNs. Many health care organizations are carefully tracking key performance measures that affect their financial bottom line in scorecards or dashboards, which are then communicated to all stakeholders, from clinical units to the board room. In many organizations, financial incentives and annual bonuses for those in strategic and operational leadership roles, as well as other key clinical staff, are based on achieving designated performance thresholds. Organizations monitor their performance against competitive market segments using comparative benchmarking systems so that they can ensure that their performance exceeds that of their peer groups. This is important not only to maintain their reputation within their community and market but also because several CMS programs, specifically the Value-Based Purchasing (VBP) and Hospital Readmission Reduction Programs, base financial incentives on the organization's ranking across approximately 3000 U.S. hospitals that are competing for incentive dollars in these programs.

The second and more compelling reason why national regulatory reporting initiatives are critical to APN outcome evaluation is because so many of the clinical processes and outcomes reflected in these performance measures are directly sensitive to APN intervention. Thus, active participation in the data collection, data analysis, and resulting performance improvement initiatives provide a rich forum to make the value added associated with the APN contribution highly visible across the organization. In many organizations, key regulatory performance metrics are included in individual provider profiles and integrated into ongoing professional practice evaluation (OPPE) activities. Although the APN has a direct and immediate opportunity to influence outcomes for many of these measures, linking APN to the performance trend is often a challenge, particularly in an acute care hospital environment in which so many providers contribute to the management of a single patient's care episode. For example, medical orders for a patient with heart failure (HF) who is eligible for angiotensin-converting enzyme (ACE) inhibitors at discharge could be written by the patient's physician, cardiac specialist, hospitalist, or acute care nurse practitioner (ACNP) who is accountable for overseeing the cardiac medical population. In the absence of a fully adopted computerized physician order entry (CPOE) system, most information or clinical documentation systems do not capture the provider responsible for ordering individual medications or nonprocedural treatments. This often causes great debate and mistrust of the data among providers.

One approach to this limitation used by many organizations is to conduct a quality review on patients who failed to receive a given standard of care. Quality specialists review the medical records for each opportunity for improvement, whereby provider attribution is assigned directly in the quality software and displayed in the provider scorecard. In this type of metric, the desired performance target is zero deficiencies versus 100% compliance. Medical providers with a recurring pattern of deficiencies are then subject to more formal peer review processes within their organizations. Another model for achieving accurate provider attribution is to select four to six records per month randomly for each provider and evaluate whether specific standards of care were met or not met. Values are tracked in a profile and reported in monthly committee meetings. APN provider groups can achieve greater levels of transparency and credibility across their organization by placing key metrics that track compliance to known best practices on department and corporate scorecards and dashboards.

Foundational Competencies in Managing Health Information Technology

At the heart of any performance measurement activity is the ability to collect data and analyze results effectively that can reliably and accurately inform and educate stakeholders about an outcome or process. In health care, these data typically consist of three types of information—clinical, financial, and administrative data. Clinical data, such as a patient's medication list or a radiology report, are generally found in the EHR (also referred to as the electronic medical record [EMR]). In some cases, clinical data may be found in specialized registries, such as the registry of the Society of Thoracic Surgeons (STS) which collects data on open heart surgical outcomes and related cardiac diseases. Financial data, such as the cost of a given hospital stay or drug, is typically tied to a cost accounting, general ledger, or billing system. Administrative data, such as a patient's age, gender, or address is typically tied to a patient registration system (often referred to as an admission-discharge-transfer [ADT] system in acute care hospitals). Collectively, the health information systems (HIS) that store these data types are generally referred to as health information technology (HIT), although the term *HIT* often has broader implications, including servers, cloud-based platforms, networks, clinical data warehouses, mobile applications, and point of care laboratory devices. Minimum informatics competencies are required before one may access the various HIT applications in an organization.

Although APNs directly engage with these technologies at various levels, not all APNs are able to manipulate independently the various HIS needed to compile the data required to evaluate outcomes. More advanced skills from nurse informatics specialists or other expert report writers may be needed to capture necessary information, such as creating a customized report or merging files from multiple databases to assemble the required information. However, stronger informatics competencies in HIT are needed by APNs to design the evaluation strategy, validate the data, and interpret the findings effectively. For APNs prepared at the Doctor of Nursing Practice (DNP) level, the expectation is that the APN is prepared to "apply new knowledge, manage individual and aggregate level information, and assess the efficacy of patient care technology appropriate to a specialized area of practice" (American Association of Colleges of Nursing [AACN], 2006, p. 12). DNP graduates also design, select, and use information systems technology to evaluate programs of care, outcomes of care, and care systems. The expectations for being fluent in the use of technology are reflected in almost every DNP competency (AACN, 2006).

TIGER Competencies for Use of Health Care Information Technology

The Technology Informatics Guiding Education Reform (TIGER) Initiative was formed in 2004 to bring together nursing stakeholders to develop a shared vision, strategies, and specific actions for improving nursing practice, education, and the delivery of patient care through the use of HIT. The TIGER Informatics Competencies Collaborative (TICC) team was formed to develop informatics recommendations for all practicing nurses and graduating nursing students, including APNs. The TIGER competency model consists of three parts—basic computer competencies, information literacy, and information management. It was the ambitious goal of the TIGER Initiative that all three million practicing and graduating nurses in the United States achieve these competencies by January 2013.

The basic computer competency requires the completion of the European Computer Driving License (ECDL) Foundation set of computer competencies. Although at first glance these competencies appear rather basic, they are comprehensive and include concepts relating to hardware, securities, networks, system performance, file compression and file transfer protocols, file management, operating systems, and a wide range of utilities. ECDL certification, already completed by over seven million Europeans, requires more than 30 hours of study and consists of seven modules—concepts of information and communication technology, file management, word processing, spreadsheets, using databases, presentation, and web browsing.

The second competency involves information literacy. Information literacy is critical to incorporating evidence-based practice into nursing practice. The APN must be able to determine what information is needed to assess outcomes of care, identify practice variation, and establish best practices. Furthermore, critical thinking and assessment skills are needed when evaluating or appraising the information and validating the source of the information. There are five components of information literacy that promote competency in the skills necessary to define what information is needed to solve a particular problem and to access, evaluate, and use that information effectively and efficiently.

The third competency involves information management, which is the underlying concept for performance measurement. This involves the process of collecting data, processing data, and presenting and communicating the processed data as meaningful information or knowledge. In addition, APNs must understand and comply with their organization's Health Insurance Portability and Accountability Act (HIPAA) policies and procedures, which provide for how and when patient protected health information (PHI) may be used and under what circumstances it must be de-identified (meaning the removal of any unique patient identifiers, such as name, birth date, medical record numbers, social security numbers, and other personal information that could potentially identify specific individuals within a data set). Breaches of information, such as an unintentional disclosure of PHI in an unencrypted e-mail or a stolen laptop or device with PHI on it, must be immediately reported to the organization's compliance officer; this can result in financial fines and

legal consequences for the health care organization. Box 24-4 lists resources for obtaining additional information about the TIGER competencies.

In addition to the TIGER competencies, APNs engaged in performance improvement activities may also require additional expertise in the information and quality management domains. These include an understanding of the various coding taxonomies and terminology sets used to classify health care data, proficiency with statistical tools, such as statistical process control charts (SPCs), which examine time-trended data, familiarity with benchmark data, data mining methods and analytics, and knowledge about any risk adjustment methodologies that may pertain to the clinical populations being evaluated.

Although organizations such as the IHI and the National Association for Healthcare Quality (NAHQ) can support the APN in achieving competency in many of the skill sets needed for successful outcome evaluation, developing such expertise in graduate programs is a challenge. Academic institutions that prepare APNs must seek alliances with practice environments that not only exemplify or aspire to the best in professional nursing practice, but also are learning organizations that are fully invested in the quality improvement process. Institutional commitments to adopting best practices are essential if health care systems are to keep pace with new developments in performance measurement and outcomes evaluation. In addition, a robust, integrated, and reliable information systems infrastructure in the clinical environment is essential to assist the APN student and graduate to achieve hands-on competencies in informatics and system evaluation.

Although most health care organizations have quality management departments with the expertise to build an outcome evaluation plan and conduct the actual data collection and reporting tasks, the APN should understand these concepts to participate in, and in some cases lead, performance measurement activities actively throughout the full data-information-knowledge continuum. Without these competencies and skill sets, APNs may find that their level of participation is often limited to routine data collection tasks that do not require critical thinking or clinical judgment. APNs should limit participation in direct data collection activities unless it is part of their professional peer review process or if the data collection process is integrated into direct patient care and clinical documentation activities. For example, the minimum data set (MDS) used in long-term care settings to capture quality indicators relating to pressure ulcers, CAUTI and CLABSI, are routinely collected from retrospective data and do not require an APN's time to abstract records and prepare reports. Rather, APNs should be validating the accuracy of the data, monitoring performance trends, and

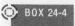 **BOX 24-4** Resources for European Computer Driving License Certification, Information Literacy, and Information Management

Technology Informatics Guiding Education Reform
This website posts the most current competencies and explains the learning curriculum and competencies in detail: www.tigersummit.com.

European Computer Driving License Foundation
The ECDL syllabus is maintained and periodically updated by the ECDL Foundation (http://ecdl.com).

Computer Skills (CS) Placement
CS Placement is the official distributor of ECDL in the United States. They offer e-learning courses and certification examinations (www.csplacement.com).

Healthcare Information Management System Society (HIMSS)
HIMSS has a certificate, Health Informatics Training System (HITS), that is substantially equivalent to ECDL (www.himss.org).

American Library Association (ALA)
The ALA's report, *Information Literacy Competency Standards for Higher Education,* lists performance indicators and outcomes for each standard (http://

www.ala.org/ala/mgrps/divs/acrl/standards/informationliteracycompetency.cfm).

Information Literacy in Technology (iLIT)
The iLIT test assesses the student's ability to access, evaluate, incorporate, and use information (http://www.ilitassessment.com).

HL7 EHR System Functional Model
The American National Standards Institute (ANSI) standard can be used by nursing instructors and educators to develop curriculum to impart the recommended information management competencies (http://www.hl7.org/EHR).

Digital Patient Record Certification (DPRC)
The DPRC program is endorsed by the American Medical Informatics Association and provides tools to assess a health care professional's ability to manage patient records in a digital environment accurately, dependably, and legally (http://dprcertification.com).

Alliance for Nursing Informatics
This organization supports the development of leaders in nursing informatics and provides programs to achieve HIT competencies (http://www.allianceni.org).

ensuring that best practices are implemented and fully adopted by the interdisciplinary team. Exemplar 24-1 illustrates a scenario of appropriate APN engagement with data collection activities associated with a professional peer review process for the purposes of outcome evaluation and performance improvement.

Coding Taxonomies and Classification Systems

As noted, APNs must understand the data-information-knowledge continuum and be able to articulate the type of data that they require to meet their information needs most effectively. In this regard, it is necessary for APNs to understand how various coding taxonomies and terminology sets are used in health information management for generating claims, and how this information can be leveraged for purposes of outcome evaluation. For inpatient settings, this would include concepts of the International Classification of Diseases (ICD; for versions 9 and 10; ICD-9 and ICD-10) codes for diagnoses and procedures. ICD codes are alphanumeric designations given to almost every diagnosis, description of symptoms, and cause of death attributed to humans and are used worldwide.

In addition, APNs practicing in acute care hospital settings must understand that for every claim there is a single principle ICD diagnosis code that indicates the primary reason for a patient's admission to the hospital. In addition, there may be multiple secondary ICD diagnosis codes that represent comorbid conditions that were present at the time of admission or conditions and complications that were acquired during the hospital stay. ICD procedure codes also have a designated principle procedure, which is typically the initial major procedure during the admission or care encounter. Many U.S. hospitals code as many as 25 to 50 secondary ICD-9 diagnoses and procedure codes in the medical claim; this number is expected to rise significantly once the transition from ICD-9-CM to ICD-10-CM is complete in October 2014. In addition, the ICD diagnosis status flag of present on admission (POA) or not present on admission (NPOA) can be used to differentiate between hospital-acquired conditions and those acquired prior to hospitalization. This is useful when evaluating phenomenon such as hospital-acquired pneumonia, pressure ulcers, acute renal failure, and sepsis. The APN should become familiar with the coding practices in their practice settings, because not all countries or organizations have adopted the use of the POA and NPOA status flags.

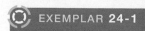 **EXEMPLAR 24-1**   **Walgreens Take Care Clinics**[SM] **Make Advanced Practice Nursing Outcomes Transparent to the World***

Walgreens Take Care Clinics has created an emerging market segment in health care delivery. The care provided is acute and episodic, family-oriented care for patients older than 18 months. Although not positioned like an emergency or urgent care clinic, in which full laboratory and imaging resources are readily available, the care provided in the Take Care Clinics help patients without immediate access to primary care providers while also providing preventive services, such as immunizations. Common complaints typically addressed with this service include upper respiratory infections (URIs), ear infections, minor sprains and injuries, school physicals, vaccinations, and screening and counseling services for hypertension, hyperlipidemia, and diabetes. More urgent conditions, such as sudden onset chest pain, active bleeding, or trauma are redirected to the nearest emergency care center. Patients can preschedule clinic visits online or walk in during hours of operation, which include extended evening and weekend hours. Clinics are located directly inside select Walgreens stores across the United States and, as of this writing, are staffed by over 1400 board-certified family nurse practitioners (FNPs).

APNs who practice in a Walgreens Take Care Clinic typically care for patients in an autonomous and technology-driven environment. Patients register at a touch screen kiosk when they arrive and services and pricing are visible via a liquid crystal display (LCD) screen outside the clinic. Patients are then seen in an examining room, which is generally located next to the pharmacy. During the visit, the APN will interview the patient, entering information into a proprietary EHR designed expressly for Walgreens, with input from APN end users. This EHR contains key information about the patient's health status and prompts the APN to inquire about selected data elements necessary to compute various health care quality outcomes. It also tracks any prescribed medications and generates discharge instructions, which are printed out and provided to the patients prior to their departure from the examination room, allowing the patient time and privacy to review instructions with the APN. Finally, patients are invited to take a brief satisfaction survey in the kiosk outside the examination room following their visit, thus ensuring feedback immediately after the visit.

As part of the Walgreens quality improvement program, Take Care Clinic uses a tool known as HEDIS (**h**ealth care **e**ffectiveness **d**ata and **i**nformation **s**et). HEDIS is a set of health care quality standards developed by the National Committee for Quality Assurance (NCQA). HEDIS is used by hospitals, physician offices, and clinics across the country to measure the quality of care they provide. Three performance measures are publicly reported at http://takecarehealth.com/Quality_And_Patient.aspx and include the following:

- Percentage of children 18 months to 18 years of age who were diagnosed and appropriately treated for an upper respiratory infection
- Percentage of patients 18 to 64 years who were diagnosed and appropriately treated for bronchitis
- Percentage of children 2 to 18 years who appropriately received a group A *Streptococcus* (strep) test when prescribed an antibiotic for pharyngitis

Every month, each APN is engaged in a professional peer review process whereby they receive randomly assigned electronic charts to review against best practice standards and quality documentation. Patient identifiers are stripped from the record, as is any information that will identify the individual APN who delivered the care. APNs then review their assigned records and enter their feedback into the computerized peer review application. In some cases, recommendations are offered to assist the growth and development of a fellow practitioner. For example, in one clinical review of a pediatric patient who presented with a URI, as well as childhood eczema, the reviewer offered a comment that it might be helpful to offer the family specific dietary counseling and skin care advice for improved management of the eczema as a comorbid condition. This recommendation later became part of a larger quality improvement strategy whereby patient educational materials on diet and skin care for pediatric eczema were developed and made available for use by all APNs across the Walgreens network.

On completion of monthly peer review activities, results of the audits are returned to the APN who completed the care; the identities of the reviewers are not disclosed. APNs may then review and validate their scores and feedback. Although occurring very rarely, there is a process for an APN to challenge their review findings by meeting with their local area APN manager and, if needed, the medical provider assigned to their practice. In addition, each APN has the ability to participate in monthly grand rounds, during which interesting and challenging cases are presented and discussed. Finally, all clinic quality and patient satisfaction scores are reported and discussed

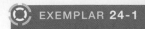

Walgreens Take Care Clinics^SM Make Advanced Practice Nursing Outcomes Transparent to the World—cont'd

in quarterly market meetings, in which attendance is required for all Walgreens APN employees nationally. Quality scores for the HEDIS measures are consistently outstanding and significantly exceed published national benchmarks, thus meeting best practice standards in the treatment of URI, bronchitis, and pharyngitis in adult and pediatric populations. Patient satisfaction is reported by region using the Gallup patient engagement score (1 to 5), in which responses typically average in the 4.4 to 4.78 range for all regions across the United States and are viewable for patients by region online.

*The author wishes to thank Walgreens and Sandra Ryan, Chief Nurse Practitioner Officer for Walgreens Take Care Clinics, for their generous time and support in describing the quality improvement process used by the APN practices at Walgreens.

APNs practicing in the US should also have a strong working knowledge of the Medicare Severity Diagnosis-Related Groups (MS-DRGs). They should understand how clinical documentation by APN and medical providers directly affect MS-DRG assignments and ultimately reimbursement. Many U.S. health care organizations are actively implementing clinical documentation improvement (CDI) programs in their institutions for purposes of coaching and training medical providers and APNs in improving their documentation skills for greater precision and accuracy in medical records coding and billing. Greater detail in the medical record can potentially lead to higher reimbursement and fewer denials and audits from payers, which are prevalent in the U.S. health care payment system. APNs should expect to have some level of inspection and chart review built into their credentialing process that reflects CDI initiatives in their organization, especially if they are practicing in an acute care setting.

Finally, it may be useful for APNs to understand other types of coding taxonomies and terminology sets that are available for purposes of quality reporting and research. Table 24-2 summarizes several common taxonomies used in inpatient and ambulatory settings.

Data such as ICD or Systematized Nomenclature of Medicine—Clinical Terms (SNOMED-CT) codes that have alphanumeric identifiers that can be easily queried from a database are termed *discrete* or *structured data*. Data containing dictated sentences and phrases, such as radiology reports, operative summaries, or history and physical dictations are termed *nondiscrete* or *unstructured*. Compiling and analyzing unstructured data is typically more challenging. Unless the organization has technology with a sophisticated reporting system containing a tool for natural language processing (NLP), with a well-developed and tested rules engine for discriminating between patients with active pneumonia and those without (e.g., the phrases "pneumonia ruled out" or "no signs of pneumonia" should not be included in a list of active

pneumonia patients), obtaining this type of data may yield too many false-positives to be a reliable and valid screening tool.

Although it is not necessary for the APN to understand the precision behind the coding processes, it is highly recommended that APNs spend time shadowing with a medical records coder (also referred to as a health information management specialist) to understand the timing and manner in which the various terminology sets are used. This is important to outcomes evaluation because some types of data are more useful than others, even though they represent similar concepts. For example, the phenomenon of pneumonia could be captured from the claim (using an ICD-9 diagnosis or CPT-4 code), laboratory culture and sensitivity report (using Logical Observation Identifiers Names and Codes [LOINC] and RxNorm codes), problem list in the EHR (using SNOMED-CT codes), chest imaging report (using natural language processing), or a dictated history and physical report (requiring manual chart abstraction). Although each source of information in the EHR may be correct, the APN may have to determine the best source of information to address the nature of the inquiry in the most timely, efficient, and accurate manner. Exemplar 24-2 illustrates the critical evaluation of the various data types that an APN would conduct when planning to deploy a new strategy to improve care, as well as the collaborative process with quality and informatics specialists that will benefit the APN in the outcome evaluation efforts.

Descriptive, Predictive, and Prescriptive Data Analytics

Another component of outcomes evaluation in which APNs need to become proficient involves understanding how data will ultimately be used to inform stakeholders about a phenomenon of interest. This may come in the form of performance metrics that describe historical trends for outcomes or processes that have happened in

TABLE 24-2	Coding Taxonomies and Terminology Sets Commonly Used in Outcomes Evaluation	
Coding Taxonomy	**Description**	**Website**
ICD-9-CM: ICD, version 9, clinical modification diagnosis codes	Approximately 13,000 codes three to five characters in length Used primarily in the United States and United Arab Emirates (UAE) to classify diagnoses for inpatient hospital claims Coding set lacks detail and laterality. Limited space for adding new codes United States targeted to sunset ICD-9 diagnosis codes October 1, 2014.	www.cms.gov/ICD9
ICD-9 procedure codes: ICD, version 9, procedure codes	Approximately 3,000 codes three or four characters in length Used primarily in the United States to classify diagnoses for inpatient hospital claims Coding set lacks detail and laterality Lacks precision to define procedures adequately. Based on outdated technology United States targeted to sunset ICD-9 procedure codes October 1, 2014.	www.cms.gov/ICD9
ICD-10-CM diagnosis codes: ICD, version 10, clinical modification diagnosis codes	Approximately 68,000 available codes three to seven alphanumeric characters in length Used by most countries worldwide (United States targeted for transition in 2014) to classify diagnoses for inpatient hospital claims Coding set is very specific and contains laterality. Flexible for adding new codes	www.cms.gov/ICD10
ICD-10 procedure codes: ICD, version 10, procedure codes	Approximately 87,000 available codes seven alphanumeric characters in length Used by most countries worldwide except the United States and UAE (United States targeted for transition in 2013) to classify procedures for inpatient hospital claims Coding set very specific, provides for precisely defined procedures and laterality.	www.cms.gov/ICD10
CPT (current procedural terminology)	Approximately 7800 available codes for reporting medical, surgical, and diagnostic services in outpatient and office settings, as well as acute care emergency settings, ambulatory surgery, and inpatient procedures done in some hospitals outside the United States. CPT is a registered trademark of the American Medical Association and is considered a proprietary terminology set requiring licensure before using inside an HIT application. New codes are released each October.	www.ama-assn.org/med-sci/cpt
HCPCS: Healthcare Common Procedure Coding System	There are two types of HCPCS codes. Level 1 HCPCS codes are identical to CPT codes used for reporting services and procedures in outpatient and office settings to Medicare, Medicaid, and private health insurers. Level II HCPCS codes are used by medical suppliers other than physicians, such as ambulance services or durable medical equipment.	www.cms.gov/HCPCSReleaseCodeSets
SNOMED-CT	Complex and highly hierarchical collection of over a million codes and medical terms that describe diseases, procedures, symptoms, findings, and more Developed by the College of American Pathologists and the National Health Service (Britain) Used extensively throughout the world, SNOMED-CT codes help organize content in the EHR and cross-walk to other terminologies such as ICD-9, ICD-10, and LOINC.	www.snomed.org
LOINC	Universal standard containing 58,000 observation terms for identifying medical laboratory tests and clinical observations, as well as nursing diagnosis, nursing interventions, outcomes classification, and patient care data sets Originally developed in the United States in 1994; international adoption expanding rapidly	http://loinc.org

Continued

TABLE 24-2   Coding Taxonomies and Terminology Sets Commonly Used in Outcomes Evaluation—*cont'd*

Coding Taxonomy	Description	Website
RxNorm	Standardized nomenclature for clinical drugs produced by the National Library of Medicine. This data set is updated monthly to stay abreast of the rapidly changing pharmaceutical industry. It contains links between national drug codes, which are used widely in EHRs and e-prescribing systems.	http://www.nlm.nih.gov/research/umls/rxnorm/docs/index.html
MS-DRGs	Each inpatient hospital stay in the United States is assigned one of over 750 MS-DRG codes, which are used for billing to Medicare and other payers. Codes are derived from ICD diagnoses and procedure codes. Many conditions are split into one, two, or three MS-DRGs based on whether any one of the secondary diagnoses has been categorized as a major complication or comorbidity (MCC), a CC, or no CC, and are weighted accordingly to reflect severity and reimbursement. Note that a separate MS-DRG code set for long-term care is used (MS-LTC-DRG). Additional coding sets apply to other areas of care (e.g., resource utilization groups [RUGs] apply to skilled nursing and rehabilitation stays).	www.cms.hhs.gov/AcuteInpatientPPS/FFD/list.asp
3M APR DRGs: (All Patient Refined Diagnosis Related Groups)	Used predominately for illness severity and risk of mortality adjustments, this proprietary coding set is commonly used to disseminate comparative performance data for hospitals and providers. APR-DRGs are derived from ICD codes; inpatients are assigned one APR-DRG code, along with a severity of illness code (1-4) and a risk of mortality code (1-4). Although APR DRGs are used internationally, 3M also supports international refined (IR-DRGs), which apply to inpatient and outpatient populations. Additional 3M methods are available to assess and forecast longitudinal resource consumption for designated populations.	http://solutions.3m.com/wps/portal/3M

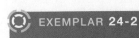 **EXEMPLAR 24-2**   Evaluating Data Types When Using Health Information Technology to Implement Practice Change

An APN working in a 400-bed, acute care setting needs to identify all inpatients with an active diagnosis of pneumonia to ensure that all best practice interventions have been implemented in a timely and appropriate manner. Although the performance in these areas is retrospectively monitored and reported periodically by the quality management department, the APN wishes to engage in the process concurrently to influence outcomes for this population. The APN's intervention is to perform clinical rounds several times a day on this population to ensure optimal delivery of best practice standards. These include antibiotic timeliness, appropriateness of antibiotic selection in intensive care unit (ICU) and non-ICU patients, smoking cessation advice and counseling, and influenza and pneumococcal vaccinations. The APN wants to leverage the hospital's information systems to create a real-time alert notification system to identify and track patients with pneumonia immediately on any nursing unit and then monitor performance trends to reflect the impact of her interventions on this population.

The APN recognizes that there are multiple taxonomies and methodologies that could be used to identify pneumonia patients in her organization and begins to inventory the pros and cons of each data type and source to create the best technology solution for her requirements. ICD-9 diagnosis codes are a typical taxonomy for identifying patients with pneumonia. Although these codes are readily available, reliable and robust population identifiers in other types of outcome evaluation measures used in her organization, such as length of stay, mortality, and readmissions, this approach would not be optimal because ICD-9 codes are typically not assigned until after the patient is discharged and the medical record is coded for the claim. Using this type of data element is too retrospective to be able to identify patients with pneumonia on a real-time basis.

The APN next considers a more concurrent coding methodology, which is based on the active problem lists in the EHR. In collaboration with a health information management specialist, a list of problem types and their corresponding SNOMED-CT codes is established,

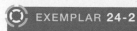

EXEMPLAR 24-2   **Evaluating Data Types When Using Health Information Technology to Implement Practice Change**—*cont'd*

which can be used to identify patients with an active diagnosis of pneumonia. However, this approach is ruled out because medical provider adoption of the new EHR has not yet fully expanded to the critical care units at her hospital. In addition, she has observed that many medical providers in the organization do not update the problem list in the EHR until the patient is being discharged, which makes a real time query unreliable.

The final option that the APN considers to create automated alerts is the use of radiology and laboratory reports with the words containing *pneumonia* or other related terms. In discussing this option with a nursing informatics specialist at her organization, she learns that the EHR has been fully implemented to report laboratory results for all clinical areas in the hospital and that this includes microbiology results. Using the LOINC (Logical Observation Identifiers Names and Codes) coding terminology set, patients with pneumonia can be identified as soon as the laboratory result transaction is received in the EHR. In addition, she learns of a pilot project in the Quality Department in which cardiac catheterization reports are being processed by an NLP engine to capture cardiac registry information. She asks about the potential to expand this pilot to include

radiology reports to identify pneumonia patients. The Quality Department agrees to expand the project scope with the help of the APN to begin formulating a list of phrases that will be used to identify pneumonia positively in a radiology report. The APN collaborates with the medical director of radiology to create the final list of terms to be used in the pilot.

After 3 months of implementing the practice change, the APN is able to demonstrate that performance in five best practice indicators for patients with pneumonia is almost 100% across the organization. She tracks the compliance rates in an SPC chart, which demonstrates a statistically significant favorable change in the process. Furthermore, she is able to use the organization's value-based purchasing calculator to demonstrate a financial contribution to the hospital's Medicare reimbursement program of almost $68,000 simply by improving performance. The APN plans to make a formal recommendation to expand similar APN interventions to other key populations influenced by so-called pay for performance initiatives, including cardiac, medical, orthopedics, and stroke. Thus, the APN is able to materially demonstrate the value-added benefit of APN clinical interventions using financial and quality analytics.

---

the past or tools that can be used real time to alert providers to a potential trends or events. Collectively, the activities of designing the measurement process, collecting and analyzing the data, and presenting the data back to stakeholders in a timely and effective manner are termed *data analytics*. As the EHR becomes more standardized and broadly adopted, the methods for performing data analytics will continue to evolve toward more automated capture and compilation of results, thus allowing data analytics to become more ingrained in every aspect of health care. Analytics in the health care industry can be organized into three main categories: descriptive, predictive, and prescriptive.

Descriptive Analytics

The term *descriptive analytics* essentially describes a retrospective trend or outcome. Typically, descriptive data are reported as percentages, rates, means, medians, ratios, or counts in which a value is assigned to inform the degree of goodness or badness against a given target or norm. For example, the graph shown in Figure 24-1 illustrates how CMS displays data about one hospital's readmission rates for a heart failure population compared with other peer

hospitals. This pattern essentially describes the performance as a static data point and informs the audience about whether their readmission rates are better, worse, or the same as those of other hospitals. Another type of descriptive analytic would be time-trended comparison data, such as shown in Figure 24-2, which also informs the audience about a hospital's performance with readmissions compared with that of other hospitals, but also shows periodic fluctuations in the hospital's performance. The limitation of both these types of charts is that they do not illuminate the reasons behind the given pattern, suggest an improvement strategy, or help the audience understand the relative stability or predictability of the process that is currently producing outcomes to date.

One of the most effective methods for demonstrating that an intervention or process modification has resulted in meaningful change over time is SPC analysis. SPC analysis examines variation within an individual process as well as the timing in which a change in process occurred. SPC uses control charts, which visually display performance data against upper and lower control limits reflective of normal variation in a system. In contrast to comparative reports illustrated in Figures 24-1 and

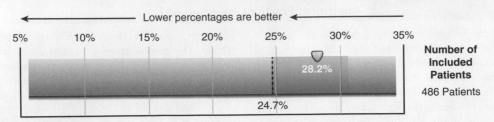

FIG 24-1 Example of a descriptive analytic used by CMS to report individual hospital performance compared the U.S. national rate of readmissions for heart failure. *(From Center for Medicare & Medicaid Services [CMS]. [2012]. Hospital compare, [www.hospitalcompare.hhs.gov]).*

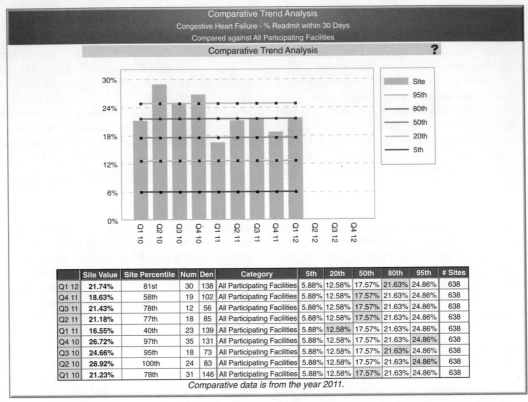

FIG 24-2 Example of a comparative benchmarking report comparing an individual hospital's quarterly performance for heart failure readmissions against 638 other hospitals. The hospital's readmission rates exceeded the 95th percentile in the second and fourth quarters in 2010 and has been under the 80th percentile for the past five quarters. *(Copyright 2013 by MidasPlus, Inc., A Xerox Company, Tucson, AZ [www.midasplus.com]).*

24-2, which display individual performance data compared with peer group performance, SPC charts display time-trended data only for individual performance data. No peer performance data are displayed in an SPC chart. Rather, the individual data is trended over time, with

mathematically computed control limits that indicate the expected ranges for random variation within a given process. When data points within the time-trended process change in a manner indicative of a statistically significant change, a special cause signal is displayed in the SPC chart. Special cause signals can occur whenever a single data points exceeds the upper or lower control limits in the SPC charts. Additional trends in the data may also designate special cause signals, such as eight data points in a row above or below the center line, or six points in a row increasing or decreasing in a single direction.

SPC charts have the added advantage of being able to distinguish results achieved during a pre-intervention process and the results achieved following a process change that occurs as a result of an innovation or practice change. This is done by inserting a phase change line between the two different processes and computing new control limits to monitor for statistical process capability moving forward. A detailed discussion of these data analysis techniques is beyond the scope of this chapter, although

a basic knowledge of control charts is useful for most situations. The reader is referred to the classic reference on SPC chart theory (Wheeler, 1993) or an online reference for basic SPC chart theory and application (Bauman, De Heck, Leonard, et al., 2006).

Figure 24-3 depicts a control chart displaying completion of breast cancer screening in women 40 to 65 years of age. The longitudinal display of data provides a more accurate and informative representation of a process change than would be evident by simply comparing completion of breast cancer screening completion rates before and after the interventions (see Exemplar 24-3, p. 672).

To understand why a hospital has fluctuations in their readmission performance data, or why a hospital's performance differs from others, the inquiry must progress

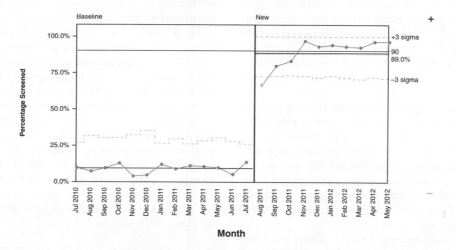

	Jul 2010	Aug 2010	Sep 2010	Oct 2010	Nov 2010	Dec 2010	Jan 2011	Feb 2011	Mar 2011	Apr 2011	May 2011	Jun 2011	Jul 2011	Aug 2011	Sep 2011	Oct 2011	Nov 2011	Dec 2011	Jan 2012	Feb 2012	Mar 2012	Apr 2012	May 2012
Numerator	4	2	3	4	1	1	5	3	5	4	3	2	6	22	28	30	34	27	33	27	25	30	37
Denominator	40	28	32	31	27	22	41	33	45	37	31	38	44	33	35	36	35	29	35	29	27	31	28
Percentage Screened	10.0%	7.1%	9.4%	12.9%	3.7%	4.5%	12.2%	9.1%	11.1%	10.8%	9.7%	5.3%	13.6%	66.7%	80.0%	83.3%	97.1%	93.1%	94.3%	93.1%	93.6%	96.8%	96.4%

The Comment/Action Plan table:

	Comment	Action Plan
Aug 2011	Mammography results were not being reported to NP's ordering diagnostic imaging from the Nurse Managed Health Clinic. Root cause traced to the fact that NP's at the NMHC were not included in the Provider Dictionary in the Imaging Center's information system.	NP's added to the Provider Dictionary in the Imaging Center's IT System. Memos and inservice provided to the imaging center's administrative staff and clinic coordinator to update them on the practice of sending reports to the ordering NP in additon to the collaborating physician.

FIG 24-3 Statistical process control chart illustrating a process phase for breast cancer screening. The process to the right of the vertical line represents the outcomes after improvement strategies. A new phase is created to monitor stability of the new process moving forward. The upper and lower control limits are reset to reflect the statistical limits of process control in the new phase. *(Copyright 2013 by MidasPlus, Inc., A Xerox Company, Tucson, AZ [www.midasplus.com]).*

further. Additional descriptive analytics may be used to look at specific details within the population, such as readmissions by gender, age, provider, payer, disease severity, and other related criteria. This type of inquiry that drills down to explore more specific patterns in data sets is termed *data mining*. APNs are likely to be engaged in this sort of activity as they evaluate outcomes for their areas of interest. Typical tools that the APN will use in this type of activity will likely involve Excel spreadsheets or other types of statistical software tools. Data patterns may then be displayed in charts to describe the patterns in the data. Table 24-3 lists several tools and techniques that are commonly used when working with descriptive analytics.

Predictive Analytics

Predictive analytics are rapidly emerging in the science of performance improvement. In contrast to descriptive analytics, which only describe a process after it has happened, predictive analytics provide insight on what might happen in the future based on past patterns or other criteria so that the appropriate interventions may be done to achieve desired outcomes. For example, a tool that would identify an individual patient's risk of readmission following discharge from a hospital would be considered a predictive analytic. CMS offers a free tool on the QualityNet web portal to predict the 30-day, all-cause readmission risk of individual patients hospitalized for pneumonia, heart failure, and acute myocardial infarction. This tool, developed by the Cooperative Cardiovascular Project initiative and under contract with CMS, uses gender, clinical history, physical examination findings, diagnostic and laboratory test results, and medications to compute an individual's overall risk of readmissions (https://www.qualitynet.org).

Currently, software engineers and clinical innovators are partnering to develop technology solutions that will help identify individual patients at highest risk for readmissions, pressure ulcers, falls, and other hospital-acquired complications. Cerner Systems and Advocate Health Care have developed a predictive analytic for hospital readmissions based on 25 variables, including payer, race, prior hospitalization and emergency department use in the past 12 months, admission source, current use of insulin or warfarin, and 17 disease-related variables (Sikk, Gagen, Crayton, et al., 2012). Most tools are not yet robust enough to have broad applicability to general populations; however this area of performance improvement will likely accelerate in the next 5 years. Such development will allow measurement of more timely and proactive interventions to ensure that best practices are delivered at the right time for more high risk patients. The reader is referred to Kansagara and colleagues (2011) for a systemic review

of predictive analytics and risk predication models pertaining to hospital readmissions as of August 2011.

Another recent application of predictive analytics is a value-based purchasing calculator. In response to the CMS VBP program, many vendors who support the HIQR reporting programs have developed online tools that will calculate the financial impact of a hospital's performance in selected clinical processes, outcomes and patient satisfaction (e.g., www.midasplus.com). These tools allow users to estimate the impact of their current performance on their Medicare reimbursement and then project what the financial impact would be if they improved performance in one or more of their key performance areas. The CMS VBP program is expected to expand rapidly to include hospital-acquired complications and additional mortality and readmission outcomes for other key populations. However, this program has come under recent scrutiny by health care leaders who have expressed concern that financial penalties for hospitals that do not perform as well as others may result in unintended negative consequences, such as bankruptcy and foreclosure of some hospitals and, in particular, hospitals serving underprivileged U.S. populations. For many larger U.S. hospitals, the VBP program can affect a hospital's financial bottom line by hundreds of thousands of dollars annually. Tools to help hospital leaders forecast their revenue and operating margins before CMS publishes the final scores for each hospital at the end of the year can be used to prioritize a hospital's quality improvement efforts and focus on initiatives that will have the greatest impact on the financial bottom line. Linking financial reimbursement to improved clinical performance for their patient populations is also a prime opportunity for APNs to demonstrate the impact of their interventions to their organization.

Prescriptive Analytics

Finally, the term *prescriptive analytics* refers tools that assist with modeling and longitudinal forecasting to inform users on how to respond to a given pattern in one's data. In prescriptive analytics, the evidence-based best practice is actually linked to the trend so that it indicates not only why there is a problem, but what the most likely solutions would be to get a trend back on a desired course. This may seem rather futuristic but, like predictive analytics, this is an area of rapid acceleration and scientific innovation, which will change how evidence-based practice is deployed in the clinical environment. The author believes that APN participation in collaborative learning with medical and nursing informatics specialists, clinical researchers, HIT vendors, and scientists may lead to transformational technologies within the next 5 to 8 years.

TABLE 24-3   Continuous Quality Improvement Tools and Techniques for Process Improvement

Tools and Techniques	Primary Function	Benefits
Flow chart	Displays the process	• Facilitates understanding of the process • Identifies stakeholders • Clarifies potential gaps and system breakdowns
Run chart	Displays performance over time	• Increases understanding of the problem • Identifies changes over time
Control chart	Displays how predictable the process is over time	• Identifies change in the process as a result of intentional or nonintentional changes in the process • Identifies opportunities for improvement
Pie chart	Displays the percentage that each variable contributes to the whole	• Identifies variables affecting process • Increases understanding of the problem
Bar chart	Compares categories of data during a single point in time	• Increases understanding of the problem • Identifies differences in variables • Compares performance with known standards
Pareto chart	Identifies the most frequent trend within a data set	• Identifies principal variables impacting the process • Identifies opportunities for improvement
Cause and effect	Displays multiple causes of a problem	• Identifies root causes • Identifies variables affecting the process • Identifies opportunities for improvement • Plans for change
Scatter diagram	Displays relationship between two variables	• Increases understanding of the relationship between multiple variables
Brainstorming	Rapidly generates multiple ideas	• Promotes stakeholder buy-in • Increases understanding of the problem • Identifies variables affecting the process
Multivoting	Consolidates ideas	• Achieves consensus among stakeholders • Prioritizes improvement strategies
Nominal group technique	Rapidly generates multiple ideas and prioritizes them	• Identifies the problem • Achieves consensus among stakeholders • Prioritizes improvement strategies • Plans for change
Root cause analysis	Identifies the cause of the problem	• Increases understanding of the problem • Identifies multicause variables affecting the process • Identifies opportunities to improve • Plans for change
Force field analysis	Identifies driving and restraining forces that impact proposed change	• Identifies and lists variables affecting process • Plans for change
Consensus	Generates agreement among stakeholders	• Increases understanding of the problem • Reduces resistance to change • Plans for change

Adapted from Powell, S. K. (2000). *Advanced case management: Outcomes and beyond.* Philadelphia: Lippincott.

Next-Generation Quality Metrics: eMeasures

Clinical quality measures that are publicly reported in the United States to CMS and other regulatory agencies such as TJC are being redesigned so that they can automatically be generated directly from the EHR and other HIT. To accomplish this, atomic data, meaning the smallest concepts that identify information in the EHR, such as a unique code that describes a specific data element (e.g., a medication), must be available in electronic clinical documentation. Assuming that all concepts in the EHR are linked to discrete codes or are available through NLP technologies, manual retrospective data collection will become a thing of the past. Definitions for existing paper-based quality measures, which are typically comprised of traditional numerator and denominator statements that define the inclusion and exclusion criteria for a particular population of patients, will need to be transformed. The new measure concepts, referred to in the U.S. meaningful use legislation as clinical quality measures (CQMs), are often referred to as electronic quality measures (eMeasures). eMeasures are a difficult concept for clinicians to master because of the unique manner in which the measure definitions are expressed in written form. Many discrete atomic data elements will be required to replicate the clinical decision making that once took place inside the "brain" of clinical data. Clinicians who review and validate data findings for eMeasures will need to become familiar with the quality data model (QDM) framework to understand the language of eMeasure development.

The Quality Data Model Framework

The QDM framework provides the basis for a standardized approach to capture data from EHRs, registries, health information exchanges (HIEs), and other data sources. All HIT vendors will eventually be required to capture and use this information in a standardized way so that information can be readily exchanged across various types of HIT systems to make health care information accessible throughout the care continuum. A QDM element is an atomic unit of information that has precise meaning to communicate the data required within a quality measure or report. A QDM element includes one of 23 categories, such as medication, procedure, laboratory test, diagnosis, family history, or care goal. Each category is accompanied by a state in which the category is expected to be found with respect to the electronic clinical data. For example, a state for a QDM element relating to the category of medication may have a state of administer, decline, order, and dispense. Similarly, a category of diagnosis may have a state of active, inactive, or resolved.

In addition, some categories may have other elements included, such as result, timing, actor, data flow, and category-specific. *Result* is used for things such as laboratory tests. *Timing* indicates the time frame in which the measurement should occur, such as admit, arrive, start, discharge, depart, or end. The *actor* attribute specifies the data source, such as a patient, clinician, or device. *Data flow* specifies whether the information is being sent or received. *Category-specific* attributes may contain additional detail depending on the category, such as facility location, route, dose, severity, or laterality.

Finally, each QDM element specifies a taxonomy that will be used to describe concepts being measured. For example, the concept of a medication would be described using RxNorm codes and the concept of a diagnosis, such as diabetes, would be described using ICD-9-CM, ICD-10, and/or SNOMED-CT codes. Each QDM element also contains a list of specific codes defined by the designated taxonomy. This code list is termed a *value set*. Figure 24-4 illustrates the concept of a simple QDM value set to describe the act of administering aspirin to a patient at discharge.

As HIT becomes more legislated and as certification bodies are established to ensure technical compliance with the evolving interoperability standards, data analytics will become an automated activity requiring increasing sophistication to design, develop, test, deploy, validate, and support. As of 2013, computerized eMeasurement technologies are still in the process of being piloted and tested; it may be some years before eMeasures completely replace manual data abstraction and become a trusted source of clinical process and outcomes data. This is an area in which APNs may find themselves engaged in collaborative projects with nurse informatics specialists and quality leaders to validate the data findings generated by eMeasures.

A full review of the QDM framework is beyond the scope of this chapter; however, these concepts are presented to give the reader an appreciation for the growing complexity behind the automated data capture of clinical metrics moving into the future. The reader is referred to NQF for more information about the QDM framework, which is expected to evolve in sophistication over the next several years (www.qualityforum.org/Projects/h/QDS_Model/Quality_Data_Model.aspx). Technical specifications for the initial set of clinical quality measures (eMeasures) used by hospitals to meet the initial stage 1 reporting requirements for meaningful use may be retrieved from the QualityNet Website (https://www.qualitynet.org/dcs/ContentServer?c=Page&pagename=QnetPublic%2FPage%2FQnetTier3&cid=12287722 17179). Additional discussion about meaningful use will be presented in the following section.

Meaningful Use of Health Information Technology and Impact on Advanced Practice Nursing

On February 17, 2009, President Obama signed the Health Information Technology for Economic and Clinical Health (HITECH) Act as part of the American Recovery and Reinvestment Act (ARRA; U.S. Congress, 2009). Under HITECH, the government financially rewards hospital providers a $2 million base payment and eligible physician providers up to $44,000 over 5 years when they purchase, implement, and make meaningful use of EHRs by the year 2015. There are three stages to

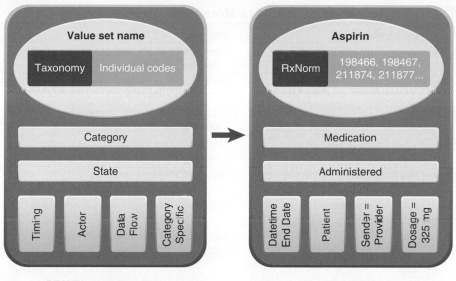

QDM Element Structure   **Example for Aspirin**

FIG 24-4 Quality data model (QDM) element structure. Shown are the components of a QDM element. *Left,* Terms used for each component of the QDM element. *Right,* Each of these components is used to describe a QDM element, indicating "Medication, administered aspirin." Each QDM element is composed of a category, the state in which the category is expected to be used, and a value set of codes in a designated taxonomy. The boxes in the lower section of the QDM element specify individual attributes to describe the QDM element. *(Adapted from the National Quality Forum. [2012]. Quality data model, December 2012 update, http://www.qualityforum.org/QualityDataModel.aspx#t=2&s=&p=3%7C. Copyright © 2012 National Quality Forum.).*

meaningful use that span 5 to 6 years and progressively expand the adoption of HIT for hospitals and providers. Each stage can last 1 to 2 years, depending on when the provider or organization initially implemented the required HIT functions. Although a detailed review of this legislation and attestation requirements for payment is beyond our scope here, it is of interest that APNs were not initially included in the HITECH legislation. However, Medicaid will pay incentives to physicians, dentists, certified nurse-midwives, NPs, and physician assistants (PAs) who are practicing in federally qualified health centers (FQHCs) or rural health clinics (RHCs) led by a NP or PA. Table 24-4 lists several resources that APNs should review to stay abreast of the evolving meaningful use requirements as their practice settings progress through the various stages of national EHR adoption in the United States.

Table 24-5 lists additional technology functions associated with the meaningful use initiative. For hospitals and eligible providers to qualify for the HITECH stimulus funding, they must implement and be able to demonstrate successfully meaningful use of each of these HIT functions. Demonstration consists of a formal attestation

process with CMS; later stages of meaningful use will require submission of data to demonstrate achievement of the full adoption of these technologies. Not only will these technologies directly affect outcome evaluation and performance management activities by making data more accessible, timely, and standardized across settings, they will theoretically allow care transitions to occur more seamlessly, reduce medical error, and ultimately improve the quality of care delivery. The manner in which APNs leverage these technologies will depend on the degree to which they develop their competencies in informatics, research, performance improvement, and systems thinking and the extent to which these competencies become embedded in APN education as these technologies continue to evolve.

Health Information Exchanges

Within the meaningful use framework there is one technology that has the potential to create a vast sharing of information across the health care continuum and, once realized, will forever change how providers practice and evaluate outcomes and that patients experience their care,

TABLE 24-4   Website Resources Related to Meaningful Use

Resource and Information Available	Website
CMS EHR Incentive Program	https://www.cms.gov/EHRIncentivePrograms/01_Overview.asp#TopOfPage
EHR Incentive Program Clinical Quality Measures	https://www.cms.gov/EHRIncentivePrograms/30_Meaningful_Use.asp#BOOKMARK5
CMS Meaningful Use FAQs	https://www.cms.gov/EHRIncentivePrograms/95_FAQ.asp#TopOfPage
CMS EHR Incentive Program Education Materials	https://www.cms.gov/EHRIncentivePrograms/55_EducationalMaterials.asp#TopOfPage
Office of the National Coordinator Meaningful Use Page	http://healthit.hhs.gov/portal/server.pt?open=512&objID=2996&mode=2
American Health Information Management Association (AHIMA) Meaningful Use Quality Measures Page	http://www.ahima.org/advocacy/arrameaningfuluse.aspx
National Quality Forum (NQF)	http://www.qualityforum.org/Home.aspx
Healthcare Information and Management Systems Meaningful Use Webpage	http://www.himss.org/ASP/topics_meaningfuluse.asp
National Rural Health Resource Center Health IT Portal	http://www.ruralcenter.org/hit
National Association of Community Health Centers HIT	http://www.nachc.org/Health%20Information%20Technologies%20%28HIT%29.cfm
Indian Health Service HIT Portal	http://www.ihs.gov/oit/index.cfm?module=dsp_oit_hit
Health Resources and Services Administration (HRSA)	http://www.hrsa.gov/healthit/meaningfuluse/MU%20Stage1%20CQM/mucqmresources.html
QualityNet Web Portal	https://www.qualitynet.org

the health information exchange. HIE can be defined in a number of ways. When used as a verb, HIE is the activity of secure health data exchange between two or more authorized parties. For example, laboratory reports from a patient's recent hospital stay could be accessed in a clinic by an APN who is conducting a follow-up assessment. Access to information in an HIE may often be viewed in a portal via the Internet so that all information is integrated in one application, even though it may be coming from multiple sources. In this example, the APN could also review information from a pharmacy about which medications the patient had filled after being discharged from the hospital, provided that the pharmacy was part of the HIE. HIE may also imply some level of data storage and warehousing.

To support data sharing among many different care settings, the concept of HIE implies a standardized file format for specific data types, regardless of the technology vendor involved in the sending or receiving applications. This concept is termed *interoperability*. It simply means that there will finally be one set of technical rules for formatting data and moving it efficiently across the health care continuum so that it can be accessed wherever and whenever it is needed for the provision of care. HIE

technologies also have the potential to make clinical information immediately accessible over the internet via mobile devices such as cell phones, tablets, or lap top computers. As technologies progress, they will enable information to be stored in a virtual environment, also referred to as a cloud platform, so that it can be pushed and pulled as needed to coordinate care effectively. APNs may find an opportunity to expand services and interventions more effectively to many nonstructured clinical settings, including nurse-managed community clinics, home care settings, church and parish nursing settings, school health areas, and retail health clinics. Using this technology will allow APNs to extend access to preventive chronic care and episodic urgent care so that the Triple Aim objectives described in the introduction of this chapter can be better achieved.

Finally, when HIE is used as a noun, it can refer to independent vendors or organizations who bring the information together on a common platform, also referred to as health information organizations (HIOs). HIEs can be created within a single health care provider system, region, or community. There has been significant growth in these organizations across the country and much debate about in which technology platforms these systems should

TABLE 24-5 Health Information Technology Functions Associated with Meaningful Use*

Objective	Description	Relevance to Outcome Evaluation
CPOE	Use of CPOE for medication orders directly entered by any licensed health care professional who can enter orders into the medical record per state, local, and professional guidelines	Allows for direct attribution of medication, treatment, and diagnostic services to APN practice
Drug screening and drug formulary checks	Implement drug-drug and drug-allergy interaction checks. Drug formulary checks optional for stage 1 meaningful use and required in stage 2.	May affect safe medication ordering practices for APNs
Electronic prescribing	Applies to eligible providers only; generate and transmit permissible prescriptions electronically	Allows for automated tracking of APN adherence to best practices for given conditions (e.g., antibiotic usage)
Demographics Recording	Record demographics—preferred language, gender, race, ethnicity, date of birth, and date and preliminary cause of death in the event of mortality in hospital or critical access hospital	Supports reporting for individual patients and populations
Problem list	Maintain up to date problem list of current and active diagnoses using structured data	Supports reporting for individual patients and populations; supports real-time alerts to identify key populations if maintained daily by all providers in the health care system
Active medication list	Maintain active medication lists for patients with at least one medication using structured data	Supports queries for patients on selected medications, predictive analytic tools, and analysis of best practice adherence
Vital signs	Record and chart vital signs, including height, weight, blood pressure, calculate and display body mass index (BMI), growth charts for children 2-20 yr old, including BMI	May be useful in demonstrating effectiveness of APN partnering with patients to manage chronic disease and prevention
Smoking status	Record smoking status for patients ≥ 13 yr	Evaluates effectiveness of APN partnering with patients
Clinical decision support	Implement at least one clinical decision support rule and the ability to track compliance with the rule	Creates automated rules to facilitate timely APN interventions
Clinical quality measures	Automated data capture and reporting of clinical quality measures to CMS or other agencies (stage 1 Meaningful Use limited to stroke, VTE, and ED populations with expansion to other clinical conditions expected to occur)	Supports reporting of APN adherence to best practice standards; directly connects APN intervention to pay for performance activities; may be used in credentialing activities
Engaging patients and families in their health care	Provide patients and families with an electronic copy of their health information (including diagnostic test results, problem list, medication lists, medication allergies, discharge summary, procedures) on request	May positively affect compliance to care regimen, readmission reduction, patient satisfaction, and patient safety
Hospital discharge instructions	Applies to hospital settings only: Provide patients with an electronic copy of their discharge instructions at time of discharge on request	May positively affect compliance to care regimen, readmission reduction, patient satisfaction, and patient safety
Clinical summaries	Applies to eligible providers only: Provide clinical summaries to patients for each office visit on request	May positively affect compliance to care regimen, readmission reduction, patient satisfaction, and patient safety
Clinical information exchange	Demonstrate capability to exchange key clinical information (e.g., problem list, medications, allergies, diagnostic test results) among providers of care and patient-authorized entities	Allows for assessment of referral patterns to and from APNs and other providers to assess appropriateness, timeliness, and efficiency of service provision

Continued

⬡ **TABLE 24-5**   **Health Information Technology Functions Associated with Meaningful Use—*cont'd***

Objective	Description	Relevance to Outcome Evaluation
Data protection	Protect electronic health information created or maintained by certified EHR technology through the implementation of appropriate technical capabilities	Allows tracking of APN adherence to HIPAA policies
Advanced directives	Applies to hospitals only: Record advance directives for patients ≥ 65 yr	May reflect APN interventions for patient partnering and ethical decision making, particularly in chronic disease populations
Laboratory results	Incorporate clinical laboratory test results into certified EHR technology as structured data	Supports real-time alerts to identify key populations for APN intervention; supports monitoring of APN adherence to best practice guidelines (e.g., antibiotics, anticoagulation management)
Patient lists	Generate lists of patients by specific conditions to use for quality improvement, reduction of disparities, research, or outreach	Supports all basic APN outcome evaluation activities
Patient reminders	Applies to eligible providers only: Send reminders to patients per patient preference for preventive and follow-up care	May be useful in demonstrating effectiveness of APN partnering with patients to manage plan of care and adherence to prevention strategies; may reduce readmissions or complications
Medication reconciliation	Medication reconciliation performed by eligible providers and hospitals when patients are received from another care setting or provider of care	May be useful in demonstrating APN compliance with organization policies; may support patient safety initiatives
Immunization	Capability to submit electronic data to immunization registries or information systems and actual submission in accordance with applicable law and practice	Supports APN adherence to best practice standards for immunization and screening
Syndromic surveillance[†]	Capability to submit electronic syndromic surveillance data to public health agencies and actual submission in accordance with applicable law and practice	May be useful in demonstrating APN skill in recognizing public health issues and adherence to policies and procedures

*Associated with Stage I Meaningful Use requirements for the electronic health record and relevance to advanced practice nursing outcome evaluation. Note that additional requirements for Stage 2 and 3 Meaningful Use may include additional functionality not listed above.
†Syndromic surveillance uses individual and population health indicators that are available before confirmed diagnoses or laboratory confirmation to identify outbreaks or health events and monitor the health status of a community. The syndromic surveillance data compiled through the meaningful use initiative not only promotes rapid response to outbreaks and health events, but provides data streams for longer term, ongoing analyses of chronic conditions such as heart disease and diabetes, injuries, and the use of health care services (http://www.cdc.gov/ehrmeaningfuluse/syndromic.html).

reside. Another source of debate has to do with the business and financial models that will support these types of endeavors. A complete discussion on HIEs is beyond the scope of this chapter, but the reader should be aware that HIE can enhance almost any of the clinical functions outlined in Table 24-5 and will likely become part of the infrastructure that supports HIT moving into the future. Additional information on HIEs may be found in the HIE Toolkit Directory (Healthcare Information and Management Systems, 2012).

Foundational Competencies in Quality Improvement

APNs must be able to participate in and lead interdisciplinary teams effectively toward data-based conclusions and process improvements. This discussion elaborates on the evidence-based practice competency described in Chapter 10. Data analysis is a specific skill for evidence-based practice. APNs are required to have the ability to manipulate and interpret raw data, query information within a database containing clinical or financial information, and use an information system to collect data and trend performance. This expectation continues to be primary work for clinical nurse specialists (CNSs). Historically APNs other than CNSs did not need this level of skill, however, the environments in which APNs now practice have changed. The purpose of this section is to elaborate on the specific skills that APNs need to be knowledgeable participants and leaders in continuous quality improvement (CQI) efforts. APN students need content on CQI knowledge and skills. Graduate APNs should seek additional CQI training through reading, continuing education, and participation in formal quality improvement (QI) training programs. A health care system's approach to CQI should be included in an APN's orientation. If such programs are not in place, APNs are strongly encouraged to include formal QI training in their performance and learning objectives within the first year of hire and to identify opportunities to initiate modest QI initiatives.

Continuous Quality Improvement Frameworks

There are numerous frameworks and related strategies for improving performance and evaluating outcomes in today's health care system. Some of these include the plan-do-study-act (PDSA) model used by the IHI, Six Sigma and Lean Manufacturing techniques (Morgan & Brenig-Jones, 2012). APNs can examine selected frameworks to understand the how-to mechanics of creating systems that are safe, effective, patient-centered, timely, efficient, and equitable. Generally, the employer will have selected a framework or philosophy that guides CQI efforts across an organization. Many of these methodologies have evolved from the work of Drs. W. Edwards Deming and Joseph M. Juran, both considered to be forefathers of modern day statistical process control theory. Although a detailed review of the various CQI frameworks is not included here, APNs are highly encouraged to contact the Quality Management Department in their organization and request an orientation to the CQI framework used in their practice settings. Marash and associates (2003) have provided a comprehensive overview of the traditional QI methodologies discussed above.

Regardless of the type of QI approach an organization selects, the APN should be competent in a variety of specific techniques, tools, and methodologies used to evaluate process performance and outcomes. Most approaches involve the use of different types of charts and analysis tools to examine findings and establish linkages. Some charts are easy to learn, such as flow charts. Other charts, such as Pareto charts, SPC charts, scatter diagrams, and cause-and-effect diagrams, also termed *fishbone* or *Ishikawa diagrams*, require specific training and expertise in statistical software. APNs may also need to become familiar with the software used in their agencies to conduct CQI analyses and reports.

APNs prepared at a master's level should achieve beginning level competencies with these tools, including the ability to interpret the data in these reports and effectively participate in teams using CQI techniques. One exception is the CNS role, which has had expectations for leading QI efforts as part of system influence expectations embedded in their role; mastery is expected for any CNS, whether master's- or DNP–prepared. Other APNs should achieve mastery of QI competencies at the DNP level, with full accountability for planning the CQI project, selecting and using appropriate tools and techniques, including being able to enter data and run the reports, synthesizing information from the reports, and coaching others in deriving meaning from the information and making decisions. QI training should also include techniques for analyzing how people and processes work. Root cause analysis is one popular approach to identifying underlying causes of problems and process failures in a particular system. This approach may be particularly useful for examining adverse events and other patient safety issues. Box 24-5 provides the reader with several website resources that

BOX 24-5 Quality Improvement and Outcome Assessment Website Resources	
Resource and Information Available	Website
Agency for Healthcare Research and Quality	www.ahrq.gov
• Supports evidence-based practice centers, outcomes and effectiveness trials, national quality measures clearinghouse	
American Society for Quality (ASQ)	http://asq.org/learn-about-quality/ quality-tools.html
• Contains tools for cause analysis, evaluation and decision-making, data collection and analysis, idea creation, project planning, and implementation	
• ASQ offers certification, training and ongoing education in QI techniques	

Continued

BOX 24-5 Quality Improvement and Outcome Assessment Website Resources—*cont'd*

Resource and Information Available	Website
Institute for Healthcare Improvement • Offers training and ongoing education in QI techniques • Promotes health care innovation through fellowships, the IHI Open School, and networking • Strong international presence	http://www.ihi.org/Pages/default.aspx
Mind Tools • Excellent site for learning skills in change management, team-building, brainstorming, straw man concept, strategy tools, leadership skills, and project management	http://www.mindtools.com
National Association for Healthcare Quality • Promotes continuous improvement of quality in health care by providing educational and development opportunities and national certification as a Certified Professional of Healthcare Quality	www.nahq.org
National Committee for Quality Assurance • Develops the HEDIS to measure quality of care delivered by U.S. health plans • Offers online training and seminars on a wide range of quality-related topics	www.ncqa.org
National Database of Nursing Quality Indicators • Collects and evaluates unit-specific nurse-sensitive data from U.S. hospitals	https://www.nursingquality.org
National Network of Public Health Institutes • Dedicated to improving public health through innovation, quality improvement (QI) and education • Website includes QI tools and frameworks (e.g., aim statements, balanced scorecard templates, brainstorming, fishbone, cause and effect diagrams, force field analysis, Kaizen, Lean, story board, radar charts, tree diagrams, interrelationship diagrams, and others that may be useful in outcome evaluation)	http://nnphi.org/tools/public-health-performance-improvement-toolkit-2?view=file&topic=59#Data%20&%20 Measurement
National Quality Forum Community Tool to Align Measurement • Excel spreadsheet inventory of NQF-endorsed measures for one or more of the national reporting programs, including the Aligning Forces for Quality Alliances in regions across the United States • Also includes drill-down to the Quality Positioning System for quick access to measure definitions of NQF-endorsed measures • These resources are in the public domain and do not require membership.	http://www.qualityforum.org/AlignmentTool/
Public Health Foundation • On-line tutorial for review of the plan-do-check-act (PDCA) process, plus additional resources for population outcomes evaluation	http://www.phf.org/quickguide/ LeftNavTwoPanel.aspx?Page=Introduction
The Joint Commission • Maintains measure definitions for hospital quality reporting programs • Provides educational offerings for quality improvement and accreditation standards • Expanding international presence	www.jointcommission.org

may be helpful in developing skills in QI methodologies and outcomes evaluation.

Organizational Structures and Cultures That Optimize Performance Improvement

APNs who practice in a hospital or an integrated delivery network (IDN) may find that their span of influence crosses many units, departments, and points of service within the system. Thus, it is important to consider carefully the reporting structures that will best support their roles. In many organizations, APNs report to nurse or medical executives. APNs with a case management component to their practice may be based in the following departments: nursing, medical group, home health, quality and performance improvement, utilization resource management, social work, or even finance or information systems, although these last three are less common. Regardless of organizational placement, APNs should seek to work within a reporting structure that supports whole-system thinking and places a high value on innovation and process improvement. Conversely, APNs should avoid reporting structures that constrain their practices to one unit's or department's interests or seem to place a particular emphasis on task-oriented activities. Optimally, the organization and its administrators should recognize that the APN is in a unique position to promote excellence in clinical practice and system performance. To achieve these outcomes, the APN may at times require the formal and tacit authority that come with the position and title of those to whom the APN reports. Those who lead APNs must be prepared to be responsible, if necessary, for changes perceived as coming from the APN. Although APNs will not need daily or even weekly supervision, they will need to be kept abreast of organizational issues that are likely to affect the practice and business environment. The APN should have routine briefing sessions scheduled with his or her immediate supervisor to clarify goals and expected outcomes, identify any resource needs, discuss any barriers, and exchange information relating to pending contracts, changes in the product line, medical practice issues, or staff education needs.

Active membership on key medical and quality oversight committees and direct access to administrative decision makers are imperative. This access affords APNs the opportunity to integrate clinical expertise with communication, negotiation, and leadership skills to promote effective and efficient clinical processes. For APNs who contract independently, becoming familiar with the organizational structure and culture and becoming a trusted insider in the organization will be critical to successful contracting and service delivery. Exemplar 24-3 illustrates an APN in a nurse-managed clinic

working collaboratively with other quality leaders within a large health care system and influencing practice and systems by exercising leadership, QI skills, systems thinking, and use of informatics.

Strategies for Designing Quality Improvement and Outcome Evaluation Plans for Advanced Practice Nursing

As noted, much of health care practice in today's economic market is data-driven, with APNs assuming greater responsibility for collecting and using clinical, economic, and quality outcomes data. In particular, interdisciplinary QI teams are increasingly charged with improving care delivery outcomes or redesigning workflow processes for greater effectiveness or efficiency. Because APNs routinely monitor and maintain clinical care delivery systems, they are in an ideal position to plan QI initiatives by leading or actively participating in interdisciplinary QI teams. As clinical experts, APNs influence practice patterns and develop meaningful standards, practice protocols, clinical guidelines, health care programs, and health care policies that promote teamwork, improve clinical outcomes, and reduce costs. Moreover, APNs' pattern recognition skills facilitate the identification of system inefficiencies, barriers to continuity of care, and other ineffective ways of delivering health care services. These in turn become opportunities for APNs to influence processes and outcomes positively at both the individual patient and system levels. With these opportunities comes the responsibility to be knowledgeable in outcome evaluation. In the remainder of this chapter, a stepwise approach is proposed to developing and implementing an outcome evaluation plan that demonstrates an APN's value and contribution to the health care setting. Although the term *outcome evaluation* is used throughout this section, these steps can be applied to impact analysis, outcomes measurement, performance evaluation, process improvement, program evaluation, and clinical research.

Phases of Preparing a Plan for Outcome Evaluation

There are three phases in the organizing framework to develop an effective outcome evaluation plan—defining the core questions that need to be answered, determining the data required to answer the questions, and interpreting the data and acting on the results. Box 24-6 lists the phases and related steps in developing and conducting an outcomes evaluation. A description of each step follows.

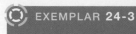 **EXEMPLAR 24-3**   **Putting It All Together: Planning and Managing Quality Reporting at a Nurse-Managed Clinic***

Nancy Lawson (NL) is an NP and clinical director of a nurse-managed health center (NMHC) in a large urban Midwestern city. Primary care services, including health promotion, preventive care, and chronic disease management are provided to a diverse population consisting of college-aged students, children, adolescents, and an increasing number of adults with chronic diseases such as hypertension and diabetes. The center's population has a mix of commercial, Medicare, and Medicaid payers, with some patients having little to no insurance. This NMHC is staffed by a practice of six primary care NPs, one administrative assistant, and a part-time information systems analyst, whose position is shared by the NMHC's sponsoring health care system. Although owned and operated by a school of nursing, the NMHC is also partnered with a large health care system, which is participating in the CMS demonstration project as a pioneering accountable care organization (ACO). The NMHC is also committed to supporting student placements at the undergraduate and graduate levels. As NL begins her annual review of the performance improvement plan, she creates a list of all quality and patient safety reporting requirements to which the NMHC must respond over the course of the next year. This year, the NMHC is planning to apply for status as an FQHC, which will expand their quality reporting requirements. NL identifies four major quality reporting initiatives:

1. CMS Shared Savings Program for ACOs (see Box 24-1)
2. HRSA Clinical and Financial Performance Measures (see Box 24-2)
3. CMS Medicaid Adult Quality Reporting Measures (see Box 24-3)
4. HIT Functions Associated with Meaningful Use (see Table 24-5)

NL downloads the NQF Community Tool to Align Measurement from the NQF website and filters the spreadsheet so that only measures associated with her clinic's programs of interest are listed. In addition, she includes a list of measures associated with the NCQA HEDIS Physician Measures and the CMS Physician Quality Reporting System (PQRS) so that she can get a complete inventory of all NQF-endorsed measures that might be applicable to the NMHC populations. In this manner, she can begin to see overlap in reporting requirements and identify any gaps in terms of what is being collected and reported in the NMHC's current performance improvement (PI) plan. Knowing this information will also be useful to NL in her planning

and prioritization for HIT enhancements that need to be implemented at the NMHC to reduce the data collection burden on her team.

Next, NL considers her professional practice team and their areas of interest. She calls a meeting to bring the stakeholders together, including her (information technology [IT]) analyst. NL then asks for input from the team to decide which measures they should select to meet their regulatory reporting requirements. She asks the stakeholders to consider the NMHC's population and mission, as well as the value of knowing versus the burden of collection. The IT analyst contributes to this assessment by advising the team on whether their EHR and IT infrastructure are currently capable of capturing this information electronically or whether manual data collection methods would need to be incorporated to collect the necessary information. The IT analyst notes areas of future expansion and prioritizes these needs relative to quality reporting initiatives at the NMHC. This information will be shared in the upcoming meeting with the health care system's corporate HIT strategy team to build their integrated health care information system to support their work as an ACO.

Finally, NL asks the team to consider any other areas of interest that they would like to focus on over the course of the next year, which are not already captured in the must measure list and which will inform them about the quality, effectiveness, efficacy, and efficiency of the group's practice. They suggest that the average waiting time to be seen by a clinic provider and the number of patients who are admitted to the emergency department (ED) or hospital within 72 hours after being seen at the NMHC would be valuable information in the year ahead. In collaboration with their IT analyst, they determine the best ways to capture waiting time to be seen and 72-hour admissions.

As the team completes their final assessment, they raise concerns that although the value of knowing the patient satisfaction and patient experience data is high, the data collection effort will be intensive and likely require the assistance of additional staff or university students to collect and analyze this information. NL and the NPs in the practice suggest including the students from the college of nursing to partner with this project. NL schedules a meeting with the Dean of Academic Affairs to discuss internship opportunities for nursing students. With enthusiasm from the Dean that these would be good learning opportunities, these measures

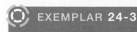 **EXEMPLAR 24-3**   **Putting It All Together: Planning and Managing Quality Reporting at a Nurse-Managed Clinic—cont'd**

and the proposed data collection plan are added to the NMHC's performance improvement plan.

Finally, for each measure, the team identifies a target for their performance. Measures in which there are known national benchmarks associated with them, such as the HEDIS process measure for diabetes care, which measures the percentage of diabetic patients receiving glycosylated hemoglobin (HbA1c) tests in the reporting year, or the outcome measure that reports the percentage of diabetic patients with a controlled HbA1c result, are set at higher percentiles of desired performance (e.g., 90%). Conversely, measures in which the relative goodness or badness of the phenomenon of interest are not established nationally, such as the number of patients admitted to the health care system's ED within 72 hours of a visit to the NMHC, may be set at lower thresholds of performance or have no specific target established until patterns in the performance data have been well established.

NL compiles the final list of measures to be reported, along with a data collection plan and schedule for periodic review and reporting to all stakeholders. She submits this PIP to the College of Nursing's Faculty Practice Plan group for feedback prior to submitting the plan to the sponsoring health care system's quality director for final review and approval. Over the course of the next year, the NMHC team monitors the results of their performance monthly. Measure rates and continuous variables are presented in a dashboard, using SPC charts so that trends can be rapidly visualized. For each measure, a target is established so that all stakeholders reviewing the monthly dashboard can see at a glance any performance trends that are falling below desired targets.

Midway through the year, the NMHC team observes that their performance in mammography screening is substantially below the national median as reported by HEDIS. The team decides to review their performance stratified by payer (commercial, Medicare, Medicaid and self-pay or uninsured) to see if any disparities might exist. No significant trends appear. However,

when reviewing the inclusion and exclusion criteria for the measure, it is observed that the primary reason for failing to meet the criterion was that the results of the mammography were not reported back to the NMHC. The team quickly realized that to understand their effectiveness in this referral metric fully, they had to correct an underlying system issue and secure the results of the mammography back to the referring NP provider.

NL organized a small team of stakeholders, which included the administrator for the contracted imaging facility, medical director of the imaging facility, oversight physician for the NMHC, and IT systems analyst. During a 1-hour meeting, it was unanimously agreed by all parties that the NP provider ordering the mammogram required a copy of the results. It was further determined that the root cause for this omission was tied to the absence of the NP providers from the hospital information systems provider dictionary. The IT analyst was able to quickly add the six NPs to the required dictionary, enabling the admissions clerk at the imaging center to select the appropriate provider and route the results to them.

The next month, the performance trend for mammography referrals from the NMHC demonstrated a statistically significant increase. Using the SPC software function to designate a phase change within a time-trended process, NL modified the SPC chart in the dashboard by inserting a phase line to distinguish between the pre- and post-process improvement periods. In this manner, she will be able to document the impact of the PI initiative to have available for potential accreditation surveys and to detect any statistically significant changes in their new process moving forward that might indicate that they are not sustaining their improvements over time (see Figure 24-3). NL makes a plan to reevaluate performance in mammography referrals monthly for the remainder of the year and at least once a quarter thereafter for the next 18 to 24 months, as long as the process appears to be stable.

*The author wishes to thank Joanne Pohl, PhD, APRN-BC, for her contribution to the development of this exemplar based on her experiences with NMHCs nationally.

Define the Core Questions

Whether the APN is designing an outcome evaluation project to assess her or his practice effectiveness, or participating on an interdisciplinary team responsible for improving the care for a given clinical population, the first step is to articulate clearly and ask "What are the questions

we are asking and why?" Clear questions will lay the foundation for an effective outcome evaluation and limit unintended project scope creep. In formulating clear core questions, it is helpful to define the target population for study, identify the relevant stakeholders, and articulate specific program goals and interventions to be evaluated.

⬡ BOX 24-6   **Summary of Outcome Evaluation Planning Process**

Phase I: Define the Core Questions

I-1. Define the target population.
  - Identify differences in patient characteristics within target population.
  - Clarify relationships between APN role behaviors and population needs and outcomes.
  - Compare target group with other groups monitored through QI activities.
  - Assess level of risk, complexity, and resource use of subpopulations within target group.

I-2. Identify the stakeholders.
  - Facilitate participation by and input from key stakeholders.
  - Isolate APN interventions and actions from those of other care providers.
  - Secure early buy-in from stakeholders.

I-3. Articulate program goals and interventions.
  - Review literature for supportive evidence.
  - Consider resources needed to implement and maintain the intervention.
  - Formulate specific questions.
  - Implement practice change or QI strategy.

Phase II: Define the Data Elements

II-1. Identify selection criteria for the population of interest.
  - Clarify inclusion and exclusion criteria.
  - Identify electronic data sources of information about the target population.

II-2. Establish performance and outcome indicators.
  - Identify measures to determine evidence of APN impact.
  - Ensure alignment among program goals, proposed interventions, and outcome indicators.
  - Consider the use of national databases for comparison and benchmarking purposes.

II-3. Identify and evaluate data elements, collection instruments, and procedures.
  - Evaluate ease of collecting data and compare with need.

  - Identify data resources available.
  - Link use of intermediate outcome indicators to target goals and outcome achievement.
  - Summarize the outcome evaluation plan.

Phase III: Derive Meaning from Data and Act on Results

III-1. Analyze data and interpret findings.
  - Seek assistance from others, as needed.
  - Select data analysis and reporting procedures.

III-2. Present and disseminate findings.
  - Prepare reports according to audience and stakeholder needs and interests.
  - Select software programs and other resources to support presentation approach.

III-3. Identify improvement opportunities.
  - Work with stakeholders to identify most appropriate opportunity for improvement.
  - Select most effective tools to facilitate performance improvement planning process.
  - Conduct pilot studies to assess new program feasibility, cost, and resource needs.

III-4. Formulate a plan for ongoing monitoring and reevaluation.
  - Summarize goals of performance improvement plan.
  - Identify proposed interventions, responsible persons, and target dates for completion.
  - Select indicators and measures based on goals and interventions identified.
  - Provide educational programs to support intervention, as needed.

III-5. Clarify the purpose of the APN's role.
  - Review organization's mission, vision, and goals.
  - Clarify role expectations.
  - Confirm clinical and reporting accountability.

It is also useful to understand any key business drivers tied to the outcome evaluation or performance improvement initiative. Once these foundational aspects have been established, the APN can progress to the mechanics of how the data for the project will be collected.

Define the Target Population for Study

APNs use a range of activities to manage heterogeneous clinical populations. When designing an outcome evaluation plan, it is necessary to focus on specific aspects of the practice with a particular patient group. This focus helps create a more manageable outcome evaluation plan and limits the impact of extraneous variables that could interfere with the interpretation of findings. Aspects of APN activities used with the target population need to be identified and included in the design. Whenever possible, the target population should be comparable to other groups monitored through quality improvement initiatives at the organizational or departmental level so that the vested interests of the organization's commitment to improving care and APN's activities are aligned. The decision to target subpopulations of patients may be based on a desire to evaluate patients who are high risk, complex, or tend to use more services than others.

Other factors to consider when defining a target population include patient satisfaction and financial performance. For example, when a large pediatric medical group hires a pediatric nurse practitioner (PNP) to provide routine physical examinations and vaccinations, parent satisfaction is likely to be an important component of the outcome evaluation plan. Patient factors such as insurance provider, age, ethnicity, or comorbid conditions also may be used to define the target population at risk for adverse outcomes. Finally, some populations are targeted because of the need for organizations to determine their level of compliance with national care delivery guidelines, best practice standards, or regulatory requirements, as illustrated in Exemplar 24-3. Frequently, APNs are involved in the care of several populations of interest and, as such, must prioritize which populations warrant first review and evaluation. APNs must be sensitive to the resource requirements of any outcome study, working closely with information systems, QI, and medical records staff for the support required to conduct the review. Figure 24-5 illustrates one example of an approach to prioritizing performance improvement initiatives in larger health care systems. The weighted scoring method used in this tool provides an objective approach to obtain input from other departments and stakeholders and identify and prioritize target populations for outcome evaluation.

Identify the Stakeholders

APNs must identify the structures and processes of care for which they share accountability. Although APNs are rarely the only or primary stakeholder in the provision of care to the populations they serve, they often serve as the glue that holds the team together. As such, they often move the team, health care agency, and/or system toward a shared vision of desired outcome. Creating this vision is not an isolated APN activity; APNs must also facilitate the contributions, ideas, and creativity of professionals who participate in the care of the target population. Stakeholders most commonly involved are physicians, PAs, other APNs, other nurses, pharmacists, administrators, and other members of the health care team. In some cases, APNs will need to include stakeholders from outside their immediate practice settings. For example, a community-based APN serving fragile older patients with chronic diseases may need to include stakeholders from managed care payers and insurers, primary care clinics, physicians' offices, skilled nursing facilities, home

health care agencies, and hospitals. Although including all stakeholders in the development of an outcome evaluation plan may not be feasible or desirable, attention to the impact of primary stakeholders on care delivery outcomes will aid in the understanding and measurement of processes and outcomes interdependent with APN practice.

Typically, APNs are only one component of a greater whole, so they cannot receive full credit for the positive results. Therefore, APNs must articulate APN-specific inputs and interventions that contribute to the team effect so that the value of the APN to the organization can be documented and demonstrated. The need to carve out additional measures of role effectiveness results in a more complex outcomes plan, requiring multiple measurement methodologies, instruments, and analytic techniques. For example, part of an outcome evaluation plan may use quantitative methods to capture specific outcomes of treatment (e.g., average number of clinic visits per year, total costs, number of diabetic patients with a normal HbA1c level within 2 months of diagnosis). Another part of the plan may use a qualitative approach, using verbal or written feedback from physician and dietitian colleagues about APN effectiveness in facilitating the development of new patient care guidelines to manage the diabetic population. Once the plan for an evaluation study has been shared with stakeholders, buy-in to any proposed change must be obtained to proceed. APNs not only will be change recipients as a result of the outcome evaluation but also will serve as change implementers and change strategists for others and their organization. Involving stakeholders early in the process facilitates ongoing communication, reduces resistance to change, and promotes adoption of recommended changes.

Articulate Program Goals and Interventions

The easiest way to demonstrate positive outcomes of care is to do the right things, at the right times, for the right patients, in the right ways. The task of evaluation becomes an artful assembly of necessary data and information that reflect the outcomes and processes associated with the intervention. Determining which interventions to implement for a given population and which to include in an outcome evaluation plan may be based in part on the resources required to accomplish these interventions and maintain them in practice. To begin, APNs should engage in a comprehensive literature review to examine all standards of care, regulatory requirements, national guidelines, and established or emerging evidence-based best practices relevant to their clinical population. The most current information may be found on websites that are relevant to the APNs clinical specialty or through specialized fee-for-service vendor services that accumulate and organize best

Proposed Population or Process: _____

	Low 1 Point	Medium 2 Points	High 3 Points
Cost	<$5,000 ❑	$5,000 - $10,000 ❑	>$10,000 ❑
Annual Volume	<50 cases ❑	50-150 cases ❑	>150 cases ❑
Risk	<1/1000 deaths ❑	<1/100 deaths ❑	>1/100 deaths ❑
Problem Prone	Minor problems infrequently reported ❑	Minor to moderate problems reported occasionally ❑	Steady stream of minor to major problems reported ❑
Regional Variation	Process of care delivery generally consistent ❑	Normal or expected variation exists ❑	Process of care delivery highly variable ❑
Improvement Opportunity	Few if any opportunities to improve exist ❑	Minor to moderate opportunities to improve exist ❑	Significant opportunities to improve exist ❑
National Guidelines	No guidelines exist and rarely discussed in the literature ❑	Topic widely discussed in the literature ❑	Guidelines exist and are recognized nationally ❑
Controversial Therapy	Process or procedure is widely accepted nationwide ❑	The literature suggests alternative approaches may be of value ❑	Process or procedure has widely accepted alternatives ❑
Market Interest	Little if any focus exists in the community ❑	Process or procedure is of general concern in the community ❑	Process of major concern to the community ❑
Physician/Staff Interest	Very few professional staff would agree this area is important ❑	Selected professional staff would agree this area is important ❑	There are many staff who would agree this area is important ❑
Total Number of Points			
	____ × 1 = [ ]	____ × 2 = [ ]	____ × 3 = [ ]

Note: Lowest possible score is 10. Highest possible score is 30.

TOTAL SCORE

FIG 24-5 Prioritization tool for performance improvement initiatives. *(Copyright 1998-2013 by MidasPlus, Inc., A Xerox Company, Tucson, AZ [www.midasplus.com]).*

practice information and a meta-analysis of the literature for selected clinical topics, such as Zynx Health (www.zynxhealth.com).

Using information from literature and experience, APNs can identify appropriate interventions for managing populations. For example, interventions may include attention to early detection and diagnostic modalities, timeliness of interventions, drug appropriateness, or patient education. The organization's needs and any political agendas should also be considered. APNs should limit the number of evaluated interventions to keep the project scope manageable. A commitment to too many interventions or unrealistic data collection activities can overwhelm available resources and undermine or stall performance improvement and outcome evaluation initiatives.

Once the program goals and interventions have been defined, the APN can begin to formulate specific questions of interest to stakeholders. Sketching out some basic questions serves as a useful exercise for establishing the outcome evaluation plan. The following are some sample questions:

- How cost-effective is this program?
- How satisfied are patients with the services that they received?
- How closely does the health care team adhere to best practice standards?
- How many patients experienced complications of care?
- What patient safety issues associated with this population should we examine?
- What can be done to reduce resource utilization for this population?
- What do we need to do differently to become a center of excellence for this population?
- How has the APN contributed to the training and development of other staff?
- What are the key business drivers behind the outcome evaluation project or performance improvement initiative?

Once the core questions have been formulated, the APN can design the data collection methodology that will be used to answer key questions. Typically, this step occurs simultaneously with the actual implementation of a practice change or quality improvement strategy. In the event that a pre-intervention baseline of performance measurement needs to be established, implementation of the improvement strategy would be deferred until after the baseline measurement has been established.

Define the Data Elements

After APNs clarify the program goals, identify the key interventions to evaluate in the outcome evaluation plan, and determine the core questions to be answered, they are ready to define the outcome indicators and data elements that they will use to measure the intervention's success. This phase in the outcome evaluation plan often poses the greatest challenge for APNs, particularly for those who have had little or no exposure to QI principles and management information systems—both of which support outcome evaluation. There are three steps in this phase. First, APNs decide how they will qualify patients or encounters of care for inclusion in the outcome evaluation; second, they identify which indicators they will use to answer the project's core questions; and third, they

determine which data elements will be collected for each indicator chosen for the study. As noted, APNs with limited expertise in these areas should seek assistance from other health care professionals with experience in CQI principles, health care statistics, nursing informatics, program evaluation, and/or nursing research.

Identify Selection Criteria for the Population of Interest

Although this may seem like an obvious step, it is important to consider which patient characteristics will be included in the evaluation. Identifying electronic data sources that contain information about the target population is generally the most efficient way to begin. For example, APNs who practice in a physician's office or clinic may be able to retrieve a list of all patients seen within a given time frame. This is possible because the APN's provider number, which identifies his or her patients in the claims database and generates the bill for services rendered, can be used to define the population of interest. The APN could further reduce this list to patients seen for a specific diagnosis or symptom through the use of ICD-9 codes, CPT-4 codes, or ambulatory payment classification (APC) codes. In behavioral health settings, the use of the *Diagnostic and Statistical Manual of Mental Disorders,* version 5(DSM-V) codes are generally more useful. Additional coding taxonomies and terminology sets relevant to this level of query are listed and described in Table 24-2.

In contrast, CNSs who practice in acute care environments may have a more difficult time obtaining a list of patients whose care they managed or influenced because CNSs do not typically bill directly for services. In this scenario, the population may be identified by non-electronic data sources, such as a log or referral list. If the CNS's influence extends to a general clinical population, specified MS-DRG or ICD-9 diagnostic or procedure codes can be used to obtain a patient list if the outcome evaluation design is retrospective. Certified registered nurse anesthetists (CRNAs) and certified nurse-midwives (CNMs) who contract with the hospital for their services may be able to identify patients for whom they have provided care from the procedure provider that corresponds to the procedure code; however, they should confirm that they are listed as the procedure provider in the final claim, rather than the medical provider assigned to their practice. This information is generally available from hospital information systems and is rapidly being enhanced through the adoption of the EHR and meaningful use technologies (see earlier). As illustrated in Exemplar 24-2, APNs should collaborate with health information management (HIM) and nursing informatics specialists for this component of their analysis to ensure that the right inclusion variables have been identified to secure their population of interest.

Establish Performance and Outcome Indicators

Once the patient population has been defined, APNs and their colleagues specify measures of performance that will be used to draw conclusions about how well the population was managed or the degree to which favorable outcomes were achieved. In general, descriptive measures are predominately classified into three types: (1) proportion measures (e.g., mortality rates, readmission rates, complication rates); (2) ratio measures (e.g., falls/1000 patient days, central line infections/1000 line days, restraint episodes per psychiatric patient days); and (3) continuous variable measures (e.g., median time to initial antibiotic, average length of stay). Some measures are direct counts of a particular phenomenon within a given time period, such as number of allergic reactions in patients receiving antibiotics. Others are sums, such as total costs of care for a given population or total patient days. For rare events, such as ventilator-acquired pneumonia in hospitals that have implemented aggressive protocols to prevent this phenomenon from occurring, the days between undesirable events may be a more effective way to track and monitor outcomes, with longer time intervals being the more desirable trend, rather than fewer events.

The type of measure selected is less important than how well it answers the core questions of the study although, ultimately, the type of measure will determine the approach required for data analysis and presentation to stakeholders. The best approach is to create a draft list of indicators and obtain feedback from stakeholders about how well the indicators address their core questions and concerns. Only after stakeholder buy-in is secured should the APN formally establish the indicators for the evaluation plan. When informing the stakeholders of the outcome evaluation plan, the APN should keep in mind that if data collection is concurrent and involves the clinical practice patterns of the clinical stakeholders, the potential exists to bias the results simply because the providers know that they are being observed and their performance is being monitored. This reaction, termed the *Hawthorne effect,* is troublesome for process measurement. The data collection period should continue for a sufficient period to ensure that the novelty of the intervention has worn off and the changes in behaviors are a true reflection of intervention effect.

Alignment among program goals, interventions, and performance and outcome indicators is another important consideration when designing the outcome evaluation plan. This process ensures that the findings of the outcome evaluation can be traced back to APN practice when

appropriate. For example, if average length of stay (ALOS) is selected as one outcome indicator for a population of acute myocardial infarction (AMI) patients under the direction of a hospital-based CNS, this variable should be linked in theory and in practice to an intervention for which the CNS has or shares accountability (e.g., discharge planning or management of complications). Measures that reflect the sub-processes of other providers, such as time from first incision for patients undergoing angioplasty to the time the wire crosses the lesion in the coronary artery, may be of interest to invasive cardiologists and other stakeholders from the cardiac catheterization laboratory; however, they may have little to do with the APN's direct practice role.

As noted earlier, APNs are often lured into coordinating data collection for other providers as part of the performance monitoring process. APNs may agree to perform these data coordination or data collection activities but must be careful not to become overburdened with tasks that diminish their own clinical effectiveness or assessment of intervention effect. If this happens, APNs should examine other potential resources in the organization so they can continue to carry out their role and provide service to the institution. Staying focused on the interventions and specific program goals for which they are responsible will assist APNs to formulate a meaningful and manageable outcome evaluation plan.

Identify and Evaluate Data Elements, Collection Instruments, and Procedures

To ensure an efficient data collection process, APNs should evaluate the effort to collect each individual data element compared with the overall usefulness of the indicator. Data available only through specialized or resource-intensive instruments, such as phone surveys, home follow-up visits, or comprehensive chart reviews, are considered difficult to obtain and should be carefully evaluated before making a final decision to include them in the outcome evaluation plan. When data are obtained electronically, the specific source for each data element needs to be identified and understood. As noted earlier, running queries and reports from the EHR may or may not become an essential part of the APN's role and, in most cases, expert resources are available in health care systems to assist APNs in retrieving the information. However, in the era of the EHR, it is especially important that data obtained electronically be validated for accuracy before it can be reliably used. APNs can collaborate with quality management and nursing informatics specialists to design a data validation strategy to ensure that data is complete, accurate, and sensitive to the issue of interest. This may involve the random review of records by expert clinicians and an inspection of an interface file by a technician in the IT department to ensure that all source systems are working as designed.

APNs can avoid duplication of effort and data collection redundancy by becoming familiar with the many sources of data and information available in their respective organizations. These may include registries, surgery scheduling systems, pharmacy or medication delivery systems, point of care laboratory devices, quality management systems, case management systems, risk management systems, infection control systems, and cost accounting systems. In some cases, information from one information system might be cross-checked against another system with a similar data set. If differences between two similar data sets are identified, they should be closely examined to understand why the differences are occurring. For example, the number of infections captured by a laboratory system might be different than those captured by an infection control practitioner using an infection control information system, and still different from those captured in a medical record coding system. Common reasons for variance among similar HIT systems include variability in the start or end dates (or times) used to run the reports, a difference in the codes used to define the population of interest, or differences in how the data were captured in the source systems. In the case of medical records coding, variation is often the result of inconsistent documentation by medical and APN providers. These types of variations should be understood during the design phase of the outcome evaluation plan so that the best data source can be selected to answer the core questions of the study.

In some cases, questions about the effective management of clinical populations can be answered only through longitudinal studies. For example, for a diabetic population, clinical outcomes such as reduced hospitalization, improved functioning, reduced evidence of retinopathy, and reduced limb amputations may be sound and reasonable for research purposes, but they are typically too long range to be useful for performance improvement or outcome evaluation activities. The link between APN practice and outcomes may be difficult to assess over long periods, making intermediate outcomes assessment more desirable for a short-term evaluation.

When collecting patient identifiable data, APNs should be cognizant of the restrictions on their use. The Health Insurance Portability and Accountability Act of 1996 (PL 104-191, 104th Congress), commonly referred to as HIPAA, includes significant restrictions on the manner in which identifiable patient information may be used for research and QI activities. Typically, information used for quality improvement and outcome evaluations is less restrictive. In some circumstances, particularly if they are contracted in a fee-for-service arrangement with the

health care agency, APNs may be required to sign a business associate agreement with the health care provider. For more information about HIPAA regulations and impact on evaluation activities, APNs should refer to their organization's policies and procedures.

The APN will have a full appreciation of the scope of the outcome evaluation project and resources required for successful completion only after all the indicators within the plan are evaluated will. Once the indicators and the individual data elements have been finalized and the sources of data secured, APNs should summarize the outcome evaluation plan in a concise document that describes the plan and communicate it to all stakeholders.

Derive Meaning from Data and Act on Results

The final phase of the outcome evaluation process involves evaluation and dissemination of the findings and identification of opportunities for improvement. In these final steps, results are transformed into meaningful information that can be used to improve quality, cost, and patient satisfaction, and to evaluate the contributions of the APN. The final step involves formulating a plan to implement and reevaluate changes that occur as a result of the study.

Analyze Data and Interpret Findings

Typically, data analysis is the responsibility of the APN, although the inclusion of other peer reviewers is useful, especially when the APN has a vested interest in the outcomes. Including others helps eliminate any perceived bias during the final data analysis and reporting phases. In some cases, the APN may wish to enlist the support and guidance of a statistician or a DNP-prepared nurse researcher to ensure that the end product is methodologically sound and contains the information necessary to convince others.

Comparing pre-intervention with post-intervention performance data is one effective way to evaluate the degree of change resulting from APN interventions. Pre-intervention performance data are commonly collected retrospectively and then compared with data collected during or after an APN intervention. Retrospective data are generally available for measures constructed from electronic data sources. When electronic data are insufficient to provide adequate baseline information, APNs may elect to collect more detailed data from non-computerized medical records. Although this approach generally requires more effort, time, and planning, it may be warranted when specific processes of care are altered as part of the APN's intervention. For example, a CRNA evaluating the frequency of intraoperative hypotensive episodes may have to review medical records because this phenomenon may not be contained in common electronic source data. In some cases, a baseline study must be conducted before the APN intervention to ensure that appropriate baseline data are available for comparison. For example, a CNM who is implementing changes in clinic protocols to reduce waiting times for prenatal patients undergoing glucose tolerance testing may have to conduct a pre-intervention time and motion study to establish a baseline against which to compare post-intervention results.

Although baseline information is useful for evaluating outcomes, not everything measured by APNs will have suitable baseline data for comparison. In these cases, performance can be evaluated against a known standard of care or benchmark, especially when an area of practice is supported by evidence-based practice. When no best practice standard of performance is known, APNs may use comparative data provided by a national database if the measures used for comparison are the same as those contained within the national database.

Present and Disseminate Findings

Effective communication of data-based findings, conclusions, and recommendations for future practice is an essential component of the outcome evaluation process. How the findings are presented depends on the audience. Nonclinical audiences with a business focus, such as boards of directors or operations teams, will require briefings that summarize pertinent findings, draw conclusions, and provide reasonable options or recommendations for consideration. Clinical audiences generally require additional detail about how the evaluation was conducted and a more extensive discussion of the clinical and statistical strengths of the evidence. Clinical audiences are becoming more sophisticated in their understanding of data analysis techniques and their assessment of the applicability of evidence to practice.

The APN may be responsible for packaging the project's findings to present to stakeholders. Assistance from the facility's media or publications department may be required, depending on the final forum for communicating findings. Findings are commonly presented in committee meetings and formal presentations, although the APN should also consider posters, newsletters, white papers, articles, bulk e-mail communications, or listserv communities as additional ways to disseminate information.

Identify Improvement Opportunities

Once the outcome evaluation findings have been interpreted, the APN begins to work closely with stakeholders to evaluate the effectiveness of the practice change or QI strategy. This step may occur very quickly following a practice change or intervention, depending on the quality improvement project. Many health care organizations are adopting a rapid cycle of learning, in which they perform

smaller tests of change, evaluate the results and then, if successful, expand to larger areas or populations. For example, an APN intervention might be pilot-tested in one nursing unit before deploying the strategy across the hospital. If the intervention does not lead to the desired outcome in a timely manner, improvement opportunities are quickly identified and implemented and the results are reevaluated, with constant scrutiny on specific aspects of the care delivery processes, technology resources, or points in time that could be altered to achieve greater efficiency or effectiveness.

For example, an APN working in an acute care hospital may identify opportunities to improve performance in teaching discharge instructions to patients with heart failure. For 1 week, the use of stickers on medication sheets may be piloted to identify patients who need heart failure instructions at discharge. The following week it is identified that during the weekends there is a gap in the use of the stickers because the APN is not available to make rounds. Rather than wait for a longer evaluation period to pass, an incremental improvement in the process is adopted whereby automated alerts are generated out of the HIT system to identify all patients with an active diagnosis of heart failure (HF) who are on the telemetry unit longer than 24 hours. Incremental improvement opportunities may be made over time until a larger and more sustaining strategy is identified and long-term adoption has been achieved. In this example, the most effective solution may ultimately be for the hospital to participate in the American Heart Association's Get With the Guidelines Program, a national demonstration of best practice performance for the treatment of AMI and HF (find it online at http://www.heart.org/HEARTORG/, retrieved February 18, 2013). With this program, comprehensive Internet-based patient education materials are available to staff nurses and other clinicians, who can quickly customize the materials to meet the specific learning needs of individual patients. This solution may not have been part of the initial strategy at the onset of the project, but the APN's stewardship of the process will assist team members to develop a shared vision of which intervention(s) to adopt and why. Bringing stakeholders together to review existing and ongoing processes of care and isolate any process failures or barriers that have contributed to suboptimal performance are essential in today's health care environment.

The process to identify opportunities for improvement is similar to any work redesign initiative. The APN should identify champions and potential opponents of change. Change theory can serve as a useful foundation for APNs responsible for preparing stakeholders and overcoming their resistance to new health care delivery practices (see Chapter 11). Issues such as level of difficulty with deploying the intervention should be addressed, as well as projected costs and the human and technology resources required to implement and sustain the plan. Consider how much time the APN will be engaged in the project and how this may affect other areas of practice. A staged pilot test approach is useful for new or large-scale projects. As noted, these smaller scale versions can help identify potential implementation problems and determine whether the intervention can achieve the desired effect.

Formulate a Plan for Ongoing Monitoring and Reevaluation

Once an acceptable outcome has been achieved and sustained for a period of time, a final summary of the performance improvement initiative should be documented. This type of documentation is useful to a health care organization during an accreditation survey so that it can demonstrate that a culture of quality has been established and that it is actively engaged in improving care. In addition, this information is also useful to demonstrate the APN's value to their organization. Each goal should specify the primary interventions that were used to reach the goal, along with who was accountable for the actions required and the dates for completion. This reevaluation then becomes the basis for future outcome evaluation plans. Once performance in a particular area is stabilized, the APN may elect to discontinue monitoring a given area of performance or periodically revisit performance through intermittent monitoring.

Clarify Purpose of the Advanced Practice Nurse's Role

A final step in the process may include a thoughtful review of the APN's role and her or his effectiveness in achieving desired outcomes. An APN's role may change as a direct result of performance improvement and outcome evaluation studies. Findings may indicate that APN interventions are better suited to other points of care across the continuum of services than originally envisioned or may reveal that care may be delivered more efficiently by other providers. Conversely, findings may support the effectiveness and efficiency of the APN intervention, which could lead to program growth and expansion to other populations or points of care. In all cases, outcome evaluation, APN role definition, and scope of practice go hand in hand. If the purposes of their roles are unclear, APNs may need to identify and discuss reasonable and appropriate expectations with administrators and collaborators. It is not possible to decide which outcomes to measure without clarity about the APN's clinical populations and their accountability for the structures and processes of care. Finally, employers may not recognize the APN's full range of services or potential benefit to the organization. In such situations, the APN may need to take the lead in identifying specific processes and areas of focus within the setting and set appropriate goals and performance objectives to meet them.

Although the strategies discussed in this chapter to evaluate outcomes and improve performance are integral to the success of the APN in any organization, it is important to remember that data are ultimately a tool that can be used to foster learning, improve quality, and assist the nursing process to achieve its ultimate goal. Exemplar 24-4 reveals a unique and powerful perspective on QI and outcomes evaluation as it pertains to nursing practice.

⊙ EXEMPLAR 24-4   A Lesson in Quality: Data as Our Tool but Not Our Master

This exemplar summarizes an interview conducted with Sean Lyon, MSN, APRN, FNP-BC, Project Director of Life Long Care, a patient-centered medical home in New London, New Hampshire. Life Long Care is the only level 3, NP-led medical home in the United States recognized by the NCQA. Staffed by four NPs, this clinic provides primary care, preventive care, and chronic disease management services to a rural community of approximately 4300 persons.

Mahn-DiNicola: Tell me about the kind of activities you and your colleagues engage in to evaluate your practice or monitor outcomes for the populations you serve.

Lyon: As part of our NCQA recognition process we selected five populations to serve as markers of our success. We used the same three populations required by most clinics: individuals with diabetes, coronary artery disease, and congestive heart failure (CHF). We also selected two additional populations—asthma, because we thought this is an important population to focus on, and what we call high-risk registry patients. For each of these populations, we collect the standard process and outcome indicators, as defined by HEDIS and PQRS (see earlier, Exemplar 24-3).

Mahn-DiNicola: Tell me more about the high-risk registry. What do you measure for this population?

Lyon: We collect patient demographics and a text-based comment about why we are placing the patient in the high-risk registry. The way this works is that any staff member at the clinic can place a patient in the high-risk registry based on their gut reaction to the patient's situation. We don't require an intensive risk assessment or analytic evaluation based on quantitative, predefined criteria. Rather, it is based on a subjective appraisal often discovered in the course of a conversation with a patient,

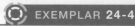 **EXEMPLAR 24-4**   **A Lesson in Quality: Data as Our Tool but Not Our Master—*cont'd***

such as a recent hospitalization, losing a job, losing a spouse, or any life change that we believe may impact the patient's well-being in a significant way.

For example, last week we had an older patient with a history of diabetes, CHF, and hepatitis whose daughter was going to Florida for several weeks on vacation. Among other things, we were concerned about this person's ability to adhere to his dietary regimen and, in particular, avoid eating foods that might impact his Coumadin (warfarin) levels. Once a patient is identified as a high-risk registry patient, we might place the patient on a daily call list or make referrals for various social supports, or even make a home visit. Our model is really a partnering with the patient model, although sometimes we call it the *do whatever it takes model*. We're trying to involve the person we are caring for in their care. For example, we give all our diabetic patients a copy of a document that lists all the periodic tests that diabetics need to be sure they undergo, such as eye examinations, foot examinations, colonoscopies or HbA1c testing. We try to foster a sense of ownership in the patient. When patients come back into the clinic, telling us it is time to schedule their tests, then we know we've created ownership in the process, but it is hard to measure the outcomes of these types of nursing practice interventions.

Mahn-DiNicola: How do you evaluate the effectiveness of your interventions?

Lyon: This is really tough to do, for several reasons. First of all, most of the NQF-endorsed measures that are used to evaluate programs like ours are based on a medical model. Although not ignoring our reporting obligations for traditional medical-oriented outcomes, such as smoking cessation advice and counseling, stable HbA1c levels for diabetics, or percentage of coronary artery disease (CAD) patients with annual lipid assessments, we elected to think about our quality program more from a nursing practice framework. One of the things we believe is that quality is not always defined by the data; in many ways, data is merely an outcome. Rather, quality is defined by the happiness of the patient and the ability to be comfortable in their own skin. I know of no NQF measures that endorse these markers of success, but Prochaska's stages of change model offers us a useful framework. We're actually working on developing some software to begin to capture this type of information.

Mahn-DiNicola: So what you are saying is that to change laboratory results such as a HbA1c or a behavior such as smoking cessation, the patient and provider go through an experiential process that doesn't lend

itself to simplistic data that's traditionally captured in an EHR.

Lyon: Exactly. In fact, in the example of smoking cessation, we actually might be doing more harm than good by forcing the patient to give up their primary coping mechanism during a time of great change or stress. But the complexity of all the data and a focus on data-driven decision making and outcomes can potentially depersonalize the process of caring that occurs between the patient and provider. Suddenly we're driven to comply with the measure mandate rather than focus on our relationship with the patient and what's really in their best interest.

Mahn-DiNicola: I think that medical providers must face many of the same challenges you are experiencing. Certainly, many measures are used to judge physicians and are often tied to privileging and recredentialing activities and, in some cases, even financial incentives. Plus, there seems to be an insurgence of the dashboard-scorecard red light, green light mentality in which provider performance, regardless of discipline, is under intense scrutiny by a myriad of stakeholders. The problem may be compounded by the fact that many nationally adopted quality metrics are often overly simplistic for patients with multiple medical conditions and polypharmacy. However, the effort to create very granular and precise measures, with all the appropriate inclusion and exclusion criteria built into them, involves the collection of so many nonstandardized and discrete data elements that it is not really feasible to do without a major restructuring of our national or even international coding taxonomies. Plus, as you have alluded to, there is the whole art of medical judgment and intuition to take into consideration.

Lyon: Certainly, there are shared concerns between both medical and nursing practice models and there will be overlap between our quality reporting systems and philosophies. The reality is that we share legislative mandates for reporting, as well as electronic information systems that will impact the patients we are ultimately serving. We need to design our measures and our measurement systems with the patient in mind.

Mahn-DiNicola: So, it sounds like you believe that mandated quality reporting and the EHR have the potential to depersonalize care to some degree.

Lyon: What I'm saying is that we're not here to enhance the data. We're here to create a place of safety, where a patient's adherence with a particular health-related behavior doesn't define their personhood. We're here to say, "I understand why you weren't able to sustain your exercise program or your smoking cessation program. It's tough to lose a spouse and it has been a really hard winter. It's OK. Let's explore some strategies to get you back on track in the spring." Instead, we tend to get too wrapped up in checking the boxes off or completing an electronic data collection form. Many times, we're not even looking at the patient; rather, we're looking at a computer screen as we're having these important conversations. So, yes, it's unfortunate, but EHRs have the potential to depersonalize care. We need to be designing person-centered data systems.

Mahn-DiNicola: So, how do we redefine the national measurement landscape to capture human responses to illness and person-centered interventions?

Lyon: Well, the problem is that we're speaking two languages. The world is asking us to measure it in French but we're speaking Italian. We need to create measures that capture the true phenomena of our concern, but we need to define our true phenomena of concern before we can create electronic information systems to capture the necessary data to measure them. For example, in the situation I described, where we give our diabetic patients the brochure from the New Hampshire Task Force, the power of the intervention isn't in giving the patient the booklet, and that's not what we should be measuring. Instead, the booklet becomes part of the nursing process;

we engage with the patient to fill it out together and create a plan that the patient ultimately owns. And, what we should be measuring is the degree of patient engagement and ownership in their health plan. I mean, if we bought a new car with an onboard computer system, we would still be accountable for scheduling our oil changes or taking it into the dealer if it developed a new squeak or leak. We wouldn't sit around and wait for the onboard computer system necessarily to tell us there is a problem or that it's time to perform routine maintenance. So why is our health care any different? Promoting and stewarding patient accountability and active engagement in their health is the ultimate end game – or at least one of them.

Mahn-DiNicola: If you could share one last thought about quality improvement and outcomes evaluation to new APN students, what would that be?

Lyon: Two thoughts, actually. First, stay actively engaged with NCQA, NQF, and other professional organizations, such as the American Academy of Nurse Practitioners. Nursing informatics specialties will also be key in creating a foundation for this work. Second, and most important, remember that we are not here to manage the data. We are here to be in a relationship with the patient and become partners for change. Data should become our tools and our guide, not our master.

Conclusion

This chapter illustrates the interconnectivity among health care information technology, information management, outcomes measurement, systems thinking, and performance improvement with every aspect of APN practice. Effective outcomes measurement and management require APNs to master information technologies, work collaboratively with others, plan and organize processes of care and assessments of quality in highly complex health services environments, and effectively manage change within their sponsoring organizations. Because reimbursement decisions are driven by evidence of organizational and individual provider performance, APNs who lack reliable and valid data to substantiate their impact will struggle for equitable reimbursement for their services, and possibly employment. For APNs to be a visible and viable resource in tomorrow's health care delivery system, they must have visible and robust outcomes that demonstrate their value. APNs in every practice setting must be willing and able to spearhead performance improvement initiatives in their institutions. Given the challenges of health care reform and the pioneering

innovations of many health care systems across the United States and internationally, there seem to be many opportunities to deploy APNs to deliver primary, preventive, acute, and chronic care and episodic care services in a quality and cost-effective manner. It may be that APNs who successfully steward safer care environments, improve clinical performance, and achieve greater efficiencies in caregiving processes will demonstrate their value more than they have ever been able to do in the past. APNs who develop robust and ongoing outcome evaluation plans place themselves in the strongest position to demonstrate their impact on outcomes of care delivery. In so doing, they also render advanced practice nursing visible to patients, other providers, administrators, payers, and communities.

Given the many quality reporting initiatives that represent so many clinical specialty domains and care delivery settings, one must wonder why it has taken so long for the nursing profession to develop a quality data set that represents the best that advanced practice nursing has to offer to those to whom we are in service. In light of emerging HIT technologies, would it now be possible to develop a robust, reliable, and highly interoperable data set of clinical outcomes that are sensitive to APN practice? Although these are important aspects of care, it seems long overdue to move beyond the traditional measurement of measures, such as pressure ulcers, falls, and medication errors, and actually examine the difference that APN practice brings to patient outcomes, the patient experience, and the entire care delivery system. Isn't it possible for APNs to make a measurable difference in conditions such as childhood obesity, diabetes management, cardiac and pulmonary disease prevention, cancer treatment, acute and episodic care, and so much more? Through advanced education and clinical expertise, APNs are in a unique position to lead the way to this new level of thought leadership and clinical practice that is sorely needed in today's health care ecosystem.

References

Agency for Healthcare Research and Quality. (2005). Patient Safety and Quality Improvement Act of 2005 (http://www.pso.ahrq.gov/statute/pl109-41.htm).

American Association of Colleges of Nursing (AACN). (2006). *Essentials of doctoral education for advanced nursing practice.* Washington, DC: Author.

Bauman, C., De Heck, J., Leonard, E., & Miranda, M. (2006). SPC: Basic control charts: Theory and construction, sample size, x-bar, r charts, s charts (https://controls.engin.umich.edu/wiki/index.php/SPC:_Basic_control_charts:_theory_and_construction,_sample_size,_x-bar,_r_charts,_s_charts).

Bisognano, M., & Kenny, C. (2012). *Pursuing the triple aim: Seven innovators show the way to better care, better health, and lower costs.* San Francisco: John Wiley & Sons.

Healthcare Information and Management Systems (HIMSS). (2012). HIE toolkit directory (http://www.himss.org/ASP/topics_FocusDynamic.asp?faid=142).

Institute of Medicine (IOM). (2011). *The future of nursing: Leading change, advancing health.* Washington, DC: National Academies Press.

Kansagara, D., Englander, H., Salanitro, A., Kagen, D., Theobald, C., Freeman, M., et al. (2011). Risk prediction models for hospital readmission: A systematic review. *Journal of the American Medical Association, 306,* 1688–1697.

Marash, S., Berman, P., & Flynn, M. (2003). *Fusion management: Harnessing the power of Six Sigma, Lean, ISO 9001:2000, Malcolm Baldrige, TQM, and other quality breakthroughs of the past century.* Fairfax, VA: QSU Publishing.

Morgan, J., & Brenig-Jones, M. (2012). *Lean Six Sigma for Dummies.* West Sussex: John Wiley & Sons, Ltd.

Powell, S. K. (2000). *Advanced case management: Outcomes and beyond.* Philadelphia: JB Lippincott.

Safriet, B. (2011). Federal options for maximizing the value of advanced practice nurses in providing quality, cost-effective health care. In Institute of Medicine (IOM). *The future of nursing: Leading change, advancing health.* (p. 2). Washington, DC: National Academies Press.

Sikka, R., Gagen, M., Crayton, M., & Esposito, T. (2012). *An administrative claims and electronic medical record derived risk prediction model for hospital readmissions.* Presented at the Academy Health Annual Research Conference, Orlando, Florida, June 24, 2012.

U.S. Congress. (2009). American Recovery and Reinvestment Act of 2009 (http://www.gpo.gov/fdsys/pkg/BILLS-111hr1enr/pdf/BILLS-111hr1enr.pdf).

U.S. Department of Health and Human Services (HHS). (2011). Patient Protection and Affordable Care Act (PPACA) (http://www.healthcare.gov/law/full/index.html).

Wheeler, D. J. (1993). *Understanding variation: The key to managing chaos.* Knoxville, TN: SPC Press.

World Health Organization. (2009). Conceptual framework for the international classification for patient safety (http://www.who.int/patientsafety/taxonomy/icps_full_report.pdf).

INDEX

Page numbers followed by "f" indicate figures, "t" indicate tables, and "b" indicate boxes.

Outcomes evaluation model *(Continued)*
  stakeholders, 675
  target population for study, 674-675
  data
    deriving meaning from, 679-681
    elements, 677-679
    results of, 679-681
  phases of, 671-681
Outcomes management, 608, 610, 620-623
Outcomes-performance contexts
  Brooten (Transitional Care) model, 618-619
  delivery of care, 612-614
    outcomes evaluation model, 612-614
    role effectiveness model, 614
  disease management, 620
  evidence-guided reviews, 614-618
    care delivery process studies, 617-618
    role description studies, 616
    role perception and acceptance studies, 616-617
  management of, 620-623
  outcome-related research strategies, 623-634
    noncomparison groups, 633-634
    physician productivity studies, 623-633
    reviews of, 607-644
    summary of, 634-635
    usual practice outcomes, 633
  performance improvement, 619-620
  processes, 619
  terminology of, 608-612
Overview concepts. *See also* Definitions/fundamentals
  of advanced practice nurse, 462-463
  of clinical nurse specialist, 359-362
  of guidance/coaching, 193
  of health policy contexts, 580-581
    politics *vs.*, 580-581
    United States *vs.* international communities, 581
OVID, 244-245
Oxford English Dictionary Online, 241

P

PAC (political action committees), 288
PainCare, 122
Pain management, 497b
Pain management clinics, 534
Pan American Health Organization, 284
Parallel communication, 300
Parallel functioning, 300
Pareto charts, 669
Part A Medicare, 450, 480, 481t, 496, 499, 516-517, 530
Part B Medicare, 14, 480, 496, 499, 501, 516-517, 530
Part C Medicare, 530
Part D Medicare, 530
Participatory, evidence-based, patient-focused process for advanced practice nursing role development, implementation and evaluation framework. *See* PEPPA (participatory, evidence-based, patient-focused process for advanced practice nursing role development, implementation and evaluation) framework
Partnerships
  cultural influences on, 154-155
  patient populations participating in, 155b
  team building and, 318

Partnerships *(Continued)*
  therapeutic
    cultural contexts and, 154-155
    interpersonal competence and, 195
Partnerships for Quality Education project, 311
Partnerships for Training project, 315
Pathophysiology, 76
Patient care policies, 239b
Patient-centered care, 184-185
Patient-centered medical home. *See* PCMH (patient-centered medical home)
Patient-centered outcomes research. *See* PCOR (patient-centered outcomes research)
Patient-Centered Outcomes Research Institute. *See* PCORI (Patient-Centered Outcomes Research Institute)
Patient-focused practice, 73-75
Patient Protection and Affordable Care Act. *See* PPACA (Patient Protection and Affordable Care Act)
Patient-provider barriers, 351-352
Patient safety organization. *See* PSO (patient safety organization)
Patient-specific contexts
  collaborations impacts, 307-312, 309b
  education, 161-162, 185
  factors related to
    consultation, 222
    contextual factors, 202
    individual, 202
  noncommunicative, 155-156
  responsibilities of, 529-530
    failure-to-pay, 529-530
    financial responsibility statement, 529
    installment plans, 529
    sliding fee scales, 529
Patterns (evolving/innovative roles), 112-128
  emerging roles (stage 3), 121-125
    interventional pain practice, 121-124
    wound, ostomy, and continence nursing, 124
  established roles (stage 4), 125-128
    advanced diabetes manager, 125-126
    genetics advanced practice nursing, 126-127
  innovative practice opportunities (stage 1), 115-117
    hospitalist practice, 115-117
  specialties in transition (stage 2), 117-121
    clinical transplant coordination, 117-118
    forensic nursing, 118-120
Pay for performance. *See* P4P (pay for performance)
Payment mechanisms, 520-533. *See also* Reimbursement mechanisms/business planning
  cash, 532
  credit card, 532
  documentation of services, 521-522
  issues related to, 593-594
  medical classification systems, 523-527
  nursing classification systems, 523-527
  for patient care services, 533
  summary, 527
  value-based purchasing, 532-533
  worldwide issues with, 142
PCMH (patient-centered medical home), 184, 397, 418, 418b
PCNP (primary care nurse practitioner), 396-428. *See also* NP (nurse practitioner)
  aging populations and, 420-421
  in Appalachia, 15-17
  barriers of, 423-424
  challenges for, 423-424